THE 5-MINUTE OBSTETRICS AND GYNECOLOGY CONSULT

THE 5-MINUTE OBSTETRICS AND GYNECOLOGY CONSULT

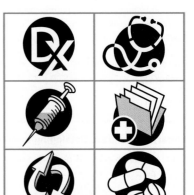

Edited by Paula J. Adams Hillard, MD

Professor, Department of Obstetrics and Gynecology
Stanford University School of Medicine
Chief, Division of Gynecologic Specialties
Stanford University Medical Center
Stanford, California

Wolters Kluwer | Lippincott Williams & Wilkins
Health

Philadelphia · Baltimore · New York · London
Buenos Aires · Hong Kong · Sydney · Tokyo

Acquisitions Editor: Sonya Seigafuse
Managing Editor: Ryan Shaw
Project Manager: Rosanne Hallowell
Manufacturing Manager: Benjamin Rivera
Marketing Manager: Kimberly Schonberger
Design Coordinator: Teresa Mallon
Cover Designer: Becky Baxendell
Production Services: Aptara, Inc.

© 2008 by LIPPINCOTT WILLIAMS & WILKINS, a Wolters Kluwer business
530 Walnut Street
Philadelphia, PA 19106
LWW.com

Printed in China

Library of Congress Cataloging-in-Publication Data

The 5-minute obstetrics & gynecology consult / edited by Paula J. Adams Hillard.
    p. ; cm.
    Includes bibliographical references and index.
    ISBN-13: 978-0-7817-6942-6
    ISBN-10: 0-7817-6942-6
  1. Obstetrics—Handbooks, manuals, etc.   2. Gynecology—Handbooks, manuals, etc.
I. Hillard, Paula Adams.   II. Title: 5-minute obstetrics and gynecology consult.
III. Title: Five-minute obstetrics & gynecology consult.
    [DNLM: 1. Obstetrics—Handbooks.   2. Female Urogenital Diseases—Handbooks.
3. Gynecology—Handbooks.   4. Pregnancy Complications—Handbooks. WQ 39 Z55 2008]
    RG110.A25 2008
    618—dc22

                               2007051064

10 9 8 7 6 5 4 3 2 1

This book is dedicated to the usual suspects:

To my husband, Arnie, who has always been incredibly supportive of my work and who sustains and nourishes me (figuratively and literally—he is a wonderfully creative chef);

To my children, Elena, Ian, and Nat, who have now flown the coop and are creating lives of their own, but who have been tolerant of, and at times even proud of, their mother's work identity as a gynecologist;

To my ever-supportive goddess of organization, Meg, without whose efforts at keeping track of the 300+ chapters, the book would never have materialized;

To my parents, Ray and Helen; my sister, Julia; and my brother, Roger, who provide the wellspring from which I draw my strength and stamina;

To the production and editing staff at Lippincott Williams & Wilkins and Aptara—Ryan, Sonya, and Max—who patiently, professionally, and calmly put up with my many, many phone calls and e-mails;

To my colleagues, who graciously shared their knowledge and expertise as chapter authors;

And finally, but not at all lastly, to the women who are and have been my patients, who have taught and inspired me more than they could ever imagine.

PREFACE

The *5-Minute Obstetrics and Gynecology Consult* joins the 5-Minute Consult series. I'd say that it's about time—literally, in the case of the busy practitioner. The specialty of Obstetrics and Gynecology and our patients deserve their own focus, and the 5-Minute format is one that works: It presents each topic within a standardized template, and the text is telegraphic and bulleted. It presents "what you need to know" about each topic. The series title of "5-Minute Consult" suggests what is truly included in the book, namely the information that you might get from a very well-organized, knowledgeable, articulate, and focused colleague/specialist when you catch her or him for 5 minutes in the hall or the physician's lounge. Of course, when you talk with your colleague in the physician's lounge, s/he may have been on call last night, may not have read the latest research paper, or may be a bit fuzzy on evidence and statistics. For these reasons, *The 5-Minute Obstetrics and Gynecology Consult* offers you the expertise of specialists, many of whom are nationally and internationally recognized in their fields. Often, these experts are writing with a junior colleague whose energy and enthusiasm for the topic perfectly balances the senior author's experience. The authors have offered you their wisdom—well-organized, essential, up-to-date information about a topic. I thank them all sincerely for their willingness to participate in this project and to provide readers with their expertise in a distilled and highly useful format. Their knowledge is at your fingertips in this text.

In the process of editing this text, I have learned a great deal from my gracious and learned colleagues. I believe the text is well suited for the bookshelf of the general ob/gyn; a resident in ob/gyn, internal medicine, family medicine, or even pediatrics; or an advanced practice nurse or other clinician who cares for women. I believe that it complements and augments the other 5-Minute texts.

HOW TO USE *THE 5-MINUTE OBSTETRICS AND GYNECOLOGY CONSULT*

The book contains some necessary redundancy, so that the practitioner can access information in a number of different ways and from different directions. **Section I: Gynecologic Signs and Symptoms** provides access to information based on the patient's concern or complaint such as abnormal bleeding, pain, vaginal discharge, etc. Such a patient might have uterine fibroids or endometriosis, both of which would be briefly listed. If the practitioner were most concerned about the possibility of uterine fibroids, this possible diagnosis could be further investigated in **Section II: Gynecologic Diseases and Conditions**. This section is organized by topics on conditions ranging from the very common (e.g., Polycystic Ovarian Syndrome (PCOS), which is present in 7% to 10% of adult women), to the very uncommon (e.g., Fallopian Tube Cancer).

Because ob/gyns provide primary health care and well-woman screening exams, I chose to include a third section, **Section III: Women's Health and Primary Care**. This section is not comprehensive, but includes basic topics such as cancer screening, contraception, and menopause. I included contraception in this section because the public health and individual impact of family planning for women deserves emphasis. Also incorporated within Women's Health and Primary Care are topics sometimes omitted from traditional texts on obstetrics or gynecology, but which are common problems for women. These topics range from domestic violence to substance use (including tobacco, alcohol, illegal substances and prescription drugs) and from eating disorders to mood disorders. Issues like the Metabolic Syndrome that have a significant overlap with women who have PCOS are also included. Topics that may receive less attention in other texts, such as preconception care and diet, are also included.

Section IV: Common Pregnancy Signs and Symptoms includes topics related to normal pregnancies and prenatal care. Establishing the estimated date of delivery, exercise in normal pregnancy, lactation, nutrition concerns, and routine prenatal laboratory testing are included in this section. Because unplanned pregnancies occur so commonly in the United States (nearly half of all pregnancies are unplanned), the section on pregnancy options counseling is included in this section.

Section V: Pregnancy-Related Conditions contains problems specific to pregnancy such as intrauterine growth restriction, multifetal pregnancy, hypertensive disorders of pregnancy, and hyperemesis gravidarum. Several topics residing at the interface between obstetrics and gynecology—in particular, early pregnancy problems, such as spontaneous abortion and ectopic pregnancy—are included in this obstetrics section, as they are truly pregnancy-related.

Section VI: Pregnancy with Underlying Medical Conditions addresses issues for consideration during pregnancy when a woman has a pre-existing medical condition such as hypertension, headaches, or thyroid disease. This section should be a reference source not only for obstetricians caring for women with these conditions, but also for clinicians who provide care for women with these conditions so that they may best advise women about what to expect with pregnancy *before* they conceive.

Section VII: Obstetric and Gynecologic Procedures focuses on common surgical and office procedures, addressing indications, informed consent, patient education, risks and benefits, medical and surgical alternatives, and complications. This section includes procedures both small and large, from vulvar biopsy to radical hysterectomy.

Section VIII addresses **Obstetric and Gynecologic Emergencies**. A routine vaginal delivery can very quickly turn life-threatening with a postpartum hemorrhage. A simple hysterectomy can precipitate intraoperative hemorrhage. Other emergencies can also be life-threatening, from an amniotic fluid embolus to a septic abortion to a necrotizing fasciitis. Because some of these conditions are extremely uncommon, the availability of a reference that succinctly describes the emergency condition, its differential diagnosis, medical, or surgical managements, prognosis, and complications in a bulleted format can be invaluable and potentially life-saving.

Finally, the **Appendices** list tables of information: cancer staging, ACOG screening guidelines, immunizations, food sources of selected nutrients, contraceptive efficacy, how to develop a patient-friendly office environment, and complementary and alternative medications used for gynecologic and women's health care. These tables offer a wealth of information, some of which is not available elsewhere, and which, in aggregate, provide added value beyond the individual chapters.

So here it is. I know that it contains up-to-date information, and I hope that the format is both useful and user-friendly. I ask readers to send me their comments. I will certainly enjoy seeing the positive ones, but regardless, all constructive critiques and suggestions will be welcome—for new or different topics, for example. I know that the comments I receive will make the next edition even better than this effort—which I happen to believe is very good!

CONTRIBUTING AUTHORS

Lisa N. Abaid, MD, MPH
Fellow, Gynecologic Oncology
Department of Obstetrics and Gynecology
University of North Carolina at Chapel Hill
Chapel Hill, North Carolina

Alison C. Agner, MD
Resident, Department of
    Obstetrics and Gynecology
University of Iowa Hospitals and Clinics
Iowa City, Iowa

Jay E. Allard, MD
Teaching Fellow
Department of Obstetrics and Gynecology
Uniformed Services University of the
    Health Sciences
F. Edward Hebert School of Medicine
Bethesda, Maryland

Raquel D. Arias, MD
Associate Professor,
    Obstetrics and Gynecology
Keck School of Medicine
University of Southern California
Los Angeles, California

Lesley Arnold, MD
Associate Professor of Psychiatry
University of Cincinnati
    College of Medicine
Cincinnati, Ohio

Mira Aubuchon, MD
Assistant Professor
Department of Obstetrics and Gynecology
University of Cincinnati College of Medicine
Attending Physician
Department of Obstetrics and Gynecology
    Center for Reproductive Health
Cincinnati, Ohio

Philippe F. Backeljauw, MD
Professor of Pediatrics
Division of Pediatric Endocrinology
Cincinnati Children's Hospital Medical
    Center
University of Cincinnati College of Medicine
Cincinnati, Ohio

Susan Ballagh, MD
Associate Professor
Department of OB/GYN
Eastern Virginia Medical School
Conrad Clinical Research Center
Norfolk, Virginia

Matthew A. Barker, MD
Fellow, Female Pelvic Medicine and
    Reconstructive Surgery
Department of Obstetrics and Gynecology
Good Samaritan Hospital
Cincinnati, Ohio

Mark A. Barone, DVM, MS
Senior Medical Associate
EngenderHealth
New York, New York

Sarah E. Bartlett, MD
Resident
Department of Obstetrics and Gynecology
University of Cincinnati
Cincinnati, Ohio

Jack Basil, MD
Associate Director, Gynecologic Oncology
Good Samaritan Hospital
Cincinnati, Ohio

Karin Batalden, MD
Pediatric Resident
Cincinnati Children's Hospital Medical
    Center
Cincinnati, Ohio

Frances Batzer, MD, MBE
Clinical Professor of Obstetrics
    & Gynecology
Jefferson University Hospital
Philadelphia, Pennsylvania

Jason K. Baxter, MD, MSCP
Assistant Professor
Department of Obstetrics and Gynecology
Thomas Jefferson University
Thomas Jefferson University Hospital
Philadelphia, Pennsylvania

F. Ariella Baylson, MD
Resident
Department of OB/GYN
Thomas Jefferson University
Philadelphia, Pennsylvania

Jyothsna Bayya, MD
Resident Obstetrics and Gynecology
Maimonides Medical Center
Brooklyn, New York

Megan N. Beatty, MD
Resident Physician
Stanford University
Stanford, California

Jonathan S. Berek, MD
Professor and Chair
Department of Obstetrics and Gynecology
Stanford University
Stanford, California

Michelle Berlin, MD, MPH
Associate Professor
Departments of Obstetrics & Gynecology,
    Public Health & Preventive Medicine,
    Clinical Epidemiology
Oregon Health & Science University
Portland, Oregon

Kelly A. Best, MD
Assistant Professor
Department of Obstetrics and Gynecology
University of Florida College of
    Medicine-Jacksonville Staff
Department of Obstetrics and Gynecology
Shands Jacksonville
Jacksonville, Florida

Snehal M. Bhoola, MD
Assistant Professor
Department of Obstetrics & Gynecology
Mercer University, Savannah Campus
Gynecologic Oncologist
Department of OB/GYN
Memorial Health University Medical Center
Savannah, Georgia

Frank M. Biro, MD
Professor of Pediatrics
Department of Pediatrics
University of Cincinnati
Division Director
Division of Adolescent Medicine
Cincinnati Children's Hospital Medical
    Center
Cincinnati, Ohio

Yair Blumenfeld, MD
Maternal-Fetal Medicine Fellow
Department of Obstetrics & Gynecology
Division of Maternal-Fetal Medicine
Stanford University
Stanford, California

Paul D. Blumenthal, MD, MPH
Professor, Obstetrics & Gynecology
Johns Hopkins University
    School of Medicine
Johns Hopkins Bayview Medical Center
Baltimore, Maryland

Annette E. Bombrys, DO
Fellow, Maternal-Fetal Medicine
Department of Obstetrics and Gynecology
University of Cincinnati
Cincinnati, Ohio

Emily Boyd, MD
Washington University in St. Louis
School of Medicine
St. Louis, Missouri

Paula K. Braverman, MD
Professor
Department of Pediatrics
University of Cincinnati
    College of Medicine
Division of Adolescent Medicine
Cincinnati Children's
    Hospital Medical Center
Cincinnati, Ohio

Lesley L. Breech, MD
Assistant Professor of Pediatrics and
    of Obstetrics & Gynecology
University of Cincinnati
    College of Medicine
Cincinnati Children's
    Hospital Medical Center
Cincinnati, Ohio

Debra L. Breneman, MD
Adjunct Associate Professor
Department of Dermatology
University of Cincinnati
Attending Staff
Department of Dermatology
University Hospital
Cincinnati, Ohio

Corinne L. Bria, MD
Resident Physician
Department of Pediatrics
Cincinnati Children's Hospital
Cincinnati, Ohio

Robert E. Bristow, MD
Associate Professor
Department of Gynecology and
    Obstetrics and Oncology
The Johns Hopkins University
    School of Medicine
Director, Gynecologic Oncology
Department of Gynecology and Obstetrics
The Johns Hopkins Hospital
Baltimore, Maryland

Jane D. Broecker, MD
Assistant Professor of
    Obstetrics & Gynecology
Ohio University College of
    Osteopathic Medicine
Athens, Ohio

Philip G. Brooks, MD
Clinical Professor
Department of Obstetrics and Gynecology
David Geffen School of Medicine at UCLA
Director, Operating Rooms for Gynecology
Department of Obstetrics and Gynecology
Cedars-Sinai Medical Center
Los Angeles, California

Rebeccah L. Brown, MD
Assistant Professor, Clinical Surgery
University of Cincinnati
    College of Medicine
Division of Pediatric Surgery
Cincinnati Children's
    Hospital Medical Center
Cincinnati, Ohio

Ronald T. Burkman, MD
Department of Obstetrics
    and Gynecology
Baystate Medical Center
Springfield, Massachusetts

Vernon T. Cannon, MD, PhD
Research Associate
Department of Obstetrics &
    Gynecology
Northwestern University
    Feinberg School of Medicine
Research Associate
Department of Obstetrics &
    Gynecology
Evanston Northwestern Healthcare
Evanston, Illinois

Lavenia B. Carpenter, MD
Assistant Professor, Obstetrics &
    Gynecology
Vanderbilt University
    Medical Center
Nashville, Tennessee

Sandra A. Carson, MD
Professor
Department of Obstetrics & Gynecology
Warren Alpert Medical
    School of Brown University
Director, Division of Reproductive
    Endocrinology & Infertility
Department of Obstetrics & Gynecology
Women & Infants' Hospital of
    Rhode Island
Providence, Rhode Island

Aaron B. Caughey, MD, PhD
Assistant Professor of Obstetrics,
    Gynecology, & Reproductive Sciences
UCSF School of Medicine
San Francisco, California

Jennifer Cavitt, MD
Assistant Professor,
    Department of Neurology
University of Cincinnati
Attending Staff
University Hospital
Cincinnati, Ohio

Weldon Chafe, MD
Professor and Head,
    Division of Gynecology Oncology
Department of Obstetrics & Gynecology
Virginia Commonwealth University
Richmond, Virginia

Linda R. Chambliss, MD, MPH
Professor, Department of Obstetrics,
    Gynecology, & Women's Health
St. Louis University School of Medicine
St. Louis, Missouri

Pauline Chang, MD
Resident
Department of OB/GYN
Stanford University
Stanford, California

Beatrice A. Chen, MD
Clinical Instructor
Department of Obstetrics,
    Gynecology, and Reproductive Sciences
University of Pittsburgh
Clinical Instructor
Department of Obstetrics,
    Gynecology, and Reproductive Sciences
Magee-Women's Hospital
Pittsburgh, Pennsylvania

Bertha H. Chen, MD
Associate Professor
Department of Obstetrics
    & Gynecology
Stanford University School of Medicine
Associate Professor/Director
    of Urodynamics Clinic
Department of OB/GYN
Stanford University Hospital
Stanford, California

Nancy Chescheir, MD
Professor & Chair,
    Department of Obstetrics
    & Gynecology
Vanderbilt University School
    of Medicine
Nashville, Tennessee

Martina Chiodi, MD
Ob/Gyn Resident
SUNY Downstate
Brooklyn, New York

Carol M. Choi, MD
Assistant Professor
Department of Obstetrics & Gynecology
University of Cincinnati
Cincinnati, Ohio

Daniel Clark-Pearson, MD
Professor & Chair, Obstetrics
& Gynecology
University of North Carolina at Chapel Hill
School of Medicine
Chapel Hill, North Carolina

Justin P. Collingham, MD
Fellow, Maternal-Fetal Medicine
Department of Obstetrics and Gynecology
Stanford University
Fellow, Maternal-Fetal Medicine
Department of Obstetrics and Gynecology
Lucile Packard Children's Hospital
Stanford, California

Joseph P. Connor, MD
Associate Professor
Department of Obstetrics & Gynecology
University of Wisconsin
Madison, Wisconsin

Susan M. Coupey, MD
Professor
Department of Pediatrics
Albert Einstein College of Medicine
Chief, Adolescent Medicine
Department of Pediatrics
Children's Hospital at Montefiore
Bronx, New York

Bryan D. Cowan, MD
Professor & Chair,
Department of Obstetrics & Gynecology
University of Mississippi Medical Center
Jackson, Mississippi

J. Thomas Cox, MD
Director, Women's Clinic
Department of Student Health Services
University of California at Santa Barbara
Santa Barbara, California

Eve S. Cunningham, MD
Assistant Professor
Department of Obstetrics and Gynecology
Olive View-UCLA Medical Center
Sylmar, California

Carrie Cwiak, MD, MPH
Assistant Professor
Department of Gynecology and Obstetrics
Emory University School of Medicine
Medical Director
Family Planning Clinic
Grady Health System
Atlanta, Georgia

Bonnie J. Dattel, MD
Professor of Obstetrics & Gynecology
Associate Director of
Maternal-Fetal Medicine
Eastern Virginia Medical School
Norfolk, Virginia

Adetokunbo Dawodu, MD
Endocrine Fellow
Department of Pediatrics & Endocrinology
University of Cincinnati
Endocrine Fellow
Department of Endocrinology
Cincinnati Children's
Hospital Medical Center
Cincinnati, Ohio

Thomas A. deHoop, MD
Associate Professor,
Obstetrics & Gynecology
University of Cincinnati
College of Medicine
Cincinnati, Ohio

Helen R. Deitch, MD
Clinical Assistant Professor
Department of Ob/Gyn
Milton S. Hershey Medical Center
Hershey, Pennsylvania
Staff Physician
Department of Ob/Gyn
Centre Medical and Surgical Associates
State College, Pennsylvania

Paul D. DePriest, MD
Division of Gynecologic Oncology
Department of Obstetrics & Gynecology
University of Kentucky
Lexington, Kentucky

Amy E. Derrow, MD
Dermatology Resident
Department of Dermatology
University of Cincinnati
College of Medicine
Cincinnati, Ohio

Laetitia Poisson De Souzy, MD
Resident
Department of Obstetrics and Gynecology
UC San Francisco
San Francisco, California

Mitchell Dombrowski, MD
Professor of Obstetrics & Gynecology
Wayne State University
School of Medicine
Chairman
Department of Obstetrics & Gynecology
St. John Hospital
Detroit, Michigan

Patricia L. Dougherty, CNM, MSN
Gynecologic Nurse-Practitioner
Department of Obstetrics and Gynecology
University of Virginia
Clinical Faculty
Department of Obstetrics and Gynecology
University of Virginia Health
Sciences Center
Charlottesville, Virginia

Angela D. Earhart, MD
Fellow
Department of Obstetrics & Gynecology
University of Texas Medical
Branch at Galveston
Galveston, Texas

Alison Edelman, MD, MPH
Assistant Professor
Department of OBGYN
Oregon Health & Science University
Portland, Oregon

M. Heather Einstein, MD
Pelvic Reconstruction Clinical
Research Fellow
Department of Surgery,
Division of Gynecology
Memorial Sloan-Kettering Cancer Center
New York, New York

Yasser Y. El-Sayed, MD
Associate Professor and Associate Chief
Division of Maternal-Fetal
Medicine and Obstetrics
Department of Obstetrics and Gynecology
Stanford University
Stanford, California

Diane E. Elas, MSN, ENRC, ARNP
ARNP
Department of Obstetrics and Gynecology
University of Iowa Hospitals and Clinics
Iowa City, Iowa

Alexandra Emery-Cohen, MD
Resident in Ob/Gyn
University of Florida College of
Medicine-Jacksonville
Jacksonville, Florida

Tania F. Esakoff, MD
Clinical Fellow
Department of Obstetrics, Gynecology,
and Reproductive Sciences
University of California, San Francisco
San Francisco, California

Eve Espey, MD, MPH
Associate Professor
Department of Obstetrics & Gynecology
University of New Mexico
Albuquerque, New Mexico

John F. Farley, MD
Associate Professor
Department of Obstetrics and Gynecology
Uniformed Services University of the
    Health Sciences
Bethesda, Maryland
Department of Obstetrics and Gynecology
Walter Reed Army Medical Center
Washington, DC

Sebastian Faro, MD, PhD
Clinical Professor of Obstetrics and
    Gynecology
University of Texas, Houston
Attending Physician
The Woman's Hospital of Texas
Houston, Texas

Judith Feinberg, MD
Professor of Medicine
University of Cincinnati College of Medicine
Holmes Hospital
Cincinnati, Ohio

Dee E. Fenner, MD
Professor of Women's Health and of
    Obstetrics & Gynecology
University of Michigan Health System
Women's Hospital
Ann Arbor, Michigan

James E. Ferguson, II, MD
The John W. Greene
    Jr. Professor and Chair
Department of Obstetrics
    and Gynecology
University of Kentucky College of Medicine
Chief
Department of Obstetrics
    and Gynecology
Chandler Medical Center,
    University of Kentucky
Lexington, Kentucky

Reinaldo Figueroa, MD
Associate Clinical Professor
Department of Obstetrics, Gynecology,
    and Reproductive Medicine
Stony Brook University, School of Medicine
Attending Physician
Department of Obstetrics, Gynecology, and
    Reproductive Medicine
Division of Maternal-Fetal Medicine
Stony Brook Medical Center
Stony Brook, New York

Paul M. Fine, MD
Associate Professor,
    Departments of Obstetrics,
    Gynecology, and Urogynecology
Baylor College of Medicine
Houston, Texas

Arin E. Ford, MD
Resident Physician
Department of Obstetrics & Gynecology
University of Kentucky
Lexington, Kentucky

Bryan E. Freeman, MD
Fellow
Department of Maternal-Fetal Medicine
University of Arizona
Tucson, Arizona

Brooke Friedman, MD
Obstetrics & Gynecology Resident
Stanford University Medical Center
Department of Obstetrics & Gynecology
Stanford, California

Rudolph P. Galask, MD, MS
Professor Emeritus
Department of Obstetrics and Gynecology
University of Iowa
Iowa City, Iowa

Donald G. Gallup, MD
Professor and Chair
Department of Obstetrics and Gynecology
Mercer University School of
    Medicine (Savannah)
Gynecologic Oncologist
Department of OB/GYN
Memorial Health University Medical Center
Savannah, Georgia

Cecilia T. Gambala, MD, MSPH
Assistant Professor
Department of Obstetrics and Gynecology
University of Illinois, Chicago
Chicago, Illinois

Margery L. S. Gass, MD
Professor Clinical Obstetrics
    & Gynecology
Department of Obstetrics and
    Gynecology
University of Cincinnati
Attending Physician
Department of Obstetrics & Gynecology
University Hospital
Cincinnati, Ohio

Verghese George, MD
Radiology Fellow
Department of Radiology
Yale University College of Medicine
New Haven, Connecticut

Aaron Goldberg, MD
Ob/Gyn Resident
Department of Obstetrics & Gynecology
Virginia Commonwealth University
Richmond, Virginia

T. Murphy Goodwin, MD
Professor and Chief, Division of
    Maternal-Fetal Medicine
Department of Obstetrics
    and Gynecology
University of Southern California
Keck School of Medicine
Los Angeles, California

Ernest M. Graham, MD
Associate Professor
Department of Gynecology and Obstetrics
Johns Hopkins University School of
    Medicine
Baltimore, Maryland

T. Brent Graham, MD
Associate Professor of Clinical Pediatrics
University of Cincinnati
    College of Medicine
Cincinnati Children's Hospital
    Medical Center
Cincinnati, Ohio

Marjorie Greenfield, MD
Associate Professor,
    Reproductive Biology
Case Western Reserve School of Medicine
Cleveland, Ohio

Donald E. Greydanus, MD
Professor of Pediatrics
    and Human Development
Michigan State University
Kalamazoo Center for Medical Studies
Kalamazoo, Michigan

Matthew Guile, MD
Resident
Department of Gynecology and Obstetrics
The Johns Hopkins Hospital
Baltimore, Maryland

Jeanne-Marie Guise, MD, MPH
Associate Professor
Division of Maternal Fetal Medicine
Departments of Obstetrics
    and Gynecology
Medical Informatics
    and Clinical Epidemiology
Public Health and Preventive Medicine
Oregon Health and Science University
Director
State Obstetric and Pediatric
    Research Collaborative (STORC)
Portland, Oregon

Mounira Habli, MD
Clinical Instructor, Fellow
Department of Obstetrics and Gynecology
University of Cincinnati
Cincinnati, Ohio

Gary D. V. Hankins, MD
Professor
Chairman
Department of Obstetrics & Gynecology
University of Texas
  Medical Branch at Galveston
Galveston, Texas

Wendy F. Hansen, MD
Associate Professor
Director of Maternal-Fetal Medicine
Department of Obstetrics and Gynecology
University of Kentucky Medical Center
Lexington, Kentucky

Zeev Harel, MD
Associate Professor
Department of Pediatrics
Brown University,
  Warren Alpert Medical School
Director of Research and Training
Division of Adolescent Medicine
Hasbro Children's Hospital/Rhode
  Island Hospital
Providence, Rhode Island

Jason N. Hashima, MD, MPH
Clinical Instructor/MFM Fellow
Department of OBGYN, Division of
  Maternal Fetal Medicine
Oregon Health and Science University
Portland, Oregon

S. Paige Hertweck, MD
Associate Professor
Pediatric and Adolescent Gynecology
Department of Obstetrics, Gynecology
  & Women's Health
University of Louisville School of Medicine
Louisville, Kentucky

Geri D. Hewitt, MD
Associate Professor, Obstetrics
  & Gynecology
Ohio State University College of
  Medicine & Public Health
Columbus, Ohio

Kimberly W. Hickey, MD
Clinical Instructor
Fellow, Maternal-Fetal Medicine
Department of Obstetrics and Gynecology
Georgetown University Hospital
Washington, DC

Paula J. Adams Hillard, MD
Professor
Department of Obstetrics and Gynecology
Stanford University School of Medicine
Chief, Division of Gynecologic Specialties
Stanford University Medical Center
Stanford, California

Jennifer B. Hillman, MD
Clinical Fellow, Adolescent Medicine
Cincinnati Children's Hospital Medical Center
Cincinnati, Ohio

Dominic Hollman, MD
Clinical Fellow
Department of Pediatrics and
  Adolescent Medicine
Albert Einstein College of Medicine
Clinical Fellow
Department of Pediatrics and
  Adolescent Medicine
Children's Hospital at Montefiore
Bronx, New York

Amanda L. Horton, MD
Clinical Instructor
Department of Obstetrics and Gynecology
UNC School of Medicine
Clinical Fellow
Department of Obstetrics and Gynecology
UNC Hospitals
Chapel Hill, North Carolina

John P. Horton, MD
Resident Physician
Department of Obstetrics and Gynecology
University of Kentucky
Lexington, Kentucky

Christopher P. Houk, MD
Assistant Professor
Department of Pediatrics
Mercer University School of Medicine
Macon, Georgia
Pediatric Endocrinologist
Department of Pediatrics
Backus Children's Hospital at Memorial
  Health University Medical Center
Savannah, Georgia

Helen How, MD
Associate Professor of Ob/Gyn
Maternal and Fetal Medicine
University of Cincinnati College of Medicine
Cincinnati, Ohio

Jill S. Huppert, MD, MPH
Research Assistant Professor of Pediatrics
University of Cincinnati College of Medicine
Cincinnati Children's
  Hospital Medical Center
Cincinnati, Ohio

Jean A. Hurteau, MD
Professor
Department of Obstetrics and Gynecology
Northwestern University Feinberg
  School of Medicine
Attending Physician
Department of OBGYN
Evanston Northwestern Healthcare
Evanston, Illinois

Amreen Husain, MD
Assistant Professor of
  Gynecologic Oncology
Department of Obstetrics and Gynecology
Stanford University School of Medicine
Stanford, California

Nader Husseinzadeh, MD
Professor, Gynecology/Oncology
University of Cincinnati College
  of Medicine
Cincinnati, Ohio

Jay Iams, MD
Professor, Department of Ob/Gyn
Division of Fetal Medicine
Ohio State University College of Medicine
Columbus, Ohio

Christine Isaacs, MD
Assistant Professors
Virginia Commonwealth
  University for Both
Department of Ob/Gyn
Richmond, Virginia

Michele M. Isley, MD
Clinical Instructor and Family
  Planning Fellow
Department of Obstetrics and Gynecology
Oregon Health and Science University
Portland, Oregon

Mary T. Jacobson, MD
Clinical Assistant Professor of Obstetrics
  & Gynecology
Stanford University School of Medicine
Stanford, California

Jeffrey T. Jensen, MD, MPH
Leon Speroff Professor of Obstetrics
  & Gynecology
Departments of Obstetrics and
  Gynecology and Public Health and
  Preventive Medicine
Oregon Health and Science University
Departments of Obstetrics
  and Gynecology
OHSU Hospital
Portland, Oregon

Christiano Jodicke, MD
Resident, Department of Obstetrics
  & Gynecology
University of Cincinnati
  College of Medicine
Cincinnati, Ohio

Susan R. Johnson, MD, MS
Associate Provost for Faculty
University of Iowa
Iowa City, Iowa

Jessica A. Kahn, MD, MPH
Associate Professor of Pediatrics
Department of Pediatrics
University of Cincinnati
   College of Medicine
Associate Professor of Pediatrics
Department of Pediatrics
Cincinnati Children's Hospital
   Medical Center
Cincinnati, Ohio

Bliss Kaneshiro, MD
Assistant Professor
Department of Obstetrics and Gynecology
University of Hawaii
Honolulu, Hawaii

Shibani Kanungo, MD, MPH
Assistant Professor
Department of Pediatrics
University of Kentucky
Attending Physician
Department of Pediatrics
Kentucky Children's Hospital
Lexington, Kentucky

Paul B. Kaplowitz, MD, PhD
Professor
Department of Pediatrics
George Washington University
   School of Medicine
Chief of Endocrinology
Department of Endocrinology
Children's National Medical Center
Washington, DC

Nicole W. Karjane, MD
Assistant Professors
Virginia Commonwealth University
   for Both
Department of Ob/Gyn
Richmond, Virginia

Beth Y. Karlan, MD
Department of Obstetrics & Gynecology
Cedars-Sinai Medical Center
Los Angeles, California

Mickey M. Karram, MD
Advanced Urogynecology & Advanced
   Pelvic Surgery
Good Samaritan Hospital
Seton Center
Cincinnati, Ohio

Jessica Kassis, MD
Resident Physician
Department of Obstetrics and Gynecology
Stanford University
Stanford University Medical Center
Stanford, California

Vern Katz, MD
Clinical Professor
Department of Obstetrics and Gynecology
Oregon Health Science University
Medical Director of Obstetrics
Department of Obstetrics and Gynecology
Sacred Heart Medical Center
Eugene, Oregon

Andrew M. Kaunitz, MD
Professor of Ob/Gyn
University of Florida College of
   Medicine-Jacksonville
Jacksonville, Florida

Angela Keating, MD
Columbia Women's Clinic
Portland, Oregon

Lisa Keder, MD, MPH
Associate Professor
Department of Obstetrics &
   Gynecology
Ohio State University
Associate Professor
Department of Obstetrics and
   Gynecology
Ohio State Medical Center
Columbus, Ohio

Rebecca S. Kightlinger, DO
Assistant Professor
Department of Obstetrics and
   Gynecology
University of Virginia
Faculty Physician
Department of Obstetrics and
   Gynecology
University of Virginia Medical Center
Charlottesville, Virginia

Sarah J. Kilpatrick, MD, PhD
Vice Dean, College of Medicine
Professor and Arends Head
Department of Obstetrics
   and Gynecology
University of Illinois
Chicago, Illinois

Merieme Klobocista, MD
Resident, Department of Obstetrics
   and Gynecology
University of Connecticut Health Center
Farmington, Connecticut

Melissa Kottke, MD
Assistant Professor
Department of Gynecology
   and Obstetrics
Emory University
Atlanta, Georgia

Stephan P. Krotz, MD
Clinical Fellow
Department of Obstetrics & Gynecology
Warren Alpert Medical
   School of Brown University
Clinical Fellow
Department of Obstetrics & Gynecology
Women & Infants' Hospital of
   Rhode Island
Providence, Rhode Island

Soo Y. Kwon, MD
Assistant Professor
Department of Obstetrics and Gynecology
Rush University
Rush University Medical Center
Chicago, Illinois

Judith Lacy, MD
Clinical Instructor, Pediatric and
   Adolescent Gynecology,
   Division of Gynecologic Specialties
Department of Obstetrics & Gynecology
Stanford University School of Medicine
Stanford, California

Inna V. Landres, MD
Resident
Department of OB/GYN
Stanford Hospital and Clinics
Palo Alto, California

Jennifer Lang, MD
Clinical Fellow, Gynecologic Oncology
Department of Obstetrics and Gynecology
UCLA Medical Center
Cedar-Sinai Medical Center
Los Angeles, California

Eduardo Lara-Torre, MD
Director Ambulatory Care
Center for Women's Medicine
Lehigh Valley Hospital
Clinical Assistant Professor of Obstetrics
   and Gynecology
Penn State University School of Medicine
Pediatric and Adolescent Gynecology
Allentown, Pennsylvania

Joel D. Larma, MD
Assistant Professor
Department of Obstetrics and Gynecology
The University of Cincinnati
Cincinnati, Ohio

Ruth Bunker Lathi, MD
Assistant Professor
Department of Obstetrics and Gynecology
Division of Reproductive Endocrinology
   and Infertility
Stanford University Medical Center
Stanford, California

Ruth A. Lawrence, MD
Professor
Department of Pediatrics and Obstetrics
and Gynecology
University of Rochester School of Medicine
and Dentistry
Attending Physician
Department of Pediatrics
Strong Memorial Hospital
Rochester, New York

Monica Hau Hien Le, MD
Fellow, Minority Health Policy
Department of Social Medicine
Harvard Medical School
Boston, Massachusetts

Catherine M. Leclair, MD
Assistant Professor
Department of Obstetrics and Gynecology
Director, Program in Vulvar Health
Center for Women's Health
Oregon Health and Science University
Portland, Oregon

Matthew A. Lederman, MD
REI Fellow
Department of OB/GYN and
Women's Health
Albert Einstein College of Medicine
Montefiore Medical Center
Bronx, New York

Nita Karnik Lee, MD, MPH
Clinical Fellow
Stanford University School
of Medicine
Stanford, California

Peter A. Lee, MD, PhD
Professor
Department of Pediatrics
Indiana University School of Medicine
Indianapolis, Indiana
Professor
Department of Pediatrics
Penn State College of Medicine
Hershey, Pennsylvania

Corinne Lehmann, MD
Associate Professor of Pediatrics
University of Cincinnati
College of Medicine
Cincinnati Children's Hospital
Medical Center
Cincinnati, Ohio

Christina Lewicky-Gaupp, MD
Instructor
University of Michigan Health System
Women's Hospital
Ann Arbor, Michigan

Valerie J. Lewis, MD, MPH
Fellow Physician
Craig Dalsimer Division of
Adolescent Medicine
Children's Hospital of Philadelphia
Philadelphia, Pennsylvania

J. Ingrid Lin, MD
Resident
Department of Obstetrics and Gynecology
University of Southern California
Women's and Children's Hospital
Los Angeles, California

Leann E. Linam, MD
Assistant Professor of Radiology
Department of Radiology
University of Cincinnati
Assistant Professor of Radiology
Department of Radiology
Cincinnati Children's Hospital
Medical Center
Cincinnati, Ohio

Daniel M. Lindberg, MD
Instructor
Department of Medicine—Emergency
Medicine
Harvard Medical School
Attending Physician
Department of Emergency Medicine
Brigham & Women's Hospital
Boston, Massachusetts

Steven R. Lindheim, MD
Associate Professor of Obstetrics
& Gynecology
University of Wisconsin Hospitals
& Clinics
University of Wisconsin Medical School
Madison, Wisconsin

Jeffrey C. Livingston, MD
Assistant Professor, Obstetrics
& Gynecology
University of Cincinnati College
of Medicine
Cincinnati, Ohio

Charles J. Lockwood, MD
Professor and Chair
Department of Obstetrics, Gynecology
and Reproductive Sciences
Yale University School of Medicine
New Haven, Connecticut

Patricia A. Lohr, MD, MPH
Medical Director
British Pregnancy Advisory Service
Stratford Upon Avon, United Kingdom

Jerry L. Lowder, MD, MSc
Assistant Professor
Assistant Clinical Professor
Division of Urogynecology
Department of Obstetrics, Gynecology,
and Reproductive Sciences
University of Pittsburgh School of Medicine
UPMC Magee-Women's Hospital
Pittsburgh, Pennsylvania

Cynthia Macri, MD
V.P. for Recruitment & Diversity Affairs
Uniformed Services University of the
Health Sciences
F. Edward Hebert School of Medicine
Bethesda, Maryland

Tessa Madden, MD, MPH
Family Planning Fellow/Clinical Instructor
Johns Hopkins University School of
Medicine
Johns Hopkins Bayview Medical Center
Department of Ob/Gyn
Baltimore, Maryland

Kathi Makoroff, MD
Assistant Professor of Pediatrics
University of Cincinnati
College of Medicine
Center for Safe & Healthy Children
Cincinnati Children's Hospital
Medical Center
Cincinnati, Ohio

Melissa Snyder Mancuso, MD
Fellow, Maternal Fetal Medicine
and Medical Genetics
Department of Obstetrics and Gynecology
Division of Maternal Fetal Medicine
University of Alabama at Birmingham
Birmingham, Alabama

Michael J. Marmura, MD
Fellow
Department of Neurology
Thomas Jefferson University Hospital
Philadelphia, Pennsylvania

Jamie A. M. Massie, MD
Resident, Obstetrics and Gynecology
Stanford University Medical Center
Stanford, California

Preeti Patel Matkins, MD
Adjunct Associate Professor of Pediatrics
UNC School of Medicine
Director, Child Maltreatment
Department of Adolescent Medicine
Levine Children's Hospital
Department of Pediatrics
Carolinas Medical Center
Charlotte, North Carolina

Donna Mazloomdoost, MD
Resident, Department of Obstetrics
& Gynecology
University of Cincinnati College of
Medicine
Cincinnati, Ohio

Shirley M. McCarthy, MD, PhD
Assistant Professor of Obstetrics and
Gynecology and Urology
University of Virginia Health System
Yale University College of Medicine
New Haven, Connecticut

C. H. McCracken III, MD
Billings Clinic
Billings, Montana

Michelle McDonald, MS
Research Assistant
Department of Obstetrics and Gynecology
University of California at Los Angeles
Los Angeles, California

Megan McGraw, MD
Child Abuse Fellow, Mayerson Center for
Safe & Healthy Children
Cincinnati Children's Hospital
Medical Center
Cincinnati, Ohio

Kelly McLean, MD
Resident, Department of Surgery
University of Cincinnati College of Medicine
Cincinnati, Ohio

Tia M. Melton, MD
Assistant Professor
Department of Reproductive Biology
Case Western Reserve University
Assistant Professor
Department of Obstetrics and Gynecology
University Hospital Case Medical Center
Cleveland, Ohio

M. Kathryn Menard, MD, MPH
Director, Maternal-Fetal Medicine
Professor and Vice Chair of Obstetrics
University of North Carolina
School of Medicine
Chapel Hill, North Carolina

Diane F. Merritt, MD
Professor
Department of Obstetrics & Gynecology
Washington University School of Medicine
Attending Physician
Director Pediatric and Adolescent
Gynecology
Barnes Jewish Hospital
Saint Louis Children's Hospital
Missouri Baptist Medical Center
St. Louis, Missouri

Jacob Meyer, MD
Resident
Oregon Health Sciences University
Eugene, Oregon

Rachel J. Miller, MD
Pediatric & Adolescent Gynecology Fellow
Cincinnati Children's Hospital
Medical Center
Cincinnati, Ohio

Leah S. Millheiser, MD
Instructor, Department of Obstetrics
& Gynecology
Stanford University School of Medicine
Stanford, California

Howard Minkoff, MD
Distinguished Professor
Department of Obstetrics and Gynecology
SUNY Downstate
Chairman
Department of Obstetrics and Gynecology
Maimonides Medical Center
Brooklyn, New York

Menachem Miodovnik
Department of Obstetrics & Gynecology
Washington Hospital Center Physicians
Washington, DC

Laurie A. P. Mitan, MD
Associate Professor of Clinical
Pediatrics-Affiliated
Department of Pediatrics
University of Cincinnati College of Medicine
Associate Professor
Department of Adolescent Medicine
Cincinnati Children's Hospital
Medical Center
Cincinnati, Ohio

Nashat Moawad, MD
Case Western Reserve University
University Hospitals
MacDonald Women's Hospital
Cleveland, Ohio

Michelle H. Moniz, BA
Fourth Year Medical Student
Department of Obstetrics and Gynecology
Washington University
School of Medicine
St. Louis, Missouri

Christopher P. Montville, MD, MS
Clinical Fellow
Department of Obstetrics and Gynecology
University of Cincinnati College of Medicine
Fellow, Reproductive Endocrinology
and Infertility
Department of Obstetrics and Gynecology
The Christ Hospital
Cincinnati, Ohio

Merry K. Moos, BSN, FNP, MPH
Research Professor
Department of Obstetrics &
Gynecology
University of North Carolina
Chapel Hill, North Carolina

Malcolm G. Munro, MD, FACOG
Professor
Department of Obstetrics & Gynecology
University of California, Los Angeles
Director, Gynecologic Services
Department of Obstetrics & Gynecology
Kaiser Permanente, Los Angeles
Medical Center
Los Angeles, California

David Muram, MD
Professor Emeritus
Department of Obstetrics &
Gynecology
University of Tennessee, Memphis
Medical Fellow
Eli Lilly and Company
Lilly Corporate Center
Indianapolis, Indiana

Stephanie J. Nahas, MD, MSEd
Instructor
Department of Neurology
Thomas Jefferson University Hospital
Philadelphia, Pennsylvania

Anita L. Nelson, MD
Professor, Department of OB/GYN
Harbor-UCLA Medical Center
Manhattan Beach, California

Lawrence M. Nelson, MD
Investigator
Investigative Reproductive Medicine Unit
National Institute of Child Health
and Human Development,
National Institutes of Health
Bethesda, Maryland

Roger B. Newman, MD
Professor of Obstetrics & Gynecology
Department of Obstetrics and Gynecology
Medical University of South Carolina
Vice Chairman for Academic Affairs and
Women's Health Research
Department of Obstetrics and Gynecology
Medical University Hospital
Charleston, South Carolina

Thuong-Thuong Nguyen, MD
Resident
Department of Obstetrics and Gynecology
Stanford Hospitals and Clinics
Stanford, California

Michael S. Nussbaum, MD, FACS
Professor of Surgery and Vice Chair,
   Clinical Affairs
Department of Surgery
University of Cincinnati
Chief of Staff
University Hospital
Cincinnati, Ohio

Meghan B. Oakes, MD
Fellow, Reproductive Endocrinology
   and Infertility
Department of Obstetrics and Gynecology
University of Michigan
Ann Arbor, Michigan

Paul L. Ogburn, Jr., MD
Director of Maternal-Fetal Medicine
Professor
Department of Obstetrics & Gynecology
Stony Brook University
Director of Maternal Fetal Medicine
Department of OB/GYN
Stony Brook University Hospital
Stony Brook, New York

Sara O'Hara, MD
Assistant Professor
Department of Radiology
Cincinnati Children's Hospital
   Medical Center
Cincinnati, Ohio

Arthur Ollendorff, MD
Associate Professor and Residency
   Program Director
Department of OB/GYN
University of Cincinnati
Chief, Section of Gynecology
VA Medical Center-Cincinnati
Cincinnati, Ohio

Hatim A. Omar, MD
Professor
Chief, Division Adolescent Medicine
Department of Pediatrics
University of Kentucky
Lexington, Kentucky

Tarita Pakrashi, MD, MPH, PGYII
PGYII Resident
Department of Obstetrics
   and Gynecology
University of Cincinnati
Cincinnati, Ohio

Lisa L. Park, MD
Clinical Fellow
Department of Adolescent Medicine
Cincinnati Children's Hospital
Cincinnati, Ohio

Willie J. Parker, MD, MPH
Clinical Lecturer
Department of Obstetrics and Gynecology
Gynecology Division, Family
   Planning Section
University of Michigan Health System
Ann Arbor, Michigan

Avinash Paupoo, MD, MA (Cantab)
REI Fellow
Department of Obstetrics and Gynecology
The University of Alabama at Birmingham
Birmingham, Alabama

Jeffrey F. Peipert, MD, PhD
Vice Chair of Clinical Research
Robert J. Terry Professor of Obstetrics
   & Gynecology
Department of OBGYN, Division of
   Clinical Research
Washington University in St. Louis
School of Medicine
St. Louis, Missouri

Carlos Perez-Cosio, MD
Resident
Department of Obstetrics and Gynecology
Rush University
Resident
Department of Obstetrics and Gynecology
Rush University Medical Center
Chicago, Illinois

Nadja Peter, MD
Assistant Professor of Pediatrics
Division of Adolescent Medicine
Children's Hospital of Philadelphia
Philadelphia, Pennsylvania

Sharon Phelan, MD
Professor, Obstetrics & Gynecology
University of New Mexico
   School of Medicine
Albuquerque, New Mexico

Amy H. Picklesimer, MD, MSPH
Clinical Fellow
Division of Maternal Fetal Medicine,
   Department of Obstetrics
   and Gynecology
University of North Carolina School
   of Medicine
Clinical Instructor
Department of Obstetrics and Gynecology
North Carolina Women's Hospital
Chapel Hill, North Carolina

JoAnn V. Pinkerton, MD
Director, Midlife Health
Professor of Obstetrics and Gynecology
University of Virginia Health Systems
Charlottesville, Virginia

Amy E. Pollack, MD, FACOG
Senior Lecturer
School of Health
Columbia University
New York, New York

William J. Polzin, MD
Director, Division of Maternal-Fetal
   Medicine
Department of Obstetrics
Good Samaritan Hospital
Cincinnati, Ohio

Vaishali B. Popat, MD, MPH
Endocrinologist
NICHD, RBMB
National Institutes of Health
Clinical Center at the National
   Institutes of Health
Bethesda, Maryland

Suzanne T. Poppema, MD
Retired Clinical Assistant Professor
Department of Family Medicine
University of Washington
Seattle, Washington
Director
International Medical Consulting
Edmonds, Washington

Jill Powell, MD
Associate Professor
Department of Obstetrics, Gynecology,
   and Women's Health
Saint Louis University
Active Staff Member
Department of Obstetrics
   and Gynecology
St. Mary's Health Center
St. Louis, Missouri

Mona R. Prasad, DO, MPH
Fellow, Maternal Fetal Medicine
Department of Obstetrics and
   Gynecology
The Ohio State University
The Ohio State University Medical Center
Columbus, Ohio

Michael Privitera, MD
Professor and Vice Chair,
   Department of Neurology
University of Cincinnati College
   of Medicine
Cincinnati, Ohio

Ruth Anne Queenan, MD
Associate Professor of Obstetrics
   & Gynecology
University of Rochester School of Medicine
   & Dentistry
Rochester, New York

Elisabeth H. Quint, MD
Professor
Department of Obstetrics & Gynecology
University of Michigan
Ann Arbor, Michigan

Kristin M. Rager, MD, MPH
Director, Adolescent Medicine
Levine Children's Hospital
Teen Health Connection
Charlotte, North Carolina

Lisa Rahangdale, MD, MPH
Instructor, Department of Ob/Gyn
Stanford University Medical Center
Stanford, California

Andrea Rapkin, MD
Professor
Department of Obstetrics and Gynecology
David Geffen School of Medicine at UCLA
Physician
Department of Obstetrics and Gynecology
UCLA Medical Center
Los Angeles, California

Kellie Rath, MD
Resident, Department of Obstetrics
& Gynecology
University of Cincinnati College of Medicine
Cincinnati, Ohio

Robert W. Rebar, MD
Executive Director
American Society for
Reproductive Medicine
Birmingham, Alabama

Kathryn L. Reed, MD
Professor
Department of Obstetrics and Gynecology
University of Arizona
Head
Department of Obstetrics and Gynecology
University Medical Center
Tucson, Arizona

Max C. Reif, MD
Clinical Professor
Internal Medicine–Nephrology
& Hypertension
University of Cincinnati College of Medicine
Cincinnati, Ohio

David R. Repaske, PhD, MD
Associate Professor
Department of Pediatrics
University of Cincinnati
Associate Professor
Division of Endocrinology
Cincinnati Children's Hospital
Medical Center
Cincinnati, Ohio

Jade Richardson, MD
Resident, Department of Obstetrics
& Gynecology
University of Cincinnati
College of Medicine
West Chester, Ohio

Charles Rittenberg, MD
Fellow, Maternal-Fetal Medicine
Department of Obstetrics and Gynecology
Medical University of South Carolina
Instructor of Obstetrics and Gynecology
Department of Obstetrics and Gynecology
MUSC Medical Center
Charleston, South Carolina

Jared C. Robins, MD
Assistant Professor
Department of Obstetrics and Gynecology
Brown University
Women & Infants Hospital
Providence, Rhode Island

Briana Robinson-Walton, MD
Director, Benign Gynecology, Associate
Residency Director
Division of Female Pelvic Medicine &
Reconstructive Surgery
Washington Hospital Center
Assistant Professor, Ob/Gyn
Georgetown University
Washington, DC

Dana Rochester, MD
Endocrinology Fellow
Division of Reproductive Endocrinology
& Fertility
Albert Einstein College of Medicine
Bronx, New York

Susan R. Rose, MD
Professor
Department of Pediatrics and
Endocrinology
University of Cincinnati
Professor
Department of Endocrinology
Cincinnati Children's Hospital
Medical Center
Cincinnati, Ohio

Barak M. Rosenn, MD
Associate Professor
Department of Obstetrics and Gynecology
Columbia College of Physicians
and Surgeons
Director of Obstetrics and
Maternal-Fetal Medicine
Department of Obstetrics and Gynecology
St. Luke's-Roosevelt Hospital Center
New York, New York

Linda S. Ross, DO, PhD
Intern
Department of Obstetrics and Gynecology
Ohio University College of Osteopathic
Medicine
Intern
Department of Obstetrics and Gynecology
O'Bleness Hospital
Athens, Ohio

Rocco A. Rossi, MD
Resident, Department of Obstetrics
and Gynecology
University of Cincinnati College of
Medicine
Cincinnati, Ohio

Nicole K. Ruddock, MD
Maternal Fetal Medicine Fellow
Department of Obstetrics and Gynecology
University of Texas Medical Branch
Galveston, Texas

Tassawan Rungruxsirivorn, MD
Instructor
Department of Obstetrics and Gynecology
Chulalongkorn University
Bangkok, Thailand

Carolyn D. Runowicz, MD
Professor of Obstetrics and Gynecology
Division of Gynecologic Oncology
University of Connecticut Health Center
The Carole and Ray Neag Comprehensive
Cancer Center
Farmington, Connecticut

Seppideh Sami, MS, RD, LDN
Lecturer
Department of Medicine-Primary Care
George Washington University
Research Coordinator
Department of Medicine
and Endocrinology
Walter Reed Army Medical Center
Washington, DC

Nanette Santoro, MD
Professor and Director
Division of Reproductive
Endocrinology & Fertility
Albert Einstein College of Medicine
Bronx, New York

Melanie R. Santos, MD
Resident, Department of Obstetrics
and Gynecology
Stanford University Medical Center
Stanford, California

Brook A. Saunders, MD
Clinical Instructor
Gynecologic Oncology
Markey Cancer Center
Whitney-Hendrickson Women's Cancer
    Facility
University of Kentucky
Lexington, Kentucky

Jonathan A. Schaffir, MD
Assistant Professor
Department of Obstetrics and Gynecology
Ohio State University College of Medicine
Attending Physician
Department of Obstetrics and Gynecology
Ohio State University Medical Center
Columbus, Ohio

Stacey A. Scheib, MD
Resident Physician
Department of Obstetrics and Gynecology
Thomas Jefferson University Hospital
Philadelphia, Pennsylvania

Michael D. Scheiber, MD, MPH
Director of Reproductive Research
Co-Director of In Vitro Fertilization
    Program
Institute for Reproductive Health
Cincinnati, Ohio

John D. Scott, MD
Assistant Professor of Surgery
Department of Surgery
University of Tennessee Graduate School
    of Medicine at Knoxville
University of Tennessee Medical
    Center at Knoxville
Knoxville, Tennessee

Julie Scott, MD
Clinical Assistant VIII
Department of Obstetrics & Gynecology
University of Arizona College of
    Medicine
Tucson, Arizona
Maternal Fetal Medicine Fellow
Department of OB/GYN
Arizona Health Sciences Center
University of Arizona
Banner Good Samaritan Medical Center
Tucson, Arizona and Phoenix, Arizona

John W. Seeds, MD
Professor and Chair
Department of Obstetrics and Gynecology
Virginia Commonwealth University
Chief of Obstetrics and Gynecology
Medical College of Virginia Hospitals
Richmond, Virginia

Vicki L. Seltzer, MD
The Edie and Marvin H. Schur Professor
Department of Obstetrics and Gynecology
    and Women's Health
Albert Einstein College of Medicine
Chairman
Department of Obstetrics and Gynecology
Long Island Jewish Medical Center and
    North Shore University Hospital
New Hyde Park, New York

Scott P. Serden, MD
Associate Professor
Department of Obstetrics
    and Gynecology
University of California,
    Los Angeles Center
Co-Director, Endoscopic Center of
    Excellence
Department of Obstetrics and Gynecology
Cedars-Sinai Medical Center
Los Angeles, California

Robert A. Shapiro, MD
Professor of Pediatrics
University of Cincinnati
    College of Medicine
Center for Safe & Healthy Children
Cincinnati Children's Hospital
    Medical Center
Cincinnati, Ohio

Howard T. Sharp, MD
Associate Professor of Obstetrics
    & Gynecology
University of Utah Health Sciences Center
Salt Lake City, Utah

Elizabeth Shaughnessy, MD, PhD
Assistant Professor
Department of Surgery, Division of
    Surgical Oncology
University of Cincinnati
    College of Medicine
Cincinnati, Ohio

Amber M. Shiflett, MD
Instructor, Obstetrics and Gynecology
University of Mississippi Medical Center
Jackson, Mississippi

Lee P. Shulman, MD
Professor, Reproductive Genetics
Department of Ob/Gyn
Northwestern University Feinberg
    School of Medicine
Chicago, Illinois

Baha Sibai, MD
Professor, Obstetrics & Gynecology
University of Cincinnati College of Medicine
Cincinnati, Ohio

Stephen D. Silberstein, MD
Jefferson Headache Center and
    Department of Neurology
Thomas Jefferson University Hospital
Philadelphia, Pennsylvania

Deborah A. Simon, MD
Staff Physician
Department of OB/Gyn
Gundersen Lutheran Medical Center
LaCrosse, Wisconsin

M. Colleen Simonelli, PhD(c), RN
Clinical Assistant Professor
Department of Maternal/Child Health
William F. Connell School of Nursing
Boston College
Chestnut Hill, Massachusetts

J. D. Sobel, MD
Professor, Division of Infectious Diseases
Wayne State University School of Medicine
Detroit Medical Center
Detroit, Michigan

Eric R. Sokol, MD
Assistant Professor
Department of Obstetrics and Gynecology
Stanford University
Stanford, California
Co-Director, Urogynecology and
    Pelvic Reconstructive Surgery
Division of Gynecologic Specialties
Stanford Hospitals and Clinics
Palo Alto, California

Michael G. Spigarelli, MD, PhD
Assistant Professor of Pediatrics
University of Cincinnati
    College of Medicine
Cincinnati Children's Hospital
    Medical Center
Cincinnati, Ohio

Sharon B. Stanford, MD
Assistant Professor
Department of Psychiatry and
    Family Medicine
University of Cincinnati
Cincinnati, Ohio

Alice M. Stek, MD
Assistant Professor of Clinical Obstetrics
    and Gynecology
University of Southern California
Venice, California

Nada L. Stotland, MD, MPH
Professor of Psychiatry and
    Obstetrics/Gynecology
Rush Medical College, Chicago
Chicago, Illinois

Naomi E. Stotland, MD
Clinical Instructor
Department of Obstetrics, Gynecology,
    & Reproductive Sciences
University of California, San Francisco
San Francisco General Hospital
San Francisco, California

Julie Strickland, MD, MPH
Professor of OB/GYN
University of Missouri Kansas City
Kansas City, Missouri

Phillip G. Stubblefield, MD
Professor of Obstetrics & Gynecology
Boston University Medical Center
Boston, Massachusetts

Joyce Fu Sung, MD
Fellow, Maternal-Fetal Medicine
Department of Obstetrics
    and Gynecology
Stanford University
Stanford, California

Victoria Surdulescu, MD
Assistant Professor, Internal
    Medicine–Pulmonary
University of Cincinnati College of
    Medicine
Cincinnati, Ohio

Edward J. Tanner III, MD
Chief Resident
Department of Gynecology and Obstetrics
Johns Hopkins University
House Staff
Department of Gynecology and
    Obstetrics
Johns Hopkins Hospital
Baltimore, Maryland

DeShawn L. Taylor, MD, MSc
Assistant Professor
Department of Obstetrics and
    Gynecology
Keck School of Medicine
University of Southern California
Physician
Department of Obstetrics and Gynecology
LAC+USC Women's and
    Children's Hospital
Los Angeles, California

Melissa D. Tepe, MD, MPH
OB/GYN PGY 3
Department of Obstetrics and Gynecology
Washington University
Barnes Jewish Hospital
St. Louis, Missouri

**Albert George Thomas, Jr., MD, MS,
    FACOG**
Associate Professor of Obstetrics
    and Gynecology
Senior Consultant Family
    Planning Services
Mount Sinai School of Medicine
Chief Obstetrics and Gynecology
North General Hospital
Bronx VA Medical Center
Ralph Lauren Center for Cancer Care
    and Prevention
New York, New York

Lisa J. Thomas, MD, FACOG
Assistant Professor of Population
    and Family Health
Heilbrunn Department of Population
    and Family Health
Columbia University, Mailman
    School of Public Health
New York, New York

Michael A. Thomas, MD
Professor of Obstetrics & Gynecology
University of Cincinnati College
    of Medicine
Cincinnati, Ohio

Loralei L. Thornburg, MD
Maternal Fetal Medicine Fellow
Department of Obstetrics and
    Gynecology
Division of Maternal Fetal Medicine
University of Rochester, Strong Memorial
    Hospital
Rochester, New York

Tracy V. Ting, MD
Clinical Fellow
Department of Rheumatology
Cincinnati Children's Hospital
    Medical Center
Cincinnati, Ohio

Jonathan D. K. Trager, MD
Assistant Clinical Professor of
    Pediatrics
Mount Sinai School of Medicine
New York, New York

Artemis K. Tsitsika, MD, PhD
Department of Pediatrics-Adolescent
    Medicine
Head of Adolescent Health Unit
Department of Pediatrics,
    Athens University
P & A Kyriakou Children's Hospital
Athens, Greece

**Gary Ventolini, MD, FACOG,
    FAAFM**
Chair and Associate Professor
Department of Obstetrics and
    Gynecology
Boonshoft School of Medicine
Wright State University
Director
Department of Obstetrics
Miami Valley Hospital
Dayton, Ohio

Jeffrey W. Wall, MD
Assistant Professor
Department of Obstetrics
    and Gynecology
University of Missouri-Kansas City,
    School of Medicine
Ambulatory Care Director
Department of Obstetrics and
    Gynecology
Truman Medical Center
Kansas City, Missouri

Shirley L. Wang, MD
Obstetrics and Gynecology
    Resident
Stanford University Medical Center
Stanford, California

Wei Wang, MPH
University of Cincinnati
    College of Medicine
Children's Hospital Medical
    Center of Cincinnati
Division of Adolescent Medicine
Cincinnati, Ohio

Alan G. Waxman, MD, MPH
Professor
Department of Obstetrics and
    Gynecology
University of New Mexico
Medical Director
University of New Mexico Health
    Sciences Center
Albuquerque, New Mexico

Anne M. Weber, MD, MS
Program Director, Female Pelvic
    Floor Disorders
NICHD, NIH
Pittsburgh, Pennsylvania

Jonathan Weeks, MD
Director, Maternal/Fetal
    Medicine
Norton Health Care
Louisville, Kentucky

Louis Weinstein, MD
Professor & Chair
Department of Obstetrics & Gynecology
Thomas Jefferson University
Chief of Service
Department of Obstetrics & Gynecology
Thomas Jefferson University Hospital
Philadelphia, Pennsylvania

Lynn Marie Westphal, MD
Associate Professor of Obstetrics
   & Gynecology
Stanford University Medical
   Center
Stanford, California

Lea E. Widdice, MD
Assistant Professor
Department of Pediatrics
University of Cincinnati
Assistant Professor
Department of Pediatrics
Cincinnati Children's Hospital
   Medical Center
Cincinnati, Ohio

Aimee M. Wilkin, MD, MPH
Assistant Professor
Section on Infectious Diseases,
   Department of Internal Medicine
Wake Forest University Health
   Sciences
Winston-Salem, North Carolina

**Barbara E. Wolfe, PhD, APRN,
   FAAN**
Professor
Department of Psychiatric-Mental
   Health
William F. Connell School of
   Nursing
Boston College
Chestnut Hill, Massachusetts
Clinical Research Associate
Department of Psychiatry
Beth Israel Deaconess Medical
   Center
Boston, Massachusetts

Kathleen Y. Yang, MD
Gynecologic Oncology Clinical Fellow
Department of Obstetrics and Gynecology
Stanford University
Stanford University Medical Center
Stanford, California

Meggan M. Zsemlye, MD
Associate Professor
Assistant Residency Program Director
Department of OB/GYN
University of New Mexico
   School of Medicine
Department of OB/GYN
University of New Mexico Hospital
Albuquerque, New Mexico

Jill M. Zurawski, MD
Clinical Assistant Professor
Department of OB/GYN
University of Arizona
Tucson, Arizona
Clinical Faculty
Department of OB/GYN
Flagstaff Medical Center
Flagstaff, Arizona

CONTENTS

Section III: Women's Health and Primary Care **227**

THE 5-MINUTE OBSTETRICS AND GYNECOLOGY CONSULT

Section I
Gynecologic Signs and Symptoms

AMENORRHEA, ABSENCE OF BLEEDING

Rachel J. Miller, MD

 BASICS

DESCRIPTION

- Amenorrhea is the absence of menses. It may be divided into primary and secondary amenorrhea:
  – Primary amenorrhea refers to the absence of menses by age 13 with no breast development, or by age 15 with normal secondary sexual development. Or absence of menses ≥5 years after thelarche.
  – Secondary amenorrhea is the absence of menses for 90 days or 3 months in females who previously menstruated.
- Amenorrhea is a sign of an underlying disease mechanism, and therapy should be directed at treating the specific condition.
- Most causes of secondary amenorrhea can also cause primary amenorrhea if the onset is prior to menarche.

EPIDEMIOLOGY

- Amenorrhea affects females during their reproductive years.
- The incidence of secondary amenorrhea is 3.3%:
  – 7.6% of females ages 15–24,
  – 3% ages 25–34, and
  – 3.7% ages 35–44 years have amenorrhea

RISK FACTORS

- Obesity
- Weight loss
- Excessive exercise
- Chronic disease

Genetics

- Amenorrhea can be associated with multiple genetic disorders but, no single mutation causes it.
- See "Gonadal dysgenesis; Ovarian Insufficiency/Premature Ovarian Failure (POF)"

PATHOPHYSIOLOGY

- Normal menstrual function requires an intact hypothalamic-pituitary-ovarian-uterine/vaginal axis.
- Normally, the hypothalamus releases pulsatile GnRH, which stimulates the pituitary to release FSH and LH.
- These gonadotropins act on the ovaries to stimulate follicular development, ovulation, and the resulting corpus luteum.
- The ovaries secrete estrogen and progesterone, which stimulate proliferation and maturation of the uterine endometrium.
- In the absence of fertilization, menstrual blood exits through a normal outflow tract.
- Any disruption or abnormality in this axis can cause amenorrhea.

ASSOCIATED CONDITIONS

Multiple, see "Differential Diagnosis"

 DIAGNOSIS

SIGNS AND SYMPTOMS

Absence of menses

History

The patient should be questioned regarding:

- Age at thelarche, pubarche, and menarche
- Menstrual history
- Sexual activity
- Pregnancy history
- History of uterine instrumentation
- Eating and exercise habits, weight loss
- Galactorrhea, headaches, anosmia, visual field defects, polyuria, polydipsia
- Symptoms of estrogen deficiency such as hot flushes or vaginal dryness
- Signs of androgen excess
- Medication use
- Illicit drug use
- Risk factors for tuberculosis or HIV
- Family history:
  – Menarche
  – Height
  – Infertility
  – Autoimmune and genetic disorders

Physical Exam

- Growth pattern
- Height and weight (BMI)
- Tanner staging
- Evidence of androgen excess, such as acne, hirsutism, clitoromegaly
- Cushing disease stigmata
- Thyroid exam
- Breast exam, especially looking for galactorrhea
- External genitalia
- Internal genitalia if developmentally appropriate

TESTS

Pregnancy must be evaluated in both primary and secondary amenorrhea.

Labs

- Urine or serum β-hCG
- TSH
- Prolactin
- If signs of hyperandrogenism:
  – Serum DHEAS and testosterone
  – 17-hydroxyprogesterone
- If symptoms or signs of hypoestrogenism:
  – FSH
  – Estradiol
- If symptoms/physical findings suggestive of genetic disorder or POF <30 years:
  – Karyotype

Imaging

- Bone age if concern for constitutional delay
- Transabdominal pelvic ultrasound to confirm presence of uterus and normal gonads or evaluate for polycystic ovaries
- If elevated prolactin levels:
  – MRI of brain to rule out pituitary tumor (i.e., prolactinoma)
- If history of uterine instrumentation:
  – Hysterosalpingogram

DIFFERENTIAL DIAGNOSIS

Infection

- Chronic disease or infection
- Uterine infectious sequelae

Metabolic/Endocrine

- POF:
  – Turner syndrome
  – Gonadal dysgenesis
- Complete androgen insensitivity
- Hyperprolactinemia:
  – Hypothyroidism
  – Prolactinoma
  – Medications
- Pituitary disease:
  – Empty sella syndrome
- Hypothalamic dysfunction:
  – Anorexia nervosa
  – Excessive exercise
  – Kallmann syndrome
- Cushing's disease:
  – Congenital adrenal hyperplasia

Immunologic

Autoimmune premature ovarian failure

Tumor/Malignancy

- Prolactinoma
- Androgen producing tumors

Trauma

See Sheehan Syndrome.

Drugs

Iatrogenic:

- Chemotherapy (i.e., cyclophosphamide)
- Radiation therapy
- Hormonal contraceptives
- Medications that induce hyperprolactinemia
- Levonorgestrel intrauterine system
- Leuprolide

Other/Miscellaneous

- Physiologic:
  – Prepubertal
  – Pregnancy and lactation
  – Menopause
- Congenital outflow tract anomalies:
  – Müllerian agenesis
  – Androgen insensitivity syndrome
  – Imperforate hymen
  – Transverse vaginal septum
- Acquired outflow tract abnormalities:
  – Uterine synechiae/Asherman syndrome
  – Cervical stenosis
- PCOS

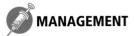 MANAGEMENT

GENERAL MEASURES
- Always treat the underlying etiology.
- Weight loss for overweight or obese patients
- Normalization of BMI and appropriate exercise behaviors for patients with excessive exercise and disordered eating

SPECIAL THERAPY
Complementary and Alternative Therapies
- Healthy, well-balanced diet to achieve normal BMI
- Appropriate, moderate exercise to achieve or maintain normal BMI

MEDICATION (DRUGS)
Always treat the underlying etiology:
- Thyroid replacement if hypothyroid
- Dopamine-agonist if hyperprolactinemia
- Metformin if PCOS and insulin resistant
- Cyclical estrogen-progesterone
- Combined estrogen-progesterone oral contraceptive pills, patches, or vaginal ring
- Patients seeking pregnancy may require ovulation induction with clomiphene citrate, exogenous gonadotropins, or pulsatile GnRH.

SURGERY
- Hymenotomy if imperforate hymen
- Resection of vaginal septum
- Tumor resection
- Lysis of intrauterine synechiae
- If gonadal dysgenesis or androgen insensitivity syndrome, consideration for gonadectomy to prevent malignant transformation

 FOLLOW-UP

DISPOSITION
The evaluation of and treatment for amenorrhea is performed in the outpatient setting.

Issues for Referral
- Many etiologies for amenorrhea can be managed by the primary care provider.
- Conditions that require the help of a specialist may include:
  - Congenital outflow tract anomaly: Pediatric gynecologist or reproductive endocrinologist
  - Uterine synechiae: Gynecologist or reproductive endocrinologist
  - POF: Endocrinologist, gynecologist, reproductive endocrinologist
  - Pituitary tumors: Neurosurgeon and endocrinologist
  - Anorexia nervosa: Psychiatrist or eating disorder specialist
  - PCOS: Endocrinologist, reproductive endocrinologist, or gynecologist
  - Other types of tumors: Oncologist, gynecologist, gynecologic or surgical oncologist
  - Infertility: Obstetrician/Gynecologist or reproductive endocrinologist

PATIENT MONITORING
- Prognosis is based on the underlying etiology.
- Many patients will begin or resume menses following therapy for the underlying condition, especially in cases of endocrine diseases, functional hypothalamic dysfunction, and PCOS.
- Prolonged hypoestrogenic states may lead to bone mineral density loss.
- Many causes of amenorrhea result in anovulation and infertility if patients remain undiagnosed and untreated.
- Women with PCOS may also have insulin resistance and should be screened for diabetes.
- Prolonged amenorrhea, particularly in obese females, is a risk factor for endometrial cancer.

BIBLIOGRAPHY

American College of Obstetrics and Gynecology Committee on Practice Bulletins-Gynecology. Management of infertility caused by ovulatory dysfunction. *Obstet Gynecol*. 2002;99(2):347–358.

Mitan LAP. Menstrual dysfunction in anorexia nervosa. *J Pediatr Adolesc Gynecol*. 2004;17:81–85.

Munster K, et al. Secondary amenorrhoea: Prevalence and medical contact: A cross sectional study from a Danish county. *Br J Obstetr Gynecol*. 1992;99: 430–433.

Pettersson F, et al. Epidemiology of secondary amenorrhea: Incidence and prevalence rates. *Am J Obstet Gynecol*. 1973;117:80–86.

The Practice Committee of the American Society for Reproductive Medicine. Current evaluation of amenorrhea. *Fertil Steril*. 2006;86(Suppl 4): S148–S155.

Speroff L, et al. *Clinical Gynecologic Endocrinology and Infertility*, 7th ed. 2004.

Welt CK, et al. Etiology, diagnosis, and treatment of primary amenorrhea. UpToDate Online 14.3, 2005.

Welt CK, et al. Etiology, diagnosis, and treatment of secondary amenorrhea. UpToDate Online 14.3, 2005.

 MISCELLANEOUS

CLINICAL PEARLS
The most common cause of amenorrhea is pregnancy.

ABBREVIATIONS
- DHEAS—Dehydroepiandrosterone
- FSH—Follicle stimulating hormone
- GnRH—Gonadotropin releasing hormone
- hCG—Human chorionic gonadotropins
- LH—Luteinizing hormone
- PCOS—Polycystic ovarian syndrome
- POF—Premature ovarian failure

CODES
ICD9-CM
- 256.8 Amenorrhea (due to ovarian dysfunction)
- 256.8 Amenorrhea (hyperhormonal)
- 626.0 Amenorrhea (primary or secondary)

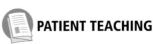 PATIENT TEACHING

PREVENTION
Amenorrhea may be prevented by:
- Treating underlying conditions
- Maintaining an appropriate body weight

BLEEDING, ABNORMAL UTERINE, IN ADOLESCENTS

Jeffrey W. Wall, MD
Julie L. Strickland, MD, MPH

 BASICS

DESCRIPTION
- Abnormal vaginal bleeding in adolescent girls can be due to a number of different etiologies and may indicate significant underlying disease. Heavy, prolonged, and recurrent bleeding episodes in adolescents do not represent normal bleeding patterns.
- Bleeding episodes lasting >7 days are statistically uncommon and require investigation.

Age-Related Factors
Cycles <21 d or >42 d are statistically uncommon, even in 1st gynecologic year and may indicate disease.

EPIDEMIOLOGY
- 55–82% of girls have anovulatory cycles in the 1st 2 years after menarche:
  - Only 20% are anovulatory after 4–5 years.
- PCOS and hyperandrogenism affect 5–10% of adults, and symptoms typically begin in adolescence.

ALERT
19–28% of girls admitted for acute bleeding have an underlying coagulation disorder.

RISK FACTORS
- Recent menarche
- Bleeding disorders
- Acne, hirsutism
- Obesity
- Pelvic pain
- STDs

PATHOPHYSIOLOGY
- The HPO axis is responsible for the orderly progression of hormones in the menstrual cycle.
- Immaturity of the HPO axis at menarche can lead to irregular and anovulatory cycles:
  - Disordered endometrium sheds irregularly and unpredictably

ASSOCIATED CONDITIONS
- Associated with hyperandrogenic states:
  - PCOS
  - CAH
- Coagulopathies:
  - vWD, ITP, hepatic dysfunction

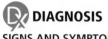 **DIAGNOSIS**

SIGNS AND SYMPTOMS
History
Obtaining a careful history may be difficult. A relaxed and nonthreatening atmosphere can aid when interviewing an anxious adolescent. Pertinent points to consider are:
- Medical history
- Pubertal milestones:
  - Breast and pubic hair development
  - Age at menarche:
    - Onset of menorrhagia with menarche is highly suspicious for a bleeding disorder.
- Sexual history
- STDs or pelvic infections
- Recent trauma
- Family history of bleeding disorders:
  - History of "easy" bleeding/bruising
  - Routine cuts and scratches
  - Surgical complications
  - Bleeding gums:
    - Dental procedures
  - Pelvic pain:
    - Consider obstructive congenital anomaly if intermenstrual bleeding
    - Endometriosis
- Menses can vary greatly and are highly subjective, a careful menstrual history should include:
  - Quantity and quality of flow:
    - Pad count
    - Number of "overflow pads"
    - Use of "double protection"—tampon+pad
    - Number of hours between pad changes
  - Presence of clots
  - Color of flow
  - Pain/Cramping
  - PMS symptoms suggest ovulatory cycles

Review of Systems
- Hair growth:
  - Facial, breasts, abdomen, back
  - Male pattern
- Weight gain or loss
- Exercise patterns
- Heat and cold tolerance

Physical Exam
- Vital signs
- Height, weight, BMI
- General exam should include:
  - Tanner staging
  - Signs of virilization:
    - Male pattern hair growth
    - Hirsutism
    - Acne
  - Ecchymoses or petechiae
  - Body habitus
  - Abdominal exam:
    - Masses
    - Pain
- Genital exam should include:
  - Inspection of external genitalia and introitus:
    - Trauma
    - Foreign bodies
    - Anomalies
  - Assessment of degree of bleeding
  - Obtain genital cultures as indicated
- Speculum exam may not be necessary:
  - If patient is virginal
  - In absence of acute heavy bleeding or pelvic pain
- Speculum exam should be performed:
  - If heavy vaginal bleeding acutely
  - Suspected vaginal trauma or foreign body
  - Use an adolescent (Pederson) or narrow-blade speculum (Huffman)
  - Consider sedation or pelvic exam under anesthesia if necessary

TESTS
Labs
- Initial blood work:
  - Pregnancy test
  - CBC
  - Platelet count
  - Fibrinogen
  - Prothrombin time
  - Partial thromboplastin time
  - Bleeding time or PFA-100
- If bleeding is severe, prolonged, or associated with menarche, also include:
  - von Willebrand factor antigen
  - Factor VIII activity
  - Factor XI antigen
  - Ristocetin C cofactor
  - Platelet aggregation studies
- If endocrinopathy or hyperandrogenism:
  - Thyroid testing
  - Testosterone, DHEA-S, 17-OHP
- All blood work should be drawn prior to initiating therapy.
- Consider endometrial biopsy:
  - If obese or PCOS

Imaging
- Transabdominal ultrasound:
  - Especially if exam is incomplete, bleeding is atypical or associated with pelvic pain
- MRI after screening ultrasound:
  - Helpful in diagnosing congenital anomalies

DIFFERENTIAL DIAGNOSIS
Pregnancy Considerations
Complications of pregnancy should always be considered and ruled out even if sexual activity is denied.
- Consequences of missing a pregnancy-related complication can be severe:
  - Miscarriage
  - Ectopic pregnancy

Infection
- STD
- Endometritis

Hematologic
Coagulation disorder:
- von Willebrand disease
- Factor XI deficiency
- ITP
- Leukemia

Metabolic/Endocrine
- Anovulation
- Endocrinopathy:
  - Polycystic ovarian syndrome
  - Congenital adrenal hyperplasia
  - Hyperthyroidism

Tumor/Malignancy
- Estrogen/Androgen secreting tumors
- Endometrial hyperplasia

Trauma
- Sexual abuse
- Straddle injury

Drugs
- Exogenous estrogen administration
- Prolonged medroxyprogesterone acetate

Other/Miscellaneous
- Systemic disease:
  - Renal disease
  - Diabetes
- Reproductive tract:
  - Leiomyoma
  - Endometriosis
  - Congenital anomalies
  - Cervical polyps

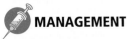 ## MANAGEMENT

GENERAL MEASURES
Treatment should be categorized according to the severity of the bleeding.

- Severe bleeding:
  - Hemoglobin <9.0, hypovolemia:
    - Hospitalization
    - IV fluid resuscitation
    - Consider blood products
  - IV CEE, 25 mg q4h for 24 hours
  - Once bleeding is controlled:
    - Oral CEE 2.5 mg/d on days 1–25 with MPA 10 mg/d on days 19–25
    - Consider long-term therapy with OCPs
    - Erythropoietin
  - Patients with bleeding disorders:
    - Desmopressin
    - Antifibrinolytics
    - Extended-cycle contraceptives for menstrual suppression
- Moderate bleeding:
  - Interfering with daily activities, mild anemia:
    - Oral CEE 2.5 mg/d on days 1–25 with MPA 10 mg/d on days 19–25
    - Alternatively, accelerated dosing of OCP may be used with 2 pills daily for 1 week followed by 1 pill daily for 3 weeks.
  - Once bleeding is controlled:
    - Combination OCP for 3–6 months
    - Iron replacement
- Mild bleeding:
  - Menses prolonged or irregular, no anemia:
    - Reassurance
    - NSAIDs
    - Consider combination OCP

MEDICATION (DRUGS)
- CEE:
  - IV for severe bleeding
  - Oral for long-term control
- MPA:
  - Usually given with CEE for cyclic control
  - May be given alone for 10 days each month to improve menstrual sloughing
- DMPA:
  - Not first-line therapy in adolescents
  - IM injection q12wk
  - 50% amenorrhea at 12 months:
    - May have prolonged breakthrough bleeding
  - Use for >2 years:
    - Increased risk of low BMD
      - May be reversible

- OCP:
  - Reliable cycle control
  - Contraceptive benefit
  - May improve acne and hirsutism
  - Low-dose combination pills
  - Most pill combinations are effective but may need to be tailored individually.
- NSAIDs:
  - Scheduled naproxen sodium or mefenamic acid given with menses decreases menstrual flow

SURGERY
- Pelvic exam under anesthesia:
  - Anxious or younger patients
  - Repair pelvic trauma
- D&C:
  - Rarely indicated in adolescents
  - May be required if failure of hormonal treatment

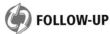 ## FOLLOW-UP

Once the bleeding has been controlled and the patient has been started on long-term therapy:
- Encourage use of menstrual diary
- Reevaluate bleeding pattern in 3–6 months

DISPOSITION
Issues for Referral
- Referral to pediatric/adolescent gynecologist:
  - Continued irregular menses
  - Suspected anomalies
  - Reproductive endocrinopathies:
    - CAH, PCOS
- Referral to hematology:
  - If patient has a bleeding disorder

PROGNOSIS
- Usually good once the source of the bleeding has been identified and adequate treatment initiated
- Continued maturation of the HPO axis usually results in regular menses within 3–5 years.
- Continued irregular menses after 4 years is associated with decreased reproductive potential.

BIBLIOGRAPHY

Bevan JA, et al. Bleeding disorders: A common cause of menorrhagia in adolescents. *J Pediatr*. 2001; 138(6):856–861.

Claessens EA, et al. Acute adolescent menorrhagia. *Am J Obstet Gynecol*. 1981;139(3):277–280.

Davis A, et al. Triphasic norgestimate-ethinyl estradiol for treating dysfunctional uterine bleeding. *Obstet Gynecol*. 2000;96(6):913–920.

DeVore GR, et al. Use of intravenous Premarin in the treatment of dysfunctional uterine bleeding: A double blind randomized control study. *Obstet Gynecol*. 1982;59(3):285–290.

Hillard P. Menstruation in young girls: A clinical perspective. *Obstet Gynecol*. 2002;99:655–662.

Hillard PJ. Adolescent and pediatric gynecology: An introduction. *Curr Opin Obstet Gynecol*. 2006;18(5):485–486.

Strickland JL, et al. Abnormal uterine bleeding in adolescents. *Infert Reprod Med Clin N Am*. 2003;14:71–85.

 ## MISCELLANEOUS

SYNONYM(S)
- Hypermenorrhea
- Ovulatory menorrhagia
- Menorrhagia

CLINICAL PEARLS
- Onset of menorrhagia with menarche is highly suspicious for a bleeding disorder.
- Speculum exam may not be necessary if the patient is virginal.
- Bleeding during hormonal contraceptive use has different etiology and management from spontaneous bleeding; patient may consider it to be similar.

ABBREVIATIONS
- BMD—Bone mineral density
- CAH—Congenital adrenal hyperplasia
- CEE—Conjugated equine estrogens
- DHEA/S—Dehydroepiandrosterone-DHEA sulfate
- DMPA—Depo medroxyprogesterone acetate
- HPO—Hypothalamic-pituitary-ovarian
- ITP—Idiopathic thrombocytopenia
- MPA—Medroxyprogesterone acetate
- OCP—Oral contraceptive pill
- PCOS—Polycystic ovarian syndrome
- STD—Sexually transmitted disease
- vWD—von Willebrand disease

CODES

ICD9-CM
- 626.2 Excessive or frequent menstruation
- 626.3 Menorrhagia, pubertal
- 626.4 Irregular menstruation
- 626.6 Metrorrhagia
- 626.8 Menstrual disorder, NEC
- 626.9 Menstrual disorder, NOS

 ## PATIENT TEACHING

- Adolescents should be encouraged to keep a menstrual diary to better track the patterns of their menses.
- Parameters of acceptable bleeding should be discussed soon after menarche.

PREVENTION
- Early diagnosis and management of PCOS can minimize menstrual dysfunction, hirsutism, acne, and psychosocial sequelae.
- Lifestyle management/weight loss may improve menstrual function if overweight/obese.

5

BLEEDING, ABNORMAL UTERINE: HEAVY MENSTRUAL BLEEDING

Malcolm G. Munro, MD
Eve S. Cunningham, MD

BASICS

DESCRIPTION
Heavy menstrual bleeding (HMB) is the symptom of excessive flow or duration of bleeding in the context of consistent and predictable menstrual cycles for >3 months. Blood loss >60–80 mL per cycle is associated with depletion of iron stores and anemia and, in research studies, has been used to quantify HMB. In clinical practice, HMB is generally self-defined, and should not require that a patient be anemic to validate the symptom.

Age-Related Factors
HMB applies only to women of reproductive age who have a uterus and one or both ovaries.

ALERT
Pediatric Considerations
Adolescents with heavy menstrual bleeding should be evaluated for an underlying systemic disorder such as vWD or other inherited disorders of hemostasis.

Pregnancy Considerations
Bleeding related to pregnancy (during or prior to the resumption of regular menses) is not HMB (see Hemorrhage: First Trimester, Third Trimester, Postpartum).

Geriatric Considerations
Postmenopausal bleeding is *not* HMB (see Bledding, Abnormal Uterine: Postmenopausal and Menopausal).

EPIDEMIOLOGY
~10–30% of menstruating women experience HMB.

RISK FACTORS
- Copper IUD
- Disorders of systemic hemostasis:
  - Inherited:
    - vWD; other
  - Acquired:
    - Idiopathic thrombocytopenic purpura; other

Genetics
Inherited disorders of hemostasis:
- vWD:
  - Autosomal dominant
  - 5 subtypes
  - Found in 13% of women with heavy menstrual bleeding
- Factor XI, XIII, and others

PATHOPHYSIOLOGY
An inability of the endometrium to adequately control menstrual flow for 1 or a combination of the following reasons:
- Disorders of local hemostasis:
  - Decreased production of endometrial vasoconstrictors:
    - PGF_2-alpha
    - Endothelin-1
  - Excess levels of endometrial vasodilators:
    - PGI
    - PGE_2
  - Increase in endometrial fibrinolysis:
    - High levels of plasminogen activator
    - Low levels of plasminogen activator inhibitor

- Systemic hemostasis:
  - Defects in the coagulation cascade may prevent formation of intravascular plugs, prevent optimal hemostasis, and result in excessive menstrual bleeding:
    - vWD
    - Factor deficiencies
- Systemic diseases including renal failure/dialysis, hepatic failure, leukemia
- Iatrogenic systemic agents such as anticoagulants and cytotoxic chemotherapy
- Local pathology:
  - Submucosal leiomyoma(s)
  - Adenomyosis
  - Chronic endometritis (?)
  - Endometrial polyps (?)
- Iatrogenic, local:
  - Copper IUD

ASSOCIATED CONDITIONS
Ovulatory DUB (idiopathic HMB):
- Abnormally heavy menstrual bleeding in the reproductive years unrelated to pregnancy, systemic disorder of hemostasis, exogenous gonadal steroids, an IUD, or structural uterine pathology
- Bleeding is predictable and cyclic.
- Estimated to affect up to 20% of reproductive aged women
- Etiology is a disorder of local hemostatic mechanisms as described in HMB (decreased vasoconstrictors, excess vasodilators, and/or increased fibrinolysis)

DIAGNOSIS

SIGNS AND SYMPTOMS
History
HMB is a symptom, not a diagnosis.
- Menstrual history:
  - Regular and predictable onset of flow with a consistent cycle length of 22–35 days (>3 months)
  - Heavy menstrual volume may include the following:
    - Frequent pad changes (q30min–2h)
    - Use of double protection (tampon and pad, or double pads)
    - Excessive duration of flow (>7 days)
    - Passage of blood clots
    - Soiling of underwear, bed linen, or upholstery
- Dizziness and lightheadedness secondary to iron-deficiency anemia
- Dysmenorrhea may or may not be present.
- Screen by history for disorders of hemostasis.
  - Positive screen if:
    - Excessive menstrual bleeding since menarche, or
    - History of one of the following: Postpartum hemorrhage, surgery-related bleeding, or bleeding associated with dental work, or
    - History of 2 or more of the following: Bruising >5 cm once or twice/month, epistaxis once or twice/month, frequent gum bleeding, family history of bleeding symptoms

Review of Systems
Fatigue related to anemia

Physical Exam
Confirm bleeding is of uterine origin:
- Pelvic exam:
  - Estimate size, shape, contour, and position of uterus.
    - An enlarged, irregular, and mobile uterus is consistent with leiomyoma; it is not possible on exam to determine relationship to the endometrial cavity.
    - A diffusely enlarged and tender uterus is consistent with adenomyosis.
- Speculum exam:
  - If examined during menstruation, should see active bleeding from cervical os.

TESTS
Endometrial sampling (endometrial biopsy or D&C):
- Consider in women >40 years, particularly if there is uncertainty regarding the predictability of the onset of menstrual flow.
- Objective tests for menorrhagia measuring blood loss >60–80 mL per cycle are not generally practicable.
- Evaluation of menstrual-related quality of life scales (Aberdeen Menorrhagia Severity Scale) are feasible but generally reserved for research.

Lab
- Pregnancy test
- CBC
- If patient fails screening by history for underlying disorder of hemostasis:
  - PT, aPTT
  - vWF antigen
  - Ristocetin cofactor
  - Factor VIII
  - ABO type
  - Bleeding time
  - PFA-100
- Other labs to consider when applicable:
  - TSH, iron studies to assess anemia; BUN/Cr to assess renal function; liver function tests

Imaging
- TVS may be used as a screening test to identify uterine leiomyomas and estimate their relationship to the endometrium. Adenomyosis may also be detected with transvaginal sonography.
- If TVS cannot confirm that the endometrial thickness is within normal limits and that leiomyomas are not impacting the endometrial cavity, 1 or more of the following procedures should be performed:
  - Sonohysterography may be used to define intracavitary lesions (i.e., polyps and myomas).
  - Hysteroscopy is a diagnostic procedure to evaluate for intracavitary lesions and in some instances allow for simultaneous removal.
  - MRI:
    - Useful in adolescent and pediatric patients to avoid vaginal manipulation
    - May distinguish between focal adenomyosis (adenomyomas) and leiomyomas
    - May be more sensitive than TVS for diffuse adenomyosis

DIFFERENTIAL DIAGNOSIS

- Infection:
  - Endometritis
- Hematologic:
  - Disorders of hemostasis (coagulopathies)
  - Congenital:
    - vWD, factor deficiencies, afibrinogenemia
    - Acquired: ITP and other platelet disorders
- Metabolic/Endocrine:
  - Renal failure
  - Hepatic failure
- Tumor/Malignancy:
  - Submucosal myoma
  - Endometrial polyps (?)
- Drugs:
  - Anticoagulants
  - Cytotoxic chemotherapy agents
- Other/Miscellaneous:
  - Copper IUD
  - Adenomyosis

 ## MANAGEMENT

GENERAL MEASURES
For HMB that is profuse requiring emergent intervention, see Hemorrhage: Acute Uterine Bleeding (Nongestational).

MEDICATION (DRUGS)
- Idiopathic HMB is presumably secondary to disorders of local hemostasis.
- Iron therapy:
  - Should be offered to all patients with HMB
  - May be only therapy that some women want/need
- Systemic:
  - NSAIDs
    - Ibuprofen, 600 mg PO t.i.d. × 5 days of cycle
    - 33–55% reduction in menstrual flow
  - Combined oral contraceptive pills:
    - 40–45% volume reduction with cyclic use
    - Consider continuous/extended cycle therapy
  - Tranexamic acid:
    - 2.5–5 g/d in divided doses (eg, 1 g q.i.d.)
    - 30–55% reduction of flow (anticipate future availability in the US)
  - Progestins:
    - Cyclical administration of progestins in the luteal phase is *not* effective.
    - Continuous may be effective. Oral norethindrone acetate 5–15 mg/d, or
    - Depomedroxyprogesterone acetate 150 mg IM q3mo (Note: associated with initiation of irregular AUB in 50% of cases in the 1st year of use)
  - GnRH agonists:
    - For special-case scenarios
    - Leuprolide acetate 3.75 mg IM monthly or 11.25 mg IM 3 monthly
    - May be used temporarily to induce a medical menopause to allow both treatment of anemia and procedure planning
  - DDAVP:
    - For severe vWD patients
    - 0.3 mcg/kg IV × 1
    - 150 mcg NAS each nostril × 1

- Local:
  - Levonorgestrel-IUS:
    - Progestin-releasing intrauterine device
    - Delivers high local levels and very low systemic levels of progestin
    - Reduces blood loss by up to 94% in 1st 3 months of use
    - Can cause light irregular bleeding/spotting that usually resolves in 3–6 months
    - Amenorrhea in 20–40+% at 1 year
    - May be used up to 5 years

SURGERY
Surgical interventions for idiopathic HMB are generally reserved for those patients who have failed or are intolerant of medical therapy and who are willing to forego fertility.

- Endometrial ablation (see topic)
- Hysterectomy (see topics):
  - 100% successful in treating HMB
- For women with HMB secondary to local pathology (e.g., leiomyomas, polyps, adenomyosis), a variety of surgical interventions is available, including those that prevent fertility (e.g., hysterectomy) and those which preserve or even enhance fertility (e.g., resectoscopic myomectomy). See related chapters for details.

 ## FOLLOW-UP

Patient should continue to be closely followed after treatment is initiated to evaluate response.

DISPOSITION
Issues for Referral
Referral to a hematologist may be appropriate for further investigation or management of a disorder of hemostasis.

PROGNOSIS
- In randomized trials comparing medical and surgical interventions, 58% of patients placed on medical therapy will undergo surgical intervention within 2 years.
- 16% of patients with LNG-IUS placed for HMB will require a surgical procedure within 1 year.
- 20% of women with HMB undergo hysterectomy by the age of 55.

PATIENT MONITORING
Recheck CBC as needed.

BIBLIOGRAPHY

Kouides P, et al. Hemostasis and menstruation: Appropriate investigation for underlying disorders of hemostasis in women with excessive menstrual bleeding. *Fertil Steril*. 2005;84:1338–1344.

Livingstone M, et al. Mechanisms of abnormal uterine bleeding. *Hum Reprod Update*. 2002;8:60–65.

Lukes A, et al. Disorders of hemostasis and excessive menstrual bleeding: Prevalence and clinical impact. *Fertil Steril*. 2005;84:1345–1351.

Marjoribanks J, et al. Surgery versus medical therapy for heavy menstrual bleeding. *Cochrane Database Syst Rev*. 2006;2.

Munro MG. Medical management of abnormal uterine bleeding. *Obstet Gynecol Clin North Am*. 2000;27: 287–304.

 ## MISCELLANEOUS

SYNONYM(S)
- Abnormal uterine bleeding
- Anovulatory bleeding
- Dysfunctional uterine bleeding

CLINICAL PEARLS
Exam of the uterine corpus may be misleadingly normal or abnormal. For example, the uterus may be palpably normal but contain a clinically relevant polyp or leiomyoma within the endometrial cavity; or, a palpable leiomyoma may not affect the endometrial cavity and therefore may not be related to the bleeding.

ABBREVIATIONS
- aPTT—Activated partial thromboplastin time
- AUB—Abnormal uterine bleeding
- BUN—Blood urea nitrogen
- Cr—Creatinine
- DDAVP—Desmopressin acetate
- DUB—Dysfunctional uterine bleeding
- GnRH—Gonadotropin releasing hormone
- HMB—Heavy menstrual bleeding
- IUD—Intrauterine device
- LNG-IUS—Levonorgestrel-releasing interuterine system
- NSAID—Nonsteroidal anti-inflammatory drug
- PFA-100®—Platelet Function Analyzer
- PGE/PGF—Prostaglandin E and F
- PGI—Prostacylcin
- PT—Prothrombin time
- TSH—Thyroid stimulating hormone
- TVS—Transvaginal sonography
- vWD—von Willebrand disease

CODES

ICD9-CM
- 626.2 Menorrhagia
- 626.3 Menorrhagia, pubertal
- 627 Premenopausal menorrhagia
- 206707 Referral vaginal bleeding

 ## PATIENT TEACHING

- Explain the relationship of blood loss to the development of anemia and the related symptoms; if anemia not present, counsel that untreated anemia will likely eventually occur.
- Explain risks, benefits of the various medical and surgical options.
- Explain to patient that HMB is generally a chronic condition that often requires further investigation and long-term management including chronic medical or even surgical intervention.

PREVENTION
Prophylactic iron therapy

BLEEDING, ABNORMAL UTERINE: WITH HORMONAL THERAPY OR CONTRACEPTION

Kelly A. Best, MD
Andrew M. Kaunitz, MD

 BASICS

DESCRIPTION
- AUB includes heavier than usual bleeding, prolonged menses, menstrual periods more frequent than every 3 weeks, bleeding/spotting between menses, bleeding after intercourse.
- BTB is used to describe spotting/bleeding in women using cyclical COC (estrogen-progestin) occurring during times other than scheduled withdrawal bleeding.
- BTB may also refer to unscheduled bleeding during continuous use of hormonal contraceptives, progestin-only methods (DMPA), progestin implants, or POPs, or menopausal hormone therapy.

ALERT
Geriatric Considerations
Atrophy and neoplasm are common causes of postmenopausal bleeding and, in the absence of hormone therapy, are NOT considered BTB. These symptoms must be evaluated. (See Bleeding, Abnormal Uterine: Postmenopausal and Menopausal.)

Pregnancy Considerations
Bleeding during pregnancy is not AUB/BTB and must be evaluated.

AGE-RELATED FACTORS
- In reproductive age women on contraception, BTB during the 1st 3 months of use of cyclic combination usually resolves without intervention after 3 months of continued use.
- Malignancy is rare in premenopausal women.
- Risk increases at ≥45 years

EPIDEMIOLOGY
BTB is the primary reason why women stop their contraceptive method of choice.

RISK FACTORS
- *Chlamydia* infection
- Imperfect contraceptive use (missed pills, late restart with new 28-day package)
- Pregnancy
- Smoking
- Obesity
- Structural anomalies (polyps, fibroids)
- Malignancy (endometrial, cervical, vaginal, ovarian)

Genetics
Genetic predisposition to anatomic anomalies such as fibroids

PATHOPHYSIOLOGY
- Benign conditions:
  - Pregnancy, fibroids (particularly those which are submucosal), polyps (endometrial, endocervical), endometriosis, cervical/vaginal infection, adenomyosis
- Systemic diseases:
  - Coagulopathies, hypothyroidism, liver/renal disease

- Neoplasia:
  - Hormone therapy
  - Hormonal contraception (oral, transdermal patch, vaginal ring, injections, implant) and intrauterine devices (copper, levonorgestrel)

ASSOCIATED CONDITIONS
See "Risk Factors" and "Pathophysiology."

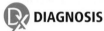 **DIAGNOSIS**

SIGNS AND SYMPTOMS
History
Complaints of spotting between predicted menstrual periods often requiring pad/panty liner. Review medications, medical/surgical and family history.

Physical Exam
Perform pelvic exam to assess cervix for lesions/infection, vaginal mucosa for atrophy/lesions or infection, uterine size/shape/mobility/tenderness, ovaries.

TESTS
- Office endometrial sampling (biopsy) to detect hyperplasia/neoplasia or atrophy:
  - >35 years has increased risk of endometrial cancer; obtain sample prior to initiating/continuing any therapy
- Pap testing to rule out dysplasia
- Cervical testing for infection such as *Chlamydia*

Labs

ALERT
- 1st, rule-out pregnancy!
- TSH, CBC, prolactin, coagulation studies used selectively

Imaging
- Transvaginal sonography:
  - Sufficient for evaluation of AUB in 65% of patients ≥39 and not clinically menopausal
  - Easy, available technology
- Saline infusion sonography:
  - Sensitivity 85.7%, specificity 95.4% for polyps/fibroids
  - May avoid need for diagnostic hysteroscopy
- Diagnostic hysteroscopy:
  - Office:
    - Safe, easy, rapid method to evaluate uterine cavity, operator dependent, increased patient discomfort, limited availability
  - Operating room:
    - Selected women with abnormal saline infusion sonography or office hysteroscopy requiring biopsy or excision of lesions

DIFFERENTIAL DIAGNOSIS
Rule out pregnancy and complications of pregnancy in reproductive-aged women such as ectopic or molar pregnancy and threatened, inevitable, complete, and incomplete abortions.

Infection
- Vulvitis and vaginitis
- Cervicitis
- Endometritis
- Pelvic inflammatory disease

Hematologic
- Coagulopathies
- Blood dyscrasias

Metabolic/Endocrine
Endocrinopathy

Tumor/Malignancy
Neoplastic disease of the vulva/vagina, cervix, uterine corpus, fallopian tube, ovary

Trauma
- Foreign body
- Trauma:
  - Direct
  - Sexual abuse/assault

Drugs
- Heparin
- Sodium warfarin
- Salicylates, other prostaglandin synthetase inhibitors
- Drugs that increase metabolism of estrogen, thus lowering serum levels:
  - Rifampin
  - Some antiepileptics
  - Certain antipsychotics including phenothiazines and risperidone

Other/Miscellaneous
Structural lesions:
- Cervical polyps
- Endometrial polyps

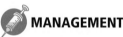 **MANAGEMENT**

GENERAL MEASURES
- Provide reassurance for 1st 3 months of contraceptive use, hormone treatment.
- Preventive guidance: Unscheduled bleeding to be expected with progestin-only methods
- Encourage smoking cessation (antiestrogen effect)
- May consider increasing estrogen component of therapy (e.g., from 20 μg estrogen to 30–35 μg formulation)
- Consistent use:
  - Avoid missed pills
  - POP q24h—unforgiving of missed pills
  - Longer-acting hormone method may be indicated if daily use is problematic.

SPECIAL THERAPY
Complementary and Alternative Therapies
- Vitamin C and estrogen are eliminated by same route. Estrogen levels may be higher in those taking contraceptive pills or hormone therapy with concomitant high-dose vitamin C.
- St. John's wort may decrease efficacy.

MEDICATION (DRUGS)

- Cycle control is an important issue for perimenopausal and reproductive-aged women. Many women are placed on OCP formulations of low estrogen doses (i.e., 20 μg). Studies have shown higher unscheduled bleeding episodes with these low-dose formulations.
- Can increase to a 35 μg OCP formulation
- Trial of 25 μg EE triphasic formulation
- Trial of extended OCP regimen (e.g., 84/7 regimen or 365-d regimen)
- Weekly transdermal patch 150 μg norelgestromin/ 20 μg EE
- 3-week vaginal ring 120 μg etonogestrel/15 μg ethinyl estradiol
- Levonorgestrel intrauterine device: This progestin-releasing IUD appears as effective as endometrial ablation (see below) in treating menorrhagia.
- 3-month DMPA injection 150 mg
- See Menopausal Symptoms and Menopause.

SURGERY

- Once a structural anomaly is identified, resection of that lesion may be appropriate (once malignancy is ruled out age >35). Expectant management may be appropriate when bleeding is associated with intramural fibroids.
- Diagnostic/Operative hysteroscopy:
  – Can resect polyps, submucosal fibroids
- Endometrial ablation is a viable option for a woman who has completed childbearing and who has failed medical management and desires conservative surgical option; because of the risk of fetal anomalies should conception occur postablation, effective contraception should be provided.
  – Roller-ball (considered gold standard)
  – Global ablation devices:
    ○ ThermaChoice (balloon)
    ○ Her Option (cryoablation)
    ○ Hydro ThermAblator HTA (heated water)
    ○ NovaSure (bipolar)
    ○ Microsulis MEA® (microwave)
- Myomectomy:
  – Most appropriate for a woman of childbearing age (and desire) who has intramural/pedunculated uterine leiomyoma:
    ○ Open or laparoscopic approach
- Uterine artery embolization (fibroid uterus):
  – Usually performed by interventional radiologists
  – Benefits include decrease in bleeding and size of fibroid(s), avoids major abdominal surgery
  – Risks include pain, fever, necrosis
- Hysterectomy

FOLLOW-UP

DISPOSITION

Issues for Referral

- Refer to gynecologic oncologist when invasive malignancy is diagnosed.
- When bleeding is found to be due to coagulopathy or liver/renal disease, refer to specialist.

PROGNOSIS

BTB not associated with identifiable pathology often subsides without treatment within 3–6 months of use of contraceptive method or hormone treatment.

PATIENT MONITORING

When placing patient on contraceptive or hormonal therapy, it is good practice to schedule a follow-up visit (with menstrual diary) to assess for success, tolerance of side effects, answer questions, provide reassurance, monitor for signs of complications.

- Avoids patient accessing inaccurate information
- Fosters discussion regarding goals of treatment
- Promotes long-term continuation of therapy

BIBLIOGRAPHY

Association of Professors of Gynecology and Obstetrics. Clinical Management of Abnormal Uterine Bleeding: Educational Series on Women's Health Issues.

Crofton MD. Association of Professors of Gynecology and Obstetrics; 2002.

De Vries LD, et al. Comparison of transvaginal sonography, saline instillation in the diagnosis of uterine pathology in pre- and postmenopausal women with abnormal uterine bleeding or suspect sonographic findings. *Ultrasound Obstet Gynecol*. 1997;9:53–58.

Kaunitz A. Gynecologic problems of the perimenopause: Evaluation and treatment. *Obstetr Gynecol Clin N Am*. 2002;29:445–473.

North American Menopause Society. Clinical challenges of perimenopause. *Consensus Opinion of the North American Menopause Society: Menopause*. 2000;7:5–13.

Stenchever M, et al., eds. *Comprehensive Gynecology* 4th ed. Philadelphia: Mosby; 2001.

MISCELLANEOUS

SYNONYM(S)

Iatrogenic bleeding

CLINICAL PEARLS

- Women frequently interpret any deviation from monthly cyclic bleeding as abnormal and will not distinguish between irregular bleeding occurring in the *absence* of hormonal treatment from that occurring *during* hormonal treatment.

- A careful history that distinguishes between bleeding while on hormonal therapy and bleeding in the absence of hormonal treatment is essential.
- A prospectively charted menstrual diary is invaluable in interpreting and managing BTB.
- Missed OCPs are a common cause of BTB.
- A careful, nonjudgmental history is required: "Many women have difficulty taking pills every day; is that a problem for you?"

ABBREVIATIONS

- AUB—Abnormal uterine bleeding
- BTB—Breakthrough bleeding
- COC—Combination oral contraceptions
- DMPA—Depot medroxyprogesterone acetate
- EE—Ethinyl estradiol
- OCP—Oral contraceptive pill
- POP—Progestin-only pill
- TSH—Thyroid-stimulating hormone

CODES

ICD9-CM

- 626.9 Uterine bleeding:
  – 627.0 Postmenopausal
  – 626.8 Dysfunctional
  – 626.6 Unrelated to menstrual cycle
  – 626.7 Postcoital
  – 628.0 Anovulatory
- 616.10 Vaginitis NOS
- 622.7 Cervical polyp
- 622.1 Cervical dysplasia, unspecified, 622.11 Mild (CIN1), 622.12 Moderate (CIN II), 233.1 Severe (CIN III/CIS)
- 621.0 Uterine polyp
- 621.2 Enlarged uterus
- 218.9 Uterine leiomyoma:
  – 218.1 Intramural
  – 218.0 Submucosal
  – 218.2 Subserosal

PATIENT TEACHING

PREVENTION

- Counseling that BTB is common in the 1st 1–3 months of use of COCs, but typically resolves spontaneously after 2–3 months may help prevent dissatisfaction and discontinuation.
- Menstrual charting/bleeding calendars can help in the evaluation of AUB/BTB.
- Counseling regarding typical unscheduled bleeding with POPs, DMPA, implants, extended cycle OCs will help women have realistic expectations about bleeding patterns.

BLEEDING, ABNORMAL UTERINE: IRREGULAR AND INTERMENSTRUAL

Eve S. Cunningham, MD
Malcolm G. Munro, MD

 BASICS

DESCRIPTION
- Intermenstrual (IM) bleeding is defined as bleeding between predictable cyclic menses during the reproductive years.
- Irregular bleeding in the reproductive years is defined as bleeding that is variable and unpredictable with respect to onset, duration, and volume.

Age-Related Factors
Irregular and IM bleeding is applied only to women in the reproductive years and not to be confused with premenarcheal, perimenopausal, and postmenopausal bleeding.

Geriatric Considerations
Always consider malignancy in differential diagnosis of older individuals with abnormal uterine bleeding.

RISK FACTORS
See "Associated Conditions."

PATHOPHYSIOLOGY
- IM bleeding:
  - Late cycle spotting:
    - Luteal phase defect
  - Mid-cycle (periovulatory) bleeding:
    - Postovulatory estradiol trough
  - Unpredictable IM bleeding secondary to local pathology:
    - Polyps
    - Leiomyomas
    - Infection (cervicitis or endometritis secondary to, for example, *Chlamydia trachomatis*)
    - Neoplasia (e.g., carcinoma cervix or endometrium)
    - Lacerations/Trauma to the genital tract.
- Irregular bleeding:
  - Unopposed estrogen:
    - Anovulation
    - Inconsistent ovulation
- Iatrogenic bleeding:
  - See Bleeding, Abnormal Uterine: with Hormonal Therapy or Contraception.
- Combination of 1 or more of the above.

ASSOCIATED CONDITIONS
- IM bleeding:
  - Local pathology (see pathophysiology)
  - Iatrogenic (See Bleeding, Abnormal Uterine: with Hormonal Therapy or Contraception.)
- Irregular bleeding:
  - Factors associated with increased risk for anovulation:
    - Perimenarcheal or perimenopausal years
    - PCOS
    - Obesity, weight change
    - Exercise
    - Pharmacologic
    - Endocrinopathies (e.g., hypothyroid, adrenal hyperplasia, hyperprolactinemia)

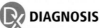 **DIAGNOSIS**

SIGNS AND SYMPTOMS
History
Irregular bleeding and IM bleeding are symptoms, not diagnoses:
- Unpredictable bleeding
- Constant use of a panty liner or pad
- Bleeding after contact or activity such as intercourse
- Soiling of undergarments
- Use of hormonal or intrauterine contraception

Physical Exam
- Vulva, perineum, and perianal areas:
  - Evaluate the vulva as well as the periurethral and perianal areas searching for lesions that may be a cause of bleeding.
- Speculum exam:
  - Look for cervical or vaginal lesions.
  - Friability of the cervix; if in combination with mucopurulent discharge consider *Chlamydia trachomatis*
- Bimanual exam:
  - Estimate size, shape, contour, and position of uterus and palpate adnexa, but the bimanual exam rarely is useful for determining the cause of either irregular or IM bleeding.

TESTS
Pregnancy Considerations
- Bleeding in pregnancy is not irregular bleeding, but any patient presenting in the reproductive years first be evaluated to rule out pregnancy complications.
- Always biopsy vulvar, vaginal, and cervical lesions.
- Consider endometrial sampling if no visible vaginal/cervical lesions are identified.

Labs
- Irregular bleeding:
  - Pregnancy test
  - CBC (if heavy bleeding)
  - TSH, free T4
  - Prolactin
  - Consider estradiol, FSH, LH, DHEAS
- IM bleeding, test for:
  - GC
  - *Chlamydia*

Imaging
- TVS may be used as a screening test to evaluate the endometrial cavity for potential polyps and leiomyomas; polyps may exist even in the presence of a normal-appearing endometrial echo complex.
- If TVS is not normal, consider evaluation of the endometrial cavity with 1 or more of the following procedures:
  - SIS may be used to define intracavitary lesions (i.e., polyps and myomas).
  - Hysteroscopy: A diagnostic procedure to evaluate for intracavitary lesions and in some instances allow for simultaneous removal.

DIFFERENTIAL DIAGNOSIS
Always evaluate for pregnancy.

Infection
- Cervicitis
- Endometritis
- Pelvic inflammatory disease

Metabolic/Endocrine
Oligo/Anovulatory cycles:
- Polycystic ovarian syndrome and other hyperandrogenic states
- Hypothyroidism and hyperthyroidism
- Hyperprolactinemia
- Perimenarcheal
- Perimenopausal

Tumor/Malignancy
- Submucosal fibroids
- Endometrial polyp
- Cervical polyp
- Endometrial neoplasia
- Cervical neoplasia
- Vaginal neoplasia
- Ovarian neoplasm:
  - Granulosa cell tumor

Trauma
- Postcoital:
  - Cervical/Vaginal lacerations
  - Exacerbation of bleeding from cervical polyps, neoplasms, or cervicitis
- Foreign body

Drugs
- Levonorgestrel IUS
- Progestin only:
  - Oral
  - Injectable/Implantable
- Combined estrogen-progestin contraceptive agents (pills, patch, vaginal ring)
- Anticoagulants

Other/Miscellaneous
Idiopathic IM bleeding:
- Not due to a demonstrable cause.

 MANAGEMENT

Directed at cause. Once a diagnosis is established, please see appropriate chapters on specific causes for therapeutic recommendations.

 FOLLOW-UP

Depends upon cause. Please see appropriate chapters on specific causes for follow-up recommendations.

BIBLIOGRAPHY

Hickey M, et al. Progestogens versus oestrogens and progestogens for irregular uterine bleeding associated with anovulation. *Cochrane Database Syst Rev*. 2007:1.

Management of Anovulatory Bleeding, ACOG Practice Bulletin. *Obstet Gynecol*. 2000:95.

 MISCELLANEOUS

SYNONYM(S)
- Oligomenorrhea
- Metrorrhagia

ABBREVIATIONS
- DHEAS—Dehydroepiandrosterone sulfate
- FSH—Follicular-stimulating hormone
- GC—*Neisseria gonorrhoeae*
- LH—Luteinizing hormone
- PCOS—Polycystic ovary syndrome
- SIS—Saline infusion sonography
- TSH—Thyroid-stimulating hormone
- TVS—Transvaginal ultrasound

CODES
ICD9-CM
- 626.1A Oligomenorrhea
- 626.6A Breakthrough bleeding
- 626.7A Postcoital bleeding
- 626.4B Irregular menstrual bleeding (irregular uterine bleeding)
- 626.8C Dysfunctional uterine bleeding
- 628.0B Anovulatory bleeding

BLEEDING, ABNORMAL UTERINE: OLIGOMENORRHEA

Rachel J. Miller, MD

BASICS

DESCRIPTION
- Oligomenorrhea refers to the absence of menses for 35–90 days or <9 cycles per year in adults, and absence of menses for 45–90 days in adolescents.
- Amenorrhea is the absence of menses in adults or adolescents for >90 days.
- Oligomenorrhea is a sign of an underlying disease mechanism, and therapy should be directed at treating the specific underlying condition.

Age-Related Factors
- Normal menstrual cycles in adolescents range from 21–45 days, even in the 1st 2 gynecologic years after menarche.
- Normal menstrual cycles in adults range from 21–35 days.
- Oligomenorrhea is more frequent during the menopausal transition.

EPIDEMIOLOGY
- Oligomenorrhea affects females during their reproductive years.
- 11.3% of college students have oligomenorrhea.

RISK FACTORS
- Obesity
- Weight loss
- Excessive exercise
- Chronic disease

Genetics
- PCOS has a strong genetic component, but genetic and phenotypic heterogeneity have made gene localization problematic.
- Specific types of thyroid dysfunction have a genetic component.
- Premature ovarian failure/ovarian insufficiency is associated with Fragile X syndrome; in women with POF, mutations of specific genes have been identified.

PATHOPHYSIOLOGY
- Normal menstrual function requires an intact hypothalamic-pituitary-ovarian-uterine/vaginal axis.
- Normally, the hypothalamus releases pulsatile GnRH, which stimulates the pituitary to release FSH and LH.
- These gonadotropins act on the ovaries to stimulate follicular development, ovulation, and the resulting corpus luteum.
- The ovaries secrete estrogen and, after ovulation, progesterone, which stimulate proliferation and maturation of the uterine endometrium.
- In the absence of fertilization, menstrual blood exits through a normal outflow tract.
- Any disruption in this axis can cause oligomenorrhea.

ASSOCIATED CONDITIONS
- Decreased bone mineral density with osteopenia and osteoporosis
- Multiple; see "Differential Diagnosis"

DIAGNOSIS

SIGNS AND SYMPTOMS
Absence of menses

History
The patient should be questioned regarding:
- Menstrual history
- Sexual activity
- Pregnancy history
- Disordered eating (anorexia or bulimia)
- Exercise habits—quantify frequency/intensity
- Weight loss
- Galactorrhea, headaches, visual field defects, polyuria, polydipsia
- Symptoms of estrogen deficiency such as hot flushes or vaginal dryness
- Medication use
- Illicit drug use

Physical Exam
- Growth pattern
- Height and weight with calculated BMI and BMI percentile for age in adolescents
- Tanner staging
- Signs of androgen excess, such as acne, hirsutism, clitoromegaly
- Cushing disease stigmata
- Thyroid exam
- Breast exam, especially looking for galactorrhea

TESTS
Pregnancy must be ruled out with a sensitive urine or serum pregnancy test.

Labs
- Urine or serum β-hCG
- TSH
- prolactin
- If signs of hyperandrogenism:
  - Serum DHEAS and testosterone
  - 17-hydroxyprogesterone
- If symptoms or signs of hypoestrogenism:
  - FSH
  - Estradiol
- If symptoms/physical findings suggestive of genetic disorder or POF in patient <30 years:
  - Karyotype

Imaging
- Transvaginal or transabdominal (in young adolescents) pelvic ultrasound to confirm normal gonads or evaluate for polycystic ovaries
- If elevated prolactin levels:
  - MRI of brain to rule out pituitary tumor (i.e., prolactinoma)

DIFFERENTIAL DIAGNOSIS

Infection
Chronic disease or infection

Metabolic/Endocrine
- POF:
  - Turner syndrome
  - Gonadal dysgenesis
- Hyperprolactinemia:
  - Hypothyroidism
  - Prolactinoma
  - Medications
- Hypothalamic dysfunction:
  - Anorexia nervosa
  - Excessive exercise
- Cushing disease
- Congenital adrenal hyperplasia

Immunologic
Autoimmune premature ovarian failure

Tumor/Malignancy
- Prolactinoma
- Androgen-producing tumors

Drugs
Iatrogenic:
- Chemotherapy (i.e., cyclophosphamide)
- Radiation therapy
- Hormonal contraceptives
- Medications that induce hyperprolactinemia
- Valproate
- Levonorgestrel IUS
- Progestin-only hormonal contraceptives (DMPA, POPs, implant)
- Leuprolide

Other/Miscellaneous
- PCOS
- Physiologic:
  - Perimenarchal
  - Perimenopausal

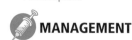

MANAGEMENT

GENERAL MEASURES
- Always treat the underlying etiology.
- Weight loss for overweight or obese patients
- Normalization of BMI and appropriate exercise behaviors for patients with excessive exercise and disordered eating

SPECIAL THERAPY

Complementary and Alternative Therapies
- Healthy, well-balanced diet to achieve normal BMI
- Appropriate, moderate exercise to achieve or maintain normal BMI

MEDICATION (DRUGS)

- Always treat the underlying etiology:
  - Thyroid replacement if hypothyroid
  - Dopamine-agonist if hyperprolactinemia
  - Metformin if PCOS and insulin resistant
  - Cyclical estrogen-progestin
  - Combined estrogen-progestin oral contraceptive pills, patches, or vaginal ring if no contraindications to estrogen therapy
- Patients seeking pregnancy may require ovulation induction with clomiphene citrate, exogenous gonadotropins, or pulsatile GnRH.

SURGERY

Tumor resection for some pituitary or ovarian tumors

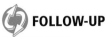 FOLLOW-UP

DISPOSITION

The evaluation of and treatment for oligomenorrhea is performed in the outpatient setting.

Issues for Referral

- Many etiologies for oligomenorrhea can be managed by the primary care provider.
- Conditions that require the help of a specialist may include:
  - POF: Endocrinologist, gynecologist, reproductive endocrinologist
  - Pituitary tumors: Neurosurgeon and endocrinologist
  - Anorexia nervosa: Eating disorder team
  - PCOS: Endocrinologist, reproductive endocrinologist, or gynecologist
  - Other types of tumors: Oncologist, gynecologist, gynecologic oncologist
  - Infertility: Obstetrician/Gynecologist or reproductive endocrinologist

PATIENT MONITORING

- Many patients will resume regular menses following therapy for the underlying condition, especially in cases of endocrine diseases, functional hypothalamic dysfunction, and PCOS.
- Prolonged hypoestrogenic states may lead to bone mineral density loss.
- Many causes of oligomenorrhea result in anovulation and infertility.
- Women with PCOS may also have insulin resistance and should be screened for diabetes.
- Prolonged oligomenorrhea, particularly in obese females, is a risk factor for endometrial hyperplasia and cancer.

BIBLIOGRAPHY

American College of Obstetrics and Gynecology Committee on Practice Bulletins-Gynecology. Management of infertility caused by ovulatory dysfunction. *Obstet Gynecol*. 2002;99(2):347–358.

Bachmann GA, et al. Prevalence of oligomenorrhea and amenorrhea in a college population. *Am J Obstet Gynecol*. 1982;144(1):98–102.

Mitan LAP. Menstrual dysfunction in anorexia nervosa. *J Pediatr Adolesc Gynecol*. 2004;17:81–85.

Paradise J. Evaluation of oligomenorrhea in adolescence. *UpToDate Online*. 2006;14:3.

The Practice Committee of the American Society for Reproductive Medicine. Current evaluation of amenorrhea. *Fertil Steril*. 2006;86(Suppl 4): S148–S155.

Speroff L, et al. *Clinical Gynecologic Endocrinology and Infertility*, 7th ed. 2004.

 MISCELLANEOUS

SYNONYM(S)

- Irregular menses
- Infrequent menses

ABBREVIATIONS

- BMI—Body mass index
- DHEAS—Dehydroepiandrosterone sulfate
- DMPA—Depot medroxyprogesterone acetate
- FSH—Follicle-stimulating hormone
- GnRH—Gonadotropin releasing hormone
- hCG—Human chorionic gonadotropins
- LH—Luteinizing hormone
- PCOS—Polycystic ovarian syndrome
- POF—Premature ovarian failure
- POP—Progestin-only pills
- TSH—Thyroid-stimulating hormone

 CODES

ICD9-CM

626.1 Oligomenorrhea

 PATIENT TEACHING

PREVENTION

- Oligomenorrhea may be prevented by treating underlying conditions.
- Maintaining an appropriate body weight minimizes the risks of irregular menses.

BLEEDING, ABNORMAL UTERINE: POSTMENOPAUSAL AND MENOPAUSAL TRANSITION

Nanette Santoro, MD
Matthew Lederman, MD

 BASICS

DESCRIPTION
- MT:
  - Previously referred to as "perimenopause"
  - Reproductive aging nomenclature defined by STRAW (Stages of Reproductive Aging Workshop) and applies to healthy, normally menstruating, nonsmoking women without anatomic abnormalities and a BMI between 18–30 kg/m². Comprised of 7 stages from −5 to +2. Perimenopause includes the MT and 12 months after the final menstrual period (FMP).
    - −5 to −3: Mid reproductive life
    - −2 to −1: Menopausal transition. Begins with first skipped menses (or >7 day variation in cycle length):
      - −2 (early stage): Menses at least once every 3 months
      - −1 (late stage): 3–11 months amenorrhea
    - 0 (menopause): 12 months after FMP
    - +1 to +2 (postmenopause):
      - +1 (early stage): 1st 5 years after FMP
      - +2 (late stage): Through remainder of life
- Postmenopausal abnormal uterine bleeding (AUB):
  - Bleeding occurring >1 year after FMP

Age-Related Factors
- Median age of onset MT = 47.5 years
- Median length of MT = 4 years
- Median age of menopause = 51.4 years
- Premature ovarian failure: Prolonged hypergonadotropic amenorrhea occurring >2 standard deviations below the mean for the reference population:
  - Generally accepted as <40 for "premature" and <45 for "early" menopause

EPIDEMIOLOGY
- AUB accounts for up to 20% of office visits and frequently seen in MT.
- <10% of cases of postmenopausal bleeding are due to endometrial cancer.

RISK FACTORS
- Factors affecting timing of natural MT:
  - Earlier transition: Current smoking, lower SES, heart disease, separated/widowed/divorced, unemployed
  - Later transition: Multiparity, prior use of OCPs, Japanese ethnicity
- See risk factors for cervicitis, endometrial hyperplasia/carcinoma, cervical carcinoma, fibroids, cervical lesions, and atrophic vaginitis/endometritis
  - In general, anatomic abnormalities increase with age.
- Endometrial polyps: Estrogen exposure, Tamoxifen
- Fibroids

Genetics
Primary determining factor influencing age of menopause

PATHOPHYSIOLOGY
- MT:
  - Shorter menstrual cycles 2° shorter follicular-phase in ovulatory cycles alternating with variable-length anovulatory cycles:
    - Cycles may get 3–7 days shorter
    - Bleeding may decrease and get lighter as menopause nears, BUT
  - Anovulatory cycles lack progesterone stabilization and cause increased endometrial vascularity without adequate stromal support, leading to endometrial fragility and occasional heavy bleeding.
  - Increased risk of hyperplasia and neoplasia with unopposed estrogen stimulation
- Postmenopausal AUB:
  - Usually related to hypoestrogenic state but depends on specific etiology; always rule out hyperplasia or carcinoma.

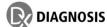 **DIAGNOSIS**

SIGNS AND SYMPTOMS
History
- Important to distinguish between a normal MT and a pathologic cause.
- Changes in bleeding patterns:
  - May be physiologic not requiring investigation
  - Prolonged bleeding >10 days or intermenstrual bleeding requires workup
- Postcoital bleeding
- Pregnancy still possible until >12 months amenorrhea
- Vaginal atrophy/pruritus/dyspareunia
- Family history of gynecologic malignancies, breast cancer, or colon cancer

Review of Systems
- Hot flashes:
  - Prevalence of 57% in late perimenopause and 49% in early menopause
- Sleep disturbances
- Symptoms of thyroid dysfunction (possible etiology for AUB in MT)
- Symptoms of anemia
- Urethritis/Cystitis
- Changes in bowel function

Physical Exam
- Vital signs:
  - Tachycardia or postural hypotension (if suspicious of anemia)
- Abdominal exam to rule out masses or ascites
- Pelvic exam assessing for:
  - Size of uterus
  - Uterine/Cervical masses or abnormalities
  - Vaginal atrophy
  - Evidence of thyroid disease (See Thyroid Disease.)
- Rectal exam

TESTS
- ACOG recommends assessment of endometrium if >35 years with anovulatory bleeding or <35 years if chronic anovulation, bleeding refractory to medical management, or risk factors for endometrial hyperplasia such as diabetes, obesity, or HTN
- EMB or EMBx (Pipelle):
  - May miss focal lesions in up to 18% of cases
- Pap smear
- +/− cervical cultures

Labs
- CBC
- TFTs
- +/− early follicular phase FSH/Estradiol
- +/− HCG

Imaging
- Clinician comfort and skill will direct workup.
- Menopausal transition AUB; use Goldstein's clinical algorithm:
  - TVS on cycle day (CD) 4–6 may be useful as triage tool:
    - EE ≤4–5 mm (bilayer) generally excludes pathology. No further workup necessary
    - +/− EMBx because rare case reports of endometrial cancer even when EE ≤4
  - EE >5 mm (bilayer) or not adequately visualized: HSN performed on CD 5–10 when bleeding has ceased:
    - If EE ≤3 mm (monolayer) with no focal abnormalities, no further workup needed
    - If EE >3 mm and symmetrical (monolayer), EMBx performed
    - If EE >3 mm and asymmetrical (monolayer) or if focal abnormality, D&C/hysteroscopy
- Postmenopausal bleeding:
  - TVS with EE ≤4 mm: No further workup usually required
    - If EE >4 mm, EMBx required
  - HSN option if TVS is suggestive of polyp or myoma; may also use in combination with EMBx in initial evaluation

DIFFERENTIAL DIAGNOSIS
Infection
Cervicitis/Chronic endometritis

Hematologic
Unlikely: Acquired von Willebrand disease

Metabolic/Endocrine
- Unlikely postmenopause unless hormone treatment used
- MT:
  - Anovulation is most likely etiology:
    - Diagnosis of exclusion termed dysfunctional uterine bleeding (DUB)
- Rule out thyroid dysfunction

Tumor/Malignancy
- Endometrial hyperplasia:
  - Simple vs. complex
  - +/− atypia
- Endometrial carcinoma:
  - Incidence increases with age
- Cervical carcinoma

Trauma
Unlikely in this age group; rule out with history

Drugs
- Hormonal therapy:
  - Breakthrough bleeding usually resolves after 6–12 months in postmenopausal women:
    - Consider endometrial evaluation if >6 months or patient anxiety
- Tamoxifen:
  - Increased risk of endometrial proliferation, hyperplasia, polyps, or carcinoma:
    - Endometrial assessment is required if AUB

Other/Miscellaneous
- Pregnancy
- Anatomic:
  - Uterine fibroids
  - Cervical/Endometrial polyps
  - Adenomyosis (MT)
  - Atrophy:
    - Most common etiology (postmenopausal)
  - Urethral caruncle (postmenopausal)

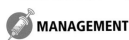

MANAGEMENT

Treatment depends on specific diagnosis

MEDICATION (DRUGS)
- DUB: Goal is to restore the stabilizing effect of luteal progesterone and prevent hyperplasia:
  - Low dose monophasic OCPs:
    - Assess contraindications and risks
  - Oral progestin 10–14 days q1–2 months:
    - Does not provide contraceptive benefit
    - Provera 10 mg daily, or Prometrium 200 mg daily, or Aygestin 2.5–10 mg/d
  - Levonorgestrel-IUD (Mirena):
    - 20 μg levonorgestrel released daily; 80% reduction of bleeding after 3 months:
    - Provides contraception
  - Combination hormonal therapy:
    - No reliable contraceptive benefit
  - NSAIDs
- Endometrial hyperplasia:
  - Medical vs. surgical treatment depends on presence of atypia
    - If no atypia, daily OCPs (perimenopausal) or cyclical Provera 10–20 mg/d for 10 days for a duration of 6 months with repeat EMBx every 3 months
- Atrophic vaginitis:
  - Oral or transdermal hormonal therapy
  - Vaginal low-dose estrogen (e.g., Estring every 3 months or Vagifem daily for 2 weeks then twice weekly)
    - Systemic absorption possible; consider intermittent progestin or endometrial surveillance if >6 months of treatment

SURGERY
- Anovulation:
  - Endometrial ablation:
    - More cost-effective than hysterectomy, less invasive, decreased morbidity, and quicker recovery
    - 1:10 women will still have hysterectomy within 5 years 2° treatment failure
  - Uterine artery embolization:
    - Alternative treatment if medical comorbidities

- Endometrial polyp: Hysteroscopic resection
- Cervical polyp: Office polypectomy
- Uterine fibroids:
  - Hysteroscopic resection if submucosal
  - Hysterectomy
  - Uterine artery embolization:
    - Alternative treatment if medical comorbidities
- Endometrial hyperplasia: Hysterectomy vs. high-dose progestin (less desirable option in this age group) if atypia present
- Endometrial carcinoma: Hysterectomy +/− surgical staging
- Cervical carcinoma: Treatment depends on stage

FOLLOW-UP

- Depends on specific diagnosis
- Hysteroscopy may be needed for persistent bleeding even if workup is negative.

DISPOSITION
Issues for Referral
May require referral to gynecological oncologist if carcinoma present or to reproductive endocrinologist for management of menopause

PROGNOSIS
- Depends on specific diagnosis
- DUB eventually remits with menopause.
- Endometrial polyps:
  - Present in 13% of women with AUB in MT:
    - Rarely associated with malignancy
- Endometrial hyperplasia:
  - Progression to carcinoma:
    - Simple hyperplasia without atypia: 1%
    - Complex hyperplasia without atypia: 3%
    - Simple hyperplasia with atypia: 8%
    - Complex hyperplasia with atypia: 29%

PATIENT MONITORING
- Depends on specific diagnosis and treatment
- Yearly office visit recommended unless change in bleeding pattern

BIBLIOGRAPHY

Gold EB, et al. Relation of demographic and lifestyle factors to symptoms in a multi-racial/ethnic population of women 40–55 years of age. *Am J Epidemiol*. 2002;152:463–473.

Goldstein SR, et al. Ultrasonography-based triage for perimenopausal patients with abnormal uterine bleeding. *Am J Obstet Gynecol*. 1997;177:102–108.

Kurman RJ, et al. The behavior of endometrial hyperplasia: A long term study of "untreated" hyperplasia in 170 patients. *Cancer*. 1985;56:403–412.

Langer RD, et al. Transvaginal ultrasonography compared with endometrial biopsy for the detection of endometrial disease. *N Engl J Med*. 1997;337:1792–1798.

McKinlay SM, et al. The normal menopausal transition. *Maturitas*. 1992;14:103–115.

Milson I, et al. A comparison of flurbiprofen, tranexamic acid, and levonorgestrel-releasing intrauterine contraceptive device in the treatment of idiopathic menorrhagia. *Am J Obstet Gynecol*. 1991;164:879–883.

O'Connor H, et al. Endometrial resection for the treatment of menorrhagia. *N Engl J Med*. 1996;335:151–156.

Practice Bulletin. ACOG. *Management of Anovulatory Bleeding*. 2006;14:623–630.

Soules MR, et al. Stages of Reproductive Aging Workshop (STRAW). *J Women Health Gender-Based Med*. 2001:10:843–848.

MISCELLANEOUS

See Menopause and Menopausal Symptoms.

SYNONYM(S)
Dysfunctional uterine bleeding

CLINICAL PEARLS
Postmenopausal bleeding is cancer until proven otherwise.

ABBREVIATIONS
- CD—Cycle day
- DUB—Dysfunctional uterine bleeding
- EE—Endometrial echo
- EMBx—Endometrial biopsy
- FMP—Final menstrual period
- FSH—Follicle-stimulating hormone
- HCG—Human chorionic gonadotropin
- HSN—Hysterosonogram
- HTN—Hypertension
- IUD—Intrauterine device
- MT—Menopausal transition
- OCP—Oral contraceptive pill
- SES—Socioeconomic status
- TFT—Thyroid function tests
- TVS—Transvaginal sonogram

CODES

ICD9-CM
- 627.0 Perimenopausal bleeding
- 627.1 Postmenopausal bleeding
- 628.8 DUB

PATIENT TEACHING

- Educate patients about normal bleeding patterns during MT and in response to HT.
- Report to physician any change in bleeding patterns after initial diagnosis established or if breakthrough bleeding >6 months on postmenopausal HT.

PREVENTION
- Goal is to prevent missing detectable early gynecologic malignancy
- Recommend yearly gynecologic exam

BLEEDING, ABNORMAL UTERINE: PREPUBERTAL

Jeffrey W. Wall, MD
Julie L. Strickland, MD, MPH

 BASICS

DESCRIPTION

Prepubertal vaginal bleeding is uncommon but can represent a varied spectrum from minor to serious medical conditions. A careful history and examination is warranted in all cases to exclude significant pathology.

- Traumatic conditions:
  - Lacerations
  - Foreign body
  - Sexual abuse
- Nontraumatic conditions:
  - Infectious
  - Endocrine
  - Medical

Age-Related Factors

- Vaginal bleeding in neonates is common:
  - Due to withdrawal from a high-estrogen maternal environment
- Precocious puberty is the onset of pubertal development prior to the age of 8 years (controversy over age) (see Puberty, Precocious).

EPIDEMIOLOGY

- Up to 50% of girls with vaginal bleeding may have a vaginal foreign body.
- 4–5% of girls exhibit precocious pubertal development using age 8 as cutoff:
  - Higher in blacks (25%) versus whites (8%)

RISK FACTORS

- Prior history of foreign bodies in other orifices
- Family history of early menses or puberty
- Participation in certain physical activities:
  - Bicycle riding
  - Gymnastics

PATHOPHYSIOLOGY

- Normal pubertal development usually follows a consistent patterns of events, the premature onset of which may lead to vaginal bleeding (see Puberty, Precocious):
  - Thelarche: Breast development:
    - Menarche typically occurs at Tanner Breast Stage 3–4
    - Bleeding with NO breast development is abnormal.
  - Pubarche: Secondary sexual characteristics:
    - Pubic hair
    - Axillary hair
  - Menarche: Onset of menses
- Premature menarche:
  - 1 or more episodes of bleeding in the absence of pubertal changes:
    - May be associated with hypothyroidism
    - Usually idiopathic
- Certain ovarian tumors may secrete estrogen:
  - Granulosa cell tumors
  - Benign follicular cysts

ASSOCIATED CONDITIONS

- Hypothyroidism
- Puberty

DIAGNOSIS

SIGNS AND SYMPTOMS

History

Obtaining a careful history may be difficult. A relaxed and nonthreatening atmosphere can aid you when interviewing an anxious young girl or preadolescent. Parent often provides historical data. Pertinent points to consider are:

- Onset and duration of bleeding
- Vaginal versus rectal bleeding
- Vaginal discharge
- Medical history
- Pubertal milestones:
  - Breast and pubic hair development
  - Growth, weight gain
- Pelvic infections
- Recent trauma or falls
- Suspicion of sexual abuse:
  - Recent behavioral changes
  - Early sexualized play/behaviors
- Family history of bleeding disorders
- Pelvic or abdominal pain

Review of Systems

- Constitutional:
  - Weight gain or loss
  - Growth, height
  - Pubertal landmarks
- Heat and cold tolerance
- Urinary complaints:
  - Dysuria, urgency, frequency
  - History of UTIs
- Constipation:
  - Hard stools

Physical Exam

- Vital signs
- Height, weight, BMI
- General exam should include:
  - Tanner staging: Breast and pubic hair
  - Body habitus
  - Abdominal exam:
    - Masses
    - Pain
- Genital exam should include:
  - Inspection of external genitalia, introitus, and urethra for:
    - Trauma
    - Foreign bodies
    - Ecchymoses
    - Excoriations
    - Discharge
  - Assessment of bleeding:
    - Vaginal, rectal, or urethral
    - Active bleeding, oozing, or hemostasis
  - Obtain genital cultures or wet mount
- Consider possible lichen sclerosus (see Vulvar Lichen Sclerosis):
  - Pale atrophic skin with hemorrhage
- Speculum exam is usually not necessary:
  - Consider sedation or pelvic exam under anesthesia
  - In absence of heavy bleeding or pelvic pain

- Speculum exam under anesthesia should be performed:
  - If heavy vaginal bleeding
  - Suspected vaginal trauma or foreign body:
    - Vulvar trauma and extent of laceration cannot be visualized
    - Deep vaginal lacerations
    - Periurethral injury
  - Use pediatric or adolescent (Huffman) narrow-blade speculum:
    - A nasal speculum works well for infants and very young girls
    - Cystoscope or hysteroscope can be used to provide vaginal visualization with magnification.
  - Consider colonoscopy if rectal involvement

TESTS

Labs

- Initial blood work:
  - CBC
  - Platelet count
- Urinary analysis
- Wet mount
- Genital cultures if sexual abuse suspected (See Rape/Sexual Assault and Sexual Abuse.)
- Cellophane tape test for pinworms
- If suspected endocrinopathy or puberty:
  - LH
  - FSH
  - GnRH stimulation test
  - Estradiol
  - If suspected bleeding disorder, consider coagulation studies
- All blood work should be drawn prior to initiating therapy

Imaging

- Ultrasound:
  - Especially if exam is incomplete
  - Assess for ovarian/uterine pathology:
    - Prepubertal uterine configuration: Size of cervix = fundus; postpubertal fundus: cervix ~2:1 size
  - Rule out pelvic hematoma from trauma
- MRI:
  - Helpful in diagnosing congenital anomalies
  - Foreign body
- X-ray:
  - May demonstrate foreign body

DIFFERENTIAL DIAGNOSIS

- Infection:
  - Vulvovaginitis
    - Candida extremely unusual in child who is not using diapers
    - Bacterial vaginitis: Group A β-strep, usually 7–10 days after URI
  - Enteric pathogens
    - With or without diarrhea
    - *Shigella*
    - *Campylobacter*
    - *E. coli*
    - *Salmonella*
  - Pinworms
  - UTI

- Hematologic:
  - Bleeding disorders alone unlikely to cause prepubertal bleeding in absence of trauma:
    - vWD
    - Factor XI deficiency
    - ITP
- Metabolic/Endocrine:
  - Postnatal estrogen withdrawal
  - Precocious puberty
  - Premature menarche
  - McCune-Albright syndrome
  - Hypothyroidism
- Tumor/Malignancy:
  - Sarcoma botryoides
  - Estrogen secreting ovarian tumors:
    - Granulosa cell tumor
    - Follicular cysts
  - Adrenal adenoma/carcinoma
- Trauma:
  - Straddle injury
  - Abuse
- Drugs
  - Exogenous estrogen exposure
- Other/Miscellaneous:
  - Foreign body
  - Urethral prolapse
  - Hemangioma
  - Dermatologic disorders:
    - Lichen sclerosis
    - Condyloma acuminata
    - Diaper rash
  - GI:
    - Diarrhea
    - Rectal bleeding: Prolapse, intussusception, anal fissures

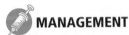 **MANAGEMENT**

GENERAL MEASURES
- If hemodynamic compromise, consider supportive measures:
  - Hospitalization
  - IV fluid resuscitation
  - Blood products
- Trauma:
  - Irrigate with warm saline
  - Superficial abrasions may be observed:
    - Pressure, ice packs
    - Topical hemostatic agents
  - Suturing may be necessary for larger or nonhemostatic lacerations
  - May need Foley catheter:
    - If large hematoma present
    - Periurethral involvement
- Vulvovaginitis:
  - Hygiene
  - Topical estrogen cream
  - Treat with appropriate antibacterial agents
  - If in diapers, may require antifungal treatment
  - Discourage scratching:
    - Sitz baths
    - Antipruritic agents and light sedation if intense pruritus

- Foreign body:
  - Remove with swab or forceps:
    - May require conscious sedation
  - If associated inflammation:
    - Sitz baths
    - Consider antibiotics
- Hemangioma:
  - Most regress spontaneously with time
- Urethral prolapse:
  - Supportive measures:
    - Sitz baths
    - Topical estrogen
    - Surgery rarely required
- Ovarian cysts:
  - Most resolve spontaneously with observation:
    - Reassurance
    - Re-examine with ultrasound in 4–6 weeks
  - Refer to gynecology for persistent cysts or solid masses
- Precocious puberty:
  - Refer to gynecology or pediatric endocrinology
- Premature menarche or premenarchal bleeding:
  - Must rule out all other etiologies
  - Reassurance
  - Follow closely for normal pubertal development
  - Consider referral to gynecology or reproductive endocrinology
- Hypothyroidism:
  - Treat with thyroid medication as appropriate
- Lichen sclerosus:
  - Topical low- to mid-potency steroid ointment:
    - Hydrocortisone
    - Betamethasone
    - Consider high-potency steroid if severe

SURGERY
Pelvic exam under anesthesia:
- Anxious or younger patients
- Repair pelvic trauma
- Removal of deep foreign objects

 FOLLOW-UP

- Traumatic lesions should be followed up in 1–2 weeks to ensure proper healing.
- Other medical conditions as appropriate to the disease process

DISPOSITION
Issues for Referral
- Referral to gynecology for:
  - Pelvic or vulvar masses
  - Extensive surgical repair
- Referral to endocrinology or gynecology:
  - Precocious puberty or premenarchal bleeding
- Referral to urology:
  - Refractory urethral prolapse
- Referral to pediatric dermatology:
  - Significant dermatoses:
    - Lichen sclerosus
- Referral to hematology:
  - Bleeding disorder

BIBLIOGRAPHY
Emans SJ, et al., eds. *Pediatric and Adolescent Gynecology*, 5th ed. Philadelphia: Lippincott; 2005.

Fishman A, et al. Vaginal bleeding in girls: A review. *Obstet Gynecol Surv*. 1991;46(7):457–460.

Lang ME, et al. Vaginal bleeding in the prepubertal child. *CMAJ*. 2005;172(10):1289–1290.

Perlman SE. Premenarchal vaginal bleeding. *J Pediatr Adolesc Gynecol*. 2001;14(3):135–136.

Pinto SM, et al. Prepubertal menarche: A defined clinical entity. *Am J Obstet Gynecol*. 2006;195(1):327–329.

Sugar NF, et al. Common gynecologic problems in prepubertal girls. *Pediatr Rev*. 2006;27:213–223.

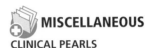 **MISCELLANEOUS**

CLINICAL PEARLS
- Accidental trauma rarely results in hymenal disruption; if present, sexual abuse should be considered.
- Benign follicular cysts may result in withdrawal bleeding as the cysts regress.
- Certain hair products used by the African-American community contain biologically active estrogens.

ABBREVIATIONS
- BMI—Body mass index
- FSH—Follicle stimulating hormone
- GI—Gastrointestinal
- GnRH—Gonadotropin releasing hormone
- ITP—Idiopathic thrombocytopenia
- LH—Luteinizing hormone
- URI—Upper respiratory tract infection
- UTI—Urinary tract infection
- vWD—von Willebrand disease

CODES
ICD9-CM
- 259.1 Precocious sexual development
- 288.0 Hemangioma
- 599.5 Prolapsed urethral mucosa
- 616.1 Vaginitis and vulvovaginitis NOS
- 620.2 Ovarian cyst NOS
- 624.0 Dystrophy of vulva (lichen sclerosus)
- 624.5 Hematoma of vulva
- 626.3 Puberty bleeding
- 878.4 Open wound, vulva NOS
- 878.6 Open wound, vagina NOS
- 939.2 Foreign body, vulva vagina

BREAST SIGNS AND SYMPTOMS: BREAST DISCHARGE AND GALACTORRHEA

Willie J. Parker, MD, MPH

 BASICS

DESCRIPTION

- Nipple discharge can be normal, or may be a sign of a significant problem.
- Galactorrhea is the secretion of breast milk in women who are not breastfeeding. Galactorrhea may be due to:
  – Prolactin-secreting pituitary adenoma (prolactinoma)—the most common hormone secreting pituitary tumor:
    ○ Microadenoma <10 mm
    ○ Macroadenoma >0 mm
  – Medications:
    ○ Methyldopa
    ○ Illicit drugs
    ○ Neuroleptics

Age-Related Factors

Nipple discharge is very common in reproductive-aged women:

- 50–80% of reproductive-aged women express a few drops of benign fluid from their breasts at some time.
- Age-related cancer risks for isolated nipple discharge (overall risk is 5%):
  – <40 years: 3%
  – 40–60 years: 10%
  – >60 years: 32%

EPIDEMIOLOGY

Incidence as high as 10–15%:

- 6.8% of women referred for evaluation of benign breast disease have nipple discharge.

RISK FACTORS

Smoking; although the relationship is unclear.

PATHOPHYSIOLOGY

Galactorrhea with elevated prolactin:

- Physiologic causes:
  – Pregnancy
  – Breast/Nipple stimulation
  – Stress
- Prolactinoma:
  – Neoplastic transformation of anterior pituitary lactotrophs resulting in excess secretion and production of prolactin
- Prolactin secretion regulated by prolactin-releasing factors and prolactin-inhibitory factors:
  – Dopamine is the principal prolactin-inhibitory factor:
    ○ Psychotropic drugs dopamine receptors
    ○ Methyldopa and reserpine antihypertensives
    ○ Disease in or near hypothalamus can interfere with domamine secretion or delivery to the hypothalamus via pituitary stalk
  – Thyrotropin-releasing hormone is likely prolactin releasing factor:
    ○ Hypothyroidism with increased TRH, TSH
  – Estrogen, including oral contraceptives can cause elevated prolactin

Other causes of nipple discharge:

- Ductal changes; ectasia
- Malignant growth with neovascularization and alteration of normal structure and physiology causing bloody discharge

ASSOCIATED CONDITIONS

- Pregnancy
- Hyperprolactinemia
- Hypothyroidism
- Renal failure
- Psychiatric conditions requiring neuroleptics

 DIAGNOSIS

SIGNS AND SYMPTOMS

History

- Complete medical history, including medication use, especially in nonlactational discharge
- One-sided or both breasts
- Color: Clear, white, gray, brown, greenish
- Milky
- Blood present
- Associated with a lump
- Tenderness
- Pregnant or nursing
- Provoked or spontaneous discharge
- Relationship to cycle
- Menstrual history

Review of Systems

- Symptoms of hypothyroidism
- Headaches, visual field changes with concern for intracranial tumor

Physical Exam

- Vital signs
- Neurologic exam with visual fields
- Complete clinical breast exam with woman sitting, lying, hand on hips and above head:
  – Elicit discharge or ask patient to do so by manual expression
  – Assess for mass, tenderness, adenopathy, skin changes, dimpling, nipple crusting

TESTS

Labs

- Labs for prolactin-related causes:
  – Thyroid function tests
  – Serum prolactin following abstinence from breast stimulation
- Discharge examination:
  – Office: Touch preparation of unstained slide:
    ○ Fat globules suggestive of galactorhea
    ○ Consider sending for cytology if negative for galactorhea, or grossly bloody
  – Specialist labs:
    ○ CEA
    ○ Occult blood test

Imaging

- Mammography should be performed in all women >30 with nonlactational, spontaneous discharge.
- Sonography:
  – Primary breast imaging for women <30, followed by mammography if nondiagnostic
- Ductography: Dye injected into a single breast duct for evaluation of bloody discharge
- Ductoscopy: Minimally invasive procedure that can obviate surgical excision
- MRI of breast: Role in nipple discharge evaluation not established
- MRI or CT of brain to identify pituitary adenoma if elevated prolactin

Diagnostic Procedures/Surgery

- Excisional breast biopsy or fine needle aspirate if mass present on exam or imaging
- Ductal lavage is of questionable value due to expense, time, and possibility of missing malignancy if mass blocks discharge.

DIFFERENTIAL DIAGNOSIS

- Presentation of discharge is helpful.
- Milky secretions:
  – Lactation
  – Medication-induced hyper-prolactinemia
  – Prolactinoma
  – Other pituitary or hypothalamic tumors
  – Thyroid disease
  – Galactorrhea in absence of hyperprolactinemia
- Straw-colored or transparent discharge:
  – Papilloma
- Grossly bloody discharge:
  – Intraductal carcinoma: 33%
  – Bleeding papillomata: 33%
  – Fibrocystic changes with an intraductal component: 33%
- Thick, sticky greenish or grayish color:
  – Ductal ectasia
- Staining of bra without obvious nipple discharge:
  – Paget disease of the nipple:
    ○ Usually has an underlying malignancy

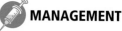 **MANAGEMENT**

GENERAL MEASURES

- Reassurance is the most common intervention *following* evaluation for breast discharge; most causes are benign.
- Anyone with findings suspicious for malignancy (unilateral, single duct, spontaneous discharge, bloody discharge) should be referred to a breast specialist for appropriate management.

MEDICATION (DRUGS)

- Indications for treatment of hyperprolactinemia due to pituitary adenoma include infertility, oligomenorrhea, amenorrhea, hypoestrogenemia. Dopamine agonists decrease prolactin secretion and reduce the size of pituitary adenomas in 90% of patients.
- Dopamine agonist therapy for medical management of galactorrhea:
  – Bromocriptine: An ergot derivative available as generic drug:
    ○ Begin 1.25 mg PO q.h.s. and increase to 15 mg/d
    ○ Give with food
    ○ Nausea, headache, fatigue common side effects
  – Cabergoline: Ergot derivative given 1–2x/wk
    ○ 0.25 mg twice weekly to 1.0 mg twice weekly; increase to every 4 weeks, based on prolactin levels
    ○ May discontinue after normal prolactin for 6 months
    ○ Less nausea than bromocriptine
- Hyperprolactinemia due to drug use:
  – Consider discontinuation or alternative drug.
  – Use dopamine agonist cautiously as it may counteract antipsychotic effects.

SURGERY

Transphenoidal surgery for pituitary adenoma can be considered for:

- Giant lactrotroph adenomas
- Consider if dopamine agonist treatment is unsuccessful in lowering prolactin, adenoma persists, or symptoms of hyperprolactinemia persist.
- Surgery is safer when performed by experienced surgeon.
- Adenoma and hyperprolactinemia may recur.

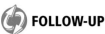 **FOLLOW-UP**

DISPOSITION

Issues for Referral

- If elevated prolactin is the cause and mass is >10 mm on neurologic imaging, neurosurgical referral for consideration of resection evaluation is warranted.
- Referral to specialist for nongalactorrhea or findings suspicious for malignancy

PROGNOSIS

- In the absence of malignant cause detected and managed by appropriate specialist, no associated mortality risk
- Control of symptoms of galactorrhea usually managed with medical therapy

PATIENT MONITORING

- As indicated. Re-evaluate if patient reports new findings.
- Mildly elevated prolactin with normal head imaging can be followed over time.
- If treating with dopamine agonists, monitor side effects and serum prolactin and titrate dose.

BIBLIOGRAPHY

Carty NJ, et al. Prospective study of outcome in women presenting with nipple discharge. *Ann R Coll Surg Engl*. 1994;76:387.

Florio MG, et al. Surgical approach to nipple discharge: A ten-year experience. *J Surg Oncol*. 1999;71:235.

Golshan M, et al. Nipple discharge. UpToDate, August 2006.

Isaacs JH. Other nipple discharge. *Clin Obstetr Gynecol*. 1994;37:898.

Santen RJ, et al. Benign breast disorders. *N Engl J Med*. 2005;353:275.

Murad TM, et al. Nipple discharge from the breast. *Ann Surg*. 1982;195:259.

Seltzer MH, et al. The significance of age in patients with nipple discharge. *Surg Gynecol Obstet*. 1970;131:519.

 MISCELLANEOUS

CLINICAL PEARLS

Galactorrhea in absence of hyperprolactiinemia is not likely the result of ongoing disease.

ABBREVIATION

CEA—Carcinoembryonic antigen

CODES

ICD9-CM

- 611.6 Galactorrhea not associated with childbirth
- 611.79 Discharge from the breast

BREAST SIGNS AND SYMPTOMS: BREAST MASS

Elizabeth A. Shaughnessy, MD, PhD
Kelly McLean, MD

BASICS

DESCRIPTION
- Breast masses are categorized as infection/abscess, benign masses, and cancer.
- Benign masses include cyst, galactocele, papilloma, fibroadenoma, phyllodes tumor, and fibrocystic change.
- Cancerous masses are usually painless, dominant masses that persist.

Age-Related Factors
- Cyst:
  - Most common in 5th decade and perimenopausal
- Galactocele:
  - Reproductive age, while gravid or postpartum
- Papilloma:
  - Usually ages 30–50 years, when solitary
  - Younger ages 20–40 years, if multiple and peripheral
- Fibroadenoma:
  - Adolescents, young adults
- Phyllodes tumor/cystosarcoma phyllodes:
  - Adolescents, young adults through middle age
- Fibrocystic changes/nodules:
  - Reproductive age
- Abscess:
  - Subareolar location:
    - 1st usually peripartum
    - Subsequent can be any age, if same location
  - Peripheral location
    - Any age, but more frequent in reproductive ages
- Cancer:
  - Average age at diagnosis is 62 years
  - Occurs as young as late teens

EPIDEMIOLOGY
- Cancer:
  - Risk continues to rise with age, never plateaus or drops
  - 20–25% of breast biopsies diagnose malignancies.
  - Age-specific incidence rises sharply after age 40 years, less sharply after menopause.
  - Incidence is rising; 1 in 7 women will be diagnosed in her lifetime.
- Fibroadenoma:
  - Most common mass in woman <40 years.

RISK FACTORS
- Breast abscess/infection:
  - Breast feeding
  - Smoking
  - History of prior subareolar abscess
  - Duct ectasia
- Galactocele:
  - Pregnancy and postpartum lactation
- Fibroadenoma, phyllodes tumor, papilloma, and fibrocystic nodules
  - Family history of papillomas or fibroadenomas or fibrocystic masses
- Cancer (See Breast Cancer.)

Genetics
- Fibroadenoma: A minority of fibroadenomas may display clonal chromosomal aberrations.
- Breast cancer (See Breast Cancer.)

PATHOPHYSIOLOGY
- Breast abscess/infection:
  - Peripartum:
    - Milk stasis
    - *Staphylococcus aureus*
  - Nonperipartum:
    - Squamous metaplasia and chronic fibrosis
    - Duct ectasia and fibrosis from periductal mastitis
    - *S. aureus* or *Streptococcus* sp.
- Galactocele:
  - Termination of lactation
  - Milk stasis
- Cyst:
  - Cyclic hormonal imbalance or fluctuation, with lobular involution, resulting in dilatation of the acinus

DIAGNOSIS

SIGNS AND SYMPTOMS
History
- Last menstrual period
- Relationship to menses
- Tenderness
- Spontaneous discharge
- Response to NSAIDs
- Termination of lactation
- Smoking
- Caffeine intake
- Family history of cancer

- Breast abscess/infection:
  - Painful mass or induration
  - Possible fever and/or chills
  - Warmth and possible erythema
  - Central fluctuance, if abscess
- Galactocele:
  - Mass during or after lactation
- Fibroadenoma and benign tumors:
  - Usually noncyclic mass, well-circumscribed
- Fibrocystic/Cystic nodules:
  - Tender nodules that wax and wane with menstrual cycle
  - Pain radiating to axilla or nipple
- Papilloma:
  - May be palpable deep to areola
  - Some with nonbloody nipple discharge, rarely bloody

Review of Systems
Fever, chills

Physical Exam
- Erythema, edema, and a tender dominant mass favor breast infection or abscess.
- Tender mass without erythema and edema favors a fibrocystic nodule or cyst.
- Discrete mobile nontender nodule favors a benign tumor; i.e., fibroadenoma.

TESTS
Labs
As indicated:
- CBC
- Culture of abscess

Imaging
- Ultrasound at any age
- Diagnostic mammogram for patients >30 or at an age 10 years younger than the age at which a 1st-degree relative developed breast cancer
- MRI for dense breasts where the clinical suspicion for cancer is high or imaging indeterminate
- Galactography/ductography if associated discharge

DIFFERENTIAL DIAGNOSIS
The diagnoses discussed represent the most common diagnoses.

MANAGEMENT

GENERAL MEASURES
- The most important intervention is accurate diagnosis.
- A benign solid mass should be followed to assure that its behavior is consistent with benignity; if it grows, suspect sampling error and excise
- Diet:
  - Cysts: Avoiding products with methylxanthines (caffeine) has been shown to decrease cyclic mastalgia, fibrocystic masses, and gross cysts.
- Nursing:
  - For galactoceles and postpartum breast abscess, maintenance of nursing is recommended.

SPECIAL THERAPY
Complementary and Alternative Therapies
Use of evening primrose oil (γ-linolenic acid) capsules has a clinical response rate of 58% at 3 g/d for cyclic mastalgia:
- Response takes at least 1 month of use, and should be discontinued after 4 months
- Symptoms of mild GI upset or nausea in <2% of patients

MEDICATION (DRUGS)
- Danocrine 100–200 mg b.i.d. is approved by the FDA for use in refractory mastalgia.
- Amoxicillin/Clavulanate or dicloxacillin for 2 weeks to treat infection, with added metronidazole if abscess:
  - Apparent breast cellulitis that fails to respond to outpatient oral antibiotic therapy may be due to resistant organism or abscess:
    - Inpatient therapy with IV vancomycin or other antibiotic may be required.
    - Re-evaluate for possible abscess.

SURGERY
- Indications for surgery:
  - Cystosarcoma phyllodes or phyllodes tumor on core biopsy:
    - Surgical excision required to assure benignity
- Fibroadenoma, hamartoma, lipoma:
  - Surgical excision for symptoms or enlargement
- Atypical cells, papilloma, or LCIS on core biopsy:
  - Excise lesion, with needle/wire localization if needed
- Breast abscess:
  - Surgical I&D for treatment
- Fibrocystic nodules and galactoceles:
  - Surgical excision not recommended unless a concern exists for missed malignancy.
- Excision if discordance among imaging, exam, and core biopsy

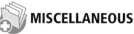 FOLLOW-UP

- Fibroadenomas and hamartomas require 6-month interval diagnostic imaging, mammogram with or without ultrasound, to document stability for 1–2 years.
- Follow-up examination of any benign mass in 3 months, then coordinate with imaging if stable:
  - Avoid examination during premenstrual phase of cycle if possible.

DISPOSITION
Issues for Referral
- Breast cellulitis fails to resolve
- Persistent mass
- Discordance between core biopsy, imaging, and exam
- Any mass with chest wall/skin fixation
- Recurrent breast abscess

PROGNOSIS
Fibroadenoma:
- Risk of recurrence is minimal with adequate excision
- For nonexcised lesion:
  - ~50% will disappear in 5 years
  - Should stabilize/diminish in postmenopausal women.

ALERT
- An enlarging fibroadenoma in a postmenopausal women should be excised; could be malignant.
- Hamartoma and lipomas have an excellent prognosis; consider excision if >5 cm, as chance of malignancy increases.
- Breast abscess definitively treated is unlikely to recur.
- Galactoceles usually resolve without surgical intervention.
- Simple cysts will regress, more than 1/2 by the 1st year and more than 2/3 by the 2nd year, leaving only 12% after 5 years.

PATIENT MONITORING
Error in diagnosis, or delayed diagnosis of cancer, is the major risk:
- Avoid by concordance evaluation of imaging, biopsy, and exam

BIBLIOGRAPHY

Brenner RJ, et al. Spontaneous regression of interval benign cysts of the breast. *Radiology.* 1994;193(2):365–368.

Cant PJ, et al. Nonoperative management of breast masses diagnosed as fibroadenoma. *Br J Surg.* 1995;82(6):792–794.

Harris JR, et al., eds. *Disease of the Breast,* 3rd ed. Philadelphia: Lippincott Williams & Wilkins; 2004.

Hindle WH, et al. Lack of utility in clinical practice of cytologic examination of nonbloody cyst fluid from palpable breast cysts. *Am J Obstet Gynecol.* 2000;182(6):1300–1305.

Mahoney MC, et al. Lobular neoplasia at 11-gauge vacuum-assisted stereotactic biopsy: Correlation with surgical excisional biopsy and mammographic follow-up. *Am J Roentgenol.* 2006;187(4):949–954.

Santeen RJ, et al. Benign breast disorders. *N Engl J Med.* 2005;353:275–285.

MISCELLANEOUS

CLINICAL PEARLS
- A dominant breast mass requires evaluation with imaging and biopsy.
- A solid breast mass can be biopsied accurately by fine needle aspiration or core biopsy.
- Simple cystic lesions must resolve completely with aspiration, or further diagnostic intervention is required.
- Most litigation against physicians is brought on behalf of women <50 years for delay in the diagnosis of breast cancer.

CODES
ICD9-CM
- 214 Lipoma
- 217 Benign neoplasm of breast
- 217 Fibroadenoma
- 238.3 Neoplasm of breast, uncertain
- 610.0 Breast cyst
- 610.4 Periductal mastitis
- 611.0 Breast abscess/mastitis
- 611.5 Galactocele
- 611.72 Breast mass
- 611.79 Nipple inversion, discharge

BREAST SIGNS AND SYMPTOMS: BREAST PAIN

Jade Richardson, MD

 BASICS

DESCRIPTION
Breast pain or mastalgia is common among women and less common among men.

Age-Related Factors
- Prepubertal:
  – Likely musculoskeletal or extramammary
  – Pubertal breast budding may be accompanied by tenderness, and may be unilateral.
- Reproductive age:
  – Any etiology possible
- Postmenopausal:
  – Malignancy more likely

EPIDEMIOLOGY
- Breast pain has been reported among up to 65% of women.
- Pain may be mild enough that it is not reported to physicians, and this may be a gross underestimate of the true incidence.
- Breast pain is more common among women but still present among men.
- Cyclic breast pain caused by hormonal fluctuations is seen in reproductive-age women.

RISK FACTORS
- Cyclic pain:
  – Use of hormonal therapies
  – Caffeine intake
  – Nicotine use
- Noncyclic:
  – Lactating women
  – BRCA/Family history of breast cancer
- Extramammary:
  – Use of pectoralis major muscle
    ○ Water skiing
    ○ Raking
    ○ Rowing
    ○ Shoveling
  – History of chest wound
  – Trauma

Genetics
BRCA genes associated with breast cancer may lead to rare cases of breast cancer presenting as breast pain.

PATHOPHYSIOLOGY
- Cyclical:
  – Estrogen stimulation of ductal elements
  – Progesterone stimulation of stromal elements
  – Prolactin stimulation of ductal secretion
- Noncyclical:
  – Mastitis/Breast abscess; obstructive lactopathy
  – Large pendulous breasts; stretching of Cooper's ligaments
  – Ductal ectasia; distention of subareolar ducts
- Extramammary:
  – Chest wall pain; use of pectoralis major muscle
  – Costochondritis
  – Spinal and paraspinal disorders; paraspinal muscle spasm or nerve impingement
  – Postthoracotomy; healing chest wound mimics breastfeeding

 DIAGNOSIS

SIGNS AND SYMPTOMS
History
- Provocative/Palliative factors:
  – Breast feeding
  – Oral contraceptive pills
- Quality of the pain:
  – Burning, aching, stabbing
  – Nipple sensitivity
- Radiation:
  – Neck, ducts, other chest wall sites
  – Systemic or other local symptoms
  – Unilateral or bilateral
- Severity
- Temporal factors:
  – Cyclic nature
  – After recent pregnancy, birth, or miscarriage

Review of Systems
- Systemic symptoms: Fever, chills, weight loss
- Other local symptoms: Erythema, nipple discharge, skin dimpling

Physical Exam
- 1st priority is to rule out malignancy:
  – Breast mass
  – Skin changes
  – Nipple discharge
  – Lymphadenopathy
- Examine breasts in seated and supine position.

TESTS
- Culture of breast discharge
- Breast biopsy as indicated if focal mass or abnormal mammogram or ultrasound

Labs
Genetic counseling if family history of breast cancer:
- BRCA 1, BRCA 2 genes

Imaging
- Mammography:
  – Screening per ACS guidelines
  – Diagnostic
- Ultrasound:
  – Can demonstrate cystic vs. solid characteristic of mass
  – Screening in young women with strong family history:
    ○ Dense breasts preclude mammography

DIFFERENTIAL DIAGNOSIS
- Hormonal fluctuation often causes cyclic breast pain:
  – Fibrocystic changes are common.
  – Hormone replacement therapy
- Pathologic processes often lead to noncyclic pain:
  – Engorgement during lactation
  – Mastitis/Breast abscess
  – Breast masses
  – Large pendulous breasts
  – Ductal ectasia
  – Hydradenitis suppurativa in axilla
- Extramammary causes:
  – Chest wall pain
  – Spinal and paraspinal disorders
- Postthoracotomy syndrome

Infection
- Mastitis
- Breast abscess

Metabolic/Endocrine
Hyperprolactinemia with galactorrhea can cause fullness and tenderness.

Tumor/Malignancy
- Breast cancer
- Inflammatory breast cancer may present similar to mastitis/breast abscess.

Trauma
- Trauma to the breast
- Trauma to the chest wall
- Trauma to the neck radiating to the breast

Drugs
- Oral contraceptive pills
- Hormone replacement therapy

Other/Miscellaneous
- Fibrocystic changes
- Large pendulous breasts
- Ductal ectasia
- Hydradenitis suppurativa

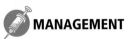 MANAGEMENT

GENERAL MEASURES
- 1st exclude malignancy and reassure patient.
- Often patients do not feel the pain is severe enough to necessitate treatment as long as cancer is ruled out.

SPECIAL THERAPY
Complementary and Alternative Therapies
- Well-fitting bra
- Stretching
- Massage
- Ice/Heating pads
- Vitamin E
- Evening primrose oil
- Chasteberry; some evidence of efficacy
- Avoidance of caffeine and nicotine

MEDICATION (DRUGS)
- NSAIDs
- Narcotics for acute cause, abscess
- Antibiotics
- Tamoxifen
- Danazol
- Bromocriptine
- Lisuride maleate

SURGERY
Used mostly for treatment of cancer etiologies.
- Lumpectomy
- Mastectomy
- Radical mastectomy

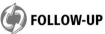 FOLLOW-UP

Dependent on etiology

DISPOSITION
Issues for Referral
Breast surgeon evaluation if malignancy suspected

PROGNOSIS
- Cyclic pain typically resolves at the end of the luteal phase of the menstrual cycle whether secondary to exogenous or endogenous hormones.
- Muscle/Joint injuries resolve.
- Breast cancer prognosis is discussed in a separate section.

PATIENT MONITORING
Follow-up mammogram or ultrasound if mass present

BIBLIOGRAPHY

Dennehy CE. The use of herbs and dietary supplements in gynecology: An evidence-based review. *J Midwifery Women's Health*. 2006;51(6):402–409.

Gumm R, et al. Evidence for the management of mastalgia. *Curr Med Res Opin*. 2004;20(5): 681–684.

Olawaiye A, et al. Mastalgia: A review of management. *J Reprod Med*. 2005;50(12): 933–939.

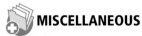 MISCELLANEOUS

CODES
ICD9-CM
- 610.1 Fibrocystic breast disease
- 611.1 Hypertrophy of the breast (gynecomastia)
- 611.71 Breast pain
- 611.72 Breast mass or lump

 PATIENT TEACHING

Monthly breast self exams

PREVENTION
- Monthly breast self exams
- Yearly clinical breast exams
- Mammography yearly after age 40

HIRSUTISM

Shibani Kanungo, MD, MPH
Hatim A. Omar, MD

 BASICS

DESCRIPTION
- From the Latin, *hirsutus* = hairy
- Symptom associated with male pattern of pigmented terminal hair growth
- Locations are assessed for research purposes in Ferriman-Gallwey score.
- Often associated with acne, irregular menstrual periods, galactorrhea, dark velvety patches of skin, central obesity, infertility

Pediatric Considerations
- Infancy to late childhood (<10 years of age): Associated with Cornelia de Lange syndrome, FAS, CAH, adrenocortical tumors, or drug-induced
- Adolescence: Associated with PCOS, late-onset CAH, HAIR-AN syndrome, steroid use, depression, pregnancy, or drug-induced
- Adulthood: Associated with PCOS, HAIR-AN syndrome, hyperprolactinemia, ovarian tumor, menopause, depression, or drug-induced

EPIDEMIOLOGY
5–10% of women, of which 20% have idiopathic hirsutism

RISK FACTORS
- Ethnicity (Mediterranean, Middle Eastern, South Asian)
- Family history
- Infertility
- Obesity

Genetics
- Can be familial or multifactorial
- Seen with:
  - Polymorphism of 5 α-reductase (SRD5A1 and SRD5A2) isomers
  - CYP21 gene mutation
  - NIPBL mutation associated with Cornelia de Lange syndrome

PATHOPHYSIOLOGY
- Caused by increased:
  - Levels of androgen secretion (DHEA, DHEAS, androstenedione and testosterone)
  - Peripheral conversion of testosterone to potent DHT
  - Sensitivity of hair follicles to androgens regulated by 5 α-reductase, which transforms testosterone or androstenedione to DHT
- Caused by decreased:
  - SHBG concentration with resultant increased free androgen

ASSOCIATED CONDITIONS
- Idiopathic hirsutism
- PCOS
- HAIR-AN syndrome
- CAH
- Cushing disease
- Hyperthecosis
- Hypothyroidism
- Hyperprolactinemia
- Adrenocortical tumors
- Ovarian tumors
- Cornelia de Lange syndrome
- Fetal alcohol syndrome
- Drugs: Corticosteroids, anabolic steroids, phenytoin, valproate, danazol, diazoxide, minoxidil
- Pregnancy
- Stress
- Male pseudohermaphroditism
- Depression

 DIAGNOSIS

SIGNS AND SYMPTOMS
- Based on the Ferriman-Gallwey score of hair growth level on 9 different locations of the body:
  - Upper lip, chin, chest, upper back, lower back, upper abdomen, lower abdomen, upper arms, and thighs
  - Hair growth is rated from 0–4, where 0 is virtually no hair at all, and 4 is completely covered with hair. The maximum score is 36. Commonly used research scale in US
  - Normal: <8
    - Light hirsutism: 8–16
    - Moderate hirsutism: 17–25
    - Severe hirsutism: >26
- The scale may vary for different ethnic groups with different levels of expected hair growth.

History
- Age of onset
- Duration
- Location
- Rate of progression
- Skin changes
- Associated symptoms of virilization
- Medication use
- Ethnic background
- Medical history
- Puberty/Menstrual history
- Family history of females with hirsutism, males with early balding
- Psychosocial history/stress, depression

Review of Systems
Other associated signs and symptoms:
- Acne
- Irregular menstrual periods
- Dark velvety patches of skin (acanthosis nigricans)
- Breast discharge
- Central obesity
- Deepening of the voice
- Increased muscle mass
- Infertility

Physical Exam
- Vitals: Increased BMI, high BP, waist circumference >30 inches
- General: Central obesity, BMI, dysmorphism, deepening of voice, male habitus
- Skin: Acne, male pattern hair, seborrhea
- HEENT: Tonsillar enlargement, thyromegaly, acanthosis nigricans, cervical fat pad, temporal balding
- Chest: Breast tenderness, galactorrhea, truncal obesity, buffalo hump
- Abdomen: Striae, tenderness
- GU: Clitoromegaly, ovarian mass

TESTS
Ferriman-Gallwey scoring for research purposes

Labs
Testing as clinically appropriate for:
- DHEA-S
- Total testosterone
- Free testosterone
- Fasting Insulin and glucose
- IGF-1
- TSH
- Free T4
- 17 OH progesterone
- Prolactin
- LH
- FSH
- ACTH
- Cortisol
- 24-hour urine cortisol

Imaging
- Pelvic ultrasound if ovarian mass suspected
- CT abdomen and pelvis if adrenal mass suspected
- MRI head if pituitary abnormality suspected

DIFFERENTIAL DIAGNOSIS
- Hypertrichosis: Excessive androgen-independent fine and soft total body hair growth in both men and women
- Idiopathic hirsutism

Metabolic/Endocrine
- PCOS
- HAIR-AN syndrome
- CAH
- Cushing disease
- Hyperthecosis
- Hypothyroidism
- Diabetes
- Hyperprolactinemia
- Male pseudohermaphroditism

Tumor/Malignancy
- Adrenocortical tumors
- Ovarian tumors

Drugs
- Corticosteroids
- Anabolic steroids
- Phenytoin
- Valproate
- Danazol
- Diazoxide
- Minoxidil

Other/Miscellaneous
- Cornelia de Lange syndrome
- Fetal alcohol syndrome
- Pregnancy
- Stress
- Depression
- Anorexia nervosa
- Obesity

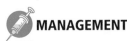 **MANAGEMENT**

GENERAL MEASURES
- Lifestyle changes/weight loss
- Topical:
  - Bleaching
  - Eflornithine HCl: Inhibits enzyme ornithine decarboxylase in skin causing decrease rate of hair growth
- Hair removal:
  - Shaving does not increase rate of hair growth.
  - Plucking
  - Waxing
  - Chemical depilatories
  - Laser epilation—not permanent
  - Electrolysis—only permanent method of hair removal

SPECIAL THERAPY
Complementary and Alternative Therapies
Aimed at pathogenesis of hirsutism:
- Photodynamic therapy (PDT) using aminolevulinic acid (ALA) decreases hair growth.
- Ethanolic extract of fennel (*Foeniculum vulgare*) decreases hair diameter and inhibits growth.
- Stinging nettle (*Urtica dioica*) roots have lignans that increase circulating SHBG.
- Saw palmetto (*Serenoa repens*) has antiandrogenic properties by reducing 5α-reductase.
- Licorice can reduce serum testosterone.

MEDICATION (DRUGS)
Aimed at primary cause of hirsutism:
- OCP reduces circulating androgen levels through suppression of circulating LH, stimulation of SHBG levels with resultant decreases in free androgens, and reduction of 5α-reductase activity
- Clomiphene induces ovulation
- Metformin promotes ovulation and reduces insulin resistance of peripheral tissue.
- Gonadotropins: Leuprolide
- Cyproterone competes with DHT for binding to the androgen receptor.
- Spironolactone competes with DHT for binding to the androgen receptor.
- Flutamide is a pure androgen receptor blocker.
- Ketoconazole reduces levels of concentration of circulating androgens.
- Finasteride inhibits activity of 5α-reductase,

SURGERY
- Hair removal with intense pulsed light irradiator system (IPL) or normal-mode ruby laser for idiopathic or familial hirsutism
- Surgery can be aimed at underlying pathology:
  - Adrenal/Ovarian tumor resection
  - Oophorectomy for androgen-producing ovarian tumor
  - Ovarian wedge resection/ovarian drilling in PCOS

 FOLLOW-UP

Depends on cause or associated condition

DISPOSITION
Issues for Referral
- Endocrinology or gynecology or genetics or surgery for hormonal or syndromic or tumor etiology
- Dermatology or cosmetology for idiopathic or familial hirsutism only

PROGNOSIS
Dependent on cause and intervention or therapy

PATIENT MONITORING
- Endocrinology or gynecology or genetics or surgery for hormonal or syndromic or tumor etiology
- Dermatology or cosmetology for idiopathic or familial hirsutism only

BIBLIOGRAPHY

Azziz R, et al. Idiopathic hirsutism. *Endocr Rev*. 2000; 21(4):347–362.

Ferriman D, et al. Clinical assessment of body hair growth in women. *J Clin Endocrinol*. 1961;21: 1440–1447.

Goodarzi MO, et al. Variants in the 5α-reductase type 1 and type 2 genes are associated with polycystic ovary syndrome and the severity of hirsutism in affected women. *J Clin Endocrinol Metabol*. 2006; 91(10):4085–4091.

Javidnia K, et al. Antihirsutism activity of fennel (fruits of *Foeniculum vulgare*) extract. A double-blind placebo controlled study. *Phytomedicine*. 2003;10(6–7):455–458.

Omar HA, et al. Clinical profiles, occurrence, and management of adolescent patients with HAIR-AN syndrome. *Sci World J*. 2004;4:507–511.

Wild RA, et al. Ferriman Gallwey Self-Scoring I: Performance assessment in women with polycystic ovary syndrome. *J Clin Endocrinol Metabol*. 2005;90(7):4112–4114.

Zakhary K, et al. Applications of aminolevulinic acid-based photodynamic therapy in cosmetic facial plastic practices. *Facial Plastic Surg*. 2005;21(2):110–116.

 MISCELLANEOUS

Virilization indicates more severe androgen effect including breast atrophy, clitoromegaly, temporal balding

CLINICAL PEARLS
- Hirsutism without menstrual irregularities or weight gain is most likely idiopathic or familial.
- Adolescents with hirsutism and early-onset, severe, and refractory acne are likely to have PCOS; OCPs can benefit self-esteem and prevent scarring from acne.
- Hirsutism can be the only clinical presentation of depression or stress in adolescents; warrants psychosocial workup.

ABBREVIATIONS
- ACTH—Adrenocorticotropic hormone
- CAH—Congenital adrenal hyperplasia
- DHEA/DHEAS—Dehydroepiandrosterone-DHEAS sulfate
- DHT—5α-dihydrotestosterone
- FAS—Fetal alcohol syndrome
- FSH—Follicular stimulating hormone
- HEENT—Head, eyes, ears, nose, throat exam
- IGF-1—Insulin–like growth factor
- LH—Luteinizing hormone
- OCP—Oral contraceptive pill
- PCOS—Polycystic ovarian syndrome
- SHBG—Sex hormone binding globulin
- TSH—Thyroid stimulating hormone

CODES

ICD9-CM
704.1 Hirsutism

 PATIENT TEACHING

- Diagnosis of idiopathic hirsutism or familial hirsutism should be considered after a thorough workup for all other causes such as hormonal, oncologic, and syndromic agents have been ruled out.
- Current medical therapies have their pros and cons. No drug is yet FDA approved. Cosmetic remediation or counseling and education may also be helpful.

PREVENTION
- Exercise for weight control and stress reduction may improve PCOS.
- Careful use of medication such as steroids, antiepileptics, vasodilators with awareness of hirsutism as side effect

MENOPAUSAL SYMPTOMS

Patricia L. Dougherty, CNM, MSN
JoAnn V. Pinkerton, MD

 BASICS

DESCRIPTION
- Menopause is defined as the cessation of menstrual bleeding secondary to decline of ovarian function.
- Retrospective diagnosis after 12 consecutive months of amenorrhea
- Spontaneous is secondary to aging of ovaries:
  - Considered premature <40 years (1%)
- Induced is secondary to bilateral oophorectomy, chemotherapy, or pelvic irradiation.
- Perimenopause includes 5–7 years preceding and 1 year after cessation of periods.
  - Cycle irregularity is common, including change in cycle frequency, duration, amount of flow.
  - Symptoms include hot flashes, menstrual disruption, sleep disturbance; vaginal dryness often precedes final menstrual period
  - Contraception is necessary until menopause is confirmed.

Age-Related Factors
Average age of menopause in US is 51.
- 5% of women menopausal <45
- Most women menopausal by age 58.

RISK FACTORS
- Advancing age
- Pelvic surgery, irradiation, chemotherapy all increase risk of induced menopause.
- Smoking increases risk of early menopause.

Genetics
Certain karyotypic abnormalities are associated with premature menopause.

PATHOPHYSIOLOGY
- Menopause is a natural biologic process.
- Signs and symptoms of menopause related to declining estrogen levels.
- Precise cause of vasomotor symptoms is not known but possibly related to narrowing in thermoregulatory zone.

ASSOCIATED CONDITIONS
All conditions associated with advancing age, especially osteoporosis, cardiovascular disease

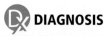 **DIAGNOSIS**

SIGNS AND SYMPTOMS
- Menstrual changes:
  - 10% of women stop cycling abruptly without menstrual pattern alterations.
  - 90% of women experience 4–8 years of cycle irregularity, including change in cycle frequency, length, amount of flow.
  - Anovulatory cycles are common, often leading to dysfunctional bleeding.
  - Diagnosis of fibroids is common in perimenopausal period.
- Vasomotor symptoms:
  - Hot flashes/night sweats hallmark of perimenopause; experienced by 75% of women
  - 25% seek medical treatment for hot flashes.
- Sleep disturbance:
  - Affects 1/3–1/2 of women 40–54 years
  - Multiple etiologies exist, including ovarian hormone changes.
- Mood lability often related to sleep disruption
- Worsening premenstrual syndrome
- Menstrual migraines may be triggered by fluctuating estrogen levels.
- Urogenital atrophy:
  - Epithelial thinning leading to fragile vaginal mucosa, decreased elasticity, decreased lubrication, increased vaginal pH
  - Vaginal shortening and narrowing
  - Itching, burning, irritation, pain with sex
  - Increase in urinary and vaginal infections in susceptible women
  - Spotting secondary to friction of atrophic tissue possible
  - Urinary frequency
- Osteoporosis:
  - Caucasian women >50 years have 40% lifetime risk for osteoporotic fracture.
  - Blacks have 1/3 fracture rate of Caucasians.
  - Risk increases with advancing age.
  - Bone loss is asymptomatic and begins in perimenopausal years.
  - Can lose up to 20% bone density in 1st 5 years of menopause

History
- Absence of menses for >12 consecutive months in a nonpregnant female ≥40 years
- In hysterectomized women, absence of menstrual bleeding makes diagnosis more difficult:
  - Vasomotor symptoms, sleep disturbance, vaginal dryness, mood lability, and cyclical headaches can assist in making diagnosis.

Physical Exam
- Annual exam including breast and thyroid
- Pelvic exam to assess urogenital atrophy:
  - Tissue appears pale, thin, dry with decreased rugae, possibly friable with petechiae
  - Vagina may be foreshortened
  - Urethral caruncles are not uncommon with pronounced atrophy
  - Vaginal pH >7 suggests atrophy

TESTS
Labs
- Typically none required, as age and symptoms are adequate to establish diagnosis:
  - Assessing hormonal status rarely impacts medical management; usually unnecessary
  - Following estradiol levels may be helpful in women with difficult-to-control hot flashes.
- Questionable diagnosis in young women:
  - FSH >30 iu/mL consistent with menopause:
    - Single measurement not adequate
    - Must be *consistently* elevated
  - Estradiol levels too erratic to use reliably
  - TSH to rule out thyroid disease leading to abnormal bleeding or vasomotor symptoms
  - Blood karyotype if <40 years may be helpful
  - Prolactin, HCG based on history
  - Endometrial biopsy if menopausal bleeding
  - Vitamin D level if osteoporosis

Imaging
- Screening:
  - Bone densitometry:
    - In all women ≥65.
    - Menopausal women ≤65 with additional risk factors
- Diagnostic:
  - Transvaginal pelvic ultrasound if postmenopausal bleeding or concern for adnexal masses

DIFFERENTIAL DIAGNOSIS
Infection
- Menstrual changes:
  - Mumps leading to POF
- Vasomotor symptoms:
  - Systemic illness (AIDS, lymphoma, TB)
- Urogenital symptoms:
  - UTI
  - Vaginal infection

Metabolic/Endocrine
Menstrual changes:
- Hypothalamic dysfunction
- Pituitary disease
- PCOS
- Thyroid disease

Tumor/Malignancy
- Menstrual changes:
  - Pituitary microadenoma
- Vasomotor symptoms:
  - Brain or spinal cord tumors
  - Carcinoid syndrome
  - Lymphoma
  - Pancreatic cancer
  - Pheochromocytoma
  - Thyroid cancer
- Urogenital symptoms:
  - Vulvar intraepithelial neoplasia

Drugs
- Menstrual changes:
  - Chemotherapy
- Vasomotor symptoms:
  - Alcohol
  - Calcium channel blockers
  - GnRH agonists
  - Niacin
  - Nitrates
  - Raloxifene
  - Tamoxifen
- Urogenital symptoms:
  - Antihistamines

Other/Miscellaneous
- Menstrual changes:
  - Asherman syndrome
  - Pelvic irradiation, surgery
  - Pregnancy
- Vasomotor symptoms:
  - MSG ingestion
  - Neurologic disorders
  - Panic attacks
  - Pelvic irradiation, surgery
  - Spinal cord injury
- Urogenital symptoms:
  - Overactive bladder
  - Vulvar dystrophy

MANAGEMENT

GENERAL MEASURES
- Education regarding menopausal process
- Identify, avoid hot-flash triggers:
  - Alcohol, spicy foods, face heat, hot baths, etc.
- Layer clothing, paced respirations, exercise
- OTC vaginal lubricants/moisturizers

SPECIAL THERAPY
Complementary and Alternative Therapies
- Vasomotor symptoms:
  - Limited data re: safety and efficacy of OTC herbal and dietary supplements
  - Black cohosh, red clover, soy, vitamin E, acupuncture
- No effect over placebo:
  - Dong Quai, ginseng, evening primrose oil, magnet therapy, reflexology

MEDICATION (DRUGS)
- Menstrual irregularity:
  - Progestin IUD or cyclic progestin therapy for perimenopausal heavy bleeding
  - OCPs for irregular or heavy cycles safe until menopause in nonsmoking, normotensive women without contraindications to OCPs
  - OCPs control hot flashes, provide contraception for premenopausal women
  - Long-cycle or 24/4 OCPs may help control many perimenopausal symptoms.
  - Check FSH level after 7 days off OCPs to diagnose menopause.
- Vasomotor symptoms:
  - Hormone therapy
    - Gold standard for relief of hot flashes
    - Contraindicated in women with hormonally mediated cancers, undiagnosed vaginal bleeding, active liver disease, increased risk clotting, coronary artery disease
    - ET for women without uteri
    - EPT for women with uterus; unopposed estrogen increases risk of endometrial cancer; progestin therapy reduces risk back to baseline
    - Per the Women's Health Initiative study, ET slightly increases risk of fatal blood clots (MI, CVA, PE), dementia; decreases risk of fractures, colon cancer
    - Per the Women's Health Initiative study, EPT slightly increases risk of fatal blood clots (MI, CVA, PE), dementia, breast cancer; decreases risk of fractures, colon cancer

- Goal is lowest effective dose for shortest time necessary to meet treatment goals
- Choice of regimen (oral vs. transdermal; continuous vs. cyclic) depends on patient preference, months of amenorrhea, comorbid conditions
  - Nonhormonal medications for women who cannot or do not wish to use hormones not FDA approved for vasomotor symptoms.
    - SSRIs/SSNRI
    - Gabapentin
    - Clonidine
- Urogenital atrophy:
  - OTC topical lubricants for sexual activity
  - OTC vaginal moisturizers for maintenance
  - Vaginal estrogen cream, tablet, or ring:
    - Local, nonsystemic therapy increases vaginal elasticity, mucosal thickness, moisture
    - Decreases vulvar/vaginal pain, dyspareunia
    - Decreases urinary frequency
    - Decreases risk of UTIs and vaginal infections
    - Can be used alone or in conjunction with systemic hormone therapy
    - Small amount absorbed systemically
- Osteoporosis:
  - 1,500 mg calcium and 800 IU vitamin D daily in divided doses through diet or supplements
  - Weight-bearing exercise
  - Estrogen indicated for prevention of osteoporosis:
    - Ultra-low dose effective for preventing bone loss in women >60
  - Oral bisphosphonates (alendronate, risedronate, ibandronate) for prevention and treatment
  - Raloxifene (SERM):
    - Decreases breast cancer risk
    - Can increase vasomotor and vaginal symptoms
    - Increases clotting and stroke risk
  - Parathyroid hormone (teriparatide):
    - Daily SC injection for patients unresponsive or intolerant to other medications
    - Approved for 18 months of use
  - Miacalcitonin nasal:
    - Less effective option for women intolerant or with contraindications to other medications
    - Mild analgesic effect

SURGERY
- Rarely required
- Endometrial ablation or hysterectomy for menorrhagia refractory to medical management
- Uterine artery embolization or hysteroscopic resection of fibroids if contributing to menorrhagia

FOLLOW-UP

PROGNOSIS
- Menstrual irregularity will cease with menopause.
- Vasomotor symptoms will lessen and often resolve over several years:
  - Taper hormone therapy after 1–2 years to determine lowest effective dose or readiness to discontinue treatment.
- Urogenital atrophy is progressive and often worsens unless local estrogen therapy is used.
- If untreated, osteoporosis often leads to fractures of the hip, vertebra, and other sites.

BIBLIOGRAPHY

North American Menopause Society. *Menopause Practice: A Clinician's Guide.* Cleveland, 2004.

North American Menopause Society, with assistance from Santoro NF, et al. Treatment of Menopause-Associated Vasomotor Symptoms: Position Statement of the North American Menopause Society. *Menopause.* 2004;11(1):11–33.

North American Menopause Society. *Menopause Core Curriculum Study Guide.* 2nd ed. Cleveland, 2002.

Santoro N, et al., eds. *Textbook of Perimenopausal Gynecology.* New York: Parthenon; 2003.

MISCELLANEOUS

See also: Osteoporosis

ABBREVIATIONS
- CVA—Cerebrovascular accident/stroke
- EPT—Estrogen plus progestin therapy
- ET—Estrogen therapy
- FSH—Follicle-stimulating hormone
- GnRH—Gonadotropin releasing hormone
- HCG—Human chorionic gonadotropin
- HPV—Human papillomavirus
- MI—Myocardial infarction
- MSG—Monosodium glutamate
- OCP—Oral contraceptive pill
- PCOS—Polycystic ovary syndrome
- PE—Pulmonary embolism
- POF—Premature ovarian failure
- SERM—Selective estrogen receptor modulator
- SSNRI—Selective serotonin norepinephrine reuptake inhibitor
- SSRI—Selective serotonin reuptake inhibitor
- TSH—Thyroid-stimulating hormone
- UTI—Urinary tract infection

CODES
ICD9-CM
- 627.2 Menopause
- 627.3 Vaginal atrophy
- 626.4 Irregular menstrual cycle
- 780.2 Vasomotor instability
- 733.00 Osteoporosis

PATIENT TEACHING

- Educational materials available at the North American Menopause Society, P.O. Box 94527, Cleveland, OH 44101
- www.menopause.org

PREVENTION
- Pap smear based on current guidelines and Pap and HPV history:
  - HPV may be more sensitive than Pap in older women in predicting risk of dysplasia
- Mammogram:
  - Every 1–2 years between age 40–50
  - Yearly after 50
- Colonoscopy:
  - Baseline at 50
  - Sooner based on family history
- Lipid levels

PAIN, CHRONIC PELVIC

Paula J. Adams Hillard, MD

BASICS

DESCRIPTION
- Chronic pelvic pain (CPP) is traditionally defined as pelvic pain that has been present for ≥6 months.
- CPP is further defined as leading to disability or requiring medical care.
- The location of CPP includes the pelvis and the lower abdomen below the umbilicus:
  – Vulvar pain is sometimes included in this category.
  – Lumbosacral pain and pain in the buttocks may also be included in this category.
- Gynecologic conditions, gastrointestinal, urologic, musculoskeletal, and psychoneurologic disorders can contribute to CPP.
- CPP includes a variety of symptoms that are described as:
  – Dysmenorrhea
  – Vulvar pain
  – Dyspareunia
  – As well as nonspecific pain of the lower abdomen, pelvic floor, adnexae, and uterus
- CPP is frequently accompanied by, associated with, and complicated by high rates of psychological dysfunction including:
  – Depression
  – History of sexual or physical abuse
- The following diagnostic subtypes of CPP have been suggested:
  – Diffuse abdominal/pelvic pain
  – Vulvovaginal pain
  – Cyclic pain
  – Neuropathic pain
  – Nonlocalized pain
  – Trigger point pain
  – Fibroid tumor pain
- Some women with CPP have neuropathic pain—pain due to abnormal neural activity which is persistent in the absence of active disease.

Age-Related Factors
- Women of all ages develop chronic pelvic pain, although the prevalence of disorders varies by age.
- Evaluation and management of chronic pelvic pain in adolescents can have long-term benefits of improving function and well-being, and avoiding chronic disability.
- Adolescents are more likely than adults to experience cycle-related pain and frequently benefit from the contraceptive and noncontraceptive benefits of COCs.
- Endometriosis does occur in adolescents and can be a cause of chronic pain.

EPIDEMIOLOGY
- Women with CPP do not differ from those without CPP by age, race or ethnicity, education, socioeconomic or employment status.
- Women with CPP may be slightly more likely to be separated or divorced.
- It has been estimated that up to 10–15% of outpatient gynecology visits include a complaint of CPP.
- CPP is the indication for ~40% of gynecologic laparoscopies in the US.
- CPP is the indication for ~20% of hysterectomies for benign disease in the US.

RISK FACTORS
History of physical and sexual abuse

PATHOPHYSIOLOGY
Multiple mechanisms of pain, depending on etiologies, although overall, the pathogenesis of chronic pelvic pain is poorly understood.

ASSOCIATED CONDITIONS
- Depression
- History of physical or sexual abuse
- Substance use or abuse
- Fibromyalgia

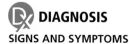

DIAGNOSIS

SIGNS AND SYMPTOMS
History
- Pain description:
  – Location
  – Intensity
  – Quality
  – Duration
  – Temporal or cyclic patterns
  – Precipitating or exacerbating factors:
    ○ Physical activity
    ○ Intercourse
    ○ Menses
  – Alleviating factors
  – Relationship to urination and defecation
- Menstrual history
- Screening for history of physical or sexual abuse
- Past therapies
- Past surgeries
- Past history of PID/STDs
- Family history of:
  – Endometriosis
  – Uterine leiomyomata

Review of Systems
- GI symptoms and function
- GU symptoms and function
- Musculoskeletal symptoms and function

Physical Exam
- Exam of abdomen:
  – Localize tenderness
  – Note surgical scars
  – Presence of hernias
  – Abdominal masses
  – Carnett sign:
    ○ After localizing point(s) of maximal tenderness, the patient is asked to do a "crunch" or bent knee sit-up during palpation of this site; myofascial pain will be increased, whereas intrapelvic or visceral pain is lessened due to splinting of the pelvis by the abdominal wall musculature.
- Careful exam of the vulva/external genitalia
- "Functional" bimanual pelvic exam with gentle careful palpation using a single vaginal finger for palpation, to assess for tenderness and reproduction of the pain, isolating:
  – Pelvic floor muscles
  – Urethra/Bladder
  – Uterus
  – Adnexae
  – Cul-de-sac/Uterosacral ligaments
- Speculum exam:
  – Cervicitis
  – Vaginitis

TESTS
Labs
- Pregnancy test
- CBC
- ESR
- Urinalysis and culture
- STD testing as indicated

Imaging
Pelvic US can be helpful in detecting:
- Uterine fibroids
- Ovarian cysts
- Other pelvic masses

DIFFERENTIAL DIAGNOSIS
Infection
PID may lead to CPP in up to 30% of women diagnosed with PID.

GI/GU
- IBS
- Constipation
- Inflammatory bowel disease
- Diverticulitis
- Interstitial cystitis
- Urethral syndrome
- Chronic or recurrent acute UTIs
- Stone/Urolithiasis

Tumor/Malignancy
- Uterine leiomyomata (fibroids)
- Adenomyosis
- Exclude malignancy if pelvic mass
- Bladder or colon malignancies
- Ovarian cancer
- Ovarian remnant syndrome
- Postoperative peritoneal cysts
- Endometrial or cervical polyps

Trauma
- History of sexual or physical abuse is associated with CPP.
- Surgical history with resultant adhesions
- Cervical stenosis

Other/Miscellaneous
- Pelvic congestion syndrome
- Genital prolapse
- Pelvic floor myalgia
- Endometriosis
- Adnexal masses
- Abdominal wall myofascial pain
- Neuralgia of iliohypogastric, ilioinguinal, and/or genitofemoral nerves
- Chronic back pain
- Abdominal cutaneous nerve entrapment in surgical scar
- Hernias: Ventral, inguinal, femoral, spigelian
- Fibromyalgia
- Abdominal migraine
- Abdominal epilepsy

 MANAGEMENT

GENERAL MEASURES
- All women with CPP deserve a nonjudgmental listener, thorough evaluation, careful history, explanations, and a commitment to work toward improving pain. It can be helpful to state that the pain may not be "cured," but can be assessed in a stepwise fashion, managed, and improved.
- One approach involves sequential drug therapy for the most likely causes of pain as assessed by the history and exam.
- Some clinicians investigate intensively, including diagnostic laparoscopy, to attempt to find a specific cause of CPP that can be treated.
- Another approach includes a combination of interventions with pharmacologic, physical, and psychological therapies. A pain management clinic may be helpful, and such a multidisciplinary approach has been shown in randomized trials to be of benefit in symptom relief.

SPECIAL THERAPY
Complementary and Alternative Therapies
- Chronic pain is one of the primary reasons given by women for the use of adjunctive or alternative therapies.
- With myofascial pain, physical therapy by a therapist trained in pelvic floor and musculo-skeletal disorders can be helpful if available.
- Although few of these therapies have been rigorously studied, treatment modalities that may prove helpful for some symptoms of CPP include:
  – Acupuncture
  – Biofeedback
  – Relaxation therapies
  – Nerve stimulation devices—TENS

MEDICATION (DRUGS)
- Scheduled NSAIDs rather than p.r.n. pain medications may be beneficial, but attention must be given to GI, CV, and renal effects.
- Menstrual or ovulation suppression with COCs may be helpful, particularly for women with cycle-related pain:
  – As a traditional 21/7 regimen of hormonally active pills followed by 7 days of placebo or
  – As an extended regimen
    ○ A formulation packaged as 84/7
    ○ 365 days of continuous pill use
- Continuous progestin therapy, given as:
  – Norethindrone acetate 5 mg/d
  – Medroxyprogesterone acetate 50 mg/d was shown to be effective in managing CPP believed due to pelvic congestion syndrome.
  – POP (norethindrone 0.35 mg/d)
  – Danazol 200–400 mg/d up to 800 mg/d
  – Levonorgestrel intrauterine system may be helpful in managing endometriosis.
- Empiric therapy with GnRH-analog may be helpful.
- Drugs that have been used in the management of neuropathic pain include:
  – Tricyclic antidepressants, such as amitriptyline, may be helpful in chronic pain syndromes.
  – SSRIs have not been shown to be helpful.
  – Anticonvulsants such as carbamazepine, valproic acid, clonazepam, gabapentin, pregabalin, lamotrigine may be beneficial.
- The use of opioids for chronic pain not due to malignancy is controversial:
  – Studies suggest benefit for intermediate intervals, even for chronic neuropathic pain.
  – Opioid therapy may be indicated after other therapies have failed:
    ○ Guidelines have been established for opioid therapy.
    ○ A single physician and pharmacy should prescribe and dispense the drugs.

SURGERY
- Trigger-point injections for abdominal wall pain may be helpful.
- Diagnostic laparoscopy is the definitive test for detecting pelvic endometriosis:
  – A normal laparoscopy does not exclude a physical cause but can exclude some specific causes.
- Laparoscopic pain mapping: Laparoscopy performed under local anesthesia with manipulation of specific sites to attempt to reproduce and localize pain
- Surgical lysis of adhesions:
  – One controlled trial in which patients were assigned to lysis or no lysis of adhesions at the time of laparoscopy showed no benefit.
  – One trial did suggest a benefit of adhesiolysis for pain relief in the presence of dense vascularized adhesions involving bowel and peritoneum.
- Interventions that have been described include nerve blocks (ilioinguinal, iliohypogastric, genitofemoral, hypogastric, presacral)
- Nerve transection procedures:
  – A Cochrane systematic review of treatments for chronic pelvic pain concluded that laparoscopic uterosacral nerve ablation (LUNA) has not been shown to be effective.
  – Presacral neurectomy may benefit midline menstrual-associated pain.
- Hysterectomy has a role in management; studies suggest ≥75% have relief at 1 year.

 FOLLOW-UP

Regularly scheduled rather than pain-dictated follow-up visits can be helpful in management.

DISPOSITION
Issues for Referral
- Referral to a comprehensive pain management team may be indicated.
- Depression is common with CPP and warrants treatment.

PROGNOSIS
The achievable goals of therapy include improved function, decreased pain by self-rating, and improved quality of life rather than "cure" of pain.

BIBLIOGRAPHY

ACOG Practice Bulletin. Chronic Pelvic Pain, #51, March 2004.

Farquhar CM, et al. A randomized controlled trial of medroxyprogesterone acetate and psychotherapy for the treatment of pelvic congestion. *Br J Obstet Gynaecol.* 1989;96(10):1153–1162.

Leserman J, et al. Identification of diagnostic subtypes of chronic pelvic pain and how subtypes differ in health status and trauma history. *Am J Obstet Gynecol* 2006;195(2):554–560; discussion 560.

Proctor M, et al. Surgical interruption of pelvic nerve pathways for primary and secondary dysmenorrhoea Cochrane Database of Syst Rev 2005. CD001896.

Stones W, et al. Interventions for treating chronic pelvic pain in women. Review. *Cochrane Database Syst Rev* 2007.

 MISCELLANEOUS

CLINICAL PEARLS
The evaluation and management of women with CPP can be challenging, and does not often result in a "cure," but can be aimed at alleviating suffering and empowering women to find management approaches that improve function and well-being.

ABBREVIATIONS
- COC—Combination oral contraceptives
- CPP—Chronic pelvic pain
- GnRH—Gonadotropin-releasing hormone
- IBS—Irritable bowel syndrome
- LUNA—Laparoscopic uterosacral nerve ablation
- PID—Pelvic inflammatory disease
- POP—Progestin-only pills
- SSRI—Selective serotonin reuptake inhibitors
- TENS—Transcutaneous electrical nerve stimulator

CODES
ICD9-CM
- 614.6 Adhesions, pelvic female
- 625 Pain and other symptoms associated with female genital organs
- 625.5 Pelvic congestion

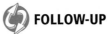 **PATIENT TEACHING**

ACOG Patient Education Pamphlet: Pelvic Pain

PAIN: DYSMENORRHEA

Zeev Harel, MD
Paula J. Adams Hillard, MD

 BASICS

DESCRIPTION
- Dysmenorrhea is the most common gynecologic complaint and the leading cause of recurrent short-term school or work absenteeism among female adolescents and young adults.
- The majority of dysmenorrhea is primary (or functional) and is associated with normal ovulatory cycles and with no pelvic pathology.
- In ~10% of adolescents and young adults with severe dysmenorrhea, pelvic abnormalities such as endometriosis and uterine anomalies may be found (secondary dysmenorrhea).

Age-Related Factors
- Dysmenorrhea is not common in the 1st 2–3 years after menarche, when most menstrual cycles are anovulatory.
- Dysmenorrhea becomes more prevalent with the establishment of ovulatory menstrual cycles during mid and late adolescence.
- The incidence of primary dysmenorrhea decreases with age, parity, and the use of hormonal contraceptives.
- Secondary dysmenorrhea increases with age.

EPIDEMIOLOGY
Prevalence
- ~70% of adolescents experience dysmenorrhea; 15% have severe symptoms.
- Among women in their 20s, 67% experience dysmenorrhea; 10% have severe symptoms.
- Secondary dysmenorrhea depends on cause.

RISK FACTORS
- Primary:
  - Nulliparity
  - Heavy menstrual flow
  - Cigarette smoking
  - Low fish intake
  - Depression/Anxiety/Sexual abuse and poor school/work performance are weaker factors.
- Secondary:
  - Pelvic infection/STDs
  - Endometriosis
  - Family history of endometriosis (risk factor for secondary dysmenorrhea)
  - Nonmedicated IUD use
  - Uterine fibroids

Genetics
Endometriosis is a genetic disorder of polygenic/multifactorial inheritance with 5–7% risk in 1st-degree relatives.

PATHOPHYSIOLOGY
- Primary dysmenorrhea:
  - After ovulation a buildup of fatty acids occur in the phospholipids of the cell membranes. The high intake of Ω-6 fatty acids in the Western diet results in a predominance of Ω-6 fatty acids in the cell wall phospholipids.
  - After the onset of progesterone withdrawal before menstruation, these Ω-6 fatty acids, particularly arachidonic acid, are released, and a cascade of prostaglandins (PG) and leukotrienes (LT) is initiated in the uterus. The inflammatory response, mediated by these PGs and LTs, produces both cramps and systemic symptoms such as nausea, vomiting, and headaches.
  - In particular, the prostaglandin F2a, COX metabolite of arachidonic acid, causes potent vasoconstriction and myometrial contractions, leading to ischemia and pain.
- Secondary dysmenorrhea—pelvic pathology:
  - External to uterus
    ○ Endometriosis (see topic)
    ○ Tumors
    ○ Pelvic adhesions
  - Uterine:
    ○ Obstructing uterovaginal anomaly in teens
    ○ Adhesions
    ○ Pelvic inflammatory disease
    ○ Adenomyosis
    ○ Uterine leiomyomas
    ○ Cervical stenosis
    ○ Uterine polyps
    ○ Nonhormonal IUDs

ASSOCIATED CONDITIONS
- Symptoms of PMDD or PMS may overlap.
- Menstrual molimina (unpleasant symptoms accompanying menstruation), including bloating, breast tenderness, headaches, nausea, vomiting, diarrhea

 DIAGNOSIS

SIGNS AND SYMPTOMS
- Primary dysmenorrhea:
  - Symptoms of lower abdominal and pelvic pain typically accompany the start of menstrual flow or occur within a few hours before or after onset, and last 24–72 hours.
  - Pain may radiate to back or thighs.
- Secondary dysmenorrhea:
  - Pain may occur 1–2 weeks before menses (chronic pelvic pain or mid cycle pain) as well as dyspareunia; pain typically throughout menstrual flow

History
- Complete menstrual, gynecologic, pain history
- Menstrual history:
  - When was menarche?
  - Frequency, duration, and amount of flow
  - Frequency of dysmenorrhea
- Pain history:
  - Onset, duration, intensity of pain (rate 0–10)
  - Does the pain occur at times other than menstruation?
  - Medications taken, including OTC; dose, frequency, efficacy
  - Other menstruation associated symptoms?
- Gynecologic history/procedures:
  - Sexual history; dyspareunia; STD history
  - Contraception
- History of physical or sexual abuse
- Past medical history:
  - Hospitalizations
  - Surgeries
  - Chronic medical conditions
- Family history:
  - Endometriosis
  - Uterine fibroids
  - Dysmenorrhea
  - Hysterectomy
- Tobacco use

Review of Systems
- Special attention to GI and GU systems
- Special attention to contraindications to hormonal contraception

Physical Exam
- Women with primary dysmenorrhea have a normal physical exam.
- Women with secondary dysmenorrhea often have a normal exam, but the clinician may find:
  - Uterine, adnexal, or rectovaginal tenderness
  - Uterine enlargement, adnexal masses
  - Cervical displacement
  - Uterosacral nodularity
  - Cervical stenosis

TESTS
- Most patients do not require extensive evaluation.
- A trial of NSAIDs is an important component of the evaluation because secondary dysmenorrhea is less likely to respond to NSAIDs than is primary dysmenorrhea.

Labs
Currently, no laboratory tests can distinguish between primary and secondary dysmenorrhea.

Imaging
- Ultrasound; transvaginal if possible:
  - Aids in the characterization of physical exam abnormalities
  - Allows the detection of uterine and adnexal lesions that may not be detectable on exam
- Pelvic MRI study is indicated in adolescents when the exam or ultrasound suggests obstructive anomaly.

DIFFERENTIAL DIAGNOSIS
Infection
- PID
- UTI

Tumor/Malignancy
- Endometrial polyp
- Uterine or ovarian neoplasm
- Cervical cancer

Other/Miscellaneous
- Congenital anomalies of the uterus or vagina
- Complications of pregnancy
- Missed or incomplete abortion
- Ectopic pregnancy
- Endometriosis
- Adenomyosis
- Pelvic adhesions
- GI pathology
- Complications of intrauterine device

 ## MANAGEMENT
GENERAL MEASURES
- Assess the patient's degree of symptoms.
- Assess whether the patient has already taken OTC medication (type, dose).

SPECIAL THERAPY
Complementary and Alternative Therapies
- Topical heat therapy:
  - Better pain relief than acetaminophen alone
  - Similar to the relief obtained by low-dose ibuprofen.
- Interventions such as herbal preparations, transcutaneous nerve stimulation, and acupuncture have been reported to improve dysmenorrhea in some studies.
- Some evidence suggests that a low-fat vegetarian diet may help some women.
- High intake of fish rich in Ω-3 fatty acids has been correlated with less dysmenorrhea symptoms.
- Some women obtain relief with aerobic exercise, although other women obtain no benefit.

MEDICATION (DRUGS)
- NSAIDs:
  - Decrease prostaglandin production, thereby decreasing the discomfort of uterine contractions
  - ~70% experience partial or total pain relief, compared to 15% with placebo
  - Ibuprofen, naproxen, and mefenamic acid are used commonly for the treatment of dysmenorrhea.
  - A loading dose of NSAID (typically twice the regular does) should be used as initial treatment, followed by a regular dose as needed.
  - A COX-2 inhibitor (Celecoxib) may be considered in patients with a history of peptic ulcer or with a history of conventional NSAID GI adverse effects.
- Hormonal therapy:
  - Combined OCPs (may be considered for first-line of therapy in a sexually active female) 21/7 or extended cycle

  - DMPA (Depo-Provera)
  - Levonorgestrel intrauterine system (Mirena)
- Other therapies for secondary dysmenorrhea:
  - GnRH agonists such as Leuprolide acetate (Lupron) +/− add back sex steroid therapy
  - Aromatase inhibitors
  - Other therapies specific to cause (e.g., antibiotics for PID)

SURGERY
- Persistent dysmenorrhea despite appropriate dose and frequency of NSAIDs and after a trial of oral contraceptives should prompt a reconsideration of the diagnosis of primary dysmenorrhea and consideration of diagnostic laparoscopy.
- Surgical correction of obstructing anomalies
- In select women, lysis of adhesions or ablation therapy for endometriosis may be indicated.
- Older women with disabling symptoms of adenomyosis or severe endometriosis may infrequently require hysterectomy.

 ## FOLLOW-UP

Patients should have an initial follow up visit in 2–3 months and periodic reassessment after.

DISPOSITION
Issues for Referral
- If a secondary cause of dysmenorrhea or if another source of chronic pelvic pain is suspected, the patient may benefit from referral to a gynecologist with expertise in dealing with pelvic pain.
- If obstructing anomalies are present, referral to a gynecologist with experience in these conditions is indicated.

PROGNOSIS
- Primary: Improves with age and parity
- Secondary: Likely to require therapy based on underlying cause

PATIENT MONITORING
- In rare cases, hospitalization may be needed for pain control or rehydration.
- If symptoms of depression or anxiety, reassess during a painfree period, as they may be independently present.

BIBLIOGRAPHY

Akin M, et al. Continuous, low-level topical heat in the treatment of primary dysmenorrhea. *Obstet Gynecol.* 2001;97:343.

Amsterdam LL. Anastrazole and oral contraceptives: A novel treatment for endometriosis. *Fertil Steril.* 2005;84:300.

Cook AS, et al. Role of laparoscopy in the treatment of endometriosis. *Fertil Steril.*1991;55:663.

Deutch B. Menstrual pain in Danish women correlated with low n-3 polyunsaturated fatty acid intake. *Eur J Clin Nutr.*1995;49:508.

Helms JM. Acupuncture for the management of primary dysmenorrhea. *Obstet Gynecol.*1987;69:51.

Hornsby PP, et al. Cigarette smoking and disturbance of menstrual function. *Epidemiology.* 1998;9:193.

Kotani N, et al. Analgesic effect of an herbal medicine for treatment of primary dysmenorrhea—a double blind study. *Am J Chin Med.* 1997;25:205.

Owen PR. Prostaglandin synthetase inhibitors in the treatment of primary dysmenorrhea. *Am J Obstet Gynecol.* 1984;148:96.

Proctor ML, et al. Combined oral contraceptive pill (OCP) as treatment for primary dysmenorrhea. *Cochrane Database Syst Rev.* 2001.

Rees MCP, et al. Prostaglandins in menstrual fluid in menorrhagia and dysmenorrhea. *Br J Obstet Gynaecol.* 1984;91:673.

Sundell G, et al. Factors influencing the prevalence and severity of dysmenorrhea in young women. *Br J Obstet Gynaecol.* 1990;97:588.

 ## MISCELLANEOUS
SYNONYM(S)
Menstrual cramps

CLINICAL PEARLS
- Adolescents with a clinical history suggestive of primary dysmenorrhea can be evaluated with a careful history and managed with NSAIDs.
- Dysmenorrhea unrelieved by NSAIDs should prompt consideration of COCs.
- Persistent dysmenorrhea after NSAIDs and COCs should prompt further evaluation.

ABBREVIATIONS
- COC—Combination oral contraceptive
- COX—Cyclooxygenase
- GnRH—Gonadotropin-releasing hormone
- OCP—Oral contraceptive pill
- PID—Pelvic inflammatory disease
- PMDD—Premenstrual dysphoric disorder
- PMS—Premenstrual syndrome
- UTI—Urinary tract infection

CODES
ICD9-CM
- 625.3 Dysmenorrhea
- 625.9 Pelvic pain

 ## PATIENT TEACHING

- Care providers should explain the physiologic etiology of dysmenorrhea.
- A review of effective treatment options should be provided.
- Discuss evidence regarding herbal, dietary, and alternative therapies. Regular exercise and heat may be beneficial.
- Reassure patient that primary dysmenorrhea is treatable with use of NSAIDs and/or OCPs, and that normal activities during menses should be the goal.
- Encourage use of NSAIDs (over-the-counter or prescription) taken prophylactically prior to expected menses on a scheduled basis.
- Discourage use of OTCs without proven efficacy.
- ACOG Patient Education pamphlet available at http://www.acog.org.

PREVENTION
- Primary dysmenorrhea: Not well established
- Secondary dysmenorrhea: Reduce risk of STDs

PAIN: DYSPAREUNIA

Diane E. Elas, MSN, ENRC, ARNP
Rudolph P. Galask, MD, MS

BASICS

DESCRIPTION
- Dyspareunia is pain with coital activity. It may occur before, during, or after intercourse. The pain can occur at the introitus and/or deep in the pelvis.

Age-Related Factors
Can occur at any age with sexual activity.

EPIDEMIOLOGY
The prevalence rate is unknown.

RISK FACTORS
- Peri- or postmenopausal status
- Prior obstetrical or surgical trauma
- Prior history of genital mutilation
- Prior history of sexual abuse/trauma
- Underlying genital dermatologic condition
- Vulvar or vaginal infection

PATHOPHYSIOLOGY
The pathophysiology of dyspareunia is influenced by many factors including but not limited to the following:
- Prior sexual experiences
- Sexual desire for partner
- Libido
- Menstrual status
- Medical conditions
- Genital dermatologic conditions
- Infections
- Medications
- Prior trauma

ASSOCIATED CONDITIONS
- Decreased libido
- Decreased vaginal lubrication
- Depression/Decreased self-esteem
- Pelvic floor muscle spasm/dysfunction

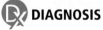

DIAGNOSIS

SIGNS AND SYMPTOMS
History
- Patient self-report of pain associated with coital activity
- The pain may occur only once.
- May be intermittent or chronic
- The pain may be partner-specific or occur with any partner.
- Assess for usual and unusual sexual practices that may contribute to the pain.
- Identify pain location:
  - Introital pain
  - Deep pelvic/thrusting pain:
    ○ Anterior pain
    ○ Posterior pain
  - Postcoital pain

Review of Systems
- GI:
  - Constipation
  - Inflammatory bowel disease
  - Irritable bowel
- Ob-Gyn:
  - Factors that affect estrogen status
  - Gyn pathology:
    ○ Endometriosis
    ○ Fibroids
  - Prior obstetric or gynecologic surgery/trauma
  - STD history
  - Vulvar/Vaginal/Pelvic infections
- Psych:
  - Anxiety
  - Depression
  - Prior sexual/physical/emotional abuse/trauma
  - Substance abuse
- Urinary:
  - Cystitis
  - Dysuria
  - Interstitial cystitis (IC)/painful bladder syndrome
  - Urinary incontinence
  - Urethral diverticulum

Physical Exam
- Abdominal examination:
  - Palpate for masses or tenderness/pain.
- Pelvic examination:
  - Assess patient's response to examination.
  - Inspect external genitalia for:
    ○ Anatomic changes/deformities
    ○ Localized erythema or tenderness at hymenal sulcus
    ○ Discharge
    ○ Lesions/Masses
    ○ Ulcerations
  - Speculum examination:
    ○ Cervical lesions/masses/discharge
    ○ Vaginal lesions/masses/discharge
  - Bimanual examination:
    ○ Cervical motion tenderness
    ○ Anterior/Posterior wall tenderness/pain
    ○ Assess resting tone of the levator muscles and pain associated with contraction, relaxation, and stretch of the muscles.
  - Rectovaginal examination:
    ○ Hemorrhoids
    ○ Masses
    ○ Pain

TESTS
- Cultures as indicated:
  - *Chlamydia*
  - HSV
  - Yeast
- Urine hCG
- Urine analysis
- Wet prep of vaginal discharge:
  - Maturation index
  - Background flora:
    ○ Clue cells
    ○ Lactobacillus, present or absent
    ○ RBCs
    ○ Trichomonads
    ○ WBCs
    ○ Yeast, buds or hyphae

Imaging
If pelvic pathology is suspected, a TVUS or CT scan is useful.

DIFFERENTIAL DIAGNOSIS
Infection
- Bacterial vaginosis
- HSV
- PID
- STD
- Trichomoniasis
- UTI
- Yeast

Metabolic/Endocrine
Hypoestrogenic state:
- Breastfeeding
- Menopause
- Medications:
  - Danazol
  - DMPA
  - GnRH agonists/antagonists
  - Leuprolide-Depot
  - Tamoxifen

Tumor/Malignancy
- Prior pelvic radiation therapy
- Underlying VIN

Trauma
- Female genital mutilation/trauma
- Obstetric trauma
- Sexual/Physical/Emotional abuse/trauma

Drugs
- Medication that decrease libido:
  - Antipsychotics
  - Cardiovascular drugs/antihypertensives
  - SSRIs
- Medications that create hypoestrogenic state:
  - See above

Other/Miscellaneous
- Substance abuse may be a sign of prior sexual, physical, or emotional abuse.
- Anatomic:
  - Congenital abnormality
  - Genital mutilation
  - Obstetrical injury
- Dermatologic:
  - Atrophic vaginitis
  - Contact vulvitis
  - Lichen sclerosus
  - Lichen planus
  - Vulvar vestibulitis
  - VIN
- Gynecologic:
  - Adnexal mass
  - Endometriosis
  - Fibroids
  - Pelvic floor muscle spasm (vaginismus)
- Other:
  - Chronic pelvic pain
  - Constipation
  - IBS
  - IC/Painful bladder syndrome
  - Trigger point

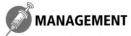 **MANAGEMENT**

GENERAL MEASURES
Treatment measures are focused on the underlying cause of the dyspareunia and the associated factors that affect desire.

SPECIAL THERAPY
Complementary and Alternative Therapies
Many products are advertised to enhance female desire; none are proven effective at this time.

MEDICATION (DRUGS)
Estrogen replacement for hypoestrogenic state:
• Systemic
• Topical/Vaginal preparations

SURGERY
As indicated for anatomic or pelvic etiology

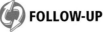 **FOLLOW-UP**

Follow-up as indicated for the underlying cause of dyspareunia.

DISPOSITION
Issues for Referral
• Gynecologist for suspected gyn/pelvic pathology
• Health psychologist/psychiatrist for associated anxiety and depression that accompany chronic dyspareunia
• Gastroenterology for dysmotility/constipation/bowel problems
• Physical therapist for pelvic floor rehabilitation
• Urology for urinary system problems

PROGNOSIS
Depends on underlying etiology of dyspareunia

BIBLIOGRAPHY

Nachtigall L, et al. Update on vaginal atrophy. *Menopause Mgmt.* 2005;September/October:17–20.
Stenchever MA, et al. Sexual dysfunction: A couples issue. *Contemp OB/GYN.* 2004;December:30–46.
Stewart I. Dyspareunia: 5 overlooked causes. *OBG Mgmt.* 2003;April:50–68.

 MISCELLANEOUS

SYNONYM(S)
• Coital discomfort
• Coital pain
• Vaginismus

CLINICAL PEARLS
Many women with dyspareunia have decreased vaginal lubrication during arousal. Encourage the use of a nonirritative lubricant such as olive oil or vegetable oil.

ABBREVIATIONS
• DMPA—Depot medroxyprogesterone acetate
• GnRH—Gonadotropin-releasing hormone
• hCG—Human chorionic gonadotropin
• HSV—Herpes simplex virus
• IBS—Irritable bowel syndrome
• IC—Interstitial cystitis
• PID—Pelvic inflammatory disease
• SSRI—Selective serotonin reuptake inhibitor
• TVUS—Transvaginal ultrasound
• UTI—Urinary tract infection
• VIN—Vulvar intraepithelial neoplasia

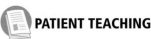 **CODES**

ICD9-CM
• 625.0 Dyspareunia
• 625.1 Vaginismus

PATIENT TEACHING

Educate the patient and her partner on the normal human sexual response. Discuss how pain with sexual activity can alter this response.

PELVIC MASSES

Nashat Moawad, MD
Tia M. Melton, MD

BASICS

DESCRIPTION
An abnormal structure or growth in the pelvic cavity, arising from:
- Pelvic organs, such as the ovaries, fallopian tubes, uterus, cervix, lymph nodes, bladder, bowel, peritoneum, and appendix
- Metastatic from extrapelvic structures, such as stomach or breast

Age-Related Factors
- Higher incidence of a neoplastic process in prepubertal and postmenopausal populations
- Higher incidence of functional and inflammatory processes in the child-bearing–age.

EPIDEMIOLOGY
The prevalence of adnexal masses ranges from 2.2–7.8% in asymptomatic women.

RISK FACTORS
- Anovulation
- Family history of breast, ovarian or colon cancer
- BRCA mutations
- Endometriosis
- Pelvic surgery: Hematoma/Abscess
- Diverticulitis/Appendicitis
- Smoking

Genetics
Genetic predisposition for ovarian cancer BRCA mutations

PATHOPHYSIOLOGY
- Functional/Physiologic: Failure of ovulation and persistence of the corpus luteum
- Inflammatory: TOA
- Neoplastic: Benign and malignant
- Postsurgical: Hematoma or abscess
- Congenital: Müllerian anomalies, teratomas
- Hormonal: Corpus luteum of pregnancy, theca-lutein cysts, struma ovarii

ASSOCIATED CONDITIONS
The following conditions can be associated with adnexal masses:
- Polycystic ovarian syndrome (PCOS)
- Endometriosis
- Pelvic kidney
- Ectopic pregnancy
- Molar pregnancy (theca-lutein cysts)
- Normal pregnancy (corpus luteum of pregnancy)
- PID/TOA
- Pedunculated fibroids

DIAGNOSIS

SIGNS AND SYMPTOMS
History
- Pelvic pain, fever, purulent cervicitis, adnexal and cervical motion tenderness are suggestive of an inflammatory etiology (PID/TOA).
- Severe acute pelvic pain can be a sign of torsion of an ovarian mass or a hemorrhagic ovarian cyst, occasionally associated with nausea and vomiting.
- Acute pelvic pain can be a sign of a ruptured ovarian cyst, occasionally caused by intercourse.
- Dyspareunia, dysmenorrhea, and infertility with a pelvic mass are suggestive of an endometrioma.
- Bloating and increased abdominal girth are common symptoms of large ovarian neoplasms or fibroids.
- Decreased appetite, nausea and vomiting, and weight loss can be associated with pelvic malignancies.

Review of Systems
- Constitutional:
  - Fever and malaise with infectious etiologies
  - Weight loss with malignant neoplasms
- GI:
  - Nausea and vomiting with ovarian torsion or malignancy
  - Decrease appetite with cancer
  - Bowel complaints with diverticular disease and Crohn's disease
  - Early satiety with large pelvic masses and ascites
- Chest:
  - Venous thromboembolism should raise suspicion for ovarian malignancies
- Endocrine:
  - Hirsutism, acne, oligomenorrhea and obesity with PCOS
  - Weight loss, heat intolerance, and other signs of hyperthyroidism with struma ovarii
  - Precocious puberty with granulosa cell tumors
  - Masculinization with Sertoli-Leydig cell tumors
- GU:
  - Hematuria and recurrent UTIs may be signs of bladder cancer.
  - Postcoital bleeding can be a sign of cervical malignancy.
  - Primary amenorrhea, cyclic pain, and hematocolpos are signs of imperforate hymen.

Physical Exam
Any of the following can be noted on physical exam:
- Fever, tachycardia, diaphoresis in inflammatory processes
- Cachexia in malignant processes
- Shock: Ruptured ectopic or hemorrhagic cyst with hemoperitoneum
- Hirsutism, acne, clitorimegaly: PCOS, androgen-secreting tumors

- Ascites can be a sign of malignant ovarian tumors; large pelvic masses can be palpated through the abdomen.
- Acute abdomen can be a sign of peritonitis due to inflammatory conditions, or hemoperitoneum due to ruptured ectopic or a ruptured hemorrhagic cyst.
- Also noted with ovarian torsion.
- Adnexal tenderness and cervical motion tenderness most often seen in inflammatory conditions.
- Vaginal bleeding with grape-like discharge are signs of molar pregnancy.
- Rectal bleeding and a mass on rectal exam can be signs of anorectal cancer.
- A cervical mass is readily visible on speculum exam and palpable on bimanual exam.
- A palpable ovary in a postmenopausal female should be evaluated for malignancy.
  - Ultrasonography and CA 125 are helpful.
- Cul-de-sac nodularity can be a sign of endometriosis or malignancy.
- A breast exam should be part of the evaluation for suspicious pelvic masses.

TESTS
- Pregnancy test
- UA and microscopy
- CBC, differential, renal panel
- CA 125 in postmenopausal women
- Pap smear, colposcopy, and biopsy if a cervical mass is suspected
- Pelvic US with Doppler flow is the mainstay of diagnosis and follow-up of adnexal masses.
- CT scan is superior in assessment of bowel and bladder masses.

Labs
- CA 125 (Normal <35 U/mL):
  - Elevated in ovarian and endometrial cancers; falsely elevated in endometriosis/endometriomas, fibroids, PID, heart, liver, and renal disease
  - Helpful for follow-up and to monitor recurrence of ovarian and endometrial cancer
- Other tumor markers are especially helpful in premenarchal patients with a suspicion for germ-cell tumor:
  - α-Fetoprotein (endodermal sinus tumor)
  - LDH (dysgerminoma)
  - hCG (nongestational choriocarcinoma)

Imaging
Pelvic ultrasound with Doppler studies:
- Test of choice for utero-ovarian masses, free fluid, and ectopic pregnancy
- Transabdominal and transvaginal
- Small, simple, follicular or luteal cysts are generally normal in premenopausal female.
- Doppler flow can help to rule out torsion and to further characterize simple, inflammatory, and neoplastic ovarian masses.

- An excellent, safe modality for follow-up and comparison
- Accurately differentiates solid from cystic masses
- A large, complex, or solid mass is concerning for malignancy.
- An ovary twice the size of the contralateral ovary in a postmenopausal female should be evaluated for cancer.
- A large ovary with multiple subcentimeter, subcapsular cysts is suggestive of PCOS.
- Papillary projections, thick septations, and low-resistance Doppler flow are markers for malignancy.
- CT scan, with contrast, is helpful to examine cervical, colorectal, appendiceal, and bladder masses and lymphadenopathy.

DIFFERENTIAL DIAGNOSIS
Infection
- TOA, appendiceal or diverticular mass
- Pelvic abscess following surgery

Hematologic
- Lymphomas
- Hematogenous spread of primary malignancy (e.g., breast cancer)
- Aneurysm of Iliac vessels

Metabolic/Endocrine
- PCOS
- Struma ovarii in teratomas

Tumor/Malignancy
- Benign
- Malignant: The risk of malignancy is high in:
  - Women with other malignancies, such as GI or breast cancer
  - Prepubertal or postmenopausal females
  - Solid or complex masses
  - Patients with ascites

Drugs
Ovulation induction medications

 ## MANAGEMENT
GENERAL MEASURES
- The decision to actively intervene versus observe is generally based on the index of suspicion and risk/benefit ratio.
- The risk of cancer, rupture, torsion, and peritonitis are usually reasons to intervene.
- Desire for future fertility should always be considered when discussing risks, benefits, and alternatives of surgical intervention with patients.
- Premenopausal simple cysts <10 cm can be followed; they usually resolve spontaneously.
- Monophasic OCPs can be used to suppress the formation of new cysts, generally used for 4–8 weeks prior to follow-up US.
- A simple cyst <3–5 cm in an asymptomatic postmenopausal female can be followed-up conservatively with serial exams, US, and CA 125 values.
- Persistent cysts, enlarging masses, or those with suspicious appearance on US should be surgically explored.
- Diagnostic/Operative laparoscopy offers the least morbidity and mortality.

MEDICATION (DRUGS)
- Monophasic OCPs
- NSAIDs

SURGERY
- Laparoscopy when risk is minimal for malignancy
- Laparotomy when risk is high for malignancy
- Consider ovarian cystectomy vs. oophorectomy for benign lesions; more radical staging procedures for malignancy

 ## FOLLOW-UP

Follow-up in 6–8 weeks with pelvic exam, pelvic US, and CA 125 as needed.

DISPOSITION
Issues for Referral
- A large postmenopausal cyst with elevated CA 125 warrants gynecologic oncology referral.
- Cervical cancer on a biopsy of a cervical mass should be referred to gynecologic oncology.
- Colorectal, appendiceal, or bladder masses should be referred to the respective specialist.
- Consider a gynecologic oncologist on stand-by during surgical exploration if malignancy is suspected.

PROGNOSIS
Prognosis depends on the etiology:
- Simple physiologic ovarian cysts generally resolve spontaneously.
- Ovarian torsion and ruptured ectopic pregnancy can be life-threatening and should be explored emergently.
- Inflammatory masses such as TOA, appendiceal, or diverticular masses generally resolve with appropriate therapy (e.g., antibiotics, drainage, excision).
- Benign tumors may remain stable or grow slowly over a long period.
- Malignant tumors grow faster and can infiltrate or encroach on other pelvic organs.

PATIENT MONITORING
Monitor symptoms, pelvic exam, US, and CA 125 as needed.

BIBLIOGRAPHY

Borgfeldt C, et al. Transvaginal sonographic ovarian findings in a random sample of women 25–40 years old. *Ultrasound Obstet Gynecol.* 1999;13(5): 345–350.

Castillo G, et al. Natural history of sonographically detected simple unilocular adnexal cysts in asymptomatic postmenopausal women. *Gynecol Oncol.* 2004;92(3):965–959.

Curtin JP. Management of the adnexal mass. *Gynecol Oncol.* 1994;55:S42.

Kinkel K, et al. US characterization of ovarian masses: A meta-analysis. *Radiology.* 2000;217:803.

 ## MISCELLANEOUS

CLINICAL PEARLS
- Ovarian masses in reproductive-age women that do not resolve after 6–8 weeks require surgical assessment, as the risk of neoplasm is high.
- Functional masses (follicular or corpus-luteum cysts) resolve without surgical intervention over 6–8 weeks.

ABBREVIATIONS
- CL—Corpus Luteum
- hCG—Human chorionic gonadotropin
- NSAIDs—Nonsteroidal anti-inflammatory drugs
- OCPs—Oral contraceptive pills
- PCOS—Polycystic ovarian syndrome
- PID—Pelvic inflammatory disease
- TOA—Tubo-ovarian abscess
- UTI—Urinary tract infection

CODES
ICD9-CM
789.3 Abdominal or pelvic swelling, mass or lump

 ## PATIENT TEACHING

PREVENTION
Combination OCPs decrease the risk of development of subsequent ovarian masses by preventing ovulation.

PUBERTY, DELAYED

Christopher P. Houk, MD
Peter A. Lee, MD, PhD

 BASICS

DESCRIPTION

- Lack of onset of physical changes of puberty (secondary sex characteristics) by age 13 years or failure to reach menarche by age 14.5 years. An abnormally slow pubertal pace after onset at a normal age may also be considered delayed.
- The time between initial breast development and menarche averages 2.5 years, and the total duration of puberty ranges from 4–5 years. Most girls with pubertal delay have pathology.
- May suggest hypothalamic-pituitary defect (hypogonadotropism) or gonadal failure (hypergonadotropism):
  - Most common form is Turner syndrome, which may be diagnosed before the age of puberty by characteristic findings at birth of because of short stature:
    ○ Turner syndrome is associated with karyotypes, including loss of key portions of 1 X chromosome, and the loss of the SHOX gene.
- May simply be a delay in normal development:
  - Constitutional
  - Secondary to chronic illness

Age-Related Factors

Ethnic differences exist:

- White: If no breast development by age 13 or pubic hair by 13.2
- African American: If no breast development by age 12.4 or pubic hair by 12.8
- Latina: If no breast development by age 12.8 or pubic hair by 13.4

ALERT

For all above ethnicities, menarche is considered to be delayed if it has not occurred by age 14.5.

EPIDEMIOLOGY

General prevalence is unknown:

- Kallmann syndrome is the most common form of permanent hypogonadotropism in 1/50,000 females.
- Turner syndrome occurs in 1/2,500 female births.

RISK FACTORS

Differ based on category:

- Constitutional delay: Family history
- Delay with normal potential: Chronic disease
- Hypogonadotropism: Anosmia, pituitary hormone deficiency, brain tumor, CNS-radiation
- Hypergonadotropism: Turner syndrome, gonadal defects (anatomic/enzyme) (disorders of sex development), gonadal radiation, chemotherapy

Genetics

Differ based on category:

- Constitutional delay: Multifactorial
- Hypogonadotropism: X-linked, autosomal dominant, autosomal recessive
- Kallmann syndrome: Kal1 (Xp22.3) and Kal2 gene (8p12) autosomal dominant form
- Other mutations resulting in hypogonadotropic hypogonadism are:
  - DAX-1 gene (Xp21) (also associated with X-linked adrenal hypoplasia congenita)
  - PROP-1 gene mutations, Prader-Willi syndrome
  - HESX1 (septo-optic dysplasia)
  - GnRH receptor mutations (4p13.1)
- Hypergonadotropism:
  - Turner syndrome
  - Noonan syndrome
  - Bardet-Biedl syndrome
  - Leptin and leptin receptor gene mutations
  - Homozygous GALT enzyme gene (9p13) resulting in galactosemia

PATHOPHYSIOLOGY

- Hypogonadotropism secondary to damage to the hypothalamus, pituitary or surrounding areas
- Hypergonadotropism secondary to damage to or defects in ovaries
- Delay with potential for normal pubertal development:
  - Malnutrition (anorexia nervosa)
  - Excessive exercise
  - Chronic disease
  - Inflammatory process (e.g., Crohn's disease)
  - Hypothyroidism
- Hypogonadotropism:
  - Midline CNS defects (septo-optic dysplasia)
  - Hemochromatosis
  - HIV
  - Craniopharyngioma and other tumors
  - Head trauma
  - Surgery
  - Infections and infiltrative diseases

ASSOCIATED CONDITIONS

Hypogonadotropic hypogonadism is associated with other anterior pituitary deficiencies (GH, TSH, ACTH).

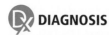 **DIAGNOSIS**

SIGNS AND SYMPTOMS

History

- General health and growth
- Radiation or chemotherapy exposure
- Psychiatric disease or disordered eating (anorexia)
- Intense exercise
- Family history of age of onset of puberty and menarche

Review of Systems

- Anosmia
- Symptoms of hypothyroidism
- Headaches
- Learning difficulties

Physical Exam

- Height, weight, BMI, upper-lower segment ratio (from sitting and standing height)
- Pubertal staging and genital inspection
- Neurologic examination including funduscopic examination and visual fields
- Assessment of subcutaneous fat, thyroid gland
- Assessment for findings of Turner syndrome including characteristic facies, micrognathia, epicanthal folds, low-set ears, low hairline, webbed neck, prominent nevi, cubitus valgus, short 4th metacarpal, spoon-shaped nails, and shield chest

TESTS

Skeletal (bone) age x-ray

Labs

- Serum LH, FSH, estradiol
- GnRH or GnRH analog stimulation testing is usually not discriminatory at presentation with delayed puberty.
  - Such a test can be used if bone age is advanced beyond the age of pubertal onset or after lack of progression of spontaneous puberty to verify low gonadotropin response.
  - Others based on history and physical findings to include DHEA-S, prolactin, ACTH, 24-hour urine free cortisol, IGF-1, TSH, free T4, CBC, electrolytes, liver functions, ESR, and karyotype

Imaging

- MRI if intracranial mass suspected
- Pelvic US for ovarian/uterine volume and description of endometrial stripe

DIFFERENTIAL DIAGNOSIS

- Generally, since skeletal age reflects biologic age, if the bone age is >10.5–11 years, the hypothalamic axis should be activated:
  - Hence, if gonadotropin levels are low, this suggests hypogonadotropism.
  - When gonadotropins are elevated, this indicates hypergonadotropism (gonadal failure).
- If skeletal age is <10.5 years, biologic immaturity is suggested, either constitutional or secondary to a chronic illness.
- In cases of primary amenorrhea, a discordance between ample breast and paucity of pubic hair development may suggest androgen insensitivity.

Differential of delayed puberty based upon the following categories:

- Hypogonadotropic hypogonadism: Hypothalamic (GnRH) and pituitary (LH, FSH) synthesis and secretory defects:
  - Defects of GnRH secretion:
    - Idiopathic hypogonadotropic hypogonadism (IHH) (1/3 familial, 2/3 sporadic)
    - Kallmann syndrome, associated with anosmia
- Hypergonadotropic hypogonadism: Hypothalamic-pituitary axis functional but no negative feedback by sex steroids indicates ovarian disease and is always pathologic.
  - Turner syndrome
  - Autoimmune
  - Mutations in gonadotropin (FSH, LH) genes or gonadotropin receptor genes
  - Galactosemia
  - Irradiation:
    - Depends on age of exposure (prepubertal less susceptible), dosage (>6 Gy associated with permanent ovarian failure) and type of chemotherapy (cyclophosphamide, busulfan, procarbazine, etoposide)
  - Infectious disease (mumps, *Shigella*, malaria, *Varicella*)

Infection
HIV infections cause both hypo- and hypergonadotropic hypogonadism (see above for other infections associated with hypergonadotropic hypogonadism).

Hematologic
Hemochromatosis may damage either the pituitary and/or the ovary resulting in hyper- or hypogonadotropic hypogonadism.

Metabolic/Endocrine
All categories of delayed puberty are a consequence of diminished function of the HPO axis, either due to low gonadotropins (pituitary or hypothalamic defects) or low sex steroids (ovarian dysfunction). Hyperprolactinemia results in hypogonadotropism.

Immunologic
- Autoimmune disease may cause hypergonadotropic and hypogonadotropic hypogonadism.
- Autoimmune polyglandular syndromes (APS): Ovarian failure (hypergonadotropism) occurs >50% of those with Type I (Addison's disease, hypoparathyroidism, mucocutaneous candidiasis) and 10% with type II (Addison's, autoimmune thyroid disease, type 1 diabetes mellitus). Presence of side chain cleavage enzyme autoantibodies in type 1 APS is a strong predictor of ovarian failure.
- Pituitary hypophysitis may be associated with hypogonadotropism.

Tumor/Malignancy
- Prolactinomas
- Craniopharyngioma

Trauma
Head trauma or severe abdominal/pelvic trauma can destroy the hypothalamic GnRH, pituitary LH and FSH, or ovarian sex steroid synthesizing ability.

Drugs
Chemotherapeutic drugs are associated with hypogonadism, particularly ovarian function.

 MANAGEMENT

GENERAL MEASURES
1st step is to establish pubertal delay by age, tempo, or developmental cutoffs. Subsequent evaluation aimed at eliminating pathologic causes.

MEDICATION (DRUGS)
- Induction of puberty using progressive doses of estrogens, generally starting with lowest available dosage
- May benefit from Provera withdrawal if normal endometrial stripe
- Progestational agent is added if breakthrough bleeding occurs or after 1–1.5 years of estrogen therapy if uterus is present. OCP preparation may be used.

SURGERY
As appropriate for brain tumors

 FOLLOW-UP

DISPOSITION
Issues for Referral
When underlying cause of delay is not apparent, or if there is no evidence of progression of puberty after skeletal age of 11 years is reached, referral is appropriate.

PROGNOSIS
- All girls with hypergonadotropism will have progressive and permanent ovarian failure.
- Outcomes in girls with hypogonadotropism depend on underlying etiology.
- Assisted fertility may be possible among those with hypogonadotropism with hormonal therapy for ovulation induction and among those with hypergonadotropism who have a competent uterus with egg donation.
- Note that patients with Turner syndrome may have cardiovascular risks making pregnancy unwise.

PATIENT MONITORING
- Patients receiving pubertal induction using progressive doses of estrogens should be monitored at intervals of 4–6 months.
- Once a diagnosis of permanent hypogonadism has been made, response to therapy and dosage adjustment is based primarily upon findings of history and physical exam.

BIBLIOGRAPHY

Reindollar RH, et al. Delayed sexual development: A study of 252 patients. *Am J Obstet Gynecol*. 1981;140:371–380.
Sedlmeyer IL, et al. Delayed puberty: Analysis of a large series from an academic center. *J Clin Endocrinol Metab*. 2002;87:1613–1620.

 MISCELLANEOUS

CLINICAL PEARLS
Referral center percentages of categories among girls presenting with pubertal delay:
- 30% constitutional delay
- 19% delay with normal potential because of systemic disease
- 20% hypogonadotropic hypogonadism
- 26% hypergonadotropic hypogonadism
- 5% other causes

ALERT
- In the majority of instances, pubertal delay in girls is not a benign entity.
- Often, time is the only method to verify whether hypogonadism or delay of pubertal hormone secretion is present.
- In a healthy patient, the maturing HPO axis will:
  - Become manifest in the patient with the potential for puberty
  - Or gonadotropins will become elevated, verifying hypergonadotropism
- It is possible within months after oncology therapy (chemotherapy and radiation therapy) that somewhat elevated gonadotropin levels suggest gonadal failure:
  - If permanent failure is present, such levels continue to rise.
  - Occasionally, normal levels suggest restoration of gonadal function. Such patients are clearly at risk of hypogonadism.
- Some patients with Turner syndrome, usually with mosaic karyotypes, may have ovarian function adequate for normal puberty.

ABBREVIATIONS
- ACTH—Adrenocorticotropic hormone
- DAX–1—Dosage sensitive sex reversal-adrenal hypoplasia congenita gene on the X chromosome, gene 1
- DHEA–S—Dehydroepiandrosterone sulfate
- FSH—Follicle stimulating hormone
- GALT—Galactose-1-phosphate uridyltransferase
- GH—Growth hormone
- GnRH—Gonadotropin-releasing hormone
- HPO—Hypothalamic-pituitary-ovarian
- IGF–1—Insulin-like growth factor 1 (aka Somatomedin C)
- LH—Luteinizing hormone
- OCP—Oral contraceptive pills
- TSH—Thyrotropin-releasing hormone

CODES
ICD9-CM
- 253.2 Hypopituitarism
- 256.3 Ovarian failure
- 259 Delayed puberty
- 307.1 Anorexia
- 626 Amenorrhea
- 758.6 Turners syndrome

 PATIENT TEACHING

- Inform the patient and her parents by disclosing knowledge of delayed puberty, together with an explanation of pubertal development and causes of delay using appropriate language.
- Consequences of hypogonadism and therapies should be discussed, including the fact that physical development and sexual function can be expected to become normal with hormonal therapy.
- Discuss fertility options.

PUBERTY, NORMAL, AND MENARCHE

Paul B. Kaplowitz, MD, PhD

BASICS

DESCRIPTION
- Puberty refers the appearance of certain physical findings, primarily a progressive increase in breast development, related to increase in estrogen secretion. It is a result of activation of the hypothalamic-pituitary-gonadal axis.
- Within 6 months of the appearance of breast development, the beginning of the pubertal growth spurt usually occurs, during which the rate of growth increases from 2 inches per year to 3–4 inches per year.
- The appearance of pubic hair and axillary odor, although occurring in many girls at about the same time, is due to *adrenarche*, or the age-related increase in adrenal androgen secretion.

Age-Related Factors
- In US girls, the average age of appearance of breast development and pubic hair is 10–10.5 years with a range of 8–13 years in whites, and earlier in blacks.
- Recent studies suggest the mean age of menarche in the US is about 12.6 years in white and 12.0 years in black girls.
- The interval between thelarche and menarche can vary from 1.5–4 years, but is between 2 and 3 years in most girls.

EPIDEMIOLOGY
- The mean age of menarche has declined from the 1800s to the mid-1900s, presumably due to improved health and nutrition.
- It is less clear how much additional decline has occurred over the last 50 years.
- In the US, evidence suggests that the age of appearance of breasts and pubic hair is occurring earlier than 30 years ago.
- Poorer, less-developed countries and countries in warmer climates show continued declines, while in northern Europe the mean age of menarche has been relatively stable at ~13 years.

RISK FACTORS
- Several studies have suggested that obesity or BMI above average for age is a risk factor for earlier onset of breast and pubic hair development and earlier menarche. Thinner girls tend to have later onset of breast development and later menarche.
- It has been suggested that estrogen-like chemicals in the environment, including metabolites of DDT, PCBs, and phthalates, as well as estrogens in meat and in hair care products, could contribute to the earlier onset of breast development, but there is no hard evidence for this.

Genetics
There is a strong genetic component to the onset of puberty, in that mothers who had early onset of breast development and early menarche are more likely to have daughters who are also early maturers.

PATHOPHYSIOLOGY
Precocious and delayed puberty are discussed in separate chapters (see Puberty, Precocious and Puberty, Delayed).

DIAGNOSIS

SIGNS AND SYMPTOMS
History
- Growth charts may be helpful.
- Pubertal growth spurt noted by parents

Physical Exam
- Appearance of breast tissue that can be palpated under the nipple is the most reliable sign of the onset of puberty.
- In chubby girls, it is easy to confuse fat tissue with breast tissue.
- Pubertal girls usually have a thickening and darkening of the nipple and areola.
- The vaginal exam may show a pink mucosa and thin mucous in the vault.
- Unlike breast development, pubic and axillary hair and body odor are not related to increased ovarian estrogen production and may appear years before the true onset of puberty.

TESTS
Labs
(See Puberty, Precocious and Puberty, Delayed.)

Imaging
(See Puberty, Precocious and Puberty, Delayed.)

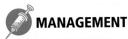 **MANAGEMENT**

GENERAL MEASURES
When breast development has progressed to Tanner stage III, parents may wish to prepare their daughter for the onset of menses, which is likely in the next 6–12 months.

MEDICATION (DRUGS)
The treatment of precocious puberty is discussed in a separate chapter. However, one may occasionally consider use of medications to prevent regular periods in girls whose timing of puberty is normal but who are so developmentally delayed that hygiene becomes a problem and they may not be willing to wear pads. The use of Depo-Provera 150 mg IM every 12 weeks is a safe, effective, and inexpensive option (see Menstrual Suppression).

 FOLLOW-UP

DISPOSITION
Issues for Referral
- Precocious or delayed puberty may prompt referral to pediatric endocrinologist.
- Menstrual suppression in girls with developmental delay may prompt gynecologic consultation (see Menstrual Suppression).

BIBLIOGRAPHY

Biro F, et al. Pubertal correlates in black and white girls. *J Pediatr*. 2006;148:234–240.

Kaplowitz PB. Pubertal development in girls: Secular trends. *Curr Opin Obstet Gynecol*. 2006;18: 487–491.

Kaplowitz PB, et al. Earlier onset of puberty in girls: Relation to increased body mass index and race. *Pediatrics*. 2001;108:347–353.

 PATIENT TEACHING

- ACOG Patient Education Pamphlet: Growing at http://www.acog.org/publications/patient˙education/bp041.cfm
- AAFP Parent Brochure: When Your Child is Close to Puberty at http://www.aafp.org/afp/990700ap/990700d.html

PUBERTY, PRECOCIOUS

Paul B. Kaplowitz, MD, PhD

 BASICS

DESCRIPTION

- The traditional definition of precocious puberty is the appearance of breast and/or pubic hair development <8 years of age.
  - Recent studies from the US suggest that, in a significant number of girls (especially black girls), breast tissue and pubic hair is already present by age 8.
  - Thus it has been suggested that age 7 might be a more appropriate age cut-off for defining when signs of puberty are precocious.
- The hormonal basis of breast development (estrogens from the ovaries) differs from that of pubic and axillary hair development (an increase in adrenal androgen secretion).
  - If a young girl has only pubic and/or axillary hair (usually accompanied by an axillary odor), it is more accurate to call this "premature adrenarche" than precocious puberty.
- True or central precocious puberty is characterized by a progressive increase in breast development over at least 4–6 months, accompanied by accelerated growth and advanced skeletal maturation.
  - In many young girls, breast development may increase briefly and then fail to progress, so a period of observation is often helpful before deciding if testing or referral is warranted.
- Breast development presenting in girls <3 rarely progresses past Tanner stage II and is rarely associated with growth acceleration. It almost always will be diagnosed as premature thelarche, which requires no treatment.

EPIDEMIOLOGY

- The frequency of precocious puberty depends on whether premature adrenarche and premature thelarche are included or only true central precocious puberty.
- Based on an analysis of cases submitted to a national Danish registry, estimated prevalence of precocious puberty was ~0.2% of girls and <0.05% of boys.
- The highest incidence was ~8 cases per 10,000 in 5–9 year old girls, which appears to be much lower than in the US, although no US studies have been done in a comparable manner.

RISK FACTORS

- Obesity or a BMI above the mean for age are risk factors for both precocious puberty and premature adrenarche.
- Girls born small for gestational age (SGA) are at higher risk for both premature adrenarche and an earlier and more rapidly progressive puberty.

Genetics

A study from Israel reported that idiopathic precocious puberty was familial in 27.5% of subjects, and that the inheritance appeared to be autosomal dominant with incomplete, sex-dependent penetrance.

PATHOPHYSIOLOGY

- Idiopathic central precocious puberty is due to an early activation of unknown cause of the hypothalamic-pituitary-gonadal axis.
- In normal girls, the HPO axis remains dormant until >8 years of age.
- When precocious puberty is due to a CNS tumor, it is believed that the tumor interrupts signals from the brain to the hypothalamus, which suppress the pulsatile secretion of GnRH, the proximal hormonal event of puberty.

DIAGNOSIS

SIGNS AND SYMPTOMS

History

- Family history:
  - Timing of menarche in the mother
  - The approximate timing of the growth spurt in the father
  - Pubertal timing in older siblings
- For girls with early breast development, the mother should be asked about the use of hair-care products containing hormones, placenta, lavender, and tea tree oil, all of which have been linked to early breast development, though the evidence is not strong.
- Menses are rarely reported at the 1st presentation of a girl with precocious puberty:
  - Occasionally, a girl with no breast development will present with vaginal spotting or bleeding, which may recur at monthly intervals:
    - Evaluation is appropriate (see Bleeding, Abnormal Uterine: Prepubertal).
    - In addition to the idiopathic and self-limited diagnosis of "premature menarche," causes can include abuse or vaginal malignancies.

Review of Systems

Symptoms and findings suggestive of CNS tumor include:

- Frequent and severe headaches
- Double vision or other visual changes
- New onset seizures

Physical Exam

- Height and growth rate:
  - Increased likelihood of central precocious puberty rather than normal variant:
    - Height >95th percentile and/or
    - A recent increase in rate of linear growth
- Breast exam and Tanner staging by both inspection in the sitting position and palpation in the supine position:
  - In the sitting position, chubby girls may appear to have breast tissue that, by palpation, is found to have the softer consistency of adipose tissue.
  - With true precocious puberty, the skin of the nipples and areola is usually thicker and darker than in the prepubertal child.
- Pubic hair assessed by Tanner staging and presence of axillary hair noted, but sexual hair may be present or absent in girls with true precocious puberty.
- The finding of café-au-lait lesions with irregular borders may be a clue to McCune Albright syndrome, which is extremely rare

TESTS

Labs

- If only a small amount of breast tissue is present, and no progress occurs over time, no testing may be needed:
  - Re-examine to determine progression.
- With progressive breast enlargement, measure LH (using sensitive 3rd-generation assay), FSH, and estradiol (NOT total estrogens).
  - If the LH is <0.1 IU/L and estradiol is low or minimally elevated, the child probably does not have precocious puberty.
  - If the LH is ≥0.3, and the estradiol is even mildly elevated, the diagnosis is likely central precocious puberty.
  - If the LH is <0.1 but the estradiol is very elevated, an ovarian tumor or cyst should be ruled out.

– FSH is generally not helpful in distinguishing between prepubertal and pubertal girls.

– If diagnosis is not clear, measure LH and FSH 30–60 minutes after a dose of GnRH or a GnRH analog.

○ In pubertal girls, the LH will generally increase to >5 IU/L.

○ In prepubertal girls, a smaller increase in LH, frequently accompanied by a larger increase in FSH, is seen.

• If pubic hair only, do NOT order the above labs.

– The only lab test likely to be abnormal is DHEA-S, which generally confirms the child has premature adrenarche.

– Other steroids, such as 17-hydroxyprogesterone, are rarely helpful, and ordering should be left to the discretion of a pediatric endocrinologist.

Imaging

• A hand X-ray for a bone age is sometimes helpful if pubertal signs seem to be progressing:

– An advance of 2 years > chronological age suggests the need for an endocrine evaluation.

• An ovarian US is usually not necessary unless LH and FSH are suppressed with estradiol elevated, as noted above, suggesting an ovarian tumor or cyst.

• With true precocious puberty, US will show bilateral ovarian enlargement with an enlarging uterus, but it is not required to make the diagnosis.

• The need for a brain MRI is controversial:

– It will be normal in the great majority of girls with central precocious puberty.

– Some experts recommend that it be done for any girl with breast development <8 years.

– Age best predicts a higher risk of a CNS cause of central precocious puberty:

○ ~20% of girls with onset of puberty <6, but only 2% with onset between the ages of 6 and 8, had a CNS lesion as the cause for precocious puberty.

– CNS signs such as headache are not always present.

DIFFERENTIAL DIAGNOSIS

The great majority of girls with precocious puberty are classified as idiopathic.

Tumor/Malignancy

• Tumors of the CNS, including hypothalamic astrocytoma and glioma, and a developmental defect called a hypothalamic hamartoma, may rarely cause precocious puberty.

• Ovarian tumors (primarily granulosa cell) are a rare cause of precocious puberty and are generally quite large by the time they are diagnosed. The rare cases generally can be suspected based on a history of rapid progression and characteristic hormonal findings (see above).

Other/Miscellaneous

McCune-Albright syndrome is an extremely rare cause of peripheral precocious puberty, and is characterized by large ovarian cysts, irregular café-au-lait pigmentation, and polyostotic fibrous dysplasia bone lesions.

 MANAGEMENT

GENERAL MEASURES

• Most girls with true precocious puberty do not require treatment, particularly if the onset is not much earlier than 8 years of age and progression is not rapid.

• Reassuring the parents that the child's maturation probably falls at the low end of the broad normal range and that most girls handle menarche well if it occurs at age 10 or later is often sufficient.

MEDICATION (DRUGS)

• For precocious puberty starting <8 and progressing rapidly, the best medication is Lupron Depot, a synthetic analog of GnRH given by monthly injection (starting dose is usually 7.5 mg per month).

• The 3-month preparation of Lupron Depot 11.25 mg, which is currently only approved for adults, has been found to be as effective as the monthly injections.

• If the goal is to suppress early menses, not slow growth and bone maturation, use a standard contraceptive dose of Depo-Provera, 150 mg every 3 months, which costs far less than Lupron.

SURGERY

Precocious puberty due to an ovarian tumor or a single large ovarian cyst is best managed by surgical removal of the tumor or cyst.

 FOLLOW-UP

For girls whose presenting signs, symptoms, and diagnostic testing do not justify treatment, follow-up at 4–6-month intervals may be indicated to assess changes in breast size and growth rate, at least until it is apparent that the child does not have progressive precocious puberty.

DISPOSITION

Issues for Referral

• After an initial assessment, any child suspected of having central precocious puberty should be referred to a pediatric endocrinologist for further evaluation.

• Girls who require treatment with GnRH analogs such as Lupron should be followed by a pediatric endocrinologist.

• Girls with an ovarian mass should be referred to a gynecologist with pediatric expertise.

BIBLIOGRAPHY

Chalumeau M, et al. Central precocious puberty in girls: An evidence-based diagnosis tree to predict central nervous system abnormalities. *Pediatrics.* 2002;109:61–67.

De Vries L, et al. Familial central precocious puberty suggests autosomal dominant inheritance. *J Clin Endocrinol Metab.* 2004;89:1794–1800.

Ibanez L, et al. Puberty after prenatal growth restraint. 2006;65 (suppl 3):112–115.

Kaplowitz PB, et al. Reexamination of the age limit for defining when puberty is precocious in girls in the United States: Implications for evaluation and treatment. *Pediatrics.* 1999;104:936–941.

Kaplowitz PB, et al. Earlier onset of puberty in girls: Relation to increased body mass index and race. *Pediatrics.* 2001;108:347–353.

Kaplowitz PB. Precocious puberty: Update on secular trends, definitions, diagnosis, and treatment. *Adv Pediatr.* 2004;51:37–62.

Teilmann G, et al. Prevalence and incidence of precocious pubertal development in Denmark: An epidemiologic study based on national registries. *Pediatrics.* 2005;116:1323–1328.

 MISCELLANEOUS

ABBREVIATIONS

• DHEA-S—Dehydroepiandrosterone sulfate
• FSH—Follicle-stimulating hormone
• GnRH—Gonadotropin releasing hormone
• HPO—Hypothalamic-pituitary-ovarian
• LH—Luteinizing hormone

CODES

ICD9-CM

259.1 Precocious sexual development and puberty, not elsewhere classified, is the only code which refers to precocious puberty and any of the normal variants that can be confused with precocious puberty.

 PATIENT TEACHING

• The Hormone Foundation: Precocious Puberty at http://www.hormone.org/pdf/Bilingual/bilingual_precocious_puberty.pdf

• Early Puberty in Girls: The Essential Guide to Coping with This Common Problem. Paul Kaplowitz, Random House, New York, 2004.

URINARY SYMPTOMS: DYSURIA

Alison C. Agner, MD

 BASICS

DESCRIPTION
- Painful urination
- Pain, tingling, or burning during or after urination

Age-Related Factors
- Incidence of cystitis is steady throughout a woman's life.
- Cervicitis is most common during adolescence and early adulthood.

EPIDEMIOLOGY
- 1 in 4 women will experience acute dysuria each year.
- 50–60% of women will have cystitis once in their life.
- 2.8 million cases of chlamydia per year
- 700,000 cases of gonorrhea per year
- 1 out of 5 adults have genital herpes.

RISK FACTORS
- History of urinary tract infection or pyelonephritis
- History of sexually transmitted infections
- High-risk sexual behavior

PATHOPHYSIOLOGY
- Inflammation:
  - Urethra or bladder trigone
  - Vulva
- Referred pain

DIAGNOSIS

SIGNS AND SYMPTOMS
History
- Timing of symptoms:
  - Onset, duration
- Associated symptoms:
  - See "Review of Systems"
- Alleviating/Aggravating factors
- Sexual history

Review of Systems
- Constitutional:
  - Fever, chills, fatigue
- GI:
  - Nausea, emesis, diarrhea
- GU:
  - Urinary frequency, hematuria, flank pain
  - Urinary incontinence
  - Abnormal vaginal discharge, pelvic pain
- Neurologic:
  - Urinary or fecal incontinence

Physical Exam
- General:
  - Fever
- Pelvic exam:
  - Through vulvar exam for lesions
  - Bladder or urethral tenderness
  - Cervical motion tenderness
  - Abnormal vaginal discharge
- Abdominal exam:
  - Suprapubic pain
  - Assess for costovertebral angle tenderness

TESTS
Labs
- UA and urine culture:
  - >100,000 organisms on a clean catch
  - >10,000 organisms on a cath specimen
- Wet prep if indicated:
  - To evaluate for yeast infect, bacterial vaginosis, or trichomoniasis
- Cervical cultures if indicated:
  - To evaluate for gonorrhea or *Chlamydia*

Imaging
- Ultrasound is not routinely needed
- Cystoscopy
  - To evaluate for nephrolithiasis or hydronephrosis
  - To evaluate for tumor or interstitial cystitis

DIFFERENTIAL DIAGNOSIS
Infection
- UTI:
  - Cystitis
  - Pyelonephritis
- Cervicitis:
  - Gonorrhea
  - *Chlamydia*
  - Herpes

Tumor/Malignancy
Bladder cancer:
- Presents with painless gross hematuria
- Irritative voiding symptoms may also be present.
- 9th most common cancer in females

Trauma
- Straddle injury
- Masturbation
- Rape/Abuse

Other/Miscellaneous
Vulvar disorders:
- Vulvitis (external dysuria)
- Contact dermatitis
- Lichen simplex
- Lichen sclerosus

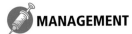 **MANAGEMENT**

MEDICATION (DRUGS)
- Pyridium:
  - For symptomatic treatment only
  - Stains urine orange
- Antibiotic to treat UTI:
  - TMP-SMX is first line therapy:
    ○ 3 days for uncomplicated UTI
    ○ 7 days for complicated UTI
  - Ciprofloxacin is second-line
  - Nitrofurantoin is used in pregnancy

SURGERY
Hydrodistention may be used to treat interstitial cystitis and for diagnosis (see topic).

 FOLLOW-UP

DISPOSITION
Issues for Referral
Consider urology referral for:
- Nephrolithiasis
- Red flag symptoms.
  - Painless hematuria

BIBLIOGRAPHY

Wrenn K. Dysuria, frequency, and urgency. In: *Clinical Methods: The History, Physical, and Laboratory Examinations*, 3rd ed. Butterworths. Available at: http://www.ncbi.nlm.nih.gov/books/bv.fcgi?indexed=google&rid=cm.chapter.5243

 MISCELLANEOUS

CLINICAL PEARLS
Asymptomatic bacteruria is more common in pregnancy:
- UA at every visit to evaluate for UTI

ABBREVIATION
UTI—Urinary tract infection
TMP-SMX—Trimethoprim/Sulfamethoxazole

CODES
ICD9-CM
- 098.15 Gonorrhea cervicitis
- 099.53 Chlamydia cervicitis
- 595.0 Cystitis
- 595.1 Interstitial cystitis
- 590.8 Pyelonephritis

 PATIENT TEACHING

PREVENTION
- Avoid bubble baths, soaps with fragrance, etc.
- Void immediately after intercourse
- ACOG—Patient Education Pamphlet—Urinary Tract Infection

URINARY SYMPTOMS: FREQUENCY

Alison C. Agner, MD

 BASICS

DESCRIPTION
- >8 voids in 24 hours and >1 void per night
- More practical definition is greater number of voids than the woman is used to.

Age-Related Factors
More common in older adults due to increased prevalence of pelvic organ prolapse.

RISK FACTORS
- History of UTI
- History of pelvic organ prolapse
- History of urinary incontinence or surgery for incontinence
- History of disorder that causes neurogenic bladder:
  - Spinal cord injury
  - Stroke
  - Multiple sclerosis

PATHOPHYSIOLOGY
4 common categories:
- Infection
- Inflammation
- Neoplasm
- Neuromuscular

ASSOCIATED CONDITIONS
- Dysuria
- Urinary incontinence
- Urinary tract infection (see topic)

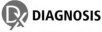 **DIAGNOSIS**

SIGNS AND SYMPTOMS
History
- Assess urinary habits carefully with urinary diary:
  - Ask about fluid intake and caffeine intake
- Assess for associated dysuria and urgency
- Assess for incontinence
  - Stress versus urge

Review of Systems
- General:
  - Fever, chills
- GI:
  - Diarrhea, nausea, emesis
- GU:
  - Dysuria, urgency, hematuria
- Neurologic:
  - Weakness or numbness
- Gynecologic:
  - Abnormal vaginal discharge

Physical Exam
- General:
  - Fever
- Pelvic exam:
  - Evaluate for bladder and urethral tenderness
  - Postvoid residual

TESTS
Labs
- UA and urine culture:
  - To evaluate for infection
- Postvoid residual volume:
  - To evaluate overflow incontinence
- Random or fasting blood glucose if other symptoms of diabetes are present
- Plasma sodium to evaluate for diabetes insipidus if other symptoms of diabetes are present
- Plasma sodium if concern exists for diabetes insipidus:
  - Expect normal or elevated sodium

Imaging
- Not routinely needed
- MRI if concern for urethral diverticulum
- Referral for urodynamics only if patient has complex incontinence symptoms

DIFFERENTIAL DIAGNOSIS
- UTI
- Stress or urge urinary incontinence
- Overactive bladder
- Urinary retention with overflow incontinence
- Interstitial cystitis
- Diabetes mellitus
- Diabetes insipidus

Infection
Most common cause:
- *Escherichia coli* is most common pathogen in otherwise healthy female
- Staph saprophyticus is nitrite negative

Metabolic/Endocrine

Diabetes may present with polyuria and polydipsia:

- Type I DM, Type II DM
- Diabetes insipidus

Tumor/Malignancy

- Urothelial tumors are uncommon:
  - Warning signs include gross hematuria
- Pelvic masses or neoplasms may also cause frequency.

Drugs

Diuretics may cause frequency, especially soon after initiation of therapy:

- Hydrochlorothiazide, furosemide

Other/Miscellaneous

- Inflammation:
  - Painful bladder syndrome (interstitial cystitis)
- Pelvic organ prolapse
- Lifestyle choices:
  - High fluid intake or fluid intake prior to bed

Pregnancy Considerations

Urinary frequency is a common symptom in early pregnancy.

MANAGEMENT

GENERAL MEASURES

Start by having patient keep a voiding diary for at least 1 week, which may be completed prior to visit.

MEDICATION (DRUGS)

- Antibiotics for UTI:
  - TMP-SMX is first-line therapy
    - 3 days for uncomplicated UTI
    - 7 days for complicated UTI
  - Ciprofloxacin is second line
  - Nitrofurantoin is used in pregnancy.
- Anticholinergics for urge urinary incontinence

SURGERY

- Useful for stress urinary incontinence
- Suprapubic catheter may be considered for neurogenic bladder with overflow incontinence.

FOLLOW-UP

DISPOSITION

Issues for Referral

Consider urology referral if:

- Infection is not present
- Lifestyle changes do not improve symptoms
- Other red-flag symptoms are present:
  - Painless hematuria, pain on exam, etc.

PROGNOSIS

UTIs are usually easily treated with oral antibiotics.

PATIENT MONITORING

Antibiotic prophylaxis is indicated if patient has recurrent UTIs.

- TMP-SMX PO daily

MISCELLANEOUS

SYNONYM(S)

Polyuria

ABBREVIATION

TMP-SMX—Trimethoprim/Sulfamethoxazole
UTI—Urinary tract infection

CODES

ICD9-CM

- 253.5 Diabetes insipidus
- 595.0 Cystitis
- 788.42 Polyuria

PATIENT TEACHING

- For recurrent UTI, advise voiding prior to and immediately after intercourse.
- Counseling on lifestyle changes:
  - Limiting fluid intake, especially 3 hours prior to bed time
  - Limiting caffeine and citrus
- ACOG Patient Education Pamphlet—Urinary Tract Infection

URINARY SYMPTOMS: INCONTINENCE

Paul M. Fine, MD

 BASICS

DESCRIPTION
- Incontinence is a complaint of any involuntary leakage of urine.
- Types of incontinence (percentage of total):
  – Stress urinary incontinence (SUI) (49%): Leakage with physical exertion
  – Urge (22%): Leakage with a strong desire to void
  – Mixed (29%): Combination of stress and urge
- See Stress Urinary Incontinence, Overactive Bladder, and Incontinence Surgeries.

Age-Related Factors
Most studies show increasing prevalence with age related to:
- Urogenital atrophy
- Hypoestrogenism
- Increasing prevalence of medical illnesses
- Increasing nocturnal diuresis
- Increasing use of medications
- Impairments in mobility
- Impairments in cognition

EPIDEMIOLOGY
- AHCPR estimates 13 million Americans are incontinent; 11 million are women.
- 15–30% in community-based population and up to 50% in long-term care are incontinent.
- Urinary incontinence is more prevalent than other chronic diseases in women including hypertension, diabetes, and depression.
- $26 billion in US annually spent on urinary incontinence, including pads and diapers.

RISK FACTORS
- Predisposing factors:
  – Female sex
  – Race: Caucasians have more stress incontinence
  – Family history of stress incontinence
- Inciting factors:
  – Childbirth
  – Hysterectomy
  – Radical pelvic surgery
  – Radiation
- Promoting factors:
  – Obesity
  – Lung disease
  – Smoking
  – Menopause
  – Constipation
  – Recreation
  – Occupation
  – Medications
- Decompensating factors:
  – Aging
  – Dementia
  – Debility
  – Environment

Genetics
- 1st-degree relative with stress incontinence increases risk
- Collagen quality, synthesis, and metabolism

PATHOPHYSIOLOGY
- Stress incontinence:
  – Insufficient urethral closure pressure:
    ○ Urethral hypermobility during Valsalva
    ○ Unequal pressure transmission from abdomen and bladder to urethra
    ○ Intrinsic urethral sphincter deficiency
- Urge incontinence:
  – Uncontrolled bladder contraction
- Mixed incontinence:
  – Combination of the above

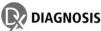 **DIAGNOSIS**

SIGNS AND SYMPTOMS
History
- How many times in the past week did you lose urine into your clothing, underwear, or pad?
  – During an activity such as coughing, sneezing, laughing, running, exercising, or lifting?
  – With such a sudden strong need to urinate that you could not reach the toilet in time?
- Do you have to (signs of overactive bladder):
  – Urinate > every 3 hours?
  – Wake up at night more than twice to urinate?
  – Have sudden strong urges to urinate and barely make it to the bathroom in time?

Review of Systems
- Complete general medical history:
  – Diabetes: Polyuria, nocturia
  – Neurologic conditions: Urinary retention and overflow incontinence
  – Prior spinal or back surgery
  – Severe arthritis; limited mobility
  – Current medications:
    ○ Diuretics: Polyuria, nocturia
    ○ Antihypertensives: Decreased urethral tone
  – Lifestyle and diet:
    ○ Alcohol: Polyuria
    ○ Caffeine: Stimulates bladder contraction
- Obstetric history:
  – Large babies
  – Vaginal versus cesarean versus forceps
- Gynecologic and urologic surgical history:
  – Prior anti-incontinence surgery
  – Prior hysterectomy
  – Prior surgery for pelvic organ prolapse
- Gynecologic symptoms indicating need for hysterectomy such as severe dysmenorrhea, menometrorrhagia, symptomatic fibroids
- Symptoms of pelvic organ prolapse such as seeing or feeling a bulge or vaginal pressure
- Associated fecal incontinence

Physical Exam
- Abdominal exam:
  – Palpate for masses causing decreased bladder capacity.
- Pelvic exam:
  – Urogenital atrophy is possible cause of decreased urethral closure.
  – Utero-vaginal prolapse (during Valsalva or with patient standing):
    ○ Distal anterior vagina: Urethral hypermobility
    ○ Apical: Cervix or vaginal cuff
    ○ Posterior vagina (rectocele, enterocele)
  – Bimanual exam:
    ○ Uterine fibroids: Decreased bladder capacity
    ○ Adnexal masses: Decreased bladder capacity
  – Ability to perform a Kegel squeeze
- Rectal exam to rule out fecal impaction
- Neurologic exam:
  – Bulbocavernosus reflex:
    ○ Stroke labia to stimulate anal contraction
    ○ Indicates intact sacral sensory and motor reflex arc for bladder and pelvic floor muscles
  – Lower extremity reflexes

TESTS
- Bladder diary may be helpful for patient to record urinary leakage, urgency, frequency, and nocturia for 1 week
- UA to rule out infection
- Post void residual volume:
  – Measure by catheter immediately after voiding
  – Should be <100 mL
  – >200 mL suggests possible urethral kinking from vaginal prolapse or poor bladder contraction due to neurologic problem.
- Q-tip test for urethral hypermobility:
  – Insert cotton swab with Xylocaine jelly into bladder, then withdraw until resistance of urethrovesical junction felt
  – Have patient perform maximal Valsalva
  – Measure angle of deflection of end of swab from horizontal:
    ○ <30° is normal
    ○ >30° indicates urethral hypermobility and loss of normal urethral anatomic support
- Standing cough stress test:
  – Fill bladder with 300 mL of sterile water/saline
  – Patient stands and coughs forcefully
  – Observe for sudden urinary leakage; this is objective confirmation of stress incontinence.

Labs

Urodynamics (patient generally referred to urologist or urogynecologist for this):

- Measures storage (cystometrogram) and emptying function (uroflow) of bladder using small catheters and electronic measurement of pressure and volume
- May demonstrate bladder muscle (detrusor) involuntary contraction (relative contraindication for anti-incontinence surgery)
- May demonstrate voiding pattern suggestive of urethral kinking or obstruction (also relative contraindication for anti-incontinence surgery)
- May demonstrate neurologic bladder dysfunction
- May demonstrate urinary leakage with Valsalva or cough, confirming SUI
- May demonstrate urinary leakage with involuntary detrusor contraction confirming urge incontinence

Imaging

Some urologists and urogynecologist use translabial ultrasonography to visualize urethral and bladder anatomic relationships.

DIFFERENTIAL DIAGNOSIS

- Type of incontinence based on symptoms:
  – Stress urinary incontinence
  – Urge urinary incontinence
  – Mixed urinary incontinence
- Type of incontinence based on urodynamics:
  – Genuine or urodynamic stress incontinence
  – Detrusor overactivity associated incontinence
  – Mixed urodynamic stress and detrusor overactivity incontinence

Infection

Suspect UTI if recent onset of incontinence, especially associated with urgency and frequency

Metabolic/Endocrine

Suspect diabetes if large volume bladder capacity or polyuria

Tumor/Malignancy

Rule out bladder tumor or cancer if hematuria without infection in patient >50 by referral for cystoscopy.

Trauma

Obstetric trauma

Drugs

- Diuretics may aggravate incontinence, urgency, and frequency.
- Antihypertensives may aggravate incontinence by lowering urethral resistance.

Other/Miscellaneous

- High-impact exercise may aggravate SUI
- Limited mobility by chronic arthritis or other chronic illness may promote urge incontinence

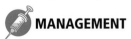 MANAGEMENT

GENERAL MEASURES

Behavioral and dietary modifications:

- Decrease caffeine
- Decrease alcohol

- Performance of pelvic floor muscle (Kegel) exercise daily is effective for all types of urinary incontinence
- Timed voiding
- Avoidance of bladder overfilling
- Avoidance of high-impact activities
- Combination of behavioral and medication therapy is synergistic (better than either alone)

MEDICATION (DRUGS)

- Anticholinergics for urge incontinence and detrusor overactivity:
  – Detrol LA 2–4 mg/day PO
  – Ditropan XL 5–15 mg/day PO
  – Enablex 7.5–15 mg/day PO
  – Vesicare 5 mg/day PO
  – Santura 20 mg b.i.d. PO
  – Oxytrol skin patch applied twice/wk
- Duloxetine (Yantreve) for stress incontinence (not available in US) 40 mg b.i.d.
- Imipramine 10–25 mg t.i.d. PO for urge, stress, and mixed incontinence. Off-label usage.

SURGERY

- Indicated for stress incontinence or mixed incontinence nonresponsive to medical therapy:
  – Generally 90% effective
  – Mid-urethral slings (minimally invasive):
    ○ Transvaginal tape (TVT) is effective for intrinsic sphincteric deficiency (ISD)
    ○ Transobturator tape (TOT)
  – Burch or Marshal-Marchetti-Krantz urethropexy (requires abdominal incision)
  – Pubovaginal sling is most effective for ISD. Requires vaginal and abdominal incision.
  – Periurethral injection of bulking agents (office procedure) especially for ISD without urethral hypermobility
- May aggravate preexisting or cause de novo urge incontinence by urethral obstruction
- May be performed with concomitant hysterectomy and/or pelvic organ prolapse repair

 FOLLOW-UP

- After surgical therapy for urinary incontinence: 6 weeks, 3 months, 1 year, then annually
- After initiating behavioral and/or medication therapy: 4–6 weeks:
  – Confirm correct Kegel squeeze by exam
  – May need to try a different anticholinergic medication depending on efficacy and side effects
  – Then in 3 months as needed, followed by annually

DISPOSITION

Issues for Referral

- Uncertain diagnosis
- Failure to respond to behavioral/medical therapy in urge incontinence
- History of prior radical pelvic surgery or radiation therapy
- History of failed prior anti-incontinence surgery

- Suspected metabolic, endocrine, or neurologic etiology for the incontinence
- Need for urodynamics to clarify diagnosis
- Need for surgical therapy beyond your scope of competency and experience

PROGNOSIS

- Medication/Behavioral therapy for urge incontinence is effective in ~70% of patients.
- Surgical therapy for stress incontinence is effective in ~90% of patients.
- Medication/Behavioral and surgical therapies are each ~50% effective in mixed incontinence. A combination of these therapies may be required to achieve 90% effectiveness.

BIBLIOGRAPHY

Bump RC, et al. Epidemiology and natural history of pelvic floor dysfunction. *Obstet Cynecol Clin North Am*. 1998;25(4):723–746.

consensus.nih.gov/2006/2006CesareanSOS027S tatementhtml.htm

Hampel C, et al. Definition of overactive bladder and epidemiology of urinary incontinence. *Urology* 1997;50(suppl 6A):4–14.

 MISCELLANEOUS

ABBREVIATIONS

- ISD—Intrinsic sphincteric deficiency
- SUI—Stress urinary incontinence
- TVT—Transvaginal tape
- TOT—Transobturator tape

CODES

ICD9-CM

788.3 Urinary incontinence
788.31 Urge incontinence
788.38 Overflow incontinence
625.6 Stress incontinence

 PATIENT TEACHING

- ACOG Patient Education Pamphlet: Urinary Incontinence
- ACOG Patient Education Pamphlet: Surgery for Urinary Incontinence

PREVENTION

- Elective primary cesarean delivery has not yet been demonstrated as efficacious in prevention of urinary incontinence.
- There is insufficient evidence to evaluate fully the benefits and risks of cesarean delivery on maternal request as compared to planned vaginal delivery, and more research is needed.
- Until quality evidence becomes available, any decision to perform a cesarean delivery on maternal request should be carefully individualized and consistent with ethical principles.

VAGINAL SIGNS AND SYMPTOMS: VAGINAL DISCHARGE

Paula J. Adams Hillard, MD

 BASICS

DESCRIPTION

- Vaginal discharge refers to the presence of vaginal secretions and fluid expelled from the vagina and visible on clothing or external genitals.
- Vaginal symptoms are extremely common in the general population and are one of the most frequent reasons for a visit to an obstetrician-gynecologist.
- The etiology of vaginal discharge includes:
  – Infectious causes—vaginal, cervical and other:
    ○ Cervicitis
    ○ Vaginitis
    ○ Pelvic inflammatory
    ○ Sexually transmitted infections
  – Other:
    ○ Chemical irritants
    ○ Hormone deficiency
    ○ Systemic disease, rarely
    ○ Malignancy
  – Physiologic (normal) discharge
  – Nonvaginal discharge:
    ○ Occasionally urine leakage can be confused with a vaginal discharge
    ○ Urethral discharge from a Skene abscess
- A vaginal discharge is a sign and not a diagnosis.

Pediatric Considerations
- A vaginal discharge in the prepubertal pediatric age group is always abnormal, but not always medically serious.
- The causes of vaginal discharge in the pediatric age group are quite distinct from the causes in the reproductive-age group.
- A vulvovaginitis in this age group is typically bacterial and related to hygiene, although other causes, including abuse and foreign body, must be considered.
- Prepubertal vulvovaginal symptoms are rarely due to yeast infection (see Vaginitis: Vulvovaginal Candidiasis).
- Vaginal discharge in adolescents is due to the causes seen in older women, but because of sexual behaviors and risk-taking, STD testing is imperative in sexually active teens.

Geriatric Considerations
- The most common cause of vaginal discharge in this age group is atrophic vaginitis (see Vaginitis, Atrophic).
- The likelihood of a discharge due to a malignancy is higher in older women.

EPIDEMIOLOGY
- The lifetime risk for yeast vaginitis may be as high as 75%:
  – Estimated $275 million annual on nonprescription antifungals
  – Antifungals among top 10 of all nonprescription medications
- Self-diagnosis frequently incorrect:
  – Recognition of classic symptoms by only 11% of those with no previous yeast diagnosis and 34% of those with previous yeast
- Causes of vaginitis include:
  – Bacterial vaginosis (BV): 22–50% of symptomatic women
  – Vulvovaginal candidiasis: 17–39%
  – Trichomoniasis vaginalis: 4–35%
  – Undiagnosed: 7–22%

PATHOPHYSIOLOGY
"Classic" descriptions of discharge:
- Yeast:
  – Thick, "curdy," white, nonodorous discharge
  – + KOH for pseudohyphae or budding yeast
  – + WBCs on wet prep
- Trichomonas:
  – Thin, frothy, odorous discharge
  – Wet mount with motile trichomonads: Sensitivity of 55–60%
  – Inflammatory vaginal and cervical changes: "Strawberry" vagina/cervix
- Bacterial vaginosis:
  – Thin, gray, homogenous discharge
  – Fishy odor
  – pH >4.5
  – Positive amine/whiff test
  – Microscopy with >20% clue cells
- Mucopurulent cervicitis:
  – Creamy, thick, yellow or greenish discharge
  – May have odor
  – Microscopy with multiple WBCs
- Physiologic discharge:
  – Thin, white, scant
  – pH <4.7
  – Absence of WBCs, clue cells, yeast, negative whiff test

RISK FACTORS
- Prepubertal and postmenopausal vagina:
  – pH ≥4.7
  – "Normal" flora includes skin and fecal flora
- Reproductive age women:
  – Glycogen in vaginal epithelial cells
  – Lactobacilli colonization
  – Lactic acid production and pH <4.7
  – Vaginal flora—heterogeneous
- Vaginal infections and discharge result from alterations of normal flora and overgrowth of bacteria or yeast

ASSOCIATED CONDITIONS
Vaginitis is often associated with vulvitis.

 DIAGNOSIS

SIGNS AND SYMPTOMS

History
- Pregnant, postpartum, nursing
- Menstrual history:
  – Menopausal
  – Relationship to timing in cycle
- Past treatment, response to treatment, self treatment, including douching
- Sexual history

Review of Systems
Symptoms that are commonly associated with vaginal discharge include:
- Itching
- Burning
- Irritation
- Odor
- Swelling
- Dyspareunia
- Dysuria

Physical Exam
- Exam is indicated if possible, rather than telephone diagnosis, given nonspecific nature of symptoms.
- Attention to the pelvic exam:
  – Vulva:
    ○ Erythema
    ○ Edema
    ○ Satellite lesions
  – Vulvar vestibule:
    ○ Vulvar vestibulitis
- Presence, characteristics of discharge:
  – Color
  – Consistency
  – Purulence
  – Odor
- Vagina:
  – Erythema
  – Rugae/Estrogenization
  – Lesion
- Cervix:
  – Discharge
  – Friability
  – Lesion
- Bimanual exam

TESTS
- Vaginal specimen obtained for the following tests:
  – Vaginal pH from mid vagina:
    ○ Elevated pH can be due to: Cervical mucous, blood, semen
  – "Whiff" test for amines on exposure to KOH
  – Microscopy if the first line for diagnosing vaginal discharge:
    ○ Wet Prep or wet mount: Saline prep
    ○ 10% KOH: Sensitivity for yeast ~50%
- Other tests (not well established):
  – Rapid tests for:
    ○ BV associated organism
    ○ Trichomonas vaginalis antigen
    ○ DNA of T vaginalis, *Gardnerella* vaginalis, and *Candida* species

- DNA amplification tests as indicated for:
  - *Neisseria gonorrhoeae*
  - *Chlamydia trachomatis*
- Cultures:
  - For yeast, indicated in cases of recurrent vulvovaginal candidiasis or possible non albicans *Candida*
  - For trichomonas if negative wet prep and suspected trichomoniasis
  - Bacterial cultures NOT indicated for diagnosing BV
  - Suspected group A streptococcal vaginitis (rare)
  - No association between group B strep and vulvovaginal symptoms in adults

DIFFERENTIAL DIAGNOSIS
Infection
- Vaginal
  - Candidal vaginitis (See Vaginitis: Vulvovaginal Candidiasis.)
  - *Trichomonas* vaginale (See Sexually Transmitted Diseases (STDs): Trichomonas.)
- Cervical:
  - *Chlamydia* cervicitis (See Sexually Transmitted Diseases (STDs): Chlamydia.)
  - Gonococcal cervicitis (See Sexually Transmitted Diseases (STDs): Gonorrhea.)
  - *Trichomonas cervicitis* (See Sexually Transmitted Diseases (STDs): Trichomonas.)
- Other:
  - BV (See Vaginitis: Bacterial Vaginosis.)

Metabolic/Endocrine
Atrophic vaginitis (See topic) due to hypoestrogenism:
- Postmenopausal
- Lactating
- Athletic-induced amenorrhea
- Anorexia nervosa

Immunologic
Uncommon graft-versus-host manifestation

Tumor/Malignancy
- Fallopian tube cancer is associated with hydrops tubae profluens in 50–60% of cases, an intermittent serosanguineous discharge that can occur as a "gush" and is associated with disappearance of the tubal mass.
- Cervical cancer can be associated with a bloody and/or purulent discharge.
- VAIN (See Vaginal Intraepithelial Neoplasia.)
- Mucositis secondary to chemotherapy

Trauma
In the prepubertal child, the presence of any vulvovaginal symptoms should lead to screening questions and consideration of the possibility of sexual abuse.

Drugs
Allergic or hypersensitivity reaction to topical treatment

Other/Miscellaneous
- Vulvar skin conditions:
  - Lichen sclerosus (see topic)
  - Psoriasis
  - Eczema
- BV
- Atrophic vaginitis
- Desquamative inflammatory vaginitis
- Erosive lichen planus

 MANAGEMENT

- Treatment is based on a specific diagnosis, which is arrived at through:
  - Careful history
  - Exam
  - Testing of vaginal discharge for:
    - pH
    - Microscopy
    - "Whiff" test
    - Cultures as needed
- Consideration of diagnoses other than vaginitis:
  - UTI
  - Vulvar vestibulitis
  - Cervicitis
  - STDs
  - Vulvar skin conditions:
    - Lichen sclerosus
    - Psoriasis
    - Eczema
    - VAIN

SPECIAL THERAPY
Complementary and Alternative Therapies
Data are insufficient regarding both the efficacy and safety of complementary and alternative therapies for vulvovaginal symptoms including:
- Lactobacilli
- Yogurt
- Garlic
- Tea tree oil
- Low-carbohydrate diet
- Desensitization to *Candida* species antigen

MEDICATION (DRUGS)
As indicated by specific diagnosis

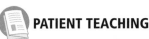 **FOLLOW-UP**

- In children, the recurrence rates of mixed bacterial vulvovaginitis are high. To assess persistent vs. recurrent vulvovaginitis, an exam documenting resolution after treatment will minimize need to evaluate for foreign body, which is required if symptoms are truly persistent, not recurrent.
- Pap tests are unreliable for diagnosing BV or trichomoniasis.

DISPOSITION
Issues for Referral
- Prepubertal girls with persistent or recurrent symptoms
- Recurrent or persistent symptoms with normal exam

PATIENT MONITORING
Annual STD testing is recommended for all sexually active adolescents, young adult women, and others at risk.

BIBLIOGRAPHY

ACOG Practice Bulletin. Clinical management guidelines for obstetrician-gynecologists, Number 72, May 2006: Vaginitis. *Obstet Gynecol.* 2006;107(5):1195–1206.

Centers for Disease Control and Prevention. Expedited partner therapy in the management of sexually transmitted diseases. 2006.

Centers for Disease Control and Prevention. Sexually transmitted diseases: Treatment guidelines, 2006. *MMWR.* 2006;55:1–100.

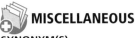 **MISCELLANEOUS**

SYNONYM(S)
- Leukorrhea
- Yeast infection

CLINICAL PEARLS
- Awareness of the presence of an abnormal vaginal discharge varies widely.
- "Asymptomatic" women:
  - Some women deny that they are having any abnormal vaginal symptoms, and yet can be found on exam to have a profuse and clearly abnormal discharge.

ABBREVIATIONS
- PID—Pelvic inflammatory disease
- STDs/STIs—Sexually transmitted diseases or infections
- UTI—Urinary tract infection
- VAIN—Vaginal intraepithelial neoplasia

CODES
ICD9-CM
623.5 Leukorrhea, not specific as infective

PATIENT TEACHING

- Women frequently use sanitary protection to cope with vaginal discharge:
  - Panty-liners
  - Tampons:
    - Patients should be cautioned against continuous use of tampons because of risk of toxic shock syndrome
    - Continuous tampon use with only scant discharge may be excessively drying
    - Tampon use is not associated with either BV or vulvovaginitis.
- Patients should be informed as to whether their symptoms are due to sexual transmission:
  - Expedited partner therapy may be indicated to treat STIs
- Douching should be discouraged:
  - No demonstrated benefit
  - Douching has been associated with increased risk of cervicitis, PID, and tubal infertility

PREVENTION
- Minimize risks of STIs by consistent use of barrier methods and condoms.
- Douching is not recommended for prevention.
- Self-diagnosis of vaginal discharge is unreliable.

VAGINAL SIGNS AND SYMPTOMS: VAGINAL LESIONS

Rebecca S. Kightlinger, DO
JoAnn V. Pinkerton, MD

BASICS

DESCRIPTION
- Vaginal lesions may be described in the following manner:
  - Epithelium:
    - Intact or disrupted
  - Number:
    - Single or multiple
  - Location(s):
    - Proximal, mid, distal, introital
    - Localized or diffuse
- Characteristics:
  - Raised (plaque) or flat
  - Smooth or rough
  - Rough
  - Indurated/Soft/Fluctuant
  - Erosive/Ulcerative
  - Margins circumscribed or diffuse
  - Mobile or fixed
  - Color:
    - Melanosis (brown or black epithelial)
    - Red
    - White
    - Clear: Vesicles or bullae
    - Blue
  - Size
  - Shape

Pediatric Considerations
- Prepubertal:
  - Vaginal adhesions, labial adhesions (See Labial Adhesions.)
  - Sarcoma botryoides
  - Mucocolpos
- Adolescent conditions:
  - Hematocolpos due to obstructing septum or imperforate hymen
  - Infection, including STIs (i.e., *Trichomonas*)
- Reproductive age:
  - Infection, including STDs
  - Endometriosis
  - Squamous cell carcinoma
  - Soft tissue neoplasms

Geriatric Considerations
- Atrophy
- Squamous cell carcinoma
- Lichen sclerosus of vulva

RISK FACTORS
- STIs:
  - Age at 1st intercourse
  - Number of sexual partners
  - Inconsistent condom usage
- Adenocarcinoma:
  - In utero DES exposure
- Cervical cancer:
  - HPV infection
- Vaginal cancer:
  - HPV infection

PATHOPHYSIOLOGY
- Atrophy:
  - Estrogen deficiency leads to thinning of mucosa and loss of collagen and elastin fibers.
- Autoimmune bullous disorders:
  - Deposition of immunoglobulins in subepithelial tissue layers

ASSOCIATED CONDITIONS
- Ulcerative lesions:
  - Crohn's disease
  - Aphthous stomatitis

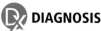

DIAGNOSIS

SIGNS AND SYMPTOMS
- Amenorrhea
- Abnormal bleeding
- Pain:
  - Dyspareunia
  - Difficulty inserting tampon
- Vaginal discharge

History
- Patients often describe vulvar lesions as "vaginal."
- STIs
- Endometriosis
- Menopause
- Trauma, domestic violence
- Depo-Provera or POP contraceptive
- Menstrual history:
  - Amenorrhea in postpubertal female
  - Menopause: Amenorrhea ≥12 months
  - Postpartum, nursing
- Medical history:
  - Crohn's disease
  - Oral or other mucosal disease
  - Immunosuppression
  - Dermatitis

Physical Exam
- Inspection:
  - Inspect anterior, posterior walls and fornices
  - Continue inspection on withdrawal of speculum
- Palpation:
  - Surface texture
  - Distensibility/Elasticity
  - Exophytic lesions
  - Submucous lesions
  - Texture: Firm, soft, fluctuant
  - Margins, size, extent
- Other:
  - Oral mucosa: Wickham's striae, ulcers, blisters
- Vulva

TESTS
- Vaginal biopsy:
  - If lesion suspicious, enlarging, or changing
  - Acetowhite lesion or areas of decreased uptake of Lugol solution on colposcopy
  - Ulcerated lesions: Biopsy the edge
- Immunofluorescence studies: Direct and indirect for ulcerative or bullous lesions

Labs
- Wet prep/KOH
- Culture:
  - Viral
  - Fungal
- RPR (syphilis)
- HIV

Imaging
- MRI:
  - Congenital duplication suspected
  - Soft tissue tumor, size indeterminate, or histologic evidence of aggressive angiomyxoma
- US:
  - Hematocolpos, mucocolpos
  - Submucosal lesion

DIFFERENTIAL DIAGNOSIS
Infection
- HSV
- Candidiasis
- HPV
- Syphilis
- Schistosomiasis

Hematologic
Petechiae:
- Thrombocytopenia

Immunologic
- Ulcerative lesions:
  - Lichen planus
  - Pemphigus
  - Crohn's disease
  - Behçet's disease
  - Eosinophilic granuloma
  - Plasma cell mucositis
  - Vulvovaginal aphthosis
- Bullous lesions:
  - Linear IgA disease
  - Pemphigus vulgaris
  - Cicatricial pemphigus
  - Epidermolysis bullosa acquisita

Tumor/Malignancy
- Preinvasive disease:
  - Vaginal intraepithelial neoplasia
  - Vaginal adenosis
- Malignancies:
  - Squamous carcinoma
  - Adenocarcinoma
  - Rare malignancies:
    - Plasmacytoma
    - Rhabdomyoma
    - Rhabdomyosarcoma
    - Granulosa cell tumor
    - Paraganglioma
    - Melanoma

Trauma
- Hematoma
- Fissure
- Laceration
- Ulceration
- Sexual abuse or assault

Drugs
- Mucositis secondary to chemotherapy
- Allergic or contact mucositis from topical preparations
- Erythema multiforme

Other/Miscellaneous
- Endometriosis
- Blue nevus
- Benign fibroepithelial polyp
- Squamous papillomatosis: Normal variant
- Vaginal stones
- Vaginal developmental anomalies:
  - Imperforate hymen (see topic)
  - Vaginal septa

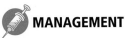 **MANAGEMENT**

GENERAL MEASURES
For control of pain, irritation:
- Loose, nonconstricting clothing with no underwear
- Control primary condition, if applicable

SPECIAL THERAPY
Complementary and Alternative Therapies
- Lubricants:
  - Astroglide, KY Jelly
- Vaginal moisturizers:
  - Replens

MEDICATION (DRUGS)
- Infection:
  - Candidiasis (See Vaginitis: Vulvovaginal Candidiasis.):
    - Topical antimycotics
    - Oral Fluconazole
  - HSV (See Sexually Transmitted Diseases (STDs): Herpes Simplex Virus.):
    - Acyclovir
    - Valacyclovir
    - Famvir
  - Syphilis:
    - Penicillin G
- Immunologic blistering and ulcerative lesion:
  - Systemic corticosteroids
  - Dapsone
  - Topical or systemic corticosteroids
- Atrophy:
  - Estrogen: Topical, if no other menopausal symptoms, using creams, tablets, rings

SURGERY
- Simple excision:
  - Vaginal polyps, if symptomatic or enlarging
- Wide local excision:
  - Melanoma
- Excision and/or repair:
  - Imperforate hymen
  - Septa
  - Vaginal duplication

 FOLLOW-UP

DISPOSITION
Issues for Referral
- Malignancy
- Vaginal atrophy with history of estrogen-dependent malignancy
- Location or size of lesion requires advanced surgical skills
- Unresponsive to treatment
- Lack of familiarity with disease
- Associated disease requires comanagement:
  - Crohn's disease
  - Immunologic disorder
  - Condition associated with chronic pain
  - Involves duplication or anomaly of urologic structures

PROGNOSIS
- Malignancy:
  - Type-, stage-, and grade-dependent
- Immunologic:
  - Prone to chronic, recurrent course
- Atrophy:
  - Excellent, if treated before significant structural changes and strictures develop

PATIENT MONITORING
- VAIN, vaginal adenosis:
  - Colposcopy
  - Pap
- Blistering, erosive diseases:
  - Frequent vaginal exam, titration of corticosteroid potency and frequency of application
- Atrophy:
  - Frequently until normal estrogenization restored, then annually or semiannually

BIBLIOGRAPHY

DeSaia P, et al., eds. *Clinical Gynecologic Oncology*, 6th ed. St. Louis: Mosby; 2002.

Fisher BK, et al., eds. *Genital Skin Disorders: Diagnosis and Treatment*. St. Louis: Mosby; 1998.

Fu YS. *Pathology of the Uterine Cervix, Vagina, and Vulva*, 2nd ed. Philadelphia: Saunders; 2002.

 MISCELLANEOUS

CLINICAL PEARLS
- Have specula of several different sizes:
  - Long (sometimes termed "large") Grave's
  - Medium Grave's
  - Pederson
  - Long Pederson
  - Huffman (narrow, sometimes termed "virginal")
- Anterior "polyps" may be urethral diverticula:
  - Evaluate for diverticulum prior to removing
- Submucous lesions of the vagina may represent soft-tissue tumors of mesenchymal origin, and therefore may require imaging studies to assess size and margins.

ABBREVIATIONS
- ACOG—American College of Obstetricians and Gynecologists
- HPV—Human papillomavirus
- HSV—Herpes simplex virus
- POP—Progestin-only pill
- RPR—Rapid plasma reagin (for syphilis)
- STD/STI—Sexually transmitted disease/infection
- VAIN—Vaginal intraepithelial neoplasia

CODES
- 617.9 Endometriosis
- 623.7 Vaginal polyp
- 627.3 Atrophic vaginitis
- 694.4 Pemphigus
- 752.42 Imperforate hymen

 PATIENT TEACHING

- American College of Obstetricians and Gynecologists (ACOG) pamphlets:
  - Vaginitis
  - Menopausal symptoms
  - Herpes infection
  - HPV infection
- North American Menopause Society: www.menopause.org:
  - Vaginal atrophy
- National Vulvodynia Association: www.nva.org:
  - Vulvodynia and chronic pain

PREVENTION
STIs:
- Limit sexual partners
- Delay sexual debut
- Condoms

VAGINAL SIGNS AND SYMPTOMS: VAGINISMUS

Catherine M. Leclair, MD
Jeffrey T. Jensen, MD, MPH

 BASICS

DESCRIPTION
- Vaginismus is defined as the recurrent, involuntary contraction of the pelvic floor muscles, leading to painful vaginal penetration.
- Primary vaginismus is described as lifelong inability to achieve vaginal penetration due to involuntary contraction of the pelvic floor muscles.
- Secondary vaginismus is defined as the inability to achieve vaginal penetration after a nonsymptomatic period. This may be situational (e.g., inability to relax muscles in clinical or sexual situation).

Age-Related Factors
Must be distinguished from anatomic factors (hymen) in young, coitally naïve women, genital atrophy in older women

EPIDEMIOLOGY
- Primary, unknown
- Secondary often due to pain response in the pelvis or vulva (See Vulvar Signs and Symptoms: Vulvodynia.)

Prevalence
- Unknown in general population
- 70% of women with localized, provoked vulvodynia (vulvar vestibulitis syndrome) have concomitant vaginismus

RISK FACTORS
- Dyspareunia (see topic)
- Pelvic pain (See Pain: Chronic Pelvic.)
- Vulvodynia (See Vulvar Signs and Symptoms: Vulvodynia.)
- Vulvar vestibulitis syndrome (see topic)
- IBS (see Irritable Bowel Syndrome)
- Interstitial cystitis (see topic)
- Sexual arousal disorder (See Sexual Dysfunction.)
- Genital atrophy (See Vaginitis: Atrophic.)
- Recurrent vaginitis

PATHOPHYSIOLOGY
Vaginistic reaction represents an involuntary, conditioned withdrawal response to vaginal penetration leading to pelvic floor contracture with subsequent pain and muscle tension.

ASSOCIATED CONDITIONS
Localized, provoked vulvodynia (vulvar vestibulitis syndrome)

 DIAGNOSIS

SIGNS AND SYMPTOMS
History
- Dyspareunia
- Painful penetration with tampon, speculum, or finger
- Constipation

Review of Systems
- GU: Dyspareunia, pelvic pain
- GI: Constipation, diarrhea

Physical Exam
Levator myalgia with increased resting tone and/or tenderness of levator ani muscle, particularly pubococcygeus muscle

TESTS
Tension readings incorporated from biofeedback (readings expressed in microvolts)

Labs
None

Imaging
None

DIFFERENTIAL DIAGNOSIS
- Localized, provoked vulvodynia (vulvar vestibulitis syndrome)
- Chronic pelvic pain
- Chronic constipation
- IBS
- Interstitial cystitis
- Vaginitis
- Vulvar dermatoses

Infection
Not associated with infection of vagina or pelvis

Metabolic/Endocrine
May be associated with vaginal atrophy in postmenopausal or lactating women

Immunologic
No autoimmune component

Tumor/Malignancy
Not associated with cancer

Trauma
Sexual abuse or surgical trauma can lead to avoidant sexual behavior, which is associated with vaginismus.

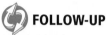 **MANAGEMENT**

GENERAL MEASURES
Most women respond well to pelvic floor physical therapy and CBT.

MEDICATION (DRUGS)
If concomitant localized, provoked vulvodynia (vulvar vestibulitis syndrome), consider using topical lidocaine with physical therapy

SURGERY
No surgical treatment

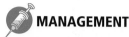 **FOLLOW-UP**

DISPOSITION
Issues for Referral
- Referral to pelvic floor physical therapist experienced with vaginismus and pelvic floor pain is the primary treatment of this disorder.
- Referral to a sex therapist familiar with CBT and vaginismus is beneficial for most.

PROGNOSIS
Most women will improve with therapy.

PATIENT MONITORING
- Home therapy often incorporates dilator therapy.
- Possible portable EMG unit

BIBLIOGRAPHY

Bergeron S, et al. A randomized comparison of group-cognitive-behavioral therapy, surface electromyographic biofeedback, and vestibulectomy in the treatment of dyspareunia resulting from vulvar vestibulitis. *Pain*. 2001;91:297–306.

Glazer HI, et al. Treatment of vulvar vestibulitis syndrome with electromyographic biofeedback of pelvic floor musculature. *J Repro Med*. 1995;40:283–290.

Romm J, et al. Incidence of vaginismus in patients evaluated in vulvar pain clinic. *North Am Society Psychosocial Obstet Gynecol*, Twenty-fourth Annual Meeting, 1996.

Seo JT, et al. Efficacy of functional electrical stimulation-biofeedback with sexual cognitive-behavioral therapy as treatment of vaginismus. *Urology*. 2005;66:77–81.

 ## MISCELLANEOUS

CLINICAL PEARLS

- Treatment of urinary incontinence with pelvic floor physical therapy is approached differently from vaginismus.
- Screen physical therapists as to their knowledge and comfort specifically with vaginismus.

ABBREVIATIONS

- CBT—Cognitive-behavioral therapy
- EMG—Electromyograph
- IBS—Irritable bowel syndrome

CODES

ICD9-CM

- 625.1 Vaginismus
- 729.1 Pelvic floor myalgia

 ## PATIENT TEACHING

- National Vulvodynia Association:
  – www.nva.org
- International Society for the Study of Vulvovaginal Disease:
  – www.issvd.org

VULVAR SIGNS AND SYMPTOMS: VULVAR MASSES

Meghan B. Oakes, MD
Elisabeth H. Quint, MD

 BASICS

DESCRIPTION

Vulvar masses have a variety of appearances and range from benign to malignant. The following categorizations can be applied. For purposes of this reference, only the most common masses will be addressed.

- Solid masses:
  - Condyloma acuminata
  - Molluscum contagiosum
  - Acrochordon "skin tags"
  - Seborrheic keratosis
  - Nevus
  - Keratoacanthoma
  - Hidradenoma
  - Vulvar intraepithelial neoplasia (VIN) (see chapter)
  - Sebaceous adenoma
  - Basal cell carcinoma
  - Squamous cell carcinoma
  - Melanoma
  - Endodermal sinus tumor
  - Embryonal rhabdomyosarcoma
  - Fibroma
  - Lipoma
  - Neurofibroma
  - Leiomyoma
  - Granular cell tumor
  - Pyogenic granuloma
  - Hemangioma
  - Lymphangioma
  - Vulvovaginal polyp
  - Bartholin mass/abscess
  - Ectopic gonad
  - Urethral caruncle
  - Urethral mucosa prolapse
- Cystic masses:
  - Epidermal inclusion cysts
  - Pilonidal cyst
  - Sebaceous cyst
  - Hidradenoma
  - Fox-Fordyce disease
  - Syringoma
  - Gartener cysts
  - Müllerian cyst
  - Urogenital sinus cyst
  - Adenosis
  - Hydrocele
  - Supernumerary mammary cyst
  - Dermoid cyst
  - Bartholin duct cyst/abscess
  - Paraurethral (Skene) cyst
  - Urethral diverticulum
  - Endometriosis
  - Cystic lymphangioma
  - Liquefied hematoma
  - Vaginitis emphysematosa

Age-Related Factors
Incidence of lesions is highly dependent on age. See "Differential Diagnosis" for further information.

EPIDEMIOLOGY
Leiomyomas are more common in African-American women, whereas hidradenomas are almost exclusively seen in white women.

RISK FACTORS
- History of STIs:
  - Condyloma acuminata
  - Molluscum contagiosum
  - Squamous cell carcinoma
- History of insulin resistance:
  - Acrochordon
- Immunosuppression:
  - Vulvar malignancy
- History of lichen sclerosus:
  - Squamous cell carcinoma
- Tobacco use:
  - Squamous cell carcinoma

Genetics
Neurofibromas are associated with von Recklinghausen disease:
- Autosomal dominant inheritance
- Gene on long arm of chromosome 17
- Examine patient for fibromas in other areas as well as café au lait spots.

PATHOPHYSIOLOGY
Dependent on specific lesion

ASSOCIATED CONDITIONS
Squamous cell carcinoma is associated with lichen sclerosus (see Vulvar Cancer and Vulvar Lichen Sclerosus).

 DIAGNOSIS

SIGNS AND SYMPTOMS
History
To narrow the differential diagnosis, it is important to consider the following:
- Onset:
  - Congenital
  - New onset
- Growth:
  - No growth
  - Slow growth
  - Rapid growth
- Associated symptoms:
  - See ROS
- Past medical history
- Family history

Review of Systems
- Fever
- Pruritus
- Dysuria
- Vaginal bleeding
- Vulvar pain

Physical Exam
- Vital signs, including temperature
- Entire body skin exam
- Abdominal exam
- Lymphadenopathy (inguinal)
- External GU exam:
  - Palpate lesion to determine if cystic
  - Measure lesion and document size and location
  - Consider photographs to document lesions and temporal progression
- Speculum exam, if indicated
- Bimanual exam, if indicated
- Rectal exam, if indicated

TESTS
Labs
- CBC and culture if infection is suspected
- Biopsy (see Vulvar Biopsy), if:
  - Uncertain diagnosis
  - Suspicion for malignancy
  - Lesion growing

Imaging
- If there is concern for malignancy, consider CT scan of pelvis.
- If unable to determine if mass is cystic or solid, consider translabial US.

DIFFERENTIAL DIAGNOSIS
Differential diagnosis based on age
Pediatric Considerations
- Premenarchal:
  - Inguinal hernia
  - Infectious:
    - Molluscum contagiosum
    - Vulvar warts (consider abuse) (See Sexual Abuse.)
  - Embryonic remnant:
    - Gartner duct cyst
    - Canal of Nuck cyst (hydrocele)
    - Bartholin duct cyst
  - Mass of mesenchymal origin:
    - Lipoma
    - Fibroma
    - Lymphangioma
    - Hemangioma
    - Neurofibroma
    - Granular cell tumor
    - Hamartoma
  - Malignant masses:
    - Embryonal rhabdomyosarcoma
    - Endodermal sinus tumor
- Reproductive years:
  - All lesions can occur in this age group
  - Infectious lesions more common
- Postmenopausal:
  - See "Geriatric Considerations"

Geriatric Considerations
- Bartholin mass associated with malignancy
- Vulvar cancer more common with aging

Infection
- HPV is a very common infection (see Sexually Transmitted Diseases (STDs): Human Papillomavirus).
- Positive HIV status can lead to VIN 3/vulvar cancer at a much younger age than usual.

Hematologic
Hemangiomas

Metabolic/Endocrine
Acrochordons are more common in those with insulin resistance and PCOS.

Immunologic
Immunosuppression can lead to premalignancies and malignancies at earlier than expected ages.

Tumor/Malignancy
- Types of malignancies are typically age dependant.
- 3% of all melanomas are located in the genital tract; 7% of invasive vulvar cancers are melanomas.
- 2–4% of vulvar neoplasms are basal cell carcinoma.

Trauma
Vulvar hematoma:
- More common in pediatric population (See Vulvar and Vaginal Trauma.)

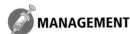 **MANAGEMENT**

GENERAL MEASURES
- For the majority of solid vulvar masses, the mainstay of therapy is excision.
- For cystic masses, the therapy may be incision and drainage or excision.
- Certain masses can be monitored over time with regular exams and photo documentation:
  – Hemangiomas
  – Neurofibromas
- Medical therapy is frequently first-line therapy for infectious masses.

MEDICATION (DRUGS)
A small number of vulvar masses, can be medically treated and/or eradicated:
- Antibiotics:
  – Bartholin gland abscess
- Immunomodulators:
  – Condyloma acuminata
  – Molluscum contagiosum
- Oral contraceptive therapy:
  – Vulvar endometriosis
- Sclerosing agents:
  – Cavernous hemangiomas
- Trichloroacetic acid:
  – Condyloma acuminata

SURGERY
Excision forms the cornerstone of therapy. Many masses do not require surgical removal, although symptoms may necessitate surgery. Simple observation should be considered if malignancy has been ruled out.
- Laser therapy:
  – Condyloma acuminata
- Cryotherapy:
  – Hemangioma of infancy
  – Senile hemangioma
- Drainage:
  – Bartholin gland cyst/abscess
  – Skene gland abscess
- Curettage of lesion:
  – Molluscum contagiosum
- Simple excision:
  – Fibroma
  – Lipoma
  – Leiomyoma
  – Pilonidal cyst
  – Hidradenoma
  – Supernumerary mammary cysts
  – Bartholin gland cyst/abscess
  – Skene gland cyst
- Wide local excision:
  – Pyogenic granuloma
  – Granular cell tumor
  – Basal cell carcinoma
  – Melanoma
- Associated surgeries:
  – Sentinel lymph node biopsy
  – Unilateral or bilateral lymphadenopathy can be necessary in cases of melanoma

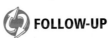 **FOLLOW-UP**

- Close follow-up for recurrence or mass growth may be indicated in certain circumstances.
- In other cases, resection is considered curative.

DISPOSITION
Issues for Referral
All histologically diagnosed cancers of the vulva should be referred to a gynecologist-oncologist or dermatologist-oncologist.

PROGNOSIS
- For the majority of vulvar masses, the prognosis is quite good, and a full recovery should be anticipated following treatment.
- Melanoma is the exception to this rule:
  – Melanoma: 5-year survival rate reported at 36–47%

PATIENT MONITORING
Please see follow-up.

BIBLIOGRAPHY

Kaufman RH, et al., eds. *Benign Diseases of the Vulva and Vagina*, 5th ed. Philadelphia: Elsevier Mosby; 2005.

Lowry DLB, et al. The vulvar mass in the prepubertal child. *J Pediat Adolesc Gynecol*. 1997;13:75–78.

Platz CE, et al. Female genital tract cancer. *Cancer*. 1996;95:270–294.

Raber G, et al. Malignant melanoma of the vulva. Report of 89 patients. *Cancer*. 1996;78(11):2353–2358.

Ragnarsson-Olding BK, et al. Malignant melanoma of the vulva in a nationwide, 25-year study of 219 Swedish females: Predictors of survival. *Cancer*. 1999;86(7):1285–1293.

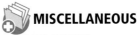 **MISCELLANEOUS**

CLINICAL PEARLS
- A histologic diagnosis is required for the majority of vulvar masses. If diagnosis is uncertain, biopsy is the rule.
- Older age is associated with an increased chance of malignancy, especially in masses that, in other age groups, are typically benign (e.g., Bartholin cyst).

ABBREVIATIONS
- HPV—Human papillomavirus
- PCOS—Polycystic ovary syndrome
- STI—Sexually transmitted infection
- VIN—Vulvar intraepithelial neoplasia

 CODES

ICD9-CM
- 616.4 Other abscess of vulva
- 616.5 Ulceration of vulva, unspecified
- 624.0 Dystrophy of vulva
- 624.8 Specified noninflammatory disorder of vulva or perineum
- 654.8 Congenital or acquired abnormality of vulva

PATIENT TEACHING

Patients, especially those with risk factors, must examine their vulva and present for regular gynecologic care.

PREVENTION
- Refrain from tobacco usage.
- Employ safe sex practices.
- Institution of widespread HPV vaccination

VULVAR SIGNS AND SYMPTOMS: VULVAR RASHES

Jonathan D. K. Trager, MD

 BASICS

DESCRIPTION

- Primary lesions:
  - Macule (flat)
  - Papule (raised, <1 cm)
  - Plaque (raised, ≥1 cm)
  - Nodule (firm, deeper papule or plaque)
  - Vesicle (fluid-filled, <1 cm)
  - Bulla (fluid-filled, ≥1 cm)
  - Pustule (vesicle or bulla with purulent exudate)
- Secondary skin changes:
  - Scale (epidermal flaking)
  - Crust (dried surface fluid)
  - Excoriation (scratch)
  - Fissure (vertical split)
  - Erosion (superficial denudation)
  - Ulcer (denudation to dermis)
  - Lichenification (skin thickening with accentuation of skin lines)
  - Atrophy (thinning of skin)
  - Scar (dense fibrotic tissue)

Age-Related Factors

- Infants: Occlusion from diapers and exposure to urine/feces (diaper dermatitis)
- Children: Poor hygiene and irritants, such as bubble bath (irritant dermatitis). (See Vaginitis: Prepubertal Vulvovaginitis.)
- Adolescents/Adults: Waxing/Shaving (folliculitis); feminine hygiene products (irritant and allergic contact dermatitis); sexual activity (contact dermatitis from latex condoms, spermicide)
- Postmenopausal women: Atrophic vulvar changes (predispose to local skin trauma)

EPIDEMIOLOGY

Common vulvar rashes during life stages:
- Infants: Seborrheic dermatitis, candidal vulvitis
- Children: Atopic dermatitis; psoriasis; pityriasis rosea; lichen sclerosus, molluscum contagiosum; vitiligo
- Adolescents/Adults: Psoriasis; candidal vulvovaginitis; hidradenitis suppurativa
- Postmenopausal women: Lichen planus; lichen sclerosus

RISK FACTORS

- Immunosuppression, diabetes, oral antibiotics, topical corticosteroid use:
  - Candidal vulvovaginitis
- Urinary and fecal incontinence:
  - Irritant dermatitis
- Lichen sclerosus and lichen planus:
  - Vulvar SCC

Genetics

Family history may be positive in:
- Atopic dermatitis
- Psoriasis
- Lichen sclerosus
- Hidradenitis suppurativa

PATHOPHYSIOLOGY

Varies, depending on etiology

ASSOCIATED CONDITIONS

Systemic or other disease:
- Crohn's disease (cutaneous vulvar Crohn's disease)
- Epstein-Barr virus (vulvar ulcers)
- Behçet's disease (vulvar ulcers)
- Streptococcal pharyngitis (toxin-mediated perineal erythema)
- HSV (erythema multiforme)

 DIAGNOSIS

SIGNS AND SYMPTOMS

History

- Acute: Contact dermatitis; infection; pityriasis rosea; medication reaction
- Chronic: Atopic dermatitis; psoriasis; lichen sclerosus; lichen planus
- Topical irritants/allergens; shaving; waxing
- Prior use of topical and systemic medications
- Extragenital skin disease

Review of Systems

- Pruritus: Common in many vulvar dermatoses
- Vaginal discharge
- Symptoms of systemic disease

Physical Exam

- Genital skin: Primary and secondary lesions
- Extragenital skin, scalp, nails, oral/ocular mucosa:
  - Atopic dermatitis: Flexural eczema
  - Psoriasis: Nail pits; scalp lesions; scaly plaques on trunk/extremities
  - Hidradenitis suppurativa: Axillary and inframammary lesions; pilonidal cyst
  - Scabies: Interdigital burrows; breast, buttock, and inframammary lesions
  - Lichen planus; Behçet's disease; autoimmune blistering diseases; erythema multiforme major; oral and ocular lesions
- Atypical appearance of vulvar rashes is common:
  - Loss of scale (due to moisture and occlusion)
  - Lichenification (scratching/rubbing)
  - Contact dermatitis (from topical treatment)
  - Masking of fungal infection (topical steroids)

TESTS

- Cultures: Bacterial, viral, fungal as needed
- Potassium hydroxide prep: Fungal rash
- Tzanck prep: HSV
- Scabies prep: Scabies
- Skin biopsy: If diagnosis difficult, results critical, treatment complicated or prolonged (See Vulvar Biopsy.)

Labs

Blood tests for underlying illness (diabetes, immunosuppression, infection, metabolic disease)

DIFFERENTIAL DIAGNOSIS

Infection

- Bacterial:
  - Folliculitis (follicular papules/pustules)
  - Impetigo (honey-crusted papules)
  - Furuncle (erythematous nodule)
  - Abscess (fluctuant nodule)

  - *Staphylococcus aureus; Streptococcus pyogenes*
  - Methicillin-resistant *S. aureus*
  - *Escherichia coli*
  - *Pseudomonas aeruginosa* (especially if large painful pustules after waxing)
  - Cellulitis: Erythema, warmth, tenderness; *S. aureus, S. pyogenes*
  - Perianal streptococcal disease: Bright red perianal erythema in young children; *S. pyogenes*
  - Toxin-mediated perineal erythema: Erythema of groin 2–3 days after streptococcal or staphylococcal pharyngitis; desquamates
  - Erythrasma: Erythematous, well-defined intriginous plaques; *Corynebacterium minutissimum*; fluoresces coral-red under Wood's light; treat with topical clindamycin, erythromycin, or oral erythromycin
- Fungal:
  - Vulvovaginal candidiasis: Vulvar erythema, edema; fissures; excoriations; maceration; lichenification; +/− vaginal discharge; pruritus
  - Candidal diaper dermatitis involves skin creases (unlike irritant diaper dermatitis); satellite papules and pustules common; consider diabetes in young girl with candidal vulvitis who has outgrown diapers, as fungal vulvitis rare until puberty
  - Tinea cruris: Erythematous plaques in groin, with or without scale; dermatophytes
- Viral:
  - Molluscum contagiosum: Skin-colored or pink umbilicated papules; sexual/nonsexual and fomite spread; treat by curettage or cryotherapy; imiquimod cream (off-label)
  - Epstein-Barr virus: May cause vulvar ulcers
  - Cytomegalovirus: Perineal ulcerative dermatitis in immunocompromised host
- Parasitic:
  - Scabies: (*Sarcoptes scabiei*); pruritic erythematous papules and vesicles; nodules if chronic; treat with topical scabicide (e.g., permethrin 5% cream) and mild topical corticosteroid for pruritus
  - Pubic lice: (*Pthirus pubis*); pruritus, excoriations, secondary infection; treat with topical pediculicide (e.g., permethrin 1% or pyrethrin shampoo; 5% permethrin cream; 1% lindane shampoo)
    - Beware lindane neurotoxicity

Metabolic/Endocrine

- Acanthosis nigricans: Velvety, hyperpigmented intriginous plaques; sign of insulin resistance
- Acrodermatitis enteropathica: Eczematous vulvar and perineal rash, diarrhea, alopecia; due to zinc deficiency; may be seen in breast-fed infants or children with immunodeficiency
- Necrolytic migratory erythema: Erosive, circinate migratory erythema in flexural and periorificial areas; seen with glucagonoma

Immunologic

Common

- Atopic dermatitis, acute: Erythematous scaly papules, plaques, crusts, excoriations
- Atopic dermatits, chronic: Lichenification
- Contact dermatitis: Pruritus, erythema, edema, blistering if severe, desquamation
  - Irritant: Direct skin irritation by caustic agent:
    - Soaps, detergents, feminine hygiene products, spermicides

– Allergic: Type IV hypersensitivity reaction:
  ○ Benzocaine, preservatives, neomycin, latex condoms, lanolin, perfume, nail polish, poison ivy
• Psoriasis: Well-demarcated pink or erythematous vulvar plaques, +/− scale
• Lichen sclerosus (see topic):
  – Pruritus, burning; rarely asymptomatic
  – Vulvar hypopigmentation, thin, wrinkled atrophic skin in figure-of-eight pattern around vulva and perineum, fissures, erosions, petechiae, purpura
  – 5% lifetime risk of SCC in women; lifetime risk of SCC in young girls with lichen sclerosus not known
  – Treatment is clobetasol propionate ointment 0.05% b.i.d. for 3 months, then wean.
  – Topical immunomodulators (tacrolimus ointment 0.1% and pimecrolimus 1% cream) have been used (off-label).
• Pityriasis rosea: "Inverse pityriasis rosea" shows erythematous oval papules and plaques concentrated in pubic area and axillae.
• Lichen simplex chronicus: Lichenified vulvar plaques often underlying pruritic dermatosis (atopic dermatitis; contact dermatitis; psoriasis)
• Hidradenitis suppurativa:
  – Recurrent cysts, nodules, abscesses, and draining sinuses in intertriginous areas
  – Treatment: Weight loss; culture fluctuant/draining lesions; topical and oral antibiotics; intralesional triamcinolone for inflamed cysts; isotretinoin or infliximab for recalcitrant hidradenitis suppurativa (both off-label); surgical excision of sinus tracts
• Erythema multiforme: Target lesions, bullae, erosions; involvement of ≥2 mucosal sites points to erythema multiforme major
• Vitiligo: Vulvar and perianal depigmentation; asymptomatic; extragenital involvement common

Less common
• Lichen planus: 3 vulvar forms:
  – Papules and plaques with generalized cutaneous disease
  – Hypertrophic disease
  – Erosive disease: Vulvovaginal gingival syndrome; vulvar and oral erosions
• Behçet's disease:
  – Oral and genital ulcers; arthritis; uveitis; neurologic disorders; arterial and venous thrombosis; pathergy
• Crohn's disease:
  – Perineal abscesses, sinuses, fistulae, tags
  – Granulomatous labial swelling (noncaseating granulomas)
• Kawasaki disease: Perineal erythema
• Autoimmune blistering diseases: Biopsy with immunofluorescence needed; treated with oral steroids and/or immunosuppressants
  – Bullous pemphigoid: Tense bullae; flexural involvement common
  – Cicatricial pemphigoid: Mimics erosive lichen planus; oral and conjunctival lesions
  – Pemphigus vulgaris: Vulvar erosions; fragile blisters on extragenital skin
  – Linear IgA bullous dermatosis: Genital involvement common in children; annular polycyclic lesions with peripheral blistering

Tumor/Malignancy
Langerhans cell histiocytosis: Vulvar and perineal ulcers and nodules; widespread lesions

Trauma
• Waxing/Shaving: Erythematous follicular papules and pustules
• Laser hair removal: Scarring, pigment changes
• Genital piercing: Infection, contact dermatitis, scarring, traumatic tearing of skin

Drugs
• Contact dermatitis (irritant and allergic)
• Fixed drug eruption: Recurrent erythematous, blistered, or eroded plaques on mucosal surfaces (trimethoprim-sulfamethoxazole, NSAIDs, others)
• Topical steroids: Atrophy, telangiectasia, striae
• Part of widespread eruption (urticaria, erythema multiforme, toxic epidermal necrolysis)

Other/Miscellaneous
Radiation vulvitis:
• Acute: Edema, violaceous discoloration, pain, burning, bullae, necrosis
• Chronic: Atrophy, hypopigmentation, scarring, telangiectasia

 MANAGEMENT

GENERAL MEASURES
• Identify and remove cause of rash
• Restore skin barrier:
  – Sitz baths, pat dry, apply petrolatum
• Relieve pruritus:
  – Cool compresses, sedating antihistamine
• Relieve inflammation
• Aluminum acetate (Burrow solution) for weeping, exudative areas

MEDICATION (DRUGS)
• Topical:
  – Corticosteroids: Low- to mid-potency usually suffice (except in lichen sclerosus and lichen planus); be aware that natural occlusion of genital area increases systemic absorption.
    ○ For atopic dermatitis; contact dermatitis; psoriasis; lichen sclerosus; lichen planus; lichen simplex chronicus; symptomatic pityriasis rosea
  – Antibiotics: Bacitracin, polymyxin B, neomycin (plus combinations); mupirocin; gentamicin
    ○ For minor cuts; fissures; impetiginized rashes
    ○ Allergy to neomycin common; any topical antibiotic may cause allergic reaction
  – Antifungal agents: Imidazoles, allylamines
    ○ For tinea cruris; tinea corporis (mons pubis); candidal vulvitis
  – Immunomodulators: Tacrolimus, pimecrolimus
    ○ For atopic dermatitis; off-label for psoriasis and lichen sclerosus
• Systemic:
  – Steroids: Prednisone or prednisolone
    ○ For severe contact dermatitis; start at 1–2 mg/kg/d for 3–5 days, taper over 14 days
  – Antibiotics:
    ○ Cover common pathogens
  – Antifungal agents:
    ○ Fluconazole: Vulvovaginal candidiasis
    ○ Itraconazole, terbinafine: Severe tinea cruris

SURGERY
May be indicated in limited situations:
• Severe scarring in lichen sclerosus
• Severe hidradenitis suppurativa

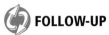 **FOLLOW-UP**

Close follow-up to determine treatment effect, accuracy of diagnosis, recurrence

DISPOSITION
Issues for Referral
• Dermatologist if diagnosis is in doubt, treatment is difficult, discomfort with doing skin biopsy, extragenital skin disease is present
• Vulvar disease specialist for chronic pain syndromes (vulvar vestibulitis, vulvodynia)
• Gynecologic oncologist for vulvar skin cancers

PROGNOSIS
Varies, depending on the cause

PATIENT MONITORING
Lifelong monitoring of patients with vulvar lichen sclerosus and lichen planus for SCC

BIBLIOGRAPHY

Margesson LJ. Vulvar disease pearls. *Dermatol Clin.* 2006;24:145.

Wojnarowska F, et al. Anogenital (nonvenereal) disease. In: Bolognia JL, et al., eds. Dermatology. Edinburgh: Mosby; 2003:1099–1113.

 MISCELLANEOUS

Psychosocial support, including addressing sexual dysfunction, is critical for chronic vulvar conditions.

CLINICAL PEARLS
Use the *morphology* of clinical lesions, not so much the location, to make the diagnosis.

ABBREVIATIONS
• HSV—Herpes simplex virus
• SCC—Squamous cell carcinoma

CODES
ICD9-CM
• 078.0 Molluscum contagiosum
• 110.3 Tinea cruris
• 112.1 Vulvovaginal candidiasis
• 691.8 Atopic dermatitis
• 692.9 Contact dermatitis
• 696.1 Psoriasis
• 696.3 Pityriasis rosea
• 697.0 Lichen planus
• 701.0 Lichen sclerosus
• 701.2 Common: Acanthosis nigricans
• 704.8 Folliculitis
• 705.83 Hidradenitis suppurativa

 PATIENT TEACHING

PREVENTION
• Avoid vulvar irritants including feminine hygiene products.
• Use unscented mild cleanser or plain water; avoid overzealous hygiene.
• Wear loose-fitting cotton underpants.
• Seek prompt care for vulvar symptoms.

VULVAR SIGNS AND SYMPTOMS: VULVODYNIA

Catherine M. Leclair, MD
Jeffrey T. Jensen, MD, MPH

 BASICS

DESCRIPTION
- Vulvodynia is defined as vulvar discomfort, most often described as burning pain, occurring in the absence of relevant visible findings or a specific, clinically identifiable, neurologic disorder.
- Classification of vulvodynia defined by site of pain:
  – Localized versus generalized
- Further classified:
  – Provoked (with touch only)
  – Unprovoked:
    ○ Mixed

Age-Related Factors
- Generalized, unprovoked vulvodynia is more common in postmenopausal women.
- Localized, provoked vulvodynia is more common in premenopausal women.

EPIDEMIOLOGY
Prevalence
15% prevalence

RISK FACTORS
Risk factors not identified

Genetics
No genetic predisposition or etiology identified

PATHOPHYSIOLOGY
- Neuropathic process with multiple etiologies suggested
- Most cases likely multifactorial

ASSOCIATED CONDITIONS
Localized, provoked vulvodynia often associated with vaginismus (See Vaginal Signs and Symptoms: Vaginismus.)

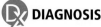 **DIAGNOSIS**

SIGNS AND SYMPTOMS
History
- Insidious onset
- Localized, provoked vulvodynia often presents as dyspareunia.

Physical Exam
- Generalized, unprovoked vulvodynia with normal vulvovaginal exam
- Localized, provoked vulvodynia with vestibular erythema and Qtip tenderness test

TESTS
- Qtip test: Localized tenderness at hymenal sulcus
- Wet mount to assess vulvovaginitis
- Vaginal pH to assess vaginitis

Labs
- Fungal culture
- Chlamydia/Gonorrhea cervical testing

Imaging
None

DIFFERENTIAL DIAGNOSIS
- Diagnosis of exclusion
- Rule out:
  – Contact vulvitis
  – Lichen sclerosus
  – Lichen planus
  – Less common vulvar dermatoses
  – HSV
  – Vaginitis
  – Vaginismus
  – Vulvar intraepithelial neoplasia (VIN)
  – Vulvar cancer

Infection
- Rule out vaginitis
- HPV testing not recommended

Metabolic/Endocrine
Generally not associated with hormonal state; however, hypoestrogenism provokes symptoms in some women.

Immunologic
Not considered autoimmune process

Tumor/Malignancy
- No association with cancer
- However VIN can present with itching and burning and must be excluded.

Trauma
No correlation with sexual abuse

Drugs
No relationship to medicines

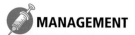 **MANAGEMENT**

GENERAL MEASURES
- Remove all contact irritants.
- Gentle care measures of the vulva advised:
  – Use hypoallergenic cleansers.
  – Avoid contact irritants.

MEDICATION (DRUGS)
- Generalized, unprovoked vulvodynia treated with oral neuromodulators for chronic pain:
  – Amitriptyline
  – Gabapentin
- Localized, provoked vulvodynia:
  – Topical lidocaine
  – Oral neuromodulators:
    ○ Amitriptyline
    ○ Gabapentin
  – Pelvic floor physical therapy with biofeedback
  – CBT

SURGERY
Complete or modified vestibulectomy for localized, provoked vulvodynia

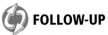 **FOLLOW-UP**

DISPOSITION
Issues for Referral
For refractory cases unresponsive to treatment, referral options are:

- Pain specialist/clinic/service
- Sexual therapist
- Physical therapist

PROGNOSIS
Most women experience improvement of symptoms.

BIBLIOGRAPHY

Bergeron S, et al. A randomized comparison of group-cognitive-behavioral therapy, surface electromyographic biofeedback, and vestibulectomy in the treatment of dyspareunia resulting from vulvar vestibulitis. *Pain*. 2001;91:297–306.

Goetsch MF. Simplified surgical revision of the vulvar vestibule for vulvar vestibulitis. *Am J Obstet Gynecol*. 1996;174:1701–1707.

Harlow BL, et al. A population-based assessment of chronic unexplained vulvar pain: Have we underestimated the prevalence of vulvodynia? *J Am Med Women's Assoc*. 2003;58:82–88.

Moyal-Borracco M, et al. 2003 ISSVD terminology and classification of vulvodynia: A historical perspective. *J Repro Med*. 2004;49:772–777.

 MISCELLANEOUS

SYNONYM(S)
- Dysthestic vulvodynia
- Essential vulvodynia
- Vulvar vestibulus syndrome

CLINICAL PEARLS
Women presenting with dyspareunia often benefit from sexual counseling.

ABBREVIATIONS
- CBT—Cognitive-behavioral therapy
- HPV—Human papillomavirus
- HSV—Herpes simplex virus
- VIN—Vulvar intraepithelial neoplasia

CODES
ICD9-CM
- 616.10 Vulvar vestibulitis
- 625.1 Vaginismus
- 625.8 Vulvodynia

 PATIENT TEACHING

- http://www.nva.org (National Vulvodynia Association)
- www.acog.org (American College of Obstetricians and Gynecologists)
- www.issvd.org (International Society for the Study of Vulvovaginal Disease)

Section II
Gynecologic Diseases and Conditions

ACANTHOSIS NIGRICANS

Kristin M. Rager, MD, MPH

 BASICS

DESCRIPTION
AN, symmetrically distributed darkening and thickening of the skin, is a cutaneous marker for insulin resistance. May be benign, which is most commonly related to obesity, or malignant, which is most commonly related to GI adenocarcinoma.

Age-Related Factors
- Low prevalence in children:
  – Prevalence increases with age.
- Malignant acanthosis nigricans (AN) occurs most commonly in those >40 years.

EPIDEMIOLOGY
- Among teens, ~40% of Native Americans, 13% of African American, 6% of Hispanic, and <1% of Caucasians are affected.
- Among obese adults, >50%

RISK FACTORS
- Obesity
- Nicotinic acid use

Genetics
Rarely may occur as an autosomal dominant trait with no obesity, associated endocrinopathies, or congenital abnormalities; may appear at birth or during childhood and is accentuated at puberty

PATHOPHYSIOLOGY
The interaction between excessive amounts of circulating insulin with IGF factor receptors on keratinocytes may lead to the development of papillary hypertrophy, hyperkeratosis, and an increased number of melanocytes in the epidermis.

ASSOCIATED CONDITIONS
- Insulin resistance (common):
  – Idiopathic
  – PCOS
  – Endocrine syndrome type A (HAIR-AN)
  – Endocrine syndrome type B (autoimmune)
  – Diabetes mellitus
- Malignancy (rare)

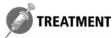 **DIAGNOSIS**

SIGNS AND SYMPTOMS
History
- Benign: Long-standing skin lesions with little progression
- Malignant: Abrupt onset and rapid progression of skin lesions

Review of Systems
- Possible pruritus
- Polydipsia, polyuria (with diabetes)
- Hirsutism, acne, dysfunctional uterine bleeding (with HAIR-AN or PCOS)
- Abdominal pain, weight loss (with malignancy)

Physical Exam
- Brown or hyperpigmented symmetric skin thickening
- Most commonly affects the axilla
- May also involve the flexural areas of the neck and groin, belt line, over dorsal surfaces of fingers, around areolae of breasts and umbilicus, vulva, and other skin folds
- Oral lesions are common in association with malignancy.
- May become leathery, papillomatous, or velvety with time

TESTS
Testing is indicated to seek out the underlying cause.
Labs
- Fasting serum insulin
- Glucose
- Consider workup for PCOS (see topic)

Imaging
- Indicated if concerned about malignancy
- Pelvic US may demonstrate multiple peripheral follicles (>12/ovary) with "string of pearls" sign, but is neither sensitive nor specific for PCOS.

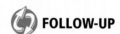 **TREATMENT**

GENERAL MEASURES
Treatment is aimed at correcting the underlying cause.

MEDICATION (DRUGS)
- Insulin sensitizers, such as metformin, may be used to correct underlying insulin resistance.
- There is little evidence that topical treatments yield significant improvement.

SURGERY
No surgical treatment

FOLLOW-UP

DISPOSITION
Issues for Referral
Consider referrals based on underlying conditions.

PROGNOSIS
Depends on underlying conditions

BIBLIOGRAPHY

Fagot-Campagna A, et al. Type 2 diabetes among North American children and adolescents: An epidemiologic review and a public health perspective. *J Pediat*. 2000;136(5):664–672.

Habif. *Clinical Dermatology,* 4th ed. Edinburgh: Mosby; 2004.

Hud JA, et al. Prevalence and significance of acanthosis nigricans in an adult obese population. *Arch Dermatol*. 1992;128(7):941–944.

Inzucchi SE, et al. The prevention of type II diabetes mellitus. *Endocrinol Metabol Clin N Am*. 2005;34(1):199–219.

MISCELLANEOUS

CLINICAL PEARLS
- Usually related to obesity and insulin resistance
- However, in a nonobese patient with rapidly progressing acanthosis nigricans, must consider malignancy.

ABBREVIATIONS
AN—Acanthosis nigricans
HAIR-AN—Hyperandrogenism, insulin resistance, and acanthosis nigricans
IGF—Insulin-like growth factor
PCOS—Polycystic ovary syndrome

CODES

ICD9-CM
701.2 Acanthosis nigricans

PATIENT TEACHING

Patients with obesity should be educated that their AN is weight-related and will therefore improve with weight loss.

PREVENTION
To prevent obesity-related AN, patients should be encouraged to maintain an appropriate weight through healthy eating and regular exercise.

Section II

ADENOMYOSIS

Jamie A. M. Massie, MD
Ruth B. Lathi, MD
Lynn M. Westphal, MD

BASICS

DESCRIPTION
The presence of endometrial glands and stroma within the uterine musculature.

Age-Related Factors
Primarily occurs in women 30–50 years old

EPIDEMIOLOGY
- Incidence difficult to determine as diagnosis based on microscopic examination of uterus and many patients are asymptomatic
- Possibly affects up to 15–20% of women
- Less common in nulliparous women

RISK FACTORS
- Age >30 years
- History of uterine surgery
- History of childbearing, although increasing parity not associated with increased risk of disease

PATHOPHYSIOLOGY
Unknown, but theories include:
- Endomyometrial invagination of the endometrium
- Activation of müllerian rests within uterine musculature

ASSOCIATED CONDITIONS
- Leiomyomas
- Endometriosis
- Endometrial polyps

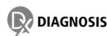

DIAGNOSIS

SIGNS AND SYMPTOMS
History
- Pelvic pain
- Excessively heavy or prolonged menstrual bleeding
- Secondary dysmenorrhea: Pain that begins after the start of menstrual flow
- ~1/3 of affected women are asymptomatic.

Review of Systems
- Lightheadedness/Dizziness
- Primary complaint not GI related
- Denies fever/chills
- Denies anorexia or nausea/vomiting
- Absence of urinary frequency or dysuria
- Absence of purulent vaginal discharge

Physical Exam
- Symmetrically enlarged and boggy uterus
- Uterus soft and tender
- Uterus is freely mobile
- No uterosacral nodularity
- No adnexal masses

TESTS
- Confirmation of clinical diagnosis can only be made by pathologic evaluation of uterus at time of hysterectomy.
- Gross appearance:
  – Diffusely enlarged uterus with thickened myometrium
  – Areas of focal involvement may appear as circumscribed adenomyomas.
- Histologic appearance:
  – Endometrial tissue within the myometrium, at least 1 low-power field from the endomyometrial junction
  – Zone of endometrial hyperplasia surrounds the adenomatous tissue

Labs
Hysterectomy specimen to pathology

Imaging
- TVS shows generally enlarged uterus:
  – Diffusely enlarged uterus with thickened uterine wall
- MRI is diagnostic modality of choice:
  – Areas of decreased signal intensity in affected areas
  – Can usually distinguish between uterine fibroids and adenomyomas (focal areas of adenomyosis)

DIFFERENTIAL DIAGNOSIS
- Uterine leiomyomata
- Endometrial polyps
- Uterine malignancy
- Primary dysmenorrhea
- Endometriosis
- Interstitial cystitis
- Pelvic adhesive disease
- PID
- Ovarian torsion
- Ectopic pregnancy

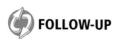

TREATMENT

GENERAL MEASURES
Only definitive treatment for adenomyosis is total hysterectomy, however, treatment is based on patient age and desire for future fertility.

MEDICATION (DRUGS)
- In women who choose to maintain their fertility or have other contraindications to surgical management, medical treatments can be utilized.
- NSAIDs
- OCPs
- Medroxyprogesterone acetate (Depo Provera)
- GnRH agonist:
  – Duration of therapy should be limited to 6 months if used alone.
  – Add-back therapy with progestins or low-dose OCPs may be utilized to minimize bone loss and limit vasomotor symptoms.

SURGERY
- Total hysterectomy, with ovarian conservation:
  – Abdominal or laparoscopic-assisted approach
  – Vaginal hysterectomy indicated if the uterus is not significantly enlarged
- Uterine artery embolization:
  – Endomyometrial ablation is useful in patients who desire conservative surgical management.
  – Laparoscopic myometrial electrocoagulation
  – Excision of adenomyomas

FOLLOW-UP

DISPOSITION
Issues for Referral
- Suspicion of uterine malignancy prior to surgical intervention or at time of planned hysterectomy necessitates referral to a gynecologic oncologist.
- Patients with adenomyosis and infertility should be referred to reproductive endocrinologist or gynecologist with expertise in infertility.

PROGNOSIS

- Hysterectomy provides definitive resolution of symptoms.
- Medical therapies result in short-term improvement, but symptoms often recur after discontinuation of therapy.
- Conservative surgical interventions, such as endomyometrial ablation or uterine artery embolization, may have benefit in patients with bleeding as primary complaint.

PATIENT MONITORING

Patients with severe menorrhagia are at risk of developing anemia:

- Preoperative CBC
- Treatment with a GnRH agonist for 3 months preoperatively can improve hematocrit and decrease need for blood transfusions intraoperatively.
- Routine CBC in symptomatic patients or those reporting persistent heavy bleeding is warranted.

BIBLIOGRAPHY

Duehold M, et al. Magnetic resonance imaging and transvaginal ultrasonography for the diagnosis of adenomyosis. *Fertil Steril*. 2001;76:588–594.

McElin TW, et al. Adenomyosis of the uterus. *Obstet Gynecol Annu*. 1974;3:425–441.

Vercellini P, et al. Adenomyosis at hysterectomy: A study on frequency distribution and patient characteristics. *Human Reprod*. 1995;10:1160–1162.

Wood C. Surgical and medical treatment of adenomyosis. *Hum Reprod Update*. 1998;4(4):323–336.

MISCELLANEOUS

ABBREVIATIONS

- GnRH—Gonadotropin-releasing hormone
- OCP—Oral contraceptive pill
- PID—Pelvic inflammatory disease
- TVS—Transvaginal ultrasound

CODES

ICD9-CM

617.0:

- Adenomyosis
- Endometriosis:
  - Cervix
  - Internal
  - Myometrium

PATIENT TEACHING

Pelvic Pain Patient Education Pamphlet, American College of Obstetricians and Gynecologists, January 2006

Section II

ANDROGEN INSENSITIVITY SYNDROME

F. Ariella Baylson, MD
Frances R. Batzer, MD, MBE

 BASICS

DESCRIPTION
• A genetic disorder of phenotypically appearing females who have XY sex chromosomes and produce normal male levels of testosterone but appear female due to a defect in androgen receptors that prevents the action of circulating androgens.

Age-Related Factors
After completion of puberty, testes should be surgically removed due to an increased risk of neoplasia and malignancy (2–5%).

Pediatric Considerations
Suspect androgen insensitivity syndrome in female infants with inguinal hernias as these may contain partially descended testes.

EPIDEMIOLOGY
• 3rd most common cause of primary amenorrhea (~10%)
• Incidence range of 1 in 13,158–64,200 live births

RISK FACTORS
Family history of similarly affected individuals

Genetics
Genetically transmitted via an X-linked recessive gene most commonly

PATHOPHYSIOLOGY
• Deletion in the gene coding for the androgen receptor
• Genetic absence of intracellular androgen receptors preventing nuclear transport of testosterone
• Testosterone is produced but has no effect due to the cell receptor defect.
• Normal phenotypic male sexual development does not occur, as androgens have no effect.
• Female external genitalia develop but antimüllerian hormone prevents the development of Müllerian duct; uterus, tubes and upper vagina.
• Incomplete forms of androgen insensitivity exist with a spectrum of clinical findings due to enzymatic defects but only account for a small fraction of total cases.

ALERT
Increased risk of neoplasia in intra-abdominal undescended testes. Testes should be removed at the completion of puberty, by the early 20s.

ASSOCIATED CONDITIONS
Primary amenorrhea

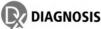 **DIAGNOSIS**

SIGNS AND SYMPTOMS
History
• Absence of menses (primary amenorrhea)
• Normal breast development
• Similarly affected family members
• History of inguinal hernia repair as an infant

Review of Systems
• Primary amenorrhea despite normal breast development
• Lack of axillary and pubic hair

Physical Exam
• Phenotypic appearing female
• Normal external female genitalia
• Blind vaginal pouch
• Absent uterus/cervix
• Scant to absent pubic and axillary hair
• Testes may be located in the abdomen or inguinal area:
  – Inguinal hernias should be evaluated as these may contain testes
• Normal to large female breast development:
  – Tanner stage II breast development; areolae are often pale and underdeveloped

TESTS
• Karyotype analysis will reveal XY sex chromosomes
• Plasma testosterone levels are elevated for female range (in the range of a normal male)
• High plasma levels of LH
• Normal to elevated FSH levels

Imaging
US, CT, MRI may help to identify location of testes and uterine absence.

DIFFERENTIAL DIAGNOSIS
• Müllerian agenesis, also called Mayer-Rokitansky-Kuster-Hauser syndrome, is a congenital absence of the vagina with variable uterine development, normal female endocrine function, and XX karyotype.
• Incomplete androgen insensitivity shows variable effects with clinical findings correlating with amount of functioning androgens.

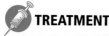 **TREATMENT**

GENERAL MEASURES
• Affected individual usually presents in late teens with primary amenorrhea, having been raised as female. Reinforce female gender identify while educating patient on diagnosis.
• Contrary to past medical thinking, chromosomal sex should not be withheld from the patient.
• Psychological counseling and treatment to aid patients in understanding diagnosis and need for eventual surgery.

MEDICATION (DRUGS)
Estrogen replacement therapy should be started after removal of testes.

SURGERY
• Surgical excision of testes (gonadectomy) should be undertaken on the completion of puberty via laparoscopy or laparotomy
• Localize gonads via imaging prior to surgery

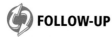 **FOLLOW-UP**

DISPOSITION
Issues for Referral
All patients with this diagnosis should be offered psychological counseling and resources; special considerations to be addressed include infertility, female gender identity

PROGNOSIS
Increased risk of neoplasia in unremoved gonads

BIBLIOGRAPHY

Griffin JE. Androgen resistance—the clinical and molecular spectrum. *N Engl J Med*. 1992;326: 611–618.

Morris JM, et al. The syndrome of testicular feminization in male pseudohermaphrodites. *Am J Obstet Gynecol*. 1953;65:1192–1211.

Speroff L, et al. *Clinical Gynecologic Endocrinology and Infertility*, 7th ed. Philadelphia: Lippincott Williams & Wilkins; 2005.

 MISCELLANEOUS

SYNONYM(S)
Testicular feminization

ABBREVIATIONS
- FSH—Follicle-stimulating hormone
- LH—Luteinizing hormone

CODES

ICD9-CM
259.5 Androgen insensitivity syndrome

 PATIENT TEACHING

Androgen insensitivity Support Group (AISSG) on the web at http://www.medhelp.org/ais/

Section II

ANEMIA

Jennifer B. Hillman, MD
Corinne Lehmann, MD

 BASICS

DESCRIPTION

- Reduction in RBC mass or blood hemoglobin (Hgb) concentration
- Hct is the fractional volume whole blood occupied by RBCs:
  - Expressed as a percent:
    - Normal Hct for adult women is 40.0 +/− 4.0.
  - Hgb is a measure of the concentration of the oxygen-carrying RBC pigment in whole blood:
    - Values may be expressed as grams of Hgb/100 mL of whole blood (g/dL) or per liter of blood (g/L).
    - Normal Hgb for adult women is 13.8 +/− 1.5.
    - WHO criteria for anemia in women defined as Hgb <12.0 g/dL
- RBC count is the number of RBCs contained in a specified volume of whole blood:
  - Expressed as millions of RBCs per μL of whole blood
  - Normal RBC count in adult women is 4.6 +/− 0.5.
- Volume status largely impacts the values for Hgb, Hct, and RBC count because these measures are all concentrations:
  - Dependent on RBC mass and plasma volume
  - Values reduced if RBC mass is decreased and/or if the plasma volume is increased
- Normal ranges not appropriate in all populations
  - At high altitudes Hgb, Hct, and RBC count are higher than for those living at sea level.
  - Hgb values for African Americans are 0.5–1.0 gm/dL lower than those in Caucasians.
- Different forms and types of anemia
- Classified based on underlying etiology:
  - Increased RBC destruction (e.g., hemolytic)
  - Blood loss
  - Decreased RBC production (e.g., bone marrow suppression or failure)
- Classified based on values of the RBC indices:
  - RBC indices include mean corpuscular volume (MCV), mean cell hemoglobin (MCH), and mean corpuscular hemoglobin concentration (MCHC):
    - MCV measured in femtoliters (fL)
  - Microcytic anemia: Decreased RBC indices:
    - MCV <80 fL
  - Normocytic anemia: Normal RBC indices:
    - MCV 80–100 fL
  - Macrocytic anemia: Elevated RBC indices:
    - MCV >100 fL

Age-Related Factors

- Normal values vary based on age in the pediatric population:
  - Use age- and sex-adjusted norms when evaluating a pediatric patient for anemia.
  - In adolescent females, 12–18 years, Hgb and Hct values are similar to those of adult women.

Geriatric Considerations

- Normal ranges may not apply to elderly populations as they are largely based on data from healthy young adults.
- Values for Hgb and Hct are generally lower in the elderly population.

EPIDEMIOLOGY

Prevalence

Prevalence rates vary by type of anemia:

- Worldwide, iron deficiency is the most common form of anemia among women.
- The prevalence among females age 12–>70 years in US ranges from 2–5%.

RISK FACTORS

Iron deficiency anemia:

- Blood loss
- Pregnancy
- Inadequate dietary intake of iron
  - Vegetarian diet
- Rapid growth spurts during adolescence

Genetics

Hereditary anemias and hemoglobinopathies

PATHOPHYSIOLOGY

Increased RBC destruction, decreased production or blood loss

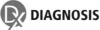 **DIAGNOSIS**

SIGNS AND SYMPTOMS

History

- Signs and symptoms depend on the severity and chronicity of the anemia:
  - Fatigue
  - Pallor
  - Reduced exercise capacity, exertional dyspnea
  - Palpitations
  - Classic findings of iron deficiency:
    - Pica (compulsive eating of nonfood items)
    - Pagophagia (compulsive eating of ice)
- Late stages of untreated and severe anemia may include the following:
  - Lethargy and confusion
  - CHF
  - Angina
  - Arrhythmia
  - Myocardial infarction
- Assess the following:
  - Bleeding from any site:
    - GI tract
    - GU tract
  - Past medical history of disease that would predispose to anemia:
    - Rheumatoid arthritis
    - SLE
    - IBD
    - Previous cancer
    - Medications
    - Peptic ulcer disease
  - Evidence of bone marrow suppression
  - Medications
  - Evidence of hemolysis (RBC destruction):
    - Jaundice
    - Tea-colored urine

Physical Exam

Depends on the stage of anemia at presentation but generally could include any of the following:

- Pallor of palms, nail beds, face, conjunctiva
- Jaundice
- Tachycardia
- Postural hypotension
- Bounding pulses
- Cheilosis (fissures at the corners of mouth)
- Koilonychia (spooning of the fingernails)
- Hepatosplenomegaly
- Lymphadenopathy
- Bone tenderness:
  - Especially over the sternum, in infiltrative diseases
- Petechiae, bruises, ecchymoses

TESTS

Labs

- CBC:
  - Includes Hgb, Hct, RBC indices, WBC
  - Platelet count
  - Thrombocytopenia (<150,000 platelets/μL) in setting of anemia is associated with the following:
    - Hypersplenism
    - TTP
    - Malignancy
    - Sepsis
    - Autoimmune platelet destruction
    - Folate or cobalamin deficiency
- WBC differential:
  - Low WBC is concerning for bone marrow suppression.
  - High WBC may reflect infection, inflammation, or hematologic malignancy.
- Reticulocyte count:
  - High reticulocyte count is more consistent with ongoing hemolysis or blood loss.
  - Low reticulocyte count in setting of stable anemia is consistent with deficient RBC production.
- Review of the peripheral smear may be indicated.
- Evaluation for iron deficiency:
  - Indicated if suspicion of chronic blood loss (e.g. menometrorrhagia, GI bleeding) and microcytic indices (low MCV, low MCH, high RDW):
    - Plasma iron, iron binding capacity, transferrin, transferrin saturation, ferritin
- Evaluation for hemolysis:
  - Consider when rapid decrease in Hgb, jaundice, elevated reticulocyte count, and abnormally shaped RBCs on peripheral smear
    - Plasma LDH, bilirubin concentrations, and haptoglobin
- Bone marrow evaluation:
  - Rarely necessary in common forms of anemia
  - Indicated in cases of pancytopenia and presence of abnormal cells on peripheral smear

DIFFERENTIAL DIAGNOSIS

- Determine if the anemia is microcytic, normocytic, or macrocytic based on the RBC indices:
  - Microcytic:
    - Consider iron deficiency anemia, thalassemias, anemia of chronic disease (typically normocytic, but may be microcytic), sideroblastic anemia, copper deficiency
    - Iron deficiency anemia is the most common form of anemia among adult women.
  - Normocytic:
    - Consider anemia of chronic disease, acute blood loss, bone marrow suppression, chronic renal insufficiency, hypothyroidism
  - Macrocytic:
    - Consider B_{12} or folate deficiency, drug-induced anemia, liver disease, ethanol abuse
    - MCV >115 fL almost exclusively seen in B12 or folic acid deficiency
    - Also consider whether the clinical history is more consistent with hemolysis, blood loss, or decreased RBC production.

Infection

- Serious bacterial or viral infections may result in temporary bone marrow suppression.
- Some infections may result in hemolysis:
  - *Bartonella*, *Babesia*, malaria
- Some infections, acute and chronic, may result in anemia of chronic disease:
  - HIV
- Parasitic infections can contribute to chronic GI blood loss:
  - Predisposition to iron deficiency anemia

Hematologic
Increased RBC destruction/Hemolytic anemias

- Intrinsic RBC defects:
  - Hereditary spherocytosis
  - Hereditary elliptocytosis
  - Glucose-6-Phosphate Dehydrogenase (G6PD) deficiency:
    - Oxidative stress of any kind results in hemolysis of RBCs
    - Triggered by infection, medications, diet
  - Hemoglobinopathies:
    - Sickle cell disease
    - Thalassemias
- TTP:
  - Includes fever, hemolytic anemia, thrombocytopenia, renal abnormality, neurologic symptoms

Decreased RBC production
Bone marrow failure or malfunction:

- Aplastic anemia
- Myelodysplasia
- Iron deficiency anemia
- Anemia of chronic disease

Metabolic/Endocrine
Hypothyroidism

Immunologic
Autoimmune hemolytic anemia

Tumor/Malignancy

- Hematologic malignancy
- GI malignancy:
  - Colon cancer in adults may lead to occult blood loss that may present solely with anemia.

Trauma
Typically leads to acute blood loss:

- Splenic fracture
- Liver laceration

Drugs

- Hydroxyurea
- AZT
- Chemotherapeutic agents

Other/Miscellaneous

- DUB may result in iron deficiency anemia.
- Hypersplenism

 ## TREATMENT

GENERAL MEASURES

- Depends on the underlying etiology for anemia
- Anemia due to blood loss:
  - Find source of bleeding and control losses
  - Restore iron stores as needed
- Anemia due to increased RBC destruction:
  - Determine underlying cause for hemolysis and treat that condition
- Anemia due to decreased RBC production:
  - Evaluate for underlying etiology, particularly work-up for malignancy

MEDICATION (DRUGS)

- Iron deficiency anemia:
  - Iron sulfate 325 mg b.i.d.–t.i.d.:
    - Equivalent to 50–60 mg elemental iron b.i.d.
    - Recommend taking iron supplements with vitamin C to increase absorption
    - May take 10–14 days to see a rise in hemoglobin
- Anemia of chronic disease:
  - Treat underlying disease
  - Use of recombinant erythropoietin controversial
- B_{12} deficiency:
  - B_{12} 1,000 μg IM daily for 1 week, then weekly for 1 month, then monthly
    - May take 2–3 months for resolution of anemia
- Folate deficiency:
  - Folic acid 1 mg/d PO

 ## FOLLOW-UP

DISPOSITION
Issues for Referral

- Drug-induced hemolytic anemia:
  - Stop offending agent
  - Refer or consult a hematologist
- Sickle cell anemia:
  - Supportive care typically with hematologist
- Anemia due to chronic renal insufficiency:
  - Typically managed by nephrologist
  - Recombinant erythropoietin replacement typically prescribed

PATIENT MONITORING

- Iron deficiency anemia:
  - Repeat CBC and reticulocyte count 2–3 weeks after beginning iron therapy
  - Normalization of Hgb typically by 2–3 months
  - Recommend continuing iron therapy for 6 months.
  - Correct underlying cause for iron deficiency, otherwise, anemia is likely to recur.

BIBLIOGRAPHY

Beutler E, et al. *Williams' Hematology*, 6th ed. New York: McGraw-Hill; 2001.

Kasper DL, et al. *Harrison's Principles of Internal Medicine*, 16th ed. New York: McGraw-Hill; 2006.

Ross E. Evaluation and treatment of iron deficiency in adults. *Nutrit Clin Care*. 2002;5:220.

Schrier S. Approach to the adult patient with anemia. Up To Date, Wellesley, MA, 2007.

Weiss G, et al. Anemia of chronic disease. *N Engl J Med*. 2005;352:1011.

 ## MISCELLANEOUS

CLINICAL PEARLS

- Use of iron sulfate turns stools dark and may cause constipation.
- Questions about stool color reveal compliance with iron therapy.
- Consider adding stool softener to treat constipation and improve compliance.

ABBREVIATIONS

- CHF—Congestive heart failure
- DUB—Dysfunctional uterine bleeding
- fL—Femtoliter
- G6PD—Glucose-6-phosphate dehydrogenase
- Hct—Hematocrit
- Hgb—Hemoglobin
- IBD—Inflammatory bowel disease
- MCH—Mean cell hemoglobin
- MCHC—Mean corpuscular hemoglobin concentration
- MCV—Mean corpuscular volume
- RBC—Red blood cell
- SLE—Systemic lupus erythematosus
- TTP—Thrombotic thrombocytopenia purpura
- WBC—White blood count

CODES
ICD9-CM

- 285.9 Anemia, unspecified
- 280.9 Iron deficiency anemia, unspecified

 ## PATIENT TEACHING

PREVENTION

- Intake of a well-balanced diet helps to avoid vitamin deficiencies and iron deficiency.
- Vegetarians should consider regular use of a multivitamin with iron.
- Strict vegans (no dairy, eggs, or meat products) should consider B_{12} replacement and regular use of a multivitamin with iron.

ASHERMAN'S SYNDROME

Philip G. Brooks, MD
Scott P. Serden, MD

 BASICS

DESCRIPTION

- The development of intrauterine adhesions (synechiae) subsequent to some traumatic intervention, and often but not always associated with amenorrhea and reduced fertility
- Categories divided by severity of the occlusion of the endometrial cavity:
  - Minimal: <1/4 of cavity involved; ostia and upper fundus relatively clear
  - Moderate: 1/4–3/4 of cavity involved; upper fundus partially occluded
  - Severe: >3/4 of cavity involved, ostia occluded
- Related Conditions: Amenorrhea; Hypomenorrhea; Postabortal amenorrhea; Postcurettage adhesions

Age-Related Factors

- Asherman syndrome is most common in the reproductive years, as it most often occurs secondary to curettage following abortion or for bleeding subsequent to delivery.
- Prognosis for fertility following treatment is age-related, with younger women having a better prognosis.

EPIDEMIOLOGY

Virtually only occurs in women during their reproductive years.

RISK FACTORS

- Pregnancy:
  - Postpartum bleeding
  - Postabortal bleeding
- Sharp curettage
- Hypoestrogenic state
- Infection/Endometritis
- Congenital uterine anomaly (uterine septum)
- Intrauterine surgery for septum, submucosus myomas, large polyps
- Abdominal metroplasty
- Abdominal myomectomy wherein the cavity is entered
- Repeated pregnancy loss
- Retained portion of placenta, adherent placenta
- Cesarean section wherein the back wall accidentally is caught in the anterior wall suture

PATHOPHYSIOLOGY

- When opposing walls of the endometrium are denuded or damaged by surgical or mechanical trauma, or infections, rapid regrowth of the normal endometrium is inhibited due to the presence of hypoestrogenicity (as with postpartum or postabortal states).
- Agglutination of only endometrial surfaces produces delicate adhesions that are easy to separate.
- Scar formation between myometrial surfaces is more avascular and prevents endometrial regrowth, resulting in dense, fibrous, and more extensive scar formation, especially in the presence of infection.
- Similarly, intrauterine surgery using scissors or with energy sources (electrosurgery, laser surgery, etc.) can result in scarring between traumatized opposing surfaces.

ASSOCIATED CONDITIONS

- Secondary amenorrhea
- Previous gynecologic surgery
- Dysmenorrhea
- Secondary infertility
- Pelvic tuberculosis

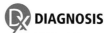 **DIAGNOSIS**

SIGNS AND SYMPTOMS

- 1st symptom usually is amenorrhea or hypomenorrhea following a pregnancy, either a term pregnancy or a miscarriage or termination, especially where sharp curettage was performed for subsequent bleeding.
- Dysmenorrhea may occur in patients wherein pockets of blood in the uterus have lost continuity with the endometrial and cervical canals.
- Unexplained infertility may occur in patients with a history of uterine surgery, even with normal menstrual patterns.
- Failure to have withdrawal bleeding after hormonal treatment

History

- A high degree of suspicion of intrauterine adhesions should be entertained in patients with menstrual abnormalities or infertility following intrauterine instrumentation of any type, especially when such instrumentation occurred after a pregnancy.
- Compare menstrual flow characteristics from before the instrumentation to those following it.
- Review of the type of instrumentation that occurred (review operative note), sharp curettage being the most dangerous in predisposing adhesion formation.
- Careful history to rule out systemic endocrine problems that can interfere with ovulation and menstruation (eating disorders, inappropriate lactation, excess exercising, hypothyroidism, androgen excess, etc.)

Physical Exam

- No physical exam findings are suspicious for or diagnostic of intrauterine adhesions.
- General physical and bimanual exams to rule out pregnancy or ovarian enlargement.

TESTS

Labs

- No laboratory findings are suggestive or diagnostic of intrauterine adhesions.
- Because of the disruption of normal menstrual pattern, urine or blood hCG may be useful to rule out pregnancy.
- Blood tests to rule out androgen excess, thyroid dysfunction, hypopituitarism, etc.

Imaging

- Transabdominal or transvaginal ultrasound, with or without saline infusion, can delineate the presence or absence of an endometrial stripe, the area of obliteration, and the area of blood accumulation, if any.
- Hysterography can show the location of the obstruction or the presence and size of synechiae.
- MRI could be used to delineate the contour and defects of the endometrial cavity, although this is not the preferred imaging modality because of expense.
- Hysteroscopy:
  - Office or hospital outpatient diagnostic hysteroscopy may be definitive to detect and define the extent of synechiae.

DIFFERENTIAL DIAGNOSIS

- Other causes of acquired amenorrhea and hypomenorrhea:
  - Pregnancy
  - Endocrine dysfunction
  - Menopause
- Other causes of intrauterine defects seen on imaging:
  - Submucous myomas
  - Endometrial polyps
  - Retained placental fragments
  - Intrauterine foreign bodies (IUD fragments, etc.)

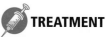 **TREATMENT**

GENERAL MEASURES

- The primary treatment of uterine synechiae is surgical.
- Scattered reports of transabdominal bivalving of the uterus in an attempt to delineate and reconstruct the endometrial cavity in severe cases have reported only minimal success.
- Operative hysteroscopy with mechanical instrumentation (scissors, flexible or rigid) is the preferred method of repair, using laparoscopic guidance in severe cases, to avoid uterine perforation.
- The goals are:
  - To restore the endometrial architecture to normal.
  - To provide continuity of the tubal lumen into the endometrial cavity for future reproduction.
  - To prevent recurrent scarring.
  - To restore normal menstruation, if possible.
  - In the case of secondary infertility, to all establishment of pregnancy.

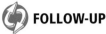

MEDICATION (DRUGS)

- No medical treatment is capable of reducing or destroying uterine adhesions.
- High-dose estrogen therapy, with sequential progesterone for withdrawal, is advocated as prevention of adhesions, to be instituted immediately after instrumentation (e.g., sharp curettage) for postpartum or postabortal bleeding, and after hysteroscopic repair of adhesions, especially when dense or extensive:
  – Conjugated estrogens 2.5 mg, once or twice daily for 2–3 cycles.
  – Medroxyprogesterone 10 mg/d 20–28 of each cycle to prevent endometrial hyperplasia.
  – Consider prophylactic antibiotics on the day of hysteroscopic surgery.

SURGERY

- Mechanical interference with adhesion reformation is important to reduce the risk of regrowth of adhesions after surgical repair:
  – Sound the uterine cavity of 1–2 weeks after hysteroscopic incision.
  – Immediately insert a Foley catheter or silastic balloon into the endometrial cavity after the surgery; prescribe antibiotics (doxycycline 100 mg b.i.d.); remove balloon after 5–7 days.
  – Immediately insert an IUD (Lippes Loop preferred over copper- or progesterone-containing IUDs due to larger surface area and lack of chemical influence on healing).

FOLLOW-UP

DISPOSITION

- Monitor menstrual function
- Menstrual calendar to note timing and quality of flow

PROGNOSIS

Reproductive outcome is related to severity of the adhesions, varying from 94% term pregnancies after resection of mild adhesion to 79% after repair of severe adhesions.

PATIENT MONITORING

Starting in the 3rd or 4th cycle after surgery and repeat periodically, depending on the resumption and quality of menses:

- Hysteroscopy, office or outpatient
- Saline-infusion sonography
- Hysterography

BIBLIOGRAPHY

March CM, et al. Hysteroscopic management of intrauterine adhesions. *Am J Obstet Gynecol*. 1978;130:653.

Sugimoto O. Diagnostic and therapeutic hysteroscopy for traumatic intrauterine adhesions. *Am J Obstet Gynecol*. 1978;131:539.

Valle RF, et al. Intrauterine adhesions: Hysteroscopic diagnosis, classification, treatment, and reproductive outcome. *Am J Obstet Gynecol*. 1998;158:1459.

MISCELLANEOUS

SYNONYM(S)

- Intrauterine adhesions
- Intrauterine synechiae

CLINICAL PEARLS

- Uterine curettage, especially for postpartum or postabortal bleeding, is at high risk for the development of Asherman syndrome.
- If bleeding requires intervention, prevention of adhesions may occur with the use of blunt or suction curettage only, the prophylactic use of antibiotics, and cyclic estrogen and progesterone treatment.
- Operative hysteroscopy is the best method of treatment for this condition.

ABBREVIATION

hCG—Human chorionic gonadotropin

CODES

ICD9-CM

- 621.5 Asherman's syndrome
- 621.5 Intrauterine adhesions
- 626.0 Amenorrhea

PATIENT TEACHING

ACOG Patient Education Pamphlet: Asherman's syndrome available at http://www.acog.org

Section II

BOWEL OBSTRUCTION

John D. Scott, MD
Michael S. Nussbaum, MD

 BASICS

DESCRIPTION
- Obstruction of the normal flow of intestinal contents due to mechanical or nonmechanical causes
- Obstruction leads to rapid increase in intraluminal enteric bacteria levels.
- Distended bowel becomes progressively more edematous and potentially ischemic.
- Closed-loop bowel obstructions in which the intestine is obstructed both proximally and distally, have a high incidence of strangulation, ischemia, and perforation.

ETIOLOGY
- Small bowel obstruction (SBO):
  - 65–75% are caused by postoperative adhesions
  - Adhesion related bowel obstructions:
    - 20% within 1 month of surgery
    - 30% within 1 year
    - 50% after 1 year
  - Other causes:
    - Neoplasms (20%)
    - Hernias (10%)
    - Crohn's disease (5%)
- Large bowel obstruction (LBO):
  - Mechanical causes:
    - Colon cancer (90%)
    - Volvulus (5%) caused by axial twisting of the bowel
    - Diverticular disease (3%)
  - Adynamic causes:
    - Colonic pseudo-obstruction (Ogilvie syndrome) is an adynamic ileus related to autonomic dysfunction and electrolyte abnormalities.

RISK FACTORS
- Previous abdominal surgery
- Hernias
- Known abdominal neoplasms
- Diverticular disease
- IBD (ulcerative colitis or Crohn's disease)
- Radiation treatment

PATHOPHYSIOLOGY
- Early:
  - Intestinal motility and contractility increase in an effort to propel enteric contents past point of obstruction.
  - As the obstruction continues, the intestine fatigues and dilates.
  - Diarrhea is common during this phase.
- Late effects:
  - As the bowel dilates, 3rd space volume losses occur.
  - Vomiting can cause hypochloremia, hypokalemia, and metabolic acidosis.
  - Increased intraluminal pressure causes decreased blood flow to affected bowel, which can lead to bowel ischemia and perforation.
  - Bacterial flora increases dramatically in obstructed bowel, increasing the risk of bacterial translocation across the bowel wall.

DIAGNOSIS

SIGNS AND SYMPTOMS
History
- Varies widely from nonspecific abdominal pain to peritoneal signs
- Most common complaints:
  - Pain
  - Nausea/Vomiting
  - Distention
  - Obstipation
  - Mass
  - Rectal bleeding

ALERT
The presence of blood in the stool indicates mucosal injury due to inflammation, cancer, or ischemia.

Physical Exam
- Vital signs:
  - Tachycardia and hypotension secondary to volume depletion
  - Fevers are associated with perforation or strangulation of bowel
- Abdominal exam:
  - Note the presence of scars on abdomen
  - Diffuse abdominal tenderness
  - Abdominal distention
  - Hyperactive and high-pitched bowel sounds
  - Peritoneal signs and rebound tenderness suggest a perforation has occurred.
  - Abdominal mass
- Hernia exam:
  - Examine for inguinal, femoral, and ventral hernias
  - Howship-Romberg sign (pain extending down medial thigh with abduction, extension, or internal rotation of the knee) for obturator hernia
- Rectal exam:
  - Presence of blood
  - Rectal mass
  - Stool present in rectal vault

TESTS
Labs
- CBC:
  - Leukocytosis is common, especially after an intestinal perforation has occurred.
- Electrolytes:
  - Hypokalemia
  - Hypochloremic metabolic acidosis
  - Prerenal azotemia
  - Electrolyte abnormalities are a potential cause for Ogilvie syndrome
- Preoperative labs:
  - Type/Crossmatch blood
  - EKG in women over 50 with risk factors

Imaging
- Plain film imaging:
  - SBO:
    - Wide range from massively dilated small bowel to small areas of small bowel air–fluid levels
    - Diagnosed as partial or complete
  - LBO:
    - Absence of rectal air with a dilated proximal colon suggests the presence of an obstructing lesion
    - Cecal volvulus: "Comma" sign
    - Cecal distention of >10–14 cm indicates pending perforation.
    - Sigmoid volvulus: "Omega" or "bent inner tube" sign

ALERT
Free air under the diaphragm on an upright chest plain film in the absence of recent (within 7–14 days) intra-abdominal surgery indicates an intestinal perforation has occurred. However, even within this time period, free air is a concern.

- CT of the abdomen and pelvis with oral, intravenous, and rectal contrast:
  - SBO:
    - Sensitivity and specificity of 90%
    - Can help define transition zone at point of obstruction
    - Detects hernias and mass lesions
    - Recognizes features of strangulation
  - LBO:
    - Can detect mass lesions
    - Useful adjunct for staging purposes
- Upper GI/small bowel follow-through:
  - Helpful in identifying the location of the obstruction
  - Disadvantage: Slow transit time in obstructed bowel
- Retrograde barium or water-soluble contrast studies:
  - Differentiate between obstruction from pseudo-obstruction
  - Cancer yields an "apple core" lesion.
  - Sigmoid volvulus reveals a "birds beak."

ALERT
Contrast enemas with barium are contraindicated with suspected perforation or peritonitis.

DIFFERENTIAL DIAGNOSIS
- Adynamic ileus
- Pseudo-obstruction (Ogilvie disease)
- Constipation/Obstipation
- Perforated peptic ulcer
- Diverticulitis
- Appendicitis
- Abdominal aortic aneurysm
- Pancreatitis
- Gallstone ileus
- Cholecystitis
- Colitis
- Acute mesenteric ischemia
- Uremia

TREATMENT

GENERAL MEASURES
- Fluid resuscitation:
  – Isotonic fluid replacement
  – Normal saline with potassium supplementation
  – May require central venous monitoring
- Correction of electrolyte abnormalities:
  – Patient with vomiting will be hypokalemic, hypochloremic, and demonstrate a metabolic alkalosis.
- Foley catheter:
  – Urine output as an index of fluid resuscitation
- Nasogastric tube:
  – Decompress stomach
  – Often brings immediate relief
  – Protects from aspiration
- Bowel rest:
  – NPO
- Antiemetics and analgesia:
  – Narcotics are necessary if patient is going to require an operation.
  – If patient is being observed, narcotics are discouraged to allow for accurate serial exams.
- Antibiotics:
  – Preoperative antibiotics are indicated in all patients for prophylaxis against wound infections.

MEDICATION (DRUGS)
- Cefazolin 1–2 g IV q8h and metronidazole 500 mg IV q8h
- Clindamycin 450–900 mg IV q6h and gentamicin 3 mg/kg IV q8h
- Hydromorphone 1–2 mg IV q2–4h p.r.n.
- Morphine sulfate 2.5–10 mg/dose IV/IM/SC q2–6h p.r.n.
- Odansetron (Zofran) 4 mg IV q4h p.r.n.
- Promethezine (Phenergan) 12.5–25.0 mg IV/IM/SC q6h p.r.n.
- Compazine 10 mg IV/IM/SC q6h p.r.n.

SURGERY
Low-grade partial bowel obstruction:
- Patients may be treated with tube decompression and resuscitation alone.
- 60–85% of partial bowel obstruction resolve without operative intervention.
- Serial abdominal exams are mandatory.

ALERT
- Clinical deterioration or increasing distension requires operative exploration:
- Virgin abdomen:
  – In patients who have no history of abdominal surgery, bowel obstructions can be due to malignancy or intussusception.
  – Surgical treatment is almost always indicated.
- Sigmoid volvulus:
  – High rate of perforation in elderly females
  – Requires decompression via rigid sigmoidoscopy and placement of rectal tube
  – After bowel preparation, a sigmoid colectomy is indicated to prevent recurrence.
  – Hartmann procedure (proximal colostomy) in face of perforation or emergency
- Complete bowel obstruction:
  – When associated with leukocytosis, fever, tachycardia, and peritoneal signs: Emergent laparotomy

ALERT
Patients with complete bowel obstructions require immediate attention due to risk of strangulation and perforation:
- Obstruction due to tumor requires prompt surgical evaluation.

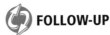 **FOLLOW-UP**

DISPOSITION
- All patients with suspected bowel obstructions should be admitted for observation or definitive surgical treatment.
- After a period of observation, patients with partial bowel obstructions can be safely discharged after return of bowel function, toleration of diet, and resolution of abdominal pain.

Issues for Referral
The general gynecologist may consider consultation with a general surgeon or gynecologic oncologist.

PROGNOSIS
- A variety of etiologies exist for partial and complete bowel obstructions, each with its own set of morbidity and mortality data depending on the condition of the patient and the nature and location of the offending lesion.
- If unrecognized, a complete bowel obstruction leading to perforation is associated with a high morbidity and mortality rate.

PATIENT MONITORING
- Elderly patients often present with hypovolemia due to fluid losses associated with diarrhea and vomiting and require close monitoring of fluid status.
- Appropriate cardiac monitoring is required if patients have a history of cardiac disease.

BIBLIOGRAPHY

Al-sunaidi M, et al. Adhesion-related bowel obstruction after hysterectomy for benign conditions. *Obstet Gynecol.* 2006;108(5):1162–1166.

Baradi H, et al. Large bowel obstruction. In Cameron ed. *Current Surgical Therapy*, 8th ed. Philadelphia: Elsevier; 2004;173–176.

Dayton MT. Small bowel obstruction. In Cameron ed. *Current Surgical Therapy*, 8th ed. Philadelphia: Elsevier; 2004;105–110.

Evers BM. Small intestine. In Townsend ed. *Sabiston Textbook of Surgery*, 17th ed. Saint Louis: Saunders; 2004.

Hayanga AJ, et al. Current management of small bowel obstruction. *Adv Surg.* 2005;39:1–33.

Lyon C, et al. Diagnosis of acute abdominal pain in older patients. *Am Fam Physician.* 2006;74(9): 1537–1544.

 MISCELLANEOUS

CLINICAL PEARLS
Keep in mind that an unrecognized bowel obstruction leading to perforation has a high morbidity and mortality rate.

ABBREVIATIONS
- IBD—Inflammatory bowel disease
- LBO—Large bowel obstruction
- SBO—Small bowel obstruction

CODES

ICD9-CM
- 552.8 Hernia with obstruction
- 552.21 Incisional hernia with obstruction
- 560.2 Volvulus
- 560 Intestinal obstruction
- 787.5 Abnormal bowel sounds

PATIENT TEACHING

Patients who have had abdominal surgery should be made aware of the signs and symptoms of bowel obstruction and seek prompt medical attention if they occur.

PREVENTION
A variety of gels, liquids and drugs have been employed to minimize postoperative adhesion formation with minimum success. Hyaluronic acid and carboxymethylcellulose absorbable barriers have been shown to decrease adhesion formation, but there is no substantive data that demonstrate a decrease in bowel obstruction rates.

BREAST CANCER

Elizabeth A. Shaughnessy, MD, PhD
Kelly McLean, MD

BASICS

DESCRIPTION
Most frequent noncutaneous cancer in women; invasive ductal carcinoma is most frequent.

Age-Related Factors
Leading cause of death in women, ages 30–70

Staging
- Primary tumor (T):
  - Tis if *in situ*, including Paget
  - T for invasive: Notes size and relation to skin or chest wall:
    - T1 ($\leq$2 cm)
    - T2 (>2 cm and $\leq$5 cm)
    - T3 (>5 cm)
    - T4 (with extension to chest or skin)
- Regional lymph nodes (N):
  - N0 denotes no regional nodal metastasis
    - Subtyped if sentinel node RT-PCR +/−, or staining by immunohistochemistry +/−
  - N1 denotes movable ipsilateral axillary nodal metastases
  - N2 denotes fixed axillary lymph nodes, or enlarged internal mammary nodes
  - N3 denotes infraclavicular, supraclavicular, or combined axillary/internal mammary nodes
- Distant metastasis (M):
  - Presence or absence (M1 or M0)

EPIDEMIOLOGY
- Average age is 61 years.
- Less frequent in women of African descent or Latinas; Asian risk rising, both native and migrant
- Lifetime risk is 1 in 7.
- Caucasian women: 115 cases/100,000 a year
- Other races: 50–101 cases/100,000 a year; African American > Asian > Latina > Native American

RISK FACTORS
- Early onset menarche <12
- Late menopause >54
- Delayed 1st full-term pregnancy after 30
- Nulliparity
- History of breast biopsy
- Excessive alcohol consumption, >20 g/d
- Use of HT for >4 years, especially combined estrogen+progestin
- Smoking influence is complex:
  - Increased with brief premenopausal use
  - Decreased with prolonged, heavy use
- Family history, maternal or paternal, with strong influence if 2 1st-degree relatives
- Personal history of breast cancer
- History of mantle radiation for Hodgkin lymphoma
- History of atypical ductal hyperplasia or lobular neoplasia (atypical lobular hyperplasia/ lobular carcinoma in situ [LCIS]) on biopsy
- BRCA1, BRCA2, or p53 mutation

- *No demonstrated risk* with implants, AIDS/organ transplants, electromagnetic fields, abortion, low-dose oral contraceptives
- Protective factors include breast-feeding >12 months, > parity, regular physical exercise

Genetics
- Genetic syndromes account for only 10–15%:
  - BRCA1 and 2 mutations constitute breast-ovarian cancer syndrome, associated with nearly 80–85% of hereditary breast cancers
  - Lifetime genetic penetrance up to 80% (BRCA1) and 31–60% (BRCA2):
    - BRCA1/2 ~40% lifetime risk ovarian cancer
  - The prevalence BRCA1/2 founder mutations in the Ashkenazi Jewish (AJ) population ~2% (1 in 47 women)
  - Early-onset breast cancer (under age 46 carries 3–13% for a BRCA1/2 mutation:
    - Up to 30% for those of AJ heritage
  - Only 45% of mutation carriers have family history of breast cancer.
- Cowden syndrome, Li-Fraumeni syndrome, ataxia-telangiectasia, and Peutz-Jeghers syndrome, CHEK2 mutation account for the remaining 15–20% genetic mutations
- A family history may constitute a genetic syndrome: Bilateral breast cancer, males with breast cancer, breast and/or ovary cancers, prostate cancer, melanoma, colon cancer, pancreas or stomach cancer, lymphoma
- Genetic inheritance may be obscured in families with few females and mutations inherited through the paternal lineage.

PATHOPHYSIOLOGY
- Phenotypic paradigm describes normal ductal epithelium with progression to hyperplasia, to atypical hyperplasia, to ductal carcinoma in situ (DCIS), and later to invasive carcinoma:
  - This does not fit all cancers.
- Research supports disease arising from different cell types (luminal A or B cells, or myoepithelial cells) with progression enhanced by stromal cell influences.
- Changes predisposing to sporadic breast cancer are felt to occur during puberty.
- Metabolic regulation likely plays a crucial role, influenced by diet and genetics.

DIAGNOSIS

SIGNS AND SYMPTOMS
History
- Painless or tender persistent breast mass
- Unilateral nipple inversion, discharge, itching
- Breast cellulitis that fails to respond/resolve
- Symptoms of systemic disease: Bone pain, cough or shortness of breath, epigastric discomfort or nausea, rarely headaches
- Family history of breast and ovary cancers
- Ethnicity: Ashkenazi Jewish, Scandinavian

Physical Exam
- Breast mass or asymmetric breast thickening:
  - Note if fixation to skin or chest wall
- Nipple thickening or scaling
- Spontaneous or elicited nipple discharge
- Nipple inversion
- Skin edema (peau d'orange), possible leather-like texture (en cuirasse changes)
- Regional lymphadenopathy: Axillary, neck, or supraclavicular
- Decreased breath sounds, dullness to percussion, with pleural effusion in advanced disease
- Hepatomegaly, in advanced disease

TESTS
Labs
Serum labs (after diagnosis):
- CBC, liver function tests

Imaging
- Diagnostic mammogram to confirm findings:
  - Architectural distortion or spiculated density
  - Lobulated or indistinct mass
  - Microcalcifications: Clustered, pleomorphic, or casting
- US of palpable or imaged mass:
  - Complex cyst needs biopsy
  - Simple cyst does not need biopsy
  - Mass with mixed echogenicity needs biopsy
- Breast MRI if exam suspicious, and either:
  - Imaging nondiagnostic
  - Dense mammogram
  - Strong family history
- Staging tests (after diagnosis), if T3 or T4:
  - Chest CT or chest x-ray
  - Bone scan
  - Abdominal/Pelvic CT

DIFFERENTIAL DIAGNOSIS
- For mass:
  - Fibroadenoma
  - Cyst
  - Radial scar (lobular malformation)
  - Mastitis
  - Fibrocystic changes
- For calcifications:
  - Sclerosing adenosis
  - Typical or atypical ductal hyperplasia

TREATMENT

GENERAL MEASURES
- Physical therapy postoperatively:
  - Massage and compression sleeve are effective in controlling lymphedema.
  - ROM and strength exercises for shoulder, if axillary node dissection

SPECIAL THERAPY
Complementary and Alternative Therapies
Support groups are linked to improve survival. The mind–body connection continues to be explored. Cognition and sexuality issues are under study.

MEDICATION (DRUGS)

- Chemotherapy
- Neoadjuvant, if chemotherapy given prior to surgery:
  - May allow for breast conservation; indicates in vivo sensitivity
  - If chest/skin fixation, inflammatory changes (skin erythema, peau d'orange)
  - Mainstay of metastatic disease; subsequent surgery may follow if highly responsive
- Adjuvant chemotherapy given after surgery if tumor >1 cm, nodal involvement, if poor prognostic indicators. Administered before radiation.
- First-line regimens:
  - AC (Adriamycin + Cytoxan):
    ○ Unless decreased cardiac function
  - CMF (Cytoxan, methotrexate and 5-fluoro-uracil) may also be used.
  - Taxane to follow if high risk of recurrence
- Endocrine therapy × 5 years for all ER+ cancers:
  - Premenopausal: Tamoxifen
  - Postmenopausal: Aromatase inhibitor or tamoxifen
- Adjuvant monoclonal antibody Herceptin if HER-2 overexpressed

SURGERY

- Breast surgery is necessary for invasive carcinoma, DCIS, or cystosarcoma phyllodes.
- Axillary assessment is necessary in invasive carcinoma.
- Breast conservation:
  - Also called lumpectomy, segmentectomy, partial mastectomy, quandrantectomy, wide local excision.
  - Neoadjuvant chemotherapy may shrink a tumor, enabling conservation in 30%.
  - Candidates must have focal or multifocal (1 quadrant) disease.
  - Multicentric disease not a candidate
  - Previous whole-breast radiation (i.e., mantle radiation for Hodgkin lymphoma) precludes breast conservation.
  - Breast conservation includes resection of the cancer with a surrounding margin of normal tissue.
- Mastectomy:
  - Can be applied to large/small tumors, multicentric disease, or if prior breast radiation
  - Often chosen by young patient with a family history of breast cancer:
    ○ Possibly with contralateral prophylactic mastectomy
  - Skin-sparing mastectomy, in conjunction with immediate reconstruction, is oncologically safe for small (<5 cm) tumors with no skin or chest wall involvement, with best cosmesis.
  - Immediate reconstruction usually delayed in patients needing chest wall radiation.
- Axillary assessment:
  - Sentinel node biopsy: A technique of labeling the "gatekeeper" node(s) before resection; a tool for determining the extent of axillary surgery.
    ○ Technetium[99] sulfur colloid and/or isosulfan blue dye, injected periareolar, around cancer, or in dermis superficial to cancer. After massage, agents are tracked to node(s).
    ○ If negative for cancer, <5% false negative. If positive, ~40% chance of additional nodal involvement, thus proceed to axillary node dissection.

- ○ 3% of patients with no dye migration get full axillary node dissection (no sentinel node).
- ○ Intraoperative testing may be performed and will detect ~70% of positive nodes, but has a false positive rate of 4%.
  - Axillary node dissection, excision of axillary lymph nodes deep and lateral to the pectoralis minor muscle, done IF:
    ○ Positive node(s) by sentinel node biopsy or prior FNA cytology
    ○ Nodes suspicious on exam
- Radiotherapy:
  - Follows breast conservation to reduce risk of local recurrence. Whole-breast external beam is the standard, delivered over 5–6 weeks.
    ○ New protocols of partial breast radiation
    ○ Elderly with good prognostic factors may be considered for observation (<1 cm, ER+)
  - Postmastectomy radiotherapy if high risk of chest wall recurrence (tumor >5 cm, >4 positive nodes, positive chest margin)

FOLLOW-UP

- Examination every 3–6 months for 5 years, if asymptomatic
- New baseline mammogram in 3–6 months
- No strong data supports testing for distant disease if asymptomatic; often checked in high-risk patients.
- Complications:
  - Surgery: Neurogenic pain, lymphedema, seroma
  - Systemic therapies: Hot flushes, vaginal discharge, neutropenic fever, bone pain, hand-foot syndrome, leukemia
  - Radiation: Scarring and tissue retraction, moist desquamation, ischemia, radionecrosis
  - Disease process: ~80% of all recurrences in 1st 2 years after diagnosis

DISPOSITION

Admission criteria (surgery is usually outpatient, unless drain included):

- Mastectomy and/or axillary node dissection may require 24–48-hour stay.
- Chemotherapy, seldom radiotherapy, complications
- Shortness of breath or disabling pain with metastatic disease

Issues for Referral

Palpable mass, even if normal mammography

PROGNOSIS

Prognosis is best reflected by stage:

- Stage I treated with the standard of care has up to 95% survival over 10 years.
- Among all resected patients, an average 85% 10-year survival.
- Patients with complete pathologic response after neoadjuvant treatment have improved survival for their stage at diagnosis.

BIBLIOGRAPHY

Cady B, et al. Mammographic screening: No longer controversial. Am J Clin Oncol. 2005;28:1–4.

Fisher B, et al. Tamoxifen for prevention of breast cancer: Report of the National Surgical Adjuvant Breast and Bowel Project P-1 Study. J Natl Cancer Inst. 1998;90:1371–1388.

Hartmann LC, et al. Efficacy of bilateral prophylactic mastectomy in women with a family history of breast cancer. N Engl J Med. 1999;340:77–84.

Hughes KS, et al. Lumpectomy plus tamoxifen with or without radiation in women 70 years of age or older with early breast cancer. N Engl J Med. 2004; 351(10):963–970.

Malone KE, et al. BRCA1 mutations and breast cancer in the general population: Analyses in women before age 35 years and in women before age 45 years with first-degree family history. JAMA. 1998;279: 922–929.

Singletary SE, et al., eds. Advanced Therapy of Breast Disease, 2nd ed. Ontario: BC Decker; 2004.

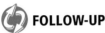

MISCELLANEOUS

CLINICAL PEARLS

- Annual breast cancer screening of women >40, a mammogram with clinical breast exam, most effectively reduces breast cancer mortality
- Breast conservation and mastectomy have equivalent survival; local recurrence less with mastectomy.
- Sentinel node biopsy is an accurate tool for the assessment of the axilla in early breast cancer.
- Neoadjuvant chemotherapy can improve chances for successful breast conservation.
- Treatment is usually multidisciplinary.

ABBREVIATIONS

- ER—Estrogen receptor
- DCIS—Ductal carcinoma in situ
- FNA—Fine needle aspiration
- HT—Hormone therapy
- LCIS—Lobular carcinoma in situ
- ROM—Range of motion

CODES

ICD9-CM

- 174.9 Breast cancer
- 233.0 DCIS
- 793.0 Abnormal mammogram
- v16.3 Family history breast cancer
- v10.3 Personal history breast cancer

PATIENT TEACHING

PREVENTION

- Tamoxifen and raloxifene reduce incidence of invasive breast cancer in NSABP P-1 and P-2 trials in high-risk women.
- Prophylactic mastectomy reduces risk by >90%.

BREAST FIBROADENOMA AND OTHER BENIGN BREAST MASSES

Donald E. Greydanus, MD
Artenmis K. Tsitsika, MD, PhD

 BASICS

DESCRIPTION
- Fibroadenoma usually presents as a rubbery, nontender breast mass that is encapsulated:
  - Typically 1–2 cm at discovery, may enlarge, up to 10–15 cm
  - Located anywhere in the breast tissue, often in upper, outer quadrants.
  - May be irregular or oval, sometimes with a hard consistency
  - No nipple discharge
  - 10–25% bilateral or multiple lesions: Fibroadenomatosis
- Associated conditions: Benign breast disease; Breast cancer (see chapter); Fibrocystic change (see Fibrocystic Breast Changes); Papilloma (see also: Breast Signs and Symptoms: Breast Mass); Phyllodes tumor

Age-Related Factors
Fibroadenoma is the most common benign palpable breast lesion of adolescents and young adults to age 25.

EPIDEMIOLOGY
- Incidence of breast mass in adolescent female: 3–5%
- Fibroadenoma represents 70–95% of breast biopsies in adolescent and young adult age group.
- Usually found in late adolescence with average age of 17 years

RISK FACTORS
- Menarche
- Late adolescence through mid-20s
- African American
- Early adolescence for giant fibroadenoma

Genetics
Not well established for this age group:
- Research has implicated chromosomes 16, 18, and 21.

PATHOPHYSIOLOGY
- Fibroadenoma is a proliferative, fibroepithelial breast lesion that is estrogen-sensitive and develops from breast lobules and stroma during adolescence.
- Estrogen receptors are found in this benign tumor.
- A number of histologic variants are found, although the typical appearance is similar to the histology of male gynecomastia and virginal hypertrophy: Fibrous stroma with elongated ducts.
- In situ cancer cells are infrequently found (2.9%), mainly in adult females.

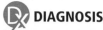 **DIAGNOSIS**

SIGNS AND SYMPTOMS
History
- Painless breast mass, slowly increasing in size over weeks to months
- Nipple discharge not noted
- Mass that doubles in size in 3–6 months suggests giant fibroadenoma.
- Cystic lesions that change with menstrual cycles suggest fibrocystic change.
- Painful mass developing during pregnancy or lactation suggests mastitis.

Physical Exam
- Rubbery mass typically from 0.5–2 cm; rarely to 10–15 cm
- Infrequently hard, oval, or irregular
- Multiple or bilateral lesions up to 25%, termed fibroadenomatosis
- Rare large lesions may have malignancy-like state with peau d'orange skin: Erythema, and enlarged veins overlying the mass.

TESTS
Imaging
- US (fibroadenoma with hypovascular appearance)
- Mammography not recommended in young women due to dense breast tissue in adolescents, unnecessary radiation, and rarity of malignancy.
- Fine needle aspiration (FNA) if diagnosis unclear
- Excisional biopsy if FNA cytologically atypical

DIFFERENTIAL DIAGNOSIS
Infection
Mastitis +/− abscess

Tumor/Malignancy
- Giant fibroadenoma (benign)
- Cystosarcoma phyllodes (phyllodes tumor)
- Adenocarcinoma

Trauma
- Fat necrosis
- Mondor disease (superficial thrombophlebitis of mammary veins)

Other/Miscellaneous
- Hyperplasia (unilateral)
- Breast cyst
- Lipoma
- Intraductal papilloma
- Hemangioma
- Lymphadenopathy
- Skin lesion
- Fat necrosis
- Sclerosis adenosis
- Ductal ectasia

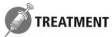 **TREATMENT**

GENERAL MEASURES
Observation and repeat examination to assess growth

MEDICATION (DRUGS)
- Medication is not of benefit
- Tamoxifen reported to be of some benefit in adult women; more research is needed.

SURGERY
- Criteria:
  - Large masses
  - Rapidly growing
  - Breast deforming or causing cosmetic defects seriously affecting the adolescent's self esteem
  - FNA cytology atypia
- Excisional biopsy for histologic identification or removal of the mass
- Mass should be removed before becoming too large, causing compression of adjacent normal tissue, overlying skin ulcerations (especially noted with a giant fibroadenoma), and need for 2nd procedure for skin closure and nipple elevation.
- If multiple tumors are present, remove the largest lesion to establish a diagnosis and prevent breast deformity.
- Minimally invasive alternatives reported in the literature:
  - Percutaneous radiofrequency-assisted excision
  - Cryotherapy

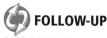 **FOLLOW-UP**

DISPOSITION
Issues for Referral
Lesions meeting criteria for surgery

PROGNOSIS
Disease prognosis variants:
- Spontaneous decrease in size
- Dormant/Stable condition
- Slow proliferation
- Rapid enlargement
- Cancer development (very rare)

PATIENT MONITORING
- Repeat exam to assess growth.
- Reassure adolescent that lesion is benign and does not lead to breast cancer.
- Single lesion does not require additional monitoring.
- Multiple lesions require close monitoring.

BIBLIOGRAPHY

Arca MJ, et al. Breast disorders in the adolescent patient. *Adolesc Med*. 2004;15:473–485.

Fine RE, et al. Percutaneous radiofrequency-assisted excision of fibroadenomas. *Am J Surg*. 2006; 192(4):545–547.

Greydanus DE, et al. Breast disorders in children and adolescents. *Prim Care Clin Office Pract*. 2006; 33:455–502.

Kaul P, et al. Breast Disorders. In: Greydanus DE, et al., eds. *Essential Adolescent Medicine*. New York: McGraw-Hill; 2006:569–590.

LIttrup PJ, et al. Cryotherapy for breast fibroadenomas. *Radiology*. 2005;234(1):63–72.

Marchant DJ. Benign breast disease. *Obstet Gynecol Clin North Am*. 2002;29:1.

Marcopoulos C, et al. Fibroadenomas of the breast: Is there any association with breast cancer. *Eur J Gynecol Oncol*. 2004;25(4):495–497.

Pacinda SJ, et al. Fine needle aspiration of breast masses: A review of its role in diagnosis and management of adolescent patients. *J Adolesc Health*. 1998;23:306.

Santen RJ, et al. Benign breast disorders. *N Engl J Med*. 2005;353:275–285.

Simmons PS. Breast disorders in adolescent females. *Curr Opin Obstet Gynecol*. 2001;13:459–461.

Templeman C, et al. Breast disorders in the pediatric and adolescent patient. *Obstet Gynecol Clin North Am*. 2000;27:19–34.

Weinstein SP, et al. Spectrum of ultrasound findings in pediatric and adolescent patients with palpable breast masses. *Radiographics*. 2000;20:1613–21.

 MISCELLANEOUS

CLINICAL PEARLS

- Fibroadenoma is the most common cause of breast mass in the adolescent.
- Presents as a slow growing, painless mass
- Management is typically observation with consideration of excisional biopsy for diagnosis and removal of the mass.

CODES

ICD9-CM

- 217. Fibroadenoma
- 610.0 Breast cyst
- 610.1 Fibrocystic breast changes
- 611.72 Breast mass

 PATIENT TEACHING

- Reassure patient that fibroadenoma is benign and does not lead to breast cancer.
- Discuss that use of complementary and alternative therapies are not proven to help.
- Discuss that NSAIDs (OTC or prescription) may help with the pain of benign breast lesions, not fibroadenoma.
- Discuss that oral contraceptives may reduce the incidence of some benign breast lesions, but not fibroadenoma.

CERVICAL CANCER
Jack Basil, MD

 BASICS

DESCRIPTION
Invasive cervical cancer is primarily a disease of 3rd world countries. The mortality from cervical cancer in the US has declined significantly over the past 50–60 years since the adoption of routine cervical cytology (Pap test) screening programs.

Age-Related Factors
- Mean age of diagnosis is 51 years
- Begin Pap screening ~3 years after onset of intercourse, but no later than 21 years of age

Staging
- Stage 0: Carcinoma in situ
- Stage Ia1: Stromal invasion <3 mm (microinvasive)
- Stage Ia2: Stromal invasion 3–5 mm
- Stage Ib1: Stromal invasion >5 mm, or gross cervical lesion <4 cm
- Stage Ib2: Gross cervical lesion >4 cm
- Stage IIa: Extending to upper 2/3 vagina
- Stage IIb: Extending into parametrium
- Stage IIIa: Extending to lower 1/3 vagina
- Stage IIIb: Extending into parametrium to pelvic sidewall or hydronephrosis
- Stage IVa: Extending to bladder/bowel mucosa
- Stage IVb: Distant metastasis

EPIDEMIOLOGY
- Estimated 9,710 new cases of invasive cervical cancer in US in 2006
- Estimated 3,700 deaths from invasive cervical cancer in US in 2006

RISK FACTORS
- Early age 1st intercourse
- Multiple sexual partners
- Infection with HPV
- Smoking
- Multiparity
- Low socioeconomic status
- Immunosuppression

Genetics
Not an inherited disease

PATHOPHYSIOLOGY
- Several high-risk HPV subtypes are responsible for the majority (99%) of invasive cervical cancers
- High-risk subtypes include: 16, 18, 31, 33, 35, 39, 45, 51, 52, 58
- Quadrivalent prophylactic vaccine against HPV subtypes (6, 11, 16, 18) FDA-approved 2006

ASSOCIATED CONDITIONS
Same high-risk HPV subtypes are also found in the majority of preinvasive high-grade dysplasias.

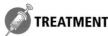 DIAGNOSIS

SIGNS AND SYMPTOMS
History
- Abnormal vaginal bleeding:
  - Menometrorrhagia
  - Postcoital
  - Postmenopausal
- Vaginal discharge
- Dyspareunia
- Pelvic pain
- Abdominal, back, or leg pain
- Shortness of breath
- Hematuria or rectal bleeding

Review of Systems
Weight loss

Physical Exam
- Pelvic exam (bimanual, rectovaginal)
- Cystoscopy
- Proctoscopy

TESTS
- Cytology Pap smear screening test
- Histology (cervical biopsies, endocervical curettage) is confirmatory test (gold standard)

Labs
- CBC
- Basic metabolic panel

Imaging
- Chest x-ray
- CT of abdomen/pelvis assesses disease status and nodal involvement and aids in treatment planning
- IVP, barium enema, lymphangiogram are optional tests

DIFFERENTIAL DIAGNOSIS
Infection
- Cervicitis
- Vaginitis
- Condyloma

Hematologic
Bleeding disorder

Immunologic
Cervical pregnancy

Tumor/Malignancy
Metastasis:
- Endometrial
- Gestational trophoblastic neoplasia
- Vulvar
- Lymphoma
- GI primary

Trauma
Cervical laceration

TREATMENT

GENERAL MEASURES
- It is important to assess the extent of disease prior to the onset of treatment.
- Surgery can be utilized in early stage-disease Ia1–IIa.
- Radiotherapy +/− chemotherapy can be utilized in all stages I–IV.

RADIOTHERAPY
- All stages can undergo radiotherapy.
- Combination of teletherapy (external beam) and brachytherapy (intracavitary)
- Chemoradiation used with locally advanced stages IIb–IVa and provides a survival advantage over radiotherapy alone
- Chemoradiation can also be used for local postsurgical recurrent disease

MEDICATION (DRUGS)
- Radiosensitizing agents include cisplatin, hydroxyurea, and 5-fluorouracil.
- Cisplatin and topotecan can be used for recurrent disease.
- Stage IVb palliative chemotherapy with cisplatin-based regimen +/− radiotherapy

SURGERY
- Cold knife cone or LEEP cone for stage Ia1 in young patients wishing to preserve fertility
- Simple hysterectomy (vaginal or abdominal) for stage Ia1 desiring definitive treatment
- Modified radical hysterectomy with bilateral pelvic lymphadenectomy for stage Ia2
- Radical hysterectomy with bilateral pelvic lymphadenectomy (para-aortic nodes optional) for stage Ib1, Ib2, IIa
- Radical trachelectomy with bilateral pelvic lymphadenectomy for smaller stage Ib1 lesions is an option in younger patients wishing to preserve fertility.
- If histologic specimen has positive margins, parametrium, or nodes then postop chemoradiation is recommended.
- Pelvic exenteration can be curative for stage IVa or centrally recurrent disease.

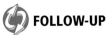 **FOLLOW-UP**

DISPOSITION

Issues for Referral

- Refer to gynecology or gynecologic oncology if diagnosis confirmed or strongly suspected by signs and symptoms.
- Refer to gynecology or gynecologic oncology if Pap suggests malignancy.
- Consider referral to palliative care or pain med consult in cases of recurrent or widely metastatic disease.

PROGNOSIS

- Directly dependent on the stage of disease
- 5-year survival:
  - Stage I: 85%
  - Stage II: 65%
  - Stage III: 35%
  - Stage IV: 10%
- Other prognostic variables:
  - Nodal involvement
  - Histologic subtype
  - Lymphvascular space invasion

PATIENT MONITORING

- After completion of treatment cancer surveillance exams with Pap/pelvic:
  - Every 3 months for 2 years
  - Every 6 months for 2 years
  - Every 12 months thereafter
- Yearly chest radiograph
- Follow closely for signs/symptoms of recurrence:
  - Vaginal bleeding
  - Pelvic pain
  - Back pain
  - Leg pain
  - Weight loss
  - Shortness of breath

BIBLIOGRAPHY

Jemal A, et al. Cancer statistics. *CA Cancer J Clin.* 2006;56:106–130.

Peters WA, et al. Concurrent chemotherapy and pelvic radiation therapy compared with pelvic radiation therapy alone as adjuvant therapy after radical surgery in high-risk early-stage cancer of the cervix. *J Clin Oncol.* 2000;18:1606–1613.

Rose PG, et al. Concurrent cisplatin-based radiotherapy and chemotherapy for locally advanced cervical cancer. *N Engl J Med.* 1999;340:1144–1153.

Smith RA, et al. American Cancer Society Guidelines for early detection of cancer. *CA Cancer J Clin.* 2006;56:11–25.

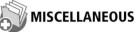 **MISCELLANEOUS**

ABBREVIATIONS

- GI—Gastrointestinal
- HPV—Human papilloma virus
- LEEP—Loop electrosurgical excision procedure

CODES

ICD9-CM

- 180.0 Endocervix, neoplasm
- 180.1 Exocervix, neoplasm
- 180.9 Primary cervix, neoplasm

 PATIENT TEACHING

It is paramount to stress the importance of cervical cancer screening guidelines. Most patients diagnosed with cervical cancer in the US have not had a Pap done in the previous 5 years.

PREVENTION

- The FDA has recently approved a prophylactic vaccine for HPV subtypes 6, 11, 16, and 18.
- Vaccine is recommended for girls and women ages 9–26.
- Highly effective in preventing infection with these HPV subtypes
- HPV subtypes 16 and 18 account for up to 70% of all cervical cancers.

CERVICAL INTRAEPITHELIAL NEOPLASIA/CERVICAL DYSPLASIA

Carol M. Choi, MD

 BASICS

DESCRIPTION
- Cervical intraepithelial neoplasia (CIN) or cervical dysplasia is the precursor to cervical carcinoma. The progression of CIN to cancer is slow (over 10–20 years).
- CIN I (mild dysplasia):
  – Confined to lower 1/3 of squamous epithelium
- CIN II (moderate dysplasia):
  – Confined to lower 2/3 of squamous epithelium
- CIN III (severe dysplasia/CIS):
  – >2/3 to full thickness of squamous epithelium

Age-Related Factors
- CIN typically diagnosed in women in their 20s.
- CIN I and II more likely to regress in adolescents than in adults
- Invasive cancer usually diagnosed in older women (40s+). Mean age at diagnosis is 47 in the US.

EPIDEMIOLOGY
- 1 million women diagnosed with CIN I/year
- 500,000 women diagnosed with CIN II-CIN III/year
- Incidence of invasive cervical cancer by age:
  – <20   0/100,000/year
  – 20–44   1.7/100,000/year
  – 45–49   16.5/100,000/year
- <10% in women ≥75

RISK FACTORS
- HPV infection
- 1st intercourse at early age
- Multiple sexual partners
- Sexual partner with multiple partners
- History of sexually transmitted infections
- Tobacco use
- HIV infection
- Immunocompromised status
- Multiparity
- Oral contraceptive use

ASSOCIATED CONDITIONS
- HPV infection:
  – Genital warts
- HIV infection
- Compromised immune status

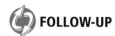 **DIAGNOSIS**

SIGNS AND SYMPTOMS
History
Abnormal Pap smear result

Physical Exam
Goal of exam is to rule-out carcinoma:
- May visualize lesion grossly or colposcopically.

TESTS
Labs
- Screening:
  – Pap smear: Conventional or liquid-based cytologic testing as *screening* test
  – HPV DNA testing for high-risk types may be used as adjunct to Pap in women >30
- Definitive diagnosis by histology:
  – Colposcopic-directed biopsies

 TREATMENT

GENERAL MEASURES
- CIN I typically regresses in the majority; follow with serial Pap smears/HPV DNA testing.
- Treatment for CIN II-CIN III is primarily surgical.

Pediatric/Adolescent Considerations
In adolescents with CIN II, consider serial colposcopy and cytology q4–6mos in lieu of surgical procedure if colposcopy is satisfactory and endocervical curettage is negative. Patient must also accept risk of occult disease.

SURGERY
- Mainstay therapy for CIN II–CIN III is surgical.
- Excision or ablation of transformation zone appropriate if colposcopy is satisfactory:
  – Satisfactory colposcopy is visualization of entire transformation zone, including the squamo-columnar junction and the entire extent of the lesion is seen.
- If colposcopy is unsatisfactory, then proceed with diagnostic excisional procedure.
- May consider ablation or conization for persistent CIN I.
- Excisional procedure:
  – LEEP
  – Cold-knife conization
  – Laser conization
- Ablation:
  – Cryotherapy
  – Laser

FOLLOW-UP

DISPOSITION
Issues for Referral
- Diagnosis of carcinoma
- Difficult colposcopic examination

PROGNOSIS
- CIN I:
  – Most lesions regress spontaneously:
    ○ Regression in 2 years, 44%; 5 years, 74%
    ○ Progression to CIN II or CIN III, 2% and 6%
- CIN II and CIN III:
  – Lesions more likely to persist or progress
  – Pregnant patients show minimal progression; lesions usually regress postpartum

PATIENT MONITORING
- CIN I:
  – Satisfactory colposcopy:
    ○ Pap q6mos for 1 year or HPV DNA testing in 12 months
  – Unsatisfactory colposcopy:
    ○ Diagnostic conization
    ○ Exception is pregnancy, adolescents
- CIN II–CIN III:
  – After treatment, Pap q4–6mos until negative × 3 or HPV DNA test at 6 months
  – Pregnant patients:
    ○ Colposcopy every trimester; postpartum with endocervical curettage

BIBLIOGRAPHY

Herbst AL. Intraepithelial Neoplasia of the Cervix: Etiology, Screening, Diagnostic Techniques, Management. In: Mishell DR Jr., et al., eds. *Comprehensive Gynecology,* 3rd ed. St Louis: Mosby-Year Book; 1997:801–833.

Holowaty P, et al. Natural history of dysplasia of the uterine cervix. *J Natl Cancer Inst.* 1999;91(3): 252–258.

Wright TC, et al. 2001 Consensus guidelines for the management of women with cervical intraepithelial neoplasia. *Am J Obstet Gynecol.* 2003;189: 295–304.

MISCELLANEOUS

SYNONYM(S)
Cervical dysplasia

CLINICAL PEARLS
Initial cervical cytology should be performed ~3 years after 1st vaginal intercourse or at age 21.

- Earlier Pap is more likely to detect clinically insignificant CIN I that will likely regress

ABBREVIATIONS
- CIN—Cervical intraepithelial neoplasia
- HPV—Human papillomavirus
- LEEP—Loop electrosurgical excision procedure

CODES

ICD9-CM
- 233.1 Severe dysplasia or CIS of cervix
- 622.10 Dysplasia of cervix, unspecified
- 622.11 Mild dysplasia of cervix
- 622.12 Moderate dysplasia of cervix

PATIENT TEACHING

ACOG Patient Education Pamphlet: Abnormal Pap Test Results

PREVENTION
Prophylactic HPV vaccine against HPV types 6, 11, 16,18, which are responsible for 90% of genital warts and 70% of cervical cancer:

- Females ages 9–26 years
- Ideally before 1st intercourse or exposure to HPV

Section II

CERVICAL LESIONS

Willie J. Parker, MD, MPH

 BASICS

DESCRIPTION

The easy accessibility of the uterine cervix by speculum exam allows for the observation of natural as well as pathologic changes to this organ. The determination of what is pathologic versus normal requires visual, tactile and, when indicated, laboratory assessment.

- Cervical lesions include:
  - Polyps
  - Condylomata
  - Nabothian cysts
  - Other:
    o Endometriosis
    o Leiomyomas
    o Papilloma
    o DES exposure
    o Epithelial tags
    o Microglandular hyperplasia

POLYPS

 BASICS

EPIDEMIOLOGY

- Common in reproductive aged women
- Peak incidence between ages 40 and 60

RISK FACTORS

Chronic inflammation

PATHOPHYSIOLOGY

- Stromal and glandular proliferation
- Often pedunculated with a stalk

ASSOCIATED CONDITIONS

- May be associated with endometrial hyperplasia
- May cause abnormal bleeding, leading to an exam in which polyps are discovered

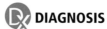 **DIAGNOSIS**

SIGNS AND SYMPTOMS

History

- Report of irregular bleeding or postcoital spotting due to trauma of prolapsed polyp
- Commonly no reported signs or symptoms (i.e., incidental finding at health maintenance exam)

Review of Systems

- Irregular bleeding
- Postcoital spotting

Physical Exam

- Flesh-colored nodule, smooth, protruding through the cervical os
- Can range from millimeters up to 3 cm in size
- May have narrow stalk, amenable to hemostatic avulsion
- May be friable

TESTS

Pelvic exam:

- Speculum for visual assessment
- Bimanual exam to palpate quality and character of the mass

Labs

Despite extremely low likelihood of malignancy, specimen should be sent to pathology for assessment.

Imaging

- None is required for cervical polyp.
- Sonohysterography is often done for evaluation of abnormal bleeding:
  - Will show endometrial polyps vs. thickened endometrium
  - Usually follows us indicated by abnormal bleeding

DIFFERENTIAL DIAGNOSIS

- Prolapsing fibroid
- Reparative changes from cervical injury; epithelial tag
- Condylomata
- Malignancy (rare)

Infection

Chronic inflammation. No overt links to infection.

Tumor/Malignancy

Polyps are seldom if ever linked to malignancy; however, any mass removed should be sent to pathology for histologic examination.

 TREATMENT

GENERAL MEASURES

- Usual treatment for a polyp is to use grasping forceps (uterine dressing forceps) to grab polyp at its stalk high in the cervical canal and avulse. This usually is hemostatic.
- If the base of the polyp is broad, hemostatic may be obtained using:
  - AgNO3 topically
  - Monsel solution (ferric subsulphate)
  - Topical Gelfoam
  - Electrocautery

 FOLLOW-UP

DISPOSITION

Issues for Referral

Usually none needed. Polyps may recur, and should be treated as needed.

PROGNOSIS

Excellent

CONDYLOMATA

 BASICS

Synonym(s): Genital warts; HPV

EPIDEMIOLOGY

- The most common viral, STD in the US, in reproductive-age women
- 67% of patients with condylomata are women.

RISK FACTORS

- Acquisition is related to sexual activity.
- Fomite transmission is controversial but theorized to be possible
- Also more common in immunosuppressed individuals

Pregnancy Considerations

- Vertical transmission possible via neonatal passage through birth canal with active viral shedding (laryngeal polyposis is exceedingly rare, whereas condylomata are exceedingly common)
  - Cesarean delivery is NOT useful in preventing the spread of HPV (ACOG)
- May enlarge during pregnancy, due to altered immune state; rarely obstructive to vaginal delivery due to mass effect and vascularity

PATHOPHYSIOLOGY

- Caused by HPV infection of sexually transmitted double-stranded DNA viruses, typically by "low-risk" types 6,11
- Incubation period after exposure ranges from ≥3 weeks to 8 months.
- Most infections are transient and cleared within 2 years.
- Viral strains that cause condylomata do not cause cancer.
- May enlarge during pregnancy

 DIAGNOSIS

SIGNS AND SYMPTOMS

History

- Usually detected at the time of a Pap smear
- May first be detected on evaluation for irregular bleeding or postcoital spotting
- Incidental finding at health maintenance exam

Physical Exam

- Presence of vulvovaginal lesions of condylomata indicate presence of HPV in the genital tract and often correlate with the presence of warts on the cervix.
- Diagnosis can usually be made by visual inspection of the affected area.
- Lesions are skin-colored or pink.
- Range from smooth, flattened papules to a verrucous, papilliform appearance

TESTS

- Pelvic exam, speculum for visual assessment, and bimanual exam to assess quality and character of the mass
- Cervical cytology

- Colposcopy and biopsy to assess for premalignant lesions (dysplasia)

Labs
- Biopsy specimens at colposcopy
- HPV viral subtyping as an adjunct to Pap testing may be indicated to assess the concomitant presence of high-risk HPV types in women >30

DIFFERENTIAL DIAGNOSIS
- Cervical carcinoma
- Epithelial tag
- Condyloma lata (secondary syphilis)

Tumor/Malignancy
Warts are not malignant, but are evidence of HPV infection. High-risk strains can coexist with the noncarcinogenic viral strains that cause warts.

 TREATMENT

GENERAL MEASURES
- Involves 1 of 3 major approaches:
  – Chemical or physical destruction
  – Immunologic therapy
  – Surgical excision
- Spontaneous regression is also possible.

 FOLLOW-UP

DISPOSITION
Issues for Referral
Monitor as needed for evidence of regression or recurrence posttreatment.

PROGNOSIS
- Excellent. In women with normal immune systems, evidence suggest HPV virus clears in the absence of ongoing reinfection with new strains.
- HPV strains causing warts may coexist with strains that cause cervical premalignant changes. Hence, the presence of warts on the cervix should prompt routine preventive health surveillance of the genital tract (screening as indicated by health status).

 MISCELLANEOUS

ABBREVIATION
HPV—Human papillomavirus

CODES

ICD9-CM
078.11 Condyloma acuminatum

 PATIENT TEACHING

PREVENTION
- Minimize number of sex partners
- Use barrier contraception/condoms

NABOTHIAN CYSTS

 BASICS

Cystic structures formed when cervical glands of columnar epithelium become covered with squamous cells by metaplasia and continue to secrete mucoid material, creating a visible and sometimes palpable "bump" on cervical palpation.

EPIDEMIOLOGY
Common in women of reproductive age, especially parous women.

PATHOPHYSIOLOGY
- Squamous metaplasia causes squamous cells to cover the opening of columnar cell-lined crypts.
- Columnar cell produces mucus that creates a small cystic structure.

 DIAGNOSIS

SIGNS AND SYMPTOMS
History
Usually detected at the time of a Pap smear under direct visualization

Review of Systems
- Often none
- May rarely give a history of spotting or irregular bleeding or discharge

Physical Exam
- Diagnosis can usually be made by visual inspection of the affected area.
- Lesions are filled with clear or whitish mucus.
- May be multiple, enough to cause cervical enlargement, making the cervix feel more prominent on exam.

TESTS
Pelvic exam, speculum for visual assessment, and bimanual exam at the time of the incidental finding is usually adequate.

Labs
None

Imaging
None required

DIFFERENTIAL DIAGNOSIS
Although the diagnosis is rarely in question, cervical biopsy will definitively confirm, as indicated.

 TREATMENT

None necessary. Any irregular-appearing areas on the cervix should be biopsied if symptoms are not explained by the findings of the exam.

OTHER CERVICAL FINDINGS

The following may be found on the cervix but are uncommon. Hence they will only be briefly described.
- Endometriosis:
  – Rare, but may present as red or blackish nodules on the cervix that do not blanch.
  – Biopsy and pathologic determination key to diagnosis
- Leiomyomas:
  – Most common tumor of the uterus but can rarely be found at or near the cervical canal.
  – May cause distortion of the cervix
  – Biopsy should be performed to rule out malignancy of the cervix.
- Papillomas:
  – Arise from the ectocervix near the squamocolumnar junction
  – May be small fingerlike projections
  – Rarely malignant but should be removed and sent to pathology

- DES exposure:
  – Deformities of the cervix consisting of transverse ridges described as hoods or cockscomb cervix.
  – No treatment required. May correlate with an increased risk of cervical insufficiency with pregnancy.
- Epithelial tags:
  – Flesh-colored, smooth epithelial appendages on the cervical portio that result from healing of cervical lacerations post childbirth or procedures.
- Microglandular hyperplasia:
  – A progesterone-related effect resulting in a polypoid growth often 1–2 cm, occurring in women who are on oral contraceptives or depo-Provera, and in pregnant or postpartum women.

 MISCELLANEOUS

SYNONYM(S)
- HPV
- Genital warts

CLINICAL PEARLS
Cervical findings are common in routine preventive care examinations, and are often asymptomatic. If a problem is present, it is often accompanied by a discharge, postcoital spotting, or bleeding. Malignancy should be excluded by cytology and/or biopsy if the diagnosis is in question.

BIBLIOGRAPHY

Aaro LA, et al. Endocervical polyps. *Obstetr Gynecol.* 1963;21:649–665.

Baker PM, et al. Superficial endometriosis of the uterine cervix: A report of 20 cases of a process that may be confused with endocervical glandular dysplasia or adenocarcinoma in situ. *Int J Gynecol Pathol.* 1999;18:198.

Ferenczy A. Anatomy and histology of the cervix. In: Blaustein A, ed. *Pathology of the Female Genital Tract.* New York: Springer Verlag; 1982:119.

Goldstein DP, et al. Congenital cervical anomalies and benign cervical lesions, UpToDate, Sept. 15, 2005.

Krantz KE. The anatomy of the human cervix, gross and histologic. In: Moghissi K, ed. *The Biology of the Cervix.* Chicago: University of Chicago Press; 1973: 1–30.

Kaminski P, et al. Benign cervical lesions. *Emedicine*, July 6, 2006.

Laufer MR, et al. Structural abnormalities of the female reproductive tract. In: Emans SJ, et al., eds. *Pediatric and Adolescent Gynecology,* 5th ed. Philadelphia: Lippincott Williams & Wilkins; 2005.

 PATIENT TEACHING

ACOG Patient Education Pamphlet: Human Papillomavirus Infection

PREVENTION
- Condom use may reduce the risk of HPV-related disease, such as genital warts and cervical neoplasia.
- Studies show that condoms may be effective in the clearance of HPV or HPV-associated lesions.

CERVICAL STENOSIS

Angela Keating, MD

 BASICS

DESCRIPTION
- Stricture of the cervical os; can be complete or incomplete

Age-Related Factors
More frequent in postmenopausal women

EPIDEMIOLOGY
Most common in hypoestrogenic women and women who have had a cervical procedure.

RISK FACTORS
- Congenital
- Acquired:
  - Operative:
    - Cervical conization
    - Cervical cauterization
    - LEEP
    - Cryotherapy
  - Radiation
  - Infection
  - Neoplasia
  - Hypoestrogenic state
  - Trauma

PATHOPHYSIOLOGY
- Diameter of normal cervix at the external os is ~5–8 mm in nulliparous women and >8 mm in most women who have had a vaginal delivery.
- Diameter of the congenital stenotic cervical os is decreased due to lack of canalization or inadequate canalization.
- Diameter of the acquired stenotic cervical canal is decreased due to adherence of raw surface within the cervical canal or contraction from scarring.
- If cervical os diameter is <2 mm, often increased fluid is present within the uterine cavity with retrograde menstruation.

ASSOCIATED CONDITIONS
- Infertility
- Dysmenorrhea
- Endometriosis

 DIAGNOSIS

SIGNS AND SYMPTOMS
History
- Symptoms depend on whether partial or complete stenosis is present and whether patient is premenopausal or postmenopausal.
- 1st sign may be inability to complete a procedure due to inability to pass the instrument through the cervical canal into the uterus (endocervical curettage, endometrial biopsy, hysteroscopy, insemination)

Review of Systems
- Premenopausal:
  - Dysmenorrhea, pelvic pain
  - Abnormal uterine bleeding (amenorrhea, oligomenorrhea, prolonged menses)
  - Hematometra, pyometra
  - Endometriosis
  - Infertility
  - Lack of cervical dilation in labor
- Postmenopausal:
  - Asymptomatic
  - Hematometra, hydrometra, pyometra

Physical Exam
- Inability to pass 1–2 mm dilator through cervical canal into uterine cavity
- Enlarged uterus, tender uterus

TESTS
Imaging
Pelvic US to assess for fluid within uterine cavity

DIFFERENTIAL DIAGNOSIS
Trauma
Asherman's syndrome (see topic)

Other/Miscellaneous
Müllerian anomaly

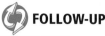 **TREATMENT**

GENERAL MEASURES
Dilate the cervix to allow access to and drainage from the uterine cavity; may be done under US guidance:
- Dilator, lacrimal duct probe, os finder
- Laminaria

MEDICATION (DRUGS)
- Misoprostol for dilation (200 μg PO or vaginally for off-label use)
- Consider menstrual suppression if recurrent hematometra

SURGERY
- Hysteroscopic canalization
- Carbon dioxide laser vaporization
- LEEP

FOLLOW-UP

DISPOSITION
Issues for Referral
- Pyometra may be associated with uterine malignancy, and thus would prompt referral to a gynecologic oncologist.
- Congenital stenosis or Müllerian anomalies may be discovered in adolescence and should prompt referral to clinician experienced in their management.

PROGNOSIS
Often recurrent if related to hypoestrogenic state or if scar tissue is not removed

PATIENT MONITORING
- Possible single intervention
- Possible serial dilations
- Consider estrogen therapy post-treatment

BIBLIOGRAPHY

Baggish MS, et al. Carbon dioxide laser treatment of cervical stenosis. *Fertil Steril*. 1987;48(1):24–28.

Darwish A, et al. Cervical priming prior to operative hysteroscopy: A randomized comparison of laminaria versus misoprostol. *Human Reprod*. 2004;19(10): 2391–2394.

Krantz KE. The anatomy of the human cervix, gross and histologic. In: Moghissi K, ed. *The Biology of the Cervix*. Chicago: University of Chicago Press; 1973;1–30.

Noyes N. Hysteroscopic cervical canal shaving: A new therapy for cervical stenosis before embryo transfer in patient undergoing in vitro fertilization. *Fertil Steril*. 1999;71(5):965–966.

Pabuccu R, et al. Successful treatment of cervical stenosis with hysteroscopic canalization before embryo transfer in patients undergoing IVF: A case series. *J Minim Invasive Gynecol*. 2005;12(5): 436–438.

MISCELLANEOUS

ABBREVIATION

LEEP—Loop electrosurgical excision procedure

CODES

ICD9-CM

- 622.4 Cervical stenosis
- 628.4 Infertility associated with congenital structural anomaly
- 654.6 Cervical stenosis in pregnancy, labor, and delivery
- 660.2 Cervical stenosis causing obstructed labor
- 752.49 Congenital stenosis of cervical canal

PATIENT TEACHING

Discuss follow-up compliance to maintain open cervical canal

CERVICITIS

Frank Biro, MD

BASICS

DESCRIPTION
- Inflammation or infection of the uterine cervix
- Often caused by sexually transmitted organisms
- Rarely related to trauma, radiation, malignancy

Age-Related Factors
~1/2 of US annual cases of STDs occur in 15–24-year-olds

EPIDEMIOLOGY
Estimated 19 million annual cases of STDs in US:
- ~1/2 in 15–24 year olds
- Estimated 7.4 million new *Trichomonas* cases/year in US (men and women)
- >975,000 cases of *Chlamydia* reported to CDC in 2005
- >330,000 cases of gonorrhea reported in 2005

RISK FACTORS
- Bacterial vaginosis
- Behavioral risk factors:
  - Unprotected intercourse
  - Inconsistent condom use
  - Sexual behaviors associated with risk of STIs including multiple partners
- Oral contraceptive use
- Epidemiologic factors:
  - Adolescence:
    - May be associated with increased biologic vulnerability with wide cervical transformation zone, active metaplasia, and possible immunologic factors
  - Young adults <25 years
  - Unmarried
  - History of STIs

PATHOPHYSIOLOGY
- Most commonly, cervicitis is the result of infectious causes, typically STDs:
  - *Chlamydia trachomatis*
  - *Neisseria gonorrhea*
  - *Trichomonas* sp.
  - Other organisms
  - HSV, streptococcus, enterococcus, *Mycoplasma*, HPV
- Inflammatory changes on a Pap smear:
  - Infectious cervicitis may cause abnormal Pap smear
  - Inflammatory changes may also be associated with cervical cancer.

ASSOCIATED CONDITIONS
PID (see topic)

DIAGNOSIS

SIGNS AND SYMPTOMS
History
- Frequently asymptomatic
- Vaginal discharge in setting of risk factors
- Pelvic pain
- Itching
- Postcoital bleeding

Review of Systems
Fever, pelvic pain suggest PID (see topic)

Physical Exam
- Mucopurulent (yellow) discharge from the cervix
- Cervical erosion or erythema
- Easily induced endocervical mucosal bleeding (friability)
- Tenderness of cervix

TESTS
Labs
- Endocervical saline preparation: >10 WBCs per high-power field suggests cervicitis
- Cervical cultures for *C. trachomatis*, *N. gonorrhoeae*
- Nucleic acid amplification tests:
  - More sensitive than culture, and may also be used on urine as well as endocervical specimens
  - Sensitivity 94%, specificity 99% for *N. gonorrhea*
  - Sensitivity 83%, specificity 99% for *Chlamydia trachomatis*
- Vaginal wet mount for *Trichomonas vaginalis*:
  - Sensitivity only 50%; consider further testing if negative microscopy
- If ulcerations are present, culture for HSV.
- VDRL or RPR to rule out concurrent syphilis
- Consider testing for concurrent HIV and Hepatitis B and C
- Lab results may be altered by a recent antibiotic treatment; DNA from nonviable organisms may persist up to 2 weeks after treatment.

DIFFERENTIAL DIAGNOSIS
- Vaginal infections with *Candida albicans* or *Trichomonas vaginalis* extending into the cervix
- Bacterial vaginosis
- Carcinoma of the cervix

TREATMENT

GENERAL MEASURES
Douching should be discouraged:
- Associated with increased risk of PID

MEDICATION (DRUGS)
First Line
- If infectious cervicitis suspected, treat without awaiting culture results:
  - Doxycycline (Vibramycin) 100 mg PO b.i.d. for 7 days or azithromycin (Zithromax) 1 g single dose; add ceftriaxone (Rocephin) if prevalence of GC is high in patient population
  - Option of Rocephin and azithromycin removes patient compliance factor, because they are 1-time doses.
- For trichomoniasis:
  - Metronidazole (Flagyl) 2-g single dose
- For herpes:
  - Acyclovir (Zovirax) 200 mg PO 5 times daily (or 400 mg t.i.d.); or valacyclovir (Valtrex) 1 g PO b.i.d. for 7 days
- Contraindications:
  - Doxycycline should not be used in pregnant or nursing mothers.
- Precautions:
  - Doxycycline should not be taken with milk, antacids, or iron-containing preparations.
- Significant possible interactions:
  - Doxycycline/Metronidazole may increase INR with warfarin (Coumadin).
- Chronic cervicitis associated with postmenopausal vaginal atrophic changes may respond to topical estrogen creams.

Second Line
- Because of the rise of gonococcal resistance to fluoroquinolones, the only alternate to ceftriaxone is cefixime 400 mg PO in a single dose; other single-dose cephalosporin therapies could be considered, but those regimens have not received recommendations by the CDC.
- Azithromycin for *Chlamydia* may be substituted with erythromycin:
  - Base or stearate 500 mg PO q.i.d.
  - Ethylsuccinate 800 mg PO q.i.d.

SURGERY
Diagnostic procedures:
- Colposcopy is indicated in chronic inflammation, with a biopsy of suspicious areas.

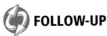 **FOLLOW-UP**

Repeat studies should be performed in 3–5 months after the index infection, because of high rates of reinfection. Follow-up nucleic acid amplification tests should not be done before 3 weeks after treatment because of false positives due to persistence of DNA from nonviable organisms.

DISPOSITION

Admission criteria:

- Only considered if refractory PID

PROGNOSIS

- Infectious cervicitis usually responds to systemic antibiotics.
- Chronic cervicitis may be resistant to treatment and should be monitored closely for cervical dysplasia.
- Complications:
  - Cervicitis due to untreated *C. trachomatis* or *N. gonorrhoeae* is associated with an 8–10% risk of developing subsequent PID.
  - Moderate to severe inflammation is associated with increased risk of HPV infection and cervical carcinoma.

PATIENT MONITORING

Repeat cultures after treatment for *Chlamydia* or gonorrhea are indicated in pregnant patients; median time to reinfection in adolescents 4–6 months.

BIBLIOGRAPHY

Centers for Disease Control and Prevention. Sexually Transmitted Diseases Treatment Guideline, 2006. *MMWR.* 2006;55:RR–11;1–94.

Geisler WM, et al. Vaginal leukocyte counts in women with bacterial vaginosis: Relation to vaginal and cervical infections. *Sex Transm Infect.* 2004;80: 401–405.

Marrazzo JM, et al. Risk factors for cervicitis among women with bacterial vaginosis. *J Infect Dis.* 2006;193:617–624.

Simpson T, et al. Urethritis and cervicitis in adolescents. *Adolescent Med Clin.* 2004;15: 153–271.

 MISCELLANEOUS

- The presence of *Trichomonas* does not rule out other concurrent infection.
- Positive results for *N. gonorrhoeae* or *Chlamydia* may need to be reported to local or state health department.
- Adolescents remain a high-risk group for STDs.
- See Cervical Intraepithelial Neoplasia, Sexually Transmitted Diseases (STDs): Chlamydia, Sexually Transmitted Diseases (STDs): Gonorrhea, Sexually Transmitted Diseases (STDs): Trichomonas, Cervical Lesions

SYNONYM(S)

Mucopurulent cervicitis

CLINICAL PEARLS

- >50% of cases of cervicitis are asymptomatic.
- The complications of untreated cervicitis include ascending infection, which can lead to infertility, and chronic pelvic pain.
- Chronic inflammation increases the risk of HPV infection and cervical cancer.
- The best empiric treatment for cervicitis (if no allergies) is azithromycin 1 g in a single dose, or doxycycline 100 mg b.i.d. for 7 days.
- Azithromycin is safe in pregnancy (pregnancy category B).
- If an organism is identified, repeat diagnostic studies in 3–5 months because of high rates of reinfection.

ABBREVIATIONS

- HPV—Human papillomavirus
- HSV—Herpes simplex virus
- PID—Pelvic inflammatory disease
- RPR—Rapid plasma reagin
- VDRL—Venereal Disease Research Laboratory

CODES

ICD9-CM

- 079.88 Chlamydia infection
- 098.15 Acute gonococcal cervicitis
- 099.53 Other venereal diseases due to *Chlamydia trachomatis*, lower genitourinary sites
- 618.9 Cervicitis

 PATIENT TEACHING

- Advise patient to use condoms consistently and include discussion of abstinence.
- If infectious etiology, advise patient to inform her partners so they can seek treatment.

PREVENTION

Patients with >1 sexual partner should be advised to use condoms at every sexual encounter.

CONGENITAL ADRENAL HYPERPLASIA

David R. Repaske, MD, PhD

 BASICS

DESCRIPTION
- Enzymatic block in cortisol production in adrenal gland leading to adrenal gland hypertrophy, cortisol deficiency, and overproduction of androgenic cortisol precursors
- Wide range of severity (partial to complete biosynthetic block) and, therefore, wide range of presentations
- 21-hydroxylase deficiency (CYP21A2 gene):
  - Most common, 95%
  - Often associated with mineralocorticoid deficiency
- 11β-hydroxylase deficiency (CYP11B1 gene):
  - Less common, 5%
  - Often associated with mineralocorticoid excess
- Other rare forms exist:
  - 17-alpha-hydroxylase deficiency (CYP17A1 gene)
  - 3-beta-hydroxysteroid dehydrogenase deficiency (HSD3B2 gene)
  - Lipoid adrenal hyperplasia (StAR or CYP11A1 gene)

Pediatric Considerations
Neonatal: Females with severe CAH have ambiguous genitalia at birth due to excess adrenal androgen production in utero. Males generally not recognized at birth.

ALERT
- Severe forms of CAH are potentially fatal if unrecognized because of salt wasting, hyponatremia, hyperkalemia, dehydration, and hypotension.
- Childhood: Mild or moderate 21-hydroxylase deficiency in males or females may present with precocious puberty, and accelerated growth and skeletal development.
- Adolescence: Girls with mild 21-hydroxylase deficiency may present with oligomenorrhea and hirsutism.
- Reproductive age: May present with infertility

EPIDEMIOLOGY
- Severe or moderate CAH is rare: ~1 case/15,000 population worldwide, with wide variation by ethnic background:
  - 1 in 300 Yapik Eskimos
  - 1 in 2,000 Reunion Island natives
  - 1 in 42,000 African Americans
- Mild or asymptomatic CYP21A2 mutations may be common:
  - As many as 1 in 3 Eastern European Jews, 1 in 4 Hispanics, and 1 in 6 random residents of New York City are carriers of a mild mutation.
  - Therefore, 1 in 27–100 are homozygous or compound heterozygous affected by mild mutations.
- Internationally, 11β-hydroxylase deficiency is most common in persons of Moroccan or Iranian Jewish descent.

RISK FACTORS
Genetics
- Autosomal-recessive.
- Heterozygotes are not affected
- CYP21A2 carrier frequency is ~1:60: Higher frequency in Hispanics, Yugoslavs, East European Jews, Eskimos.
- CYP21A2 alleles can be deleted or have point mutations. Severity of disease is correlated with least affected allele.

PATHOPHYSIOLOGY
- Presentation depends on severity of cortisol biosynthetic block.
- 100% block is associated with most severe "salt wasting" disease:
  - Cortisol and mineralocorticoid cannot be synthesized.
  - Absence of cortisol feedback inhibition of CRH and ACTH release from pituitary leads to elevated ACTH and hyperstimulation of adrenal gland.
  - Beginning in fetal adrenal at 8–10 weeks, androgenic precursors are produced in excess and secreted as they cannot be converted into cortisol and aldosterone.
  - Androgen excess occurs during period of formation of external genitalia, leading to virilization of female.
  - Absence of mineralocorticoid leads to hyperkalemia and dehydration and shock at 7–14 days of life.
  - Absence of cortisol compromises ability to respond to shock, with fulminant deterioration and potential death.
- A 98% biosynthetic block still allows adequate mineralocorticoid production to prevent dehydration and may present with "simple virilization" only.
- Less block may cause milder hyperandrogenemia associated with "late presentation" that may manifest as hirsutism, acne, PCOS, and/or infertility.

ASSOCIATED CONDITIONS
- Virilization
- Hirsutism
- Acne
- Infertility

 DIAGNOSIS

SIGNS AND SYMPTOMS
History
- Presentation depends on severity of gene defect.
- Symptoms may relate to mineralocorticoid deficiency, cortisol deficiency, and/or androgen excess.
- Severe "salt wasting" disease presents in neonatal period:
  - Feeding difficulty
  - Weight loss
  - Emesis
  - Shock and dehydration
  - Females with ambiguous genitalia
- Moderate "simple virilizing" disease may present in neonatal period or childhood:
  - Growth spurt
  - Acne
  - Body odor
- Mild "late presentation" disease may present as adolescent or young adult:
  - Menstrual irregularity
  - Infertility
  - PCOS symptoms
  - Acne or oily skin

Physical Exam
- Abnormal physical findings are due to androgen excess and will be more remarkable in females than in males.
- Salt wasting:
  - Virilization or genital ambiguity in newborn females:
    - Clitoromegaly
    - Posterior labial fusion
    - "Female pseudohermaphrodite"; proposed terminology 46XX,DSD (disorder of sex development)
  - Subtle abnormality in newborn male:
    - Hyperpigmented scrotum
    - Generous phallus
- Simple virilizing:
  - Mild virilization or genital ambiguity in newborn females
  - Normal physical exam in newborn males
  - Male and female children may develop premature pubic hair, adult body odor, accelerated growth velocity, tall stature, hirsutism, precocious puberty.
  - Hyperpigmentation may develop from elevated ACTH levels.
- Late presentation:
  - No physical findings as newborn
  - Premature puberty
  - Intractable acne, male pattern baldness, hirsutism as adolescent or young adult

TESTS
Labs
- Diagnosis:
  - Elevated 17-hydroxyprogesterone for salt wasting or simple virilizing:
    - Age and prematurity adjustment is necessary to interpret 17-hydroxyprogesterone for neonates.
  - Abnormal 17-hydroxyprogesterone 60 minutes after high dose (250 mcg) ACTH injection for late presentation
  - Hyperkalemia and hyponatremia for salt waster
- Molecular diagnosis:
  - Diagnosis can be confirmed by molecular analysis of the CYP21A2 gene that is commercially available.

Imaging
US diagnostic of male infertility due to adrenal rests within testes.

DIFFERENTIAL DIAGNOSIS
Metabolic/Endocrine
- Congenital Adrenal Hypoplasia, also known as Adrenal Hypoplasia Congenita (AHC):
  - Hypoplastic adrenal glands
  - Cortisol and mineralocorticoid deficiency present, but no androgen excess
  - 17-hydroxyprogesterone is low.
- Adrenal tumors:
  - Often androgen-producing
  - 17-hydroxyprogesterone may be elevated but DHEA-S tends to be very elevated.
- PCOS:
  - 17-hydroxyprogesterone response to ACTH is normal.

Drugs
Maternal exposure to androgens in first trimester of pregnancy

Other/Miscellaneous
Neonates:
- Other causes of failure to thrive
- Other disorders of sex development
- Maternal androgen producing tumor

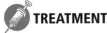

TREATMENT
GENERAL MEASURES
- Replace missing hormone
- Reduce inappropriate androgen production
- Repair genital ambiguity

MEDICATION (DRUGS)
- Salt wasting disease with shock, dehydration, and hyperkalemia in neonate:
  - Dexamethasone, fludrocortisone, potassium-binding resins, IV fluid
- Salt wasting and simple virilizing disease:
  - Cortisol for children (less likely to suppress growth):
    - 10–25 mg/m^2/d in 2 or 3 divided doses
    - Monitor and adjust therapy by suppression of testosterone and androstenedione to normal levels, and by suppression of 17-hydroxyprogesterone to near normal levels.

- Monitor bone age and height velocity.
- Avoid overtreatment which will inhibit growth and cause Cushing syndrome.
  - Dexamethasone after completion of growth:
    - 0.25–0.75 mg at HS
    - Monitor and adjust therapy by suppression of testosterone and androstenedione to normal levels and/or by improvement in hirsutism symptoms.
    - Avoid overtreatment which will cause Cushing syndrome.
  - Fludrocortisone for all:
    - 0.1 mg/d
    - Helps suppress androgen production even in non–salt wasters
    - Monitor and adjust therapy by suppression of plasma renin to normal range
- Late presentation:
  - Cortisol or dexamethasone, as above
  - Or, spironolactone (plus OCP) as androgen blocker
  - Fludrocortisone generally not needed

ALERT
- Salt wasters (and perhaps simple virilizers) will not be able to produce the extra burst of cortisol required to fight physiologic stress. For fever, fasting, trauma, surgery, or other physiologic stress, the dose of glucocorticoid must be increased. Typically, the whole day's dose is administered q8h by mouth or by injection if unable to take PO for the duration of stress.
- Chronic glucocorticoid therapy in late presenters may lead to adrenal suppression, necessitating similar stress dosing of glucocorticoid.

SURGERY
Reconstructive surgery (clitoroplasty and/or vaginoplasty) to treat the in utero genital virilization of salt wasting and simple virilizing girls. Increasing consensus to delay surgery to allow affected person input into decision making, when possible.

FOLLOW-UP
PROGNOSIS
- Risk of death from physiologic stress that is not appropriately treated with stress dose of glucocorticoid
- Excess androgen signs and symptoms can usually be successfully treated by appropriate therapy.
- Fertility in both females and males can generally be restored, although this may require a period of careful monitoring of therapy.

PATIENT MONITORING
Medical therapy is typically monitored every 4 months in growing children and every 12 months in adults.

BIBLIOGRAPHY
Joint LWPES/ESPE CAH Working Group, Consensus statement on 21-hydroxylase deficiency from the Lawson Wilkins Pediatric Endocrine Society and the European Society for Paediatric Endocrinology. *J Clin Endo Metabol.* 2002;87:4048–4053.

Moran C, et al. 21-hydroxylase deficient nonclassical adrenal hyperplasia is a progressive disorder: A multicenter study. *Am J Ob Gyn.* 2000;183: 1468–1474.

White PC, et al. Congenital adrenal hyperplasia. *N Engl J Med.* 2003;349:776–788.

MISCELLANEOUS
SYNONYM(S)
21-hydroxylase deficiency

CLINICAL PEARLS
Intrauterine therapy can successfully prevent female genital virilization if:
- The diagnosis is suspected (e.g., because of an affected sib)
- Therapy is started before 8 weeks gestation
- Pregnant mother takes 20 mg/kg/d dexamethasone (typically 0.5 mg q12h)
- Sex and genotype of fetus are determined by amniocentesis or CVS. Therapy is stopped for male fetus or unaffected fetus.
- Many states now screen for 21-hydroxylase deficiency on the newborn screen.

ABBREVIATIONS
ACTH—Adrenocorticotropic hormone
AHC—Adrenal Hypoplasia Congenita
CAH—Congenital adrenal hyperplasia
CRH—Corticotropin-releasing hormone
DHEA-S—Dehydroepiandrosterone-sulfate
PCOS—Polycystic ovary syndrome

CODES
ICD9-CM
255.2 Adrenogenital disorder

PATIENT TEACHING
- Genetic counseling:
  - If one child is affected, 25% chance of subsequent child from same parents being affected.
  - If one parent is affected, and the status of the other parent is unknown, risk is ~0.4% that a child will be affected.
- Medication:
  - Do not stop taking glucocorticoid abruptly.

DEVELOPMENTAL DELAY, INCLUDING DOWN SYNDROME

Jane D. Broecker, MD
Linda S. Ross, DO, PhD

 BASICS

DESCRIPTION

- Gynecologic care of patients with Down syndrome and developmental delay can be facilitated by understanding the special needs of those with mental retardation (MR).
- The American Association on Mental Retardation defines MR as a disability characterized by significant limitations both in intellectual functioning and in adaptive behavior as expressed in conceptual, social, and practical adaptive skills.
- This disability originates before age 18.
- Developmental disability is a broader term used to describe MR, cerebral palsy, epilepsy, autism, and other neurologic conditions.

Age-Related Factors

Many patients with MR appear child-like, but the clinician must keep in mind that puberty and reproductive function occur normally for most.

- Staging using the DSM IV based on IQ:
  - Mild (IQ 50–70)
  - Moderate (IQ 35–50)
  - Severe (IQ 20–35)
  - Profound (IQ <20)

EPIDEMIOLOGY

2.5% of the population has MR.

RISK FACTORS

Genetics

- Down syndrome is associated with the presence of all or part of an extra chromosome 21; also described as trisomy 21.
- Other genetic causes of MR include:
  - Fragile X syndrome
  - Other trisomies, 18 and 13
  - Genetic neurologic and metabolic conditions

ASSOCIATED CONDITIONS

- Limited verbal skills may affect ability to express concern about symptoms or pain and discomfort with menses or during exams.
- Associated physical disabilities such as limb contracture and spasticity may limit mobility and complicate evaluation and physical exam.
- Patients may express a variety of emotions.
- MR patients are at high risk for sexual abuse (see chapter and see below), and prior sexual abuse or trauma may cause extreme fear of the pelvic exam.
- Premenstrual syndrome may be severe or debilitating in patients with severe MR.
  - Symptoms appear up to 7 days prior to menses and may be:
    - Physical (weight gain, cramping, seizures)
    - Behavioral (aggression, tantrums, crying spells, self-abusive behaviors)
- Menstrual hygiene may be a problem in patients with severe MR:
  - Most women with mild or moderate MR will learn good menstrual hygiene with effective instruction and behavior-modification training.
  - In severe cases, menstrual suppression may be used (see chapter and see below).

DIAGNOSIS

SIGNS AND SYMPTOMS

History

- Obtain a thorough history as you would for any other patient, keeping in mind the unique needs of these patients.
- Patients may be nonverbal, and if verbal, may be inappropriate, tangential, or difficult to understand.
- Assess level of functioning, being aware that MR patients are more likely to have associated neurologic disorders and medical illness.
- Establish trust.
- Try to take a complete history, utilizing family and caregivers as necessary.
- It may be appropriate to spend 1-on-1 time with both patient and caregiver.
- Document whether patient, caregiver, or both give history.
- Evaluate for contraindications to hormonal management of menstruation or menopause.
- CC and HPI
- Past medical, surgical, gyn, OB history
- Medications (institutionalized patients often have a printed list)
- Social history (guardianship, current living arrangements, substances)
- Sexual history:
  - Obtain a confidential history if possible
  - Sexual preference
  - Physical, sexual abuse

Review of Systems

Include questions related to:

- Behavior changes related to menses
- Acne
- Unwanted facial hair
- Pain
- Weight fluctuations

Physical Exam

- Patient education:
  - Done prior to the exam, this is essential to decrease anxiety and facilitate process.
  - Wear a white coat to indicate to the patient you are a medical professional.
  - Schedule one or more counseling sessions.
  - Use clear, concise language.
  - Explain why exam is necessary.
  - Discuss anatomy and physiology to make patient comfortable with her body.
  - Use anatomic dolls, visual graphics, models, or movies to demonstrate breast, abdominal, and pelvic exams.
  - Allow patient to hold and examine speculum.
  - Demonstrate positions used during exam.
  - Encourage questions.
  - Encourage patient to have a caregiver/friend present during exam.

- Physical exam: Associated neurologic conditions and physical disabilities may make positioning for gyn exam difficult. Past abuse may increase anxiety during exam. Remember that a successful exam will increase the likelihood of successful subsequent exams:
  - Utilize extra staff for assistance in positioning.
  - Use automatic bed.
  - Consider alternative positions: Frog leg, knee to chest, side-lying position.
  - Explain each step of the procedure before doing it, and use a reassuring voice.
  - Use smallest appropriate speculum and run the speculum under warm water for a few seconds before insertion.
  - Encourage patient to breathe deeply to help her relax.
  - Use diversion strategies such as riddles, songs, during exam if appropriate.
  - Never use force, and tell the patient that if she needs you to stop she should signify her need by saying stop, or using some other sign. In this way you give her a sense of control over the situation.
  - Note hirsutism if present.
  - Document ability to communicate and general level of function (ambulatory, etc.)
- Alternatives to traditional pelvic exam:
  - Bimanual exam without speculum (Q-tip Pap method) reserved for patients with extreme fear of speculum:
    - Q-tip method: Palpate cervix with lubricated index finger, slide swab alongside finger and rotate against cervix several times. Adequate specimens can be obtained.
  - Sedation: Oral dosage of 2–8 mg/kg of ketamine or 0.2–0.4 mg/kg midazolam. Should only be used with appropriate protocol for conscious sedation and emergency care backup.

TESTS

Labs

- Pap test (follow current guidelines)
- HPV testing as option with Pap smear
- CBC if menorrhagia
- Urine hCG if indicated
- STI testing:
  - Trichomoniasis
  - *Chlamydia* and *Gonorrhea*
  - DNA probe with amplification is most sensitive, but genital culture with special culture media is imperative for legal (abuse) issues. Consider obtaining both.
  - Syphilis, HIV, hepatitis, HSV: Genital culture or serum antibodies as indicated
- Androgen levels if signs of hirsutism.

Imaging

- Transabdominal US: Noninvasive, may be used to identify problems such as uterine fibroids, ovarian cysts, or if exam unsatisfactory
- Mammogram (as indicated)
- Bone density (as indicated)

DIFFERENTIAL DIAGNOSIS

Metabolic/Endocrine

- Patients with developmental delay should have normal onset of puberty and develop a normal menstrual pattern. If they do not, the usual evaluation should be done to uncover the cause of any menstrual abnormality.

- Abnormal uterine bleeding may be due to thyroid disease (high prevalence among patients with Down syndrome), antiseizure/neuroleptic medication.
- Older MR women may be at increased risk for osteoporosis due to amenorrhea, earlier menopause, inactivity, prolonged treatment with DMPA. Consider DEXA.

Trauma
- Sexual abuse: Mild-to-moderately retarded patients are at high risk for physical and sexual abuse.
- Abuse is usually committed by a known or trusted person.
- Lack of education about sexuality may increase the risk for abuse.
- Be vigilant for unexplained bruises.
- Patients with STIs in the absence of a history of consensual sexual activity should be evaluated for sexual abuse.
- Sexuality education and abuse-prevention strategies should be given to both patient and caregivers.
- Refer patients and caregivers to community resources for counseling and support groups.
- Physicians are mandatory reporters of suspected physical and sexual abuse.

Drugs
- Many patients with MR are on multiple medications to control behavior and/or seizures.
- Neuroleptics may cause hyperprolactinemia, with resulting amenorrhea and/or galactorrhea.

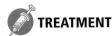
TREATMENT

GENERAL MEASURES
- Provide care in the best interest of the patient.
- Treat each patient as a unique individual with distinct concerns.
- Be aware of the interplay of medical and social issues.
- Use the least harmful option whenever possible.
- Be sensitive to widely shared societal views; use an ethics committee if necessary.
- Educate caregiver to monitor reproductive health on regular basis.

MEDICATION (DRUGS)
- Menstrual suppression (see topic):
  - Can be used to improve menstrual hygiene, lessen dysmenorrhea, or treat heavy bleeding
  - Also provides contraception.
  - DMPA is one of the best-studied methods of menstrual suppression in patients with MR, but issues around weight gain and black box warning regarding bone density should be weighed.
  - Levonorgestrel IUS: Compliance-independent, but may be associated with initial BTB, unrecognized expulsion, or perforation. Patient's ability to vocalize complaints must be considered.
  - Implantable rod containing progestin, with 3-year contraception, but with unscheduled bleeding.
  - Combination hormonal methods in the form of pills, patches, or rings, may be used cyclically or continuously. Benefits include contraception as well as noncontraceptive benefits for acne, dysmenorrhea, menorrhagia, dysfunctional uterine bleeding, and PMDD.

- Contraception:
  - To be used in sexually active patients.
  - Parents and caregivers may be reluctant to acknowledge sexuality and needs of MR patient.
  - Assess sexual behaviors before choosing contraceptive plan.
  - Parents of mildly MR patients ranked IUD > Depo-Provera > OCPs on satisfaction with method.
  - OCPs also decrease menstrual flow and dysmenorrhea, but require daily compliance. Encourage caregiver to monitor medication use.
  - Consider interaction with neuroleptics and antiseizure medications.
  - Long-acting progestins such as DMPA and Implanon: Unscheduled bleeding may be poorly tolerated, especially if menstrual hygiene difficult.
  - Barrier methods require planning and manual dexterity.

SURGERY
- Both surgical sterilization and hysterectomy are procedures often requested by family members of retarded patients. Both are surgical procedures that prevent pregnancy. Hysterectomy carries the added benefit of cessation of menses, but should be performed only when all other reasonable alternatives have been considered or when other gynecologic conditions would mandate. Consider:
  - Surgical risks (including risk of general anesthesia, as many Down patients have congenital cardiac and pulmonary abnormalities.
  - Gynecologic indications (fibroids, menorrhagia, pelvic pain, others)
  - Route (many can be done vaginally by a skilled surgeon)
  - Removal or preservation of ovarian function
  - With MR patients, informed consent may be limited, and autonomy may be impaired. To determine ability to give informed consent, determine if the patient is deemed legally competent, and assess her level of capacity (ability to make choices on her own behalf)
- Regarding sterilization, discuss:
  - Risks and benefits of sterilization
  - Reversible alternatives
  - Risk of regret
  - Types of surgical sterilization
  - Endometrial ablation options may be considered at the time of surgical sterilization.
  - Discussion with sexual partner
  - Consult laws of jurisdiction involved. Local laws for determination of competency vary greatly.
  - Consider language, culture, quality of information provided, setting of counseling (privacy), changes in level of comprehension.
  - Consult professionals trained to communicate with mentally disabled to help determine capacity to understand options.
  - Court approval may be necessary in difficult cases and depends on state laws.
- If patient cannot give informed consent, use these guidelines:
  - Conform to patient's expressed values and beliefs, and discuss alternatives.
  - Be vigilant for undue pressure from family members whose interests differ from patient's interests. Interview the patient without family members present when possible.
  - Discuss noninvasive modalities such as socialization training, supportive family therapy, sexuality education, sexual abuse avoidance training, and contraception with family members and caregivers.

- Consider likelihood of adverse outcomes if surgical sterilization is not performed: How likely is it that the patient will become pregnant or be sexually abused? Does the patient have health problems that will be worsened by pregnancy (heart disease or advanced diabetes)?
- Consider well-being of a potentially conceived child.
- Utilize hospital ethics committee to discuss difficult or complicated cases.

BIBLIOGRAPHY

Chamberlain A, et al. Issues in fertility control for mentally retarded female adolescents: I. Sexual activity, sexual abuse, and contraception. *Pediatrics*. 1984;73:445–450.

Elkins TE. Providing gynecological care for women with mental retardation. *Med Aspects Hum Sex*. 1991;56–62.

Morano JP. Sexual abuse of the mentally retarded patient: Medical and legal analysis for the primary care physician. *Prim Care Companion J Clin Psychiatry*. 2001;3:126–135.

Pulcini J, et al. The relationship between characteristics of women with mental retardation and outcomes of the gynecologic examination. *Clin Excell Nurse Pract*. 1999;3:221–229.

Quint EH. Gynecological health care for adolescents with developmental disabilities. *Adolesc Med*. 1999;10:221–229.

Reproductive Health Care for Women with Mental Handicaps. *The Contraception Report*. 1997;8:1–11.

Sterilization of women, including those with mental disabilities. In: *Ethics in Obstetrics and Gynecology/the American College of Obstetricians and Gynecologists*, 2nd ed. Washington DC: ACOG; 2004:56–59.

MISCELLANEOUS

CLINICAL PEARLS
- Girls who have learned to toilet themselves can usually be taught to cope with menses.
- Parents may be apprehensive about the child's approaching puberty. Preventive guidance can be helpful.

ABBREVIATIONS
- BTB—Breakthrough bleeding
- DEXA—Dual energy X-ray absorptiometry
- DMPA—Depot medroxyprogesterone acetate
- HPV—Human papillomavirus
- HSV—Herpes simplex virus
- IUS—Intrauterine system
- MR—Mental retardation
- OCP—Oral contraceptive pill
- PMDD—Premenstrual dysphoric disorder
- STD/STI—Sexually transmitted disease/infection

CODES

ICD9-CM
626.8 Menstrual suppression

PATIENT TEACHING

PREVENTION
Consider all preventative vaccines, including HPV vaccine.

ENDOMETRIAL CANCER

Kathleen Y. Yang, MD

 BASICS

DESCRIPTION
- Endometrial adenocarcinomas comprise 95% of uterine cancers, with the remaining 5% sarcomas.
- Type I endometrial adenocarcinoma:
  – Estrogen-dependent
  – More common, 90%
  – Associated with endometrial hyperplasia
  – More indolent course, better prognosis
- Type II endometrial cancer:
  – Estrogen-independent
  – Less common, 10%
  – More aggressive, worse prognosis

Age-Related Factors
- Predominantly seen in older women with average age 55–65.
- May be seen in younger women with a history of chronic anovulation.

Staging
Surgical staging:
- Stage I: Uterus only:
  – 1A: Endometrium only
  – 1B: <50% myometrial invasion
  – 1C: >50% myometrial invasion
- Stage II: Uterus + cervix:
  – 2A: Endocervical glands
  – 2B: Cervical stromal involvement
- Stage III: Local/Regional spread:
  – 3A: Uterine serosa +/– adnexa/pelvic washing
  – 3B: Vagina
  – 3C: Inguinal +/– para-aortic lymph nodes
- Stage IV: Metastases:
  – 4A: Bladder or bowel
  – 4B: Distant metastasis

EPIDEMIOLOGY
- The most common gynecologic malignancy
- 4th most common cancer in US women
- 2.6% lifetime risk in a woman in the general population
- 40,000+ cases diagnosed each year
- In US, 74,000 deaths estimated for 2007
- More common in Caucasians than African Americans

RISK FACTORS
- Unopposed estrogen:
  – Increased risks for endometrial hyperplasia and endometrial cancer
  – Risk associated with dose and duration of estrogen exposure
  – Risk can be decreased by use progestin
- Endogenous estrogen:
  – Estrogen-producing tumor
  – PCOS
- Tamoxifen: 2–3-fold risk
- Obesity

- Diabetes mellitus/hypertension
- Chronic anovulation (i.e., PCOS)
- BRCA1: 2-fold risk
- Lynch syndrome/hereditary nonpolyposis colorectal cancer (40–60% lifetime risk)
- Nulliparity
- Early menarche, late age of menopause
- Older age

Genetics
- Gene expression represents a proliferative pattern.
- Microsatellite instability (Lynch syndrome/hereditary nonpolyposis colorectal cancer)

PATHOPHYSIOLOGY
- Excessive endogenous or exogenous estrogen unopposed by progestin leading to endometrial hyperplasia followed by cancer
- Histologic types:
  – Endometrioid adenocarcinoma (75–80%)
  – Villoglandular adenocarcinoma
  – Adenocarcinoma
  – Mucinous adenocarcinoma
  – Papillary serous adenocarcinoma (UPSC)
  – Clear-cell adenocarcinoma
  – Squamous cell carcinoma
  – Undifferentiated carcinoma
  – Malignant mixed mesodermal carcinoma

ASSOCIATED CONDITIONS
- Obesity
- Type 2 diabetes
- Hypertension
- Infertility
- Anovulation
- PCOS
- Endometrial hyperplasia
- Colorectal cancer
- Tamoxifen use

 DIAGNOSIS

SIGNS AND SYMPTOMS
- Postmenopausal vaginal bleeding
- Endometrial cells on Pap smear in postmenopausal women
- Intermenstrual bleeding or heavy prolonged bleeding in premenopausal or anovulatory premenopausal women
- Obese, hypertensive women

History
- Complete gynecologic, past medical, family history
- Menstrual history:
  – Menarche
  – Frequency, duration, and amount of flow
  – Menopause
- Gynecologic history/procedures:
  – History of endometrial polyps or fibroid uterus
  – Recent Pap smear result
- Past medical history:
  – Hospitalizations
  – Surgeries
  – Chronic medical conditions
  – History of breast cancer and/or Tamoxifen use

- Family history:
  – Breast cancer
  – Colon cancer
  – Ovarian cancer
  – Uterine cancer
  – Degree of relatives affected
  – Age of diagnosis in relatives

Review of Systems
- Special attention to GI and GU systems
- Weight loss or weight gain

Physical Exam
- General:
  – Appearance
  – VS
  – BMI
  – BP
- Abdominal exam:
  – Masses
  – Hepatomegaly
  – Tenderness, rebound, guarding
- Pelvic exam:
  – Bimanual exam to assess uterine size, shape, position, mobility, and tenderness
  – Bimanual exam to assess adnexal mass, tenderness, mobility
  – Bimanual exam to palpate the vulva, vagina, and cervix
  – Rectovaginal exam to assess any mass in the rectum, or cul-de-sac

TESTS
- Endometrial biopsy:
  – First-line diagnostic modality
  – Fractional curettage if endometrial biopsy is negative
- Hysteroscopy:
  – Used if endometrial biopsy is nondiagnostic but suspicion is high
  – Does not increase the yield of diagnosis in endometrial cancer in meta-analysis
- Pap smear is not a reliable screening test for endometrial cancer.

Labs
CA 125:
- Useful in predicting extrauterine metastasis and monitor response to treatment
- Not a diagnostic or screening test

Imaging
- TVU:
  – Stripe thickness <5 mm in postmenopausal woman is typically low risk for endometrial hyperplasia or cancer.
  – If stripe thickness >5 mm (postmenopausal), then tissue diagnosis is still required.
  – Persistent postmenopausal bleeding warrants endometrial biopsy even if US is negative.
  – Not a screening test for endometrial cancer
  – Used in patients who cannot tolerate office endometrial biopsy or who has structural abnormalities of the uterine cavity (i.e., fibroids) that make endometrial biopsy difficult
- MRI:
  – Helpful in evaluating myometrial invasion and cervical invasion
  – Not necessary if surgery is planned

- CT:
  - Evaluating extent of metastasis if suspected
  - Not necessary if surgery is planned

DIFFERENTIAL DIAGNOSIS
- Atrophic endometritis/Vaginitis
- Endometrial/Cervical polyps
- Endometrial hyperplasia
- Cervical cancer, uterine sarcoma

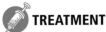

TREATMENT
GENERAL MEASURES
- Initially treat with surgery
- Postoperative management depends on risk of recurrence:
  - Low risk:
    - Grade 1 or 2, and stage IA or Ib, or grade 3 without myometrial invasion
    - No lymphovascular space involvement
    - No lymph node involvement
  - Intermediate risk:
    - Grade 1 or 2, stage IC, or cervical/isthmus involvement
    - No lymphovascular space involvement
    - No lymph node involvement
  - High risk:
    - Grade 3 and any myometrial invasion
    - Adnexal/Pelvic metastasis
    - Grade 2 and >50% myometrial invasion, and cervix/isthmus involvement
    - Lymphovascular space involvement

SPECIAL THERAPY
- For stage I disease, adjuvant radiation therapy can reduce the risk of local recurrence, but it does not improve survival or reduce distant metastasis.
- For stage II disease, options include:
  - Neoadjuvant radiation combined with total hysterectomy
  - Radical hysterectomy with lymphadenectomy followed by adjuvant chemotherapy or radiation directed toward known sites of disease
- For stage III or IV, adjuvant therapy is indicated:
  - Adjuvant chemotherapy, or radiation, or both are all reasonable options.
  - Adjuvant pelvic radiation improves disease-free survival rate.
  - Para-aortic radiation is associated with improved survival for those who have para-aortic lymph node involvement and complete resection of the nodes.
  - Concomitant chemotherapy may be beneficial.

MEDICATION (DRUGS)
Progestin therapy:
- Candidates are women with atypical endometrial hyperplasia and stage 1A grade 1 endometrial cancer who desire to maintain their fertility.
- Optimal dose/duration is unclear.
- Serial complete intrauterine evaluation with dilation and curettage is indicated every 3 months to document response.
- High-dose oral progestins or
- Levonorgestrel IUS has also been reported to be effective in young women.

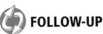

SURGERY
Surgical staging (including bilateral pelvic and paraaortic lymphadenectomy):
- Exceptions are young women with grade 1 endometrioid adenocarcinoma associated with atypical endometrial hyperplasia and women at increased risk of mortality secondary to comorbidities.
- Lymphadenectomy is helpful in guiding adjuvant therapy.
- Palpation of retroperitoneum or lymph node sampling are inaccurate assessments of lymph nodes.

FOLLOW-UP
DISPOSITION
Issues for Referral
A referral to a gynecologic oncologist is recommended if:
- The ability to surgically stage the patient adequately is not readily available at the time of initial procedure.
- Preoperative histology (grade 3, papillary serous, clear-cell, carcinosarcoma) suggests a high risk for extrauterine spread.
- Unexpected cancer diagnosis on final pathology report
- Suspicious for extrauterine metastasis

PROGNOSIS
- Stage is the most important prognostic factor.
- Other prognostic factors are grade, histologic subtype.
- 5-year survival rates:
  - Localized (stage IA or IB): 96%
  - Regional: 65%
  - Metastatic: 26%

PATIENT MONITORING
- Pelvic exam every 3–4 months for 2–3 years, then twice yearly
- CA 125, vaginal Pap smear, speculum exam, and rectovaginal exam at each follow up visit
- For women who have received radiotherapy, less frequent surveillance for recurrence is appropriate.
- For women who have not received radiotherapy, vaginal and pelvic recurrence can be successfully treated with salvage radiotherapy.

BIBLIOGRAPHY

Aalder J, et al. Postoperative external irradiation and prognostic parameters in stage I endometrial carcinoma: Clinical and histopathologic study of 540 patients. *Obstet Gynecol*. 1980;56:419–427.

Creutzberg CL, et al. Surgery and postoperative radiotherapy versus surgery alone for patients with stage 1 endometrial carcinoma: Multicentre randomized trial. PORTEC Study Group. Postoperative Radiation Therapy in Endometrial Carcinoma. *Lancet*. 2000;355:1404–1411.

Creutzberg CL, et al. Outcome of high-risk stage IC, grade 3, compared with stage I endometrial carcinoma patients: The Postoperative Radiation Therapy in Endometrial Carcinoma Trial. *J Clin Oncol*. 2004;22:1234–1241.

Gershenson DM, et al., eds. *Gynecologic Cancer: Controversies in Management*. Philadelphia: Elsevier; 2004:833–845.

Kilgore LC, et al. Adenocarcinoma of the endometrium: Survival comparisons of patients with and without pelvic node sampling. *Gynecol Oncol*. 1995;56:29–33.

Orr J, et al. ACOG Practice Bulletin No. 65: Management of endometrial cancer. August 2005.

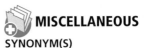

MISCELLANEOUS
SYNONYM(S)
- Adenocarcinoma of the endometrium/uterus
- Cancer, uterine
- Corpus cancer/carcinoma
- Endometrial/Uterine adenocarcinoma
- Fundal carcinoma
- Uterine cancer

CLINICAL PEARLS
Tissue diagnosis is the gold standard in women presented with postmenopausal vaginal bleeding.

ABBREVIATIONS
- COC—Combined oral contraceptives
- IUS—Intrauterine system
- PCOS—Polycystic ovary syndrome
- TVU—Transvaginal ultrasound
- UPSC—Uterine papillary serous carcinoma

CODES
ICD9-CM
182.0 Malignant neoplasm of the body of uterus

PATIENT TEACHING
- ACOG Patient Education Pamphlet: Cancer of the Uterus
- NCI patient education session www.cancer.gov/cancertopics/pdq/treatment/endometrial/patient

PREVENTION
- Based on solid evidence, giving progestin in combination with estrogen therapy for menopause eliminates the excess risk of endometrial cancer associated with unopposed estrogen.
- Use of COCs is associated with a reduced risk of endometrial cancer from 50–72%.
- There is inadequate evidence to state that weight reduction decreases the incidence of endometrial cancer.

ENDOMETRIAL HYPERPLASIA

Carol M. Choi, MD

BASICS

DESCRIPTION
- Endometrial hyperplasia is characterized by proliferation of endometrial glands, which results in greater gland-to-stroma ratio compared to normal endometrium.
- Architecture (glandular/stromal pattern):
  – Simple or complex
- Nuclear atypia:
  – Present or absent:
    ○ Single most important predictor of malignant transformation and resistance to progestin therapy

Age-Related Factors
Endometrial hyperplasia is associated with increasing age, although it can be diagnosed in young women.

EPIDEMIOLOGY
Endometrial hyperplasia typically affects perimenopausal and postmenopausal women, although it can affect younger women.

RISK FACTORS
- Increasing age
- Unopposed estrogen therapy
- Nulliparity
- Early menarche/late menopause
- Chronic anovulation
- Obesity
- Diabetes mellitus
- Hereditary nonpolyposis colorectal cancer (HNPCC)
- Tamoxifen therapy
- Estrogen-secreting tumor

Genetics
- Caucasian women are more likely than African American women to develop endometrial cancer and its precursors.
- HNPCC syndrome is characterized by a predisposition for endometrial, ovarian, and colorectal cancers.
- Genetic molecular factors are likely in at least some endometrial cancers and their precursor lesions.

PATHOPHYSIOLOGY
Unopposed estrogen exposure of the endometrium in the absence of progesterone leads to the development of endometrial hyperplasia.

ASSOCIATED CONDITIONS
See "Risk Factors."

DIAGNOSIS

SIGNS AND SYMPTOMS
History
- Abnormal uterine bleeding
- Infertility due to anovulation

Review of Systems
Abnormal uterine bleeding

Physical Exam
- BMI
- "Apple" body morphology versus "Pear"
- Pelvic exam may be normal

TESTS
Endometrial hyperplasia is a histologic diagnosis and thus requires endometrial sampling.

Labs
Endometrial tissue sample is the gold standard:
- Office biopsy or D&C

Imaging
TVU to measure endometrial stripe (consider in postmenopausal women not on HRT):
- Endometrial sampling if stripe >4 mm in postmenopausal woman

DIFFERENTIAL DIAGNOSIS
Infection
- Endometritis
- Cervicitis

Hematologic
Coagulopathy

Metabolic/Endocrine
- Hypothyroidism
- Chronic anovulation

Tumor/Malignancy
- Endometrial cancer
- Uterine leiomyomata

Trauma
Genital tract trauma

Drugs
- Unopposed estrogen
- Tamoxifen

Other/Miscellaneous
- Endometrial polyp
- Endocervical polyp
- Atrophy

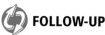 TREATMENT

GENERAL MEASURES
Goal of treatment is to control abnormal uterine bleeding and, more importantly, to prevent progression to endometrial cancer.

MEDICATION (DRUGS)
- Progestin therapy is mainstay of treatment. Type of progestin, dose, and duration of treatment varies (usually 3–6 months):
  – Medroxyprogesterone acetate
  – Megestrol acetate
  – Norethindrone acetate
  – DMPA
  – Levonorgestrel IUS
  – Micronized progesterone vaginal cream
- In younger women desiring contraception, a COC pill is appropriate.
- If pregnancy is desired, ovulation is induced with clomiphene citrate.

SURGERY
Hysterectomy is appropriate if:
- Atypia present and patient no longer desires childbearing potential
- Patient is unable to comply with medical therapy
- Persistent hyperplasia

FOLLOW-UP

DISPOSITION
Issues for Referral
Endometrial carcinoma

PROGNOSIS
If left untreated, endometrial hyperplasia progresses to endometrial cancer at the following rates:
- Simple 1%
- Complex 3%
- Simple atypical 8%
- Complex atypical 29%

PATIENT MONITORING
- Repeat endometrial sampling every 6 months for women treated with medical/progestin therapy
- Consider also for women with history of atypia that decline hysterectomy

BIBLIOGRAPHY

Herbst AL. Neoplastic Diseases of the Uterus: Endometrial Hyperplasia, Endometrial Carcinoma, Sarcoma: Diagnosis and Management. In: Mishell Jr. DR, et al., ed. *Comprehensive Gynecology,* 3rd ed. St Louis: Mosby–Year Book; 1997:865–899.

Kurman RJ, et al. The behavior of endometrial hyperplasia: a long-term study of "untreated" hyperplasia in 170 patients. *Cancer.* 1985;56:403–412.

Woodruff JD, et al. Incidence of endometrial hyperplasia in postmenopausal women taking conjugated estrogens (Premarin) with medroxyprogesterone acetate or conjugated estrogens alone. *Am J Obstet Gynecol.* 1994;170:1213–1223.

 ## MISCELLANEOUS

SYNONYM(S)
Endometrial intraepithelial neoplasia (EIN)

ABBREVIATIONS
- COC—Combined oral contraceptive
- DMPA—Depot medroxyprogesterone acetate
- EIN—Endometrial intraepithelial neoplasia
- HNPCC—Hereditary nonpolyposis colorectal cancer
- HT—Hormone therapy
- PCOS—Polycystic ovary syndrome
- IUS—Intrauterine system
- TVU—Transvaginal ultrasound

CODES
ICD9-CM
- 621.30 Endometrial hyperplasia, unspecified
- 621.31 Simple endometrial hyperplasia without atypia
- 621.32 Complex endometrial hyperplasia without atypia
- 621.33 Endometrial hyperplasia with atypia

 ## PATIENT TEACHING

PREVENTION
- Avoidance of unopposed estrogen therapy (HT) in women with intact uterus
- Weight loss in overweight women
- Management of PCOS with oral contraceptives or regular withdrawal bleeding with progestins

Section II

ENDOMETRIOSIS

Jamie A. M. Massie, MD
Ruth B. Lathi, MD
Lynn M. Westphal, MD

 BASICS

DESCRIPTION
The presence of endometrial glands and stroma at any site outside the uterine cavity.

Age-Related Factors
- Occurs during the active reproductive period
- Rare in postmenopausal women

Pediatric Considerations
- Rare in pre- or recently postmenarchal girls, but can occur
- 25–38% of adolescents with chronic pelvic pain affected
- The development of endometriosis during childhood or adolescence may indicate some degree of genital tract obstruction (i.e., uterine or vaginal septum).

Staging
Staging is based on site(s) and severity of involvement at the time of surgery:
- Stage I (minimal): Isolated implants, no significant adhesions
- Stage II (mild): Superficial implants with <5 cm of total disease, no significant adhesions
- Stage III (moderate): Multiple superficial and deep implants, with or without peritubal and periovarian adhesions
- Stage IV (severe): Multiple superficial and deep implants, large ovarian endometrioma(s), with presence of adhesions

EPIDEMIOLOGY
Present in 7–10% of women in the general population

RISK FACTORS
- Delayed childbearing
- 1st-degree relative with endometriosis
- Short menstrual cycles
- Delayed parity may increase risk
- Increased incidence in women with uterine anomalies leading to outflow obstruction (i.e., transverse vaginal septum)

Genetics
- Familial disposition is suggested by current data.
- Concordance in twins has been observed.

PATHOPHYSIOLOGY
Controversial, but theories include:
- Retrograde menstruation (Sampson's theory)
- Dissemination of endometrial cells through lymphatics/blood vessels (Halban's theory)
- Direct transplantation
- Coelomic metaplasia

ASSOCIATED CONDITIONS
- Adenomyosis
- Uterine leiomyomata
- Chronic pain syndromes
- Infertility
- Müllerian anomalies
- Autoimmune diseases (i.e., hypothyroidism)
- Ovarian cancer (independent risk factor for epithelial ovarian cancer)

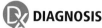 **DIAGNOSIS**

SIGNS AND SYMPTOMS
History
- Dysmenorrhea and/or back pain: Cyclic
- Dysmenorrhea is usually secondary; pain typically begins before the onset of menstrual flow and may be severe
- Deep dyspareunia
- Premenstrual spotting
- Infertility

Review of Systems
- Primary complaint not GI related
- Denies fever/chills
- Denies anorexia or nausea/vomiting
- Absence of urinary frequency or dysuria
- Absence of purulent vaginal discharge

Physical Exam
- Pelvic exam is nonspecific. The following may be present:
  - Uterus of normal size, but mobility limited
  - Uterosacral nodularity and tenderness
  - Adnexal mass
- Abdominal exam usually benign, unless ruptured endometrioma produces peritoneal signs

TESTS
- Direct visualization via laparoscopy with biopsy confirmation of endometriosis is required for definitive diagnosis.
- Vesicular lesions on peritoneal surfaces may be black, brown, red, clear, or white.
- Clear or red flame lesions ("atypical" lesions) are more common in adolescents.
- Lesions outside of the pelvis can be present (e.g., appendix, diaphragm, bowel).
- Pelvic adhesions vary from none to severe.

Labs
Serum CA-125:
- May be elevated (>35 IU/mL) in women with endometriosis
- Sensitivity and specificity are low
- Also elevated in other gynecologic disorders (i.e., ovarian cancer)

Imaging
- Rarely helpful in diagnosis of disease
- Vaginal/Abdominal US can be used to diagnose endometrioma.
- MRI can be used to map extent of disease if bladder or bowel involvement is suspected.
- Hysterosalpingography is useful only in evaluation of fallopian tube occlusion.

DIFFERENTIAL DIAGNOSIS
- Adenomyosis
- Uterine leiomyomata
- Interstitial cystitis
- Pelvic adhesive disease
- PID
- Primary dysmenorrhea
- Ovarian torsion
- Ectopic pregnancy
- IBS
- Appendicitis
- Diverticulitis

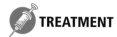 **TREATMENT**

GENERAL MEASURES
Treatment plans should be individualized and based on patient age and desire for future fertility.

MEDICATION (DRUGS)
- First-line therapies below should be combined with NSAIDs to obtain maximum benefit:
  - COCs daily
  - Medroxyprogesterone acetate (MPA) 150 mg IM every 3 months
- If symptoms persist after 3 months of OCPs or MPA and NSAIDs:
  - Empiric therapy with a 3-month course of GnRH agonist may be initiated:
    - Duration of therapy should be limited to 6 months unless add-back therapy is started
  - Danazol 600–800 mg/d for a course of 6 months is a lower-cost option than GnRH agonist, however side-effect profile less favorable
- Levonorgestrel IUS: Limited data suggest improvement in dysmenorrhea and menorrhagia with use

SURGERY

- Patients with persistent pain despite appropriate medical therapies or those with infertility should pursue surgical treatment.
- Laparoscopy with destruction of identifiable lesions via one of the following mechanisms:
  - Excision
  - Laser vaporization
  - Electrocautery
  - Endocoagulation
- Hysterectomy with/without bilateral salpingo-oophorectomy can be offered to women who have completed childbearing.
- Postoperatively, use of GnRH agonists for a period of 3–6 months may extend the painfree interval.

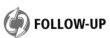

FOLLOW-UP

DISPOSITION

Issues for Referral

- Patients with unexplained infertility should be referred to board-certified reproductive endocrinologist or gynecologist with expertise in infertility.
- Patients with endometriosis resulting in severe adhesive disease with significant distortion of the pelvic anatomy may benefit from referral to a gynecologic oncologist or laparoscopic specialist for surgical treatment.
- Patients with persistent or inadequately treated pain may benefit from consultation with an interdisciplinary pain management team or service.

PROGNOSIS

- Up to 80% of women have improvement in pain with medical treatment alone, although there is a high rate of recurrent symptoms after cessation of therapy.
- 80–90% of women have improvement in pain after surgery.
- Pregnancy rates are improved after surgical treatment of endometriosis in patients with infertility.
- Endometriosis often improves or resolves after pregnancy.

PATIENT MONITORING

- For those patients on extended therapy with a GnRH agonist, vasomotor symptoms and/or bone loss can develop.
- Add-back therapy with progestins or low-dose OCPs may be utilized to minimize bone loss and limit vasomotor symptoms.

BIBLIOGRAPHY

ACOG Practice Bulletin. Medical management of endometriosis. Clinical Management Guidelines for Obstetrician-Gynecologists. Number 11, December 1999.

Kennedy S, et al. ESHRE guideline for the diagnosis and treatment of endometriosis. *Hum Reprod.* 2005;20(10):2698–2704.

Schenken RS. Pathogenesis. In: Schenken RS, ed. *Endometriosis: Contemporary Concepts in Clinical Management.* Philadelphia: JB Lippincott; 1989.

Vercellini P, et al. Endometriosis and pelvic pain: Relation to disease stage and localization. *Fertil Steril.* 1996;65(2):299–304.

 MISCELLANEOUS

ABBREVIATIONS

- COC—Combined oral contraceptives
- GnRH—Gonadotropin releasing hormone
- IBS—Irritable bowel syndrome
- IUS—Intrauterine system
- MPA—Medroxyprogesterone acetate
- NSAIDs—Nonsteroidal anti-inflammatory drugs
- OCP—Oral contraceptive pill
- PID—Pelvic inflammatory disease

CODES

ICD9-CM

- 617.0 Endometriosis of uterus
- 617.1 Endometriosis of ovary
- 617.3 Endometriosis of pelvic peritoneum
- 617.5 Endometriosis of intestine
- 617.9 Endometriosis, site unspecified

 PATIENT TEACHING

- Endometriosis Patient Education Pamphlet, American College of Obstetricians and Gynecologists, November 2001
- The Endometriosis Association www.endo-online.org

ENDOMETRITIS

Melissa D. Tepe, MD, MPH
Jeffrey F. Peipert, MD, MPH

 BASICS

DESCRIPTION
- Endometritis is inflammation of the endometrium or lining of the uterus; it often divided into acute and chronic:
  - Acute: Associated with neutrophils within the endometrial glands; often accompanied by pelvic pain and/or abnormal uterine bleeding
  - Chronic: Associated with plasma cells within the endometrial stroma
- 4 common categories:
  - Acute nonobstetric:
    - PID
    - Postinvasive gynecologic procedures
  - Acute obstetric:
    - Post cesarean or vaginal delivery
  - Chronic nonobstetric:
    - Chronic PID or tuberculosis
    - IUDs
    - Intrauterine pathology such as leiomyoma or polyp
    - Radiation therapy
    - Idiopathic
  - Chronic obstetric:
    - Retained products of conception post delivery or termination
    - Late onset postpartum
- See Pelvic Inflammatory Disease and Postpartum Fever.
- Subclinical endometritis is common among women with lower genital tract infection including *Chlamydia trachomatis*, *Neisseria gonorrhoeae*, bacterial vaginosis, and trichomoniasis. The impact of this silent endometritis is currently unknown.

Age-Related Factors
Most cases are in women of reproductive age, given risk factors associated with pregnancy and PID; however, any woman with a uterus may get endometritis.

EPIDEMIOLOGY
- Endometritis is uncommon after invasive transcervical procedures. One sample found only 2 in 927 hysteroscopies were complicated by infection.
- As many as 45–50% of nonpregnant women with lower genital traction infections with *C. trachomatis*, *N. gonorrhoea*, or bacterial vaginosis may have histologic evidence of upper genital tract inflammation (endometritis).

RISK FACTORS
- Infection:
  - *C. trachomatis*
  - *N. gonorrhoeae*
  - Bacterial vaginosis
  - Trichomonis
  - HSV-2
- Intrauterine foreign bodies or pathology
- Transcervical procedures:
  - Hysterosalpingogram
  - Sonohysterography
  - IUD insertion
  - Endometrial biopsy
  - D&C
  - Hysteroscopy: Diagnostic and operative
- Pregnancy, especially if complicated by retained products of conception, prolonged labor, rupture of membranes, multiple vaginal exams, or entry into the uterine cavity of anaerobic bacteria or group B streptococci

PATHOPHYSIOLOGY
- Any cause of endometrial inflammation, ranging from idiopathic to infection with microorganisms, foreign bodies, and/or uterine pathology
- Increased risk of endometritis with breach of the cervical mucous, which acts as a protective barrier from ascending infection
- Ascending infection often polymicrobial

ASSOCIATED CONDITIONS
- Increased risk of infertility if associated with PID, especially salpingitis
- Increased risk of ectopic pregnancy
- Recurrent PID
- Chronic pelvic pain

DIAGNOSIS

SIGNS AND SYMPTOMS
History
- Recent IUD insertion
- Recent transcervical procedure
- Diagnosis of lower genital tract infection

Review of Systems
- May be asymptomatic
- Sharp-to-crampy pelvic pain
- Dysmenorrhea and/or dyspareunia
- Fever, malaise, nausea, vomiting
- Abnormal uterine bleeding
- Signs of lower genital tract infection:
  - Vaginal discharge, malodor, pruritus

Physical Exam
- Tender abdomen/pelvis:
  - Symptoms may be vague and/or mild
- Cervical motion tenderness
- Palpable adnexal swelling (more likely if associated with salpingitis)
- Vaginal discharge
- Mucopurulent endocervicitis
- Leukorrhea:
  - WBCs greater than epithelial cells

TESTS
Labs
- Vaginal wet mount with findings such as clue cells associated with bacterial vaginosis, trichomoniasis, WBCs associated with vaginitis/cervicitis
- Cervical culture for *C. trachomatis* and/or *N. gonorrhoeae*
- Endometrial biopsy with neutrophils or plasma cells as well as fragments of polyp/fibroids or infectious agent
- Leukocytosis
- Elevated C-reactive protein (CRP) or ESR

Imaging
- Consider abdominal/transvaginal US or MRI:
  - May demonstrate thickened, fluid-filled fallopian tubes with or without free fluid
  - To rule out other pelvic pathology such as tubo-ovarian abscess and/or retained products of conception
- CT scan to rule out other sources of pelvic masses, including PID-associated and postoperative tubo-ovarian abscess

DIFFERENTIAL DIAGNOSIS
Infection
- PID (see topic)
- Lower genital tract infection (See topics on Sexually Transmitted Diseases.)
- Tubo-ovarian abscess (See Pelvic Abscess.)
- UTI (see topic):
  - Pyelonephritis
  - Cystitis

Tumor/Malignancy
Endometrial hyperplasia or cancer (see topics)

Trauma
Post–sexual assault (See Rape/Sexual Assault and Sexual Abuse.)

Other/Miscellaneous
- Ectopic pregnancy (see topics)
- Missed, inevitable, incomplete abortion (See Spontaneous Abortion and Septic Abortion.)
- Retained products of conception post abortion or delivery (See Hemorrhage: Postpartum.)
- Endometriosis (see topic)
- Pelvic adhesions
- Ruptured ovarian cyst (See Ovarian Cyst Rupture.)
- Nephrolithiasis
- Appendicitis
- IBS (see topic)
- Ulcerative colitis
- Crohn's disease

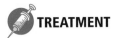 ## TREATMENT

GENERAL MEASURES
Evaluate for the cause of endometritis whether postprocedure, PID or lower genital tract infection, or peripartum and treat accordingly with supportive measures and the appropriate antibiotics.

MEDICATION (DRUGS)
- Prophylactic antibiotics prior to transcervical procedures:
  - Hysterosalpingography:
    - Doxycycline 100 mg PO b.i.d. for 5 days if HSG shows dilated fallopian tubes
  - Sonohysterography:
    - Routine use of prophylactic antibiotics is not recommended
  - Hysteroscopic surgery:
    - Routine use of prophylactic antibiotics is not recommended
  - IUD insertion:
    - No antibiotic prophylaxis is needed if negative screen for *N. gonorrhoeae* and *C. trachomatis*
  - Endometrial biopsy:
    - Routine use of prophylactic antibiotics is not recommended
  - Induced surgical abortion:
    - Consider treatment with doxycycline 100 mg PO 1 hour before procedure and 200 mg PO after procedure
    - OR metronidazole 500 mg PO b.i.d. for 5 days
    - OR doxycycline 100 mg PO b.i.d. for 7 days
  - Incomplete abortion:
    - Routine use of prophylactic antibiotics is not recommended
  - Medical abortion:
    - Routine use of prophylactic antibiotics is not required
    - Some facilities treat with doxycycline 100 mg PO b.i.d. for 7 days
- See Pelvic Inflammatory Disease for on inpatient and outpatient treatment regimens for PID
  - Note that metronidazole has been added to most regimens given the association of anaerobic bacteria with PID
- See Postpartum Fever for treatment of obstetric endometritis

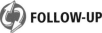 ## FOLLOW-UP

DISPOSITION
Issues for Referral
- Refer to inpatient setting with unstable vitals or if need for IV antibiotics arises
- Guidelines for inpatient treatment of PID:
  - Cannot rule-out a surgical emergency
  - Pregnancy
  - Unresponsive to oral antibiotics
  - Unable to take outpatient oral antibiotics
  - Severe illness, nausea and vomiting, or high fever
  - Tubo-ovarian abscess

PROGNOSIS
Prognosis is good with prompt antibiotic treatment of infectious causes.

PATIENT MONITORING
After antibiotic treatment, patients with documented *C. trachomatis* and *N. gonorrhoeae* infection may be retested in 3 months. All women with documented infections should be offered HIV testing.

BIBLIOGRAPHY

American College of Obstetricians and Gynecologists. Medical Management of Abortion. ACOG Practice Bulletin 67. Washington, DC: American College of Obstetricians and Gynecologists; 2005.

American College of Obstetricians and Gynecologists. Antibiotic Prophylaxis for Gynecologic Procedures. ACOG Practice Bulletin 74. Washington, DC: American College of Obstetricians and Gynecologists; 2006.

Centers for Disease Control and Prevention. Sexually Transmitted Disease Guidelines, 2006. *MMWR*. 2006;55(No. RR–11):50–52.

Haggerty CL, et al. Bacterial vaginosis and anaerobic bacteria are associated with endometritis. *Clin Infect Dis.* 2004;39:990–995.

Korn AP, Hessol NA, Padian NS, et al. Risk factors for plasma cell endometritis among women with cervical Neisseria gonorrhoea, cervical Chlamydia trachomatis, or bacterial vaginosis. *Am J Obstet Gynecol*. 1998;178:987–90.

Propst AM, et al. Complications of hysteroscopic surgery predicting patients at risk. *Obstet Gynecol*. 2000;96:517.

Wiesenfeld HC, et al. Lower genital tract infection and endometritis: Insight into subclinical pelvic inflammatory disease. *Obstet Gynecol*. 2002;100: 456–463.

 ## MISCELLANEOUS

ABBREVIATIONS
- HSV-2—Herpes simplex virus type 2
- IBS—Irritable bowel syndrome
- PID—Pelvic inflammatory disease
- STD/STI—Sexually transmitted disease/infection
- UTI—Urinary tract infection

CODES
ICD9-CM
- 615.0 Acute Inflammatory disease of the uterus
- 615.1 Chronic Inflammatory disease of the uterus
- 615.9 Unspecified Inflammatory disease of the uterus
- 634-638 with .0 Inflammatory disease of the uterus complicating an abortion
- 639.0 Inflammatory disease of the uterus complicating an ectopic or molar pregnancy
- 646.6 Inflammatory disease of the uterus complicating pregnancy or labor
- 670.0 Major puerperal infection including endometritis

 ## PATIENT TEACHING

- Prevention and treatment of STDs
- Report signs or symptoms of vaginal infection before any operative procedure.
- Risk and benefits of planned transcervical procedures including any recommended prophylactic antibiotics

PREVENTION
Safe sex practices including condoms for the prevention of STIs

FALLOPIAN TUBE CANCER

Kathleen Y. Yang, MD

 BASICS

DESCRIPTION
- Primary carcinoma: Rare
- Secondary carcinoma: Metastatic disease from the ovaries, endometrium, gastrointestinal tract, or breast

Age-Related Factors
Mean age of diagnosis is 55–60 years.

Staging
Surgical staging:
- Stage 0: Carcinoma in situ
- Stage I: Tubes only
  - 1A: 1 tube
  - 1B: Both tubes
  - 1C: Tubal serosa, malignant ascites or pelvic washing
- Stage II: Pelvic metastasis
  - 2A: Uterus and ovaries
  - 2B: Other pelvic tissues
  - 2C: Pelvic metastasis plus malignant ascites or pelvic washing
- Stage III: Abdominal metastasis, and/or positive lymph nodes:
  - 3A: Microscopic abdominal seeding
  - 3B: Abdominal seeding <2 cm
  - 3C: Abdominal seeding >2 cm, and/or positive lymph nodes
- Stage IV: Distant metastasis, or malignant pleural effusion, or liver parenchymal involvement

EPIDEMIOLOGY
- Primary carcinoma is rare (0.2–0.5% of malignant neoplasm of the female genital tract).
- Estimated annual incidence in US is 3.6/1,000,000 women.
- Tubal metastasis from other cancer is more common.
- 10–25% of fallopian tube cancer cases are bilateral.
- At the time of diagnosis, stage distribution is:
  - 37% in stage I
  - 20% in stage II
  - 31% in stage III
  - 10% in stage IV

RISK FACTORS
- BRCA 1 or 2 germline mutations carry a 120-fold increased risk compared to general population.
- Unclear association with *Chlamydia* infection, or pelvic inflammatory disease, or infertility, or sterilization

Genetics
- High proportion of BRCA 1 mutation identified in women diagnosed with primary fallopian tube carcinoma
- If primary fallopian tube cancer is diagnosed, then BRCA testing/genetic counseling should be offered.

PATHOPHYSIOLOGY
Histological types include:
- Papillary serous adenocarcinoma (most common)
- Endometrioid
- Clear cell
- Adenosquamous
- Squamous cell carcinoma
- Sarcoma
- Choriocarcinoma
- Malignant teratoma

ASSOCIATED CONDITIONS
Breast, colon, endometrial, ovarian cancers

 DIAGNOSIS

SIGNS AND SYMPTOMS
- Classic triad:
  - Hydrops tubae profluens (intermittent serosanguinous vaginal discharge)
  - Pelvic pain secondary to tubal distension: Colicky or dull
  - Pelvic mass
- Abdominal discomfort/pressure/bloating
- Dyspepsia, early satiety
- Leukorrhea (clear vaginal discharge) and vaginal bleeding after a negative endometrial biopsy
- Abnormal cervical cytology with a negative colposcopy and biopsies
- Urinary frequency and/or urgency with negative workup for UTI, sensation of incomplete emptying of bladder

History
- Complete gynecologic, pain, family history
- Gynecologic history/procedures:
  - STD history
  - PID
  - Menopause
  - Sexual activity: Number of partners, use of local estrogen, dyspareunia
  - History of cervical dysplasia or Human papillomavirus infection
  - Recent pap smear result
- Pain history:
  - Onset, quality, frequency, duration, intensity of pain (use pain scale of 0–10)
  - Pain medication taken, including OTC: Name, dose, frequency, efficacy
  - Any history of chronic pelvic pain
- Past medical history:
  - Hospitalizations
  - Surgeries
  - Chronic medical conditions
  - Personal history of breast cancer
- Family history:
  - Breast cancer
  - Ovarian cancer
  - Uterine cancer
  - Degree of relatives affected
  - Age of diagnosis in relatives

Review of Systems
- Special attention to GI and GU systems
- Weight loss or weight gain
- Night sweats
- Change of waist line in normal clothing (ascites)

Physical Exam
- General:
  - Appearance
  - VS
  - BMI
  - BP
- Abdominal exam:
  - Masses
  - Ascites: Shifting dullness, fluid wave
  - Hepatomegaly
  - Tenderness, rebound, guarding
- Pelvic exam:
  - Speculum exam to observe any clear or serosanguineous discharge from the cervix
  - Bimanual exam to assess uterine size, shape, position, mobility, and tenderness
  - Bimanual exam to assess adnexal mass, tenderness, mobility
  - Rectovaginal exam to assess any mass in the rectum or cul-de-sac

TESTS
Labs
- CA 125:
  - Usually elevated in fallopian tube cancer patients
  - CA 125 alone is not diagnostic
  - Preoperative CA 125 has prognostic value
  - Can be used serially to follow the course of disease, response to treatment, and recurrence surveillance
- Urine analysis if indicated by symptoms
- Pap smear
- Vaginal wet mount, STD testing if indicated

Imaging
- TVU with color Doppler:
  - Pelvic mass
  - Cystic vs. solid
  - Simple vs. complex
  - Septations or implants
  - Doppler flow or not
  - Ascites
- CT/MRI:
  - Poor diagnostic value
  - Used to assess metastasis, lymph node involvement, surgical planning, and recurrence surveillance
- PET: Assess metastasis

DIFFERENTIAL DIAGNOSIS
Infection
- Tubo-ovarian complex/abscess
- Hydrosalpinx
- PID
- Pelvic tuberculosis
- UTI

Tumor/Malignancy
- Uterine, ovarian, or peritoneal neoplasm
- Metastatic breast cancer or gastrointestinal neoplasm
- Cervical cancer

Other/Miscellaneous
- Endometrioma
- Ovarian cysts
- Paratubal cysts
- Fibroid uterus

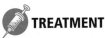 **TREATMENT**

GENERAL MEASURES
- Surgery is required to obtain tissue for definitive diagnosis.
- Treatment guidelines are similar to those for epithelial ovarian cancer.
- Mainstay of treatment is initial surgery, followed by chemotherapy, and possibly radiotherapy.

SPECIAL THERAPY
Adjuvant radiotherapy:
- No established standards on mode of delivery, radiation field, and dosage
- Whole abdominal radiotherapy may be necessary given the pattern of metastasis involved the upper abdomen.

MEDICATION (DRUGS)
Adjuvant chemotherapy:
- No data from prospective RCTs secondary to the rarity of the disease
- Advanced stage cancer:
  – Current recommendation is combination chemotherapy with paclitaxel and carboplatin.
- Early stage cancer:
  – Role of chemotherapy is unclear.

SURGERY
- Optimal tumor debulking is the key to improving survival rate.
- Exploratory laparotomy
- Total abdominal hysterectomy and bilateral salpingo-oophorectomy
- Retroperitoneal lymph node dissection
- Omentectomy
- Pelvic washing
- Tumor debulking

 FOLLOW-UP

DISPOSITION
Issues for Referral
A patient with diagnosis of fallopian tube cancer should follow-up with a gynecologic oncologist.

PROGNOSIS
- Stage is the most important prognostic factor.
- Overall prognosis is better than for ovarian cancer, likely secondary to a more favorable stage distribution at the time of the diagnosis.
- 5-year survival:
  – Stage I: 95%
  – Stage II: 75%
  – Stage III: 69%
  – Stage IV: 45%

PATIENT MONITORING
- Guidelines for recurrence surveillance are similar to those of ovarian cancer.
- Surveillance visits and physical exam every 3 months for the 1st year, then every 4 months for the 2nd year, then every 6 months for the 3rd–5th year, then annually.
- Annual CXR for the 1st–3rd year
- CA 125 every 3 months for 1st–2nd year, then every 6 months for 3rd–5th year
- CT/ MRI/PET as indicated
- Annual mammography for patients >50 years of age
- Colonoscopy every 10 years if age >50

BIBLIOGRAPHY

Berek JS, et al., eds. *Practical Gynecologic Oncology*, 4th ed. Baltimore: Williams & Wilkins; 2005: 533–541.

Brose MS, et al. Cancer risk estimates for BRCA1 mutation carriers identified in a risk evaluation program. *J Natl Cancer Inst*. 2002;94:1365.

Cormio G. Experience at the Memorial Sloan-Kettering Cancer Center with paclitaxel-based combination chemotherapy following primary cytoreductive surgery in carcinoma of the fallopian tube. *Gynecol Oncol*. 2002;84(1):185–186.

Eddy GL, et al. Fallopian tube carcinoma. *Obstet Gynecol*. 1984;64:546.

Kosary C, et al. Treatment and survival for women with fallopian tube carcinoma: A population-based study. *Gynecol Oncol*. 2002;86:190.

Pecorelli S, et al. Carcinoma of the fallopian tube: FIGO annual report on the results of treatment in gynecological cancer. *J Epidemiol Biostat*. 1998;3:363–374.

Rauthe G, et al. Primary cancer of the fallopian tube. Treatment and results of 37 cases. *Eur J Gynaecol Oncol*. 1998;19:356.

 MISCELLANEOUS

SYNONYM(S)
- Tubal cancer
- Fallopian tube neoplasm
- Cancer of the oviduct

ABBREVIATIONS
- BMI—Body mass index
- PID—Pelvic inflammatory disease
- RCT—Random clinical trial
- STD—Sexually transmitted disease
- TVU—Transvaginal ultrasound
- UTI—Urinary tract infection

CODES
ICD9-CM
183.2 Malignant neoplasm of fallopian tube

PATIENT TEACHING
- ACS Patient Education pamphlet available at http://www.cancer.org
- MD Anderson Cancer Center Patient Education Q&A "What to know about fallopian tube cancer" at http://www.cancerwise.org

PREVENTION
Not established

Paula J. Adams Hillard, MD

 BASICS

DESCRIPTION

- 5–6% of all breast cancers are associated with inherited genetic mutations.
- 2 susceptibility genes, BRCA1 and BRCA2, are among several known susceptibility genes associated with both breast and ovarian cancer:
  - Several hundred mutations of these genes reported.
  - Autosomal dominant inheritance
- Mutations of BRCA1 (80%) and BRCA2 (15%) genes account for the majority of inherited breast and ovarian cancers.

Age-Related Factors
For women with a family history of breast or ovarian cancer, age at the time of diagnosis will help guide the initiation of screening.

EPIDEMIOLOGY

- Mutations in BRCA1 or BRCA2 are rare, affecting 0.1–0.8% of general population:
  - Mutations of these genes account for <1/5 of the familial risk of breast cancer.
  - Mutations of BRCA1/2 are more common in women of Ashkenazi Jewish (Eastern European) descent:
    - 2.3% to 12–30%, respectively, of breast cancer in this is group attributable to BRCA mutations
- Cancer risks with BRCA1/2:

PATHOPHYSIOLOGY

- BRCA genes appear to act as tumor suppressor genes.
- Mutations interfere with DNA repair, with resultant accumulation of chromosomal abnormalities and risk of cancer.
- Inherited BRCA gene abnormalities have a high penetrance.
- Mechanism by which BRCA mutations predispose to breast and ovarian cancers is not clear.

ASSOCIATED CONDITIONS
Ovarian, pancreatic, colon cancer, family history of prostate cancer, male breast cancer

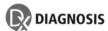 **DIAGNOSIS**

SIGNS AND SYMPTOMS
History
- Family and personal history are important:
  - Ashkenazi Jewish heritage
  - Family history of breast cancer:
    - 12% of women have a family history, which provides a 2-fold higher risk compared to the general population.
  - Relatedness:
    - 1st-degree relative: RR, 2.1
    - 2nd-degree relative: RR, 1.5

- Number of relatives:
  - 1 1st-degree relative: RR, 2.1
  - 2 1st-degree relatives: RR, 3.6
- Age at diagnosis:
  - 1st-degree <50: RR, 2.3
  - 1st-degree >50: RR, 1.8
- 1st-degree relative with bilateral breast cancer RR: 9.8
- 1st-degree relative with ovarian cancer: RR 1.27
- Genetic testing of relatives and results
- Family history of ovarian cancer
- BRCA testing recommended if estimated risk >10%:
  - Breast Cancer Risk Assessment Tool developed by the National Cancer Institute (NCI)

TESTS
- Because inherited mutations are rare, most women, even those with a family history of breast and ovarian cancer, do not require genetic testing.
- Testing should be considered if risk of having a BRCA mutation is at least 10%.
- Risks of routine testing in all women:
  - Risk of indeterminate or false-positive results
  - Psychologic and social risks of testing
  - False reassurance if genetic testing is negative
- Genetic counseling should be considered:
  - Pretest counseling address factors that enter into the decision to have testing:
    - Medical, emotional, practical, financial factors
  - Posttest counseling is recommended
- BRCA genes are large, with hundreds of mutations, and thus full testing is expensive.
- Once a mutation is identified in affected individual, testing of that specific mutation can be performed on family members.
- Analysis of 3 specific mutations most commonly seen in Ashkenazi Jewish individuals can be performed.
- In individuals with negative testing, but high-risk family history, possible undetected BRCA1/2 mutation may be present.
- Most insurance will cover a percentage of costs.
- True negative test result if tested for specific mutation previously identified in family member:
  - The risks are approximately the same as risk in general population
- If individual is the 1st in family to be tested, negative test results could mean:
  - BRCA mutation present, but not detected by currently available methods.
  - A mutation may be present in another gene that is rare or not yet isolated.
  - The tested individual could have developed sporadic, not hereditary cancer.
- Psychological issues:
  - "Survivor's guilt" if testing is negative
  - If positive, implications for prophylactic surgery or fertility

Pediatric Considerations
Decisions regarding genetic testing for BRCA mutations in the adolescent are complex and should include consideration of the medical and psychological implication of testing for the individual and her family.

Cancer	Lifetime risk in general population	Lifetime risk in BRCA1 carrier	Lifetime risk in BRCA2 carrier
Breast	12.5%	55–85%	50–85%
Contralateral breast	0.5–1%/yr	Up to 6%	Up to 50%
Ovarian	1.5%	40–50%	15–25%
Colon	5%	? slight increase	? slight increase
Prostate	15%	Incr	35–40%
Male breast	0.1%	5–10%	5–10%
Pancreatic	1.3%	<10%	<10%

RISK FACTORS
Genetics
- Other genes, associated syndrome, and chromosome sites:

Gene	Syndrome	Chromosome site
BRCA1	Hereditary breast ovarian cancer syndrome	17q21
BRCA2	"	13q12–13
p53	LI–FRAUMENI	17P13.1
PTEN	Cowden	10q22–23
ATM	Ataxia–telangiectasia	11q22–23
STK11	Peutz-Jeghers	19p13.3

Imaging
With family history of ovarian cancer, screening has not been shown to prevent ovarian cancer deaths, nor is routine screening recommended.
- TVU has been used.
- CA-125 testing may be performed in postmenopausal women.

TREATMENT

MEDICATION (DRUGS)
- OCPs are associated with a decreased risk of ovarian cancer in the general population, and studies suggest a benefit in BRCA mutation carriers as well.
- Tamoxifen in BRCA mutation carriers reduces the risk of 2nd breast cancer in opposite breast by ~40–50%:
  – Risks of Tamoxifen, particularly in women >50 include: endometrial cancer, stroke, DVT, PE

SURGERY
Some high-risk women consider prophylactic surgery:

- Tubal sterilization may decrease the risks of ovarian cancer.
- Prophylactic bilateral mastectomy provides ~90% reduction in risk of breast cancer for high-risk women, including those with BRCA mutations.
- Prophylactic BSO for women with BRCA mutation provides:
  – ~5–95% reduction of ovarian cancer
  – 40–50% reduction in breast cancer for premenopausal women
  – BSO recommended by age 35 or once childbearing complete

FOLLOW-UP

DISPOSITION
Issues for Referral
Genetics counseling may be appropriate for an individual in assessing risk of breast or ovarian cancer and in considering testing for BRCA mutations.

PROGNOSIS
Depends of family history, mutation, screening, early diagnosis

PATIENT MONITORING
- For women with a family history of breast cancer, mammography should be combined with clinical breast exams, breast self-examination, and consideration of MRI screening:
  – ACS expert panel recommend MRI imaging for annual screening in addition to mammography for women with a 20–25% or greater lifetime risk.
- For women with a family history of ovarian cancer, counseling and discussion of monitoring techniques is indicated, with consideration of CA-125 and TVU.

BIBLIOGRAPHY

ACOG Committee Opinion No. 350, November 2006: Breast concerns in the adolescent. *Obstetrics and Gynecology.* 2006;108(5):1329–1336.

Bermejo-Perez MJ, et al. Effectiveness of preventive interventions in BRCA1/2 gene mutation carriers: A systematic review. *Intern J Cancer.* 2007;121(2):225–231.

Calculator for risk of BRCA inherited breast cancer at http://astor.som.jhmi.edu/BayesMendel/brcapro.html

Fletcher SW. Overview of genetics in breast and ovarian cancer. UpToDate http://uptodate.com. Accessed 09/22/07.

Lux MP, et al. Hereditary breast and ovarian cancer: Review and future perspectives. *J Mol Med.* 2006;84(1):16–28.

U.S. Preventive Services Task Force. Screening for Ovarian Cancer: Recommendation statement. *Ann Fam Med.* 2004;2:260–262.

MISCELLANEOUS

CLINICAL PEARLS
A careful complete family history is essential in initiating an assessment of risk.

ABBREVIATIONS
- BSO—Bilateral salpingo–oophorectomy
- DVT—Deep vein thrombosis
- OCP—Oral contraceptive pill
- PE—Pulmonary embolism
- RR—Relative risk
- TVU—Transvaginal ultrasound

CODES
ICD9-CM
- V16.3 Family history of breast cancer
- V16.41 Family history of ovarian cancer
- V84.01 Gentic susceptibility to malignant neoplasm, breast
- V84.09 Gentic susceptibility to other malignant neoplasm

PATIENT TEACHING

Understanding Cancer Risk from NCI at http://understandingrisk.cancer.gov/

PREVENTION
See Medication (Oral contraceptives) and Surgery (Prophylactic surgery) within this topic.

FECAL INCONTINENCE

Christina Lewicky-Gaupp, MD
Dee E. Fenner, MD

ALERT

Obstetric trauma is the most common cause of fecal incontinence in young women. However, aging and diarrheal states have the greatest impact on bowel control in women >40. Fecal incontinence is a disease with profound social and psychologic stigma that is underreported by patients to their physicians.

 BASICS

DESCRIPTION

Fecal incontinence is defined as the inability to control the passage of liquid or solid stool.

Age-Related Factors

- Prevalence of fecal incontinence increases with older age:
  - Ages 30–50, ~4%
  - 50–60, 7%
  - 60–70, 12%
  - 70–80, 11%
  - 80–90, 15%

Geriatric Considerations

Fecal incontinence is one of the primary reasons (outnumbering senile dementia) for nursing home placement.

Pregnancy Considerations

In women who have had a sphincter laceration in the past and are symptomatic, Cesarean section is recommended.

EPIDEMIOLOGY

- Prevalence varies according to what definition of incontinence is used.
- Prevalence rates of fecal incontinence may be as high as 15% in women >50.
- Highest incidence rate in adults >65.
- 60–70% of fecally incontinent people are women.
- <50% of women with fecal incontinence seek professional help.
- >$400 million is spent annually on adult diapers.

RISK FACTORS

- Direct obstetric trauma to sphincter muscle from normal spontaneous vaginal delivery, episiotomy, or forceps-assisted vaginal delivery
- Obstetric trauma resulting in damage to pudendal nerve
- Diarrheal states
- Diabetes resulting in neuropathy
- Prior anorectal surgery resulting in iatrogenic injury
- Increasing age
- Depression
- Other medical comorbidities
- Urinary incontinence

Genetics

Congenital abnormalities and hereditary conditions such as familial polyposis may cause fecal incontinence.

PATHOPHYSIOLOGY

- Obstetric trauma:
  - Direct injury to anal sphincter muscle or damage to motor innervation of the pelvic floor
  - Chronic 3rd- and 4th-degree lacerations
  - Rectovaginal fistula
- Surgical injury, such as incidental sphincterotomy or low anterior resection
- Diarrheal states including IBS, radiation enteritis, infectious enteritis, laxative abuse
- Neurologic conditions such as diabetic neuropathy, spinal cord injury, congenital anomalies, dementia
- Congenital anorectal malformation
- Pelvic floor denervation resulting in rectal prolapse, chronic straining

ASSOCIATED CONDITIONS

- Rectovaginal fistulas (see topic)
- Pelvic organ prolapse/rectocele (see topic)
- Urinary incontinence (see topic)

DIAGNOSIS

SIGNS AND SYMPTOMS

History

- Onset of incontinence:
  - Correlation with prior surgeries
  - Correlation with obstetric history
- Degree of incontinence and degree of bother
- Type of incontinence: Solid or liquid stool
- Presence or absence of sensation of need to defecate
- Incomplete evacuation
- Presence of concurrent urinary incontinence
- Detailed history of comorbidities

Review of Systems

Standard review of symptoms is appropriate with a focus on *when* incontinence began, *how long* for symptoms to worsen, and *how bothersome* are the symptoms.

Physical Exam

- Inspection of anal area: Hemorrhoids present? Patulous anus? Dovetailing?
- Examination for concurrent prolapse
- Examination for prior obstetric scarring
- Digital rectal exam: Low resting tone? Concentric squeeze? Early fatigability?
- Neurologic assessment: Anal wink present?

TESTS

- Rectal examination is accurate in assessing neuromuscular function in 85% of patients:
  - Consider pudendal nerve terminal motor latency in suspected neurogenic incontinence.
  - Consider electromyography to delineate extent of denervation and reinnervation of anal sphincter.
- Consider a colonic transit study if impaction or overflow incontinence is suspected.
- Consider anorectal manometry in patients with decreased anal sensation:
  - Resting tone correlates with internal sphincter function
  - Squeeze tone correlates with external sphincter function

Labs

- Fecal occult blood testing
- Stool cultures
- TSH
- Basic metabolic panel
- Serum glucose
- Lactose intolerance:
  - Hydrogen breath test
- Celiac sprue:
  - IgA antiendomysium antibodies
  - IgA antigliadin antibodies
  - IgG antigliadin antibodies
  - IgA antitissue transglutaminase

Imaging

- Transanal US:
  - Assess sphincter defects and atrophy
- MRI with endoanal coil:
  - Measures volume of sphincter, thus degree of defect and atrophy
  - Dynamic MRI useful in also evaluating pelvic floor support and concurrent prolapse
- Defecogram:
  - Dynamic evaluation of defecation process
  - Assess concomitant perineal descent, paradoxic levator contraction leading to obstruction, rectocele and/or enterocele
- Colonoscopy

DIFFERENTIAL DIAGNOSIS

Infection

Infectious diarrhea from virus, bacteria, or parasite

Metabolic/Endocrine

- Hyper- or hypothyroidism (See Thyroid Disease.)
- Diabetes

Immunologic

Gluten enteropathy or celiac sprue

Tumor/Malignancy

Colonic or rectal tumors

Trauma

Obstetric, surgical, fistula, anorectal trauma

Drugs

Laxative abuse

Other/Miscellaneous

- Overflow incontinence
- Neurogenic incontinence

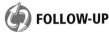 **TREATMENT**

GENERAL MEASURES
- Treat underlying disease.
- Protective skin care measures
- Psychologic and social support
- Maximization of nonsurgical therapy is vital with dietary modification.

SPECIAL THERAPY
Complementary and Alternative Therapies
- Biofeedback:
  – Efferent training: Enhances voluntary contraction of the external anal sphincter
  – Afferent training: Improves sensation in the anorectal canal
- Pelvic muscle floor exercises:
  – Kegel exercises may benefit patients with early fatigability of the sphincter on digital exam.
- Dietary management:
  – Increasing stool bulk and avoiding highly spicy foods and other irritants like coffee, beer, dairy

MEDICATION (DRUGS)
- Fiber: Increases stool bulk with 25–35 g/d
- Loperamide: Retards transit time and stimulates anal sphincter
- Hyoscyamine sulfate: Anticholinergic
- Diphenoxylate with atropine: Decreases peristalsis

SURGERY
- Anal sphincteroplasty:
  – Overlapping vs. end-to-end technique; likely no difference in success rates
- Muscle transposition procedures:
  – Gracilis, gluteus maximus
- Artificial anal sphincter placement:
  – Implanted device with inflatable balloon that occludes anus
  – Very specialized procedure with high risk of infection

- Sacral nerve stimulation:
  – Remodulates sacral reflexes
  – Not FDA approved for this indication but widely used in Europe with good success
- Diversion as a final resort:
  – Colostomy or ileostomy

 FOLLOW-UP

DISPOSITION
Issues for Referral
- Gastroenterology for colonoscopy/evaluation
- Urogynecology for evaluation of surgical management and concurrent urinary incontinence
- Colorectal surgery for surgical evaluation

PROGNOSIS
- Up to 60% of patients report improved continence with dietary and medical management alone.
- Up to 90% of patients with concomitant pelvic floor dysfunction report improved continence after biofeedback therapy.
- 20–50% of patients report improved continence after anal sphincteroplasty.

PATIENT MONITORING
- Postoperatively, patients should be seen within 4–6 weeks for evaluation.
- In patients who are following dietary and behavioral modification programs, periodic assessments of bowel habits and symptom improvement are important.

BIBLIOGRAPHY

Melville JL, et al. Fecal incontinence in US women: A population-based study. *Am J Obstet Gynecol.* 2005;193(6):2071–2076.

Nirhira MA, et al. Fecal incontinence. In: Bent A, et al., eds. *Ostergard's Urogynecology and Pelvic Floor Dysfunction*, 5th ed. Philadelphia: Lippincott & Wilkins; 2003:341–353.

Stenchever M, et al. Anatomic defects of the abdominal wall and pelvic floor. In: Stenchever MA, et al., eds. *Comprehensive Gynecology*, 4th ed. St. Louis: Mosby; 2001:565–606.

 MISCELLANEOUS

SYNONYM(S)
- Anal incontinence
- Bowel incontinence

CLINICAL PEARLS
- As the population ages, it is vital for clinicians to recognize and treat this debilitating and socially isolating condition.
- In patients with fecal incontinence, concurrent screening for other medical and psychiatric comorbidities is important.
- Maximization of dietary and behavior therapy should occur prior to surgical therapy for fecal incontinence.
- Health care providers and patients must treat impaired bowel function as a chronic condition.
- In most cases, improvements in fecal incontinence can be made but absolute cures are infrequent.

ABBREVIATIONS
- FI—Fecal incontinence
- IBS—Irritable bowel syndrome
- TSH—Thyroid-stimulating hormone

CODES
ICD9-CM
787.6 Fecal incontinence

 PATIENT TEACHING

PREVENTION
- In women with a history of a birth-related sphincter laceration, subsequent Cesarean sections may prevent the recurrence or worsening of fecal incontinence in women who are symptomatic.
- Maintain healthy bowel habits with adequate fiber and water intake.
- Appropriately manage symptoms of other illnesses such as IBS and celiac sprue.
- Colonoscopy screening for all women ≥50 and for any woman with new onset of GI symptoms regardless of age is recommended as a Grade A recommendation from the US Preventive Services task force (USPSTF).

FIBROCYSTIC BREAST CHANGES

Eduardo Lara-Torre, MD

 BASICS

DESCRIPTION
- A fibrocystic change of the breast is a term used to describe benign breast disorders causing a fluid-filled breast mass and pain.
- Because of their common occurrence and spontaneous resolution, they are not considered a true disease.
- Characterized by ductal lobular proliferation, duct dilatation and elongation, and terminal duct cyst formation
- In addition to clear fluid cysts, other common lesions in this category include:
  – Fibrosis
  – Non-atypical ductal or lobular hyperplasia
  – Adenosis
  – Apocrine metaplasia
  – Fibroadenoma
  – Papilloma

Age-Related Factors
- These changes are generally present in menstruating premenopausal women.
- Postmenopausal women on HRT may carry this disease to the later years.

Pediatric Considerations
2nd most common lesion in teenagers after fibroadenomas

EPIDEMIOLOGY
- >90% of women have these changes during their lifetime.
- Mostly reserved to menstruating premenopausal women
- May appear in those postmenopausal women on HRT

RISK FACTORS
- Mechanism for appearance not understood
- Old association with caffeine intake now very weak
- Young age in menstruating women appears to be a risk factor

Genetics
No definitive association found.

PATHOPHYSIOLOGY
- Not completely understood
- Not considered a true pathologic disorder

ASSOCIATED CONDITIONS
Those with atypical ductal or lobular hyperplasia may have an increased risk of breast cancer.

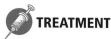 **DIAGNOSIS**

SIGNS AND SYMPTOMS
History
- May be asymptomatic and presents as a mass
- Breast pain or tenderness premenstrually
- Common resolution of pain after menses
- Occasional clear nipple discharge
- May be localized, diffuse, or bilateral
- May take 2 or 3 menstrual cycles to disappear

Review of Systems
- No fever or erythema
- No trauma
- Unlikely to have skin changes

Physical Exam
- Palpable mass
- Sometimes fluctuant
- Tenderness over the mass

TESTS
Labs
- Not necessary unless galactorrhea present
- If galactorrhea:
  – TSH, free T4, and prolactin may be helpful.
  – Instruct patient to not touch breast for at least 72 hours prior to testing.
- Needle aspiration:
  – May be of assistance in making diagnosis.
  – Provides therapeutic relief
  – Provides diagnostic sample for cytology
  – Determines cystic nature of the mass

Imaging
- US considered best in differentiating solid vs. cystic
- Mammogram lacks sensitivity or specificity but may identify other lesions

Pediatric Considerations
US is the only sensitive test in adolescents, given increased breast density.

DIFFERENTIAL DIAGNOSIS
- Fibrosis
- Atypical and non-atypical ductal or lobular hyperplasia
- Adenosis
- Apocrine metaplasia
- Fibroadenoma
- Papilloma

Infection
Abscess

Tumor/Malignancy
Breast cancer

Trauma
Trauma

Other/Miscellaneous
Non–breast disease:
- Gastroesophageal reflux
- Skin disorders
- Muscle or bone pain (costochondritis)

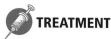 **TREATMENT**

GENERAL MEASURES
- Proper evaluation to rule out malignant breast disease in the adult
- Generally resolves spontaneously and requires no intervention
- Persistent mastalgia may benefit from:
  – Proper breast support, such as sports bra
  – Cold compresses

SPECIAL THERAPY
Complementary and Alternative Therapies
- The use of primrose oil is well studied and effective at 3–4 g/d.
- Vitamin E and calcium have no evidence of efficacy.
- Limiting caffeine has not been shown to be efficacious.

MEDICATION (DRUGS)
- NSAIDs commonly used with good result.
- Other FDA products approved for the treatment of mastalgia:
  – Tamoxifen
  – Bromocriptine
  – Danazol

SURGERY
Only reserved for those cases suspicious for malignancy and recurrent or persistent cysts after aspiration.

Pediatric Considerations
- Biopsy should no be performed in the pediatric or adolescent patient to determine the cystic nature; an US should confirm the diagnosis.
- Biopsy in the pediatric patient may result in poor breast bud development and should not be done.

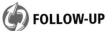 **FOLLOW-UP**

DISPOSITION

Issues for Referral
- Nonresolving or persistent cysts after aspiration
- General surgeon when diagnosis is in question

PROGNOSIS
Generally good, as cyst resolves spontaneously

PATIENT MONITORING
- Should be performed depending on the diagnosis of the initial evaluation
- If benign fibrocystic changes confirmed, monitoring for recurrence or persistence after aspiration recommended

BIBLIOGRAPHY

Breast concerns in the adolescent. ACOG Committee Opinion No. 350. American College of Obstetricians and Gynecologists. *Obstet Gynecol* 2006;108: 1329–1336.

Carpenter SE, et al, eds. *Pediatric and Adolescent Gynecology,* 2nd ed. Philadelphia: Lippincott-Williams; 2000.

Neinstein LS. Review of breast masses in adolescents. *Adolesc Pediatr Gynecol.* 1994;7:119.

Nemoto T. In: *Ferri's Clinical Advisor: Instant Diagnosis and Treatment,* 8th ed. Chicago: Mosby; 2006.

Vorherr H. Fibrocystic breast disease: Pathophysiology, pathomorphology, clinical picture, and management. *Am J Obstet Gynecol.* 1986;154:161–179.

 MISCELLANEOUS

SYNONYM(S)
- Fibrocystic disease of the breast
- Mammary dysplasia
- Cystic changes

CLINICAL PEARLS
- US very useful in differentiating cyst vs. solid.
- FNA is good office technique for diagnostic and treatment approach.

ABBREVIATIONS
- HRT—Hormone replacement therapy
- T4—Thyroxine
- TSH—Thyroid-stimulating hormone
- US—Ultrasound

 CODES

ICD9-CM
- 610.0 Solitary cyst of the breast
- 610.1 Fibrocystic disease of the breast
- 610.11 Breast lump

PATIENT TEACHING

- Self breast examination in adult women and annual clinical breast examination
- Available patient education at www.acog.org, www.cancer.org, and the National Cancer Institute

Section II

FITZ-HUGH-CURTIS SYNDROME

Valerie Lewis, MD, MPH
Nadja Peter, MD

 BASICS

DESCRIPTION
- Fitz-Hugh-Curtis (FHC) is the syndrome (FHCS) of perihepatitis, an inflammation of the liver capsule, associated with PID in the reproductive-aged female.
- Characterized laparoscopically by "violin-string" adhesions between the liver capsule and abdominal wall.
- Characterized clinically by acute or subacute onset of RUQ pain at the time of genital tract infection (may be asymptomatic) with *Chlamydia trachomatis* or *Neisseria Gonorrhea*.
- RUQ pain can be persistent in the chronic phase of the disorder.

Age-Related Factors
- Rates of FHCS are higher among adolescent females than adult women with PID.
- The higher rates among adolescents may be related to their immature cervical ectropion (presence of columnar cells on the ectocervix), making them biologically more susceptible to cervicitis.

EPIDEMIOLOGY
The incidence of FHCS (perihepatitis in presence of PID) is higher among adolescent girls (27%) when compared to adult women (4–13.8%).

RISK FACTORS
Those factors which place an individual at risk for acquiring a genital infection with *Chlamydia* or *Gonorrhea* resulting in pelvic inflammation:
- Unprotected intercourse
- Early sexual debut
- Multiple sexual partners
- In adult women, recent IUD placement may be a risk factor in the development of PID.

PATHOPHYSIOLOGY
- The pathophysiology of this disorder is poorly understood, but the following mechanisms have been proposed (some with conflicting or controversial evidence, and maybe with different mechanisms in operation for *Chlamydia* vs. *Gonorrhea*):
  - Direct bacterial spread from the fallopian tubes to the liver via the pericolic gutters:
    - Although it is possible that pelvic fluid can be tracked to the RUQ, the causative bacteria has seldom been isolated from the liver surface.
  - Hematogenous or lymphatic spread:
    - Some evidence for these mechanisms for *Gonorrhea* but very little for *Chlamydia*.
- Exaggerated immune response to *C. trachomatis* is the most likely explanation, given what is known to date.
  - Higher anti-*Chlamydial* IgG titers have been found in those with both perihepatitis and salpingitis than with salpingitis alone.
  - Antigenic proteins from *Chlamydia* may cross-react with host tissue proteins, resulting in an exaggerated inflammatory response.

ASSOCIATED CONDITIONS
- PID
- Salpingitis

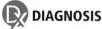 **DIAGNOSIS**

SIGNS AND SYMPTOMS
History
- The acute phase is characterized by:
  - Sharp, pleuritic pain located in the RUQ of the abdomen, or pain referred to the ipsilateral shoulder
  - Symptoms are usually associated with acute salpingitis, but signs or symptoms of PID may be absent, especially with *Chlamydia*.
- The chronic phase is characterized by persistent RUQ pain.
- Pericapsular adhesions can occur in the absence of RUQ pain or salpingitis, which can make the diagnosis challenging.

Review of Systems
May be associated with nausea, vomiting, hiccups, fever, chills, malaise, or signs of salpingitis (lower abdominal pain and abnormal vaginal discharge)

Physical Exam
- No pathognomonic exam findings, making FHCS a diagnosis of exclusion
- Examination will demonstrate RUQ tenderness, or rarely a friction rub is heard over the same area.
- In patients with concurrent salpingitis, cervical motion or adnexal tenderness may be present.

TESTS
Laboratory tests and imaging studies are often nonspecific.

Labs
- Liver enzyme levels: Typically, normal, but may be elevated. (Transaminase elevations are more likely in the setting of gonococcal rather than *Chlamydial* perihepatitis.)
- ESR and/or C-reactive protein may be elevated.
- WBC count may be normal or elevated.
- Isolation of either *Chlamydia* and/or *Gonorrhea* from the cervix using a variety of testing techniques including culture, direct immunofluorescent smears, enzyme immunoassays, DNA probes, or nucleic acid amplification tests.
- *Chlamydia*-specific serology tests
- If high clinical suspicion for STDs exists, samples should also be obtained from the rectum, urethra, and pharynx.
- Obtain studies to rule out other gastrointestinal or renal causes of RUQ pain: Amylase, lipase, stool guaiac, and urinalysis/urine culture.

Imaging
- Imaging studies are useful in ruling out or eliminating other potential causes of RUQ pain.
- Chest and abdominal radiographs to evaluate for pneumonia or subdiaphragmatic free air:
  - A right-sided hemidiaphragm elevation or small reactive pleural effusion may be seen in FHCS.
- US to evaluate the liver, the gallbladder for cholelithiasis or cholecystitis, or the ovaries for a tubo-ovarian abscess or other signs of PID:
  - Rarely, ascites in the hepatorenal space, loculated fluid in the pelvis or abdomen or adhesions between the liver and abdominal wall may be seen in FHCS.
- CT occasionally demonstrates liver capsule enhancement.

DIFFERENTIAL DIAGNOSIS
- FHCS can mimic other conditions making the diagnosis difficult.
- Cholelithiasis/cholecystitis
- Pneumonia
- Pulmonary embolism
- Rib fracture/abdominal trauma
- Pyelonephritis
- Hepatitis/Peritonitis
- Nephrolithiasis
- Subphrenic abscess
- Pancreatitis
- Appendicitis
- Herpes zoster
- Enteroviral epidemic pleurodynia (Burnhold disease)/pleurisy

Infection
C. trachomatis is more likely to be the etiologic agent than *N. gonorrhea*, although both have been implicated in FHCS.

 TREATMENT

GENERAL MEASURES
- Antibiotic therapy is indicated in the management of FHCS.
- The same agents directed against *Chlamydia* and *Gonorrhea* are used to treat PID and FHCS.
- One should not await confirmatory lab results to treat if clinical suspicion is high.
- Pain control can be achieved with NSAIDs or narcotic agents.
- Sexual activity should be avoided until 1 week after both the patient and partner(s) have completed treatment.

MEDICATION (DRUGS)

- Treatment regimen as per CDC Guidelines for treatment of PID
- Oral regimens:
  - Ceftriaxone 250 mg IM in a single dose PLUS doxycycline** 100 mg PO b.i.d. for 14 days WITH OR WITHOUT Metronidazole 500 mg PO b.i.d. for 14 days
  - Alternative: OR cefoxitin 2 g IM in a single dose and probenecid 1 g PO administered concurrently in a single dose, OR other parenteral 3rd-generation cephalosporin PLUS doxycycline 100 mg PO b.i.d. for 14 days WITH OR WITHOUT metronidazole 500 mg PO b.i.d. for 14 days
- Parenteral regimens:
  - Cefotetan 2 g IV q12h OR cefoxitin 2 g IV q6h PLUS doxycycline** 100 mg PO or IV q12h
  - Clindamycin 900 mg IV q8h PLUS gentamicin loading dose IV or IM (2 mg/kg of body weight), followed by a maintenance dose (1.5 mg/kg) q8h. Single daily dosing may be substituted.
  - Alternative: OR ampicillin/sulbactam 3 g IV q6h PLUS doxycycline** 100 mg PO or IV q12h
  - Fluoroquinolones should only be used in persons with intolerance to other aforementioned antibiotics and with low individual risk and low community prevalence of *Gonorrhea*. If testing for *Gonorrhea* is positive, the antibiotic should be changed or susceptibility testing done.

Pediatric Considerations
Fluoroquinolones should be used sparingly in those younger than 18 years secondary to concerns about interference with bone development.

Pregnancy Considerations
Fluoroquinolones and doxycycline should be avoided during pregnancy.

SURGERY

- Laparoscopic exploration can be used to assist in making the diagnosis of PID and FHCS.
- Surgical intervention is indicated only in the event that symptoms do not resolve after antibiotic therapy:
  - Laparoscopy can be used to lyse perihepatic adhesions in the case of chronic RUQ pain following an episode of FHCS.

 FOLLOW-UP

DISPOSITION

- Hospital admission criteria for FHCS are similar to those for PID and include:
  - Inability to rule out a surgical emergency
  - Inability to tolerate an oral regimen
  - The presence of a complication of PID such as tubo-ovarian abscess
  - Pregnancy
- Discharge when the patient's symptoms of salpingitis have resolved.

Issues for Referral
Consider gynecologic surgical referral for lysis of perihepatic adhesions in individuals with chronic RUQ pain.

PROGNOSIS
Excellent

PATIENT MONITORING

- Monitor for resolution of RUQ pain, as well as signs and symptoms of salpingitis.
- An association may exist between FHCS and fallopian tube dysfunction that results in infertility. Severity of the tubal abnormality is determined by the host's reactivity to *Chlamydia*.

BIBLIOGRAPHY

Centers for Disease Control and Prevention, Updated recommended treatment regimens for gonococcal infections and associated conditions – United States, April 2007. http//www.cdc.gov/std/treatment/2006/updated-regimens.htm

Kobayashi Y, et al. Pathological study of Fitz-Hugh-Curtis syndrome evaluated from fallopian tube damage. *J Obstet Gynaecol*. 2006;32(3): 280–285.

Litt IF, et al. Perihepatitis associated with salpingitis in adolescents. *JAMA*. 1978;240:1253–1254.

Peter NG, et al. Fitz-Hugh-Curtis syndrome: A diagnosis to consider in women with right upper quadrant pain. *Cleve Clin J Med*. 2004;71(3): 233–239.

Tsubuku M, et al. Fitz-Hugh-Curtis syndrome: Linear contrast enhancement of the surface of the liver on CT. *J Comput Assist Tomogr*. 2002;26:456–458.

 MISCELLANEOUS

SYNONYM(S)

- Gonococcal perihepatitis
- Perihepatitis syndrome

CLINICAL PEARLS

- *C. trachomatis* and *N. gonorrhea* are the main causative agents implicated in FHCS.
- Among those with PID, FHCS occurs more commonly among adolescent females (27%) than adult women (4–14%).
- FHCS is usually a clinical diagnosis based on exclusion of other causes of RUQ pain and isolation of the bacterial pathogen.
- Treatment is with antibiotics directed against *C. trachomatis* and *N. gonorrhea*. Can consider lysis of perihepatic adhesions if RUQ pain persists.

ABBREVIATIONS

- FHCS—Fitz-Hugh Curtis syndrome
- PID—Pelvic inflammatory disease
- RUQ—Right upper quadrant
- STD/STI—Sexually transmitted disease/infection

CODES

ICD9-CM

- 99.56 Perihepatitis
- 614.9 Pelvic inflammatory disease

PATIENT TEACHING

- Educate about safer sex practices including consistent condom use.
- Encourage testing for other STIs, including HIV and syphilis.
- Counsel about the importance of partner notification to prevent spread or reinfection.
- Frequent STI screening and testing among sexually active populations

PREVENTION
Reduction of high-risk sexual behaviors

GESTATIONAL TROPHOBLASTIC NEOPLASM

Nader Husseinzadeh, MD

 BASICS

DESCRIPTION
- GTD can be divided into 4 categories:
  - Hydatidiform mole
  - Invasive mole
  - Choriocarcinoma
  - Placenta site trophoblastic tumor
- These tumors are relatively rare and are distinguished by three unique features:
  - Secretion of hCG
  - Sensitivity to chemotherapy
  - The immunologic relationship between the tumor and its host
- Classification of molar pregnancy:
  - Complete mole: Abnormal conceptus characterized by gross villi swelling without embryo, membrane, or cord development
  - Incomplete mole: Invariably associated with an embryo, fetus, or cord membrane. Embryo dies by 8–10 weeks of gestation or may survive into 2nd trimester.
  - Transitional mole: Blighted ovum hydropic villi. The hydropic villi are generally inconspicuous and never affect all villi. The trophoblast are normal or hydropic. Amnion and embryo are present.
- Gestational trophoblastic neoplasia (GTN) or gestational trophoblastic tumor (GTT) comprises invasive mole, choriocarcinoma, and placental site trophoblastic tumor:
  - Invasive mole:
    - Benign tumor arising from hydatidiform mole, invades the myometrium by direct extension or by venous channels and may metastasize to distant sites.
    - Incidence of invasive mole estimated to be:
      - 1/15,000 pregnancies or
      - 1–15% of molar pregnancy
  - Choriocarcinoma:
    - Gestational choriocarcinoma may arise in association with any type of pregnancy:
      - 50% follow hydatidiform mole and ~2–3% of hydatidiform moles progress to choriocarcinoma
      - 25% follow abortion or tubal pregnancy.
      - 25% follow term gestation.
    - The incidence of choriocarcinoma is ~1/40,000 pregnancies.
- Placental site trophoblastic tumor (PSTT) (trophoblastic pseudotumor)
  - Originally described by Kurman et al. (1976); rare.
  - Pathologically, the tumor is polypoid, the trophoblastic cells infiltrate the myometrium and grow between smooth muscle cells, and there is vascular invasion.
  - PSTT occurs in women of reproductive age.
    - The average age is 28 years.
    - The patient presents with vaginal bleeding, usually after amenorrhea.
    - The uterus is usually enlarged (8–16 weeks)
    - β-hCG is usually <3,000 mL/IU.

Staging
- When the diagnosis of GTT has been made, it is important to determine the extent of disease. A variety of classification and scoring systems are used:
- FIGO:
  - Stage 0: Molar pregnancy, low or high risk
  - Stage I: Confined to uterine corpus
  - Stage II: Metastasis to pelvis and vagina
  - Stage III: Metastasis to lung
  - Stage IV: Metastasis to liver, brain, etc
- Good prognosis metastatic GTN (Low Risk Group):
  - Urinary hCG excretion <100,000 IU/24 h
  - Serum hCG <40,000 mLU/mL
  - Duration of disease <4 months
  - Lung or vaginal metastasis
  - No prior chemotherapy
- Poor prognosis metastatic GTN (High Risk Group):
  - Urinary hCG excretion >100,000 IU/24 h
  - Serum hCG >40,000 mLU/mL
  - Duration of disease >4 months
  - Brain or liver metastasis
  - Failed prior chemotherapy
  - Term pregnancy

EPIDEMIOLOGY
- The reported incidence of hydatidiform mole varies throughout the world.
- In the US and Europe, the incidence is ~1/1,800 pregnancy terminations.
- In other parts of the world, ~1/85 normal pregnancy.
  - ~0.5–2.5% chance of molar pregnancy in subsequent pregnancies (US)

RISK FACTORS
High-risk criteria for management:
- Uterus large for dates
- hCG >100,000 mIU/mL
- Theca-lutein cysts >5 cm
- Maternal age >40 years
- Prior trophoblastic tumor

Genetics
Cytogenetics:
- Karyotyping in complete mole is 95% 46XX (reduplication of 23X sperm haploid) and 5% 46XY.

PATHOPHYSIOLOGY
Hydatidiform moles are histologically characterized by:
- Swelling of placental villi
- Trophoblastic proliferations

ASSOCIATED CONDITIONS
- Hyperemesis gravidarum
- Theca lutein cysts
- Toxemia
- Coagulopathy
- Hyperthyroidism
- Trophoblastic embolization

 DIAGNOSIS

SIGNS AND SYMPTOMS
History
- Hydatidiform mole most commonly presents with uterine bleeding, usually during 1st trimester.
- Severe nausea and vomiting

Review of Systems
- Signs of hyperthyroidism
- Signs suggesting metastatic disease

Physical Exam
- Vital signs:
  - Rarely presents with pregnancy-induced hypertension in 1st trimester
  - Rarely with tachycardia associated with hyperthyroidism
- Thyroid
- Pulmonary
- Abdomen: Assess uterine size
- Pelvic exam:
  - Uterine size > dates
  - Absent fetal heart tones
  - Cystic enlargement of ovaries

TESTS
Labs
- Serum quantitative hCG elevated
- Once diagnosis of molar pregnancy is made, the following labs are indicated:
  - CBC with platelets
  - Clotting function studies
  - Blood type with antibody screen
  - Baseline pre-evacuation chest x-ray
- If diagnosis of malignant GTN is made, the following studies are recommended:
  - CBC with platelets
  - CXR or CT of chest
  - Pelvic US
  - Brain MRI or CT scan
  - Abdominopelvic CT with contrast or MRI

Imaging
Molar pregnancy may be found on routine US for pregnancy dating:
- "Snow storm" pattern representing blood and fluid in the villi

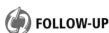

TREATMENT

MEDICATION (DRUGS)

- For GTN, nonmetastatic:
  - Single agent chemotherapy with:
    - Methotrexate 0.4 mg/kg IV days 1–5 OR
    - Actinomycin-D 10–12 μg/kg IV days 1–5
    - Methotrexate 40 mg/m^2 every week
- Patients with metastatic GTN:
  - With low-risk metastatic disease:
    - Treat with single-agent chemotherapy, either methotrexate or actinomycin-D, sequentially or alternately, with expected overall remission of 80%.
    - ~15–20% of patients treated for low-risk metastatic disease with single-agent chemotherapy require combination chemotherapy, with or without surgery, to achieve complete remission.
    - Chemotherapy is continued for 2 or 3 courses after normal hCG value.
    - Cure rates should approach 100% in this group of patients if treatment is administered properly.
  - High-risk or poor prognosis metastatic disease:
    - Treated more aggressively initially with combination chemotherapy with or without adjuvant radiation therapy or surgery.
    - Traditionally, the primary multidrug regimen used in these patients has been MAC, consisting of: Actinomycin-D, 8–10 μg/kg/d IV for days 1–5; methotrexate 0.3 mg/kg/d IV for days 1–5; AND cyclophosphamide 3–5 mg/kg/d IV for days 1–5
  - Brain metastasis occurs in ~10% of women with metastatic GTT. Whole-brain radiation in combination with systemic chemotherapy has been successful in improving survival in 50% of patients with brain involvement. One report of a cure rate of 72% in 25 patients with CNS metastasis using EMA/CO plus intrathecal MTX.
  - Liver metastasis:
    - The major issue in managing choriocarcinoma with liver metastases is the role of radiation therapy, which has been advocated.
    - Usually a dose of 2,000 cGY over 10 days to diminish the risk of liver hemorrhage, although some experts do not recommend.

SURGERY

For molar pregnancy:

- Suction evacuation of uterus as soon as possible after assessing and stabilizing any medical complications
- If uterus is large, perform procedure in a facility with ICU, blood bank, and anesthesia services.
- Rh-negative patients should be treated with anti-D immune globulin.
- Pulmonary complications, especially with large uterus, can include:
  - Trophoblastic embolization and RDS
  - High-output CHF
- Theca lutein cysts typically resolve over several months, with surgery reserved for rupture or torsion (rare).

FOLLOW-UP

DISPOSITION

Issues for Referral

- Referral to clinician experienced with D&E procedures or suction uterine evacuation as appropriate
- Gyn oncologist for management of GTN

PROGNOSIS

- Medical complications of hydatidiform moles are seen in ~25% of patients with uterine size >14–16 weeks, and include:
  - Anemia
  - Infection
  - Hyperthyroidism
  - Pregnancy-induced hypertension
  - Coagulopathy
  - Trophoblastic embolism
- All cases of nonmetastatic GTN are considered curable
- Factors primarily responsible for treatment failures in patients with metastatic disease are:
  - Presence of extensive disease at the time of initial treatment
  - Inadequate initial treatment
  - Failure of presently used chemotherapy protocols in advanced disease

PATIENT MONITORING

After evacuation of molar pregnancy, the following labs are indicated:

- Effective contraception is indicated to preclude confusion with followup hCG
- The following labs are indicated:
  - Weekly quantitative hCG assay until 3 negative results
  - Then monthly for 3 months
  - Then every 3 months for 1 year
  - If hCG levels decreasing, no role for chemotherapy
  - If plateau or increasing levels, treatment for GTN is indicated

ALERT

False-positive hCG values ("phantom hCG") may rarely occur resulting from interference with hCG assays, usually caused by nonspecific heterophilic antibodies in patient's serum.

BIBLIOGRAPHY

ACOG Practice Bulletin #53, June 2004: Diagnosis and treatment of Gestational Trophoblastic Disease.

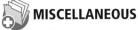

MISCELLANEOUS

ABBREVIATIONS

- CHF—Congestive heart failure
- GTD—Gestational trophoblastic disease
- hCG—Human chorionic gonadotropin
- PSTT—Placental site trophoblastic tumor
- RDS—Respiratory distress syndrome

CODES

ICD9-CM

630 Gestational trophoblastic disease

PATIENT TEACHING

ACOG Patient Education Pamphlet: *Early Pregnancy Loss: Miscarriage and Molar Pregnancy*

PREVENTION

Effective contraception is indicated after evacuation of molar pregnancy to avoid confusing new pregnancy with worrisome rise in hCG associated with GTN.

GONADAL DYSGENESIS

Peter A. Lee, MD, PhD
Christopher P. Houk, MD

 BASICS

DESCRIPTION

Gonadal dysgenesis is a condition in which gonadal development is abnormal, with presentation depending upon features.

Pediatric Considerations

- Diagnosis may be made:
  - After prenatal karyotype
  - At birth if phenotypic genital developmental problem or phenotype inconsistent with karyotype
  - With growth failure during childhood
  - With lack of puberty
- Testing revealing hypogonadism, elevated gonadotropins, and low sex steroids can be done during early infancy or at the age of usual pubertal onset.
- If findings do not lead to testing in the neonatal period, the diagnosis is often delayed until abnormal or lack of pubertal development.
- Phenotypic findings and short stature may lead to the diagnosis during childhood among those with Turner syndrome and its variants, but not among the other categories as outlined below.
- Categories include:
  - Turner syndrome and variants:
    - May be diagnosed prenatally based on karyotype or prenatal ultrasonography, in the newborn period based on somatic anomalies. Features in the newborn, more common among 45,X that other karyotypes, include lymphedema and redundant skin folds over the back of the neck.
    - Consequences of severe prenatal edema result in anomalies that may be noted during childhood including low-set rotated ears, low hairline, webbed neck, widely spaced nipples, hyperconvex nails, with risk of renal and cardiac malformations such as coarctation of the aorta. Such occur primarily among those with 45,X.
    - Those with other karyotypes may present during childhood with only short stature.
  - XX gonadal dysgenesis (pure gonadal agenesis):
    - Failure of ovarian development is accompanied by female external and internal genital development since this is the constitutive differentiation.
    - Because of continued growth in height, such patients may be tall when presenting with lack of puberty (in contrast to the typical Turner patient).
  - XY gonadal dysgenesis (pure gonadal agenesis or Swyer syndrome):
    - Constitutive development is female phenotype.
    - The SRY gene is missing or mutated, thus failure of testis formation.
    - Lack of anti-Müllerian hormone allows development of female internal reproductive organs.

- Mixed gonadal dysgenesis (abnormal and asymmetrical gonadal development):
  - Karyotype commonly 45,X/46,XY
  - Presentation usually female phenotype, but ranging from a Turner-like to male phenotype with empty scrotum or single palpable testis
  - Hence, phenotype may fit the definition for gonadal dysgenesis presenting as female, while instances may present with ambiguous genitalia or a male phenotype.
  - In these later instances, if adequate Leydig cell function is present to produce androgens, virilization may occur at puberty.

ALERT

- Although gonadal dysgenesis among females is usually thought of as synonymous to Turner syndrome, other more uncommon forms of gonadal dysgenesis present with a female phenotype. Also, gonadal dysgenesis may be used to include both dysgenesis (partial but dysfunctional development of the gonads) and agenesis, in which no gonadal development occurs. Patients with gonadal dysgenesis generally have gonadal streaks, whereas agenesis indicates no gonads. A gonadal streak anatomically contains the connective tissue stroma characteristic of an ovary without follicles.
- Dysgenetic gonads, primarily those from patients with a 46,XY karyotype, have an increased risk of development of gonadal neoplasms, including gonadoblastoma, germinomas, and teratomas. Tumor propensity is not recognized among those with 45,X or 46,XX gonadal dysgenesis although must be considered among those who have a fragment of a Y chromosome on karyotype.
- Prophylactic gonadectomy should be considered among those at high risk by the age of puberty, because the risk increases considerably by young adulthood.

Age-Related Factors

- Usually presents at puberty with lack of pubertal development
- If prenatal karyotype or phenotypic abnormalities, may be diagnosed at birth
- Turner syndrome may be diagnosed prenatally or during childhood.

EPIDEMIOLOGY

- Turner syndrome occurs in ~1 of 2,500 births of a child with a female phenotype.
- Other forms are very rare, some being identified with genetic mutations.

RISK FACTORS

- Specific risk factors for the development of gonadal dysgenesis are unknown.
- Occurrence is sporadic, whereas an association with advanced maternal and paternal age has been suggested for Turner syndrome.
- 46,XX gonadal dysgenesis occurs in familial cases as autosomal recessive.
- 46,XY familial cases may be X-linked or male-limited autosomal dominant.

Genetics

- Gonadal dysgenesis patients have different karyotypes.
- Turner syndrome—consequence of loss of part of all of an X chromosome:
  - Karyotype 45,X;46,XrXp-; 45,X,46XX, etc.
- Pure gonadal agenesis:
  - Karyotype 46,XX and 46,XY (Swyer syndrome)
  - 46,XX gonadal dysgenesis may be associated with FSH receptor mutations.
- Swyer syndrome results from mutations or deletion of the SRY (sex-determining region of the Y chromosome) gene in ~15% of instances.
- Mixed gonadal dysgenesis:
  - 45,X/46,XY; 45,X/47,XXX; 45,X/46,XX,47,XXX

PATHOPHYSIOLOGY

- Lack of pubertal development is a consequence of failure of gonadal development, in some instances as a consequence of mutations of crucial genes.
- Agenesis indicates no gonadal development, whereas dysgenesis indicates severely defective development.

ASSOCIATED CONDITIONS

- Turner syndrome is associated with an increased incidence of autoimmune disorders, particularly autoimmune thyroiditis.
- An increased incidence of carbohydrate intolerance with an increased incidence of type 2 diabetes mellitus, Addison's disease, chronic liver disease, Crohn's disease and ulcerative colitis
- Because of renal anomalies, pyelonephritis and obstructive uropathy may occur.
- Otitis media and hearing loss occur more commonly and severely during childhood.

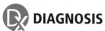 **DIAGNOSIS**

SIGNS AND SYMPTOMS

History

If not diagnosed because of prenatal or subsequent karyotype, syndromic features or associated findings, gonadal dysgenesis presents with lack of development of the physical changes of puberty.

Review of Systems

Except among Turner patients, those with gonadal dysgenesis are healthy except for conditions related to hypogonadism.

Physical Exam

- Physical exam ranges from normal, to phenotypic findings associated with Turner syndrome, to genital abnormalities associated with mixed gonadal dysgenesis.
- Turner syndrome may present at birth with lymphedema, and consequential webbed neck, low posterior hairline, and broadly spaced nipples; findings noted at older ages include hypertension, short stature, increased nevi, and lack of puberty.
- Pure gonadal agenesis typically presents with a normal female phenotype, if presenting with delay of puberty, may have tall stature.
- Mixed gonadal dysgenesis phenotype ranges from female, to female with Turner features to male:
  - Genitalia at birth may be ambiguous, female or male with nonpalpable or a single high testis.

TESTS

- Hypogonadism can be documented by elevated LH and FSH levels and low estradiol levels during infancy and after the years approaching the age of puberty:
  – FSH levels rise 1st.
  – Such elevated FSH levels are indicative of gonadal failure.
- Other testing is based on potential defects associated with the form of gonadal dysgenesis.

Labs

- Tests include:
  – LH, FSH, and estradiol levels
- For Turner syndrome:
  – Karyotype of leukocytes, echocardiogram, thyroid function tests, glucose

Imaging

- Pelvic US, renal ultrasound and, during teen years, bone density
- Presence or absence of internal reproductive system development is based on US, CT, or MRI.

DIFFERENTIAL DIAGNOSIS

- The categories of gonadal dysgenesis are listed under the basic description section, each being an instance of congenital failure of gonadal development.
- Lack of gonadal function, hypergonadotropic hypogonadism, may occur as a consequence of autoimmune disease, chemotherapy or radiation therapy, infection, or infiltration.

Tumor/Malignancy

Gonadal tumors, most commonly gonadoblastoma, occur in ~25% of those with Swyer syndrome, 46,XY gonadal dysgenesis.

 TREATMENT

GENERAL MEASURES

- General education of the patient and family concerning the need of HRT, expected development with puberty, and potential for fertility or pregnancy is indicated.
- Turner patients should have cardiovascular risks assessed.
- Psychological counseling should be provided at diagnosis and available thereafter concerning the impact of hypogonadism.

SPECIAL THERAPY

Complementary and Alternative Therapies

Among those with well-developed uteri and general good health, pregnancy may be possible using assisted fertility techniques and donated ova.

MEDICATION (DRUGS)

- Estrogen should be used to stimulate development of pubertal changes, followed by progesterone and cycling of medications if uterus present.
- After full growth and development, frequency of cycling can vary as with other indications for HRT.

SURGERY

Turner syndrome: Corrective surgery may be indicated for cardiovascular or renal abnormalities, cosmetic surgery for webbed neck, low-set ears, etc., with varying success.

 FOLLOW-UP

DISPOSITION

Pregnancy Considerations

- With current techniques of assisted fertility, patients with gonadal dysgenesis who have a uterus can be considered to receive fertilized donated ova.
- Those with Turner syndrome appear to have an increased risk of cardiovascular complications, specifically aortic dissection during pregnancy.

PROGNOSIS

- Patients with Turner syndrome have risks as outlined above for cardiovascular, renal, thyroid, and glucose-tolerance problems.
- Appropriate sex steroid therapy should avoid problems associated with hypogonadism, such as osteoporosis.
- Pregnancy may be possible using assisted fertility techniques among those with adequately developed uteri, although cardiac status must be carefully assessed among those with Turner syndrome.
- Mixed gonadal dysgenesis carries a risk of development of gonadoblastoma with presence of Y chromosome and dysgenetic (vs. agenetic) gonadal tissue carrying indication for gonadectomy.

PATIENT MONITORING

- Children with diagnoses or suspected diagnoses of gonadal failure should have growth monitored
- FSH measurement beginning at age 6–7 to document failure.
- Puberty can be initiated with estrogen at the age of pubertal onset, usually 10 years.
- If short stature is present, as may occur with Turner and mixed gonadal dysgenesis, GH therapy can be considered, to begin during childhood as soon as growth failure is noted.

BIBLIOGRAPHY

Alvarez-Nava F, et al. Mixed gonadal dysgenesis: A syndrome of broad clinical, cytogenetic and histopathologic spectrum. *Genet Couns*. 1999:10: 233–243.

Bondy CA, Turner Syndrome Study Group. Care of girls and women with Turner syndrome: A guideline of the Turner Syndrome Study Group. *J Clin Endocrinol Metab*. 2007;92:10–25.

Grumbach MM, et al. Disorders of Sex Differentiation. In: Larsen PR, et al., eds. *Williams Textbook of Endocrinology*, 10th ed. Philadelphia: Saunders; 2003:842–1002.

Saenger P, et al. Fifth International Symposium on Turner Syndrome. *J Clin Endocrinol Metab*. 2001;86:3061–3069.

 MISCELLANEOUS

ABBREVIATIONS

- FSH—Follicle-stimulating hormone
- GH—Growth hormone
- HRT—Hormone replacement therapy
- LH—Luteinizing hormone

CODES

ICD9-CM

- 256.3 Ovarian failure
- 725.0 Anomalies of ovaries
- 752.7 Pure gonadal dysgenesis/Sawyer's syndrome
- 758.6 Gonadal dysgenesis/Turner syndrome

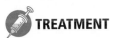 **PATIENT TEACHING**

As with all disorders that involve genital development, sexuality, or the reproductive system, it is crucial that patients understand the basic pathophysiology of their condition and understand that they can be well-adjusted and live productive, satisfying lives.

ILEUS

Rebeccah L. Brown, MD

 BASICS

DESCRIPTION

- Profound disturbance of bowel motility resulting in marked diminution or cessation of bowel peristalsis
- Failure of antegrade propulsion of intestinal contents leads to luminal distension with subsequent nausea, vomiting, and pain
- May be difficult to distinguish from bowel obstruction
- Generally divided into 2 major categories:
  - Postoperative ileus
  - Ileus without antecedent operation

Age-Related Factors

Most studies show increasing prevalence with age related to:

- Urogenital atrophy
- Hypoestrogenism
- Increasing prevalence of medical illnesses
- Increasing nocturnal diuresis
- Increasing use of medications
- Impairments in mobility
- Impairments in cognition

RISK FACTORS

- Abdominal/Pelvic surgery
- Spinal surgery
- Infection/Abscess
- Metabolic disturbances
- Opiates

PATHOPHYSIOLOGY

- Neurogenic disturbances:
  - Decreased parasympathetic tone (via vagus nerves) → decreased bowel motility
  - Increased sympathetic nerve tone (via splanchnic nerves) → decreased bowel motility
- Inflammatory mediators:
  - Tissue trauma → release of cytokines and other inflammatory mediators → decreased bowel motility
- Hormonal mediators:
  - Motilin
  - Vasoactive intestinal peptide
  - Substance P
  - Endogenous opiates
  - Nitric oxide

ASSOCIATED CONDITIONS

- Intra-abdominal:
  - Intra-peritoneal:
    - Operative tissue trauma
    - Peritonitis
    - Abscess
    - Intestinal ischemia
  - Retroperitoneal:
    - Pancreatitis
    - Retroperitoneal hematoma
    - Spinal cord injury/fracture
    - Aortic surgery
    - Pyelonephritis
    - Metastases
- Extra-abdominal:
  - Thoracic:
    - Myocardial infarction
    - Pneumonia
    - CHF
    - Rib fractures
  - Metabolic abnormalities:
    - Electrolyte imbalance
    - Sepsis
    - Hypothyroidism
    - Uremia
  - Drugs:
    - Opiates
    - Anticholinergics
    - α-Agonists
    - Antihistamines
    - Catecholamines
- Chemotherapy

 DIAGNOSIS

SIGNS AND SYMPTOMS

History

- Previous surgery
- Previous episodes of bowel obstruction
- Abdominal or pelvic cancer
- Inflammatory abdominal conditions (i.e., pancreatitis, IBD, PID, trauma)
- UTIs
- Opiate use

Review of Systems

- Anorexia
- Nausea and vomiting
- Crampy abdominal pain
- Abdominal bloating
- Absence of flatus
- Obstipation
- Fever/Tachycardia/Hypotension worrisome for obstruction/strangulation

Physical Exam

- Abdominal distension
- Absence of bowel sounds
- Tympany to percussion
- Mild, diffuse tenderness to palpation
- Absence of peritoneal signs

TESTS

Labs

- CBC with differential
- Renal, calcium, phosphorous, magnesium:
  - Hypokalemia
  - Hypochloremia
  - Alkalosis
  - Hypocalcemia
  - Hypophosphatemia
  - Hypomagnesemia
- UA/culture:
  - Rule out UTI as source of ileus

Imaging

- CXR:
  - Rule out pneumonia, free air
- Abdominal plain films (2 views):
  - Dilated loops of small and large bowel
  - Air-fluid levels
- CT of abdomen/pelvis if prolonged ileus >3–4 days or clinical deterioration:
  - Differentiate between ileus versus mechanical obstruction
  - Exclude intra-abdominal abscess as cause of ileus
- Upper GI series if prolonged ileus >3–4 days:
  - Differentiate between ileus versus mechanical obstruction

DIFFERENTIAL DIAGNOSIS

- Mechanical bowel obstruction
- Intestinal pseudo-obstruction:
  - Small bowel pseudo-obstruction
  - Colonic pseudo-obstruction (Ogilvie syndrome)

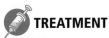 **TREATMENT**

GENERAL MEASURES
- NPO if nausea and vomiting
- Intravenous fluid hydration
- Consider nasogastric decompression if profound nausea, vomiting, abdominal distension
- Consider insertion of urinary catheter to guide fluid resuscitation
- Correct electrolytes, calcium, phosphorus, and magnesium
- Minimize or discontinue opiates
- Consider epidural analgesia
- Treat underlying infection

SPECIAL THERAPY
Complementary and Alternative Therapies
Colonoscopy and placement of rectal tube for massive colonic ileus

MEDICATION (DRUGS)
- Antiemetics (i.e., odansetron, promethazine)
- NSAIDS (i.e., ketorolac):
  - Reduce inflammatory response contributing to ileus
  - Reduce need for opioid analgesics
- Rectal suppository (i.e., Dulcolax) to stimulate bowel movement
- Nasogastric administration of water-soluble contrast agents (i.e., diatrizoate meglumine, diatrizoate sodium)
- μ-Agonist (i.e., alvimopan)

SURGERY
- Not generally indicated
- May be necessary to exclude mechanical cause of obstruction

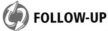 **FOLLOW-UP**

DISPOSITION
Discharge home once tolerating regular diet

PROGNOSIS
Usually resolves spontaneously within a few days if underlying cause is appropriately treated

PATIENT MONITORING
Attention to fluid and electrolyte balance

BIBLIOGRAPHY

Delaney CP, et al. Alvimopan postoperative ileus study group. Phase III trial of alvimopan, a novel, peripherally acting, mu opioid antagonist, for postoperative ileus after major abdominal surgery. *Dis Colon Rectum*. 2005;48(6):1114–1125.

Helton WS. Intestinal obstruction. In: Wilmore DW, ed. *ACS Surgery Principles and Practice*. New York: WebMD Corporation; 2002:263–281.

Kehlet H, et al. Care after colonic operation – is it evidence-based? Results from a multinational survey in Europe and the United States. *J Am Coll Surg*. 2006 202(1):45–54. Epub 2005, Oct 20.

Mattei P, et al. Review of the pathophysiology and management of postoperative ileus. *World J Surg*. 2006;30(8):1382–1391.

Nelson R, et al. Prophylactic nasogastric decompression after abdominal surgery. *Cochrane Database Syst Rev*. 2005;25(1):CD004929.

 MISCELLANEOUS

SYNONYM(S)
- Adynamic ileus
- Paralytic ileus

ABBREVIATIONS
- CHF—Congestive heart failure
- IBD—Inflammatory bowel disease
- NPO—Nil per os (nothing by mouth)
- NSAIDS—Nonsteroidal anti-inflammatory drugs
- PID—Pelvic inflammatory disease
- UTI—Urinary tract infection

 CODES

ICD9-CM
560.1 Paralytic ileus

 PATIENT TEACHING

PREVENTION
Fast-track surgery to minimize postoperative ileus:
- Minimally invasive surgical techniques whenever possible
- Epidural analgesia
- Minimize opiates
- Use of NSAIDs
- Early enteral feedings
- Early ambulation
- Limited, selective use of nasogastric tubes
- Avoid overhydration:
  - May result in bowel edema and ileus

IMPERFORATE HYMEN

Judith Lacy, MD

 BASICS

DESCRIPTION
- Imperforate hymen is among the most common obstructive anomaly of the female reproductive tract.
- The hymen represents the epithelial junction between the sinovaginal bulbs and the urogenital sinus.
- Typically, the connective tissue of the central portion of the hymen degenerates spontaneously prior to birth. If this event does not occur, the hymen remains intact at birth.
- An imperforate hymen is easily visible in the 1st few days of life, as the influence of maternal estrogens accentuate the genital anatomy.
- However, the diagnosis is frequently missed and not discovered until after the expected time of menarche.
- Hymenal abnormalities occur as a result of incomplete resorption of the hymenal tissue. Variants of hymenal configuration include:
  - Imperforate
  - Microperforate
  - Septate
  - Cribriform

Age-Related Factors
In the neonate, a bulging hymen due to mucocolpos may result as a consequence of maternal estrogen stimulation. If undiagnosed, the retained mucus secretions resorb and the bulge resolves. The imperforate hymen will persist undiagnosed, until after the onset of menarche, when a variably-sized hematocolpos forms due to an obstructed outflow tract.

EPIDEMIOLOGY
Imperforate hymen is a relatively rare diagnosis, with a reported incidence of 0.014–0.1% or ~1 in 2,000 females.

RISK FACTORS
Genetics
Although familial occurrences have been reported, typically, most cases of imperforate hymen are isolated events.

PATHOPHYSIOLOGY
- Embryologically, the female genital tract develops from ~3 weeks gestation through the 2nd trimester.
- The ovaries develop independently from the vagina, and thus vaginal anomalies are typically NOT associated with ovarian anomalies.
- The uterus and upper vagina develop from the caudal portion of the fused müllerian ducts, which subsequently canalize to form the uterus and upper vagina.
- The distal vagina forms from evaginations of the urogenital sinus as a solid vaginal plate that degenerates centrally. Canalization is complete by 20 weeks of development.

ASSOCIATED CONDITIONS
Reported anomalies associated with imperforate hymen include:
- Polydactyly
- Bifid clitoris
- Ureteral duplication
- Ectopic ureter
- Hypoplastic kidney
- Multicystic dysplastic kidney
- Urethral membrane
- Imperforate anus
- Law anorectal anomaly

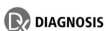 **DIAGNOSIS**

SIGNS AND SYMPTOMS
History
- If the imperforate hymen is undiagnosed in the neonatal period, the adolescent female will typically present with:
  - Cyclic abdomino-pelvic pain
  - Primary amenorrhea
- Additional complaints associated with an expanding hematocolpos and/or hematometra include:
  - Voiding difficulties
  - Constipation
  - Back pain
  - Nausea
  - Vomiting
  - Diarrhea
- In extreme cases, ureteral obstruction secondary to the grossly enlarged fluid-filled vagina could lead to hydronephrosis.

Physical Exam
- Tanner staging:
  - Normal secondary sexual characteristics
- Abdominal exam:
  - Palpable pelvic or abdominal mass
- Perineal exam:
  - Frog-leg or knee-chest position
  - Gentle labial traction:
    - Premenarchal: No vaginal opening
    - Classically, if undetected prior to accumulation of blood in vagina (hematocolpos), a tense, bulging, bluish membrane is visualized at the vaginal introitus
- Rectal exam, if hematocolpos:
  - Palpable mass that extends to the level of the hymen

Imaging
- Typically, when the diagnosis has been delayed and a hematocolpos has accumulated, the diagnosis is made on the basis of the physical exam alone.
- A distal transverse vaginal septum or vaginal agenesis can have a somewhat similar appearance if the vagina is not distended by hematocolpos.
- An accurate diagnosis prior to surgical intervention is imperative.

- Transabdominal, transperineal, or transrectal US imaging is indicated if the diagnosis is in question. Findings on imaging may include:
  - Hematocolpos
  - Hematometra
  - Dilated and distended cervix
- The diagnosis is more difficult to confirm in a prepubertal child, as a microperforate hymen may have a similar appearance.
  - Reexam should be performed once the child is pubertal (after the onset of breast development).
  - US exam at this time will establish the presence or absence of a uterus, although the distinction between a vaginal septum and imperforate hymen is difficult in the absence of a hematocolpos.

DIFFERENTIAL DIAGNOSIS
- Labial agglutination:
  - Labial traction allows visualization of the area of labial fusion
- Transverse vaginal septum:
  - External genitalia appear normal
  - Hymenal tissue present
  - US/MRI used to evaluate location and thickness of vaginal septum
  - Usually no associated renal anomalies
- Obstructed hemivagina with longitudinal vaginal septum:
  - May be associated with bulging mass at introitus
  - Normal menses present from contralateral side
- Vaginal agenesis associated with Mayer-Rokitansky-Küster-Hauser (MRKH) syndrome:
  - External genitalia appear normal
  - Hymenal tissue usually present
  - Blind vaginal dimple may be present
  - US/MRI usually reveals absence of the uterus, although uterine tissue with endometrium may be present in up to 10%
  - Frequently associated renal anomalies
- Absent vagina associated with androgen insensitivity syndrome:
  - Elevated serum testosterone
  - Karyotype XY
  - Gonadectomy indicated to prevent malignant transformation

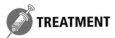 TREATMENT

ALERT
To avoid introducing bacteria and the development of an ascending infection, never attempt needle drainage or aspiration of an obstructive anomaly unless prepared to immediately proceed to definitive surgical management.

GENERAL MEASURES
- Repair of the imperforate hymen is best timed once estrogenization of the vaginal tissue has occurred after the onset of pubertal breast development, but prior to the accumulation of a hematocolpos.
- If time is needed to complete a thorough preoperative workup, menstrual suppression with continuous OCPs is recommended:
  – Allows cessation of menses and consequently decreases the symptoms associated with vaginal distension.
- NSAIDs can be given for pain relief.

MEDICATION (DRUGS)
Use of vaginally applied Premarin cream twice daily for the 1st week postoperatively may assist in healing of the vaginal mucosa.

SURGERY
- Hymenectomy/Hymenotomy:
  – Diagonal cruciate incisions
  – Elliptical incision
- Drainage and evacuation of hematocolpos:
  – Have 2 suction devices available as drainage is viscous
- Excise excess hymenal tissue
- If hymen tissue/distal septum is thick, suture vaginal mucosa to hymenal ring:
  – Circumferentially placed interrupted 2–0 Vicryl sutures allows hemostasis

 FOLLOW-UP

DISPOSITION
Issues for Referral
If diagnosis is not well established, refer to clinician with experience in evaluating and managing genital anomalies, such as a pediatric/adolescent gynecologist or reproductive endocrinologist.

PROGNOSIS
- Retrospective studies reveal that females with a history of imperforate hymen and repair generally go on to have subsequently normal menstrual behavior, sexual function, and fertility.
- Retrograde menstruation associated with obstructive anomalies is traditionally said to resolve quickly without persistent symptoms of endometriosis, although evidence is anecdotal.

BIBLIOGRAPHY

Liang CC, et al. Long-term follow-up of women who underwent surgical correction of imperforate hymen. *Arch Obstet Gynecol*. 2003;269:5–8.

Pokorny SF. Genital examination of prepubertal and peripubertal females. In: Sanfilippo JS, et al. *Pediatric and Adolescent Gynecology*, 2nd ed. Philadelphia: W.B. Saunders Company; 2001: 188–193.

Posner JC, et al. Early detection of imperforate hymen prevents morbidity from delays in diagnosis. *Pediatrics*. 2005;115:1008–1012.

Schillings WJ, et al. Amenorrhea. In: *Berek and Novak's*, 14th ed. Philadelphia: Lippincott Williams and Wilkins; 2007:1049.

Wachtel SS, et al. Molecular biology and genetic aspects. In: Sanfilippo JS, et al. *Pediatric and Adolescent Gynecology*, 2nd ed. Philadelphia: W.B. Saunders Company; 2001:175.

 MISCELLANEOUS

ABBREVIATIONS
- MRKH—Mayer-Rokitansky-Küster-Hauser syndrome
- NSAIDs—Nonsteroidal anti-inflammatory drugs
- OCPs—Oral contraceptive pills

CLINICAL PEARLS
Diagnosis of imperforate hymen should be made in the delivery room or nursery for all female neonates, as the influence of maternal estrogens accentuates the genital anatomy.

CODES
ICD9-CM/CPT
- 70.11 Hymenotomy
- 70.31 Hymenectomy
- 752.42 Imperforate hymen

 PATIENT TEACHING

The use of drawings can facilitate patient understanding of genital anatomy.

PREVENTION
The severe cyclic pain associated with an imperforate hymen with hematocolpos and hematometra can be prevented by the routine genital exam of female infants and children with appropriate diagnosis and timely management of imperforate hymen after the onset of puberty but before expected menarche.

INFERTILITY

Christopher P. Montville, MD, MS
Michael A. Thomas, MD

 BASICS

DESCRIPTION

- Inability to conceive after ≥12 months of regular, unprotected, intercourse. 85% of general population will conceive without medical assistance in this time period.
- Fecundability: Probability of conception within 1 menstrual cycle
- Fecundity: Probability of pregnancy resulting in live birth during 1 menstrual cycle
- Chemical pregnancy: Positive blood or urine pregnancy test with clinical suspicion of pregnancy

Age-Related Factors

- Ability to conceive decreases as maternal age increases.
- Oocyte number and quality decrease with time.
- Accelerated loss after age 35.
- Oocytes less sensitive to FSH stimulation
- Oocyte chromosomal abnormalities
- Increased rate of aneuploidy in embryos
- Decreased IVF success rates:
  - ↓ Pregnancy rates
  - ↑ SAB: Age <40 (18–20%), Age >40 (>35%)

EPIDEMIOLOGY

- Fecundability of general population approximately 20%. In general, declines in populations with time.
- Diagnoses in infertile couples:
  - Ovulatory disorder: 25–27%
  - Tubal disease/defect: 22–35%
  - Male factor: 25–40%
  - Endometriosis: 5%
  - Other: 4%
  - Unexplained: 17%

RISK FACTORS

- Any etiology that can cause abnormalities in gamete production, gamete transport, or embryo implantation
- Infectious:
  - PID
  - Endometritis
  - Epididymitis
- Pelvic adhesive disease:
  - PID
  - Prior pelvic/abdominal surgery
  - D&C (septic abortion)
- Chemical exposure:
  - Smoking
  - Work environment (semen parameters)

Genetics

Genetic defects associated with infertility are primarily associated with chromosomal abnormalities in the oocytes and embryos of women of advanced maternal age. Maternal genetic defects include:

- Turner syndrome (45 XO) or Turner mosaicism
- X chromosome translocations/deletions (premature ovarian failure)
- Identified mutated genes affecting:
  - FSH receptor; LH receptor
  - FMR1 (Fragile X syndrome)

PATHOPHYSIOLOGY

- Abnormal gamete (oocyte/sperm) production
- Reproductive tract defects resulting in abnormal gamete/embryo transport
- Dysfunctional implantation
- Abnormal embryo development
- Other: Genetics, immunologic factors, lifestyle

ASSOCIATED CONDITIONS

Iatrogenic causes of infertility with cytotoxic chemotherapy or pelvic radiation for malignancy

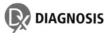 **DIAGNOSIS**

SIGNS AND SYMPTOMS

Menstrual irregularities most common. Absence of 22–35 day cycles, breast tenderness, dysmenorrhea or bloating (moliminal symptoms) suggests ovulatory dysfunction.

History

Complete history, female and male:

- Obstetric, menstrual, surgical (especially history of pelvic/abdominal surgery).
- Infectious disease; GYN (pap smear, endometriosis, etc)
- Endocrinologic (thyroid; prolactin)
- Male partner: Chemical exposure, history of mumps, testicular trauma, inguinal hernia, past paternal history, family history (genetic and reproductive), sibling history

Review of Systems

Menstrual cycle characteristics:

- Moliminal symptoms, dysmenorrhea, menorrhagia, vasomotor symptoms
- Abnormal nipple discharge
- Palpitations, constipation, diarrhea
- Dyspareunia
- Male:
  - Erectile dysfunction, testicular lesions

Physical Exam

- Particular attention to thyroid, breasts, abdomen, and pelvis:
  - BMI
  - Hirsutism, acanthosis nigricans
  - Thyroid size and contour
  - Nipple discharge
- Pelvic exam:
  - Size of uterus and adnexa
  - Utero-sacral ligament/cul-de-sac nodularity
- Male:
  - Usually defer to urologist
  - Hernia and varicocele evaluation

TESTS

- Goal is to identify cause of infertility.
- Ovulatory dysfunction
  - Basal body temperature (biphasic normal)
  - Ovulation predictor assay:
    - Urine LH assay for presence of LH surge
  - Serum progesterone:
    - >3 ng/mL: Positive ovulation
    - >10 ng/mL: Correlates with in-phase endometrium

- Clomiphene citrate challenge:
  - FSH cycle day #3 → 100 mg PO cycle days 5–9 → day 10 FSH
  - Elevated FSH on day 3 or 10 (10–20 ng/mL) indicates poor ovarian reserve
- Anatomic factors (see "Imaging"):
  - Postcoital test and endometrial biopsy rarely performed.
- Male factor:
  - Semen analysis (see "Labs")

Labs

- Day 3 FSH (if age >35 or question of ovarian reserve)
- Midluteal progesterone
- TSH; prolactin
- Total testosterone (if hyperandrogenism/PCOS suspected)
- LFTs, renal panel (if considering metformin)
- Semen analysis:
  - Normal: >50% motile; >20 million; >14% normal forms

Imaging

- Pelvic US and hysterosalpingogram mainstays of diagnostic imaging
- Pelvic US:
  - Appearance of ovaries; follicular development
  - Corpus luteum formation
  - Adnexal mass/endometrioma
  - Hydrosalpinx
  - Uterine leiomyoma; endometrial stripe measurement
- Sonohysterogram (saline infusion sonography):
  - Distention of uterine cavity with saline with concomitant pelvic US. Valuable for identification of uterine leiomyoma/polyps
- Hysterosalpingogram (HSG):
  - Fluoroscopy with contrast dye injected into uterus. Evaluation of tubal patency, tubal lumen diameter, peritubal adhesions, endometrial contour, presence of endometrial adhesions
- Hysteroscopy:
  - Office-based or in operating room. Evaluation of uterine cavity, tubal ostia
  - Potential for cannulation of ostia
- Laparoscopy:
  - Direct visualization of pelvic anatomy and peritoneal structures. Advised in women with unexplained infertility, history of endometriosis, prior pelvic surgery and/or infection; tubal occlusion on HSG.
- Chromopertubation:
  - Injection of methylene blue or indigo carmine through cervix into uterus to evaluate tubal patency
  - Concomitant adhesiolysis and tubal surgery
- MRI is useful to delineate uterine leiomyoma prior to myomectomy.

DIFFERENTIAL DIAGNOSIS

Ovulatory dysfunction:

- Anovulation/Oligo-ovulation:
  - PCOS most common (70%)

Infection
Tubal disease (occlusion/adhesions):
- PID/STDs
- Ruptured appendix

Metabolic/Endocrine
- Ovulatory dysfunction/oligo-ovulation:
  – PCOS most common (70%)
- Thyroid dysfunction
- Hyperprolactinemia
- Hypothalamic dysfunction:
  – Eating disorders
- Athletic induction amenorrhea
- Hypothalamic hypogonadism
- Poor oocyte quality:
  – POF
  – Prior ovarian surgery
  – Age-related factors
- Extremes in BMI (<20; >27)

Immunologic
Ovarian insufficiency/POF

Trauma
- Tubal occlusion/adhesions
- Pelvic surgery

Drugs
- Cytotoxic chemotherapy with ovarian failure
- Drug induced hyperprolactinemia

Other/Miscellaneous
- Endometriosis (tubal damage, inflammation)
- Male factor (azoospermia/oligospermia)
- Uterine anomalies (fibroids, polyps, septum)
- Asherman's syndrome

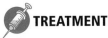 TREATMENT

GENERAL MEASURES
Treatment should be centered on specific diagnosis, patient safety, and patient preference. Adequate counseling and informed consent of vital importance.

Ovulatory Dysfunction
- Weight loss (if PCOS), smoking cessation, timed intercourse
- Clomiphene citrate:
  – 50–100 mg PO for 5 days (cycle day 3–7)
  – 50% will ovulate with 50 mg dose:
    ○ In PCOS, 8–25% fecundability with 3–6 cycles
    ○ Metformin 500 mg t.i.d. improves success in PCOS
  – Antiestrogen effect on endometrium possible
- Aromatase inhibitor: Controversial; off label
- Gonadotropin therapy:
  – Indications: Hypothalamic hypopituitarism; PCOS following failed clomiphene therapy; decreased ovarian reserve; IVF:
    ○ Multifollicular development and ovulation
    ○ 80% ovulation rate; 10–40% fecundability
    ○ Risk of multiple gestation and OHSS

Tubal Factor
- Tubal surgery (See Fallopian Tube Surgery.):
  – Adhesiolysis; fimbrioplasty; salpingotomy (hydrosalpinx); tubal cannulation (proximal occlusion):
    ○ Success rates depend on indication and severity of disease
- If significant tubal disease → IVF

Endometriosis
Adhesiolysis; endometrioma resection:
- Pretreatment with GnRH agonists/antagonists helpful prior to ovulation induction

Uterine Factors
- Myomectomy (abdominal/hysteroscopic):
  – Success dependent on leiomyoma size; proximity to endometrium, iatrogenic endometrial damage.
- Hysteroscopic polypectomy
- Hysteroscopic septum resection
- Adhesiolysis (Asherman syndrome)

Male Factor
- Varicocele repair
- IVF → intracytoplasmic sperm injection (ICSI)

Endocrinologic
- Medical treatment of hyper-/hypothyroid
- Hyperprolactinemia:
  – Bromocriptine (2.5–7.5 mg PO daily)
  – Growth of microprolactinoma unlikely during pregnancy

IVF
- Patient selection depends on diagnosis and prior medical therapy.
- Gonadotropin ovulation induction with transvaginal oocyte aspiration

SURGERY
- Majority of procedures associated with tubal disease/occlusion (See Fallopian Tube Surgery.)
- Ovarian drilling:
  – In PCOS, thermal destruction of cortex and stroma associated with increased ovulation:
    ○ Temporary improvement in ovulation

 FOLLOW-UP

DISPOSITION
Issues for Referral
Referral to fertility center based on past history and current treatment, duration of infertility, extent of possible treatment. Expedited referral:
- Female age >35
- History of known tubal disease including PID
- Known male infertility
- Prior history of cancer, genetic disease, or immunologic disease

PROGNOSIS
- Success rates depend on etiology of infertility and presence of coexisting factors
- Ovulatory dysfunction: 5–20%
- Tubal factor: 10–60%:
  – Risk of ectopic (s/p surgery) 4–21%
- Unexplained: 4–23%
- Male factor: Success dependent on oocyte quality and female factors:
  – ICSI: ~25%

PATIENT MONITORING
- Therapy should be tailored to patient preferences, costs, and etiologic factors.
- Follicle monitoring with US should be performed with ovulation induction in addition to:
  – Estradiol levels with gonadotropin use
  – Attention to development of OHSS
  – Increased vascular permeability due to elevated estradiol:
    ○ Risks include ascites, VTE, pulmonary edema

- Treatment guidelines:
  – Clomiphene: 3–6 cycles
  – Gonadotropins: 3–6 cycles
  – Reevaluation of patient expectations and desire for further, more intensive therapy necessary

BIBLIOGRAPHY
ACOG Committee on Practice Bulletins. Management of infertility caused by ovulatory dysfunction. Practice Bulletin No. 34. *Obstet Gynecol.* 2002;99:347–358.

Adamson GD, et al. Subfertility: Causes, treatment, and outcome. *Best Pract Res Clin Obstet Gynaecol.* 2003;17(2):169–185.

Barbieri RL. Female infertility. In: Stauss JF, et al., eds. *Yen and Jaffe's Reproductive Endocrinology: Physiology, pathophysiology, and clinical management*, 5th ed. Philadelphia: Elsiver; 2004: 633–668.

The Practice Committee of the American Society for Reproductive Medicine. Optimal evaluation of the infertile female. *Fertil Steril.* 2006;86(Suppl 4): S264–S267.

The Practice Committee of the American Society for Reproductive Medicine. Effectiveness and treatment for unexplained infertility. *Fertil Steril.* 2004;82(Suppl 1):S160–S163.

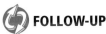 MISCELLANEOUS

ABBREVIATIONS
- BMI—Body mass index
- FSH—Follicle-stimulating hormone
- GnRH—Gonadotropin-releasing hormone
- ICSI—Intracytoplasmic sperm injection
- IVF—In vitro fertilization
- LH—Luteinizing hormone
- OHSS—Ovarian hyperstimulation syndrome
- PCOS—Polycystic ovarian syndrome
- PID—Pelvic inflammatory disease
- POF—Premature ovarian failure
- SAB—Spontaneous abortion
- STI—Sexually transmitted infection

CODES
ICD9-CM
- 256.39 Polycystic ovaries (PCOS)
- 628.0 Infertility, anovulatory
- 628.2 Infertility, tubal origin
- 628.9 Infertility, unexplained origin

 PATIENT TEACHING

- Smoking cessation, normal weight maintenance, limit chemical exposures
- Effects of age on fertility. Preconception counseling in women >35
- Attention to emotional health; counseling if needed

PREVENTION
STI prevention

INTERSTITIAL CYSTITIS

Ronald T. Burkman, MD

 BASICS

DESCRIPTION
- Interstitial cystitis (IC) is a multifactorial, chronic condition of unknown etiology.
- Exact prevalence is unknown due to lack of definitive diagnostic tests.
- Estimated that between 25% and 85% of women presenting with chronic pelvic pain may have IC
- Characterized by various combinations of urinary frequency, urgency, incontinence, or pelvic pain including dyspareunia
- ~15% of women with the condition will not have urinary symptoms.
- Consider diagnosis in women with a history of frequent UTIs not substantiated by positive cultures.
- Can both mimic and be associated with endometriosis.

Age-Related Factors
- The condition is most frequently diagnosed in Caucasian women age 25–55.
- May be seen in children <10 years of age, manifested as enuresis, symptoms of UTI, or daytime "accidents." Symptoms may regress then reappear at ages 13–17.
- Mean age at diagnosis in all women was 42 years in 1 series.

EPIDEMIOLOGY
- Prevalence and demographics difficult to estimate due to misdiagnosis and lack of standardized testing
- As many as 1 in 4.5 women in the US have findings suggestive of IC.
- The Nurses Health Study suggests the prevalence may be increasing perhaps due to increased awareness and testing.
- IC and endometriosis may coexist frequently.

RISK FACTORS
There are no known risk factors.

Genetics
Genetic factors have not been identified in association with this disorder.

PATHOPHYSIOLOGY
- Abnormal bladder epithelial permeability:
  - Damage to bladder surface; GAG epithelium
  - Damage due to prior bladder infections, vascular insufficiency, or alterations in factors such as APF or THP
  - Potassium ions pass to muscularis to produce symptoms
- Increased activation of sensory nerves:
  - Upregulation of sensory nerve fibers
  - Activation produces both pain and urgency.
- Potassium, mast cells, and other mediators:
  - Potassium and mast cells could be causative.
  - Can see elevated levels of kallikrein and substance P; may reflect an inflammatory response and increased nerve activity, respectively.

ASSOCIATED CONDITIONS
- Endometriosis
- Chronic pelvic pain
- Fibromyalgia
- Depression
- Chronic fatigue
- IBS

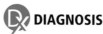 **DIAGNOSIS**

SIGNS AND SYMPTOMS
History
- Progressive disorder, can be mild or severe; symptoms often wax and wane
- Urinary urgency and occasional urge incontinence
- Urinary frequency including nocturia
- Dyspareunia
- Pelvic pain
- Bladder pain, sometimes relieved after voiding
- Depression

Review of Systems
- Dysmenorrhea
- Vaginal discharge
- Hematuria
- Bowel habits

Physical Exam
- Suprapubic tenderness
- Anterior vaginal wall and bladder base tenderness
- Levator muscle spasm

TESTS
- Pelvic Pain and Urgency/Frequency (PUF) Symptom Scale quantitates symptoms by severity with higher scores correlating highly with the likelihood of a positive Potassium Sensitivity Test (PST).
- Voiding diary with intake and output for 3 days: Urinary frequency >12 times daily in absence of other causes may suggest IC.
- PST involves instilling a potassium solution into the bladder; IC patients experience pain or urgency:
  - Test positive in 78% of women with abnormal bladder permeability
  - Due to intermittent nature of IC, negative test does not exclude diagnosis.
- Cystoscopy has limited use with IC:
  - Ulcers seen with advanced disease
  - Glomerulations may be seen with IC and in normal individuals.
  - Primarily used to exclude other pathology

Labs
- UA and culture to exclude infection
- Urine cytology to exclude bladder cancer

Imaging
IVP occasionally is used to exclude other pathology when hematuria is present.

DIFFERENTIAL DIAGNOSIS
Infection
- UTI
- STDs (e.g., chlamydial urethritis)
- Vaginitis

Tumor/Malignancy
Bladder cancer

Other/Miscellaneous
- Endometriosis
- Overactive bladder
- Vulvodynia
- Urethral diverticula
- Pelvic relaxation (e.g., uterine prolapse)
- Urethral syndrome

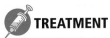 TREATMENT

GENERAL MEASURES
- Dietary modification with elimination of foods that cause symptoms: Chocolate, caffeine, high-acidity items (e.g., tomatoes, citrus fruits, carbonated beverages), alcohol, spicy foods
- Eliminate cigarette smoking
- Bladder training with scheduled voids
- Physical therapy with pelvic relaxation techniques
- Warm sitz baths, heating pads, ice packs after intercourse

SPECIAL THERAPY
Complementary and Alternative Therapies
No known alternative therapies appear effective.

MEDICATION (DRUGS)
- Several medications may relieve the symptoms of IC.
- Oral medications:
  - Pentosan polysulfate sodium: ~30% of IC patients experience relief; may take months
  - Amitriptyline
  - Cimetidine: Small studies suggest some benefit for IC patients.
  - Hydroxyzine: Controls allergies in IC patients whose symptoms are triggered during allergy seasons.
  - Second-line medications include analgesics and antispasmodics.
- Intravesical therapy:
  - DMSO: Instillations improve symptoms in up to 50% of IC patients; requires instillations every 2 weeks for several months.
  - Heparin, pentosan polysulfate sodium, and lidocaine: ~80% of IC patients achieve some relief within 2 weeks.

SURGERY
Limited surgical approaches are available:
- Hydrodistention provides relief in 20–90% of IC patients for several months.
- Cystectomy is performed as a last resort for IC patients who are refractory to other treatments and who have severe symptoms.

 FOLLOW-UP

DISPOSITION
Issues for Referral
Consultation with a urogynecologist or urologist with interest in managing chronic pelvic pain may be helpful.

PROGNOSIS
- Mild forms of disorder may wax and wane with little progression.
- Severe forms of IC may require multiple modalities to control symptoms.

PATIENT MONITORING
Psychologic support may be helpful in managing chronic pelvic pain and urinary symptoms.

BIBLIOGRAPHY

Burkman RT. Chronic pelvic pain of bladder origin: Epidemiology, pathogenesis and quality of life. *J Reprod Med*. 2004;49:225–229.

Parsons CL, et al. Increased prevalence of interstitial cystitis: Previously unrecognized urologic and gynecologic cases using a new symptom questionnaire. *Urology*. 2000;60:573–578.

Sant GR, et al. A pilot clinical trial of oral pentosan polysulphate and oral hydroxyzine in patients with interstitial cystitis. *J Urol*. 2003;170:810–816.

van Ophoven A, et al. Long-term results of amitriptyline treatment for interstitial cystitis. *J Urol*. 2005;174:1837–1843.

 MISCELLANEOUS

ABBREVIATIONS
APF—Antiproliferative factor
DMSO—Dimethyl sulfoxide
GAG—Glycosaminoglycan
IBS—Irritable bowel syndrome
IC—Interstitial cystitis
IVP—Intravenous pyelogram
PST—Potassium sensitivity test
PUF—Pelvic pain, urgency, frequency syndrome
STD—Sexually transmitted disease
THP—Tamm–Horsfall protein
UTI—Urinary tract infection

CODES
ICD9-CM
595.1 Chronic interstitial cystitis

 PATIENT TEACHING

Interstitial Cystitis Association, 110 Washington St., Rockville, MD 20850; 1–800–HELPICA; http://www.ichelp.org

PREVENTION
No known prevention, other than avoidance of foods that trigger symptoms.

LABIAL ADHESIONS

Jane E. D. Broecker, MD

 BASICS

DESCRIPTION
- Labial adhesions occur when the labia fuse in the midline, causing partial or complete obstruction of the opening to the vagina and/or urethra.
- It is typically seen in infants >3 months of age, prepubertal girls, and menopausal women.

Age-Related Factors
- Incidence of labial adhesions is related to tissue estrogen exposure.
- Never present at birth due to intrauterine exposure to maternal estrogen.
- Most common between 13 and 23 months of age, with an incidence of 3.3% in this age group.
- Occur in 1.8% of prepubertal girls
- With pubertal estrogen production, labial adhesions become less common.
- Rare in pubertal girls and reproductive-age women.
- Occasionally noted in postpartum women.
- Occasionally noted in postmenopausal women.
- May be secondary to lichen sclerosis at any age.

RISK FACTORS
- Low estrogen levels:
  - Infants (but not neonates)
  - Prepubertal or menopausal status
  - Postpartum (rare)
- Inflammatory conditions:
  - VV
  - Lichen sclerosis
  - Chronic urine exposure secondary to diapers
- Trauma:
  - Genital trauma of any kind:
    - Untreated straddle injuries
    - Female circumcision
    - Sexual abuse

PATHOPHYSIOLOGY
The delicate epithelium of the nonestrogenized vulva is vulnerable to inflammation and trauma, with fusion of the epithelium of labia minora forming a bridge between the labia.

ASSOCIATED CONDITIONS
Once adhesions occur, efflux of urine and vaginal secretions may become blocked, causing:
- VV
- UTI
- Severe inflammation due to chronic urine exposure
- Rarely, complete obstruction with urinary retention (a surgical emergency)

 DIAGNOSIS

SIGNS AND SYMPTOMS

History
- Often labial adhesions are asymptomatic, but when symptoms do occur, common complaints are related to the vulva and urinary systems.
- Burning on urination, dribbling, vulvar discomfort itching and pain, and vagina odor

Review of Systems
- Pubertal development
- Hygiene:
  - Baths vs. showers, cotton vs. nylon undergarments, diaper/toileting habits
- Genital trauma:
  - Straddle injuries, female circumcision
- Infection:
  - Bacterial VV
  - UTI
  - Pinworms
  - Yeast
- Prior treatment (prescribed or OTC)
- Sexual abuse with confidential questioning as appropriate
- Home/Care situation:
  - Divorced parents (inconsistent parenting)
  - Day care/school situation
  - Institution (nursing home)

Physical Exam
- Age-appropriate exam with Tanner staging
- Wear a white coat to signal that you are a medical professional and have a female assistant with you during the examination.
- Guidelines for genital exam in young girls:
  - Positioning of infant and small child:
    - Child on parent's lap. Grasp labial fat pads pull gently laterally and inferiorly, providing visualization of the hymen and urethral meatus if no adhesions are present.
  - Positioning of older premenarchal girl:
    - Ask the girl if she would like female parent present and honor her request. If accompanied by male family member, may ask him to step out.
    - Ask the girl to recline in frog-legged position, or assume knee-chest position.
    - Tell her how and where you are going to touch before you examine her.
    - As appropriate, use a mirror to help her see her anatomy and explain what you are doing using medically accurate language.
    - Examine labia as with infant or small child
- For postmenarchal or menopausal female:
  - Most mature girls and older women will feel comfortable in stirrups for genital exam.
  - Use a mirror, as appropriate, and explain anatomy and findings.

- Document significant findings of exam:
  - Thickness of and extent of any adhesions. A drawing in the chart can be very helpful.
  - Shape and estrogen status of hymen.
  - Note exam position and who was present.
  - Document level of cooperation of the patient and whether or not exam was optimal.
  - Note conditions: VV, excoriations, hygiene, lichen sclerosis, rectal abnormalities or other lesions

Lab
- Lab testing is typically not needed unless the diagnosis is unclear or there are associated conditions such as UTI, vulvar lesions, others.
- Wet prep/KOH exam and possibly genital cultures if history or exam indicate VV.
- Urinalysis and culture if symptoms of UTI
- See Sexual Abuse, if suspected abuse
- Scotch tape test or empiric pinworm treatment if history and exam suggestive
- Vulvar punch biopsy rarely needed:
  - Lichen sclerosis diagnosed based on exam

Imaging
If findings suggest absent vagina, US

DIFFERENTIAL DIAGNOSIS
- By history alone, labial adhesions may be incorrectly diagnosed as a UTI or a yeast infection when symptoms are treated without appropriate physical exam.
- UTI
- Yeast infection (rare in prepubertal girls)
- Trauma
- Abuse
- Imperforate hymen
- Müllerian agenesis
- Transverse vaginal septum
- Labial adhesions (in which labia are fused over a normal hymen) vs. imperforate hymen (in which labia minora are normal, and hymen is visible, but is not patent.)

Infection
- Labial adhesions may be due to a VV or may precipitate VV due to pooling of secretions.
- With both labial adhesions and VV, the primary causative agent will be unclear, and both should be treated.
- Occasionally, a UTI causing incontinence and dribbling will cause adhesions.

Trauma
Differentiate from scarring after abuse or trauma.

TREATMENT

GENERAL MEASURES

- Minimal asymptomatic labial adhesions may be observed, and usually resolve spontaneously.
- Symptomatic adhesions can be treated with topical estrogen cream or emollients (petroleum or A&D).
- Untreated adhesions may lead to UTI or VV.
- Surgical separation is rarely necessary, but may be indicated if urethra is completely obstructed.
- Hygiene:
  - Poor hygiene or improper bathing contributes to formation or recurrence of labial adhesions.
  - Encourage wiping from "front to back."
  - Encourage baths (in plain warm water) over showers.
  - Discourage use of all soaps, perfumes, or bubble baths in bath water.
  - Encourage unscented and dyefree clothing detergents.
  - Encourage clean white cotton undergarments.
  - Avoid moist conditions, such as wet bathing suits.
  - Encourage potty training to avoid overuse of diapers and pull-ups, with chronic urine exposure to the delicate vulvar tissues.
  - Ensure that all caregivers are consistently involved in encouraging hygiene measures.

SPECIAL THERAPY

Complementary and Alternative Therapies

- Emollients can prevent recurrence and are recommended after successful treatment with estrogens.
- Vaseline or A & D ointment:
  - Apply nightly
  - Girls can be taught to apply it themselves.
  - Emollient use following resolution of adhesions may be recommended for a long period of time, from months to years.
  - Some clinicians recommend emollient use to prevent recurrence until onset of puberty.
- Emollients alone may help resolve thin or only partially obstructing labial adhesions.

MEDICATION (DRUGS)

Estrogen cream is first-line therapy for most cases of labial adhesions. Estrogen cream causes adhesions to 1st thin and then separate over a period of days to weeks. Resolution of adhesions with topical estrogen cream has been reported in 79–100% of patients

- Apply b.i.d.–t.i.d. (or after each diaper change) and reassess every 2 weeks with an office exam.
- Apply a "pea-sized" amount of cream to the adhesion, providing a small amount of pressure to the adhesion at the time of cream application.
  - Patients of appropriate age may apply the cream themselves with parental supervision.
- Thin or minor adhesions typically resolve within 2 weeks, whereas thicker or more extensive adhesions may require 1–3 months of use.
- Use cream until 3 days after complete separation of the adhesions and then encourage use of an emollient to prevent recurrence.
- Discuss common side effects of local estrogen effects:
  - Erythema, pigmentation, and estrogenization of the hymen and vulva.
- Discuss rare side effects with longer duration of therapy:
  - Vaginal bleeding from stimulation of uterus
  - Breast tenderness
  - Breast budding in a prepubertal child

- Estrogen side effects are self-limited, reversible, and harmless.
- When topical estrogen has thinned and decreased the extent of the adhesions, some clinicians will gently separate the labia in the office using a lidocaine-jelly–soaked cotton swab or gentle manual traction. Care must be used to avoid patient discomfort.

SURGERY

- Surgical separation of labial adhesions is rarely necessary, but can result in immediate resolution of adhesions and is essential in certain circumstances:

  - Dense adhesions are more likely to be refractory to estrogen cream and necessitate treatment.
  - Topical estrogen application is essential for days to weeks following surgical separation.
- Surgical separation is performed under sedation or general anesthesia.
- Recurrence ≥10%, as a result of formation of "raw" edges
- Surgical separation is essential in certain situations:
  - Complete fusion of labia causing obstruction to the flow of urine or vaginal secretions:
    - Complete urinary outflow obstruction may cause severe distention of the bladder and is a surgical emergency.
    - Complete vaginal obstruction may rarely result in distention of the vagina and uterus with fluid and mucous.
  - Severe VV refractory to antibiotic treatment due to extensive adhesions
  - When topical application of estrogen is impractical or socially prohibited

 FOLLOW-UP

DISPOSITION

Issues for Referral

Referral to pediatric gynecologist for complicated cases:

- If diagnosis is unclear
- If adhesions are refractory to 6–12 weeks of estrogen therapy
- If recurrences occur
- If surgical separation is necessary
- If physical or sexual abuse is suspected

PROGNOSIS

- Labial adhesions are rarely symptomatic and, when need for treatment arises, local application of estrogen cream is usually successful, with surgical separation reserved for refractory or emergency cases.
- General hygiene practices and emollient therapy may prevent recurrence, but recurrence is common.
- Reformation of adhesions may be seen in up to 0–41% of girls treated with estrogen cream.
  - Most recurrences resolve with a repeat course of estrogen cream.
- Reseparation of adhesions is necessary in ~10% of surgically managed patients.

PATIENT MONITORING

- Initial diagnosis is typically made by primary care physicians on routine genital exam, or in those who present with VV symptoms.
- An external genital exam is part of a complete physical for the pediatric age group as well as for adult women.
- Once labial adhesions have resolved, patients need only be examined annually or if symptoms recur.

BIBLIOGRAPHY

Leung A, et al. Treatment of labial fusion with topical estrogen therapy. *J Pediatr*. 2005;44:245–247.

Leung A, et al. The incidence of labial fusion in children. *J Pediatr Child Health*. 1993;29:235–236.

Nurzia M, et al. The surgical treatment of labial adhesions in pre-pubertal girls. *J Pediatr Adolesc Gynecol*. 2003;16:21–23.

Schober J, et al. Significance of topical estrogens to labial fusion and vaginal introital integrity. *J Pediatr Adolesc Gynecol*. 2006;19:337–339.

 MISCELLANEOUS

SYNONYM(S)

- Labial agglutination
- Labial fusion

CLINICAL PEARLS

- Mothers may become anxious about potential cancer or other risks from topical estrogen after reading the patient package insert; reassure regarding the nonapplicability of these risks to children.
- Recurrences of adhesions are likely more frequent than series report; parents may become frustrated with ongoing treatment and discontinue or use only intermittently.

ABBREVIATIONS

- US—Ultrasound
- UTI—Urinary tract infection
- VV—Vulvovaginitis

CODES

ICD9-CM

623.2 Labial adhesion

PATIENT TEACHING

Patients should be educated about:

- Hygiene (see "General Measures")
- Normal vulvar anatomy
- Effectiveness of topical emollients for prevention of recurrence
- Symptoms and signs of vulvovaginal infections and UTI
- Signs and symptoms of abuse
- Topical estrogens should not be used p.r.n., but require consistent daily use

PREVENTION

- Practicing good hygiene and identifying and treating any inflammatory conditions may help prevent formation of adhesions.
- Recurrences may be prevented with attention to hygiene and consistent use of emollients:
  - Emollients may be necessary until the patient has adequate estrogen levels (as signified by breast development in a girl, or consistent hormone therapy for a menopausal woman).
- Some patients will form adhesions with no identifiable cause, and many patients will have recurrence despite attention to hygiene and use of emollient therapy.

LUTEAL PHASE DEFECT

Stacey A. Scheib, MD
Frances Batzer, MD, MBE

 BASICS

DESCRIPTION
- Luteal phase defect (LPD) is characterized by the failure to develop a fully mature secretory endometrium.
- An inability of the corpus luteum to secrete progesterone in high enough amounts or for long enough duration results in an inadequate or out-of-phase transformation of the endometrium that prevents embryo implantation
- Controversial as to whether or not LPD is a real entity

Age-Related Factors
Potential increased incidence age >40 years

Staging
- Type I or classical defect:
  - Histologic endometrial maturation is delayed by ≥2 days
  - Common condition even in fertile women
- Type II defect:
  - Endometrial histology is within normal limits but impairment in the expression of integrin cell adhesion molecules as markers of maturation needed for embryo implantation

EPIDEMIOLOGY
- 3–10% of primary or secondary infertility in women is associated with LPD.
- Up to 35% of those who have recurrent spontaneous abortion are found to have a LPD.
- No statistically significant difference between fertile and infertile women in the incidence of LPD

RISK FACTORS
- Idiopathic
- Systemic disease:
  - Stress
  - Exercise
  - Weight loss
  - Dieting
  - Eating disorders
  - Chronic disease
- Endocrinopathies:
  - Hyperprolactinemia
  - Thyroid dysfunction
  - Hyperandrogenism
- Drugs:
  - Clomiphene citrate
  - Gonadotropins
  - GnRH agonists and antagonists
  - Opioids
  - NSAIDs
  - Phenothiazines
- Miscellaneous:
  - Menstrual cycles at the onset of puberty or perimenopause
  - Inadequate progesterone (P) receptors
  - Subclinical endometritis
  - Endometriosis
  - Early luteolysis
  - Inhibin abnormalities

PATHOPHYSIOLOGY
- Dysfunctional follicular phase:
  - Poor follicular development secondary to GnRH pattern, FSH/LH pattern, obesity, hyperprolactinemia, thyroid dysfunction
  - Presentation: Inadequate E2 production, poor follicular growth, inadequate LH surge, inadequate induction of LH receptors, lack of follicular rupture, elevated prolactin levels, decreased inhibin levels:
    - Elevated prolactin levels interfere with GnRH secretion, which results in a decrease in LH pulses that impairs luteal function.
    - Failure of small luteal cells in the ovary to respond to LH
    - Decreased levels of FSH in follicular phase; conflicting data to support this
    - Abnormal LH pulsatility
    - Decreased levels of LH and FSH during the ovulatory surge
- Dysfunctional luteal phase after ovulation:
  - Inadequate production of, or endometrial response to progesterone
  - Presentation: Inadequate maturation of the endometrium to decreased progesterone production, decreased number of P receptors, and decreased number of E2 receptors
- Dysfunctional early pregnancy after ovulation:
  - Inadequate maturation of the corpus luteum
  - Presentation: Short luteal phase, early occult miscarriage, low progesterone levels in early pregnancy, accelerated luteolysis

ASSOCIATED CONDITIONS
- Recurrent spontaneous abortions: Loss of ≥3 consecutive pregnancies before the 20th week of gestation
- Primary infertility
- Secondary infertility
- Luteal suppression in assisted reproduction

 DIAGNOSIS

SIGNS AND SYMPTOMS
History
- Recurrent spontaneous abortions
- Primary infertility
- Secondary infertility
- Assisted reproduction
- Change in menstrual cycles

Review of Systems
- Frequently no symptoms
- Stress
- Exercise
- Weight loss

Physical Exam
Normal physical exam in most cases

TESTS
- Basal body temperature (BBT) chart monitors the patient's daily temperature before rising in the morning during the menstrual cycle:
  - BBT correlates with serum progesterone
  - Normally, a sustained elevation of 0.4–0.6°C in temperature occurs for 12–15 days secondary to elevated progesterone during the secretory phase of the menstrual cycle
  - Abnormal when the temperature elevation lasts <11 days
  - Not reliable enough to be a diagnostic tool, but is a simple initial screening tool to identify women with a shortened secretory phase
- Luteal phase endometrial biopsy:
  - Usually taken 10 days after LH surge
  - A histologic determination is made to determine the degree of differentiation of the endometrial sample and to see if it corresponds to the cycle day on which the biopsy was performed.
  - LPD present when a >2–3 day lag occurs in the endometrial maturation
  - 2 out-of-phase endometrial biopsies from 2 cycles is more reliable than 1 biopsy to make diagnosis of LPD
  - Retrospective dating method uses calculation based on the determination of LH surge.
  - Prospective dating method uses calculation based on the next menstrual period.

Labs
- Midluteal serum progesterone:
  - A single level taken 5–9 days after ovulation or a sum of 3 random luteal serum measurements
  - A single measurement <10 ng/mL or a sum of 3 random luteal measurements that is <30 ng/mL correlates with a LPD.
- The following tests are useful to evaluate other underlying causes of infertility:
  - TSH: Either elevated or decreased
  - Prolactin: >20 ng/mL
  - Testosterone: Increased in female hyperandrogenism and PCOS
  - FSH and LH level:
    - Both decreased in hypopituitarism
    - LH/FSH ratio >2.5 associated with PCOS
  - Maternal karyotype: Turner syndrome and Turner syndrome mosaics
  - Elevated 17 OH progesterone: Late-onset congenital adrenal hyperplasia
  - Elevated DHEA-S: Adrenal disease

Imaging
TVU:

- A maximum mean preovulatory follicle diameter of <17 mm may indicate a LPD, but the evidence is inconclusive.

DIFFERENTIAL DIAGNOSIS
Infection
Endometritis

Hematologic

- Thrombophilia:
  - Activated protein C resistance
  - Factor V Leiden (FVL) mutation
  - Protein S deficiency
  - Protein C deficiency
  - Antithrombin III deficiency
  - Prothrombin factor II mutation
  - Hyperhomocysteinanemia
- Prothrombotic/Hypofibrinolytic disorders

Metabolic/Endocrine

- PCOS
- Insulin resistance
- Obesity
- Hyperprolactinemia
- Uncontrolled diabetes mellitus
- Thyroid dysfunction

Immunologic

- Antiphospholipid syndrome
- Antinuclear antibodies
- Presence of antithyroid antibodies
- SLE
- Sjögren syndrome

Trauma

Intrauterine adhesions

Other/Miscellaneous

Structural abnormalities:

- Incompetent cervix
- Uterine fibroids
- Congenital uterine abnormalities

TREATMENT

SPECIAL THERAPY

Complementary and Alternative Therapies

- NOT evidence-based
- Stress reduction
- Vitamin B_6 50–300 mg/d
- Natural progesterone cream: 1/4–1/2 teaspoon spread on the inner arm, inner thigh, neck, and chest b.i.d. from ovulation to menstruation or until the 10th week of pregnancy:
  - Skin does not absorb natural progesterone
- Vitamin C 750 mg/d

MEDICATION (DRUGS)

- Ovulation induction:
  - Clomiphene citrate:
    - Estrogen antagonist that binds to receptors in the hypothalamus and pituitary and stimulates increased release of GnRH, leading to increased secretion of FSH and LH from the pituitary
    - Typical dose: 50 mg/d for 5 days on days 5–9 of cycle, but can increase dose up to 150 mg/d.
    - Side effects: OHSS) ovarian cyst, multiple pregnancy, hot flashes, cervical mucus thickening

- Gonadotropins:
  - Human menopausal gonadotropins, recombinant FSH, urofollitropin
  - Side effects: OHSS, ovarian cysts, multiple pregnancy, injection site reactions, headaches, mastalgias, dizziness
- GnRH antagonists:
  - Ganirelix, cetrorelix
  - Side effects: hot flashes, injection site reaction
- Aromatase inhibitors:
  - Letrozole and anastrozole
  - Side effects: Hot flushes, headaches, leg cramps
- hCG:
  - Timed injection given with evidence of a mature follicle by TVU or with LH surge
  - May be used in conjunction with progesterone, clomiphene citrate, and gonadotropins
- The role of estradiol is controversial, with conflicting data for its support.
- GnRH pulse therapy
- Luteal-phase support:
  - IM, oral, or intravaginal progesterone:
    - Administer from start of luteal phase until 10–12 weeks of gestation
    - IM progesterone is 50 mg/d
    - Intravaginal progesterone is given 200 mg once or twice daily.
    - Oral progesterone is less effective than intravaginal or intramuscular progesterone due to variable absorption.
    - Oral progesterone is associated with a higher rate of side effects secondary to the metabolites, drowsiness.
    - Side effects of IM progesterone: Sterile abscesses, severe inflammatory reactions, discomfort
    - Side effects of intravaginal progesterone: Vaginal discharge, vaginal irritation
  - Bromocriptine/cabergoline:
    - For persistent LPD associated with hyperprolactinemia
    - Side effects: Headaches, nausea, lightheadedness, orthostatic hypotension
  - Propylthiouracil/Methimazole:
    - For persistent LPD associated with hyperthyroidism
    - Side effects: Fever, rash, urticaria, arthralgias, agranulocytosis, hepatotoxicity
  - Levothyroxine:
    - For persistent LPD associated with hypothyroidism
    - Side effects: Signs of hyperthyroidism, hair loss, insomnia, headache, irritability or nervousness, sweating or fever, change in menstrual cycle, weight or appetite changes, tremor, diarrhea

Pregnancy Considerations

Progestin treatment of luteal phase into early pregnancy should only be with natural progesterone support until the luteal placental shift after 8 weeks.

FOLLOW-UP

DISPOSITION

Issues for Referral

Family physician or general ob-gyn may consider referral to specialist in infertility.

PROGNOSIS

- Good with treatment
- Controversy over the significance of LPD impacts assessment of management.

BIBLIOGRAPHY

Bukulmez O, et al. Luteal phase defect: Myth or reality. *Obstet Gynecol Clin N Am.* 2004;31:727–744.

Daly D. Treatment strategies for luteal phase deficiency. *Clin Obstet Gynecol.* 1991;31(1): 222–232.

Daya S, et al. Luteal phase support in assisted reproduction cycles [Cochrane Review]. In: *The Cochrane Library,* Issue 3. Chichester, UK: John Wiley and Sons Ltd., 2004.

Lessey BA, et al. Integrins as markers of uterine receptivity in women with primary unexplained infertility. *Fertil Steril.* 1995;63(3):535–542.

Noyes RW, et al. Dating the endometrial biopsy. *Fertil Steril.* 1950;1:3.

Wallach EE, et al., eds. *Reproductive Medicine and Surgery.* St. Louis: C.V. Mosby; 1995.

MISCELLANEOUS

SYNONYM(S)

- Luteal-phase dysfunction
- Luteal-phase deficiency
- Inadequate luteal phase

ABBREVIATIONS

- DHEA-S—Dehydroepiandrosterone sulphate
- E2—Estradiol
- FSH—Follicle-stimulating hormone
- GnRH—Gonadotropin-releasing hormone
- hCG—Human chorionic gonadotropin
- LH—Luteinizing hormone
- LPD—Luteal phase defect
- OHSS—Ovarian hyperstimulation syndrome
- PCOS—Polycystic ovarian syndrome
- TVU—Transvaginal ultrasound

CODES

ICD9-CM

628.9 Female infertility of unspecified origin

PATIENT TEACHING

Web sites:

- www.asrm.org
- www.resolve.org
- infertility.about.com
- www.emedicine.com

MENSTRUAL SUPPRESSION

Anita L. Nelson, MD
Monica Hau Hien Le, MD

 ## BASICS

DESCRIPTION
- Withdrawal bleeding with hormonal contraceptives has no medical benefit and often causes physical suffering and significant inconvenience.
- Most of the physical discomforts with COC use occur during the hormone-free week of placebo pills.
- Extended use of combined hormonal contraceptives (pills or rings) or progestin-only methods (DMPA or LNG IUS) prevents endometrial proliferation and reduces or eliminates the need for periodic endometrial sloughing and withdrawal bleeding.
  - 2 FDA-approved OCP products are currently available with 84/7 patterns, 1 with 7 placebo pills, the other with 7 pills of 10 μg EE
  - 1 product with 28 active pills/packet is intended for 12 months of continuous use.
  - Off-label continuous use of monophasic pills with strong progestin is also possible.
  - Vaginal contraceptive ring has been used as consecutive 3-week cycles for up to 13 cycles.
  - 1 documented study of 1-time use of weekly patches without interruption for 91 days.
  - DMPA and DMPA Sub Q 104 used for menstrual suppression for prolonged periods despite black box warning (see Contraception, Hormonal: Injectable).
  - LNG IUS causes amenorrhea in 20% of women by 1 year.

Age-Related Factors
- Adolescents with 1^0 dysmenorrhea benefit from fewer withdrawal bleeding episodes.
- Women with decreased productivity due to monthly bleeding can benefit.
- Premenopausal women with menorrhagia from adenomyosis or fibroid uteri can use menstrual suppression to avoid surgery.
- Hysterectomies for menorrhagia may be avoided by menstrual suppression.

EPIDEMIOLOGY
- Up to 85% of reproductive-aged US women suffer premenstrual symptoms.
- 3–8% suffer PMDD
- Menstruation is the single greatest cause of lost days of school and work for women <25

MECHANISMS OF ACTION
- High-dose progestin directly suppresses endometrial proliferation even when combined with estrogen.
- The average endometrial stripe on cycle day 21 of conventional OCP pack is 2.8 mm.
- The average endometrial stripe on cycle day 84 of extended cycle OCP pack is 2.1 mm.
- DMPA suppresses ovarian steroidogenesis.
- LNG IUS does not reduce ovarian E2 production but prevents endometrial stimulation.

EFFICACY
- Progestin-only injections and the LNG IUS are in the top tier of contraceptive efficacy.
- LNG IUS reduces menstrual blood loss by 70–90% after 12 months of use.
- >50% women achieve amenorrhea by their 3rd injection of DMPA.
- Extended-cycle OCPs did not demonstrate contraceptive superiority in clinical trials but have that potential in typical use. Without frequent placebo periods to allow ovarian follicular recruitment, extended-cycle OCPs may be more forgiving of missed pills.
- Use of 84/7 products reduces the median number of scheduled days bleeding from 36 to 10 each year; total days of bleeding and spotting are reduced 49–36 days a year.
- Extended cycle vaginal ring can be used for up to 12 months.

 ## EVALUATION

SIGNS AND SYMPTOMS
History
- As with conventional hormonal methods.
- Document reason(s) patient desires menstrual suppression (e.g., anemia, dysmenorrhea, PMS, and/or quality of life benefits).
- Family history should be documented as with conventional hormonal methods.
- Medications/Drug interactions should be documented as with conventional hormonal methods.

TESTS
As with conventional hormonal methods.

Physical Exam
- Measure BP.
- Perhaps do a breast exam.
- No pelvic exam necessary before prescribing any hormonal contraceptive (except LNG IUS)

TESTS
Labs
None routinely needed.

Imaging
None routinely needed.

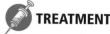 ## TREATMENT

PATIENT SELECTION
- Every woman who qualifies for and selects OCPs or vaginal rings should be advised of health and quality-of-life benefits of menstrual suppression with extended cycle products.
- Document why the woman wants monthly menstrual bleeding if she declines extended cycle use. Provide education to dispel myths.
- Women selecting DMPA or LNG IUS will also benefit from discussion of health benefits of method-induced oligomenorrhea or amenorrhea.

INDICATIONS
- All women using hormonal contraceptives may benefit from extended cycle use to suppress withdrawal bleeding.
- Medical indications:
  - Dysmenorrhea from endometriosis, adenomyosis
  - Menorrhagia due to bleeding diathesis, fibroid uterus, mediations such as anticonvulsants
  - PCOS
  - Extended cycles with COCs or vaginal rings suppresses circulating androgens without monthly menses.
  - PMS, PMDD
  - Menstrual migraines without aura
  - Catamenial exacerbation of conditions such as seizures, asthma attacks, etc.
- Quality of life:
  - Menstruation can interfere with routine and special activities, such as work, sports, social, sex

CONTRAINDICATIONS
Same as for cyclic use of OCs with exception of menstrual migraines.

INFORMED CONSENT
No special consent is needed for FDA-approved products or off-label use of other hormonal contraceptives for menstrual suppression.

PATIENT EDUCATION
- Early unpredictable spotting and bleeding is reduced over time.
- Amenorrhea with these methods is not cause for concerns that would arise if women were amenorrheic spontaneously.

Risks
As with conventional hormonal methods.

Benefits, Including Noncontraceptive
- Menstrual suppression eliminates or minimizes menstrually related problems of dysmenorrhea, menorrhagia, PMS, PMDD, menstrual migraine, etc.
- Continuous or extended-cycle use of estrogen-containing contraceptives suppresses ovarian follicle recruitment, which may decrease breakthrough ovulation and pregnancy rates.
- All noncontraceptive benefits from cyclic use apply to extended-cycle use.

Alternatives

- Menstrual suppression can be achieved with a variety of hormonal methods: Extended-cycle use of OCPs, vaginal rings, DMPA, and LNG IUS.
- LNG IUS does not suppress ovulation.
- Alternatives depend upon indication for menstrual suppression.
- Endometriosis: GnRH agonists, danazol, hysterectomy
- Menorrhagia: Endometrial ablation, hysterectomy
- PMS/PMDD: 24/4 EE/drospirenone pills, SSRIs

SPECIAL GROUPS

Mentally Retarded/Developmental Delay

- Provides more secure pregnancy protection
- Prevents hygiene challenges caused by menses
- Prevents fear some women experience with bleeding they do not understand

Adolescents

- Treats primary dysmenorrhea
- Prevents disruptions in teen's life with menses (lost school days, inability to participate in sports, etc.)
- Provides teen with PCOS needed progestin and estrogen without increasing her number of bleeding episodes.
- Does not encourage sexual activity.

Women with Chronic Illness

- Women with bleeding disorders (vWD, platelet disorder)
- Women experiencing renal failure (especially, LNG IUS and DMPA)
- Women using anticoagulants and anticonvulsants (except LNG IUS)

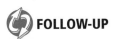 FOLLOW-UP

DISPOSITION

Issues for Referral

Same as for LNG IUS, DMPA, and cyclic OCs (see Contraception: Intrauterine Contraceptives; Contraception, Hormonal: Injectable; and Contraception, Hormonal: Combination Oral Contraceptives).

PROGNOSIS

With appropriate counseling, the unscheduled bleeding and spotting experienced early in use will be better tolerated.

COMPLICATIONS

Same as listed in LNG IUS, DMPA, and cyclic OCs: Unscheduled spotting/bleeding occurs more frequently in early cycles than later.

PATIENT MONITORING

Same as listed in LNG IUS, DMPA, and cyclic OCs

BIBLIOGRAPHY

Anderson FD, et al. Safety and efficacy of an extended-regimen oral contraceptive utilizing continuous low-dose ethinyl estradiol. *Contraception.* 2006;73:229–234.

Birtch RL, et al. Ovarian follicular dynamics during conventional vs. continuous oral contraceptive use. *Contraception.* 2006;73:235–243.

Canto De Cetina TE, et al. Effect of counseling to improve compliance in Mexican women receiving depot-medroxyprogesterone acetate. *Contraception.* 2001;63:143–146.

Miller L, et al. Extended regimens of the contraceptive vaginal ring: A randomized trial. *Obstet Gynecol.* 2005;106:473–482.

Sulak PJ, et al. Hormone withdrawal symptoms in oral contraceptive users. *Obstet Gynecol.* 2000;95: 261–266.

 MISCELLANEOUS

SYNONYM(S)

- Extended cycle pills
- Extended cycle vaginal contraceptive rings
- Menstrual elimination

CLINICAL PEARLS

- In suggesting use of extended-cycle contraception, it is important to validate the patient's concerns that lack of regular menses when not using hormonal contraception is "not normal," and to explain that the situation with hormonal contraception is different.
- Management of unscheduled bleeding/spotting (off-label) with vaginal rings or OCPs: After at least 1 pack of OCPs or 1 vaginal ring, if spotting/bleeding not controlled with high-dose NSAIDs, may interrupt use for 2 days to establish menstrual flow, then restart use and progressively increase uninterrupted use over time.

ABBREVIATIONS

DMPA—Depo-medroxyprogesterone acetate
E2—Estradiol
EE—Ethinyl estradiol
LNG IUS—Levonorgestrel intrauterine system
OCP—Oral contraceptive pill
PMDD—Premenstrual dysphoric disorder
PMS—Premenstrual syndrome

LEGAL ISSUES

Age/Consent or Notification for Minors

No requirements needed beyond those for conventional use of hormonal contraceptive

Emergency Contraception

Can be used in conjunction with any method at time of initiation when not on menses if indicated or with lapse in use of method.

ACCESS ISSUES

- Many insurance plans do not cover 84/7 products but provision of 3-month supply of contraceptive at a time increases contraceptive continuation rates, compared to providing only 1–2 month supplies at a time.
- Insurance coverage for LNG IUS for treatment of menorrhagia may require preauthorization.

CODES

ICD9-CM

626.8 Menstruation, suppression of

 PATIENT TEACHING

- Menstrual suppression is healthy.
- Withdrawal bleeding with hormonal contraceptives is not normal menstruation; it is bleeding that is artificially induced by the placebo pills.
- The use of 7 days of placebo pills with low-dose pills may increase risk of pregnancy.
- The unscheduled bleeding women have with extended cycle (84/7) pills is lighter and lasts fewer days than the bleeding episodes women have each month with 21/7 pill use.
- Women who use extended-cycle pills or vaginal rings, DMPA or LNG IUS suffer less from pain, nausea, and other complaints of PMS related to bleeding.
- There are no known medical risks from taking extended cycle pills or vaginal rings compared to their monthly use.

PREVENTION

The use of extended hormonal contraceptives and menstrual suppression can prevent significant menstrual morbidity.

MITTELSCHMERZ

Jill M. Zurawski, MD

 BASICS

DESCRIPTION
- Literally, "middle pain": Mid-cycle pain in ovulatory patients
- Proposed etiologies:
  - Enlargement of ovarian follicle just prior to ovulation (capsular distention)
  - Bleeding following rupture of ovum

Age-Related Factors
Theoretically, less likely to occur at extremes of reproductive age—adolescence and menopausal transition—as anovulatory cycles are more common at these ages.

EPIDEMIOLOGY
- ~20% of menstruating women experience some degree of discomfort with ovulation.
- Rarely, women seek treatment for consistent pain each month.

RISK FACTORS
Normal ovulation

PATHOPHYSIOLOGY
- Growth and rupture of the ovarian follicle may cause awareness of mild to severe discomfort.
- Ovarian capsular distention:
  - Hemorrhage from rupture site may result in peritoneal irritation and pain.

ASSOCIATED CONDITIONS
Hemorrhagic corpus luteum

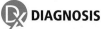 **DIAGNOSIS**

SIGNS AND SYMPTOMS

History
- Menstrual history: Ovulatory cycles (regular monthly menses with menstrual molimina)
- Pain is unilateral.
- Degree of pain varies from mild twinge to pressure to stabbing.
- Duration is several hours to several days.

Review of Systems
- Normal bowel, bladder history
- Intercourse may exacerbate pain

Physical Exam
- Unilateral pelvic and/or lower abdominal pain without mass
- No evidence of infection or PID
- Normal bowel sounds

TESTS
- Pregnancy test and STD tests are negative.
- CBC may reflect hemorrhagic anemia if bleeding from ovulation is massive (rare).
- Pelvic US may show follicular cyst, or collapsed follicular cyst and small free fluid representing recent ovulation.
- Adnexa have normal Doppler blood flow.

Labs
Pregnancy test, *Gonorrhea/Chlamydia*, possibly hematocrit:
- Used to rule out more worrisome diagnoses such as ectopic pregnancy and PID

Imaging
Pelvic US:
- Not always necessary but may confirm diagnosis
- May reassure patient of absence of more serious pathology (mass, PID)

DIFFERENTIAL DIAGNOSIS

Infection
Appendicitis

Hematologic
Women on anticoagulants are more likely to develop hemoperitoneum with corpus luteum cyst rupture.

Metabolic/Endocrine
Normal ovulation

Immunologic
IBD

Trauma
Intercourse may exacerbate discomfort.

Other/Miscellaneous
- Ectopic pregnancy
- Hemorrhagic corpus luteum
- Ovarian/Adnexal torsion
- Renal colic

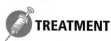 **TREATMENT**

GENERAL MEASURES
- Rest
- NSAIDs, acetaminophen
- Heating pad
- Avoid intercourse for several days

SPECIAL THERAPY

Complementary and Alternative Therapies
Castor oil packs (castor oil on cotton cloth covered with heating pad)

MEDICATION (DRUGS)
- NSAIDs (ibuprofen, naproxen, ASA)
- Acetaminophen
- COCs prevent functional cyst formation.

SURGERY
Rarely necessary except as diagnostic confirmation if pain is excessive (laparoscopy)

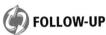 FOLLOW-UP

PROGNOSIS
Generally excellent

PATIENT MONITORING
- Menstrual calendar may predict/confirm future episodes.
- Diagnosis may be confirmed in retrospect with onset of menses in ~14 days.

BIBLIOGRAPHY

Berek JS, *Novak's Gynecology*. 13th ed. Philadelphia: Lippincott, Williams & Wilkins; 2002.

Speroff L, et al. *Clinical Gynecology Endocrinology and Infertility*. Philadelphia: Lippincott, Williams & Wilkins; 2005.

 MISCELLANEOUS

SYNONYM(S)
Ovulation

CLINICAL PEARLS
- Mittelschmerz can be suspected as a cause of pelvic pain, but if pain is severe, it is important to rule out other causes of pain listed above.
- Occurrence of menses 14 days after onset of pain strongly suggests mittelschmerz—a diagnosis made in retrospect.

ABBREVIATIONS
- ASA—Acetylsalicylic acid (aspirin)
- COC—Combined oral contraceptive
- IBD—Inflammatory bowel disease
- NSAIDs—Nonsteroidal anti-inflammatory drugs
- PID—Pelvic inflammatory disease
- STD—Sexually transmitted disease

 CODES

ICD9-CM
625.2 Mittelschmerz

 PATIENT TEACHING

Encourage charting of menses in relation to episodes of pain or discomfort.

PREVENTION
Hormonal contraception to prevent ovulation

Section II

OSTEOPOROSIS AND OSTEOPENIA

Avinash Paupoo, MD, MA
Margery L. S. Gass, MD

 BASICS

DESCRIPTION
- Skeletal disorder characterized by impaired bone strength that increases the risk of fracture
- Bone strength is a composite of bone density and bone quality, the latter not fully understood.

Age-Related Factors
Incidence increases with increasing age:
- Each decade has a 1.4–1.8-fold increase

Staging
- The severity of bone loss is characterized relative to the mean bone mineral density in young healthy women (T-score):
  – A 1–unit change in T-score corresponds to a 1 standard deviation difference from the reference population
- WHO definition is based on T-scores:
  – Normal: ≥ -1
  – Osteopenia: Between -1 and -2.5
  – Osteoporosis: ≤ -2.5
  – Severe osteoporosis: < -2.5 and ≥ 1 fragility fractures

EPIDEMIOLOGY
- Osteoporosis prevalence in the US:
  – 26% of women aged ≥ 65 years
  – >50% of women aged ≥ 85 years
- Health care implications per year:
  – >1.5 million osteoporotic fractures
  – 300,000 hip fractures
  – 180,000 nursing home placements
  – \$12–18 billion in direct healthcare costs

RISK FACTORS
- For osteoporosis:
  – Age
  – Low peak bone mineral density
  – Premature menopause; low estrogen states
  – Low body weight
  – History of anorexia nervosa
  – Asian or Caucasian ethnic origin
  – Glucocorticoid therapy
  – Hyperthyroidism, hyperparathyroidism
  – Lifelong low dietary calcium intake
  – Vitamin D deficiency
  – Long-term immobilization
  – Cigarette smoking
- For hip fractures:
  – Previous low trauma fracture
  – Family history of hip fracture
  – Poor health, low body mass index
  – Increased risk of falling: Excessive alcohol intake, poor visual acuity, neuromuscular disorders, poor balance, use of sedatives/narcotics/antihypertensives

Genetics
- Familial predisposition
- More common in Caucasians and Asians

PATHOPHYSIOLOGY
- Bone-remodeling cycle consists of bone resorption and bone formation:
  – Osteoclasts dissolve bone mineral and proteins.
  – Osteoblasts create a collagen matrix that calcifies to produce mineralized bone.
- Osteoporosis results when an imbalance favors bone resorption:
  – Estrogen deficiency leads to overexpression of osteoclasts.
  – Osteoclast activity predominates with aging.
- Failure to attain peak BMD may predispose to earlier osteoporosis.
- Primary osteoporosis: Inadequate bone-remodeling process, mainly due to aging
- Secondary osteoporosis: The result of a medical condition or drug effect (see "Differential Diagnosis")

ASSOCIATED CONDITIONS
Kyphosis

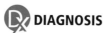 **DIAGNOSIS**

SIGNS AND SYMPTOMS
History
- Goal of treatment is to determine if substantial risk for osteoporosis or fracture exists.
- Review risk factors
- Past medical history:
  – Chronic medical conditions (see "Differential Diagnosis")
  – Number of years of low estrogen
  – History of low trauma fracture
- Medications (see "Differential Diagnosis," "Drugs")
- Family history:
  – Osteoporosis (clarify not osteoarthritis)
  – Compression fractures, hip fractures
  – Significant height loss with age, kyphosis

Review of Systems
Usually asymptomatic until a fracture occurs

Physical Exam
- Height: Historical and actual measured, preferably with stadiometer
- Weight
- Calculated BMI
- Kyphosis
- Signs of systemic disease

TESTS
Labs
Evaluate for secondary causes when BMD is more severe than expected or when failure to respond to treatment occurs:
- Complete metabolic panel, CBC, TSH, 24-hour urinary calcium excretion, urinary free cortisol, serum 25-hydroxyvitamin D, serum protein electrophoresis
- Serum intact parathyroid hormone if serum calcium is elevated
- Antiendomysial antibodies (celiac disease) if all else is negative

Imaging
- Most guidelines recommend BMD testing in:
  – All women aged ≥ 65 years
  – Younger postmenopausal women with ≥ 1 risk factor
  – Postmenopausal women who present with fractures
- DEXA of hip and spine is the gold standard for measuring BMD and establishing a diagnosis of osteoporosis.
- Single-photon absorptiometry or US of calcaneus if DEXA is not available. Bone loss occurs later in the heel.
- Lateral spine radiograph to diagnose compression fractures if significant height loss

DIFFERENTIAL DIAGNOSIS
Metabolic/Endocrine
- Cushing' syndrome
- Insulin-dependent diabetes mellitus
- Hypogonadism
- Hyperthyroidism, hyperparathyroidism

Tumor/Malignancy
- Multiple myeloma
- Lymphoma
- Leukemia

Drugs
- Glucocorticoids
- Alcohol excess
- Heparin
- Lithium
- GnRH agonists
- Anticonvulsants
- Excess thyroid hormone
- Chemotherapy

Other/Miscellaneous
- GI: Malabsorption syndrome (e.g., celiac disease, Crohn's disease), liver disease, gastrectomy/bypass procedures
- Systemic disease: Rheumatoid arthritis, ankylosing spondylitis, sarcoidosis, chronic renal failure
- Anorexia nervosa
- Genetic: Hemophilia, hemochromatosis, thalassemia

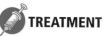 **TREATMENT**

GENERAL MEASURES
- Physical activity is necessary for bone formation and maintenance throughout life:
  – Exercise-associated improvements in mobility, muscle function, and balance may reduce fractures by decreasing the risk of falling.
  – Weight training induces a small increase in BMD at some skeletal sites.
- Adequate calcium intake is essential for attaining and maintaining adequate bone mass. Recommended calcium intake:
  – Age ≤ 50 years: 1,000 mg/d
  – Age >50 years: 1,200 mg/d

- Vitamin D is essential for intestinal absorption of calcium. Recommended vitamin D intake:
  - Age 51–70 years: 400 IU/d
  - Age ≥71 years: 600 IU/d
  - 800 IU/d for women at risk of deficiency due to inadequate sunlight exposure
  - Vitamin D_3 may be preferable.
- 30% of people aged ≥60 years fall at least once a year. Preventing falls is crucial:
  - Recommend canes or walkers to those at risk of falling (see "Risk Factors, Falling").
  - Make environment safe (e.g., remove obstacles on floor, install handrails, improve poor lighting)
  - Hip protectors reduce risk of hip fracture for those who fall (available on Internet)

SPECIAL THERAPY
Complementary and Alternative Therapies
- Chiropractic manipulations:
  - Potential risks with chiropractic adjustments for patients with osteoporosis or risk factors
- Omega-3 fatty acids dietary supplement:
  - Agency for Healthcare Research and Quality (AHRQ) Evidence report 2004:
    ○ Variable results of studies on BMD
    ○ No studies on fracture
- Studies of other therapies to prevent and treat osteoporosis are underway or recently completed:
  - Soy/Isoflavone supplement
  - Kudzu
  - High-phytoestrogen diet:
    ○ Flax seed
    ○ Macrobiotic diet
  - Therapeutic touch for wrist fractures
- Insufficient evidence to conclude benefit:
  - Red clover

MEDICATION (DRUGS)
- Treatment recommended in:
  - Women with T-scores <-2 by hip DEXA with no risk factors
  - Women with a prior vertebral or hip fracture
  - The NOF includes women with T-scores <−1.5 by hip DEXA with ≥1 risk factor
- Goals of therapy:
  - Prevention of fracture
  - Stabilization or increase in BMD
  - Maximizing physical function
- Bisphosphonates:
  - Alendronate, risedronate, ibandronate (PO or IV), zoledronic acid (IV q yr). Oral forms are taken on an empty stomach, 1st thing in the morning, with 8 oz. of water, ≥30 minutes before eating or drinking (1 hour for ibandronate). Caution if low creatinine clearance.
  - Patients should remain upright during this interval.

- Side effects: Gastroesophageal irritation; a very rare occurrence of osteonecrosis of the jaw seen primarily in cancer patients receiving IV bisphosphonates and undergoing dental procedures
  - Alendronate:
    ○ 10 mg/d, 70 mg weekly
    ○ Reduces hip and vertebral fractures
  - Risedronate:
    ○ 5 mg/d, 35 mg weekly
    ○ Reduces vertebral and non-vertebral fractures
  - Ibandronate:
    ○ 2.5 mg/d, 150 mg monthly, 3 mg IV q3mos
    ○ Reduces vertebral fractures
  - Zoledronic acid:
    ○ 5 mg IV q yr
- SERMs:
  - Raloxifene:
    ○ 60 mg/d
    ○ Reduces vertebral fractures
    ○ Side effects: Venous thrombosis, leg cramps
- Other osteoporosis treatments:
  - Teriparatide:
    ○ Daily subcutaneous injection 20 μg
    ○ No fracture data
    ○ Recommended for 2 years only and probably needs to be followed by a bisphosphonate to preserve gain in bone density. Expensive
    ○ Side effects: Hypercalcemia, hypotension
  - Calcitonin:
    ○ 1 spray in 1 nostril per day
    ○ Reduces vertebral fractures
    ○ Side effects: Nasal irritation
- Postmenopausal hormone therapy:
  - Approved for prevention only
  - Many products available
  - Side effects: Venous thrombosis, stroke, breast cancer

SURGERY
- Surgical treatment is reserved for the management for osteoporotic fractures.
- Vertebroplasty or kyphoplasty using percutaneous bone cement injections for treatment of persistently painful compression fractures

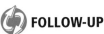 FOLLOW-UP

DISPOSITION
Issues for Referral
Referral to an osteoporosis specialist is recommended for patients who:
- Have a T-score <−3.0
- Do not respond to treatment
- Are intolerant of approved therapies
- Have osteoporosis at a young age
- Have fractures despite having borderline or normal BMD
- Have secondary osteoporosis
- Are candidates for teriparatide or combination therapy
- Would benefit from vertebroplasty or kyphoplasty

PROGNOSIS
- Osteoporosis responds to treatment.
- Treatment reduces fracture rate.
- Little can be done for severe kyphosis.

PATIENT MONITORING
- Monitor calcium, vitamin D, exercise, and medication compliance
- BMD measurement in 2 years to monitor efficacy of treatment

BIBLIOGRAPHY

Gass M, et al. Preventing osteoporosis-related fractures: An overview. *Am J Med.* 2006;119(4A): 3S–11S.

McClung MR. Do current management strategies and guidelines adequately address fracture risk? *Bone.* 2006;38(2 Suppl 2):S13–S17.

National Osteoporosis Foundation. Building Strength Together Program. Available at: http://www.nof.org/patientinfo/support_groups

Primer on the Metabolic Bone Diseases and Disorders of Mineral Metabolism, 6th ed. The American Society for Bone and Mineral Research, 2006.

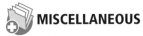 MISCELLANEOUS

CLINICAL PEARLS
- Target treatment to patients at high risk for fracture. Future treatment intervention may be based on the patient's estimated fracture risk for the next 5–10 years, rather than bone density alone.
- Stress fractures are not considered osteoporotic fractures.
- Patient education is essential to ensure compliance with medication.

ABBREVIATIONS
- BMD—Bone mineral density
- DEXA—Dual energy X-ray absorptiometry
- GnRH—Gonadotropin-releasing hormone
- NOF—National Osteoporosis Foundation
- SERMs—Selective estrogen receptor modulators
- TSH—Thyroid-stimulating hormone
- US—Ultrasound
- WHO—World Health Organization

CODES
ICD9-CM
- 256.31 Ovarian failure, premature
- 733.01 Osteoporosis, postmenopausal
- 733.09 Osteoporosis, drug-induced
- V58.65 Long-term (current) use of corticosteroids

 PATIENT TEACHING

- ACOG Patient Education pamphlet available at http://www.acog.org
- National Osteoporosis Foundation (NOF) support groups: http://www.nof.org

PREVENTION
- See "General Measures."
- Eliminate factors potentially harmful to bone.

OVARIAN CYSTS, FUNCTIONAL

Paula J. Adams Hillard, MD

 BASICS

DESCRIPTION
- Functional or physiologic cysts are non-neoplastic ovarian masses that result from an exaggeration of the physiologic cyclic ovarian function in premenopausal women.
- The vast majority of functional cysts resolve within 6–10 weeks or 1–2 cycles. Functional cysts include:
  - Follicular:
    - Follicular cysts result when ovulation does not occur and follicular cyst fluid accumulates.
    - US appearance is that of thin-walled, smooth, unilocular mass.
    - Because a normal follicle may be as large as 25–30 mm, a cystic area should not be defined as a "cyst" unless larger than these dimensions.
    - Functional cysts are typically described as being <5–10 cm in size.
  - Corpus luteum (CL):
    - Typically present in luteal phase of cycle
    - A ruptured CL cyst can cause significant intraperitoneal bleeding.
    - CL cysts can cause acute pain without rupture, presumably due to bleeding into the enclosed cyst cavity (a hemorrhagic CL cyst).
    - US characteristics:
      - Mixed echogenicity (solid and cystic)
      - Typically with septa
      - May be "reticular" or "spongelike" pattern
    - May be confused with ectopic pregnancy
  - Pregnancy luteoma:
    - Rare
    - Hyperandrogenemia with maternal virilization
    - Fetal masculinization of female fetus (50%)
    - Typically asymptomatic and discovered incidentally at time of Cesarean delivery or postpartum tubal sterilization
    - May be unilateral or bilateral
    - May be up to 20 cm in diameter
    - Solid, but can have cystic areas
    - May be difficult to differentiate from hyperreactio luteinalis because of presence of multiple benign theca lutein cysts.

Age-Related Factors
The majority occur in women of reproductive age.

Pediatric Considerations
Benign, functional ovarian cysts can occur in prepubertal girls and even fetuses and, if unilocular and small, can be observed to demonstrate resolution or lack or growth.

Geriatric Considerations
Although the presence of a mass in a postmenopausal woman was once considered evidence of neoplasm, increasing use of US frequently demonstrates transient or nonenlarging cysts:
- An autopsy study demonstrated 54% with benign adnexal cysts and concluded that small (<50 mm) cysts are so common that their presence may be regarded as normal.

EPIDEMIOLOGY
- Ovarian cysts were demonstrated in 7.8% of a random sample of asymptomatic women:
  - 83% resolved, indicating functional cysts
- Pregnancy luteomas:
  - <200 cases described

RISK FACTORS
- Progestin-only contraceptives
- Sterilization associated with increased risk
- Smokers with relative risk of 2.0 in 1 study
- Risk of malignancy increased:
  - In prepubertal or postmenopausal women
  - If the mass is complex or solid
  - Ascites is present
  - Past history of breast, colon, gastric cancer

ASSOCIATED CONDITIONS
- Ovulatory dysfunction
- Pregnancy luteomas reported with hydronephrosis, UTI from ureteral obstruction, maternal and fetal virilization, ascites

 DIAGNOSIS

SIGNS AND SYMPTOMS
History
- Functional cysts may be asymptomatic and an incidental finding.
- Functional cysts can cause acute pain due to:
  - Torsion: A cystic ovary is more likely to torse than a normal ovary.
  - Rupture with intraperitoneal bleeding that can be life-threatening
  - Bleeding into the enclosed space of the cyst
- Functional cysts can cause:
  - Symptoms of pressure
  - Subacute pain over several weeks:
    - Often described as dull, achy
    - Pain with intercourse
    - Pain with a bowel movement
    - Bloating
  - Abnormal bleeding:
    - Shorter or longer menstrual cycle
    - Irregular bleeding
- Timing in relationship to menses should be correlated with US characteristics
  - Unilocular thin-walled cyst in follicular phase
  - Complex or mixed-echogenicity in luteal phase

Physical Exam
- General exam:
  - Hirsutism or virilization
- Abdominal exam: Tenderness or rebound
- Pelvic exam:
  - An adnexal mass may be palpable:
    - Ability to palpate mass depends on cyst size, patient's body weight or habitus

TESTS
Labs
- hCG essential
- CA-125 in premenopause not helpful in distinguishing benign from malignant masses, as many conditions, including endometriosis and functional cysts can cause an elevation
- Pregnancy luteomas can be associated with:
  - Hyperandrogenism:
    - Testosterone
  - CA-125 may be elevated
  - AFP

Imaging
- US imaging is the modality most commonly used when an adnexal mass is suspected.
- CT will demonstrate mass, but is US better for distinguishing cystic vs. solid characteristic.
- MRI not frequently indicated.

DIFFERENTIAL DIAGNOSIS
- Benign ovarian neoplasm:
  - Serous and mucinous cystadenoma
  - Dermoid cyst (mature cystic teratoma)
- Malignant neoplasm:
  - Epithelial ovarian cancer
  - Germ cell tumor
  - Fallopian tube carcinoma
  - Metastatic disease of breast or GI tract
- Pedunculated uterine leiomyoma
- Endometrioma
- PCOS
- Inflammatory lesions, acute or chronic:
  - PID with TOA or tubo-ovarian complex
  - Hydrosalpinx
- Paratubal cyst
- Ectopic pregnancy
- Appendicitis
- Hyperandrogenism in pregnancy:
  - Pregnancy luteomas, solid, bilateral:
    - Hyperreactio luteinalis, usually bilateral, associated with high hCG, including molar pregnancy, multiple pregnancies, erythroblastosis fetalis, and gestational diabetes
  - Hyperthecosis
  - PCOS
  - Leydig cell tumor
  - Other malignant ovarian tumors

TREATMENT

GENERAL MEASURES

- The primary management issue is distinguishing which ovarian masses are likely malignant and require surgical excision.
- If likely benign (young patient, benign characteristics on US, no evidence of ascites, metastasis, or intra-abdominal spread), then functional cysts must be distinguished from benign neoplasms.
- The characteristics of the mass on US and the clinical presentation determine management:
  – If US suggests follicular cyst (unilocular, thin walled, no septations, <10 cm) or CL cyst, observe mass for 1–2 cycles and repeat US.
    ○ Functional cysts will be smaller or resolved.
    ○ Other masses require surgery.
  – If patient presents with acute pain, consider:
    ○ Timing in cycle and US characteristics
    ○ Possibility of torsion (see Adnexal Torsion).
    ○ Possible rupture with hemodynamic instability
- Management of ovarian cysts presenting with acute pain, late in cycle, and suspected to be CL:
  – Avoid surgery and manage expectantly:
    ○ Adequate analgesia, including narcotics
    ○ Reassess within a week; pain should be markedly improved and onset of menses is likely.
    ○ If pain is persistently severe or worsens, reconsider torsion.
    ○ Repeat US in ~6 weeks (not sooner).
    ○ Enlarging or persistent cysts may be neoplastic.
- Ovary-sparing procedures are generally indicated if surgery required and if possible; avoid oophorectomy if likely benign:
  – Ovarian cystectomy if dermoid
- The management of ovarian masses in pregnancy can be difficult or challenging in differentiating between possible malignancy requiring surgery and benign masses that can be managed expectantly.

MEDICATION (DRUGS)

- OCPs do not hasten the resolution of functional ovarian cysts.
- NSAIDs and narcotics if acute pain

SURGERY

- Surgery should be avoided if possible; Expectant management is indicated as functional cysts resolve spontaneously.
- Needle aspiration, via laparoscopy or using interventional radiologic techniques frequently results in recurrence, and is seldom required.
- Laparoscopy indicated if possible torsion:
  – Detorsion alone, with follow-up to assess resolution of mass (likely if functional)
- Surgery indicated for enlarging or persistent mass after 1–2 cycles:
  – Laparoscopic vs. laparotomy
  – If appears benign, cystectomy if possible
  – Approach as if possible malignancy: Pelvic washings, exploration, peritoneal biopsies

FOLLOW-UP

DISPOSITION

Issues for Referral

Referral to gyn oncologist may be indicated if malignancy considered likely on the basis of US characteristics.

PROGNOSIS

- Follicular and CL cysts will resolve without surgical intervention over a period of 1–2 cycles or 6–10 weeks:
  – Failure of resolution suggests neoplastic, rather than functional cyst, and should prompt consideration of surgery.
- Pregnancy luteomas resolve spontaneously after delivery.
- Recurrence risks for symptomatic functional ovarian cysts are unknown, although this is a clinically important question:
  – Consider OCPs to prevent subsequent functional cysts.

PATIENT MONITORING

- Regular exams
- US not routinely required

BIBLIOGRAPHY

Borgfeldt C, et al. Transvaginal sonographic ovarian findings in a random sample of women 25–40 years old. *Ultrasound Obstet Gynecol*. 1999;13(5): 345–350.

Grimes DA, et al. Oral contraceptives for functional ovarian cysts. *Cochrane Database Syst Rev*. 2006;(4):CD006134.

Hallatt JG, et al. Ruptured corpus luteum with hemoperitoneum: A study of 173 surgical cases. *Am J Obstet Gynecol*. 1984;149(1):55–59.

Helmrath MA, et al. Ovarian cysts in the pediatric population. *Semin Pediatr Surg*. 1998;7(1):19–28.

Manganiello PD, et al. Virilization during pregnancy with spontaneous resolution postpartum: A case report and review of the English literature. *Obstetric Gynecol Survey*. 1995;50(5):404–410.

Muram D, et al. Functional ovarian cysts in patients cured of ovarian neoplasms. *Obstet Gynecol*. 1990;75(4):680–683.

Valentin L, et al. Frequency and type of adnexal lesions in autopsy material from postmenopausal women: Ultrasound study with histological correlation. *Ultrasound Obstet Gynecol*. 2003;22(3):284–289.

MISCELLANEOUS

SYNONYM(S)

- Benign cysts
- Simple cysts
- Physiologic cysts

CLINICAL PEARLS

- Functional cysts resolve with time alone; COCs do not lead to a more rapid regression.
- Avoid surgery for functional cysts if possible because sequelae, including adhesions, hampering fertility.
- Do not assume that patient will always have the contralateral ovary.
- Avoid oophorectomy if possible.

ABBREVIATIONS

- AFP—α-Fetoprotein
- CL—Corpus luteum
- COC—Combination oral contraceptive
- hCG—Human chorionic gonadotropin
- OCP—Oral contraceptive pill
- PCOS—Polycystic ovarian syndrome
- PID—Pelvic inflammatory disease
- TOA—Tubo-ovarian abscess
- UTI—Urinary tract infection

CODES

ICD9-CM

- 620.0 Follicular (atretic) cyst
- 620.1 Corpus luteal cyst
- 620.2 Other and unspecified ovarian cyst

PATIENT TEACHING

- Patient anxiety is almost always high, with specter of cancer or infertility.
- Reassure concerning low likelihood of malignancy with typical presentation and US characteristics
- ACOG patient education pamphlet: Ovarian Cysts

PREVENTION

- OCPs, by preventing ovulation, markedly decrease the risks of CL cysts.
- Current low-dose COCs decrease the risk of follicular cysts, but may not prevent their formation as effectively as did previous higher-dose pills.
- COCs can be helpful in girls and women with a previous malignant ovarian neoplasm by preventing the occurrence of functional cysts that lead to concern about recurrent malignancy.

OVARIAN INSUFFICIENCY/PREMATURE OVARIAN FAILURE

Vaishali B. Popat, MD, MPH
Lawrence M. Nelson, MD

 BASICS

DESCRIPTION

- Premature ovarian failure (POF) is defined as the development of hypergonadotropic hypogonadism in women <40 years.
- The diagnosis is made if a patient has at least 3 months of oligomenorrhea and 2 serum FSH levels in the menopausal range, confirmed on 2 separate occasions.
- In reality the term "premature ovarian failure" is problematic because it implies the permanent cessation of ovarian function:
  - In fact, many women with this condition experience intermittent ovarian function that may last for decades after the diagnosis.
  - Pregnancy may even occur in some women years after the diagnosis.
- Our preferred term for this condition is "primary ovarian insufficiency," as 1st introduced by Fuller Albright in 1942.

Age-Related Factors
The age-specific incidence of spontaneous POF is ~1 in 1,000 by age 30, 1 in 250 by age 35, and 1 in 100 by age 40.

Staging
- Spontaneous POF is characterized by intermittent and unpredictable ovarian function.
- Staging is not possible due to the variable natural history of the disorder.

EPIDEMIOLOGY
- POF is the mechanism identified in ~10–30% of cases of primary amenorrhea and 5–20% of cases of secondary amenorrhea.
- ~90% of women with POF present with secondary amenorrhea; 10% present with primary amenorrhea.

RISK FACTORS
- A premutation in the *FMR1* gene
- Autoimmune adrenal insufficiency
- Smoking has been associated with a slightly earlier age of menopause but not with POF.

Genetics
May occur on the basis of the *FMR1* premutation, galactosemia, or X-chromosomal abnormalities that can be detected by karyotype.

PATHOPHYSIOLOGY
- In 90% of cases, the pathogenesis of spontaneous POF remains unknown even after thorough evaluation.
- 2 mechanisms are presumed to playa role in the pathophysiology: Ovarian follicle depletion and ovarian follicle dysfunction.
- X-chromosomal abnormalities are a mechanism of follicle depletion.
- Ovarian follicle dysfunction may be on the basis of autoimmune oophoritis, low follicle cohort number, or rarely due to steroidogenic enzyme defects such as 17–alpha-hydroxylase deficiency.

ASSOCIATED CONDITIONS
- Vasomotor symptoms
- Vaginal dryness and dyspareunia
- Infertility
- Emotional distress
- Osteoporosis
- Hypothyroidism
- Addison disease

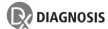 DIAGNOSIS

SIGNS AND SYMPTOMS
History
The onset of menstrual irregularity is the most common initial symptom. In some cases regular menses are never established after menarche, in other cases the onset may be acute, develop postpartum, or make initial appearance after discontinuation of OCPs. In as many as 50% of cases, a long history of oligomenorrhea or polymenorrhea, with or without menopausal symptoms, is present.

Review of Systems
- The most commonly encountered symptoms are a result of hypoestrogenism such as hot flashes, sweats, irritability, vaginal dryness, discomfort and pain during sexual intercourse, decreased libido, and decreased energy.
- Symptoms of hypothyroidism and adrenal insufficiency may also be present.

Physical Exam
- Aside from signs of estrogen deficiency, generally, women with spontaneous POF have unremarkable clinical findings.
- Clinicians should look for the signs of Turner syndrome, hypothyroidism, Addison disease, or other autoimmune diseases.

TESTS
Labs
- A pregnancy test should be the 1st study performed in women of reproductive age who presents with amenorrhea.
- Test to establish diagnosis of premature ovarian failure: FSH, LH, estradiol:
  - As a rule, serum estradiol is low and FSH is high, in the postmenopausal range.
  - Occasionally, women with POF may have spontaneous follicular activity; if hormonal tests are performed during such episodes, results may be normal or only mildly abnormal:
    - In these cases, repeat tests in 1 month.
- To clarify the etiology: Test for adrenal antibodies to detect women who have autoimmune oophoritis. Offer testing for the *FMR1* premutation and karyotype analysis.
- Screen for autoimmune conditions only as clinically indicated by signs and symptoms.

Imaging
- Bone density by DEXA scan should be performed to evaluate bone health, as estrogen deficiency causes high bone turnover.
- Transvaginal/transabdominal US has little practical value in the evaluation.

DIFFERENTIAL DIAGNOSIS
Pregnancy

Infection
A definite cause-and-effect relationship between POF and infection has not been established.

Metabolic/Endocrine
- Secondary (central) ovarian insufficiency/failure due to:
  - Eating disorder, excessive physical exercise, stress, hyperprolactinemia, pituitary and hypothalamic tumors, hypothalamic and pituitary infiltrative and inflammatory processes, pituitary hemorrhage, gonadotropin-producing pituitary adenoma
- Hyperandrogenic conditions such as PCOS, CAH, ovarian or adrenal androgen-producing tumors
- Enzyme deficiencies such as 17-α-hydroxylase deficiency/17-20-desmolase deficiency and galactosemia

Tumor/Malignancy
- Most gonadotropin-producing pituitary adenomas do not secrete gonadotropins. These generally present in postmenopausal aged women who develop symptoms of a CNS mass lesion and have inappropriately low gonadotropins.
- FSH-secreting pituitary adenomas are exceedingly rare in premenopausal women and can be distinguished from POF by the associated elevated serum estradiol levels.
- In rare cases, tumors of the thymus (thymoma) can be associated with POF.

Other/Miscellaneous

Autosomal recessive syndromes associated with ovarian failure, such as Cockayne syndrome, Nijmegen breakage syndrome, Werner syndrome, thymic hypoplasia/aplasia or tumor, pseudohypoparathyroidism

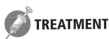 TREATMENT

GENERAL MEASURES

- The diagnosis of spontaneous POF raises issues that must be addressed related to emotional, endocrine, and reproductive health.
- Discuss the test results at a special visit with extra time set aside (not by phone). At the visit, warn the patient that you have information about her ovarian function that she may find emotionally troubling. The diagnosis of POF can be particularly traumatic for young women. Provide information in a manner that permits the patient enough time to process what you are saying.
- Referral for emotional support may be indicated.
- The ovary is not only a reproductive organ but also is a source of important hormones that help maintain strong bones. Adequate replacement of these missing hormones, a healthy lifestyle that includes regular exercise, and a diet rich in calcium are essential.
- Inform the patient that POF is not menopause. Return of ovarian function and even unexpected pregnancies are possible.
- Restoration of fertility: No intervention has been proven to restore ovarian function and fertility in patients with POF:
  – Currently available options include a change of family building plans such as childfree living, adoption, foster care, ovum donation, or embryo adoption.

SPECIAL THERAPY

Complementary and Alternative Therapies

- No proven therapies exist to restore fertility.
- Herbal therapies as a means to maintain bone density and relieve symptoms of estrogen deficiency are unproven in this population.
- Unproven therapies should be administered under a review board-approved research protocol.

MEDICATION (DRUGS)

- HRT should be offered to all women with POF. Cyclical HRT with estrogen and progestin is needed to relieve the symptoms of estrogen deficiency and to maintain bone density.
- First-line approach can use transdermal estradiol (100 μg/d) and 10 mg of oral medroxyprogesterone acetate for 12 days each month.
- Patients should keep a menstrual calendar while on HRT and obtain a pregnancy test if an expected menses fails to occur.

- Contraceptive doses of steroids should be avoided as they deliver a higher dose than is required for replacement.
- Women with this condition who desire to avoid conception should use a barrier method. OCPs have not been demonstrated to be effective in women who have high gonadotropin levels and intermittent ovarian function.

Pediatric Considerations

- ~50% of children who present with primary amenorrhea and failure of pubertal development will be found to have an abnormal karyotype.
- Estradiol replacement should be started at a lower dose and gradually increased over 1–3 years to mimic normal puberty and before adding progestin.
- Discussions regarding the associated infertility should be handled delicately, individualized, and may benefit from the special expertise of an adolescent psychologist.

SURGERY

Ovarian biopsy is not clinically indicated.

 FOLLOW-UP

- Symptoms and signs of thyroid disease and adrenal insufficiency should be sought during the annual follow-up visits.
- TSH levels should be checked every 3–5 years (every year if antiperoxidase antibody test is positive).
- Those with positive adrenal antibodies on initial evaluation should have a baseline and annual ACTH stimulation test to detect the development of asymptomatic adrenal insufficiency.

DISPOSITION

Issues for Referral

- Patients with infertility due to POF usually have a grief response after hearing the diagnosis. They may benefit from a baseline psychological evaluation and appropriate counseling.
- Consultation with an endocrinologist may be indicated in some cases because of concerns of hypothyroidism or adrenal insufficiency.
- Genetic counseling in cases related to the *FMR1* premutation or a family history of fragile-X syndrome.

PROGNOSIS

- At present, no studies clarify the long-term prognosis.
- These women are generally young and otherwise healthy when they present to clinicians.
- They have higher incidence of hypothyroidism, adrenal insufficiency, and osteoporosis.

PATIENT MONITORING

Patients with ovarian failure should be seen annually to monitor their HRT and to detect the development of other associated conditions.

BIBLIOGRAPHY

Nelson LM, et al. Development of luteinized Graafian follicles in patients with karyotypically normal spontaneous premature ovarian failure. *J Clin Endocrinol Metab*. 1994;79(5):1470–1475.

Nelson LM, et al. An update: spontaneous premature ovarian failure is not an early menopause. *Fertil Steril*. 2005;83(5):1327–1332.

Popat V, et al. Spontaneous primary ovarian insufficiency and premature ovarian failure. in emedicine updated June 1, 2007. Accessed July 15, 2007 at http://www.emedicine.com/med/topic1700.htm

 MISCELLANEOUS

SYNONYM(S)

- Primary ovarian insufficiency
- Primary ovarian failure
- Premature menopause

CLINICAL PEARLS

- The diagnosis of POF can be particularly traumatic for young women.
- All women with POF should be offered estradiol/progestin replacement.
- This work supported by the Intramural Research Program of the National Institutes of Child Health and Human Development, NIH

ABBREVIATIONS

- ACTH—Adrenocorticotropic hormone
- CAH—Congenital adrenal hyperplasia
- DEXA—Dual-energy x-ray absorptiometry
- FSH—Follicle stimulating hormone
- HRT—Hormone replacement therapy
- LH—Luteinizing hormone
- OCP—Oral contraceptive pill
- PCOS—Polycystic ovary syndrome
- POF—Premature ovarian failure
- TSH—Thyroid-stimulating hormone

CODES

ICD9-CM

- 156.3 Premature ovarian failure
- 259.9 Estrogen deficiency
- 156.39 Other ovarian failure

 PATIENT TEACHING

- POF is not menopause. Patients have 5–10% chance of spontaneous pregnancy even many years after the diagnosis.
- Women with POF should be educated on the nature of their disorder. The mere understanding of the disorder helps patients cope better.
- Information for women with POF available at: http://pof.nichd.nih.gov/

PREVENTION

No effective strategies for prevention have been identified.

OVARIAN TUMORS, BENIGN

Paula J. Adams Hillard, MD

 BASICS

DESCRIPTION
Benign ovarian tumors are common in women of reproductive age. Most ovarian tumors (80–85%) are benign. Ovarian masses may be:

- Functional cysts, benign, usually asymptomatic, and usually do not require surgery:
  - Follicular cyst
  - Corpus luteum cyst
- Endometriomas "chocolate cysts" may develop in women with endometriosis (see "Endometriosis" chapter).
- Benign cystic teratomas "dermoid cysts" are benign germ cell tumors:
  - Most common ovarian tumor in adolescents
  - ~60% of ovarian neoplasms in women <40
- Epithelial tumors:
  - Serous tumors:
    - Generally benign
    - 5–10% are low malignant potential (LMP) or borderline tumors
    - 20–25% are malignant
    - Often multilocular, +/−papillary components
  - Mucinous tumors:
    - Can grown to large dimensions
    - Multiloculated, bilateral ~10%
    - 5–10% are malignant
  - Other benign tumors: Endometrioid, clear cell, Brenner, mixed epithelial, fibromas

Age-Related Factors
The majority of benign ovarian tumors occur in women of reproductive age.

Pediatric Considerations
- Unilocular small ovarian cysts in the pediatric age group are most often benign functional cysts.
- Solid masses in this age group are likely to be malignant; germ cell tumors are the most common.
- Benign ovarian masses other than functional cysts are uncommon in this age group.

Geriatric Considerations
- With the increasing use of pelvic US, small ovarian cysts are discovered incidentally in postmenopausal women.
- If asymptomatic, small (<5 cm), unilocular, thin-walled with normal CA-125, the risk of malignancy is low, and these masses can be followed conservatively without surgery.
- A mass that does not meet these criteria (is complex or enlarges while under observation) requires surgical excision to rule out ovarian cancer.

Staging
Benign ovarian tumors do not have a staging system.

EPIDEMIOLOGY
- True incidence not known
- ~44,000 female inpatients with discharge diagnosis of benign ovarian neoplasm
- 2/3 of benign ovarian tumors occur in women 20–44.
- The chance if primary ovarian malignancy in a patient <45 years old is <1 in 15

RISK FACTORS
Possible risk factors for benign serous and mucinous epithelial ovarian tumors have been described, and include:

- A 3-fold increase in risk of mucinous tumors in smokers.
- Recent obesity and obesity at age 20 associated with increased risk of benign serous ovarian tumors
- Ever having had a term pregnancy was *inversely* associated with both tumor types.

Genetics
Familial breast and ovarian cancers should be assessed by screening history (see Familial Breast and Ovarian Cancer Syndromes).

PATHOPHYSIOLOGY
- Epithelial ovarian tumors comprise ~80% of ovarian tumors, and are classified as:
  - Benign
  - Malignant
  - Tumors of LMP (borderline malignancy)
- The diagnosis is based on pathologic exam after surgical excision.
  - Intraoperatively, a benign tumor typically *lacks* characteristics of malignancy:
    - Ascites
    - Excrescences on surface of ovary
    - Peritoneal tumor studding
  - A frozen section exam helps to determine the extent of the surgical procedure (see Laparotomy for Ovarian Malignancy).
- The natural history of the development of ovarian epithelial cancers is not well established, although it has been suggested that a benign ovarian tumor may be associated with an increased risk of ovarian cancer later in life.

ASSOCIATED CONDITIONS
Ovarian torsion (see Adnexal Torsion) can present with acute onset of pain, frequently accompanied by nausea and vomiting:

- It is uncommon for a normal ovary to torse.
- Benign ovarian masses are more likely to torse than malignancies.

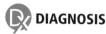 **DIAGNOSIS**

SIGNS AND SYMPTOMS
- A thorough history and exam are important, although most often imaging is required to suggest a diagnosis, which is then ultimately confirmed with histologic exam after surgical excision if indicated.
- The pooled sensitivity and specificity (respectively) for diagnostic assessment has been reviewed, including symptomatic and asymptomatic pre- and postmenopausal women:
  - Bimanual exam (45% and 90%)
  - US morphology (86–91% and 68–83%)
  - MRI (91% and 87%)
  - CT (90% and 75%)
  - PET scan (67% and 79%)
  - CA-125 (78% and 78%)

History
- Ovarian tumors are often asymptomatic, but symptoms may include:
  - Chronic aching pelvic or lower abdominal pain
  - Dyspareunia
  - Menstrual irregularities
- Nonspecific GI complaints:
  - Bloating
  - Nausea and vomiting
  - Indigestion
  - Constipation
- Early satiety
- Urinary urgency or frequency
- Increased abdominal girth
- Nonspecific symptoms:
  - Fatigue
  - Weight loss

Review of Systems
- Personal history of breast cancer
- Particular attention to GI/GU symptoms

Physical Exam
- Breast exam
- Abdomen:
  - Ascites
  - Palpable mass
  - Hepatomegaly
- Pelvic exam, noting:
  - Presence of pelvic tenderness
  - Pelvic mass:
    - Size >8–10 cm suggests neoplasm
    - Bilaterality
    - Mobile vs. fixed
    - Nodularity of rectovaginal septum

TESTS
Lab
- β-hCG should be obtained on all reproductive-age women to exclude pregnancy or pregnancy-related complications.

- CBC when PID is considered
- Tumor markers can suggest the possibility of malignancy, but are most helpful for postoperative surveillance for recurrence or response to therapy:
  – CA-125 helpful in postmenopausal women; high in epithelial ovarian malignancy
  – CA-125 in premenopausal women not useful as diagnostic test, as it can be elevated in a number of benign conditions, including:
    ○ Endometriosis
    ○ Leiomyomata
    ○ PID
    ○ Renal and liver disease
  – Other tumor markers such as AFP and hCG may be useful in following malignant germ cell tumors.

Imaging
- US exam is the imaging modality most often used to evaluate pelvic masses. US morphology may help to assess the probability of benign vs. malignant ovarian disease.
- Characteristics suggesting a benign mass:
  – Anechoic fluid-filled cyst:
    ○ <2–3 cm in reproductive age woman likely represent normal follicles
  – Homogeneous low- or medium echogenicity in thick-walled cyst suggests endometrioma
  – "Fishnet" or reticular internal echoes suggests hemorrhagic cyst
  – Hyperechoic nodule with shadowing suggest a dermoid/teratoma
  – Fat-fluid level with more echogenic fluid component being superior suggests dermoid
- PCOS is characterize by the presence of ≥12 follicles in each ovary (2–9 mm in diameter) or increased ovarian volume (>10 mL)
- Characteristics suggesting malignant mass:
  – Absence of above characteristics
  – Solid component, especially if nodular or papillary
  – Thick septations
  – Color Doppler flow in the solid component
  – Presence of ascites
  – Peritoneal masses, lymphadenopathy, matted bowel

DIFFERENTIAL DIAGNOSIS
A number of conditions can be confused on exam or US with an ovarian mass

Infection
TOA or complex

Metabolic/Endocrine
PCOS

Tumor/Malignancy
- Ovarian malignancy
- Fallopian tube carcinoma
- Metastatic carcinoma
- Benign ovarian functional cysts
- Ovarian tumors of low malignant potential

Other/Miscellaneous
Gynecologic conditions:
- Hydrosalpinx
- Pedunculated uterine fibroid
- Paraovarian cyst
- Peritoneal cyst

TREATMENT
GENERAL MEASURES
- Although the possibility of an ovarian malignancy must always be kept in mind, and is typically a concern of a woman who is found to have an ovarian mass, a stepwise approach is appropriate, as the majority of ovarian masses in women of reproductive age are benign.
- Observation for a period of 6–8 weeks may be appropriate if the characteristics of the mass on US and exam are benign.
- Decisions for surgical management based on:
  – Age
  – US characteristics
  – Presence of pain, and thus likelihood of rupture or torsion
  – Persistence or growth over time

MEDICATION (DRUGS)
Combination hormonal contraceptives, by inhibiting ovulation, minimize the development of functional, but not neoplastic ovarian masses, but do not hasten the resolution of functional cysts.

SURGERY
- In the absence of concerns of torsion, surgery should generally be avoided for masses that exhibit the US characteristics of a functional cyst (follicular or corpus luteum).
- Ovarian masses that do not resolve or that enlarge over time warrant surgical assessment.
- Based on the likelihood of malignancy, the planned surgical approach may be via laparoscopy or laparotomy:
  – Combinations of laparoscopy and minilaparotomy have been described, allowing a laparoscopic assessment for characteristics of malignancy (surface excrescences, peritoneal studding).
  – Minilaparotomy techniques involving cyst decompression have also been described.
- For benign cystic teratomas, ovarian cystectomy can almost always be accomplished, with ovarian preservation.
  – Controversy exists over the benefits of a laparoscopic approach balanced with the risks of spillage of cyst contents, with subsequent granulomatous (chemical) peritonitis.
- For solid or mixed masses, the surgical approach should include:
  – Obtaining pelvic washings
  – Methodical survey of the abdomen (diaphragm, bowel, liver, omentum, appendix), pelvis (ovaries, tubes, uterus, cul de sac), and peritoneal surfaces
  – Removal of ovarian mass and fallopian tube
  – Frozen section for pathologic exam, with subsequent management including lymph node sampling, biopsies, and careful assessment of the abdomen and pelvis if malignant
  – Assessment of contralateral ovary
- Frozen section to distinguish benign, borderline, malignant tumors
- Appropriate staging if malignant, with consultation as required from a gynecologic oncologist or general surgeon as available

FOLLOW-UP
DISPOSITION
Issues for Referral
Careful surgical staging and optimal debulking impact survival for ovarian malignancies. Intraoperative consultation from a gyn or surgical oncologist is appropriate for borderline or malignant ovarian tumors.

PROGNOSIS
If the final pathologic exam is benign, prognosis is excellent.

PATIENT MONITORING
- Following the excision of an ovarian neoplasm, regular pelvic exams will provide appropriate monitoring.
- Routine pelvic US exams are not required.

BIBLIOGRAPHY
Jordan SJ, et al. Risk factors for benign serous and mucinous epithelial ovarian tumors. *Obstet Gynecol.* 2007;109(3):647–654.

Myers ER, et al. Management of Adnexal Mass. Evidence Report/Technology Assessment No.130 (Prepared by the Duke Evidence-based Practice Center under Contract No. 290-0–02-2–0025.) AHRQ Publication No. 06-6–E004. Rockville, MD: Agency for Healthcare Research and Quality; February 2006.

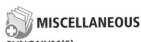
MISCELLANEOUS
SYNONYM(S)
- Ovarian cyst, tumor, mass
- Adnexal mass

CLINICAL PEARLS
OCPs suppress the development of functional cysts, and may be appropriate treatment after the management of ovarian masses to avoid unnecessary confusion with subsequent follicular and corpus luteal cysts.

ABBREVIATIONS
- AFP—α-Fetoprotein
- COC—Combined oral contraceptive
- hCG—Human chorionic gonadotropin
- LMP—Low malignant potential
- OCP—Oral contraceptive pill
- PID—Pelvic inflammatory disease
- TOA—Tubo-ovarian abscess

CODES
ICD9-CM
220 Benign neoplasm of ovary

PATIENT TEACHING

ACOG Patient Education—Ovarian Cysts

PREVENTION
- Some studies suggest a decreased risk of benign ovarian tumors in users of COCs.
- The recently described association between obesity or smoking and an increased risk of benign epithelial serous or mucinous tumors suggests the potential for prevention.

OVARIAN TUMORS, BORDERLINE MALIGNANCIES

Robert E. Bristow, MD
Edward J. Tanner, III, MD

 BASICS

DESCRIPTION

- Neoplasms of the ovary characterized by a less aggressive course than carcinoma but with the potential to metastasize and recur
- Generally occur in younger women and at an earlier stage than ovarian carcinoma
- Also know as tumors of low malignant potential (LMP)

Age-Related Factors

- Peak incidence ~10–20 years earlier than ovarian cancer
- Fertility preservation may impact treatment in early-stage disease.

Staging

- Requires surgical exploration of the abdomen to determine extent of disease
- Surgical staging based on International Federation of Gynecologic Oncologists (FIGO) recommendations and requiring at a minimum:
  - Excision of the involved ovary (or cystectomy if bilateral ovarian involvement and fertility preservation desired)
  - Omentectomy
  - Pelvic and para-aortic lymph node dissection
  - Pelvic washings or ascites for cytology
  - Multiple biopsies of peritoneal surfaces
  - If evidence of extraovarian disease, removal of all involved tumor should also be performed.
- FIGO stages of ovarian carcinoma and borderline tumors:
  - Stage 1: Tumor limited to the ovaries (70%):
    - Stage 1A: Growth limited to one ovary; no surface tumor involvement, capsule rupture, or malignant ascites
    - Stage 1B: Growth limited to both ovaries; no surface tumor involvement, capsule rupture, or malignant ascites
    - Stage 1C: Tumor either stage 1A or 1B but with surface tumor involvement, capsule rupture, or malignant ascites
  - Stage 2: Pelvic extension of tumor (10%):
    - Stage 2A: Extension/metastasis to uterus or fallopian tubes
    - Stage 2B: Extension to other pelvic tissues
    - Stage 2C: Tumor either stage 2A or 2B but with surface tumor involvement, capsule rupture, or malignant ascites
  - Stage 3: Tumor implants in abdominal cavity or inguinal/retroperitoneal lymph nodes (20%):
    - Stage 3A: Microscopic peritoneal surface implants
    - Stage 3B: Visible peritoneal surface implants, none >2 cm in diameter
    - Stage 3C: Visible peritoneal implants >2 cm in diameter or positive retroperitoneal/inguinal lymph nodes
  - Stage 4: Distant metastasis including malignant pleural effusions, parenchymal liver or brain metastasis (<1%)

EPIDEMIOLOGY

- Peak incidence in mid-40s
- Most cases occur from 30s–50s
- Represent 15% of all epithelial ovarian malignancies (~3000 cases per year)

RISK FACTORS

- Nulliparity (OR 0.79)
- Unlike ovarian carcinoma, the following factors do not reduce risk:
  - OCPs
  - Bilateral tubal ligation
  - Nonsmoker
- Unlike ovarian cancer, the following factors do not increase risk:
  - BRCA-1 and -2 germline mutations
  - Family history of ovarian cancer

Genetics

No familial association has been identified

PATHOPHYSIOLOGY

- WHO criteria for diagnosis:
  - Epithelial proliferation with papillary formation and pseudostratification
  - Nuclear atypia and increased mitotic activity
  - Absence of true stromal proliferation
- Presence of stromal invasion in metastatic implants increases the risk of progression or recurrence
- Histologic subtypes:
  - Serous (65%)
  - Mucinous (30%)
  - Endometrioid
  - Clear cell
  - Brenner cell
  - Mixed
- Pattern of spread:
  - Exfoliation and implantation of cells within peritoneal cavity
  - Lymphatic spread to pelvic and para-aortic lymph nodes
  - Hematogenous spread to distant organs (liver and spleen parenchyma, lung, brain)

DIAGNOSIS

SIGNS AND SYMPTOMS

History

Gradual onset of often vague signs and symptoms

Review of Systems

- GI: Abdominal pain, constipation, bloating, distension, nausea, decreased appetite, weight changes
- GU: Dysuria
- Gyn: Irregular menses

Physical Exam

- Solid or fixed mass on pelvic exam
- Ascites or palpable mass on abdominal exam
- Palpable inguinal adenopathy (rare)

TESTS

Labs

- CA-125 should not be used for screening.
- CA-125 elevated in many benign conditions especially in premenopausal women (i.e., endometriosis, PID, liver disease)
- CA-125 often normal in early-stage disease

Imaging

- To differentiate between benign and malignant gynecologic conditions:
  - Pelvic US
  - CT
- Findings suspicious of ovarian malignancies include:
  - Persistence of pelvic mass on serial imaging
  - Size >8 cm
  - Bilateral ovarian involvement
  - Multiple septations
  - Solid components
  - Increased vascularity
  - Abdominal implants (carcinomatosis)
  - Retroperitoneal lymphadenopathy

DIFFERENTIAL DIAGNOSIS

Infection

TOA may mimic pelvic malignancy

Tumor/Malignancy

- Benign gynecologic masses:
  - Benign ovarian neoplasms
  - Endometriosis/Endometriomas
  - Pedunculated uterine fibroids
- Malignant gynecologic neoplasms:
  - Epithelial ovarian carcinoma
  - Nonepithelial ovarian carcinoma
  - Fallopian tube carcinoma
- Metastatic nongynecologic malignancies:
  - Ovarian metastasis of breast, colon, or other GI sources (Krukenberg tumors)

Other/Miscellaneous

Pelvic kidney may mimic a gynecologic malignancy

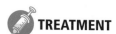 **TREATMENT**

GENERAL MEASURES

- Surgical excision of all visible disease
- Additional treatment (i.e., chemotherapy or radiation) is unlikely to be of benefit even in advanced disease.

MEDICATION (DRUGS)

Generally nonresponsive to chemotherapy due to slow growth rate

SURGERY

- Surgery is both diagnostic and primary treatment.
- If a borderline tumor is diagnosed on frozen section, intraoperative consultation by a gynecologic oncologist is recommended to ensure proper staging and complete removal of disease
- Survival greatly improved if all visible disease removed
- If fertility is not desired, surgical treatment should include hysterectomy, bilateral salpingo-oophorectomy, omentectomy, pelvic/para-aortic lymphadenectomy, and excision of all visible disease
- If fertility is desired and disease appears to be confined to one ovary, conservative surgery including unilateral oophorectomy, omentectomy, and multiple peritoneal biopsies may be performed:
  - Although risk of recurrence is higher with conservative management, long-term survival appears to be equivalent with close surveillance.
  - Removal of contralateral ovary is generally recommended upon completion of childbearing but is of unclear benefit.
- Appendectomy should be performed if mucinous histology
- Recurrences are generally treated with repeat surgical excision.

Pregnancy Considerations

- Surgery should be considered in the 2nd trimester of pregnancy if findings on imaging are highly suspicious for malignancy; complete staging may be performed at this time.
- If surgery deferred, educate patient regarding symptoms of ovarian torsion (surgical emergency!).

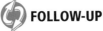 **FOLLOW-UP**

DISPOSITION

Issues for Referral

Patients are often diagnosed with borderline tumors following oophorectomy for suspected benign conditions:

- Complete staging procedure often not performed
- If pathology reveals disease confined to the ovary, no further surgery is recommended.
- Consultation by gynecologic oncologist for close monitoring and any further treatment is recommended.

PROGNOSIS

- Recurrences often late (10–15 years later)
- Gradual decrease in overall survival for advanced stage or high-risk disease
- Survival for stage 1 or 2 disease:
  - 5 years: 98–99%
  - 20 years: 96–99%
- Survival for stage 3:
  - 5 years: 90%
  - 20 -years: 45%
- Invasive implants, especially in the setting of micropapillary architecture, have negative impact on survival.
- A small percentage of serous borderline tumors will progress to low-grade serous carcinoma (~6%); prognosis is poor.
- Fertility following conservative management of early-stage tumors is excellent.

PATIENT MONITORING

- No consensus regarding interval of monitoring; generally:
  - Physical exam every 3 months for 2 years, then every 6–12 months thereafter
  - Imaging (CT scan) every 6 months for 2–3 years, then annually thereafter
  - CA-125 every 3 months for 2 years then every 6 months for 3 years if elevated at diagnosis

BIBLIOGRAPHY

Cadron I, et al. The management of borderline tumours of the ovary. *Curr Opin Oncol*. 2006;18:488–493.

Giuntoli RL, et al. Evaluation and management of adnexal masses in pregnancy. *Clin Obstet Gynecol*. 2006;49(3):492–505.

Longacre TA, et al. Ovarian serous tumors of low malignant potential (borderline tumors). *Am J Surg Pathol*. 2005;29(6):707–723.

Seracchioli R, et al. Fertility and tumor recurrence rate after conservative laparoscopic management of young women with early-stage borderline ovarian tumors. *Fertil Steril*. 2001;76(5):999–1004.

Tinelli R, et al. Conservative surgery for borderline ovarian tumors: A review. *Gynecol Oncol*. 2006;100:185–191.

 MISCELLANEOUS

CLINICAL PEARLS

- Conservative surgery is safe in early-stage disease if fertility-preservation is desired.
- Recurrences often occur late; therefore, patients should be counseled regarding the need for long-term follow-up.

ABBREVIATIONS

- LMP—Low malignant potential
- OCP—Oral contraceptive pill
- PID—Pelvic inflammatory disease
- TOA—Tubo-ovarian abscess
- WHO—World Health Organization

CODES

ICD9-CM

236.2 Neoplasm of uncertain behavior of ovary

 PATIENT TEACHING

Counsel regarding the risk of late recurrence and need for long-term follow-up

OVARIAN TUMORS, GERM CELL

Vernon T. Cannon, MD, PhD
Jean A. Hurteau, MD

 BASICS

DESCRIPTION
- Malignant germ-cell tumors are derived from the primordial germ cells of the ovary:
  - <5–7% of ovarian cancers
  - Mainly occur in young women and adolescent girls
  - The most common germ-cell tumor is the benign mature cystic teratoma ("dermoid" tumor)

Age-Related Factors
Median age 16–20 with a range of 6–46 years

Staging
- FIGO (International Federation of Gynecology and Obstetrics) staging used for *malignant* ovarian germ-cell tumors.
- Stage I: Tumor limited to the ovary:
  - IA: Tumor limited to 1 ovary, no ascites, intact capsule
  - IB: Tumor limited to both ovaries, no ascites, intact capsule
  - IC: Tumor either stage IA or IB, but with ascites present containing malignant cells or with ovarian capsule involvement or rupture or with positive peritoneal washings
- Stage II: Tumor involving 1 or both ovaries with extension to the pelvis:
  - IIA: Extension to the uterus or tubes
  - IIB: Involvement of both ovaries with extension to other pelvic tissues.
  - IIC: Tumor either stage IIA or IIB, but with ascites present containing malignant cells or with ovarian capsule involvement or rupture or with positive peritoneal washings
- Stage III: Tumor involving 1 or both ovaries with tumor implants outside the pelvis or with positive retroperitoneal or inguinal nodes. Superficial liver metastases qualify as stage III:
  - IIIA: Tumor limited to the pelvis with negative nodes but with microscopic seeding of the abdominal peritoneal surface
  - IIIB: Negative nodes, tumor implants in the abdominal cavity ≤2 cm
  - IIIC: Positive nodes or tumor implants in the abdominal cavity >2 cm
- Stage IV: Distant metastases present

EPIDEMIOLOGY
- Germ-cell tumors account for up to 60% of ovarian tumors occurring <20 years of age.
- 1/3 of these are malignant.

Pregnancy Considerations
Account for 25% of all malignant tumors in pregnancy:
- Stage IA, dysgerminomas can be removed and the pregnancy continued.
- In patients with advanced dysgerminomas, continuation of the pregnancy depends on gestational age.
- Chemotherapy can be used to treat dysgerminomas in the 2nd and 3rd trimesters.

RISK FACTORS
Young female

Genetics
Karyotypic abnormalities are common, and an association between dysgerminoma and dysgenic gonads is well recognized.

PATHOPHYSIOLOGY
- WHO Classification of ovarian germ-cell tumors.
- Dysgerminoma:
  - Variant: With syncytiotrophoblast cells
- Yolk sac tumor (endodermal sinus tumor):
  - Variant: Polyvesicular vitelline tumor:
    ○ Hepatopoid
    ○ Glandular: Variant, endometrioid
- Embryonal carcinoma
- Polyembryoma
- Choriocarcinoma
- Teratomas:
  - Immature
  - Mature:
    ○ Solid
    ○ Cystic (dermoid cyst) with and without secondary tumor formation
    ○ Fetiform (homunculus)
  - Monodermal and highly specialized:
    ○ Struma ovarii: With or without thyroid tumor
    ○ Carcinoid (insular, trabecular)
    ○ Strumal carcinoid
    ○ Mucinous carcinoid
    ○ Neuroectodermal tumors
    ○ Sebaceous tumors
    ○ Others
- Mixed (specify types)

Dermoid Cyst (Mature Cystic Teratomas)
- Occur bilaterally in 12% of cases
- Most contain sebaceous material and hair but can contain elements of all 3 germ-cell layers (endoderm, mesoderm, and ectoderm).
- In older patients (>40) malignant transformation of dermoids should be ruled out.
- Squamous carcinoma is found in 1% of dermoid cysts.

Dysgerminoma
- Comprise ~50% of ovarian germ-cell tumors
- Bilateral in 10% of cases
- Dysgerminomas may be present in 10% of normal-appearing contralateral ovaries.
- Predilection for lymphatic spread
- Elevated serum LDH
- 5% contain multinucleated syncytiotrophoblastic giant cells that can produce hCG
- *C-kit* expression may be targeted for treatment with inhibitors of *c-kit*, such a Gleevec.

Yolk-Sac Tumors (Endodermal Sinus Tumors)
- Bilateral in <5% of cases
- Account for ~25% of ovarian germ-cell tumors
- More friable on examination than dysgerminomas
- Distinct reticular pattern with Schiller-Duval bodies on microscopic examination
- Commonly contains periodic acid-Schiff (PAS)-positive hyaline bodies
- Cells stain positive for AFP and secrete AFP in serum.

Immature Teratomas
- ~20% of ovarian germ-cell tumors
- Bilateral in <5% of cases but contralateral ovary may contain a dermoid cyst in 10% of cases
- Contains all 3 primordial germ cell layers.
- Graded from 1–3 based on content of primitive neuroectodermal tissue
- May be associated with mature glial peritoneal implants (gliomatosis peritonei)
- May experience *growing teratoma syndrome* during chemotherapy due to glial implants

Embryonal Carcinomas and Choriocarcinomas
- May produce hCG
- May have irregular uterine bleeding

ASSOCIATED CONDITIONS
- Hyperthyroidism
- Carcinoid syndrome
- Ovarian torsion
- Isosexual precocity related to hCG production
- Primary amenorrhea, virilization, developmental abnormalities of the genitalia ± pelvic mass

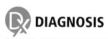 **DIAGNOSIS**

SIGNS AND SYMPTOMS
History
- Menstrual history
- Symptoms of pelvic mass

Review of Systems
- Abdominal pain/acute abdomen usually caused by:

  - Rupture
  - Hemorrhage
  - Torsion
- Abdominal distention
- Fever
- Vaginal bleeding
- Symptoms of hyperthyroidism (Struma ovarii)
- Symptoms of carcinoid syndrome

Physical Exam
- Abdominal/Pelvic mass
- Acute abdomen
- Isosexual precocity due to hCG secretion
- Primary amenorrhea, virilization, developmental abnormalities of the genitalia ± pelvic mass

TESTS
Lab
- hCG
- AFP
- LDH
- CA-125

Imaging
- CXR (PA and lateral)
- CT of abdomen and pelvis
- Pelvic US:
  – Characteristics of mature cystic teratoma include:

    ○ Hyperechoic, may have distal acoustic shadowing
    ○ Fat-fluid levels
    ○ Calcification (teeth, bone)

DIFFERENTIAL DIAGNOSIS
- Appendicitis
- Ectopic pregnancy
- Ovarian torsion

Tumor/Malignancy
- Other benign or malignant ovarian tumors:
  – Epithelial ovarian tumors
  – Adrenal tumor causing virilization
- Other pelvic mass:
  – Uterine leiomyoma

 TREATMENT

GENERAL MEASURES
- Ovarian germ-cell tumors mainly affect young women and adolescent girls, and consideration is given to preserving fertility.
- Radiation therapy is no longer commonly used as first-line therapy due to fertility issues.
- ~70% of all malignant germ-cell tumors are stage I at presentation.

MEDICATION (DRUGS)
- Bleomycin, etoposide (VP16), cisplatin (BEP) is main chemotherapy regimen for treatment of ovarian germ-cell tumors:
  – BEP 3 cycles for completely resected tumors
  – BEP 4 cycles for incompletely resected tumors
- Other regimens: Vincristine, actinomycin D, cyclophosphamide (VAC)

SURGERY
Benign Cystic Teratoma
Ovarian cystectomy:
- Risk of chemical peritonitis if spill
- Laparoscopy vs. laparotomy

Dysgerminoma
- Unilateral oophorectomy with complete staging is appropriate if fertility desired:
  – Stage IA requires no further treatment.
  – All other stages require BEP.
  – Tumor is extremely sensitive to BEP.

- Total abdominal hysterectomy with bilateral salpingo-oophorectomy:
  – If fertility is not necessary
- Bilateral salpingo-oophorectomy:
  – If karyotype has Y chromosome then uterus can be left in situ for fertility procedures.
- Staging operation:
  – As for epithelial ovarian tumors however, unilateral oophorectomy acceptable if fertility is desired
- Cytoreductive surgery:
  – Recommended; benefit not clearly defined

Nondysgerminomatous Tumors
- Staging and cytoreductive surgery as above
- Immature teratoma:
  – Stage IA Grade I require no adjuvant treatment.
- Yolk sac tumor:
  – Potentially aggressive, and any stage requires adjuvant chemotherapy.
- All other nondysgerminomatous tumors:
  – Any stage requires adjuvant chemotherapy

 FOLLOW-UP

DISPOSITION
Issues for Referral
Complex pelvic mass in patient of reproductive age with elevated hCG, AFP, LDH, or CA125

PROGNOSIS
- Dysgerminoma:
  – Stage IA dysgerminomas completely staged: No adjuvant treatment: 10-year survival approaches 100%
  – 15% recur: Can be retreated successfully with a high likelihood of cure
- Immature teratoma:
  – Most important indicator of survival is the grade of the tumor.
  – 5-year survival rates:
    ○ Grade 1: 82%
    ○ Grade 2: 62%
    ○ Grade 3: 30%
- Yolk sac tumor:
  – Poor prognosis without adjuvant chemotherapy
  – 5–20% survival with surgery alone
  – Therefore, all stages require adjuvant chemotherapy

PATIENT MONITORING
- Can recur rapidly; therefore, follow-up:
  – 4–6 weeks for 1st 2 years
  – 8–12 weeks for year 3
  – 3–4 months for year 4–5
- LDH, hCG, AFP, CA125
- CT scan if symptoms
- US contralateral ovary if conserved

BIBLIOGRAPHY

Hurteau JA, et al. Ovarian germ cell tumors. In: Sutton GP, et al., eds. *Ovarian Cancer,* 2nd ed. New York: McGraw-Hill; 2001:371–382.

Lu KH, et al. Update on the management of ovarian germ cell tumor. *J Reprod Med.* 2005;50(6): 417–425.

 MISCELLANEOUS

SYNONYM(S)
- Benign cystic teratoma
- Dermoid cyst

CLINICAL PEARLS
- Completely stage IA dysgerminoma and stage I, grade I, immature teratoma require no adjuvant treatment.
- All other malignant germ-cell tumors require adjuvant chemotherapy.
  – BEP is recommended:
    ○ 3 cycles for completely resected
    ○ 4 cycles for incompletely resected

ABBREVIATIONS
- AFP—α-Fetoprotein
- BEP—Bleomycin, etoposide (VP16), cisplatin
- FIGO—International Federation of Gynecology and Obstetrics
- hCG—Human chorionic gonadotropin
- LDH—Lactate dehydrogenase
- VAC—Vincristine, actinomycin D, cyclophosphamide
- WHO—World Health Organization

CODES
ICD9-CM
- 183 Malignant neoplasm of ovary
- 220 Benign neoplasm of the ovary

 PATIENT TEACHING

- National Cancer Institute patient information on ovarian germ-cell tumors at http://www.cancer.gov/cancertopics/pdq/treatment/ovarian-germ-cell/patient
- ACOG Patient Education Pamphlets: Ovarian Cancer at http://www.acog.org/publications/patient_education/bp096.cfm
- ACOG Patient Education Pamphlets: Ovarian Cysts at http://www.acog.org/publications/patient_education/bp075.cfm

OVARIAN TUMORS, MALIGNANT EPITHELIAL

Nita Karnik Lee, MD, MPH
Jonathan S. Berek, MD

 BASICS

DESCRIPTION
- Epithelial ovarian cancer (EOC) is the leading cause of death among all gynecologic cancers and is the 4th leading cause of all cancer deaths in women in the US.
- 90% of all ovarian cancers are of epithelial origin from the surface (coelomic) epithelium.

Age-Related Factors
- Epithelial ovarian cancer primarily affects postmenopausal women.
- The mean age at diagnosis is 60–63.

Staging
- All malignant ovarian tumors should be surgically staged when feasible to accurately assess prognosis and guide appropriate treatment.
- Federation of Gynecologic Oncologists (FIGO) stages are listed below:
  - Stage I: Limited to ovaries:
    - Ia: Limited to 1 ovary; negative cytology; no external tumor, capsule intact
    - Ib: Limited to both ovaries; negative cytology; no external tumor, capsule intact
    - Ic: Ia or Ib with ruptured capsule, tumor on ovarian surface, malignant ascites or cytology
  - Stage II: Involving ovaries with pelvic extension:
    - IIa: Involvement of uterus or fallopian tubes
    - IIb: Extension to other pelvic tissues
    - IIc: IIa or IIb with ruptured capsule, tumor on ovarian surface, malignant ascites or cytology
  - Stage III: Involves ovaries with peritoneal implants outside the pelvis and/or retroperitoneal or inguinal lymph nodes:
    - IIIa: Tumor confined grossly to pelvis, negative nodes, microscopic seeding of peritoneal surfaces:
      - Most often microscopic omental metastasis
    - IIIb: Negative nodes; tumor implants in abdomen <2 cm
    - IIIc: Abdominal implants >2 cm or positive retroperitoneal or inguinal nodes:
      - This is the most common stage at presentation
  - Stage IV: Involvement of ovaries with distant metastasis:
    - Pleural effusions must be sent for cytology and confirmed to be malignant.
    - Parenchymal liver metastasis, not only surface implants, equals Stage IV.

EPIDEMIOLOGY
- In the US, the annual incidence of new cases of ovarian cancers is estimated to be 22,000. >16,000 women will die annually of their disease.
- The lifetime risk of developing ovarian cancer is ~1.4%.

RISK FACTORS
- Early menarche
- Late age of menopause
- Low parity
- Infertility
- Talc use
- Protective factors include: Pregnancy, breastfeeding, OCP use, tubal ligation, and hysterectomy.

Genetics
- The majority of epithelial ovarian cancer cases are sporadic but 5–10% are hereditary. Hereditary cancers generally occur 10 years earlier than those in the general population.
- BRCA1 (chr 17) mutations are associated with 20–45% lifetime risk of ovarian cancer.
- BRCA2 (chr 13) mutations are thought to have up to a 20–25% risk of ovarian cancer.
- Higher rates of BRCA mutations are seen in Ashkenazi Jewish (1 in 40 women; 2.5%) and Icelandic populations.
- Patients with known hereditary mutations should be offered risk-reducing surgery.

 DIAGNOSIS

SIGNS AND SYMPTOMS
History
- The majority of patients with malignant epithelial ovarian tumors are asymptomatic and do not present until they have advanced disease.
- Abdominal fullness or bloating (often vague)
- Early satiety
- Pelvic pressure
- Urinary frequency and pressure
- Increased abdominal girth
- Constipation
- Abdominal pain
- Abnormal vaginal bleeding

Review of Systems
Symptoms are often nonspecific and can include:
- Abdominal pain, bloating, pelvic pressure, urinary changes, or constipation.

Physical Exam
- A complete physical exam should be performed to look for localized and metastatic disease.
- Lungs:
  - Decreased breath sounds may be a sign of pleural effusions.
- Lymph nodes:
  - Observe for the presence of any palpable or suspicious lymph nodes.
- Abdominal exam:
  - Observe for ascites or palpable masses
- Pelvic exam:
  - Palpate for pelvic mass; solid, irregular, or fixed masses are more likely to be malignant.

TESTS
Lab
- Serum CA-125 levels can used to help assess preoperative risk of malignancy and to monitor response to therapy and recurrence in patients with known cancers.
- CA-125 should not be used for screening of asymptomatic low-risk women.
- CEA (if colonic primary suspected)
- CA19–9 (if pancreatic or other upper GI tumor suspected)
- CBC
- Metabolic panel

Imaging
- US:
  - May show complex mass with nodularity, ascites, or free pelvic fluid
- Chest radiograph:
  - May demonstrate pleural effusion or nodules
- CT:
  - May demonstrate pelvic/abdominal masses, omental disease, peritoneal implants, ascites, or lymphadenopathy
- Mammogram/Colonoscopy

DIFFERENTIAL DIAGNOSIS

Infection
Infectious causes presenting with abdominal masses and elevated CA-125 include:

- TOA
- Diverticulitis with abscess
- Appendicitis

Metabolic/Endocrine
Women with underlying liver disease, including cirrhosis of different etiologies, may present with ascites and elevated CA-125.

Tumor/Malignancy
- Nonmalignant neoplasms of ovary:
  – Meigs syndrome: Benign ovarian fibroma presenting with ascites and/or pleural effusion
  – Endometriomas
- Borderline tumors of ovary
- Malignant neoplasms metastatic to ovary from breast, colon, or other GI primaries

 ## TREATMENT

GENERAL MEASURES
- Patients with a clinical suspicion for ovarian cancer should undergo laparotomy and staging procedure.
- If a cancer is found, the goals of the surgery should also be maximal cytoreductive surgery as this has a well-established impact on improving overall survival.
- Primary surgery followed by adjuvant chemotherapy is the standard of care for most patients with ovarian cancer.

MEDICATION (DRUGS)
- Patients with advanced-stage ovarian cancer and patients with early-stage disease with risk factors including high grade, malignant cytology, or ascites should receive adjuvant chemotherapy.
- Standard primary chemotherapy consists of a 2-drug regimen of a platinum agent (carboplatin or cisplatin) and a taxane (paclitaxel or docetaxel).
- In women with advanced disease that is optimally cytoreduced, regimens with intraperitoneal chemotherapy may offer improved recurrencefree and overall survival. Combination intraperitoneal/intravenous chemotherapy should be considered for appropriate patient as an individualized decision.
- Neoadjuvant chemotherapy can be considered for patients with extensive metastatic disease, such as those with stage IV disease (e.g., hepatic metastasis) or for patients unable to undergo surgery for medical reasons.
- For patients who develop recurrent disease, several agents can be used as either monotherapy or in combination. These drugs may offer response rates up to 10–25%, and are not curative.

SURGERY
- Surgical staging should be performed via a midline vertical or paramedian incision to ensure adequate visualization and access to the upper abdomen.
- Peritoneal washings for cytology
- Total abdominal hysterectomy
- Bilateral salpingo-oophorectomy
- Infracolic omentectomy
- Peritoneal biopsies
- Retroperitoneal exploration including lymphadenectomy if no other evidence of extraovarian disease
- Diaphragmatic sampling by biopsy or scraping
- Metastatic tumor resection for advanced disease with the goal of primary maximum cytoreductive surgery
- Consideration for intraperitoneal port placement
- Young women with early-stage disease who desire maintaining fertility may opt to undergo unilateral salpingo-oophorectomy and staging with preservation of the uterus and opposite ovary. These patients must be appropriately counseled regarding recurrence risk and future fertility.

 ## FOLLOW-UP

DISPOSITION
Issues for Referral
- Patients with a high clinical suspicion for ovarian cancer should be referred to a gynecologic oncologist when possible for complete evaluation and surgical management.
- This should be done in a hospital that has the necessary support and consultative services to optimize the outcome.
- When a general ob-gyn discovers a malignant ovarian tumor, and the appropriate surgical staging and debulking cannot be performed, a gynecologic oncologist should be consulted.

PROGNOSIS
Overall survival for all patients with ovarian cancer is estimated to be 48.6%. Patients with early-stage/localized disease (Stage I) have a 5-year survival of 80–90%, whereas advanced-stage patients have a 5-year survival of ~20–30%.

- Prognostic factors for improved survival include younger age, early stage, favorable histologic types, low-grade tumors, and undergoing standard cytoreductive surgery.

PATIENT MONITORING
- Patients who are free of disease after primary treatment are followed by CA-125 and clinical exam every 3 months initially (1–2 years).
- CT and other imaging may be used.
- The majority of recurrences occur in the 1st 2–3 years after treatment. After this time, the interval for monitoring may be increased.

BIBLIOGRAPHY

ACOG Committee Opinion. The Role of Generalist Obstetrician-Gynecologist in the Early Detection of Ovarian Cancer #280, December 2002.

Berek JS. Epithelial ovarian cancer. In: Berek JS, et al., eds. *Practical Gynecologic Oncology*, 4th ed. Philadelphia: Lippincott, Williams and Wilkins; 2005:443–509.

Berek JS, et al. Ovarian and fallopian tube cancer. In: *Berek & Novak's Gynecology*, 14th ed., Philadelphia: Lippincott Williams & Wilkins; 2007:1457–1547.

Chan JK, et al. Patterns and progress in ovarian cancer over 14 years. *Obstet Gynecol*. 2006;108:521–528.

Franceschi S, et al. Pooled analysis of three European case control studies of epithelial ovarian cancer: Oral contraceptive use. *Int J Cancer*. 1991;49:61–65.

Jemal A, et al. Cancer Statistics, 2007. *CA Cancer J Clin*. 2007;57(1):43–66.

Kauff ND, et al. Risk-reducing salpingo-oophorectomy in women with BRCA1 and BRCA2 mutation. *N Engl J Med*. 2002;346:1616–1622.

 ## MISCELLANEOUS

ABBREVIATIONS
- EOC—Epithelial ovarian cancer
- OCP—Oral contraceptive pill
- TOA—Tubo-ovarian abscess

CODES

ICD9-CM
183.0 Malignant neoplasm of ovary and other uterine adnexa

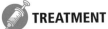 ## PATIENT TEACHING

PREVENTION
- Combination OCPs are associated with a proven risk reduction for ovarian cancer. Studies have demonstrated a 50% reduction in the risk of ovarian cancer in women who use OCPs for ≥5 years.
- Several studies have demonstrated a significant reduction in ovarian cancer in BRCA mutation carriers who undergo risk-reducing bilateral salpingo-oophorectomy.

OVARIAN TUMORS, VIRILIZING

Jay E. Allard, MD
John Farley, MD
Cynthia Macri, MD

BASICS

DESCRIPTION
- Virilizing tumors of the ovary are a subset of ovarian sex cord-stromal tumors that produce excess androgenic steroid hormones.
- Many of these tumors secrete other proteins that can serve as diagnostic markers. These tumors include:
  - Sertoli-stromal cell tumors, androblastomas:
    - Well-differentiated
    - Intermediate differentiation
    - Poorly differentiated (sarcomatoid)
    - Retiform
  - Gynandroblastoma
  - Steroid (lipid) cell tumors:
    - Stromal luteoma
    - Leydig cell tumor
    - Unclassified

Pregnancy Considerations
Virilizing tumors during pregnancy include, in descending order of frequency:
- Luteoma of pregnancy
- Krukenberg tumors
- Mucinous cystic tumors
- Brenner tumors
- Serous cystadenomas
- Endodermal sinus tumors
- Dermoid cysts

Age-Related Factors
- Sertoli-Leydig cell tumors:
  - ~75% occur in women under the age of 40
  - Mean age at diagnosis is 25
- Gynandroblastomas:
  - Age at diagnosis ranges from 16–65 years
  - Mean age at diagnosis is 30
- Steroid (lipid) cell tumors:
  - Similar age range as above

Pediatric Considerations
In prepubertal girls with signs of heterosexual precocious puberty, consider a virilizing tumor as a causative factor.

Staging
- Typically, these tumors are unilateral and Stage I. Surgical staging system as with other primary ovarian carcinomas.
- Stage I: Growth limited to the ovaries:
  - Stage IA: Growth limited to 1 ovary, no ascites containing malignant cells. No tumor on the external surface, capsule intact.
  - Stage IB: Growth limited to both ovaries, no ascites containing malignant cells. No tumor on the external surfaces, capsules intact.
  - Stage IC: Tumor either stage IA or IB, but with tumor on the surface of 1 or both ovaries, or with capsule ruptured, or with ascites present containing malignant cells, or with positive peritoneal washings.
- Stage II: Growth involving 1 or both ovaries with pelvic extension:
  - Stage IIA: Extension and/or metastases to the uterus and/or fallopian tubes.
  - Stage IIB: Extension to other pelvic tissues.
  - Stage IIC: Tumor either stage IIA or IIB, but with tumor on the surface of 1 or both ovaries, or with capsule(s) ruptured, or with ascites present containing malignant cells, or with positive peritoneal washings
- Stage III: Tumor involving 1 or both ovaries with peritoneal implants outside the pelvis and/or positive retroperitoneal or inguinal nodes. Superficial liver metastases. Tumor is limited to the true pelvis, but with histologically proven malignant extension to small bowel or omentum.
  - Stage IIIA: Tumor grossly limited to the true pelvis with negative nodes, but with histologically confirmed microscopic seeding of abdominal peritoneal surfaces.
  - Stage IIIB: Tumor of 1 or both ovaries with histologically confirmed implants of abdominal peritoneal surfaces, none exceeding 2 cm in diameter, nodes negative.
  - Stage IIIC: Abdominal implants >2 cm in diameter and/or positive retroperitoneal or inguinal nodes.
- Stage IV: Growth involving 1 or both ovaries with distant metastasis. Must have positive cytologic test results on pleural effusion to allot case to stage IV based on pleural effusion. Parenchymal liver metastases equates to stage IV.

EPIDEMIOLOGY
- Rare; ~0.5% of primary ovarian neoplasms.
- Most occur in the 2nd and 3rd decades of life, but can occur in any age group.
- ~2–3% of Sertoli-stromal cell tumors demonstrate extraovarian spread at time of diagnosis.
- <20% demonstrate malignant behavior.
- Recurrences most commonly occur with poorly differentiated tumors
- If recurrence does occur, it typically occurs in 1st few years after surgery.

RISK FACTORS
None known

Genetics
Not known

PATHOPHYSIOLOGY
- Develop from the cells surrounding the oocytes
- May be benign or malignant
- Tumors are typically a firm, solid, lobulated mass with smooth external surface
- Well-differentiated tumors may be soft and spongy; poorly differentiated tumors may show hemorrhage and necrosis
- Most tumors are of low-grade histology
- Microscopically, well-differentiated tumors are composed of hollow or solid tubules surrounded by fibrous stroma; intermediate and poorly differentiated tumors tend to contain dense cellular areas with increasing numbers of mitoses
- The presence of nonepithelial tissues is associated with poorer prognosis

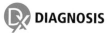

DIAGNOSIS

SIGNS AND SYMPTOMS
History
- Age of onset
- Rapid rate of progression of virilization
- Abdominal pain
- Increasing abdominal girth

Review of Systems
Persistent nonspecific symptoms may suggest ovarian cancer:
- Bloating, pelvic or abdominal pain, difficulty eating or feeling full quickly, urinary frequency or urgency

Physical Exam
- Palpable adnexal mass
- Signs of virilization including:
  - Atrophic breasts
  - Hirsutism
  - Deep voice
  - Male pattern baldness
  - Acne on face and/or back
  - Enlarged clitoris

TESTS
Labs
- Inhibin
- Total testosterone
- DHEA
- Androstenedione
- 17–hydroxyprogesterone
- α-Fetoprotein
- If oligomenorrhea, consider:
  - LH
  - FSH
  - Prolactin
  - TSH
- If Cushing syndrome is suspected:
  - 24-hour urinary cortisol

Imaging
- Pelvic US
- CT scan of chest, abdomen, pelvis

DIFFERENTIAL DIAGNOSIS
Metabolic/Endocrine
- PCOS
- Cushing syndrome

Tumor/Malignancy
- Virilization distinguishes these tumors from epithelial ovarian cancer, germ cell tumors of the ovary, and the uncommon small-cell carcinoma of the ovary.
- Adrenal neoplasm

Drugs
Anabolic/Exogenous steroid use

Other/Miscellaneous
- CAH
- Ovarian stromal hyperplasia and hyperthecosis

TREATMENT
MEDICATION (DRUGS)
- Chemotherapy for metastatic disease:
  - Typically bleomycin, etoposide, cisplatin (BEP)
- Metastatic disease and/or nonmetastatic poorly differentiated tumors or with heterologous elements, surgery, with addition of:
  - Platinum-based combination chemotherapy

SURGERY
- Surgery is the mainstay of treatment.
- Sertoli-stromal cell tumors:
  - For women who have completed childbearing:
    - Total abdominal hysterectomy with bilateral salpingo-oophorectomy (TAH-BSO)
  - For women who would like to preserve fertility or who would like to avoid exogenous hormone replacement:
    - Unilateral salpingo-oophorectomy
  - For women with advanced stage disease:
    - TAH-BSO, lymph node dissection, and adjuvant therapy
- Gynandroblastoma:
  - Unilateral oophorectomy or salpingo-oophorectomy is typically sufficient, as this is a benign tumor.

FOLLOW-UP
DISPOSITION
Issues for Referral
- Follow-up with surgeon, typically gynecologic oncologist, 2–4 weeks post-discharge. Then, continue to follow-up with physical examination and testosterone levels every 3–4 months for the 1st 2 years, and every 6 months for the subsequent 3 years.
- CT scan should be reserved for evaluation of recurrent symptoms or increasing testosterone level.

PROGNOSIS
- Overall 5-year survival is 70–90%.
- Related to stage and histologic differentiation

PATIENT MONITORING
- Physical exam and testosterone levels every 3–4 months for the 1st 2 years, and every 6 months for the subsequent 3 years.
- CT scan should be reserved for evaluation of recurrent symptoms or increasing testosterone level.

BIBLIOGRAPHY
American Joint Committee on Cancer Staging Manual, 6th ed. New York: Springer-Verlag; 2002.

Berek JS, et al, eds. Novak's Gynecology, 12th ed. Baltimore: Williams & Wilkins; 1996.

Berek JS, et al, eds. Practical Gynecologic Oncology, 4th ed. Philadelphia: Lippincott Williams & Wilkins; 2005.

Dorigo O, et al. Sex cord-stromal tumors of the ovary. UpToDate Online, 2006; version 14.2.

Hoskins WJ, Young et al, eds. Principles and Practice of Gynecologic Oncology, 4th ed. Philadelphia: Lippincott Williams & Wilkins; 2005.

MISCELLANEOUS
ABBREVIATIONS
- CAH—Congenital adrenal hyperplasia
- DHEA—Dehydroepiandrosterone
- FSH—Follicle-stimulating hormone
- LH—Luteinizing hormone
- PCOS—Polycystic ovary syndrome
- TSH—Thyroid-stimulating hormone

CODES
ICD9-CM
- 183 Malignant neoplasm of ovary and other uterine adnexa
- 220 Benign neoplasm of ovary:
  - Use additional code to identify any functional activity (256.0–256.1)
- 256.1 Other ovarian hyperfunction:
  - Hypersecretion of ovarian androgens

PATIENT TEACHING
- After surgery avoid:
  - Deep tub baths for 2 weeks
  - Strenuous exercise for 6 weeks
  - Heavy lifting (>15 lbs) or straining for 6 weeks
  - Intercourse for 6 weeks
- Additionally, call your physician if you develop:
  - Worsening abdominal/pelvic pain that is not relieved by pain medication
  - Persistent nausea or vomiting
  - Temperature >38°C (100.4°F)
  - Bleeding, separation, or drainage from your incision site
  - Worsening redness or swelling around your incision site

OVERACTIVE BLADDER

Bertha H. Chen, MD

BASICS

DESCRIPTION
- Overactive bladder is a symptom syndrome consisting of urgency, with or without urge incontinence, usually associated with frequency and nocturia, in the absence of infection or other pathology.

Age-Related Factors
Overactive bladder can occur in women of all ages.

EPIDEMIOLOGY
- In US, estimated 33 million adults
- 16.9% of women
- 16% of men
- Overall prevalence tends to increase with age:
  – Women > Men <60 years
  – Men > Women >60 years

RISK FACTORS
- Aging
- Neurologic problems
- Spinal injury
- Diabetes

Genetics
No data at this time

PATHOPHYSIOLOGY
- Several theories exist on the etiology of overactive bladder but the precise cause has not been identified, possibly because overactive bladder is a clinical and symptom diagnosis.
- Currently 3 main theories regarding overactive bladder:
  – The myogenic theory relies on changes in smooth muscle to explain the involuntary detrusor contractions.
  – The neurogenic theory suggests that damage to central inhibitory pathways in the brain or spinal cord or sensitization of the peripheral afferent terminal in the bladder can unmask primitive voiding reflex, thus triggering detrusor overactivity.
  – The autonomous bladder theory hypothesizes that the detrusor is modular, with each module defined by the area supplied by a node of interstitial cells called the *myovesical plexus*. During normal bladder filling, autonomous activity occurs with nonmicturition activity and phasic sensory discharge. This mechanism is modified in pathologic conditions, causing an imbalance in excitatory inputs and inhibitory outputs, leading to detrusor overactivity.

ASSOCIATED CONDITIONS
- MS
- Parkinson disease
- Stroke
- Spinal injury
- Diabetes

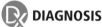

DIAGNOSIS

SIGNS AND SYMPTOMS
History
- Urinary urgency, urgency with incontinence, frequency, and nocturia
- Past medical history of diabetes, neurologic compromise (stroke, spinal injury/surgery, MS, Parkinson disease), and medications are important
- History of dietary habits, such as caffeine and fluid intake, will help with treatment and evaluation.

Review of Systems
Should focus on general medical conditions/health to elicit neurologic conditions, diabetes, kidney problems, mobility issues, and quality-of-life impediments.

Physical Exam
- In addition to routine physical exam, a neurologic exam should be performed.
- Pelvic exam should evaluation for prolapse and evidence of genital focus on vaginal atrophy.

TESTS
- A 24–hour voiding diary should be obtained for 3 days. This chart is invaluable in the management of overactive bladder for:
  – Quantifying frequency episodes
  – Quantifying fluid input and output
  – Estimating bladder capacity
  – Excluding 24–hour polyuria
  – Excluding nocturnal polyuria
- Urine analysis helps to exclude:
  – Infection
  – Hematuria
  – Glucosuria
- Postvoid residual to rule out:
  – Urinary retention
  – Overflow incontinence
- Quality-of-life questionnaire/assessment to document the effect of overactive bladder on the patient and to follow treatment

Labs
- In severe cases, urodynamic testing to assess for concurrent SUI, impaired detrusor contractility, or detrusor sphincter dyssynergia

DIFFERENTIAL DIAGNOSIS
- UTI
- Chronic cystitis
- Interstitial cystitis
- Radiation cystitis
- Overflow incontinence
- Urethritis
- Urethral syndrome
- Spinal injury
- Stroke
- Diuretic use
- Diabetes/Glucosuria
- MS
- Parkinson disease
- Diabetes insipidus
- Foreign body in the bladder
- Vaginal atrophy
- Idiopathic

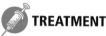

TREATMENT

GENERAL MEASURES
- Decrease caffeine intake and avoid smoking
- For patients with nocturia, avoid fluid intake 4 hours before bedtime
- Pelvic floor muscle exercises (Kegel exercises)
- Fluid reduction
- Empty bladder before going to bed
- Bladder training

SPECIAL THERAPY
Complementary and Alternative Therapies
- Bladder training
- Pelvic floor muscle exercises (biofeedback therapy)

MEDICATION (DRUGS)
Medications: Antimuscarinic agents are the mainstay of pharmacotherapy for overactive bladder:
- Oxybutynin
- Tolterodine
- Solifenacin
- Trospium chloride
- Darifenacin

SURGERY
- Botulinum toxin detrusor injections
- Sacral nerve neuromodulation

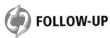

FOLLOW-UP

DISPOSITION

Issues for Referral

Patients should be referred to the appropriate specialists if any of the following is identified:

- Neurologic problems
- Severe prolapse
- Hematuria (gross or microscopic)
- Elevated PVRs
- Glucosuria
- Urinary/Fecal incontinence

PROGNOSIS

70–80% of patients treated for overactive bladder experience an improvement in their symptoms.

PATIENT MONITORING

The following can be done every 3–6 months, depending on the severity of the patient's condition:

- Quality-of-life assessment
- Renal function
- Postvoid residuals:
  – 24-hour diaries

BIBLIOGRAPHY

Abrams P, et al. Recommendations of the International Scientific Committee: Evaluation and treatment of urinary incontinence, pelvic organ prolapse and faecal incontinence. In: Abrams P, et al., eds. *Incontinence. 3rd Internation Consultation on Incontinence*. Paris: Health Publication Ltd.; 2005:1589–1630.

Abrams P, et al. The standardization of terminology of lower urinary tract function: Report from the Standardization Subcommittee of the International Continence Society. *Neurourol Urodyn*. 2002;21: 167–178.

Andersson KE, et al., eds. Incontinence. *3rd International Consultation on Incontinence*. Paris: Health Publication Ltd.; 2005:809–854.

Brown JS, et al. Comorbidities associated with overactive bladder. *Am J Mang Care*. 2000; 6(11 Suppl):S574–S579.

Bulmer P, et al. Does cigarette smoking cause detrusor instability in women? *J Obstet Gynaecol*. 2001;21: 528–589.

Burgio KL. Current perspectives on management of urgency using bladder and behavior training. *J Am Acad Nurse Pract*. 2004;16(10 Suppl):4–7.

Chapple CR, et al. The role of urinary urgency and its measurement in the overactive bladder symptom syndrome: Current concepts and future prospects. *BJU Int*. 2005;95:335–340.

Dmochowski RR, et al. Bladder-health diaries: An assessment of 3-day vs 7-day entries. *BJU Int*. 2005;96:1049–1054.

Irwin DE, et al. Population-based survey of urinary incontinence, overactive bladder, and other lower urinary tract symptoms in five countries: Results of the EPIC study. *Eur Urol*. 2006;50:1306–1314.

Milson I, et al. How widespread are the symptoms of an overactive bladder and how are they managed? A population-based prevalence study. *BJU Int*. 2001;87:760–766.

Nixon A, et al. A validated patient reported measure of urinary urgency severity in overactive bladder for use in clinical trials. *J Urol*. 2005;174:604–607.

Sellers DJ, et al. Developments in the pharmacotherapy of the overactive bladder. *Curr Opin Urol*. 2007;17:223–230.

Swithinbank L, et al. The effect of fluid intake on urinary symptoms in women. *J Urol*. 2005;174: 187–189.

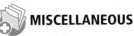

MISCELLANEOUS

SYNONYM(S)

- Urge syndrome
- Urgency-frequency syndrome

CLINICAL PEARLS

- Rule out overflow incontinence and abnormally elevated PVR, as these could signify impending or existing renal compromise.
- Treat associated vulvar skin rashes (resulting from urinary incontinence) with routine baby diaper rash cream application to protect the vulvar skin.
- Monitor PVR after starting anticholinergic medications to avoid retention problems.

ABBREVIATIONS

- MS—Multiple sclerosis
- PVR—Postvoid residual
- SUI—Stress urinary incontinence

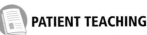

CODES

ICD9-CM

596.51 Hypertonicity of bladder (overactive bladder)

PATIENT TEACHING

- Bladder training
- Timed fluid intake
- ACOG Patient Education Pamphlet: Urinary incontinence
- Kegel exercises are described online at http://www.Wikipedia.com

PREVENTION

For women with only occasional urinary incontinence due to overactive bladder, incontinence may be minimized by regular voiding and avoidance of overly full bladder.

PARATUBAL AND PARAOVARIAN CYSTS

Bliss Kaneshiro, MD
Alison Edelman, MD, MPH

 BASICS

DESCRIPTION
- Thin-walled, fluid-filled, clear cysts
- Found alongside the fallopian tube
- Single or multiple
- Small, <1–2 cm in diameter but can be >20 cm in diameter
- Larger cysts can contain papillary excrescences on the internal surface.

Age-Related Factors
- Usually discovered in the 3rd and 4th decade of life
- Children are rarely affected although it has been reported in the literature.

Staging
Borderline and malignant tumors of serous origin have been reported but are rare.

EPIDEMIOLOGY
- Present in 50% of women in some case series
- Incidence of torsion among patients with paratubal cysts is 2.1–16%.

PATHOPHYSIOLOGY
- Arise from embryonic remnants
- Mesonephric or paramesonephric origin:
  - Cysts of mesonephric origin are found in broad ligament or lateral to ovary.
  - Cysts of paramesonephric origin are found adjacent to tube or its subserosal aspect.
- Slowly accumulate fluid and grow after adolescence due to secretory activity of tubal epithelium
- Larger cysts can undergo torsion and hemorrhage.

Pregnancy Considerations
- Paratubal cysts can grow rapidly during pregnancy.
- Most cases of torsion occur during pregnancy or the puerperium.

ASSOCIATED CONDITIONS
Although an association with tubal infertility has been hypothesized, no evidence supports this.

 DIAGNOSIS

SIGNS AND SYMPTOMS
Review of Systems
- Usually asymptomatic, often found incidentally:
  - In one series, only 3 of 79 paratubal cysts were symptomatic.
- Occasionally cause dull abdominal pain
- Cysts that have undergone torsion or hemorrhage can present with symptoms similar to ovarian torsion:
  - Lower quadrant, acute, colicky pain
  - Nausea and vomiting
  - Mild fever

Physical Exam
- Difficult to distinguish between a paratubal cyst and an ovarian mass on bimanual examination
- If torsion or hemorrhage occurs, cysts can cause pronounced local sensitivity deep in the pelvis.

TESTS
Labs
- Pregnancy test to rule out ectopic pregnancy
- CA-125 if ovarian malignancy is suspected

Imaging
- US:
  - Because of small size, paratubal cysts may be more easily identified by transvaginal than by transabdominal ultrasound.
  - Doppler flow studies if torsion suspected
  - Difficult to distinguish between paratubal cyst and ovarian cyst on ultrasound
- MRI may be useful in select situations.

DIFFERENTIAL DIAGNOSIS
Infection
- Acute appendicitis (See Appendicitis in Pregnancy.)
- Diverticular abscess
- TOA (See Pelvic Abscess.)

Tumor/Malignancy
- Ovarian neoplasm (benign or malignant) (See Ovarian Cysts and Ovarian Tumors.)
- Fallopian tube carcinoma (see topic)
- Pedunculated fibroids (See Uterine Fibroids.)

Other/Miscellaneous
- Ectopic pregnancy (see topic)
- Ovarian or tubal torsion (See Ectoptic Pregnancy.)
- Physiologic/Functional ovarian cyst (See Ovarian Cysts, Functional.)
- Hydrosalpinx

TREATMENT

GENERAL MEASURES
- Premenopausal women with asymptomatic simple cysts <10 cm can be followed conservatively.
- Surgery is recommended for large (>10 cm), persistent, enlarging, or symptomatic cysts.
- Fine needle aspiration (FNA) of cysts is not recommended because of high rate of recurrence and potential dissemination of malignant cells.

SURGERY
- Laparoscopic removal is the mainstay of treatment if surgery is required.
- Laparotomy can be also used depending on the size of the cyst and the patient's history and clinical presentation.
- Goal is to preserve fallopian tube even if it is stretched over a large paratubal cyst because it will return to its normal shape after the cyst is excised.
- Differentiation between benign and malignant masses cannot be made by examination at the time of surgery:
  - Do not aspirate cyst because of the potential for missing or disseminating malignant disease.
- If paratubal cyst is discovered incidentally at the time of surgery it should be excised to prevent possible enlargement or torsion.

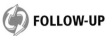

FOLLOW-UP

DISPOSITION
Issues for Referral
- No need for referral if cysts are asymptomatic and small (<10 cm)
- Refer to a gynecologist if cysts are symptomatic and/or large (>10 cm).
- Refer to gynecologic oncologist if malignancy is strongly suspected.

PROGNOSIS
- If cyst is completely excised it is unlikely to recur, although new cysts can form.
- Fenestrated or aspirated paratubal cysts can recur.

PATIENT MONITORING
Postoperative follow-up depends upon surgical course.

BIBLIOGRAPHY

Okada T, et al. , Paratubal cyst with torsion in children. *J Pediat Surg*. 2002;37:937–940.

Rutledge RH. Torsion of a hydatid of Morgagni. *Texas Med*. 1966;62:66–67.

Samaha M, et al. Paratubal cysts: Frequency, histogenesis, and associated clinical features. *Obstet Gynecol*. 1985;65:691–693.

Stenchever MA, et al., eds. *Comprehensive Gynecology*. St. Louis: Mosby; 2001.

 MISCELLANEOUS

SYNONYM(S)
- Parovarian cyst
- Paraovarian cyst
- Paratubal cyst

CLINICAL PEARLS
Hydatid cysts of Morgagni are pedunculated paratubal cysts arising at the fimbrial end of the fallopian tube.

ABBREVIATION
TOA—Tubo-ovarian abscess

CODES
ICD9-CM
- 620.8K Cyst of fallopian tube
- 620.08N Cyst of broad ligament
- 620.08T Cyst of broad ligament or fallopian tube
- 752.11D Parovarian cyst

Section II

PELVIC ABSCESS

Arthur Ollendorff, MD

 ## BASICS

DESCRIPTION
- A pelvic abscess is a cavity of infectious debris within the pelvis due to a variety of causes and, if untreated, can be deadly.

Age-Related Factors
- Pelvic abscesses is women <25 years are usually due to untreated PID.
- When pelvic abscess occurs in postmenopausal women, it is usually associated with an underlying gynecologic malignancy.

Geriatric Considerations
Geriatric patients with PID are at high risk of having an underlying gynecologic malignancy.

EPIDEMIOLOGY
- ~10% of women with PID may develop a TOA
- The risk of developing a pelvic abscess as a postoperative complication after hysterectomy is ~2–3

Pregnancy Considerations
Pelvic abscess is uncommon in pregnancy; other etiologies for a pregnant patient's pain or infection must be considered.

> **ALERT**
> Because of the high risk for morbidity and for preterm delivery, pregnant women with suspected pelvic abscess should be hospitalized and treated with parenteral antibiotics.

RISK FACTORS
- PID (TOA)
- History of diverticulosis
- Recent pelvic surgery
- Immunosuppression
- Recent instrumentation of genital tract:
  - Endometrial biopsy
  - IUD placement

PATHOPHYSIOLOGY
- Infection ascends from bacterial colonization of the cervix and extends to the uterus, fallopian tubes, and ovaries, or may develop from tissue injury following pelvic surgery.
- *Gonorrhea* and *Chlamydia* species are typically isolated from the cervix in cases of TOA, but these pathogens are rarely isolated in the abscess cavity.
- Micro-organisms that comprise the vaginal and rectal flora have been associated with pelvic abscess:
  - Anaerobes
  - *G. vaginalis*
  - *Haemophilus influenzae*
  - Gram-negative rods
  - *Enterococcus*
  - *Escherichia coli*
  - *Peptostreptococcus*
  - *U. urealyticum*
  - *Bacteroides*

ASSOCIATED CONDITIONS
- Oophoritis
- TOA
- Inflammation of the ovary
- Infection of the ovaries
- Ectopic pregnancy
- Pelvic adhesions
- Tubal infertility
- Chronic pelvic pain

 ## DIAGNOSIS

SIGNS AND SYMPTOMS
History
- Abdominal pain
- Pelvic pain
- Dyspareunia
- Fever
- Chills
- Nausea/Vomiting

Review of Systems
GI symptoms:
- Diverticulitis

Physical Exam
- Temperature >38°C
- Abdominal tenderness in lower quadrants
- Possible rebound tenderness on pelvic exam
- Cervical motion tenderness
- Adnexal tenderness
- Adnexal mass

TESTS
- Diagnostic laparoscopy is the definitive test.
- The diagnosis is difficult because of the wide variation in symptoms and signs, which may be subtle.

Labs
- Elevation of the WBC count to >10,000/μL is a nonspecific indicator of infection; however, the count may be within reference ranges soon after onset.
- UA is used to exclude cystitis.
- Urine pregnancy testing is used to exclude ectopic pregnancy.
- Cervical testing/cultures for gonococcal and chlamydial species are used to help exclude, diagnose, and treat infection with these organisms.

Imaging
- Pelvic US or CT scan of the abdomen and pelvis is needed to confirm the presence of a possible abscess.
- May allow visualization of appendix if appendicitis is considered in the differential

DIFFERENTIAL DIAGNOSIS
Infection
- Appendicitis
- Diverticulitis

Tumor/Malignancy
- Associated with gynecologic malignancies when seen in older patients
- Adnexal tumors

 ## TREATMENT

GENERAL MEASURES
- Determine extent of disease and severity to assess if the patient has a ruptured pelvic abscess.
- Hospitalization is required and should be continued until the patient is afebrile and clinically stable for at least 24–48 hours.

MEDICATION (DRUGS)
- Inpatient parenteral management:
  - Option 1:
    - Clindamycin 900 mg IV q8h PLUS
    - Gentamicin loading dose (2 mg/kg) IV or IM then maintenance 1.5 mg/kg q8h OR
    - Metronidazole 500 mg IV q12h
  - Option 2:
    - Ampicillin/Sulbactam 3 gm IV q6h PLUS
    - Doxycycline 100 mg IV q12h WITH OR WITHOUT
    - Metronidazole 500 mg PO b.i.d. 14 days
- Oral antibiotics should be given at hospital discharge to complete a 14-day course of antibiotic therapy. Options include:
  - Metronidazole 500 mg PO b.i.d.
  - Doxycycline 100 mg PO b.i.d.
  - Ofloxacin 400 mg PO b.i.d.

SURGERY
- Diagnostic laparoscopy if diagnosis unsure
- Exploratory laparotomy if ruptured TOA
- Interventional radiology drainage should be considered to improve the efficacy of antibiotic treatment.

 ## FOLLOW-UP

DISPOSITION
Issues for Referral
Refer to gynecologist if:
- Diagnosis unclear
- Clinically unstable
- Failure of medical management of PID:
  - Possible TOA

PROGNOSIS
Pelvic abscess can lead to infertility and ectopic pregnancy in future pregnancies and chronic pelvic pain.

PATIENT MONITORING
- Patients treated as outpatients must be seen within 7 days of hospital discharge to monitor efficacy of treatment.
- Clinical decline should prompt consideration of rehospitalization, additional diagnostic tests, or abscess drainage.
- In a clinically stable patient, radiographic imaging should be performed in 6 weeks to monitor the size of the abscess.

BIBLIOGRAPHY

Centers for Disease Control. 2006 guidelines for treatment of sexually transmitted diseases. *MMWR*. 2006;55(RR11):1–100.

Gjelland K, et al. Transvaginal ultrasound-guided aspiration for treatment of tubo-ovarian abscess: A study of 302 cases. *Obstet Gynecol*. 2005;193: 1323–1330.

Stenchever M, et al. *Comprehensive Gynecology*. 4th ed. Chicago: Mosby Year Book; 2001: 708–731.

 ## MISCELLANEOUS

SYNONYM(S)
Tubo-ovarian abscess (TOA)

CLINICAL PEARLS
- PID is a major cause of infertility and chronic pelvic pain and is better overtreated than undertreated.
- 20% of patients with PID do not have cervical cultures with *Gonorrhea* or *Chlamydia*.

ABBREVIATIONS
- PID—Pelvic inflammatory disease
- TOA—Tubo-ovarian abscess

CODES
ICD9-CM
- 614.4 Chronic or unspecific parametritis and pelvic cellulitis
- 614.3 Acute parametritis and pelvic cellulitis

PELVIC INFLAMMATORY DISEASE

Arthur Ollendorff, MD

 BASICS

DESCRIPTION
- PID is an ascending infection of the ovaries and a major cause of female infectious morbidity, ectopic pregnancy, infertility, and of chronic abdominal pain.

Age-Related Factors
- Most commonly occurs in women <25 years.
- When oophoritis occurs in postmenopausal women, it is usually associated with an underlying gynecologic malignancy.

Geriatric Considerations
Geriatric patients with PID are at high risk of having an underlying gynecologic malignancy.

EPIDEMIOLOGY
- 1 million women experience an episode of acute PID.
- >100,000 women become infertile each year as a result of PID, and a large proportion of the ectopic pregnancies occurring every year are due to the consequences of PID.
- Annually, >150 women die from PID or its complications.

Pregnancy Considerations
PID is uncommon in pregnancy, and other etiologies for a pregnant patient's pain or infection must be considered.

> **ALERT**
> Because of the high risk for morbidity and for preterm delivery, pregnant women with suspected PID should be hospitalized and treated with parenteral antibiotics.

RISK FACTORS
- Multiple sexual partners
- Non-use of barrier methods of contraception
- Concurrent *Gonorrhea* or *Chlamydia* infection
- Immunosuppression
- Recent instrumentation of genital tract:
  - Endometrial biopsy
  - IUD placement

PATHOPHYSIOLOGY
- Infection ascends from bacterial colonization of the cervix and extends to the uterus, fallopian tubes, and ovaries.
- *Gonorrhea* and *Chlamydia* species are typically isolated from the cervix in cases of PID, but these pathogens are rarely isolated in ovarian tissue:
  - These organisms instead facilitate infection of the adnexa by other bacteria.
- Micro-organisms that comprise the vaginal flora have been associated with PID:
  - Anaerobes
  - *Gardnerella vaginalis*
  - *Haemophilus influenzae*
  - Gram-negative rods
  - *Streptococcus agalactiae*
- Other organisms have been associated with PID:
  - Cytomegalovirus
  - *Mycoplasma hominis*
  - *Ureaplasma urealyticum*
  - *Mycoplasma genitalium*
- If left untreated, an abscess may form around the fallopian tubes and ovaries, a condition known as a TOA.

ASSOCIATED CONDITIONS
- Oophoritis
- TOA (See Pelvic Abscess.)
- Inflammation of the ovary
- Infection of the ovaries
- Ectopic pregnancy
- Pelvic adhesions
- Tubal infertility
- Chronic pelvic pain

DIAGNOSIS

SIGNS AND SYMPTOMS
History
- Abdominal pain
- Pelvic pain
- Vaginal discharge
- Dyspareunia
- Fever
- Chills
- Nausea/Vomiting

Review of Systems
Right upper quadrant pain:
- Fitz-Hugh Curtis syndrome (see topic)

Physical Exam
- Temperature >38°C
- Abdominal tenderness in lower quadrants
- Possible rebound tenderness on pelvic exam
- Mucopurulent discharge
- Cervical motion tenderness
- Adnexal tenderness
- Adnexal mass (if a TOA is present)

TESTS
- Diagnostic laparoscopy is the definitive test.
- The diagnosis is difficult because of the wide variation in symptoms and signs, which may be subtle.
- The diagnosis is usually made clinically, although a clinical diagnosis is imprecise, with no single historical, physical, or lab finding that is both sensitive and specific for the diagnosis.
- Many episodes of PID are not recognized.

Labs
- Elevation of the WBC count to >10,000/mL is a nonspecific indicator of infection; however, the count may be within reference ranges soon after onset.
- UA is used to exclude cystitis.
- Urine pregnancy testing is used to exclude ectopic pregnancy.
- Wet preparation of cervical discharge shows numerous WBCs and bacteria.
- Cervical testing/cultures for gonococcal and chlamydial species are used to help exclude, diagnose, and treat infection with these organisms. All women diagnosed with PID should be treated for these organisms.
- All women with PID should be screened for HIV infection.

Imaging
- Pelvic US may be needed if the patient cannot tolerate a thorough palpation of the adnexa because of pain.
- An US exam can exclude the presence of a TOA.
- May allow visualization of appendix if appendicitis is considered in the differential.

DIFFERENTIAL DIAGNOSIS

Infection
- Appendicitis
- Diverticulitis
- Gastroenteritis
- Cystitis
- Mesenteric lymphadenitis

Tumor/Malignancy
- Associated with gynecologic malignancies when seen in older patients
- Adnexal tumors

Other/Miscellaneous
- Ectopic pregnancy
- Adnexal torsion

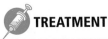

TREATMENT

GENERAL MEASURES
- Determine extent of disease and severity to assess whether patient requires inpatient or outpatient management.
- Because the diagnosis of PID is imprecise, empiric treatment should be used in sexually active young women and other women at risk for STDs who experience pelvic or lower abdominal pain if no other cause can be identified and with one or more of the following:
  – Cervical motion tenderness on exam OR
  – Uterine tenderness OR
  – Adnexal tenderness
- Suggested CDC criteria for hospitalization include:
  – Surgical emergencies (appendicitis) cannot be excluded.
  – The patient is pregnant.
  – The patient does not respond clinically to oral antimicrobial therapy.
  – The patient is unable to follow or tolerate an outpatient oral regimen.
  – The patient has severe illness, nausea and vomiting, or high fever.
  – The patient has a TOA.

MEDICATION (DRUGS)
- For women with mild or moderate PID parenteral and oral therapy has similar efficacy.
- Oral outpatient management:
  – Regimen A:
    ○ Levofloxacin 500 mg/d PO for 14 days OR
    ○ Ofloxacin 400 mg PO b.i.d. for 14 days WITH OR WITHOUT
    ○ Metronidazole 500 mg b.i.d. for 14 days
  – Regimen B:
    ○ Ceftriaxone 250 mg IM OR cefoxitin 2g IM plus 1 g PO probenecid concurrently PLUS
    ○ Doxycycline 100 mg PO b.i.d. for 14 days WITH OR WITHOUT
    ○ Metronidazole 500 mg PO b.i.d. for 14 days
- Inpatient parenteral management:
  – Regimen A:
    ○ Cefotetan 2g IV q12h OR cefoxitin 2g IV q6h PLUS
    ○ Doxycycline 100 mg PO or IV q12h
  – Regimen B:
    ○ Clindamycin 900 mg IV q8h PLUS
    ○ Gentamicin loading dose (2 mg/kg) IV or IM then maintenance 1.5 mg/kg q8h

SURGERY
- Diagnostic laparoscopy if diagnosis unsure
- Exploratory laparotomy if ruptured TOA
- Salpingo-oophorectomy if failure of medical management
- Interventional radiology drainage may be considered if abscess present.

FOLLOW-UP

DISPOSITION

> **ALERT**
> Sex partners should be treated empirically with regimens effective against both *C. trachomatis* and *N. gonorrhoeae*.

Issues for Referral
- Refer to gynecologist if:
  – Diagnosis unclear
  – Clinically unstable
  – Failure of medical management:
    ○ Persistent TOA
- Gynecologist should ensure that sex partners are referred for appropriate treatment or should make arrangements to provide expedited partner treatment (EPT) for male partners.

PROGNOSIS
PID can lead to infertility and ectopic pregnancy in future pregnancies.

PATIENT MONITORING
- Patients treated as outpatients must be seen within 72 hours of initial treatment to monitor efficacy of treatment.
- No improvement should prompt consideration of hospitalization, additional diagnostic test, or surgical intervention.

BIBLIOGRAPHY

Beigi RH, et al. Pelvic inflammatory disease: New diagnostic criteria and treatment. *Obstet Gynecol Clin North Am*. 2003;30(4):777–793.

Centers for Disease Control. 2006 guidelines for treatment of sexually transmitted diseases. *MMWR*. 2006;55(RR11):1–100.

Stenchever M, et al. *Comprehensive Gynecology*, 4th ed. Chicago: Mosby Year Book; 2001:708–731.

MISCELLANEOUS

SYNONYM(S)
- Salpingitis
- Oophoritis
- Salpingo-oophoritis

CLINICAL PEARLS
- PID is a major cause of infertility and chronic pelvic pain and is better overtreated than under-treated.
- 20% of patients with PID do not have positive cervical cultures with gonorrhea or chlamydia.

ABBREVIATIONS
- EPT—Expedited partner treatment
- PID—Pelvic inflammatory disease
- STD—Sexually transmitted disease
- TOA—Tubo-ovarian abscess
- US—Ultrasound

CODES

ICD9-CM
- 614.3 Acute parametritis and pelvic cellulitis
- 614.4 Chronic or unspecified parametritis and pelvic cellulitis
- 614.9 Unspecified inflammatory disease of female pelvic organs and tissues

PATIENT TEACHING

Reinforce need for safer sex practices

PREVENTION
- Barrier methods of contraception
- Limit number of sexual partners

PELVIC RELAXATION/PELVIC ORGAN PROLAPSE

Briana Robinson-Walton, MD

 BASICS

DESCRIPTION
- Pelvic organ prolapse (POP) is a condition in which descent of a pelvic organ into or beyond the vagina, perineum, or anal canal has occurred. This relaxation can occur in one or multiple areas of the vagina.
- The following terms are used to describe where the prolapse can arise:
- Anterior wall prolapse:
  – Cystocele (bladder)
  – Urethrocele (urethra)
- Posterior wall prolapse:
  – Rectocele (rectum)
  – Enterocele(small/large bowel)
- Apical prolapse:
  – Uterine prolapse (uterus)
  – Vaginal vault prolapse (vaginal cuff)

Age-Related Factors
Advancing age is commonly associated with POP, with an 11% lifetime risk for surgery by age 80.

Pediatric Considerations
POP in adolescents may warrant an evaluation of a connective tissue disorder such as Marfan's or Ehlers-Danlos syndromes.

Staging
Prolapse is assessed by the Pelvic Organ Prolapse Quantification (POPQ) exam. The staging system utilizes objective measurements to assign severity (see "Physical Exam"):
- Stage 0: No prolapse is demonstrated:
  – Aa, Ba, Ap, Bp are −3
  – C and D are ≤TVL − 2 cm
- Stage 1: Most distal portion of prolapse is >1 cm above the level of the hymen:
  – Points <−1 cm
- Stage 2: Most distal portion of prolapse is within 1 cm of the hymen:
  – Point ≥−1 cm and ≤+1 cm
- Stage 3: Most distal portion of prolapse is 1 cm past the introitus:
  – >+1 cm and ≤TVL − 2 cm
- Stage 4: Complete eversion of uterus or vaginal vault:
  – >TVL −2

EPIDEMIOLOGY
POP is highly prevalent among postmenopausal women. The lifetime prevalence is between 30% and 50%. Most women are not symptomatic. However, 1 in 10 women will require surgery for this condition and ~29% will undergo reoperation. The actual incidence of POP is unknown.

RISK FACTORS
- Obstetric risks:
  – Multiparity
  – Operative vaginal delivery
- Surgical risks:
  – Hysterectomy
  – Prolapse surgery
  – Prior colposuspension

- Biologic risks:
  – Menopause
  – Hypoestrogenemia
  – Obesity
  – Weak pelvic musculature
  – Large diameter of bony pelvis
  – Collagen abnormalities
- Lifestyle:
  – Occupational (heavy lifting)
  – Chronic constipation/straining

Genetics
Pregnancy, parturition, aging, and menopause affect each woman differently. Genetic predisposition is one aspect of the development and severity of POP. The encoded metabolism of extracellular matrix proteins (collagen, elastin and fibronectin) and enzymes (matrix metalloproteinases) may help to explain why prolapse occurs in some women and not others.

PATHOPHYSIOLOGY
- Prolapse results from a combination of anatomical factors, pelvic floor trauma, inadequate surveillance, and limited intervention.
- Anatomical/Genetic factors:
  – Collagen disorder/defect
- Pelvic floor trauma from vaginal delivery or surgery:
  – Injury to tissue, muscles, and nerves
- Inadequate surveillance:
  – Lack of recognition of early stage/grade POP
- Limited intervention:
  – Unmodified risk factors (i.e., untreated constipation)
  – Pessary or surgical management

ASSOCIATED CONDITIONS
- POP can occur in conjunction with other pelvic floor disorders and result in a detrimental effect on quality of life.
- Incontinence:
  – Urinary
  – Fecal

DIAGNOSIS

SIGNS AND SYMPTOMS
History
- Patients are generally asymptomatic with early stages of POP. As the prolapse progresses, the patient may present with a number of complaints
- Prolapse:
  – Pressure/pain:
    ○ Vagina
    ○ Lower back
- Urinary:
  – Incontinence
  – Hesitancy/Retention
- Bowel:
  – Fecal incontinence
  – Constipation/Impaction
- Sexual:
  – Dyspareunia
  – Decreased pleasure/satisfaction

Physical Exam
Perform a general exam to evaluate health status and impact of comorbidities.
- Pelvic exam includes:
  – Vagina:
    ○ Suburethral mass/tenderness (diverticulum)
    ○ Bladder mass/tenderness (interstitial cystitis)
    ○ Atrophy (mild, moderate, severe)
    ○ Pelvic musculature: atrophy, Kegel exam
  – Cervix (mass, elongation)
  – Uterus (enlargement ,mobility, descent)
  – Adnexa
  – Rectal (mass, exacerbation of rectocele, presence of enterocele)
  – Prolapse evaluation and staging
    ○ Perform exam during Valsalva, with a half speculum and in the standing position.
    ○ POPQ measurements are made relative to the hymen in 0.5 cm increments.

Point	Measurement	Range
Aa	Anterior vaginal wall 3 cm proximal to urethral meatus	−3 to +3
Ba	Most distal point on the anterior wall prolapse	+3 to tvl
C	Most distal edge of cervix or cuff	+/− tvl
D	Most distal position of posterior fornix	+/− tvl
Ap	Posterior vaginal wall 3 cm proximal to hymen	−3 to +3
Bp	Most distal point on the posterior wall prolapse	+3 to tvl
gh*	Middle urethral meatus to posterior midline of hymen	No limit
pb^	Posterior midline of hymen to mid-anal opening	No limit
tvl°	Posterior hymen to the posterior fornix or vaginal cuff	No limit

*genital hiatus
^perineal body
°total vaginal length

- Points measured inside of the hymen are negative, whereas points outside the hymen are positive.
- The hymen is assigned a value of zero.
- All measurements, except the total vaginal length are obtained with Valsalva.
- The measurements recorded on 9 point grid:

Aa	Ba	C
gh	pb	tvl
Ap	Bp	D*

*Is not measured in patients without a cervix

TESTS

- Urinary incontinence:
  - Urodynamic testing
  - +/− Cystoscopy (hematuria, smoking history)
- Constipation:
  - Colonoscopy
  - Marker studies for transit time
  - Defecography
- Fecal incontinence:
  - Anal sonography
  - Manometry
  - Pudendal nerve motor latency

Imaging
Consider contrast CT of upper urinary tract with abnormal cystoscopy findings:

- Negative exam for hematuria evaluation
- Lack or abnormal ureteral patency

DIFFERENTIAL DIAGNOSIS
- Urethral diverticulum or suburethral cyst
- Fibroids in the lower uterine segment
- Cervical elongation
- Rectovaginal mass

TREATMENT

GENERAL MEASURES
- Observation is appropriate for stage 1 prolapse or asymptomatic stage 2 prolapse:
  - Interval POPQ exams repeated to evaluate for progression, regression, or stability
  - Topical estrogens and pelvic floor exercises
- Pessaries if nonsurgical management is desired or poor operative candidate.
  - Prior to fitting, a POPQ exam and correction of vaginal atrophy are performed.
  - Pessary selection based on location and severity of POP. A knob with the pessary addresses concurrent stress incontinence.

Anterior	Posterior	Apical
Ring	Ring	Ring
Gehrung	Gehrung	Gelhorn
Mar-Land		Donut

- Initial fitting:
  - Assess vaginal length and select pessary size (i.e., use pessary with length ≤70 mm for TVL 8 cm)
  - Assess comfort, ability to retain during Valsalva, ambulation, and voiding after placement.
  - Instruct patient to remove nightly to weekly independently
  - Provider-dependent checks every 1–3 months
  - Use Trimo-San ointment to decrease discharge
  - Evaluation of infection, lacerations/erosions, and satisfaction at every visit

MEDICATION (DRUGS)
- Most patients who have POP will require treatment of vaginal atrophy.
- Vaginal creams:
  - Estradiol cream 0.01% (Estrace)
  - Conjugated estrogens 0.625 mg/gm (Premarin)
- Vaginal tablet:
  - Estradiol 25 μg (VagiFem)
- Vaginal ring:
  - Estradiol 2 mg (Estring)

SURGERY
- The goals of surgical correction are to restore anatomy and correct symptoms while respecting desire for sexual function.
- The type of repair is based on these goals as well as concurrent incontinence issues.
- Generally, POP is approached through the vagina; however, abdominal and laparoscopic approaches may be appropriate in certain cases.
- Biologic materials and synthetic meshes are proposed to decrease the risk of recurrence.
- Successful repair addresses each defect and involves selection of the appropriate surgery.
- Performance of hysterectomy and/or incontinence procedure is based on concurrent conditions, patient preference, and surgical route.
- Compartment defect/ common procedures:
  - Anterior prolapse (cystocele, urethrocele):
    - Anterior repair
    - Paravaginal repair
  - Posterior prolapse (rectocele/enterocele):
    - Posterior repair/colporrhaphy
    - Enterocele repair (culdoplasty)
  - Apical prolapse (uterine prolapse, vaginal vault prolapse or enterocele):
    - Uterosacral ligament suspension (McCall, modified McCall, suspension)
    - Sacrospinous ligament fixation
    - Ileococcygeus suspension
    - Sacrocolpopexy/Sacrocervicopexy
  - Perineal prolapse:
    - Perineorrhaphy

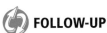

FOLLOW-UP

DISPOSITION
Issues for Referral
Consultation with a urogynecologist is necessary for the following reasons:

- Concurrent problem with incontinence
- Recurrent prolapse
- Unable to properly assess POP
- Inability to properly manage POP

PROGNOSIS
- Women with pessaries may discontinue use due to infection, discharge, bleeding, or the desire for definitive therapy.
- Women who elect surgical management should be counseled that the recurrence rates are variable depending on the procedure performed:
  - Recurrence in the anterior compartment is the highest, 20–40%, and more common with vaginal procedures.
  - The need for another procedure is as high as 30%.

PATIENT MONITORING
- Pessary evaluation every 1–3 months if woman doesn't remove the pessary on her own.
- Annual reevaluation of POP in women who remove the pessary independently.
- The POPQ evaluation of surgical outcomes is executed annually after the 1st year.

BIBLIOGRAPHY

Bump RC, et al. Epidemiology and natural history of pelvic floor dysfunction. *Obstet Gynecol Clin*. 1998;25:723–746.

Bump RC, et al. The standardization of terminology of female pelvic organ prolapse and pelvic floor dysfunction. *Am J Obstet Gynecol*. 1996;175:10–17.

MISCELLANEOUS

SYNONYM(S)
Pelvic or vaginal relaxation

CLINICAL PEARLS
- Severe atrophy:
  - Burning symptoms may be initially encountered with use of topical estradiol.
  - Pretreatment with petroleum jelly may help.
- Pessary use:
  - Deflate donut pessary with 18-gauge needle and 30-cc syringe to ease insertion and placement.
  - May have higher failure rates with pessary with a large GH (≥6 cm) or shortened vagina (TVL <8 cm)
- Surgery:
  - Bowel prep all patients prior to surgery and prevent constipation postoperatively.

ABBREVIATIONS
- POP—Pelvic organ prolapse
- GH—Genital hiatus
- PB—Perineal body
- TVL—Total vaginal length

CODES

ICD9-CM
- 618.00 Prolapse, vaginal walls
- 618.01 Cystocele, midline
- 618.02 Cystocele, lateral
- 618.03 Urethrocele
- 618.04 Rectocele
- 618.05 Perineocele
- 618.1 Prolapse, uterine
- 618.2 Uterovaginal prolapse, incomplete
- 618.3 Uterovaginal prolapse, complete
- 618.5 Vaginal vault prolapse hysterectomy
- 618.6 Enterocele

PATIENT TEACHING

PREVENTION
- POP is multifactorial, and the inability to predict who will develop symptomatic pelvic floor relaxation prevents modification of inciting factors among reproductive-age women.
- The strongest risk factors for development of POP are obstetric: Multiparity and vaginal delivery. Prevention of POP with cesarean delivery is controversial. Once recognized, certain factors may be modified to improve or prevent worsening of POP:
  - Constipation
  - Occupational and recreations stress
  - Obesity
  - Chronic lung disease
  - Smoking
  - Vaginal estrogen

PITUITARY ADENOMA
Robert W. Rebar, MD

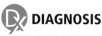 BASICS

DESCRIPTION
Pituitary adenomas are virtually always benign and may arise at any time in life. Because they are thought to arise by clonal expansion from a single pituitary cell, they may secrete 1, or less commonly, >1 pituitary hormone. They also may appear to be nonfunctioning.

Age-Related Factors
The highest incidence is in women aged 15–44.

Staging
- Microadenomas are <10 mm in diameter.
- Macroadenomas are ≥10 mm in diameter.

EPIDEMIOLOGY
- Incidence ranges from 0.5–7.4 per 100,000 persons per year depending on age and sex.
- Autopsy studies indicate that pituitary tumors are quite common, with a prevalence of ≥10%:
  – Almost all are microadenomas.
- Prolactin-secreting pituitary adenomas are most frequent in women.

PATHOPHYSIOLOGY
- Adenomas that hypersecrete corticotropin, GH, TSH, and prolactin result in the clinical syndromes of Cushing disease, acromegaly, secondary hyperthyroidism, and hyperprolactinemia, respectively.
- The most common adenomas in women of reproductive age cause hyperprolactinemia.
- Most of the nonfunctioning tumors arise from gonadotropes and commonly secrete either α or β subunits which are not biologically active; less commonly, small quantities of FSH or LH.

ASSOCIATED CONDITIONS
- Stalk compression from macroadenomas can lead to hyperprolactinemia, and partial or complete hypopituitarism may be present as well.
- If the posterior pituitary is compromised, diabetes insipidus may be present.
- Visual field defects, typically bitemporal hemianopsia, may result from compression of the optic chiasm.

DIAGNOSIS

SIGNS AND SYMPTOMS
History
- The most common symptoms are galactorrhea and/or oligo- or amenorrhea due to hyperprolactinemia.
- Headache may result from an enlarging adenoma.
- Patients may report visual problems if the macroadenoma impinges on the optic tracts.
- Coarsening of features and enlargement of hands and feet may be reported in acromegaly.
- Women with Cushing's disease often give a history of:
  – Weakness and fatigue, centripetal weight gain, recent onset hypertension, increased facial hair, oligo- or amenorrhea.

- Pituitary apoplexy, acute infarction of the pituitary gland, is rare and occurs more commonly in macroadenomas:
  – This medical emergency presents with sudden onset of severe retro-orbital headache, visual disturbances, and nausea and vomiting, sometimes followed by lethargy and loss of consciousness, which evolves over hours to days.

Physical Exam
- Evidence of hyper- or hyposecretion of pituitary hormones should be sought.
- Signs of acromegaly and Cushing disease are usually apparent.
- Gross visual field exam is always indicated if a pituitary adenoma is being considered.
- Hypothyroidism may be subtle and may not always be apparent on exam.
- Galactorrhea is most easily identified with the patient seated. The examiner should stand behind the patient and attempt to express any fluid toward the nipple. If fluid is expressed, it should be placed on a glass slide, covered with a coverslip, and examined under low to medium power under the microscope.
  – Perfectly round thick-walled globules of various sizes indicate fat and are typical of milk.
- Evidence of hypopituitarism may manifest as hypoestrogenism, documented by atrophic vaginal mucosa and scanty cervical mucus.

TESTS
The diagnosis is established by using a combination of laboratory tests and imaging studies.

Lab
- Regardless of whether galactorrhea is present or not, all amenorrheic women should have basal levels of FSH, TSH, and prolactin measured.
- If the prolactin level is >20 ng/mL, a basal fasting sample should be measured at 0800 to document hyperprolactinemia.
- Estradiol can be measured in women of reproductive age if the FSH level is normal or low to confirm hypoestrogenism.
- Other pituitary hormones should be measured depending on the history and physical findings.
- Goldman perimetry visual fields are warranted if there is any suggestion of visual difficulties and in all women with macroadenomas.

Imaging
- MRI is the most sensitive test to document the presence of a pituitary adenoma. Lesions that are ≥3 mm in diameter are easily visualized, and compromise of the optic chiasm and/or tracts can be identified as well.
- CT scanning is acceptable as well:
  – Although coned-down views of the sella turcica will be abnormal in the presence of macroadenomas, they cannot identify small microadenomas.
- Emergency imaging is required if pituitary apoplexy is suspected.
- In amenorrheic women with evidence of hypoestrogenism, measurement of BMD is warranted.

DIFFERENTIAL DIAGNOSIS
- Galactorrhea:
  – Primary hypothyroidism.
  – Fibrocystic breast disease may be associated with breast discharge, but the discharge will not contain fat globules on microscopic exam.
  – After miscarriage, fetal demise, or delivery, galactorrhea will persist if the milk is expressed on a regular basis.
  – Various medications, especially psychotropic agents and some antihypertensives, may result in hyperprolactinemia:
    ○ In general, the higher the basal levels of prolactin, the more likely is it that the patient has a prolactinoma.
- Levels of prolactin that are only mildly increased in the presence of an adenoma should suggest the possibility that the tumor is not a prolactinoma.

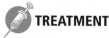 TREATMENT

GENERAL MEASURES
Therapy depends on type and size of adenoma and the desires of the patient.

MEDICATION (DRUGS)
- Initial therapy for prolactin-secreting micro- or macroadenomas is a dopamine agonist:
  – Either bromocriptine mesylate (Parlodel) or cabergoline (Dostinex) can be used.
  – In general, both medications should be started at low dose levels and increased weekly until prolactin levels fall into the normal range:
    ○ Nausea, headache, and nasal congestion are common side effects.
    ○ Bromocriptine especially can cause postural hypotension.
    ○ Doses should be divided and may be taken after meals to reduce side effects.
    ○ Studies indicate that side effects can be reduced by vaginal administration of bromocriptine (not FDA approved).
    ○ As much as 30 mg/d of bromocriptine in divided doses or 1 mg of cabergoline twice a week may be required to lower prolactin levels in macroadenomas.
    ○ A dopamine agonist may be effective in reducing tumor size and reversing any space-occupying effects of a macroadenoma.
- Because of the side effects of dopamine agonists, some clinicians advocate observation only for women with *micro*prolactinomas who do not have significant problems with galactorrhea and who do not desire pregnancy.
- Women with hypoestrogenic amenorrhea can be provided exogenous estrogen without concern that microadenomas will increase in size.

- If contraception is desired, low-dose OCPs can be administered.
- In normal individuals, dopamine agonists raise GH levels, but in patients with acromegaly, paradoxically, lower them:
  – Bromocriptine and cabergoline suppress GH levels in ~70% of patients with acromegaly but rarely reduce them to normal.
  – Somatostatin agonists such as octreotide and lanreotide and GH-receptor antagonists such as pegvisomant may be effective in reducing GH levels in some patients.
  – Valvular heart disease has been reported with use of cabergoline for treatment of Parkinson disease at 10-fold the dosage used for hyperprolactinemia and acromegaly.

SURGERY

- For non–prolactin-secreting macroadenomas, surgical resection is often the treatment of choice:
  – Transsphenoidal resection is the approach of choice.
  – SIADH transiently can follow surgery, especially for macroadenomas, and permanent hypopituitarism can result.
- Surgery is generally indicated for Cushing disease and acromegaly, even though the tumors are generally quite small.
- Surgical resection also can be offered to women with macroprolactinomas and should be recommended to those in whom suprasellar extension persists after treatment with a dopamine agonist.
- Early transsphenoidal surgical decompression is generally required for pituitary apoplexy.
  – High-dose corticosteroids should be provided before surgery to provide coverage for acute adrenal insufficiency and to alleviate intracranial swelling. Vigorous supportive measures will be required as well.

RADIOTHERAPY

- Postoperative radiation therapy can be used in the unusual patient in whom the tumor has extended into the cavernous sinus or other brain structures such that total resection is not possible.
- Radiotherapy may be used in patients who suffer from recurrences:
  – Radiation to the pituitary usually results in eventual hypopituitarism, and this may occur years after completion of therapy.
  – If too much radiation is delivered to the optic chiasm, fibrosis and eventual blindness may result.

Pregnancy Considerations

- ~3/4 of women with prolactinomas who desire pregnancy do conceive during therapy with dopamine agonists:
  – In women with microadenomas, it is reasonable to stop the dopamine agonist when pregnancy is confirmed.
  – Women with macroadenomas may continue the dopamine agonist throughout the pregnancy.
  – No evidence of any adverse effects on either the pregnancy or the fetus in pregnancies in which therapy is continued.
- <5% of women with microadenomas will develop signs and symptoms suggestive of tumor expansion during pregnancy.

- ~15% of women with macroadenomas will develop tumor enlargement during pregnancy.
- Because prolactin levels typically increase dramatically during pregnancy, measurement of prolactin during pregnancy is not helpful in monitoring patients for tumor expansion.
- Recurrent headaches usually precede any visual changes and indicate tumor enlargement.
- Symptoms establish the need for sellar imaging and visual field testing.
- Surgery is rarely required; usually increasing the dose of dopamine agonist is sufficient. If surgery is needed, it almost invariably is for women with large macroadenomas.
- Life-threatening hemorrhage into the tumor or permanent visual impairment is possible.
- Women who develop hypopituitarism can conceive following administration of gonadotropins to induce ovulation. Pituitary hormone replacement will need to be continued during and following the pregnancy.

FOLLOW-UP

DISPOSITION
Issues for Referral
Women who present with macroadenomas or signs and symptoms indicative of pituitary over- or underactivity should be evaluated and followed by clinicians familiar with the care of these challenging patients.

PROGNOSIS
- Therapy with a dopamine agonist may result in resolution of microadenomas:
  – It may be possible to discontinue the dopamine agonist after 1–2 years in women with microadenomas to determine if the prolactin increases again.
- Women with macroprolactinomas treated medically generally require therapy for the remainder of their lives, as will those undergoing surgery and/or radiation therapy.

PATIENT MONITORING
- Periodic monitoring of prolactin levels is required for women treated with a dopamine agonist for hyperprolactinemia.
- After successful surgery, women should be evaluated at least yearly for evidence of any recurrence.
- After radiation therapy, evaluate at least annually for evidence of hypopituitarism.

BIBLIOGRAPHY

Bevan JS, et al. Dopamine agonists and pituitary tumor shrinkage. *Endocr Rev*. 1992;13:220.

Chanson P. Pituitary tumors: Overview of therapeutic options. In: Becker KL, et al., eds. *Principles and Practice of Endocrinology and Metabolism*, 3rd ed. Philadelphia: Lippincott Williams & Wilkins; 2001: 264–276.

Roth BL. Drugs and valvular heart disease. *N Engl J Med*. 2007;356:6–9.

Schlechte J, et al. The natural history of untreated hyperprolactinemia: A prospective analysis. *J Clin Endocrinol Metab*. 1989;68:412.

Vance ML. Hypopituitarism. *N Engl J Med*. 1994;330: 1651–1662.

Webster J, et al. A comparison of cabergoline and bromocriptine in the treatment of hyperprolactinemic amenorrhea. Cabergoline Comparative Study Group. *N Engl J Med*. 1994;331:904–909.

MISCELLANEOUS

ABBREVIATIONS
- BMD—Bone mineral density
- FSH—Follicle-stimulating hormone
- GH—Growth hormone
- LH—Luteinizing hormone
- OCP—Oral contraceptive pill
- TSH—Thyroid-stimulating hormone

CODES
ICD9-CM
- 237.0 Neoplasm of uncertain behavior of endocrine glands and nervous system
  – 237.0 Pituitary gland and craniopharyngeal duct
- 253 Disorders of the pituitary gland and its hypothalamic control
  – 253.0 Acromegaly and gigantism
  – 253.1 Other and unspecified anterior pituitary function hyperfunction
  – 253.2 Panhypopituitarism
  – 253.4 Other anterior pituitary disorders
  – 253.5 Diabetes insipidus
  – 253.6 Other disorders of neurohypophysis
  – 253.7 Iatrogenic pituitary disorders
  – 253.8 Other disorders of the pituitary and other syndromes of diencephalohypophysial origin
- 628 Infertility, female
  – 628.1 Of pituitary-hypothalamic origin

PATIENT TEACHING

- Patients desiring pregnancy should not attempt to conceive until resumption of normal menstrual periods.
- Patients should be cautioned about the side effects of medications.
- Patients should be cautioned to seek care should they develop any visual symptoms or develop recurrent headaches.
- Women treated for hypopituitarism must be instructed on seeking care for any illness and should always carry information with them about the medications (especially adrenocorticoids) they are taking:
  – They should be instructed to double or triple their corticosteroid dosage when under stress, as typified by infection, trauma, and major surgery.

POLYCYSTIC OVARIAN SYNDROME (PCOS)

Mira Aubuchon, MD

 BASICS

DESCRIPTION
The cardinal features of PCOS have been described by international consensus and consist of ovarian dysfunction along with hyperandrogenism and polycystic ovary (PCO) morphology. PCOS is a syndrome and, as such, no single diagnostic criterion is sufficient for clinical diagnosis.
- Chronic hyperandrogenic anovulation
- Insulin-resistant state

Age-Related Factors
Usually postmenarchal and premenopausal

EPIDEMIOLOGY
- 5–10% of reproductive-age women
- 75% obese, 25% lean

RISK FACTORS
- Largely unknown
- Weight gain
- Familial/Genetic component

Genetics
- High association of PCOS in sisters of PCOS patients
- Possible altered gene near insulin receptor (chromosome 19p13.2)

PATHOPHYSIOLOGY
- Altered GnRH secretion, disordered pituitary LH and FSH:
  – Impaired ovarian folliculogenesis and anovulation, unopposed estrogen
  – Hyperandrogenism and hirsutism:
    ○ Decreased liver SHBG
    ○ Adipose aromatizes to estrogen, endometrial hyperplasia risk
- Insulin resistance and pancreatic cell dysfunction:
  – Increased theca cell androgens perpetuate ovarian dysfunction
  – Increased IGF1 decreases liver SHBG, worsens hirsutism

ASSOCIATED CONDITIONS
- Obesity (See Diet: Obesity.)
- Infertility (see topic)
- Hirsutism (see topic)
- Acne
- Endometrial hyperplasia and cancer (See Endometrial Hyperplasia and Endometrial Cancer.)
- Depression
- Sleep disorders (see topic)
- Hypertension (see topic)
- Insulin resistance
- DM Type 2
- Metabolic syndrome (see topic)
- Cardiovascular disease

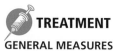 **DIAGNOSIS**

SIGNS AND SYMPTOMS
History
- Oligo-ovulation:
  – Amenorrhea (see chapter)
  – Oligomenorrhea (See Bleeding, Abnormal Uterine: Oligomenorrhea.)
  – Menorrhagia/Heavy bleeding (See Bleeding, Abnormal Uterine: Heavy Menstrual Bleeding.)
- Midline hair growth, acne, hair thinning or loss, voice changes
- Infertility, desire for fertility
- History of gestational DM or HTN
- Overweight/Obesity/Weight gain
- Family history DM or cardiovascular disease
- Individual goals for treatment

Review of Systems
- Mood, appetite, energy, sleep
- Weight and diet

Physical Exam
- BP, pulse, height, weight, BMI, waist circumference, hip circumference, waist:hip ratio
- Thyroid: Nodules, enlargement
- Skin:
  – Acanthosis nigricans, acne, hirsutism, balding, skin tags
- Breast: Galactorrhea
- Abdomen: Masses or organomegaly
- Extremities: Edema, DTRs
- GU: Clitoromegaly, adnexal masses

TESTS
Rotterdam Criteria (2/3 with other causes of hyperandrogenism excluded):
- Oligo- or anovulation
- Clinical and/or biochemical signs of hyperandrogenism
- PCO (on US)

Labs
- Pregnancy test
- Clinical criteria may be sufficient, with labs to rule out other causes
- TSH, Free T4, prolactin, DHEAS, total testosterone, 17-hydroxyprogesterone
- Fasting lipids, glucose and 2-hour GTT after 75-gm load
- No longer considered useful:
  – LH:FSH ratio (pulsatile, can be normal in PCOS)
  – Fasting glucose:insulin ratio (can miss glucose tolerance aberrations)

Imaging
- TVU: >12 antral (<10 mm) follicles on a single ovary or ovarian volume >10 cm^3
- Endometrial thickness

DIFFERENTIAL DIAGNOSIS
- Pregnancy
- Prolactinoma
- Thyroid dysfunction (See Thyroid Disease.)
- Androgen-secreting tumor (See Ovarian Tumors, Virilizing.)
- Adrenal enzyme defect:
  – Late onset CAH (See Congenital Adrenal Hyperplasia.)
- Cushing's disease

Metabolic/Endocrine
- Impaired fasting glucose (IFG):
  – >100 mg/dL
- Impaired glucose tolerance (IGT):
  – 2-hour glucose >140 mg/dL
- DM:
  – Glucose fasting >126 mg/dL or 2-hour >200 mg/dL
- Metabolic syndrome (3 or more of):
  – WC >85 cm (35 in)
  – IGT or IFG
  – SBP ≥140 mm Hg or DBP ≥85 mm Hg
  – Triglycerides ≥150 mg/dL
  – HDL cholesterol <50 mg/dL

Tumor/Malignancy
- Risk of endometrial hyperplasia and malignancy
- Consider endometrial biopsy:
  – US EC >9 mm
  – <2 menses/year

TREATMENT

GENERAL MEASURES
If overweight or obese:
- 5–10% weight loss to improve ovulation, hirsutism, fertility, pregnancy safety
- Calorie restriction, 30 minutes of vigorous exercise 5 times a week
- If IGT, lifestyle modification better than medication at preventing DM and metabolic syndrome

MEDICATION (DRUGS)
- Endometrial protection: OCPs (monitor lipids and BP) or progestin withdrawal every 3–4 months
- Hirsutism control (try modalities for 6 months)
  – OCPs
  – Antiandrogens (use contraception)
    ○ Spironolactone 100–200 mg/d (monitor electrolytes)
    ○ Flutamide 130–500 mg/d (hepatotoxicity)
  – Eflornithine cream (Vaniqa): b.i.d. only on face
  – Rosiglitazone (4–8 mg/d): Mild improvement:
    ○ Monitor electrolytes, kidney, liver function
    ○ ± Weight gain (water retention)

- Metabolic (controversial for adolescents):
  – Metformin HCl 1,500 mg–2,000 mg/d for prevention of DM and metabolic syndrome if IGT:
    ○ Nausea, diarrhea, fatigue, ± weight loss; start 500 mg and increase slowly
    ○ Rare-lactic acidosis; Monitor electrolytes, liver, kidney every 6–12 months
    ○ Hold drug for surgery or contrast dye

Pregnancy Considerations
- Ovulation Induction with timed intercourse, intrauterine insemination, or IVF
- Insulin sensitizers, alone or with clomiphene:
  – Metformin 1,500 mg/d (Category B):
    ○ May improve miscarriage rate if continued during pregnancy (but studies are small)
  – Rosiglitazone 4–8 mg/d (Category C)
- Clomiphene citrate, 50–200 mg/d, 4–6 cycles:
  – Cycle days 3–7 or 5–9
  – Alone or with insulin sensitizer
  – 8–10% multiple pregnancy rate
  – Vasomotor effects, visual symptoms (d/c)
- Aromatase inhibitors (Letrozole): 5 mg/d, 4–6 cycles (use instead of clomiphene controversial)
- Gonadotropin injections, FSH or LH:
  – 20–30% multiple pregnancy rate
  – Higher risk of ovarian hyperstimulation syndrome

SURGERY
Ovarian drilling/diathermy via laparoscopy:
- Similar live birth rates to gonadotropin injections
  – Temporary (6 months) spontaneous ovulation
  – Risk of adhesion formation

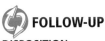 FOLLOW-UP

DISPOSITION
Issues for Referral
- Consider referral for nutrition/dietary counseling
- May need specialist for management of cardiovascular risks:
  – Hyperlipidemia
  – HTN
  – DM
- May need to consult dermatology:
  – Moderate-severe acne with scarring
- Hair removal:
  – Electrolysis is only permanent method
  – Laser is long-lasting
  – Depilatories, bleaching, waxing, shaving for hirsutism

PROGNOSIS
- With appropriate diagnosis and management, symptoms can be controlled.
- Surveillance and active management may minimize cardiovascular risks.
- Treatment with OCPs or progestin can minimize menstrual irregularities and decrease risks of endometrial cancer.

PATIENT MONITORING
- Lipids every year if abnormal
- Fasting glucose and 2-hour GTT every 3 years
- Monitor menses, BP, weight, WC every 6 months to 1 year

BIBLIOGRAPHY

Legro RS, et al. Detecting insulin resistance in polycystic ovary syndrome: Purposes and pitfalls. *Obstetrical*. 2004;59(2):141–154.

Cheung AP. Ultrasound and menstrual history in predicting endometrial hyperplasia in polycystic ovary syndrome. *Obstet Gynecol*. 2001;98(2): 325–331.

Ehrmann DA. Polycystic ovary syndrome. *N Engl J Med*. 2005;352(12):1223–1236.

Guzick DS. Polycystic ovary syndrome. *Obstet Gynecol*. 2004;103(1):181–193.

Orchard TJ, et al. The effect of metformin and intensive lifestyle intervention on the metabolic syndrome: The Diabetes Prevention Program randomized trial. *Ann Intern Med*. 2005;142(8):611–619.

Revised 2003 consensus on diagnostic criteria and long-term health risks related to polycystic ovary syndrome (PCOS). *Hum Reprod*. 2004;19(1):41–47.

Urbanek M, et al. Candidate gene region for polycystic ovary syndrome on chromosome 19p13.2. *J Clin Endocrinol Metab*. 2005;90(12):6623–6629.

 MISCELLANEOUS

SYNONYM(S)
- Syndrome XX
- Stein-Leventhal syndrome

CLINICAL PEARLS
- Signs and symptoms of PCOS may begin in adolescence. Severely irregular menses with moderate to severe acne and/or hirsutism should not be dismissed as "normal adolescence."
- Coordination of care between primary care, dermatology, endocrinology, and gynecology is essential.

ABBREVIATIONS
- CAH—Congenital adrenal hyperplasia
- DBP—Diastolic blood pressure
- DHEAS—Dehydroepiandrosterone sulfate
- DM—Diabetes mellitus
- DTR—Deep tendon reflexes
- FSH—Follicle-stimulating hormone
- GnRH—Gonadotropin-releasing hormone
- GTT—Glucose tolerance test
- HTN—Hypertension
- IFG—Impaired fasting glucose
- IGT—Impaired glucose tolerance
- IVF—In vitro fertilization
- LH—Luteinizing hormone
- OCP—Oral contraceptive pills
- SBP—Systolic blood pressure
- SHBG—Sex hormone binding globulin
- T4—Thyroxine
- TSH—Thyroid-stimulating hormone
- US EC—Ultrasound endometrial complex
- WC—Waist circumference

CODES
ICD9-CM
628.0, 256.4 Polycystic ovarian syndrome

 PATIENT TEACHING

- Lifestyle modification is key
- Focus on chronic disease management and prevention of cardiovascular risks
- http://www.asrm.org/Patients/FactSheets/PCOS.pdf
- http://4women.gov/faq/pcos.htm
- http://www.acog.org/publications/patient_education/bp121.cfm

PREMENSTRUAL SYNDROME (PMS) AND PREMENSTRUAL DYSPHORIC DISORDER (PMDD)

Michelle McDonald, MS
Andrea Rapkin, MD

BASICS

DESCRIPTION
Premenstrual syndrome (PMS) and premenstrual dysphoric disorder (PMDD) comprise a spectrum of premenstrual disorders. The disorders include affective, somatic and behavioral symptoms that occur during the luteal phase of the menstrual cycle and abate soon after onset of menses.
- PMS includes a constellation of bothersome emotional or physical symptoms that affect but tend not to significantly impair level of functioning.
- PMDD is a severe form of PMS encompassing emotional and physical symptoms, with at least one severe emotional symptom causing a marked degree of impairment in woman's social and occupational activities:
  - Affective/Behavioral symptoms: Mood swings, depression, anxiety, irritability, tension, difficulty concentrating, feeling out of control
  - Physical symptoms: Abdominal bloating, breast tenderness, headache, fatigue, increased appetite and food cravings

Age-Related Factors
Symptoms are present in ovulatory, postmenarchal females, and cease during pregnancy and after menopause.

EPIDEMIOLOGY
- Prevalence: An estimated 20–40% of reproductive age women experience PMS.
- 3–8% of reproductive-age women meet criteria for PMDD.
- Prevalence does not appear to depend on socioeconomic, cultural, or ethnic factors.

RISK FACTORS
- Increases with age within the reproductive years (peak late 30s).
- Personal or family history of past psychiatric disorder:
  - History of depressive disorder appears to increase severity and duration of depressive premenstrual mood changes
- History of sexual abuse or domestic violence.
- Stress may precipitate condition.

Genetics
- Concordance rate is 2 times higher in monozygotic vs. dizygotic twins.
- Genetic tendency toward developing PMDD and other psychiatric disorders

PATHOPHYSIOLOGY
- Results from interaction between cyclic changes in ovarian steroids with central neurotransmitters
- Changes in hormone levels affect neurotransmitters in the CNS.
- Serotonin is the most implicated neurotransmitter.

- γ-Aminobutyric acid (GABA):
  - Major inhibitory neurotransmitter
  - The progesterone metabolite, allopregnanolone is a potent neuroactive steroid that binds $GABA_A$ receptors and modulates GABA-ergic transmission
  - A malfunctioning $GABA_A$ receptor system may result in altered neuroactive steroid sensitivity during the luteal phase in women with PMS/PMDD.

ASSOCIATED CONDITIONS
- Affective disorders
- Anxiety disorders

DIAGNOSIS

SIGNS AND SYMPTOMS
History
- Symptoms must be cyclical and begin in the luteal phase with cessation by end of menses.
- Obtain record of symptoms, including severity and timing
- Regularity of cycle (21–35 days), suggesting ovulation
- History of mood or anxiety disorder may be a "red flag" for premenstrual exacerbation of underlying psychiatric diagnosis
- PMDD and PMS diagnostic criteria:
- Comprehensive assessment of symptoms with patient's daily rating of symptoms for at least two consecutive menstrual cycles:
  - Based on symptoms, severity, timing and exclusion of other diagnoses.
  - Criteria must be confirmed by prospective daily ratings.*
  - Symptoms emerge in second half of menstrual cycle and subside shortly after onset of menstruation OR symptoms must occur within the 5 days before onset of menses and not recur until after day 13 of the cycle.*
  - Interference with work/school and social activities/relationships (subjective impairment for PMDD and bothersome for PMS).*
  - May be superimposed on other psychiatric or medical disorders provided it is not merely an exacerbation of that disorder.*
  - Most commonly used diagnostic criteria are the American Psychiatric Association (DSM-IV) criteria for PMDD and the ACOG criteria for PMS.
- DSM-IV criteria for PMDD: At least 5 symptoms, including 1 of the 1st 4, with moderate to severe intensity, plus above:*
  - Depressed mood
  - Anxiety, tension
  - Labile mood
  - Irritability, anger
  - Decreased interest in usual activities
  - Difficulty concentrating
  - Fatigue, tiredness
  - Appetite changes (overeating/cravings)
  - Hypersomnia/Insomnia
  - Feeling out of control/overwhelmed
  - Physical symptoms: Breast tenderness, bloating, headache, joint/muscle pain

- ACOG Criteria for PMS:
  - 1 or more bothersome affective or somatic symptoms, plus above*
- *Necessary for both PMDD and PMS diagnosis

Review of Systems
Rule out other medical or psychiatric disorders in the differential diagnosis

Physical Exam
Normal

TESTS
- No definitive diagnostic test exists.
- The patient's report of her experience is the only source of information on which to base a diagnosis.
- Diagnosis based on prospective rating. Severity rating must be an integral part of daily rating scales. For example a scale of 0–4 (0 = no symptoms, 4 = severe symptoms).
- Validated prospective questions include (but not limited to): Visual Analog Scale (VAS) and Daily Record of Severity of Problems (DRSP)
  - DRSP includes symptoms needed for DSM-IV PMDD diagnostic criteria.
  - Sample available at www.pmdd.factsforhealth.org/drsp/drsp_month.pdf

Labs
Limited to screening for other medical disorders in differential diagnosis:
- CBC, chemistry profile, TSH, day 3 FSH if indicated by history and exam

Imaging
Imaging is not used in diagnosis

DIFFERENTIAL DIAGNOSIS
Exclude other disorders including:
- Breast disorders
- PCOS
- Postpartum disorders
- Perimenopause
- Chronic pelvic pain, endometriosis
- Anemia
- Connective tissue disease
- Chronic fatigue syndrome
- Thyroid disease
- Depressive, anxiety, panic disorder,
- Drug or alcohol abuse

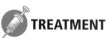

TREATMENT

GENERAL MEASURES
- Initial treatment for PMS should be nonpharmacologic and geared toward lifestyle changes. PMDD usually requires pharmacologic treatment.
- Nonpharmacologic therapy can ensue during prospective recording months.

Diet
- Limit caffeine, alcohol, and sodium intake
- Increase consumption of dairy and complex carbohydrates:
  - No RCT to support this

Activity
Aerobic activity at least 30 minutes, a least 3 times a week:
- No RCT to support this

Dietary Supplementation
- Vitamin B_6 50–100 mg/d:
  - Meta-analysis shows there may be a reduction in physical and depressive symptoms. Doses of 200 mg/d or greater are associated with peripheral neuropathy
- Calcium carbonate 1,200 mg/d in luteal phase

SPECIAL THERAPY
Complementary and Alternative Therapies
- CBT and relaxation therapy. Studies of efficacy generally positive.
- Herbal preparations are not studied adequately:
  - Chaste berry fruit (*Vitex agnus castus*): 20 mg/d more effective than placebo in small trial

ALERT
Chaste berry fruit is unsafe during pregnancy.

MEDICATION (DRUGS)
- For more severe symptoms of PMS or PMDD SSRIs are drug of choice:
  - Should be given an adequate trial of 2 months before initiating another SSRI for treatment failure
  - Many RCTs have shown that SSRIs are superior to placebo
  - Continuous dosing or dosing only during luteal phase may be equally effective
  - Fluoxetine 10–20 mg/d*, sertraline 50–150 mg/d*, paroxetine 10–30 mg/d*, or paroxetine CR 12.5–25 mg/d*, citalopram 20–40 mg/d
- Other antidepressants:
  - Fluvoxamine 25–50 mg/d
  - Venlafaxine 75–150 mg/d
- Anxiolytics (luteal phase only):
  - Buspirone: 5 HT-1 agonist, 10 mg/d to t.i.d.:
    - Try 1st, as no addictive potential
  - Alprazolam: Benzodiazepine, 0.5–1 mg t.i.d.:
    - Results contradictory; limited by an abuse potential
- Ovulation suppression:
  - OCPs:
    - Most OCPs do not affect premenstrual mood but can help with somatic symptoms.
    - OC formulation containing 20 μg EE and 3 mg drospirenone with 24-day hormonal interval followed by a 4-day hormone free interval has been shown to be effective for the treatment of PMDD.
    - Drospirenone, a new progestin, is an analogue of spirolactone; US FDA indication for PMDD.
    - Continuous low-dose OCPs may prove effective.

- GnRH agonists:
  - Try after SSRIs, OCPs, anxiolytics have failed
  - Leuprolide 3.75 mg IM every month or 11.25 mg IM every 3 months:
    - Hypoestrogenic effects limit use.
  - Danazol 200–600 mg/d:
    - Androgenic effects limits use; risk of virilization of fetus if women becomes pregnant
- Diuretics:
  - Spironolactone 25–100 mg/d during luteal phase improves bloating and weight gain. May improve emotional symptoms
  - NSAIDs helpful for physical symptoms.

SURGERY
- Hysterectomy with bilateral oophorectomy is curative as demonstrated in RTC.
- Indications for surgery:
  - Recalcitrant cases: Previous therapies have been adequately pursued but failed
  - Evaluate by a psychiatrist to preclude psychiatric comorbidities
  - Completed childbearing
  - Consider diagnostic trial of GnRH agonist with estrogen add-back for 3–6 months

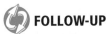 ## FOLLOW-UP

DISPOSITION
Issues for Referral
- Patients should record symptoms during 2 consecutive menstrual cycles:
  - Ascertain diagnosis and begin treatment based on symptom complex.
  - Re-evaluate therapy after 2 months.
  - If stable, monitor patient every 4–6 months.
  - Continue effective treatment for at least 9–12 months, but long-term therapy usually necessary.
- Consider psychiatric referral when:
  - Treatment ineffective and mood symptoms are severe
  - Suicidal ideation

PROGNOSIS
- Treatment response rate 65–85% for each modality
- Symptoms recur upon cessation of treatment but cease with pregnancy or menopause.
- Concern and risk for postpartum and perimenopausal depression

PATIENT MONITORING
Complications may include side effects of medical treatment.

BIBLIOGRAPHY
ACOG Practice Bulletin. Premenstrual syndrome. *Obstet Gynecol*. 2000;95:4.

Grady-Weliky TA. Clinical practice. Premenstrual dysphoric disorder. *N Engl J Med*. 2003;348(5): 433–438.

Johnson S. Premenstrual syndrome, premenstrual dysphoric disorder, and beyond: A clinical primer for practitioners. *Obstet Gynecol*. 2004;104(4): 845–859.

Pearlstein TB. Hormonal and nonpharmacologic treatments for premenstrual syndrome and premenstrual dysphoric disorder. *Prim Psychiatry*. 2004;11:48–52.

Premenstrual dysphoric disorder. In: *Diagnostic and Statistical Manual of Mental Disorders*, 4th ed., Text Rev. Washington, DC: American Psychiatric Association; 2004:771–774.

Winer SA, et al. Premenstrual disorders: Prevalence, etiology and impact. *J Reprod Med*. 2006; 51(4 Suppl):229–347.

Yonkers KA, et al. Efficacy of a new low-dose oral contraceptive with drospirenone in premenstrual dysphoric disorder. *Obstet Gynecol*. 2005; 106(3):492–501.

 ## MISCELLANEOUS
SYNONYM(S)
- Menstrually related mood disorders
- Premenstrual disorders

ABBREVIATIONS
- ACOG—American College of Obstetricians and Gynecologists
- CBT—Cognitive behavioral therapy
- CNS—Central nervous system
- DSM-IV—Diagnostic and Statistical Manual of Mental Disorders, 4th ed.
- EE—Ethynyl estradiol
- FSH—Follicle-stimulating hormone
- GABA—γ-Aminobutyric acid
- GnRH—Gonadotropin-releasing hormone
- NSAIDs—Nonsteroidal anti-inflammatory drugs
- OCPs—Oral contraceptive pills
- PCOS—Polycystic ovary syndrome
- RCT—Randomized controlled trial
- SSRI—Selective serotonin reuptake inhibitor
- TSH—Thyroid-stimulating hormone

CODES
ICD9-CM
625.4 PMS or PMDD

 ## PATIENT TEACHING

- Cycle and symptom monitoring
- Stress reduction

RECTO-VAGINAL FISTULA

Amreen Husain, MD
Melanie Santos, MD

 BASICS

DESCRIPTION
Abnormal epithelial-lined tract between rectum and vagina

Pediatric Considerations
Rare except as sequelae of sexual abuse with penetration and vaginal trauma

Pregnancy Considerations
Obstetric trauma is the most common cause (see below).

Staging
- Location:
  - Low: Vaginal opening near posterior fourchette
  - Mid: From level of cervix to superior to posterior fourchette
  - High: Area of posterior fornix
- Size:
  - Small: <0.5 cm in diameter
  - Medium: 0.5–2.5 cm in diameter
  - Large: >2.5 cm in diameter

EPIDEMIOLOGY
- Incidence is specific to etiology.
- Obstetric trauma:
  - Most common cause; up to 88%
  - ~5% of vaginal deliveries result in 3rd- or 4th-degree tears:
    ○ 1–2% lead to rectovaginal fistulas
- Radiation-induced:
  - Second most common cause
  - Occurs in <2% of patients
  - Incidence increases when radiation dose exceeds 5,000 cGy

RISK FACTORS
- Congenital anorectal anomalies
- Obstetric trauma
- Operative trauma
- Violent trauma
- IBD
- Infectious
- Radiation
- Carcinoma

PATHOPHYSIOLOGY
- Congenital:
  - Rare, and associated with imperforate anus and other anorectal anomalies
- Obstetric trauma:
  - Associated with prolonged labor, difficult forceps delivery, shoulder dystocia, midline episiotomy
  - Failed recognition of 4th-degree injury postpartum
  - Secondary infection of wound with breakdown of repair
  - Usually appears 7–10 days after delivery, though can develop immediately

- Operative trauma:
  - Vaginal, rectal, or pelvic operations
  - May be aggravated by extensive adhesions in the rectovaginal septum associated with endometriosis, PID, or pelvic malignancy
- Violent trauma:
  - Blunt instrumentation or penetrating trauma
  - Sexual assault
- IBD:
  - Most often Crohn's disease
  - In relation to perirectal abscess, manifesting as complicated perianal sepsis
- Infectious:
  - Cryptoglandular infections of the anorectal region
  - Most commonly associated with perianal abscess and diverticulitis
  - Less often associated with tuberculosis, lymphogranuloma venereum, and Bartholin gland abscess
- Radiation:
  - Complication of therapy
  - Increased risk with diabetes, hypertension, smoking, prior abdominal or pelvic surgery
  - Usually appears 6 months to 2 years after completion of therapy
  - Fistulas occurring during therapy are usually due to tumor regression.
- Carcinoma:
  - Include tumors of the anal canal, rectum, and gynecologic organs
  - Can be primary, recurrent, or metastatic disease

ASSOCIATED CONDITIONS
Fecal/Flatal incontinence:
- Incidence up to 48%

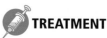 **DIAGNOSIS**

SIGNS AND SYMPTOMS
History
- Prior history of complicated vaginal delivery, anorectal surgery, IBD, malignancy, and/or radiation therapy
- Degree of fecal/flatal continence

Review of Systems
- Uncontrolled passage of gas and/or stool through vagina
- Foul-smelling vagina
- Vaginitis or cystitis
- Bloody or mucous-rich diarrhea
- Rectal bleeding
- Few patients are asymptomatic.

Physical Exam
- Inspection of vagina, rectum, perineum
- Identification of location, size, and number of openings:
  - Thin probe from vagina through fistulous tract
  - Rigid proctoscopy for identification if difficult
- Assess anal continence
- Proctosigmoidoscopy:
  - Assess rectal compliance and health of rectal mucosa

TESTS
- Anal manometry
- Pudendal nerve terminal motor latency testing (less commonly used)

Labs
Primarily to assess for sepsis and establish preoperative baseline:
- CBC, blood cultures, metabolic panel, type and screen

Imaging
- Endo-anal US
- Contrast studies:
  - Vaginography
  - Barium enema
  - CT scan of abdomen and pelvis

DIFFERENTIAL DIAGNOSIS
- Enterovaginal fistula
- Colovaginal fistula

TREATMENT

GENERAL MEASURES
- Most small fistulas, especially those associated with IBD, may be managed with a conservative medical approach to allow spontaneous closure of fistula.
- Delay surgical treatment several weeks after development of fistula to allow surrounding inflammation to resolve.
- With large fistulas, consider initial diverting colostomy followed by repair of fistula with subsequent colostomy takedown once fistula closure is well healed.
- If a malignancy is suspected, perform biopsy.

SPECIAL THERAPY
Complementary and Alternative Therapies
Conservative medical therapy:
- Local care
- Drainage of abscesses
- Directed antibiotic therapy
- Allow 6–12 weeks for proper tissue healing
- Include dietary modification and fiber supplementation

MEDICATION (DRUGS)
- All patients should be placed on directed antibiotic therapy and proper bowel regimen to reduce the fecal stream.
- IBD:
  - Initiate appropriate medical therapy
  - Increased risk of failure of fistula repair in patient on steroids
  - Repair can be maintained while on 6-mercaptopurine or azathioprine.
  - Use of infliximab associated with poor healing of fistula but dramatic improvement of symptoms

SURGERY
- Preoperative details:
  - Complete mechanical bowel preparation
  - IV antibiotic prophylaxis
  - Thorough vaginal preparation with antiseptic solution
- Low rectovaginal fistula: Transvaginal approach:
  - Transvaginal circular excision around fistula
  - Separate vagina from underlying rectal wall via sharp dissection
  - Excise fistula after mobilization of vagina
  - Placement of 3-0 delayed absorbable interrupted sutures through muscularis and mucosa of anterior anal canal, with suture line 5–8 mm above and below site of fistulous tract
  - 2nd layer placed 5 mm above and below primary suture line, inverting initial suture line into rectum
  - Approximate puborectalis muscle and external anal sphincter for 3rd layer of anal wall closure
  - Approximate vaginal wall
- Low rectovaginal fistula with associated sphincter defect: Transperineal approach:
  - Divide bridge of skin, sphincter, and perineal body to convert to 4th-degree tear
  - Excise fistulous tract and mobilize posterior vaginal wall from anterior anal wall
  - Reconstruct anal canal with interrupted or running fine delayed absorbable sutures in 2 layers as above
  - Reapproximate retracted ends of external anal sphincter in midline in end-to-end fashion
  - Alternatively, may perform overlapping sphincteroplasty
  - Consider transanal/endorectal flap, involving lower portion of rectovaginal septum
  - Complete repair as a 4th-degree tear
- Repair of radiation-induced fistula:
  - Requires aggressive excision of surrounding radiation-damaged tissues with utilization of pedicled bulbocavernosus muscle with overlying labial fat pad (Martius procedure)
  - Determine sites for bilateral pedicled bulbocavernosus flaps
  - Circumferentially separate scarred vagina from underlying anterior rectal wall
  - Excise edge of scarred vaginal epithelium adjacent to edge of rectal mucosa
  - Create subcutaneous tunnel with Mayo scissors from labium majus to fistula under labium and vaginal mucosa
  - Guide flap through tunnel
  - Suture edge of squamous epithelium from vulvar graft to edge of rectal mucosa with 4-0 delayed absorbable sutures
  - Suture muscle and subcutaneous tissue of graft to surrounding connective tissue
  - Develop simple pedicled graft from opposite labium and approximate skin of vulva to skin of vagina
  - Small suction catheter placed between the 2 pedicled grafts and brought out through stab wound to perineal incision
  - Reapproximate vulvar incisions with fine delayed absorbable sutures
  - May also consider sartorius or gracilis free flaps
  - Consider fecal diversion
- Repair of fistula with severe Crohn disease:
  - Proctectomy
- Transanal approach:
  - Preferred by colorectal surgeons

FOLLOW-UP

DISPOSITION
Issues for Referral
With fistula involving the upper rectum or other complicated fistula, consult specialist

PROGNOSIS
- With proper repair, small fistulae heal in 90–95% of cases.
- ~50% of small fistulae may heal spontaneously.
- Prognosis is poor with recurrent fistulas.
- With radiation-induced fistulae, repair may compromise vagina with significant colpocleisis, with further contracture and stenosis of vagina, resulting in significant dyspareunia.

PATIENT MONITORING
- Immediately postoperative care:
  - Follow patient's bowel habits because constipation and diarrhea can disrupt the repair; the goal is soft, formed stools.
  - Counsel patient on diet, high fluid intake, use of stool softeners.
  - Consider use of bulking agents.
  - Oral broad-spectrum antibiotics
  - Monitor for bleeding, signs of infection.
- 2 weeks postoperative:
  - Evaluate wounds and bowel habits.
  - Evaluate for bleeding, signs of infection, increased risk of recurrence.

BIBLIOGRAPHY
Berek JS, ed. *Berek & Novak's Gynecology*. 14th ed. Philadelphia: Lippincott Williams & Wilkins; 2007.

Rock JA, et al., eds. *TeLinde's Operative Gynecology* 9th ed. Philadelphia: Lippincott Williams & Wilkins; 2003.

Saclarides TJ. Rectovaginal fistula. *Surg Clin N Am*. 2002;82:1261–1272.

Tsang CBS, et al. Anal sphincter integrity and function influences outcome in rectovaginal fistula repair. *Dis Colon Rectum*. 1998;41:1141–1146.

Venkatesh KS, et al. Anorectal complications of vaginal delivery. *Dis Colon Rectum*. 1989;32:1039–1041.

MISCELLANEOUS

ABBREVIATIONS
- IBD—Inflammatory bowel disease
- PID—Pelvic inflammatory disease

CODES
ICD9-CM
619.1 Recto-vaginal fistula

PATIENT TEACHING

- Dietary modifications:
  - High fluid intake
  - Fiber supplementation
- Bowel habits:
  - Use of stool softeners
  - Consider bulking agents
- Hygiene:
  - Local care with sitz baths

PREVENTION
Prevention is etiology-specific:
- Avoid trauma
- With disease-associated fistula development, control of disease is essential (IBD, infections, malignancy).
- With radiation-induced fistulas, importance of control/cessation of comorbidities (diabetes, hypertension, smoking)

Tarita Pakrashi, MD, MPH

 BASICS

DESCRIPTION
- Chlamydia is a common STI caused by the bacterium *Chlamydia trachomatis*.
- Can be transmitted during vaginal, anal, or oral sex
- Asymptomatic infection is common.

Age-Related Factors
Highest prevalence of infection in persons aged ≤25 years

Pediatric Considerations
- Chlamydia is transmitted via the birth canal of an infected mother, and neonates exposed to chlamydia at birth may develop conjunctivitis 5–13 days later.
- Neonates who have been exposed to an infected birth canal can also develop chlamydial pneumonia.

Pregnancy Considerations
Screening should occur during routine prenatal care.

EPIDEMIOLOGY
- Highest rates among females 15–19 years, followed by females 20–24 years.
  - Screening in family planning clinics: ~6% infected
  - More common among young women than young men:
    ○ Related in part to more screening in women
- African American women more likely to have Chlamydia (1,729.0/100,000) than American Indian/Alaska Native women (1,177.7/100,000); Hispanic females (733.2/100,000) > white females (237.2/100,000) > Asian/Pacific Islander women (222.3/100,000)
- Most frequently reported infectious disease in the US
- Most frequently reported bacterial STD in the US
- In 2005, >975,000 cases were reported in U.S.
- Most chlamydial infections go undiagnosed
- CDC estimate ~2.8 million new cases in the US each year

RISK FACTORS
- Sexually active women ≤25 years
- Women with new sex partner(s)
- Women with multiple sexual partners
- Inconsistent use of barrier contraception
- Unmarried status
- Women with a prior history of sexually transmitted disease

PATHOPHYSIOLOGY
- *C. trachomatis* is an obligate, intracellular bacterium with a biphasic life cycle.
- Metabolically inactive infectious particles are called elementary bodies.
- In a host cell, the elementary bodies transform into reticulate bodies.
- Reticulate bodies use the ATP from the host cell and after some time they transform back into elementary bodies and then exit the cell to continue propagating the infection.
- With infection a humoral response is evoked with IgA, IgM and IgG.

ASSOCIATED CONDITIONS
- Other STDs such as HIV and Gonorrhea
- Health consequences for women:
  - PID:
    ○ Up to 40% of those with untreated chlamydia
  - Ectopic pregnancy
  - Infertility
    ○ Up to 20% of those with PID

 DIAGNOSIS

SIGNS AND SYMPTOMS
History
- Most often asymptomatic in both men and women
- Mucopurulent endocervical discharge
- Dysuria
- Dyspareunia
- Intermenstrual spotting
- Sexual history:
  - Number of partners (male, female, or both within last 2 months, last 12 months)
  - Contraceptive methods/protection against STD's
  - Sexual practices (oral sex, vaginal intercourse, anal intercourse)
  - Specific questions about use of condoms
- Past history of STD/PID
- History of sexual abuse

Review of Systems
Special attention to GI and GU systems

Physical Exam
- Abdominal:
  - Masses
  - Tenderness, including guarding, rebound tenderness

- Pelvic:
  - Pelvic exam in older adolescent or adult.
    ○ Speculum exam with cervical testing for STDs
    ○ Bimanual exam to assess uterine size, shape, position, mobility, and tenderness including cervical motion tenderness
    ○ Bimanual exam to assess adnexal enlargement or tenderness

TESTS
Lab
- Urine hCG to rule out pregnancy
- Vaginal wet mount, STD testing by testing urine or swab specimens either by culture, direct immunofluorescence, EIA, nucleic acid hybridization or NAAT's
- PAP smear as indicated
- Urinalysis, if indicated by symptoms

Imaging
Ultrasound to define anatomy as indicated

DIFFERENTIAL DIAGNOSIS
Infection
- Gonorrhea, trichomoniasis, ureaplasma infection, mycoplasma genitalium, bacterial vaginosis (See Sexually Transmitted Diseases (STDs): Gonorrhea, Sexually Transmitted Diseases (STDs): Trichomonas, and Vaginitis: Bacterial Vaginosis.)
- Urinary tract infection (See Urinary Tract Infection, Urinary Symptoms: Dysuria, and Urinary Symptoms: Frequency.)

Other/Miscellaneous
Vaginal foreign body:
- Retained tampon

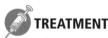 **TREATMENT**

GENERAL MEASURES
- Notification and presumptive treatment of sex partners, workup for other common STDs and providing barrier contraceptives as well as counseling about safer sex practices.
- Advise patient to abstain from sexual intercourse until they and their sex partners are completely treated.
- Abstinence for 7 days after a single-dose regimen or after completion of a 7-day regimen.
- Patients who have gonococcal infection are frequently coinfected with *C. trachomatis* and hence presumptive treatment for Chlamydial infection in a setting of gonorrhea may be appropriate while awaiting test results.

MEDICATION (DRUGS)

- For nonpregnant women and adolescents, recommended regimen by CDC:
  - Azithromycin 1 g PO
  - Doxycycline 100 mg PO b.i.d. for 7 days
- Alternative regimens:
  - Erythromycin base 500 mg PO q.i.d. for 7 days
  - Erythromycin ethylsuccinate 800 mg PO q.i.d. for 7 days
  - Ofloxacin 300 mg PO b.i.d. for 7 days
  - Levofloxacin 500 mg PO once a day for 7 days

Pregnancy Considerations

- During pregnancy, Erythromycin estolate, doxycycline and fluoroquinolones are contraindicated, and hence the recommended regimens are:
  - Azithromycin 1g PO in a single dose
  - Amoxicillin 500 mg PO t.i.d. times a day for 7 days
- Alternative regimens:
  - Erythromycin base 500 mg PO q.i.d.for 7 days
  - Erythromycin base 250 mg PO q.i.d. for 14 days
  - Erythromycin ethylsuccinate 800 mg PO q.i.d. for 7 days
  - Erythromycin ethylsuccinate 400 mg PO q.i.d. for 14 days

 FOLLOW-UP

- Repeat testing (test-of-cure) in 3–4 weeks after completion of therapy is indicated only in:
  - Pregnant women
  - Cases of questionable compliance to therapy
  - Persistent symptoms or reinfection
- Repeat infections increase the risk of PID and hence the CDC advises repeat testing of women diagnosed with chlamydia in ~3 months after treatment.

PROGNOSIS

Untreated Chlamydia: PID in up to 40% of women and its sequelae such as chronic pelvic pain, infertility or ectopic pregnancies

PATIENT MONITORING

- Regular gynecologic evaluation and examination
- Annual screening women ≤25 years of age

BIBLIOGRAPHY

Brocklehurst P, et al. Interventions for treating genital chlamydia trachomatis infection in pregnancy. *Cochrane Database Syst Rev.* 1998;4:CD000054.

Centers for Disease Control and Prevention. Sexually transmitted diseases treatment guidelines, 2006. *MMWR.* 2006;55:2–3, 38–48.

Gaydos CA, et al. Chlamydia trachomatis infections in female military recruits. *N Engl J Med.* 1998;339: 739.

Cook RL, et al. Screening for Chlamydia trachomatis infection in college women with a polymerase chain reaction assay. *Clin Infect Dis.* 1999;28:1002.

Immunization of health-care workers: Recommendations of the Advisory Committee on Immunization Practices (ACIP) and the Hospital Infection Control Practices Advisory Committee (HICPAC). *MMWR Recomm Rep.* 1997;46:1.

Recommendations of the International Task Force for Disease Eradication. *MMWR Recomm Rep.* 1993;42:1.

Phillips RS, et al. Chlamydia trachomatis cervical infection in women seeking routine gynecologic: Criteria for selected testing. *Am J Med.* 1989;86: 515.

 MISCELLANEOUS

SYNONYM(S)

- Cervicitis
- Nongonococcal urethritis
- Sexually transmitted disease

CLINICAL PEARLS

- Sexual abuse must always be considered as a cause of chlamydial infection in children and adolescents.
- Differentiate between test-of-cure and repeat testing

ABBREVIATIONS

- STI—Sexually transmitted (or transmissible) infection
- STD—Sexually transmitted disease
- PID—Pelvic inflammatory disease
- NAAT—Nuclein acid amplification technology
- EPT—Expedited partner therapy

 CODES

ICD9-CM

- 099.41 Chlamydia trachomatis
- 099.50–099.59 Other venereal diseases due to Chlamydia trachomatis, by site

PATIENT TEACHING

- Encourage safe-sex practices, especially consistent use of barrier contraception.
- Discuss PID and its sequelae.
- ACOG Patient Education pamphlet available at http://www.acog.org

PREVENTION

- Primary: Safe-sex practices with consistent and correct use of latex male condoms
- Secondary: Screening:
  - Prenatal screening
  - Annual screening of all sexually active women ≤25 years of age
  - Screening for older women with risk factors:
    - New sexual partner
    - Multiple sex partners
- Expedited partner therapy (EPT) is the clinical practice of treating the sex partners of patients with Chlamydia or gonorrhea by providing prescriptions or medications to the patient to take to her/his partner without the health care provider 1st examining the partner. See http://www.cdc.gov/std/treatment/EPTFinalReport2006.pdf

SEXUALLY TRANSMITTED DISEASES (STDs): CONDYLOMA

J. Thomas Cox, MD

BASICS

DESCRIPTION
- Genital HPV is the most common STI.
- Condyloma (genital warts) are the most common external genital lesion of HPV.
- Most HPV infections do not have symptoms and their presence is unknown.

Age-Related Factors
Highest prevalence in persons aged ≤25

Pediatric Considerations

ALERT
- Genital warts raise concern of possible sexual abuse.
- Other causes of genital warts in children:
  – Perinatal transmission (rare but possible in children younger than 2–3 years old)
  – Warts caused by nongenital HPV types (uncommon)
  – Transmission during diaper care (unproven)
  – Possible fomite transmission or other unproven pathways
- Treatment options should be least traumatic:
  – Off-label imiquimod in children <12
  – Can cause irritation
  – Application at home is advantage

Pregnancy Considerations
- Reduced immune response of pregnancy may promote viral expression:
  – Not uncommon to appear for the 1st time
  – May be more difficult to clear with treatment
- Important to try to reduce wart volume before delivery, but Imiquimod, podophyllin, and Podofilox should not be used during pregnancy
- HPV-6 or -11 can be transmitted to fetal oropharynx in utero or to neonate during delivery.
  – Recurrent respiratory papillomatosis (RRP) of the larynx ~0.4–1.1/100,000 live births
- Unclear if cesarean section prevents RRP

ALERT
- The only indication for caesarian delivery is if warts obstruct the pelvic outlet, or trauma from delivery through the warts would risk hemorrhage.
- RRP is a rare but serious problem, often resulting in multiple laser treatments.

EPIDEMIOLOGY
- >100 HPV types; ~30 infect the genital area.
- Genital types divided into 2 groups defined by association with specific epithelial cancers:
  – 12 HPV types are "low risk":
    ○ Rarely, if ever, found in cervical cancer.
    ○ Most important are HPV-6, -11, -30, -42, -43, -44
    ○ ~90% of condyloma caused by HPV-6 or -11
  – 15 types are "high risk":
    ○ Associated with cervical cancer
    ○ Most important high-risk types are HPV-16, -18, -31, -33, -35, -39, -51, -52, -58, -61.
    ○ 20–50% of women with condyloma are coinfected with high-risk HPV types.

- ~1% of the adult population has symptomatic external genital warts (EGWs):
  – Vulva, perineal, perianal, and crural folds
  – Each year 1 million new cases of EGWs
  – 2/3 of these in women
- Incidence of EGWs increased from 13/100,000–106/100,000 from 1950–1978
- 450% increase in reports between 1966 and 1984.
- Prevalence of EGWs estimated to be 15%.
- Condyloma, if persistent, may rarely progress to invasive cancer (Buschke-Lowenstein tumors).

RISK FACTORS
- All sexually active women and men
- Women and men with new sex partner(s)
- Women and men with multiple sexual partners
- Inconsistent use of condoms
- Cigarette smoking (both behavioral and reduction in the cellular immune response)

PATHOPHYSIOLOGY
Transmission
- Almost solely through external genital-to-genital contact, and vaginal and anal intercourse
- Genital-oral sex speculated but not proven
- Fomites speculated but even less sure
- ~2/3 of exposed partners will develop EGWs

Proliferation
- HPV infects basal epithelial cells, most often gaining access through fissures and abrasions common in posterior fourchette, peri hymenal area, and labia. EGWs most common in those sites
- After infection and variable latency period, accelerated HPV DNA replication in differentiating epithelial cells (keratinocytes), results in warts.
- Latency typically 3 weeks to 8 months, with most EGWs developing within 2–3 months.

Immune Response
- Optimal treatment strategies based on the immune response
- Skin cells are not good at antigen presentation; the immune system often does not recognize its presence; HPV does not kill these cells. Hence, some EGWs do not trigger an immune response for months or years.
- Evidence for spontaneous immune recognition of HPV in genital warts varies from 0–40%.
- Treatment leaves lysed cells and viral DNA, increasing opportunity for immune recognition
- Primary immune response to HPV is cellular; dendritic, CD4 and CD8 cells are important.

ASSOCIATED CONDITIONS
- HIV and other immune suppression:
  – Increases risk of HPV expression if infected
  – Reduces likelihood of spontaneous immune suppression
  – Reduces the effectiveness of therapy
- Anything that increases access of HPV to the basal epithelium (vulvovaginal candidiasis, genital herpes, vulvar eczema), increases the chance that exposure leads to EGWs.

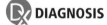
DIAGNOSIS

SIGNS AND SYMPTOMS
Physical Exam
- Most often based on physical findings

- Most common presenting complaint is "vaginal bumps" or partner known to have EGWs.
- Rarely, irritation or bleeding with intercourse secondary to a friable introital or cervical wart
- Found on pelvic exam (patient unaware)
- EGWs come in many different shapes and colors:
  – Majority are "cauliflowerlike" condyloma acuminata or genital papillomas.
  – Can also be dome-shaped papules, pedunculated, or flat
  – Single lesions, or in clusters, or as plaques
  – Flesh-colored, or pigmented; red or white, depending on whether the virus induces keratin, making the lesions white and hiding underlying color (hiding flesh-colored or red due to angiogenesis)
  – May have increased pigmentation from stimulation of melanocytes
  – Condyloma, papillomas, and nonpigmented papules most often caused by HPV-6 or -11.
  – Pigmented papules or papules with extensive angiogenesis (red papules) are most commonly secondary to HPV-16.
  – Genital warts can also be found on the cervix and vagina, in the anus and oral cavity (rare), and at the urethral meatus.

TESTS
Only valid test for EGW diagnosis is biopsy:
- Biopsy only rarely necessary if exam or lack of response to treatment raises concern of malignancy; or if appearance not definitive

ALERT
- HPV testing not helpful in diagnosis of EGWs and should not be done solely for this reason.
- STD testing for *Chlamydia*, gonorrhea, HIV, and syphilis as appropriate
- Pap only if due for routine cervical screening

DIFFERENTIAL DIAGNOSIS
Infection
Molluscum contagiosum

Other/Miscellaneous
- Normal skin appendages: Nevi, sebaceous hyperplasia, labial micropapillae
- Other abnormal findings: Condyloma lata, seborrheic keratoses, dysplastic nevi, bowenoid papulosis (high-grade VIN-3); invasive vulvar cancer (squamous cell, Buscke-Lowenstein tumors)

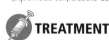
TREATMENT

GENERAL MEASURES
- No current options that directly treat the virus
- Spontaneous resolution can occur; thus observation is an acceptable alternative, with treatment only if lesions persist or enlarge.
- Most women want treatment, with expectation of accelerated clearance; reduced infectivity with treatment is not established
- Partner(s) exam not necessary; no evidence that reinfection plays a role in recurrence
- Counsel partner(s); evaluate for other STDs

MEDICATION (DRUGS)

- Home (patient-applied) for EGWs; Podofilox and imiquimod are CDC-recommended as first-line treatment.
- Podofilox:
  - Purified derivative of podophyllin resin
  - Supplied in 0.5% gel or solution, relatively inexpensive, easy to apply, safe
  - B.i.d. for 3 days, then 4 days with no therapy.
  - Can be repeated weekly for 2–4 cycles.
  - Total area not >10 cm^2; volume <0.5 mL/d
  - Clearance within 4–6 weeks: 37–77%
  - Recurrences reported in 4–38%
  - Side effects: Itching, burning, pain, erosion
- Imiquimod 5% cream:
  - Immune response modifier
  - May be used with provider-applied therapies
  - Enhances HPV immune recognition by inducing cytokines and toll-like receptors
  - Applied 3 times a week, ideally q.o.d., up to 16 weeks
  - Washed off 6–10 hours after application
  - Response is usually seen within 8 weeks.
  - In 3 RCTs, 50% complete clearance in 16 weeks
  - Adverse effects: Mild to severe erythema, itching, erosion, burning are common; usually resolve within a few days of stopping meds
  - Lower recurrence rates ~13–19%
- Kunecatechin 15% cream: Botanical drug product extracted from green tea leaves:
  - Newly FDA-approved
  - Partially purified fraction of the water extract; a mix of catechins and other components
  - Catechins are bioflavonoids, polyphenols, and powerful antioxidants shown to enhance immune system function and fight tumors.
  - Specific indication is the topical treatment of EGWs including perianal warts in immunocompetent patients ≥18 years
  - 0.5-cm strand applied in a thin layer over all EGWs t.i.d. for up to 16 weeks.
  - 53.6% complete clearance vs. 35.3% placebo
  - 16 weeks median time to complete clearance
  - Side effects: Erythema, pruritus, burning, pain/discomfort, erosion/ulceration, edema, induration, vesicular rash
- In-office (clinician-applied) for EGWs: BCA, TCA, cryotherapy, and podophyllin resin are CDC-approved first-line treatment.
- Bi-, trichloroacetic acid (BCA, TCA):
  - Most common in-office therapies
  - Usually applied as an 85% solution
  - Can apply weekly as needed
  - RCT and case series show BCA/TCA and cryotherapy have similar efficacy.
  - Wart clearance 63–70%; recurrence not evaluated
  - Very safe; apply sparingly, minimize acid on adjacent normal skin (causes increased pain, potential ulceration)
- Cryotherapy:
  - Liquid nitrogen (LN$_2$) sprayed from dermatologic canister or application of frozen Q-tips pulled from a canister of LN$_2$.
  - Nitrous oxide thin-pointed cryoprobe
  - Necrosis and scarring can occur with cryoprobe; care not to freeze too deeply
  - LN$_2$ methods very safe and rarely cause necrosis into the dermis
  - Response rates similar to other treatments
  - Recurrence rates up to 38–73% by 6 months

- Podophyllin resin 10–25% in benzoin:
  - Antimitotic induces tissue necrosis
  - Serious side-effects reported with excessive application: Bone marrow suppression, hepatocellular dysfunction, neurologic compromise, hallucinations, psychosis, nausea, vomiting, diarrhea, acute abdominal pain
  - Toxicity due to absorption of resin, therefore restrict to <10 cm^2 and a volume of <0.5 mL
  - Wash off in 1–4 hours
  - May be applied in office weekly
  - Do not apply to area with increased capacity for absorption; e.g., denuded, fissured skin.

Pregnancy Considerations
- NO: Podofilox, podophyllin resin, kunecatechin and Imiquimod
- YES: Cryotherapy and BCA/TCA
- Treatment of genital warts in other areas:
  - Cervical warts:
    - Always biopsy 1st to rule out high-grade precancer or cancer
    - BCA or TCA, or cryotherapy
  - Vaginal warts:
    - Cryotherapy with LN$_2$
    - BCA or TCA
  - Urethral warts:
    - Cryotherapy with LN$_2$
    - Podophyllin 10–25%
    - Imiquimod 5% cream
  - Anal warts:
    - Cryotherapy with LN$_2$
    - BCA or TCA
    - Surgical removal
    - Inspect rectum for warts

 ## FOLLOW-UP

Recurrences most common in 1st 3 months after clearance; 3 month follow-up to assess resolution, then as needed

DISPOSITION
Issues for Referral
Surgical therapy, if large volume or failure of topical therapy

PROGNOSIS
- Lack of recurrence within 6 months usually indicates either viral clearance or long-term HPV suppression, following which recurrence is rare.
- Immune suppression may prolong treatment and may result in persistence.
- Median time for complete clearance 5.9 months but many clear much more quickly

PATIENT MONITORING
- Regular annual gynecologic evaluation
- No change in cervical screening intervals

BIBLIOGRAPHY

Baseman JG, et al. The epidemiology of human papillomavirus infections. *J Clin Virol.* 2005;32(Suppl 1):S16–S24.

Beutner KR, et al. Genital warts and their treatment. *Clin Infect Dis.* 1999;28(Suppl 1):S37–S56.

Centers for Disease Control and Prevention Sexually Transmitted Diseases Treatment Guidelines. *MMWR.* 2006;55(No. RR-11):62–69.

Chow HH, et al. Effects of dosing condition on the oral bioavailability of green tea catechins after single-dose administration of Polyphenon E in healthy individuals. *Clin Cancer Res.* 2005; 11(12):4627–4633.

Markowitz LE, et al. Centers for Disease Control and Prevention (CDC); Advisory Committee on Immunization Practices (ACIP). Quadrivalent human papillomavirus vaccine: Recommendations of the Advisory Committee on Immunization Practices (ACIP). *MMWR Recomm Rep.* 2007;56(RR-2):1–24.

Scheinfeld N, et al. An evidence-based review of medical and surgical treatments of genital warts. *Dermatol Online J.* 2006;12:5.

Wiley DJ, et al. External genital warts: Diagnosis, treatment, and prevention. *Clin Infect Dis.* 2002;35(Suppl 2):S210–S224.

Winer RL, et al. Genital human papilloma-virus infection: Incidence and risk factors in a cohort of female university students. *Am J Epidemiol.* 2003;157:218–226.

 ## MISCELLANEOUS

CLINICAL PEARLS
- Sex partners almost always share the virus; ongoing sexual intimacy doesn't prolong infection.
- Folic acid may help promote an immune response: Higher serum folic acid levels promotes quicker clearance of HPV, more rapid return of normal Pap test, < high-grade CIN.
- Smoking is known suppressor of the immune response to HPV; encourage smoking cessation.

ABBREVIATIONS
- BCA—Bichloroacetic acid
- CIN—Cervical intraepithelial neoplasia
- EGW—External genital warts
- HPV—Human papillomavirus
- LN$_2$—Liquid nitrogen
- RCT—Randomized controlled trial
- RRP—Recurrent respiratory papillomatosis
- STD/STI—Sexually transmitted disease/infection
- TCA—Trichloroacetic acid
- VIN—Vulvar intraepithelial neoplasia

CODES
ICD9-CM
- 078.10 Viral wart, unspecified
- 078.11 Condyloma acuminata
- 078.19 Other unspecified viral wart

 ## PATIENT TEACHING

PREVENTION
- Abstinence
- Quadrivalent HPV vaccine before exposed to HPV-6 and -11. Recommended for females 9–26.
- Consistent use of condoms reduces the risk of EGWs by 60–70%.
- Counseling on HPV infection:
  - HPV is very common, almost all sexually active individuals get HPV at some point during their lifetime.
  - The interval between infection and exposure is very variable, hence most do not know for sure when they were exposed.
  - Most HPV infections resolve on their own.

Angela Keating, MD

 BASICS

DESCRIPTION
- Gonorrhea is an STI that can involve the urogenital tract, the oropharynx, or rarely can become disseminated.

Age-Related Factors
- Highest prevalence in females: 15–19 years
- Highest prevalence in males: 20–24 years

Pediatric Considerations
Sexual abuse must be considered if gonorrhea is diagnosed in a prepubertal child (almost 100% of cases are acquired by sexual contact if beyond the newborn period).

EPIDEMIOLOGY
- *Neisseria gonorrhea* is a gram-negative oxidase-positive diplococcus that causes infections only in humans.
- Second most commonly reported bacterial STD in US.
- CDC estimates >700,000 people get gonorrhea each year in US
- From 1975–1997, rates in US declined, with slight increase in 1998 and slight decline since

RISK FACTORS
- New sexual partner
- Multiple sexual partners
- <25 years old
- Commercial sex work
- Drug use
- Prior STD

Genetics
The genetics of drug resistance in the *N. gonorrhoeae* organism is an area of active study.

PATHOPHYSIOLOGY
- Transmission is almost always from sexual contact or from intimate contact with infected mucosal surfaces of the urogenital tract or oropharynx.
- Incubation period usually is 2–7 days.
- Cervix is the most common site of mucosal infection.
- Infection usually begins at the cervix and then may ascend to the uterus, tubes, and ovaries leading to PID if not treated:
  – PID occurs in 10–30% of women with gonococcal cervicitis.
- Infection can rarely become disseminated.
- Acute gonococcal infection can lead to:
  – Cervicitis
  – Vaginitis (usually premenarchal girls)
  – Urethritis
  – Anorectal infection
  – Pharyngitis
  – PID
  – Fitz-Hugh-Curtis syndrome (perihepatitis)
  – Arthritis
  – Disseminated gonococcal infection (arthritis-dermatitis syndrome)
  – Endocarditis or meningitis rarely

Pregnancy Considerations
- Maternal–fetal transmission at time of birth is possible due to exposure to infected cervical exudate.
- Fetal infection in utero is associated with spontaneous abortion, fetal demise, neonatal ophthalmia, neonatal arthritis, or neonatal sepsis.

ASSOCIATED CONDITIONS
Possible sequelae:
- Chronic pelvic pain
- Infertility
- Ectopic pregnancy

 DIAGNOSIS

SIGNS AND SYMPTOMS
History
- Majority of infections are asymptomatic.
- Symptoms may be acute or chronic.

Review of Systems
- Cervicitis:
  – Abnormal vaginal discharge; irritation
  – Abnormal vaginal bleeding
  – Postcoital bleeding
  – Dyspareunia
- Vaginitis:
  – Most common symptom in prepubertal girls
  – Vaginal pruritus/irritation/vaginal bleeding
- Urethritis:
  – Urinary urgency/frequency/dysuria
- Anorectal infection:
  – Anal itching/irritation/painful defecation
  – Bloody stools/rectal discharge
- PID:
  – Dysmenorrhea/Pelvic pain/Dyspareunia
  – Abdominal pain
  – Abnormal uterine bleeding
  – Fever
- Oropharyngeal infection:
  – Sore throat, cough
- Disseminated gonococcal infection (arthritis-dermatitis syndrome):
  – Petechial or pustular acral skin lesions
  – Asymmetrical arthralgia; joint swelling
  – Signs of meningitis or endocarditis

Physical Exam
- Friable cervical mucosa
- Mucopurulent cervical discharge
- Friable vaginal mucosa
- Friable anal mucosa
- Cervical motion tenderness
- Uterine tenderness/adnexal tenderness
- Abdominal pain
- Painful joint
- Fever

TESTS
- Diagnostic tests for gonorrhea are via swabs from the endocervix, vagina, urethra, anus, pharynx, or urine.
- PID is a clinical diagnosis.

Lab
- Nucleic acid amplification techniques:
  – Recommended by CDC
  – Most sensitive and specific (98–100%)
  – Can be done via cervical, vaginal, or urine swabs or via liquid Pap specimen
  – Results within a few hours
  – Good for up to 7 days at room temperature
  – Most expensive
- Culture:
  – Gold standard
  – Should be done for medicolegal purposes if sexual abuse is considered
  – 85–95% sensitive; 100% specific
  – Results within 48 hrs
  – Must be sent to lab within 24 hours
- Gram stain:
  – Intracellular Gram-negative oxidase positive diplococci
  – Not to be used for oropharyngeal testing due to other *Neisseria* species at this site
  – 60% sensitive

Imaging
If diagnosis of PID is considered, imaging may be warranted to delineate abscess or rule out other causes of pelvic pain:
- Pelvic US
- CT scan

DIFFERENTIAL DIAGNOSIS
Infection
- *Chlamydia*
- Trichomoniasis
- Bacterial vaginosis
- Appendicitis
- Diverticulitis

Metabolic/Endocrine
Ovarian cyst:
- Ovarian torsion

Tumor/Malignancy
Ovarian/Adnexal mass as cause of pelvic pain

Other/Miscellaneous
Endometriosis

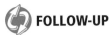

TREATMENT

GENERAL MEASURES

- Patient should be tested for other STDs.
- Recommend no resumption of sexual relations until patient and partner have been treated and are without symptoms (asymptomatic patients should wait at least a week).

ALERT

- Due to common coinfection with *Chlamydia trachotomatis*, CDC recommends treating for both when gonorrhea is diagnosed and *Chlamydia* cannot be ruled out by nucleic acid amplification test.
- CDC no longer recommends quinolones due to the high level of resistance to quinolones.

MEDICATION (DRUGS)

- Cervical, urethral, anorectal infection:
  - Recommended regimens:
    - Ceftriaxone 125 mg IM single dose
    - Cefixime 400 mg PO single dose
  - Alternative regimens:
    - Spectinomycin 2 g IM single dose (not available in US)
    - 3rd-generation cephalosporin single dose
- Pharyngeal infection (more difficult to eradicate):
  - Recommended regimen:
    - Ceftriaxone 125 mg IM single dose
- PID:
  - Recommended regimens:
    - Gentamicin 2 mg/kg IV, then 1.5 mg/kg q8h + clindamycin 900 mg IV q8h until 24–48 hrs after improvement and then PO regimen for 14 days
    - Cefotetan 2 g IV q12h or cefoxitin 2 g IV q6h + doxycycline 100 mg PO or IV q12h until 24–48 hours after improvement, then PO regimen for 14 days
    - PO treatment for mild to moderate PID: Ceftriaxone 250 mg IM single dose + doxycycline 100 mg b.i.d. PO for 14 days +/– metronidazole 500 mg b.i.d. for 14 days (may substitute ceftriaxone with another parenteral 3rd-generation cephalosporin or cefoxitin 2 g IM + probenecid 1 g PO)
- Disseminated gonococcal infection:
  - Recommended regimen:
    - Ceftriaxone 1 g IV q24h for 24–48 hours after improvement, then PO regimen for 1 week with cefixime

Pregnancy Considerations

Hospitalize if PID in pregnancy; use IV regimen (rare in pregnancy)

SURGERY

Only with persistent symptomatic PID/pelvic TOA despite antibiotic treatment or concern for surgical process (e.g., torsion)

FOLLOW-UP

- Reevaluation needed if persistent symptoms
- Consider retest to verify no reinfection

DISPOSITION

Issues for Referral

Referral to a gynecologic surgeon if torsion or ovarian mass remain a consideration

PROGNOSIS

- Effective cure in 98.9% of uncomplicated urogenital and anorectal gonorrhea infections if recommended treatment regimen used. 90% cure in pharyngeal infections
- Chronic pain possible with untreated gonorrhea infections or with delayed treatment
- Increased risk of infertility and ectopic pregnancy with untreated gonorrhea infections or with delayed treatment

PATIENT MONITORING

- No test of cure needed unless concern regarding compliance, pregnancy, pharyngeal infection, complicated infection, or persistent symptoms
- Consider retesting at 3 months to verify no reinfection of gonorrhea
- Patients should be instructed to have their sexual partners evaluated and treated.
- All cases of gonorrhea in the US must be reported to local health department.

BIBLIOGRAPHY

Beers M, ed. *The Merck Manual of Diagnosis and Therapy*, 18th ed. Whitehouse Station, NJ: Merck Research Laboratories; 2006;1381–1664.

Committee on Infectious Diseases, American Academy of Pediatrics. Red Book: 2006 Report of the Committee on Infectious Diseases. 27th ed. USA; 2006:301–308.

Kouman EH, et al. Laboratory testing for N. gonorrhea by recently introduced nonculture tests: A performance review with clinical and public health considerations. *Clin Infect Dis*. 1998;27:1171–1180.

US Preventive Services Task Force. Screening for gonorrhea: Recommendation statement. *Ann Fam Med*. 2005;3:263–267.

Workowski KA, et al. Sexually transmitted diseases treatment guidelines, 2006. *MMWR Recomm Rep*. 2006;55(RR-11):1–10, 37–49, 56–61.

MISCELLANEOUS

SYNONYM(S)

- GC
- Clap
- Drip

ABBREVIATIONS

- PID—Pelvic inflammatory disease
- STD/STI—Sexually transmitted disease/infection
- TOA—Tubo-ovarian abscess

CODES

ICD9-CM

- 098.0 Gonorrhea
- Gonococcal infection:
  - 098.10 Upper urogenital tract, acute
  - 098.15 Cervix, acute
  - 098.19 Fallopian tubes, acute
  - 098.5 Joint
  - 098.7 Anus
  - 098.6 Pharyngitis
  - 098.89 Septicemia

PATIENT TEACHING

- Discuss medication compliance
- Instruct patient to have partners get evaluated and treated.
- Review safe-sex practices.

PREVENTION

- Counseling regarding safe sex practices (latex condoms and minimize sexual exposures)
- All at-risk patients should be screened regularly.
- All patients with symptoms consistent with possible gonorrhea should be tested.
- All pregnant women should be screened at the 1st prenatal visit; women at high risk for gonorrhea should be screened again in the 3rd trimester.
- All newborns get routine prophylaxis for neonatal ophthalmia with erythromycin or tetracycline eye ointment.

SEXUALLY TRANSMITTED DISEASES (STDs): HERPES SIMPLEX VIRUS

Corinne Bria, MD
Karin Batalden, MD
Frank M. Biro, MD

BASICS

DESCRIPTION
- Most common etiology of genital ulcers
- Genital disease may be from HSV type 1 or type 2
- Recurrent disease more likely from HSV type 2.
- Initial infection presents with waves of vesicles, pustules, ulcers, lasting 2–6 weeks
- Median number of recurrences 4 per year

Pregnancy Considerations
- A primary outbreak in the 1st trimester of pregnancy has been associated with neonatal chorioretinitis, microcephaly, and rarely, skin lesions. Recent studies do not confirm an increased risk for spontaneous abortion.
- The risk of fetal transmission of HSV with a primary infection at the time of delivery is 30–60%.
- Antiviral treatment may be administered for an initial outbreak to reduce the duration and severity of symptoms and to reduce the duration of viral shedding.
- A randomized trial of acyclovir vs. placebo from 36 weeks until delivery for 1st episode of genital herpes found:
  - A significant reduction in clinical recurrences at delivery and a reduction in cesarean delivery for recurrence
  - An insufficient number of deliveries to assess the efficacy of antiviral treatment in preventing neonatal HSV
  - Evidence is insufficient to support scheduled cesarean delivery before labor for the prevention of transmission.

ALERT
- Presence of an active lesion of genital HSV at the time of labor onset is an indication for cesarean delivery:
  - Cesarean delivery is not indicated in women with a history of HSV in the absence of active genital lesions or prodromes.
- Among women with recurrent lesions at the time of delivery, the rate of transmission at vaginal delivery is 3%

Pediatric Considerations
- ~1,200–1,500 cases of neonatal herpes infection occur each year in the US.
- Neonatal infection is classified as:
  - Disseminated disease: 25%; mortality of 30%
  - CNS disease: 30%; mortality of 4%
  - Disease limited to skin, eyes, or mouth: 45%
- ~20% of survivors of neonatal herpes have long-term neurologic sequelae.
- Neonatal herpes is typically acquired during vaginal delivery, although in utero and postnatal infection may rarely occur:
  - 80% of mothers of infected infants report no history of HSV

Age-Related Factors
- May present as:
  - Neonatal infection (acquired at time of birth)
  - 1st episode genital infection with initiation of sexual activity
- Prevalence of HSV-2 antibody is 1–5% (mean 1.6%) in teens, and 11% in young adults 20–29.

EPIDEMIOLOGY
- Attack rate among sexually active female teens is 4.4/100 person years.
- Attack rates are higher in those without pre-existing HSV type 1 antibodies.
- Seroprevalence rates vary with:
  - Gender (higher in females)
  - Age (increases from age 14 to 40s)
  - Race and ethnicity (higher in persons of color)
- ~200,000 office visits for newly diagnosed cases of genital herpes
- The annual incidence (newly diagnoses cases) of genital herpes among those 15–24 years of age is 640,000 cases.
- The majority of infections are transmitted by those who unaware of having herpes.
- Recent data suggest that a greater proportion of new cases of genital herpes are due to HSV type 1 rather than type 2.

RISK FACTORS
- Serologic attack rates higher in those without previous HSV type 1 antibody
- Clinical genital herpes infections also higher in those without previous HSV type 1 antibody
- Recurrent disease is more common in those with HSV type 2 genital infections as contrasted to those with HSV type 1 genital herpes.

PATHOPHYSIOLOGY
- HSV types 1 and 2 are members of the Herpesviridae family.
- Large (100 nm in diameter), DNA-containing enveloped viruses, composed of outer envelope, tegument, nucleocapsid, and internal core

ASSOCIATED CONDITIONS
Previous genital HSV infection is associated with an increased risk of HIV acquisition, and new genital HSV infection has a greater association with HIV acquisition than previous HSV infection.

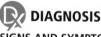

DIAGNOSIS

SIGNS AND SYMPTOMS
History
- The majority (84%) of people with antibody to HSV type 2 are unaware of a history of genital ulcers.
- The likelihood of asymptomatic infection is even greater (94%) among those with antibodies to both HSV type 1 and type 2.
- Typically, symptomatic initial genital infections include:
  - Genital pain and itching
  - Dysuria
  - Painful adenopathy
  - Systemic symptoms:
    - Systemic symptoms include headache, fever, and malaise.
- Initial primary infections (as contrasted to initial nonprimary genital infections or recurrent infections) have greater number of lesions, and longer duration of lesions.

Physical Exam
- Lesions initially appear as vesicles, followed 2–3 days later by pustules, then ulcers and subsequently crusted lesions.
- Lesions may be isolated or coalesced.
- Of note, lesions may appear as fissures rather than ulcers.
- New lesions may form up to 10 days after the initial lesion in primary infection.
- Lesions are often associated with tender adenopathy.
- Other findings associated with primary genital herpes infection include:
  - Meningitis
  - Urinary retention from transverse myelitis
  - Autonomic nervous dysfunction
  - Proctitis

TESTS

Labs

- The standard for diagnosis of genital herpes has been culture:
  - The sensitivity of lesion culture is greatest when a vesicle is unroofed; declines sharply 3 days after the onset of the ulcer
- PCR is more sensitive than culture, but many laboratories have HSV-PCR available only for CSF samples.
- Type-specific serology is available, but controversies exist regarding its utility:
  - The specificity of serology is 96–97%.
  - Because the overall seroprevalence of HSV type 2 in adolescents is 2%, many of those receiving a positive result on a "screening test" (rather than a clinical evaluation of a suspicious lesion) will receive a false-positive result.

DIFFERENTIAL DIAGNOSIS

- Other infectious etiologies of genital ulcers include:
  - Syphilis
  - Chancroid
  - LGV
  - Granuloma inguinale
  - Although the incidence of most common of these infections, syphilis, is <2% the incidence of genital herpes.
- Noninfectious etiologies of genital ulcers include:
  - Aphthosis (See Vulvar Ulcers: Aphthosis.)
  - Behçet's disease
  - Allergic dermatitis

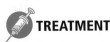 TREATMENT

GENERAL MEASURES

- Although the primary approach to genital herpes is medical management, the care provider should be aware of the psychological distress associated with the diagnosis.
- Genital herpes interferes with sexual relations, and those infected report a lower health quality of life.

MEDICATION (DRUGS)

- 1st episode of genital herpes is managed for 7–10 days with the following regimens. Of note, treatment can be extended if the lesions are not healed:
  - Acyclovir 400 mg PO t.i.d.
  - Acyclovir 200 mg PO 5 times daily
  - Famciclovir 250 mg PO t.i.d.
  - Valacyclovir 1 g PO b.i.d.

- Episodic therapy, if begun during the prodrome, or within 1 day of symptom onset, has been shown to abort an outbreak as well as decrease duration of lesions.
  - Episodic treatment does not reduce the number of outbreaks.
  - These regimens are often of shorter duration than previously recommended regimens:
  - Acyclovir 400 mg PO t.i.d. 5 days
  - Acyclovir 800 mg PO b.i.d. 5 days
  - Acyclovir 800 mg PO t.i.d. 2 days
  - Famciclovir 125 mg PO b.i.d. 5 days
  - Famciclovir 1 g PO b.i.d. 1 day
- Suppressive therapy can reduce the frequency of infections, decrease the risk of transmission, and may provide psychological benefits as well as improve quality of life.
  - Studies have shown that low rates exist in the development of resistance in immunocompetent patients on continuous suppressive therapy:
    - ○ Valacyclovir: 500 mg PO daily
    - ○ Acyclovir: 400 mg PO b.i.d.
    - ○ Famciclovir: 250 mg PO b.i.d.
    - ○ Valacyclovir: 1 gm PO daily

 FOLLOW-UP

DISPOSITION

Issues for Referral

- Health care provider must be aware of the psychological trauma associated with HSV infection.
- Given decreased rate of transmission to partners, decrease in frequency of recurrences, and improved psychological outcomes, those with 1st episode of genital herpes should be offered suppressive therapy.

PROGNOSIS

The recurrence rate of HSV type 2 > HSV type 1:

- In patients with HSV type 2 followed for an average of 13 months, >1/3 had at least 6 recurrences, and 1/5 had ≥10 recurrences.
- Recurrence rate in HSV type 1 is much lower.

BIBLIOGRAPHY

ACOG Practice Bulletin #82 June 2007—Management of Herpes in Pregnancy.

Benedetti J, et al. Recurrence rates in genital herpes after symptomatic first episode infection. *Ann Intern Med.* 1994;121:847–854.

Centers for Disease Control and Prevention. Sexually transmitted diseases treatment guideline, 2006. *MMWR.* 2006;55:RR-11;1–94.

Corey L, et al. Once-daily valacyclovir to reduce the risk of transmission of genital herpes. *N Engl J Med.* 2004;350:11–20.

Patel R, et al. Impact of suppressive antiviral therapy on the health related quality of life of patients with recurrent genital herpes infection. *Sex Transm Inf.* 1999;75:398–402.

Roberts CM, et al. Increasing proportion of herpes simplex virus type 1 as a cause of genital herpes infection in college students. *Sex Transm Dis.* 2003;30:797–800.

Stanberry LR, et al. Longitudinal risk of herpes simplex virus (HSV) type 1, HSV type 2, and cytomegalovirus infections among young adolescent girls. *Clin Infect Dis.* 2004;39:1433–1438.

Xu F, et al. Trends in herpes simplex virus type 1 and type 2 seroprevalence in the United States. *JAMA* 2006;296:964–973.

 MISCELLANEOUS

CLINICAL PEARLS

- The vast majority of cases presenting with genital ulcers are due to genital herpes infections.
- The majority of people with herpes type 2 antibodies are unaware of a previous episode of genital herpes.
- Suppressive antiviral therapy can reduce the frequency of recurrent genital herpes infections, decrease the risk of transmission, and may provide psychological benefits as well as improve quality of life.

ABBREVIATIONS

- CSF—Cerebrospinal fluid
- HSV—Herpes simplex virus
- LGV—Lymphogranuloma venereum
- PCR—Polymerase chain reaction

CODES

ICD9-CM
054.1 Genital herpes

 PATIENT TEACHING

ACOG Patient Education Pamphlets: Genital Herpes

PREVENTION

Consistent use of condoms can minimize but not eliminate the risk of acquiring HPV.

SEXUALLY TRANSMITTED DISEASES (STDs): HIV/AIDS

Aimee Wilkin, MD, MPH
Judith Feinberg, MD

 BASICS

DESCRIPTION

- HIV is a retrovirus, leading to AIDS through progressive destruction of immune function.
- Chronic infection that can alter or exacerbate many other conditions; clinical course variable:
  - HIV testing is critical to early diagnosis:
    ○ Improved morbidity and mortality with early treatment
    ○ Decreased transmission with treatment
    ○ Per CDC, all persons 13–64 who have been sexually active should be tested for HIV as part of routine medical care

Age-Related Factors

- More rapid disease progression in older adults
- Biologic factors, such as immature vaginal tract in adolescent girls and vaginal dryness in postmenopausal women, facilitate HIV acquisition
- Risk of infection compounded by failure of women to perceive that they are at risk

Staging

- CD4+ (T helper) lymphocyte count and HIV viral load define stage.
- Acute HIV syndrome (seroconversion):
  - Usually within 1st 2 months of infection
  - Asymptomatic or nonspecific "viral syndrome"
- Chronic infection (not AIDS) with CD4+ counts >200 cells/mm^3:
  - Lasts 2–10 years with wide variation
  - Mild symptoms or associated conditions that are not CDC-defined opportunistic infections
- AIDS: CD4+ count <200 cells/mm^3 and/or a CDC-defined opportunistic infection or malignancy

EPIDEMIOLOGY

Worldwide, 39.5 million people living with HIV (2006) with 4.3 million new infections/year and 2.9 million deaths/year

Incidence

In the US:

- ~40,000–45,000 new infections per year
- 25% of new cases and those living with HIV are women
- Risk of infection:
  - Black women 21 times >whites
  - Hispanic women 6 times >whites

Prevalence

- In US:
  - ~1.2 million people living with HIV/AIDS
  - 25–33% do not know they are infected

RISK FACTORS

Male-to-female transmission more effective than female-to-male; sharing needles/syringes; vertical transmission from HIV+ mother to neonate perinatally or by breast-feeding

Genetics

- Homozygotes with delta 32 deletion in CCR5 coreceptor confers resistance to HIV infection.
- Heterozygotes can be infected but may have slower disease progression.

PATHOPHYSIOLOGY

- HIV Infection alters normal immune function through CD4 lymphocyte destruction, disruption of normal cytokine responses, and alteration of B-cell responses.
- Initial infection:
  - Enters genital mucosa, attaches to dendritic cells, and travels to lymph nodes
- Chronic infection:
  - Proliferates in lymph nodes and blood
  - Destruction of CD4+ cells
  - Latent infection in quiescent CD4+ cells and other protected sites

ASSOCIATED CONDITIONS

- AIDS-defining opportunistic infections/malignancies:
  - Cervical cancer, invasive
  - Candidiasis, esophageal (or pulmonary)
  - Coccidioidomycosis
  - Cryptococcosis
  - Cryptosporidiosis
  - CMV end organ disease
  - Encephalopathy, HIV-related
  - Herpes simplex, chronic ulcer >1 month
  - Histoplasmosis
  - Isosporiasis
  - Kaposi sarcoma
  - Lymphoma: Burkitt, immunoblastic, or brain (primary CNS)
  - *Mycobacterium avium* complex
  - *Mycobacterium* tuberculosis
  - Other species of *Mycobacterium*
  - *Pneumocystis* pneumonia
  - Recurrent bacterial pneumonia
  - Progressive multifocal leukoencephalopathy
  - *Salmonella septicemia*
  - Toxoplasmosis
  - Wasting syndrome
- Other associated conditions:
  - Candidiasis, oropharyngeal (thrush)
  - Candidiasis, vulvovaginal
  - Cervical dysplasia
  - PID, TOA
  - Bacillary angiomatosis
  - Herpes zoster
  - ITP
  - Listeriosis
  - Invasive pneumococcal infection
  - Amenorrhea, menorrhagia and infertility

DIAGNOSIS

SIGNS AND SYMPTOMS

ALERT

Acute HIV syndrome (seroconversion) often is not recognized and is misdiagnosed as flu-like illness. Chronic HIV may be asymptomatic until the conditions described above start to occur.

History

- Review: Risk factors, sexual history (STDs such as hepatitis B or C), previous HIV testing.
- Consider recent versus chronic infection
- Acute HIV syndrome may mimic mononucleosis, with broad range of presentations:
  - Fever, rash, lymphadenopathy, pharyngitis

- Chronic infection:
  - Fatigue, weight loss, lymphadenopathy, skin disorders, pneumonia, fevers, night sweats, chronic diarrhea, headaches, mental status changes

Review of Systems

Perform a multisystem review. Plus:

- Psychiatric history and symptoms
- Substance abuse history, signs and symptoms
- Neurologic signs and symptoms

Physical Exam

- Complete physical exam indicated. Key findings:
- General appearance:
  - Vital signs, weight, signs of wasting
- Skin findings:
  - Folliculitis
  - Eczema, xerosis
  - Seborrheic dermatitis
  - Kaposi sarcoma (purplish papules, plaques, nodules)
- HEENT:
  - White plaques on buccal mucosa, tongue and/or palate that can be scraped off most typical; erythema (oral candidiasis)
  - Oral hairy leukoplakia
  - Gingivitis
- Abdominal findings:
  - Hepatosplenomegaly (with late stage complications)
- GU:
  - Pelvic exam with Pap, STD screening, wet prep for associated infections or neoplasia
- Neurologic findings:
  - Peripheral neuropathy
  - Dementia (loss of memory, concentration; motor retardation)
  - Weakness (focal or generalized)
- Lymphatic/Hematologic:
  - Lymphadenopathy
  - Petechiae, bruising

TESTS

- Screening ELISA or EIA is confirmed by Western blot. Current assays can distinguish HIV-1 from HIV-2 (a much more slowly progressive infection).
- Serologic testing can be negative during acute infection (seroconversion):
  - "Window period," although patients will have a high HIV viral load
  - Repeat serology in 1 and 2 months

Labs

- CBC
- CD4 cell count (T cell subsets) and HIV viral load by RNA PCR or branched-chain DNA (bDNA) assays useful for staging; determine need for anti-HIV therapy
- Other initial lab tests:
  - Serologic tests for hepatitis B and C, syphilis; renal and hepatic

Imaging

Imaging useful for complications, but not diagnosis

DIFFERENTIAL DIAGNOSIS

Many medical conditions are exacerbated by or related to HIV, often with symptoms that overlap with HIV; diagnosis may be missed without testing.

Infection
- Acute HIV:
  - Mononucleosis
  - Strep pharyngitis
  - CMV
  - Nonspecific "viral syndrome"
  - Other STDs: Syphilis, Chlamydia, gonorrhea, HSV, trichomoniasis
  - Hepatitis (viral)
- Chronic HIV:
  - Pneumonia
  - Infectious diarrhea: Parasitic, bacterial
  - Bacterial vaginosis
  - Other STDs: Syphilis, Chlamydia, gonorrhea, HSV, trichomoniasis
  - Hepatitis A, B and C

Hematologic
- Thrombocytopenia
- Hypergammaglobulinemia

Metabolic/Endocrine
- Hyperthyroidism
- Diabetes

Immunologic
- Sarcoidosis
- Collagen vascular disease
- Reiter syndrome

Tumor/Malignancy
- Specific cancers are associated with HIV/AIDS*; other cancers may occur more often in HIV+ patients.
- Lymphoma*:
  - Non-Hodgkin's (EBV-associated)
  - Primary CNS lymphoma
  - Hodgkin disease
- Cervical cancer and dysplasia*
- Kaposi sarcoma*
- Skin cancers
- Lung cancer
- Colon cancer
- Breast cancer

Trauma
High rates of domestic violence and substance abuse may increase risk of traumatic injuries.

Drugs
Higher rates of substance abuse, including IV drug use: Consider testing for HIV

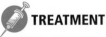

TREATMENT
GENERAL MEASURES
- Baseline assessment is important to assess disease stage and possible related conditions.
- CD4+ lymphocyte count relates to degree of immunosuppression:
  - Drops with acute HIV, then rises and stabilizes with seroconversion; later declines slowly over time
  - May drop excessively during acute illness of any cause and then return to baseline
- HIV viral load is rate of disease progression; increases with higher viral loads:
  - Easier to transmit HIV with higher viral load
- CBC, chemistry panel with liver and renal function, lipid profile
- Drug-resistance testing (genotype prior to starting HIV therapy) (12–14% have resistant HIV)
- Tuberculin skin test: Positive is >5 mm
- Screening for hepatitis A, B, C:
  - Vaccinate for hepatitis A and B if needed

- Screen for exposure to toxoplasmosis (IgG)
- G6PD deficiency screening if at risk for this
- Syphilis testing (annually)
- Pap testing every 6 mos for 2 years, then yearly if normal
- Other STD screening: HSV type II, Chlamydia, gonorrhea, trichomoniasis

SPECIAL THERAPY
Complementary and Alternative Therapies
Monitor for usage: Known and predicted drug interactions occur between many HIV drugs and herbal or other natural supplements

MEDICATION (DRUGS)
- Drugs for antiretroviral therapies, opportunistic infections, and for associated conditions
- ART:
  - Currently, a combination of ≥3 drugs, to include 2 NRTIs and a NNRTI or PI
  - Therapy should be initiated with input from HIV specialist because of complex drug interactions and need to individualize treatment.
  - Avoid interruptions in ART if possible to minimize drug resistance risk.
  - Multiple drug–drug interactions with ART, particularly with PIs, NNRTIs, including hormonal birth control. Review new medications for potential interactions.
- Opportunistic infection prophylaxis:
  - Pneumocystis pneumonia when CD4+ count <200 cells/mm^3 (trimethoprim/sulfamethoxazole, dapsone)
  - Mycobacterium avium complex when CD4 count ≤50 cells/mm^3 (azithromycin)
  - Toxoplasmosis when CD4+ count <200 cells/mm^3 (trimethoprim/sulfamethoxazole)
- Associated conditions:
  - Pneumococcal vaccination every 5 years
  - Influenza vaccine annually
  - Consider suppressive treatment of HSV-2 to decrease recurrence and transmission

Pregnancy Considerations
- ART goal is maximal viral suppression to decrease risk of perinatal transmission and maximize maternal health:
  - Combination ART selected in conjunction with HIV specialist during pregnancy, usually started after 1st trimester
  - Intravenous AZT during delivery
  - Consider scheduled caesarian delivery if viral load >1,000 near time of delivery
  - NNRTI efavirenz associated with risk of birth defects
  - HIV+ mothers should not breast-feed

SURGERY
As indicated; recovery not affected.

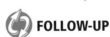

FOLLOW-UP
DISPOSITION
Issues for Referral
Consider referral to HIV specialist; ART is complex and a wide range of comorbid conditions is possible.

PROGNOSIS
Excellent with adherence to ART and as above.

PATIENT MONITORING
CD4 cell count and HIV viral load every 3–4 months; other tests as indicated. Pap and STD testing as above.

BIBLIOGRAPHY
Anderson J, ed. A Guide to the Clinical Care of Women with HIV/AIDS 2005 ed. Rockville, MD: DHHS Health Resources and Services Administration HIV/AIDS Bureau, 2005. http://hab.hrsa.gov/publications/womencare05/index.htm

Centers for Disease Control and Prevention. Revised Recommendations for HIV testing of adults, adolescents, and pregnant women in health-care settings. MMWR. 2006;55(RR14);1–17.

Hoffman C, et al., eds. HIV Medicine 2006. Paris: Flying Publishers; 2006. http://www.hivmedicine.com

Panel on Antiretroviral Guidelines for Adults and Adolescents. Guidelines for the use of antiretroviral agents in HIV-1 Infected adults and adolescents. DHHS. October 10, 2006;1–113. http://aidsinfo.nih.gov/ContentFiles/AdultandAdolescentGL.pdf

Perinatal HIV Guidelines Working Group. PHS Task Force Recommendations for Use of Antiretroviral Drugs in Pregnant HIV-1 Infected Women for Maternal Health and Interventions to Reduce Perinatal HIV-1 Transmission in the United States. October 12, 2006; 1–65. http://aidsinfo.nih.gov/ContentFiles/PerinatalGL.pdf

 MISCELLANEOUS

CLINICAL PEARLS
- Monogamous women can contract HIV from their husband or partner.
- Recurrent vaginal candidiasis may be 1st sign of HIV.
- History of STDs should prompt testing for HIV.

ABBREVIATIONS
ART—Antiretroviral therapy
CMV—Cytomegalovirus
EBV—Epstein-Barr virus
EIA/ELISA—Enzyme-linked immunosorbent assay
HEENT—Head, eyes, ears, nose, throat
HSV—Herpes simplex virus
ITP—Idiopathic thrombocytopenia purpura
NNRTI—Nonnucleoside reverse transcriptase inhibitor
NRTI—Nucleoside/tide reverse transcriptase inhibitors
PCR—Polymerase chain reaction
PI—Protease inhibitor
PID—Pelvic inflammatory disease
TOA—Tubo-ovarian abscess

CODES
ICD9-CM
042 Human immunodeficiency virus disease

 PATIENT TEACHING

HIV transmission, safer sex, adherence to therapy

PREVENTION
- Safer sex methods: Consistent and proper use of latex condoms, use of bleach to clean IV drug paraphernalia; not sharing needles/syringes
- Limiting numbers of sexual partners or abstinence
- Pregnant HIV+ women can prevent vertical transmission by use of ART during pregnancy from at least the 2nd trimester on and during labor and delivery, with avoidance of breastfeeding postpartum.

SEXUALLY TRANSMITTED DISEASES (STDs): HUMAN PAPILLOMAVIRUS (HPV)

Lea E. Widdice, MD
Jessica A. Kahn, MD, MPH

 BASICS

DESCRIPTION
- HPV:
  - Papillomaviridae family
  - Papillomaviruses widespread in higher vertebrates, species specific
  - HPV infects only humans
- Virion structure:
  - Double stranded, circular DNA genome surrounded by protein capsid
  - Protein capsid consists of 2 proteins (L1 and L2)
  - The L1 capsid protein is immunogenic in humans
- Genotypes (types) and classification:
  - A unique type is defined as a papillomavirus with >10% difference in a defined region of the viral DNA.
  - >100 HPV types exist that have tropism for mucosal or cutaneous epithelium.
  - >40 HPV types infect mucosal epithelium (aerodigestive and genital tracts):
    - High-risk types (e.g., 16, 18) cause cervical cancer and are associated with head, neck, genital, anal cancers.
    - Low-risk types (e.g., 6, 11) cause genital warts, respiratory warts, low-grade intraepithelial lesions of the cervix, vagina, vulva but are not associated with cancer of the genital tract.
  - >60 types infect cutaneous epithelium and cause palmar and plantar warts (e.g., types 1, 2, 4).

Age-Related Factors
- Infants and children may acquire HPV without sexual contact, but sexual abuse must be ruled out.
- Squamous metaplasia of the transformation zone may increase adolescent's vulnerability to HPV.
- 74% of infections occur among 15–24-year-olds

EPIDEMIOLOGY
- HPV infection:
  - Estimated prevalence of HPV infection in reproductive age women in the US is 28%, and estimated annual incidence is 6.2 million per year; thus HPV is the most common STI in the US.
  - In general, genital HPV is a transient infection:
    - Most (70%) infections will clear by 1 year, 90% by 2 years in young women.
- Transmission of genital HPV:
  - Most often by genital skin-to-skin contact
  - Typically through vaginal or anal intercourse
  - Less commonly through hand-genital or mouth-genital contact (oral sex)
  - Condom use may decrease transmission

Pediatric Considerations
HPV can be transmitted:
- Vertically from mother to infant, which may lead to RRP (rare)
- Horizontally from caregivers to children, resulting in anogenital warts
- Sexually through abuse
- Incubation period of HPV in children with perinatal transmission has not been conclusively determined but ranges from 6 months–3 years.

Pregnancy Considerations
- HPV may be transmitted from mother to infant perinatally.
- Pregnancy may affect the natural history of HPV infection, anogenital warts, and cervical dysplasia.

RISK FACTORS
- Number of sexual partners
- Sexual partner's number of partners
- Impaired cellular immunity
- Cervical ectopy
- Tobacco smoking
- Poverty

Genetics
2 inherited disorders are associated with an increased risk of HPV-related disease:
- Epidermodysplasia verruciformis: Rare autosomal recessive disorder associated with defect in cell-mediated immunity leading to increased susceptibility to warts and squamous cell carcinomas of sun-exposed epithelium with extensive and unusual HPV types
- Fanconi anemia: Rare autosomal recessive disorder with congenital malformations, bone marrow failure, and predisposition to cancers including HPV-associated SCC

PATHOPHYSIOLOGY
- HPV infects basal cells of the epithelium via trauma or microtrauma.
- Viral life cycle depends on differentiation of epithelium.
- Proteins transcribed from HPV E6 and E7 viral genome open-reading frames foster replication of viral DNA within host cell. These proteins also disrupt tumor suppressor genes (p53 and retinoblastoma protein), which leads to cell proliferation, chromosomal abnormalities, and aneuploidy and may lead to cell immortalization.

- Persistent infection with high-risk HPV is the primary risk factor for development of severe cervical dysplasia, which ultimately may progress to cervical carcinoma-in-situ and cervical cancer.
- The 2 main types of cervical cancer are SCC and adenocarcinoma.

ASSOCIATED CONDITIONS
- Clinical manifestations of HPV infections:
  - Cutaneous warts
  - Papillomas of the conjunctiva, oral and nasal mucosa
  - RRP, a rare but serious manifestation of HPV 6 or 11 infection of the airway mucosa
  - Genital warts
  - Abnormal cervical cytology (Pap tests)
  - Intraepithelial neoplasia of the cervix, vagina, and vulva
  - SCC, adenocarcinoma
  - Anal intraepithelial neoplasia and anal cancer
  - Bowen disease: HPV-associated intraepithelial neoplasia
  - Buschke-Lowenstein tumor: Rare semimalignant growth that can transform to SCC

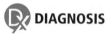 **DIAGNOSIS**

SIGNS AND SYMPTOMS
History
- Sexual and gynecologic history:
  - Sexual risk factors
  - Genital lesions with or without bleeding, mild pain or pruritus
  - Abnormal vaginal bleeding
- Medications:
  - Hormonal contraceptive use
  - Medications used in genital area
  - Immunosuppressive therapy
- Past medical history:
  - STD history and treatments
  - Chronic medical conditions
  - Immunosuppression
- HPV immunization history
- Social history:
  - History of sexual abuse
  - Potential barriers to screening and treatment

Review of Systems
- Special attention to GU and dermatology systems
- Special attention to immune status

Physical Exam
- HEENT:
  - Oral lesions
  - Hoarseness, aphonia, respiratory distress
- Skin:
  - Condylomata and other lesions
- GU:
  - Vulva, vagina, and cervix for the presence of warts and other lesions

TESTS

- Acetic acid applied to genital area results in whitening of areas of HPV infection; other infections or inflammation may cause false-positive findings.
- Cervical cytology (Pap) for cervical cancer screening

Labs

- HPV DNA detection:
  - Digene Hybrid Capture2 (HC2) High-Risk HPV DNA Test:
    - FDA approved for the detection of 18 HPV types in cervical specimens
    - Differentiates between low- and high-risk but does not determine the specific HPV type
    - Some labs using HC2 HPV DNA test may test only for presence or absence of high-risk, not low-risk types.
    - Current guidelines recommend its use in conjunction with cytology for primary cervical cancer screening in women >30 years and triage of women with atypia on Pap test results.
  - Other HPV DNA detection tests have been developed but are not commercially available in the US.
- No serologic test for HPV is used clinically.
- HPV cannot be cultured.

Imaging

Colposcopy is used to evaluate abnormal cytology findings and obtain biopsies for histologic exam to diagnose precancerous lesions (CIN 2, 3), carcinoma-in-situ and invasive cancer.

DIFFERENTIAL DIAGNOSIS

Infection

- Condylomata lata of secondary syphilis
- Molluscum contagiosum
- HSV

Tumor/Malignancy

Non-HPV-associated oropharyngeal or anogenital cancers

Other/Miscellaneous

- Normal anatomy:
  - Micropapillomatosis labialis
  - Sebaceous glands
- Dermatologic:
  - Fibroepithelial polyps
  - Skin tags
  - Seborrheic keratosis

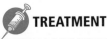 ## TREATMENT

GENERAL MEASURES

- HPV infection without clinical manifestations is not treated.
- Treatment is directed toward clinical manifestation of HPV infections.

MEDICATION (DRUGS)

- Topical treatments for genital warts:
  - Patient applied:
    - Imiquimod 5% cream
    - Podofilox 0.5% solution or gel
  - Provider applied:
    - Cryotherapy
    - BCA/TCA
    - Podophyllin resin 10–25%
- Podofilox, imiquimod, podophyllin should not be used during pregnancy.

SURGERY

- Surgical excision is indicated for management of persistent, extensive, large condylomata.
- Biopsy may be indicated for condylomata if the diagnosis is uncertain or lesions are pigmented, indurated, fixed, bleeding, ulcerated, or not responding to treatment.

 ## FOLLOW-UP

DISPOSITION

Issues for Referral
Condylomata requiring surgical therapy or on rectal mucosa

Pediatric Considerations
A diagnosis of HPV warrants an evaluation for sexual abuse.

PROGNOSIS

- Majority of genital HPV infections will clear spontaneously.
- Warts often recur, even with treatment.
- The risk of progression of CIN in healthy women after HPV infection is low.
  - Clearance of infection is the norm.
  - Persistent infection with a high-risk HPV type is the strongest risk for development of HSIL.

PATIENT MONITORING

- No monitoring for asymptomatic HPV infection is necessary.
- Monitoring of HPV-related disease is tailored to the specific condition. Guidelines are available for treatment and monitoring of genital warts, abnormal cervical cytology, cervical dysplasia, and cervical cancer.

BIBLIOGRAPHY

ACOG. Management of abnormal cervical cytology and histology. *Obstet Gynecol*. 2005;106(3):645–664.

Centers for Disease Control. Sexually transmitted diseases treatment guidelines. *MMWR*. 2006; 55(RR-11):1–93. Available at: http://www.cdc.gov/std/treatment/

Saslow D, et al. American Cancer Society guideline for the early detection of cervical neoplasia and cancer. *CA Cancer J Clin*. 2002;52(6):342–362. Available at: http://caonline.amcancersoc.org/cgi/content/full/52/6/342

USPSTF. Screening for Cervical Cancer. 2003. Available at: http://www.ahcpr.gov/clinic/uspstf/uspscerv.htm

Wright TC, Jr., et al. 2001 Consensus Guidelines for the management of women with cervical cytological abnormalities. *JAMA*. 2002;287(16):2120–2129. Available at: http://www.asccp.org/consensus.shtml

Wright TJ, et al. 2001 consensus guidelines for the management of women with cervical intraepithelial neoplasia. *Am J Obstet Gynecol*. 2003;189(1): 295–304. http://www.asccp.org/consensus.shtml

 ## MISCELLANEOUS

SYNONYM(S)

- Genital warts:
  - Condylomata acuminata
  - Venereal warts
- Premalignant lesions:
  - High-grade squamous intraepithelial neoplasia (HSIL)
  - Dysplasia
  - Carcinoma in-situ (CIS)
  - Cervical intraepithelial neoplasia (CIN)
  - Vaginal intraepithelial neoplasia (VAIN)
  - Vulvar intraepithelial neoplasia (VIN)

ABBREVIATIONS

- BCA—Bichloracetic acid
- CIN—Cervical intraepithelial neoplasia
- HEENT—Head, ears, eyes, nose, throat
- HSIL—High-grade squamous intraepithelial lesion
- HSV—Herpes simplex virus
- RRP—Recurrent respiratory papillomatosis
- SCC—Squamous cell carcinoma
- STD/STI—Sexually transmitted disease/infection
- TCA—Trichloroacetic acid
- VAIN—Vaginal intraepithelial neoplasia
- VIN—Vulvar intraepithelial neoplasia

CODES

ICD9-CM
079.4 HPV infection

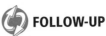 ## PATIENT TEACHING

PREVENTION

- Primary:
  - Vaccination:
    - Against HPV type 16 and 18 can prevent precancerous and cervical, vulvar and vaginal lesions caused by 16 and 18
    - Against HPV types 6 and 11 can prevent genital warts
    - Most effective if completed prior to sexual initiation but women with a history of sexual contact, abnormal Pap tests, or warts can receive the vaccine
  - Patient education:
    - Abstinence and limiting number of sexual partners
    - Correct and consistent condom use
    - Avoid tobacco use
- Secondary:
  - Regular cytology screening (Pap):
    - Screen regardless of HPV vaccination since ~30% of cervical cancers are caused by high-risk HPV types other than 16 and 18
    - Follow current recommendations
  - HPV is not a reportable infection to public health departments.
  - Sex partner notification is not required as a public health measure after diagnosis of genital warts, abnormal Pap findings, or cervical cancer.
  - If sex partners present for care:
    - Examine for genital warts
    - Provide education about HPV and other STDs
    - Educate female partners of the importance of cervical cancer screening regardless of known HPV infection or sexual orientation.

SEXUALLY TRANSMITTED DISEASES (STDs), OTHER: LYMPHOGRANULOMA VENEREUM (LGV), GRANULOMA INGUINALE, MOLLUSCUM CONTAGIOSUM, PUBIC LICE

Wei Wang, MPH

Jill S. Huppert, MD, MPH

 BASICS

DESCRIPTION

- Lymphogranuloma venereum (LGV) is a genital ulcer disease caused by serovars L1, L2, L3 of Chlamydia trachomatis:
  - Transmission is primarily sexual.
  - Endemic in east and west Africa, India, southeast Asia, South America, Caribbean
- Granuloma inguinale (GI) is an STD caused by Klebsiella granulomatis, a pleomorphic gram-negative bacillus:
  - It produces indolent, granulomatous, and progressive genital ulceration.
  - Endemic in western New Guinea, Caribbean, southern India, southeast Asia, Australia, Brazil
  - Transmission may be sexual, fecal, or by passage through infected birth canal.
- Molluscum contagiosum (MC) is a benign superficial skin disease caused by a poxvirus of the same name that causes a chronic localized infection producing characteristic flesh-colored, dome-shaped papules on the skin:
  - Common in the US, ~1% of all diagnosed skin disorders
  - Infection is usually self-limited and spontaneously resolves in the immunocompetent
  - Transmission may be through direct skin-to-skin contact, fomites, or autoinoculation; is considered an STD if genital lesions are found.
- Pubic lice (PL) is an STD involving the skin caused by a small 2–3-mm long translucent parasite Phthirus pubis, or the crab louse:
  - Characterized by itching and pale bluish spots (maculae caeruleae)
  - May involve pubic area as well as axillae, anus, abdomen, chest, and eyelashes or eyebrows
  - Transmitted by close physical contact, sexual contact, or fomites

Age-Related Factors

- LGV is most common in adults in their 3rd or 4th decade.
- If LGV or GI is seen in children, sexual abuse should be strongly considered.
- MC and PL can affect women of all ages due to nonsexual transmission.

EPIDEMIOLOGY

- Cases of LGV or GI in developed countries such as the US are rare and predominantly found in individuals who traveled to endemic areas:
  - LGV in developed countries is most prevalent in men who have sex with men. 5 cases reported in 2005 in association with HIV have raised concerns.
  - <100 cases of GI are reported annually in US.
  - GI is higher among African Americans in the US than among whites.
  - GI is considered mildly contagious, and repeated exposure may be necessary for clinical symptoms.
- Because MC and PL can be transmitted fairly easily through skin-to-skin contact, infection occurs in all age groups and both genders.
- PL is more common in women than men.

RISK FACTORS

As with all STDs, sexual promiscuity and unsafe practices, such as lack of condom use, increase the risk of LGV, GI, MC, and PL. Other risk factors include:

- For LGV/GI:
  - HIV seropositivity
  - Concurrent ulcerative disease
  - Unprotected receptive anal sex
- For molluscum contagiosum:
  - Cellular immunodeficiency (e.g., HIV infection, chemotherapy or corticosteroid therapy)
- For pubic lice:
  - Overcrowding
  - Poor hygiene

PATHOPHYSIOLOGY

- LGV is primarily a disease of lymphatic tissue:
  - C. trachomatis is an obligate intracellular bacterium.
    - Unlike most mucosal chlamydial infections, LGV serovars induce a lymphoproliferative reaction.
    - Organism enters lymphatics through contact with skin or mucous membranes.
  - The 3 stages of LGV include:
    - 1st or primary LGV (3–30 day post inoculation): Begins as small, painless papule or pustule that may erode to form asymptomatic herpetiform ulcer that heals without scarring.
    - 2nd or secondary LGV (2–6 weeks after primary lesion):
      - Painful regional lymphadenopathy occurs in 20–30% of females, although most present with nonspecific back or abdominal pain.
      - Includes fever, chills, myalgia and malaise
    - Tertiary LGV or genitoanorectal:
      - More common in women
      - Includes malaise, weight loss, bloody purulent discharge, fever, rectal pain, and tenesmus

- GI is caused by K. granulomatis, which causes granulomatous ulcerations:
  - Women may develop lesions on labia minora, mons veneris, fourchette, and/or cervix (10%).
  - Extragenital involvement may involve oral cavity or GI tract.
  - Incubation period: 1 week–3 months.
- MC poxvirus infects only the basal layer of the epidermis:
  - Latent period can be up to 6 months.
  - Clinical lesions appear as single or multiple discrete, painless, dome-shaped papules with an umbilicated center and a white curd-like core:
    - Infection is often mild and may spontaneously resolve without notice.
    - With superinfection, lesions present as pustules that may be painful.
    - No systemic symptoms
- PL usually presents as itching, sometimes with maculae caeruleae around the hair follicles:
  - Secondary bacterial infection or inflammation may be caused by scratching.

ASSOCIATED CONDITIONS

HIV and other STDs should be considered.

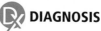 **DIAGNOSIS**

SIGNS AND SYMPTOMS

History

- Enquire about sexual risk behaviors such as new sexual partners and inconsistent use of condoms.
- Enquire about travel to endemic areas

Review of Systems

- Skin lesions:
  - Location, duration, amount of pain or itching, description
- Constitutional symptoms:
  - Pain, fever, malaise, weight loss
- GI symptoms:
  - Nausea, vomiting, diarrhea, or tenesmus

Physical Exam

- A comprehensive general physical exam is indicated, including skin and lymph nodes.
- On pelvic exam, the following findings may be seen:
  - LGV: Large fluctuant buboes or unexplained perianal deformity usually suggests LGV diagnosis.
    - 1st stage: Painless, small papule or shallow ulcer on external vulva.
    - 2nd stage: Painful, usually unilateral inguinal lymphadenopathy. Large fluctuant nodes or draining fistulas can be seen.
    - 3rd stage: Proctocolitis, enlargement, thickening and fibrosis of the labia.

- GI: 4 types of skin lesions occur on the vulva:
  - Ulcerovegetative (most common): Large, red, painless, ulcerative lesions with friable bases and distinct raised margins that bleed easily.
  - Nodular type: Soft, sometimes pruritic red nodules that may have a bright red, granulating surface.
  - Cicatricial type: Dry ulcers that become plaques, associated with lymphedema.
  - Hypertrophic or verrucous type (rare): Resemble genital warts.
- MC: Painless, flesh-colored, umbilicated papules ~2–6 mm in diameter (up to 10–15 mm in immunocompromised patients)
- PL: Lice firmly attached to the pubic hair:
  - Also look for bluish-grey maculae caeruleae on the abdomen or thighs.

TESTS

- Diagnosis of LGV, GI, MC, and PL is usually made clinically after excluding other causes.
- Tests for common ulcerative diseases (HSV, syphilis) and comprehensive STD testing (*Chlamydia*, gonorrhea, and trichomonas) should be performed.
- HIV testing is mandated if LGV or GI suspected.

Labs

- LV:
  - Culture from ulcer or lymph node aspirates is difficult, as yield is low.
  - Serologic tests, nucleic acid amplification testing, microimmunofluorescence, or complement fixation can be used but are not available in most settings.
  - For suspected cases, contact the CDC: http://www.cdc.gov/std/lgv/default.htm. cdclgvinfo@cdc.gov
- GI:
  - Direct visualization of the intracytoplasmic inclusion Donovan bodies in macrophages in biopsy or cytology specimens is the best method of diagnosis.
  - Isolation of *K. granulomatis* is possible but culture of the fastidious organism is difficult.
  - Pap smears can be used to demonstrate Donovan bodies in cervical cells.
- MC:
  - Diagnosis is usually made clinically.
  - Biopsy or staining of thin smears with Giemsa, Gram, or Wright can reveal infected cells.
  - MC viral antigens can be detected by fluorescent antibody.
- PL:
  - Microscopy can confirm nits/lice attached to pubic hair.

DIFFERENTIAL DIAGNOSIS

Infection

- Other ulcerative genital lesions:
  - HSV
  - Syphilis
  - Fungal infection
  - Mycobacterial infection

- Other skin lesions similar to MC:
  - Dermatitis
  - Granuloma
  - Herpes zoster
  - HPV/Genital warts

Immunologic

- Other autoimmune genital ulcers:
  - Crohn's disease
  - Behçet's disease
  - Aphthosis major

Tumor/Malignancy

Lymphadenopathy may also be associated with:

- Hodgkin disease
- Other cancers

 ## TREATMENT

GENERAL MEASURES

- Complete all prescribed medication.
- Avoid all sexual contact until 7 days after medical treatment is completed and lesions healed.

MEDICATION (DRUGS)

- LGV: Antibiotics required:
  - Doxycycline 100 mg PO b.i.d. for 21 days
  - Erythromycin base 500 mg PO q.i.d. for 21 days
- GI: Antibiotics required:
  - Doxycycline 100 mg PO b.i.d. for 21 days
  - Azithromycin 1 g/wk PO for 3 doses
- MC: Treatment is optional; no evidence that any treatment is better than placebo:
  - Oral therapy: Cimetidine
  - Topical therapy: Salicylic acid, tretinoin, cantharidin, imiquimod
- PL: Topical chemical pediculicides required:
  - Permethrin 1% lotion
  - Pyrethrins

SURGERY

- LGV: Needle aspiration or incision and drainage of inguinal nodes may be necessary.
- GI: Genital scars may need to be surgically corrected.
- MC: Each lesion can be unroofed with a needle or cuvette, but this is time consuming.

 ## FOLLOW-UP

DISPOSITION

Issues for Referral

MC and PL are common and self-limited. LGV and GI are rare and, if suspected, HIV testing is strongly recommended and referral to a vulvar or infectious disease specialist could be helpful.

PROGNOSIS

- LGV: Excellent prognosis with prompt and appropriate antibiotic.
- GI: Untreated lesions may continue to expand for years:
  - Relapse may occur up to 18 months after treatment.
- MC: Usually self-limited:
  - Recurrence in up to 35% of patients.
- PL: >90% cure rate with treatment.

PATIENT MONITORING

- All sexual partners of infected women should be evaluated.

BIBLIOGRAPHY

Centers for Disease Control and Prevention. 2006 Guidelines for treatment of sexually transmitted diseases. Diseases Characterized by Genital Ulcers. *MMWR*. 2006;55(RR-11):14–21.

Moodley P, et al. Association between HIV-1 infection, the etiology of genital ulcer disease, and response to syndromic management. *Sex Transm Dis*. 2003; 30(3):241–245.

Richens J. Donovanosis (granuloma inguinale). *Sex Transm Infect*. 2006;82(Suppl 4):iv21–iv22.

van der Wouden JC, et al. Interventions for cutaneous molluscum contagiosum. *Cochrane Database Syst Rev*. 2006(2):CD004767.

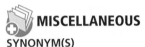 ## MISCELLANEOUS

SYNONYM(S)

- LGV: Tropical bubo; poradenitis inguinales
- GI: Donovanosis
- PL: Crabs

ABBREVIATION

- GI—Granuloma inguinale
- HSV—Herpes simplex virus
- LGV—Lymphogranuloma venereum
- MC—Molluscum contagiosum
- PL—Pubic Lice
- STD—Sexually transmitted disease

CODES

ICD9-CM

- 078.0 Molluscum contagiosum
- 099.1 Lymphogranuloma venereum
- 099.2 Granuloma inguinale
- 132.2 Pubic lice (pediculus pubis)

PATIENT TEACHING

- Notify all sexual partners that they need to be treated.
- Complete all medication and avoid sexual contact until all partners have been treated.
- Get tested for all other STDs, including HIV.

PREVENTION

- Abstinence, monogamy, and consistent use of condoms with each episode of sexual intercourse will decrease the risk of infection.
- Good hygiene may reduce the risk of nonsexual transmission of MC and PL.

SEXUALLY TRANSMITTED DISEASES (STDs): SYPHILIS

Sarah E. Bartlett, MD

 BASICS

DESCRIPTION

- Sexually transmitted chronic infection, with characteristic sequential changes:
  - Primary and secondary stages (infectious)
  - Latent syphilis
  - Tertiary stage
  - Congenital syphilis
- Infectious organism: A spirochete, *Treponema pallidum*
- Early syphilis is defined as the stages of primary, secondary, and early latent syphilis; typically within 1st year of infection.
- Late syphilis suggests cardiovascular, gummatous, and CNS syphilis.

Pediatric Considerations
If not congenital, consider sexual abuse as source.

Pregnancy Considerations
- Vertical transmission leads to stillbirth, nonimmune hydrops, neonatal death, prematurity, low birth weight, and the sequelae of congenital syphilis.
- Cervical changes (hyperemia, friability) in pregnancy may facilitate entry of *T. pallidum*.
- Early detection is key:
  - Universal 1st trimester screening recommended to identify asymptomatic patients.
  - If high risk of exposure, consider repeat tests later in pregnancy, at delivery.
- Neonates can also acquire syphilis from contact with active lesions.
- No risk of transmission with breast-feeding unless lesions are present.
- Monitor for Jarisch-Herxheimer reaction:
  - Can lead to contractions, preterm labor
  - Only supportive treatment

EPIDEMIOLOGY

- Predominantly in sexually active age groups
- In the US, rate declined by 90% from 1990–2000, but rates increased between 2000–2004.
- Higher rates with men who have sex with men
- Higher rates in blacks and Hispanics
- High rate of HIV coinfection
- 1 million pregnancies per year are affected by maternal syphilis worldwide.

Incidence
Early syphilis:

- Peaked in 1990: 20.3 cases/100,000 population
- In 2004: 2.7 cases/100,000 population

RISK FACTORS

- Multiple sexual partners
- Infants of infected mothers
- Men who have sex with men
- HIV

PATHOPHYSIOLOGY

- Mostly sexually transmitted via inoculation with *T. pallidum* at disrupted epithelium from minor trauma:
  - Initial local response with erosion
  - Wider spread via regional lymph nodes and hematogenous spread
- Primary pathology is vasculitis.
- Cellular immunity is likely involved in late syphilis.
- Slow evolution of infectious process due to long dividing time of organism

ASSOCIATED CONDITIONS

- Other STIs
- HIV and hepatitis B:
  - Syphilis promotes transmission of HIV

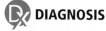 **DIAGNOSIS**

SIGNS AND SYMPTOMS

- Primary syphilis (infectious):
  - Indurated, painless ulcer (chancre) begins 9–90 days after exposure; anogenital
  - Also found on lips, tongue, tonsils, nipples, fingers
  - Chancre heals with scarring in 3–6 weeks regardless of treatment
- Secondary syphilis (infectious):
  - Generalized rash on palms and soles
  - Generalized lymphadenopathy, plus orogenital mucosal lesions
  - Rash usually resolves spontaneously in 2–6 weeks
  - Contact with broken skin can spread infection
  - Condyloma lata:
    - Large gray-white lesions involving warm, moist areas of body (mucous membranes, perineum, etc.)
  - Also mild hepatosplenomegaly at this stage
  - Alopecia ("moth-eaten")
  - Wide variety of neurologic manifestations
- Latent syphilis:
  - Positive serology without signs or symptoms
  - After 1 year, patients no longer infectious but might relapse to infectious stage if untreated
- Tertiary syphilis:
  - Characterized by gummatous lesions, cardiovascular and neurologic involvement
  - 1/3 of patients with secondary syphilis progress to this stage.
  - Cardiovascular involvement most commonly affects aortic root:
    - Signs include murmur, left heart failure, ascending aorta aneurysms, AV regurgitation
  - Deep cutaneous gummas are destructive granulomatous pockets, found in skin, bones, or internal organs.
  - Neurosyphilis includes stroke, parenchymal disease leading to general paresis, tabes dorsalis.

- Congenital syphilis:
  - Infant symptoms:
    - Snuffles (mucopurulent rhinitis)
    - Failure to thrive
    - Lymphadenopathy
    - Jaundice
    - Anemia
    - Meningitis
    - Rash
  - Childhood symptoms:
    - Hutchinson teeth
    - Saber shins
    - Charcot joints
    - Deafness
    - Interstitial keratitis

History
- Always ascertain sexual practices and potential exposures
- Keep in mind latent periods as well as potential for decades-long infections

Physical Exam
See "Signs and Symptoms."

TESTS
- Screening tests:
  - VDRL or RPR
- Confirmation tests:
  - FTA-ABS and TPHA

Labs
- Dark-field microscopy, using samples from lesions; high false-negative rate
- *T. pallidum* cannot be cultured.
- Nontreponemal tests (VDRL and RPR):
  - Used as primary screening tests
  - Positive within 7 days of exposure
  - Also used to quantify response to treatment (titers decrease)
  - False-positives common, especially with pregnancy, malignancy, EBV, hepatitis, autoimmune diseases
- Treponemal tests (FTA-ABS and MHA-TP):
  - Become reactive earlier, remain positive indefinitely (despite treatment)
  - Expensive
- New diagnostic tests include EIA/ELISA and immunoblotting to detect *T. pallidum* IgG and IgM. Also, PCR to detect bacterial DNA
- Lumbar puncture for CSF serologies whenever tertiary syphilis is suspected or HIV present

Imaging
Brain and cardiac imaging as indicated in tertiary cases

DIFFERENTIAL DIAGNOSIS
- Primary:
  - Chancroid, lymphogranuloma venereum, granuloma inguinale, herpes, Behçet's syndrome, trauma
- Secondary:
  - Pityriasis rosea, guttate psoriasis, drug eruption
- Positive serology, no symptoms:
  - Previously treated syphilis, biologic false positive, other spirochetal disease (e.g., yaws, pinta)

 ## TREATMENT

GENERAL MEASURES
Early diagnosis is key.

MEDICATION (DRUGS)
- Parenteral penicillin G is drug of choice.
- Primary, secondary, and early latent:
  - Benzathine PCN G 2.4 million units IM single dose
- Late latent and tertiary (not neurosyphilis):
  - Benzathine PCN G 2.4 million units IM weekly in 3 doses
- Neurosyphilis:
  - Pen G 3–4 million units IV q4h or 24 million units continuous IV infusion for 10–14 days
- Consider desensitization for penicillin allergy, especially with pregnant patients:
  - Can also use tetracyclines, macrolides, and ceftriaxone, although data are limited.
  - Can only use PCN for neurosyphilis.
- Congenital:
  - Pen G 50,000 U/kg q8–12h for 10–14 days, or Pen G procaine 50,000 U/kg IM daily for 10–14 days
  - If negative CSF cultures, 50,000 U/kg benzathine Pen G IM single dose

 ## FOLLOW-UP

DISPOSITION
Issues for Referral
Penicillin allergy, especially for desensitization during pregnancy

PROGNOSIS
Excellent prognosis with most except late syphilis and HIV

PATIENT MONITORING
- Follow treatment efficacy with VDRL or RPR.
- Reassess all patients clinically and serologically at 6 and 12 months post treatment for primary and secondary disease.
- Reassess every 3, 6, 12 months for tertiary disease.
- 4–fold reduction in titer of nontreponemal test suggests adequate treatment.
- Monitor for Jarisch-Herxheimer reaction during antibiotic treatment.

BIBLIOGRAPHY

Centers for Disease Control and Prevention. Primary and Secondary syphilis United States, 2002. *MMWR Morb Wkly Rep.* 2003;21:117–120.

Centers for Disease Control and Prevention. Sexually transmitted disease surveillance 2003 supplement, syphilis surveillance report, December 2004.

Doroshenko A, et al. Syphilis in pregnancy and the neonatal period. *Intern J STD AIDS.* 2006;17: 221–228.

Goh BT. Syphilis in adults. *Sex Transm Inf.* 2005;81: 448–452.

 ## MISCELLANEOUS

SYNONYM(S)
- Lues
- The Great Imitator

ABBREVIATIONS
- CSF—Cerebrospinal fluid
- EBV—Epstein-Barr virus
- ELISA—Enzyme-linked immunosorbent assay
- FTA-ABS—Fluorescent treponemal antibody, absorbed
- PCN—Penicillin
- PCR—Polymerase chain reaction
- RPR—Rapid plasma reagin
- TPHA—Treponema pallidum hemagglutination assay
- VDRL—Venereal Disease Research Laboratory

CODES
ICD9-CM
097.9 Syphilis, unspecified

 ## PATIENT TEACHING

- Early diagnosis and full treatment is critical.
- All sexual contacts must be traced.
- Safe sex always!

PREVENTION
Safe sex always!

SEXUALLY TRANSMITTED DISEASES (STDs): TRICHOMONAS

Jill S. Huppert, MD, MPH

BASICS

DESCRIPTION
- The causative agent of trichomoniasis or trichomonas vaginitis is *Trichomonas vaginalis* (Tv), a pear-shaped, motile protozoa.
- A parasite with no nonhuman or environmental reservoir
- Infects both human male and female GU tract
- Transmitted via sexual intercourse and intimate sexual contact
- In addition to heterosexual contact, female-to-female transmission has been reported.

Age-Related Factors
- Sexual contact: Affects women of all ages, most commonly between 20 and 45 years
- Nonsexual contact: Intrapartum transmission to neonates has been rarely described.

EPIDEMIOLOGY
- An estimated 180 million cases of Tv in the world each year.
- Estimated to be the most common treatable STD in the US
- Not a reportable STD
- Incidence and prevalence estimates are limited by poor diagnostic methods and lack of a screening program.
- Prevalence estimates in symptomatic women range from 5–30%, and depend on the population studied.
- Currently, only 1 population based prevalence study: Among asymptomatic sexually active females age 18–26, 2.8% have Tv.
- In 1 incidence study, 23% of adolescent women age 14–17 acquired Tv within 3 months.

RISK FACTORS
- High-risk sexual behaviors, such as multiple partners and lack of condom use, increase risk of infection.
- In the US, prevalence is higher in southern states.
- African Americans have higher prevalence.
- Other risks: Incarcerated women, history of prior STDs

PATHOPHYSIOLOGY
- Tv preferentially infects the vagina, but can also infect the urethra or perivaginal glands.
- After inoculation, Tv must adhere to the vaginal epithelium.
- Tv damages the epithelial mucosa and provokes an inflammatory response.
- To ensure prolonged survival, it alters host flora and increases the vaginal pH.
- These changes increase susceptibility to other infections and increase the risk of morbidity, especially HIV infection.
- Typically, symptoms occur 4–28 days after sexual contact.
- Because of its growth requirements and adaptation to the vaginal environment, Tv has rarely been isolated from other body sites such as the pharynx and lungs.

ASSOCIATED CONDITIONS
Other STDs are often found to coexist with Tv.

DIAGNOSIS

SIGNS AND SYMPTOMS
History
- Enquire about sexual risk behaviors such as new sexual partners and inconsistent use of condoms.
- >90% of infected women have no symptoms.
- Some infected women report:
  - Vaginal discharge, itching or odor
  - Dysuria
  - Abnormal vaginal bleeding or spotting

Physical Exam
- General physical exam may be performed if indicated.
- Pelvic exam is recommended but is normal in >90% of infections
- Inspect external vulva: Normal or may have erythema, excoriations, and notable discharge
- Speculum exam:
  - Vagina may appear inflamed or normal.
  - Vaginal discharge may be normal, frothy, green, or pink-tinged.
  - Cervix may be normal or friable. Punctuate hemorrhage (also described as a "strawberry cervix") is seen in <2% of infections.
- Bimanual exam: Normal or tender

TESTS
- All sexually active women at risk for STDs should be offered Tv testing.
- Available diagnostic tests are highly specific but vary in sensitivity, cost, availability.
- Tests that support, but do not make the diagnosis of Tv include:
  - Elevated vaginal pH >4.5
  - Elevated WBCs (≥10 per high-powered field) on wet-mount microscopy

Lab
- The most commonly used test is office microscopy of a saline preparation of vaginal fluid or "wet mount":
  - Requires visualizing *motile* trichomonads
  - Requires microscopy skills
  - 60% sensitive compared to culture
- Culture using selective media is the gold standard (75–90% sensitive), but often not available
- Rapid antigen test is point of care, equivalent to culture, and inexpensive (83–90% sensitive)
- Nucleic acid amplification tests are not yet commercially available (>95% sensitive).
- Above tests have high specificity (100%), so any positive wet-mount, culture, or rapid antigen test should be treated as a true positive.
- Tv may be seen on Pap smear, but lower specificity increases the rate of false-positives.
- Some Tv tests may be performed on self-obtained vaginal swabs if resources are not available for a complete pelvic exam.
- Tests of cure are not indicated.

DIFFERENTIAL DIAGNOSIS
Many women who complain of vaginal discharge have no diagnostic abnormality, and can be reassured that their discharge is physiologic.

Infection
- Other agents can cause a range of vaginal symptoms:
  - *Candida albicans* and other yeast species:
    - Itching is usually more prominent with candida
- Other STDs such as gonorrhea and herpes
- Bacterial vaginosis shares many nonspecific signs and symptoms with Tv; However, it should be considered only if Tv is excluded by culture or rapid antigen test.

Trauma
Mechanical irritation, such as due to friction from condoms, may cause vaginal erythema and discharge.

Drugs
Allergic reaction to topical vaginal products or latex (as in condoms) may cause redness and discharge.

Other/Miscellaneous
- A foreign body, such as a retained tampon, can cause vaginal discharge and odor.
- Vulvar vestibulitis can cause poorly characterized symptoms.

TREATMENT

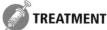

GENERAL MEASURES
- Complete all prescribed medication.
- Avoid all sexual contact until 7 days after medical treatment is completed.

MEDICATION (DRUGS)
First Line
- Metronidazole 2 g, or tinidazole 2 g, as a single PO dose
- Alternate: Metronidazole 500 mg PO b.i.d. for 7 days
- Both are imidazoles and cause a disulfiram-like effect if taken with alcohol.
- GI side effects such as nausea, vomiting, and metallic taste are reduced with tinidazole.
- The multiday regimen may be used for resistant or recurrent cases, but has more side effects and poorer compliance.
- For resistant cases where reinfection has been ruled out, the dose of metronidazole or tinidazole can be increased to 2 g PO for 5 days.
- Contraindications: Documented allergy to imidazoles
- Patients with a true allergy may be managed with metronidazole desensitization in consultation with a specialist.
- Precautions: Avoid alcohol during treatment and for 24–48 hours after completion of medication.
- Topical treatment with metronidazole vaginal cream or other topical antibiotics are less efficacious (<50% cure rate) than oral imidazoles, and are discouraged.

Pediatric Considerations
- Tv has been detected in the pediatric age group among victims of sexual assault.
- In these cases, Tv culture may be obtained using a "blind" vaginal swab rather than speculum exam.

Geriatric Considerations
- Tv may affect older women; some estimate that it can persist for up to 5 years.
- Tv infects the vagina, so sexually active women without a cervix (i.e., posthysterectomy) remain at risk.

Pregnancy Considerations
- Knowledge regarding the relationship between Tv and pregnancy complications continues to evolve.
- Large studies have failed to show consistent improvement in pregnancy outcomes when Tv is detected and treated in mid-trimester.
- Smaller studies suggest a decrease in 1st trimester miscarriages when Tv is detected and treated early in pregnancy.
- In 2006, the CDC recommended that routine Tv screening of pregnant women did not change pregnancy outcomes.
- However, Tv detected and treated during pregnancy can reduce vaginal symptoms and reduce sexual transmission as a public health measure.
- Metronidazole is pregnancy category B, and the usual 2-g dose may be given.
- Tinidazole is pregnancy category C, and its safety in pregnant women has not been studied.

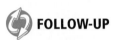

FOLLOW-UP

DISPOSITION
Issues for Referral
- Those positive for Tv should be offered/referred for comprehensive STD testing, including HIV testing.
- Tv-positive patients should be counseled regarding HIV risk reduction.
- Those with recurrent infections should be counseled regarding compliance with therapy and treatment of all partners.
- If drug resistance is suspected, contact the CDC for guidance (www.cdc.gov/std) or 770-488-4115.

PROGNOSIS
- 95% of Tv infections are cured with single-dose treatment.
- Poor compliance with therapy is a frequent cause of "recurrent" infections.
- Partner treatment improves cure rates.
- Complications: Women infected with Tv who are not treated are at higher risk for the following:
  – Concurrent infection with other STDs.
  – Acquiring other STDs such as HSV, HPV, and HIV.
  – Developing cervical dysplasia due to persistence of HPV.
  – Possible pregnancy complications such as preterm delivery and postpartum endometritis
  – In HIV-positive women, increased shedding of HIV virus

PATIENT MONITORING
- All sexual partners of infected women should be treated, as Tv testing for males is considerably less sensitive than for females.
- Adolescents who test positive for Tv should be retested in 3 months due to the high incidence of reinfection.
- All others should be tested at least yearly or with any new high-risk sexual behavior.

BIBLIOGRAPHY

Huppert JS, et al. Use of an immunochromatographic assay for rapid detection of *Trichomonas vaginalis* in vaginal specimens. *J Clin Microbiol*. 2005;43(2):684–687.

Miller WC, et al. The prevalence of trichomoniasis in young adults in the United States. *Sex Transm Dis*. 2005;32(10):593–598.

Petrin D, et al. Clinical and microbiological aspects of Trichomonas vaginalis. *Clin Microbiol Rev*. 1998;11(2):300–317.

Soper D. Trichomoniasis: under control or undercontrolled? *Am J Obstet Gynecol*. 2004;190(1):281–290.

Van Der Pol B, et al. Prevalence, incidence, natural history, and response to treatment of trichomonas vaginalis infection among adolescent women. *J Infect Dis*. 2005;192(12):2039–2044.

MISCELLANEOUS

SYNONYM(S)
Trick or Trich

CLINICAL PEARLS
- Unlike *Chlamydia*, the prevalence of Tv does not decrease in women >25.
- Asymptomatic infection can persist for months to years.
- Relying upon the wet-mount for diagnosis will miss 40–50% of infections, unless culture or rapid test is used as a back-up for those who are wet-mount negative.

ABBREVIATIONS
- GI—Gastrointestinal
- HIV—Human immunodeficiency virus
- HPV—Human papillomavirus
- HSV—Herpes simplex virus
- STD—Sexually transmitted disease
- Tv—*Trichomonas vaginalis*

CODES

ICD9-CM
- 131.0 Urogenital trichomoniasis
- 131.01 Trichomonal vulvovaginitis
- 131.02 Trichomonal urethritis

PATIENT TEACHING

- Notify all sexual partners that they need to be treated.
- Complete all medication and avoid sexual contact until all partners have been treated.
- Get tested for all other STDs, including HIV.

PREVENTION
Abstinence, monogamy, and consistent use of condoms with each episode of sexual intercourse decreases risk of infection.

SHEEHAN SYNDROME

Robert W. Rebar, MD

 BASICS

DESCRIPTION

- Sheehan syndrome is caused by infarction and necrosis of the pituitary gland as a result of severe obstetric hemorrhage and shock. Most commonly, only involvement of the anterior pituitary gland is present, but it is possible for the posterior pituitary to be involved and for the patient to have diabetes insipidus.

EPIDEMIOLOGY

Although Sheehan syndrome is said to be the most common cause of panhypopituitarism in women of child-bearing age, it is extremely rare and is decreasing as a result of improvements in peripartum care.

RISK FACTORS

The incidence appears increased following:

- Multiple pregnancies
- With placental abnormalities such as placenta accreta, placenta previa, and abruption
- Disseminated intravascular coagulation (as may occur with amniotic fluid embolus)
- In women with diabetes mellitus (perhaps as much as 10-fold)

PATHOPHYSIOLOGY

The anterior pituitary gland almost doubles in size during pregnancy, largely because of hypertrophy and hyperplasia of the lactotropes. The enlarged gland is particularly susceptible to ischemia because the oxygen supply depends on an intact arterial blood supply and the low-pressure portal venous system connecting the gland to the hypothalamus. With hypotension and hypovolemia as a result of hemorrhage and shock, blood flow to the anterior pituitary is markedly reduced. Arterial spasm and intravascular coagulation also may play roles in producing ischemia and necrosis.

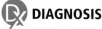 **DIAGNOSIS**

SIGNS AND SYMPTOMS

History

- The clinical presentation is variable but affected women may complain of:
  - Inability to breastfeed
  - Loss of pubic and axillary hair
  - Fatigue
  - Weakness
  - Dizziness
  - Nausea and vomiting
  - Amenorrhea
- Symptoms may arise acutely after delivery or even months or years later.
- Rarely symptoms have even appeared for the 1st time during a subsequent pregnancy.
- Up to 70% of the time following severe hemorrhage, pituitary mass is lost without development of any symptoms; conversely, perhaps 70% or more of the anterior pituitary must be destroyed before hypopituitarism results.
- Although amenorrhea and loss of libido are common even in the chronic form of Sheehan syndrome, some women menstruate and ovulate normally, and spontaneous pregnancies have been reported.
- Some of these women recall transient polydipsia and polyuria in the immediate postpartum period due to transient diabetes insipidus.

Physical Exam

Physical signs of hypopituitarism may be obvious or subtle:

- Hypotension, sometimes postural
- Slowed reflexes
- Breast involution
- Diminished axillary and pubic hair
- Atrophic vaginal mucosa
- Diminished cervical mucus

TESTS

Sheehan syndrome is confirmed by laboratory testing.

Labs

- In severe cases, confirmation is not difficult.
- Fasting blood sugar may be low due to a combination of growth hormone deficiency and hypoadrenalism.
- Hyponatremia may exist due to hypoadrenalism and diabetes insipidus.
- Secondary hypothyroidism may be documented by measurement of TSH.
- Cortisol and corticotropin levels may be very low in hypoadrenalism.
- Basal levels of LH and FSH and estradiol may be low.
- Basal levels of prolactin may be <5 ng/mL.
- A corticotropin stimulation test is of no value in the postpartum period because the adrenal gland will not yet have atrophied.
- Similarly, T4 levels may not be decreased because of the 7-day half-life of the hormone:
  - More subtle cases may require provocative testing of anterior pituitary functions to document hypopituitarism.
- Although most women have no symptoms when seen in later years, many demonstrate impaired urinary concentrating ability and deficient vasopressin secretion if subjected to dehydration testing of posterior pituitary function.

Imaging

MRI or CT of the sella turcica can rule out other causes of hypopituitarism. These tests may show a partially or completely empty sella turcica due to the destruction of the pituitary gland.

DIFFERENTIAL DIAGNOSIS

Hematologic

Pituitary infarction can occur in individuals with sickle cell disease, independent of profound blood loss at delivery.

Metabolic/Endocrine
Pituitary infarction can occur in individuals with diabetes, independent of profound blood loss at delivery.

Tumor/Malignancy
- Pituitary neoplasms must be ruled out in women whose symptoms arise slowly several months or years after delivery.
- Pituitary infarction also can occur in individuals with pituitary tumors, independent of profound blood loss at delivery.
- Hypopituitarism resulting from infarction or hemorrhage of undiagnosed silent pituitary tumor during CABG has been described.

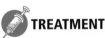 TREATMENT

GENERAL MEASURES
- For the patient presenting with hypotension and lethargy in the immediate postpartum period:
  - Immediate parenteral administration of corticosteroids.
  - Once the patient is stabilized, oral corticosteroids can be administered at maintenance dosage.
  - Corticosteroid therapy should be initiated before thyroid hormone therapy begins to prevent circulatory collapse secondary to adrenal crisis:
    - T4 should be given slowly, beginning with 25 μg/d PO increasing slowly at 1-week intervals until full replacement doses are achieved.
    - TSH levels may not be helpful in adjusting the dose of T4, and free T4 levels and resting pulse rate may be more helpful in assuring appropriate thyroid replacement.
- Estrogen and progestogen therapy are needed in women who remain amenorrheic.

Pregnancy Considerations
Many cases of successful pregnancy in women with Sheehan syndrome have been reported:
- Gonadotropin therapy is required to induce ovulation in women who remain amenorrheic.
- Replacement therapy (except for estrogen and progestogen) must be continued during the entire pregnancy.

 FOLLOW-UP

DISPOSITION
Issues for Referral
Women with Sheehan syndrome should be evaluated and cared for by clinicians familiar with the use of hormones for the treatment of hypopituitarism.

PROGNOSIS
With early diagnosis and treatment, prognosis for women with Sheehan syndrome is excellent, but life-long therapy for hypopituitarism is typically required.

PATIENT MONITORING
Patients with hypopituitarism should be seen frequently and checked for adequate replacement by appropriate laboratory tests at least yearly.

BIBLIOGRAPHY

Boulanger E, et al. Sheehan syndrome presenting as early post-partum hyponatremia. *Nephrol Dial Transplant*. 1999;14:2714–2715.

Dejager S, et al. Sheehan's syndrome: Differential diagnosis in the acute phase. *J Intern Med*. 1998;244:261–266.

Molitch ME. Pituitary disease in pregnancy. *Semin Perinatol*. 1998;22:457–470.

Sheehan HL. The recognition of chronic hypopituitarism resulting from postpartum pituitary necrosis. *Am J Obstet Gynecol*. 1971;111:852–854.

Sheehan HL, et al. Pituitary necrosis. *Br Med Bull*. 1968;24:59–70.

 MISCELLANEOUS

SYNONYM(S)
- Postpartum pituitary necrosis
- Postpartum pituitary insufficiency
- Postpartum hypopituitarism
- Simmond disease

CODES
ICD9-CM
- 253 Disorders of the pituitary gland and its hypothalamic control
- 253.2 Panhypopituitarism
- 253.4 Other anterior pituitary disorders
- 253.5 Diabetes insipidus

 PATIENT TEACHING

- Patients should be instructed to double or triple the dose of corticosteroids under stressful circumstances, such as infection, trauma, or major surgery.
- Patients should be instructed to wear a medical alert bracelet and always carry with them information about the replacement drugs they are taking.

PREVENTION
Prevention of extreme hemorrhage and hypovolemia at and following delivery reduces the incidence of this rare disorder.

Section II

STRESS URINARY INCONTINENCE

Soo Y. Kwon, MD
Carlos Perez-Cosio, MD

BASICS

DESCRIPTION
- According to International Continence Society (ICS) definition, the complaint of involuntary leakage of urine during effort or exertion (coughing, sneezing), in the absence of a bladder contraction.
- The term *stress urinary incontinence* also describes that the leakage from the urethra must be synchronous with the increase in the abdominal pressure.
- When SUI is confirmed by urodynamics, it is defined as urodynamic stress incontinence (UDSUI).

Age-Related Factors
Most studies show increasing prevalence with age:
- 5–40% in women 30–60 years of age
- 5–45% >60 years of age

Pregnancy Considerations
The incidence of SUI during pregnancy can be as high as 32%; by 1 year postpartum, only 3% of patients reported SUI.

Geriatric Considerations
The prevalence of SUI rises with age and can be associated with pelvic organ prolapse in the elderly.

EPIDEMIOLOGY
Affects both sexes but particularly adult women:
- 10–43% of community-dwelling female population
- Up to 50% of nursing home population

RISK FACTORS
- Obesity
- Caucasian
- Vaginal delivery
- Prolonged 2nd stage of labor
- Strenuous physical exercise
- Chronic coughing
- Obstructive pulmonary disease
- Increasing age
- Menopause
- Multiparity
- Dementia
- Neurologic disorder
- Functional impairment

Genetics
Increased prevalence between 1st-degree relatives

PATHOPHYSIOLOGY
- Weakening or damage to vaginal wall and the endopelvic fascia, which provide support to the urethra and bladder neck
- With increases in intra-abdominal pressure, intravesical pressure rises as well
- This pressure may overcome urethral resistance, resulting in leakage
- Damage to neuromuscular function of pelvic floor
- Damage to supporting tissue of urethra and bladder neck
- Possible loss of intrinsic urethral tone
- Other factors:
  - Hypovascularity
  - Tissue atrophy
  - Local scarring

ETIOLOGY
- SUI is a result of impaired urethral support from the pelvic endofascia, nerves, and muscles.
- Most commonly during childbirh
- Less commonly due to failure of urethral closure, called *intrinsic sphincter deficiency*:
  - This usually results from operative trauma, scarring
  - May also occur with muscular atrophy in postmenopausal women

DIAGNOSIS

SIGNS AND SYMPTOMS
The most important tools in the diagnosis are a complete history with a voiding diary and physical exam including a cough stress test and a PVR urine volume.

History
- Voiding frequency including nocturia
- Voided volume
- Frequency and volume of incontinence episodes
- Duration of symptoms
- Precipitating factors
- Fluid and caffeine intake
- Tobacco and alcohol use
- Impact on daily life
- Incomplete emptying
- Use of pads
- Obstetric history
- History of pelvic surgeries, hysterectomy, prior incontinence procedures
- Medications

Review of Systems
- Chronic illnesses, cough, COPD, DM
- Vaginal bulge or pressure in the vagina
- Recurrent UTIs or symptoms of urgency, frequency, dysuria, hematuria, pain with full bladder
- Anal incontinence and defecatory dysfunction

Physical Exam
- Evaluate for pelvic masses, pelvic organ prolapse, and vaginal atrophy.
- Assess neurologic function.
- Cough stress test
- Demonstrating hypermobility of the bladder neck (Q-tip test) is helpful when planning a surgical procedure.
- Systematic exam for cystocele, rectocele, enerocele, and perineal integrity
- Pelvic Organ Prolapse Quantitative (POP-Q) is an objective, site-specific system for describing, quantifying, and staging pelvic support in women and notes degree of relaxation and measures prolapse above or below hymen.

TESTS
- The role of routine urodynamics is controversial.
- Indications for urodynamics include:
  - Prior to surgical treatment of SUI
  - Unclear history
  - Symptoms not consistent with physical exam
  - Symptoms not improved with conservative treatment
  - History of prior anti-incontinent surgery
- The use of routine cystoscopy is recommended for patients with:
  - Sterile hematuria
  - Bladder pain
  - Suspected mass

Labs
- UA to rule out diabetes, infection, and tumor
- Urine culture

Imaging
Pelvic US if pelvic mass is suspected

DIFFERENTIAL DIAGNOSIS
- SUI vs. overactive bladder vs. mixed urinary incontinence
- 7% of those with symptoms of SUI have stress-induced detrusor instability

TREATMENT

GENERAL MEASURES
- Lifestyle interventions can decrease SUI in many women:
  - Weight loss
  - Smoking cessation
  - Decreasing caffeinated and carbonated intake
  - Treatment of constipation and fecal impaction
- Pelvic floor training "Kegel exercises" when done 3–4 times per week with 3 repetitions of 8–10 sustained contractions lasting 8–12 seconds are an effective treatment for SUI compared to placebo in RCTs.
- Electro stimulation of the pelvic floor muscles
- Pessaries:
  - Experience with fitting and sizing
  - Easy to insert but require removal for cleaning

SPECIAL THERAPY
Minimally invasive procedures, like injectable bulking agents

MEDICATION (DRUGS)
- Duloxetine has shown limited improvement in SUI symptoms compared to placebo 59% (40 mg/d), 64% (80 mg/d) vs. 40% in the placebo group.
- Estrogens had been used to treat SUI although more recent data does not show improvement of symptoms.

SURGERY
- Bladder neck suspension surgery such as Marshall-Marchetti-Krantz (MMK) and Burch remain gold standard surgeries for SUI. Burch has a 48-month cure/dry rate of 84%.
- Midurethral slings:
  - The 48-month cure/dry rate for slings is 83%.
  - More clinical studies are necessary to evaluate the long-term efficacy of TOT.
  - Autologous: From rectus fascia or fascia lata
  - Xenograft: Dermal or small intestine-porcine
  - Synthetics:
    - Tension free TVT
    - Tension free TOT

 FOLLOW-UP

DISPOSITION
Issues for Referral
- Recurrent UTIs
- Failed conservative treatment
- Prior gynecologic-urologic surgery
- Associated pelvic organ prolapse

BIBLIOGRAPHY

Gilleran JP, et al. An evidence-based approach to the evaluation and management of stress incontinence in women. *Curr Opin Urol.* 2005;15(4):236–243.

Kirby M. Managing stress urinary incontinence: A primary care issue. *Int J Clin Pract.* 2006;60(2):184–189.

Miller KL. Stress urinary incontinence in women and update on neurological control. *J Womens Health.* 2005;14:595–608.

Norton P, et al. Urinary incontinence in women. *Lancet.* 2006;367:57–67.

Nygaard IE, et al. Stress urinary incontinence. *Obstet Gynecol.* 2004;104:607–620.

 MISCELLANEOUS

ABBREVIATIONS
- COPD—Chronic obstructive pulmonary disease
- DM—Diabetes mellitus
- ICS—International Continence Society
- POP–Q—Pelvic organ prolapse–quantative
- PVR—Postvoid residual
- RCT—Randomized controlled trial
- SUI—Stress urinary incontinence
- TOT—Transobdurator tape
- TVT—Transvaginal tape
- UDSUI—Urodynamic stress urinary incontinence
- US—Ultrasound
- UTI—Urinary tract infection

CODES
ICD9-CM
- 625.6 Stress urinary incontinence
- 788.33 Mixed incontinence

PATIENT TEACHING

- Recommend pelvic floor (Kegel) exercises:
  - http://patients.uptodate.com/topic.asp?file= wom_issu/3002
- Include instructions regarding good nutrition and exercise practices.
- Address the need for easy access to toilet facilities.
- Recommend bladder training to ensure regular and complete bladder emptying.

PREVENTION
- It has been suggested that cesarean delivery will minimize the risks or prevent SUI.
  - Studies demonstrating prevention are few and controversial.
  - In one randomized trial, the cesarean delivery group reported less stress urinary incontinence than vaginal birth (4.5% vs. 7.3%).
- Episiotomy not protective
- Pelvic floor muscle training has shown to be effective in both treatment and prevention.

TURNER SYNDROME

Philippe F. Backeljauw, MD

BASICS

DESCRIPTION
- TS describes phenotypic females with short stature, gonadal failure, and infertility.
- It is caused by the loss of all or part of the X-chromosome.
- TS is associated with varying degrees of skeletal, cardiovascular, renal, endocrine, lymphatic, and neurologic anomalies.
- Karyotype analysis shows either complete or partial absence of 1 sex chromosome, or mosaicism with 2 or more cell lines.
- 1st described as a syndrome of sexual infantilism, cubitus valgus, and congenital webbing of the neck by Henry Turner, in 1938.

Age-Related Factors
- Mean age at diagnosis is 4.2 years, but range is from prenatal life to 16 years.
- Within the different age groups, the keys to diagnosis of TS are different:
  – Prenatally: Incidental diagnosis after amniocentesis or chorionic villus sampling
  – Infancy: Lymphedema and congenital heart disease (coarctation of the aorta)
  – Childhood: Growth failure
  – Adolescence: Delayed puberty, amenorrhea, and growth failure
- Rarely, patients are diagnosed in adulthood as part of an infertility evaluation.

EPIDEMIOLOGY
- Prevalence: ~1 in 1,900 female live births (may be higher with increasing prenatal diagnosis of TS mosaicism).
- 3% of all females conceived have TS, but nearly 99% of all TS conceptions do not survive beyond 28 weeks of gestation.

RISK FACTORS
- Sporadic event due to faulty chromosome distribution (often nondisjunction during paternal meiosis, or postfertilization mitotic error leading to TS mosaicism)
- Rare cases of familial TS are associated with an inherited X-chromosome anomaly or hereditary mosaicism.

Genetics
- Most frequent genotypes include 45,X, karyotypes with an isochromosome of X, the mosaic karyotype 45,X/46,XX, and karyotypes containing part of or the entire Y chromosome.
- Many other types of mosaicism have been described, including with ring chromosome X and X chromosome deletions.

PATHOPHYSIOLOGY
TS phenotypic characteristics are related to:
- Haploinsufficiency of pseudoautosomal genes, such as the SHOX gene (leading to short stature)
- Extent of chromosome imbalance
- Aneuploidy
- Other mechanisms, such as imprinting- and X-inactivation abnormalities

ASSOCIATED CONDITIONS
- Growth failure and short stature
- Gonadal dysgenesis: Delayed puberty and infertility (≥98%)

- Chronic estrogen deficiency in the presence of streak ovaries
- Cardiac anomalies (40%): Bicuspid aortic valve, coarctation, and other left-sided defects
- Renal anomalies (25%): Horseshoe kidney and duplication of the collecting system
- Endocrine disturbances: Glucose intolerance, diabetes, and autoimmune hypothyroidism
- Skeletal abnormalities: Short neck, scoliosis, cubitus valgus, and Madelung deformity
- Psychosocial issues, including specific learning disorders and ADD.
- Other:
  – Hearing and vision problems
  – Hypertension (up to 40% of TS adults)
  – Osteopenia and osteoporosis
  – GI problems
  – Orthodontic problems

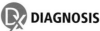

DIAGNOSIS

SIGNS AND SYMPTOMS
Physical Exam
- Short stature: Height <5th percentile (95–100%)
- Delayed puberty (≥85%)
- Lymphedema at birth (or later) (25–50%)
- Low-set ears (>60%)
- High-arched palate (>70%)
- Micrognathia (>60%)
- Short neck (>40%)
- Low hairline (40–60%)
- Webbing of neck (25–44%)
- Broad chest with widely spaced nipples
- Cubitus valgus (50%)
- Short 4th metacarpal (35%)
- Nail hypoplasia (common/variable)
- Many pigmented nevi (25–44%)
- Feeding difficulties in infancy
- Heart murmur
- Recurrent otitis media (>60%)
- Deficits in neurodevelopmental and psychosocial functioning

TESTS
Once TS has been diagnosed:
- Anthropometric measurements to monitor growth carefully; track weight gain closely
- BP and peripheral pulses; compare arm and leg systolic pressures
- Annual hearing screen
- Dental/Orthodontic evaluation in childhood
- Psycho-educational evaluation for any perceived scholastic problems

Lab
- Determination of karyotype by cytogenetic chromosome analysis is the key to TS diagnosis:
  – Minimum of 25 cells in metaphases should be evaluated (more if suspecting low-level of mosaicism).
  – Evaluate marker chromosomes for presence of Y material (using FISH probes).
- Measurement of gonadotropins during the adolescent years and thereafter may reveal elevated FSH and LH indicative of gonadal failure.
- Annual (or biannual) thyroid function testing (TSH, T4) after TS diagnosis, to screen for autoimmune hypothyroidism

- Fasting glucose and/or OGTT in patients at increased risk for type 2 diabetes mellitus

Imaging
Once TS has been diagnosed:
- Echocardiography (and/or cardiac MRI)
- Renal US
- Consider scoliosis/kyphosis films as needed
- Skeletal age determination
- Pelvic US can be considered if there remain uncertainties about the gonadal anatomy

DIFFERENTIAL DIAGNOSIS
- Noonan syndrome:
  – Usually occurs sporadically, occasionally autosomal dominant; associated with right-sided congenital heart disease
- Any growth failure/short stature in females:
  – Normal short stature variations, hypothyroidism, GH-deficiency, skeletal dysplasias, and short stature due to chronic illness can usually be distinguished from TS clinically.
- Girls with delayed puberty and amenorrhea:
  – Exclude TS 1st if also short stature. POF (e.g., autoimmune oophoritis), is rare in adolescence.
  – POF due to irradiation or chemotherapy injury of the ovaries is becoming increasingly more frequent in long-term survivors of childhood neoplasia.

Tumor/Malignancy
- ~5–12% of TS patients are found to have Y chromosome material. Most often the karyotype is the mosaic 45,X/46,XY.
- An estimated 15–25% of TS patients with Y material may develop a gonadoblastoma. Recent population studies appear to indicate a lower risk.
- Gonadoblastomas do not metastasize, but can give rise to germinomas through local ovarian stroma invasion.
  – Gonadoblastomas are often microscopic.
  – Some gonadoblastomas have been reported in early childhood.
- Karyotyping done >10 years ago should be repeated with present standards.
- Prophylactic gonadectomy is recommended for TS patients with Y material diagnosed by karyotype or FISH (not by PCR).

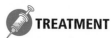

TREATMENT

SPECIAL THERAPY
- Management of short stature:
  – Use of TS-specific growth charts is recommended to monitor linear growth.
  – GH therapy should be offered for all TS patients predicted to have a subnormal adult height (<5th percentile).
  – Routine testing of the GH secretory status is not necessary prior to therapy.
  – GH therapy should be initiated once growth failure can be documented.
  – Standard GH therapy in TS patients in the US uses a dosage of 0.375 mg/kg/wk, divided into 7 daily SC injections. Individual dosing should be considered based on the patient's response; higher doses may lead to improved growth response.
  – GH therapy started at an earlier age will lead to greater improvements in adult height.

– The age at initiation of estrogen therapy also is an important determinant of the overall growth response to GH therapy.
– Adjunct therapy with the anabolic steroid oxandrolone (0.5 mg/kg/d) can be offered at ~11 years, especially for girls with a late diagnosis of TS.
– Follow GH response using specific TS growth charts.
– Therapy is continued until a satisfactory height is achieved or the bone age is >14 years.
• Management of gonadal failure:
– Exclude the possibility of delayed spontaneous puberty (measure FSH, LH).
– Sex steroids are usually initiated between 12 and 15 years, based on achieved growth and future growth potential at that time.
– Begin with 12–18 months of unopposed low-dose estrogen, with gradually increasing dosages.
– Initial estrogen supplementation can use either conjugated estrogens, oral EE, or estrogen patches.
– This is followed by larger-dose estrogens cycled with progesterone (e.g., 5–10 mg medroxyprogesterone acetate). Administer the estrogens from days 1–26 of each month, while progestin is given from day 17–26 only.
– Maintenance therapy with transdermal estrogen plus micronized progesterone or OCPs, after menses onset and secondary sexual characteristics are fully established
– Continue into patient's 5th decade.
– Routine gynecologic evaluation is recommended, and, as with all other adolescents, counseling for STD prevention as well.

Complementary and Alternative Therapies
• Cardiovascular abnormalities:
– If a structural cardiac anomaly is found, a cardiologist will direct additional care.
– ECG (and/or cardiac MRI) is repeated in adolescence and every 3–5 years thereafter in adulthood, because of the increased risk of aortic root dilatation and aortic dissection/rupture.
– Close monitoring for hypertension
– Monitoring for dyslipidemia
• Thyroid disease:
– After the adolescent period, monitor thyroid anti-antibodies every 3–5 years.
– When positive, do annual screening of TSH and thyroxin.
• Hearing:
– Annual audiology testing because of risk for sensorineural hearing loss
• Other issues:
– Screen for osteoporosis and optimize physical activity, calcium, and vitamin D intake.
– Screen for UTI if known renal collecting system anomaly.
– Monitor for obesity and diabetes.
– Evaluate and treat developmental difficulties and learning disorders.
– Address problems with psychosexual development and social adjustment in collaboration with clinical psychologists.
– Assist in career and vocational planning.

SURGERY
• Prophylactic gonadectomy is recommended for TS patients with Y material diagnosed by karyotype or FISH (not by PCR).
• Cosmetic plastic surgery may be contemplated for correction of neck webbing.
• Counsel about increased risk for keloid scar formation with surgical procedures.
• Prophylactic tympanostomy for patients with recurrent otitis media in childhood.

 FOLLOW-UP

DISPOSITION
Issues for Referral
• Referral to a pediatric endocrinologist is imperative for optimal TS care, preferably in a center with a multidisciplinary team approach.
• Additional genetic counseling may be necessary in specific cases and with prenatal diagnosis; still involve pediatric endocrinology.

Pregnancy Considerations
Referral to reproductive endocrinology:
• Cryopreservation of ovarian tissue and immature oocytes is currently under intensive investigation.
• Oocyte or embryo donation can be considered if a TS woman desires to carry a pregnancy.
• Pregnancy rate achieved in TS women after embryo transfer is similar to recipients with POF, but the TS recipients have a higher (40%) percentage of miscarriage.
• Any pregnancy in a TS woman is considered high-risk, including for the development of aortic dissection.
• <1% of TS women have unassisted pregnancies. Their children are at much higher risk for chromosomal disorders (≥20%); therefore, prenatal amniocentesis is recommended. These pregnancies also carry a higher risk of spontaneous abortion.

PROGNOSIS
• Many TS patients can be expected to lead a relatively normal life, despite the fact that almost every system in the body can be affected.
• Comorbidities vary significantly between patients, often without genotype-phenotype correlation.
• Multisystem and multidisciplinary approach to TS care is instrumental to optimize the quality of life. Despite this, overall mortality is increased, leading to a decrease in life expectancy for the TS population as a whole.

BIBLIOGRAPHY

Gravholt CH. Epidemiological, endocrine and metabolic features in Turner syndrome. *Eur J Endocrinol*. 2004;151(6):657–687.

Lippe BM, et al. Turner syndrome. In: Sperling MA, ed. *Pediatric Endocrinology*, 2nd ed. Philadelphia: Saunders; 2002:519–564.

Saenger P, et al. Recommendations for the diagnosis and management of Turner syndrome. *J Clin Endocrinol Metab*. 2001;(867):3061–3069.

Savendahl L, et al. Delayed diagnoses of Turner syndrome: Proposed guidelines for change. *J Pediatr*. 2000;137(4):455–459.

Sybert VP, et al. Turner syndrome. *N Engl J Med*. 2004;(351)12:1227–1238.

MISCELLANEOUS

SYNONYM(S)
• Gonadal dysgenesis
• Ullrich-Turner syndrome
• Bonnevie-Ullrich syndrome
• 45X karyotype
• 45X syndrome
• Monosomy X
• XO syndrome

CLINICAL PEARLS
• ~50% girls with TS have the 45,X karyotype. TS girls with the 45,X/46,XX karyotype often have a milder phenotype, especially if there is a higher percentage of the 46,XX cell line. They may only have short stature.
• Evaluate for gonadal dysgenesis if no breast development by age 12 or no menses by 14 with FSH/LH. Karyotype if elevated.
• Short stature is the most common clinical feature in TS, and TS must be considered in any girl who is growing significantly below her genetic expectation.
• Consider chromosome analysis in any short girl. Webbed neck, peripheral lymphedema, and coarctation of the aorta should also lead the clinician to consider chromosome analysis.
• Gonadal failure occurs due to an accelerated reduction of the oocyte pool in dysgenetic ovaries.
• Cardiac- and renal-associated structural abnormalities are common in TS.
• Intelligence is relatively normal, but nonverbal learning disorder is common.

ABBREVIATIONS
• ADD—Attention deficit disorder
• BP—Blood pressure
• ECG—Echocardiography
• EE—Ethinyl estradiol
• FISH—Fluorescence in situ hybridization
• FSH—Follicle-stimulating hormone
• GH—Growth hormone
• LH—Luteinizing hormone
• OGTT—Oral glucose tolerance test
• OCP—Oral contraceptive pill
• POF—Primary ovary failure
• PCR—Polymerase chain reaction
• STD—Sexually transmitted disease
• T4—Thyroxine
• TS—Turner syndrome
• TSH—Thyroid-stimulating hormone
• UTI—Urinary tract infection

CODES
ICD9-CM
758.6 Turner syndrome (disorder)

 PATIENT TEACHING

Families can be referred for additional reading to:
• http://www.turner-syndrome-us.org/
• http://www.hgfound.org/
• http://www.magicfoundation.org/www

URETHRAL DIVERTICULUM

Matthew A. Barker, MD
Mickey M. Karram, MD

 BASICS

DESCRIPTION
- Urethral diverticula are urothelial mucosal-lined sacs that lie outside the urethra, but within the periurethral fascia, and lack surrounding muscle.
- Pseudo-diverticula occur when there is prolapse of urethral mucosa through a discontinuity in the urethrovaginal connective tissue.
- Congenital urethral diverticula are rare and most likely arise from cloagenic rests, remnants of Gartner duct, müllerian cell rests, or due to faulty union of primordial urogenital sinus folds.
- Majority of urethral diverticula are acquired from urethral trauma.

Pregnancy Considerations
Urethral diverticula diagnosed in pregnancy should be treated conservatively with antibiotics or aspiration, avoiding surgical therapy until after delivery.

Age-Related Factors
- Congenital urethral diverticula are rare and rarely diagnosed before the age of 20.
- Most diagnosed 3rd–6th decade.

Staging
- Leng & McGuire classification based on presence or absence of a preserved periurethral fascial layer
- Leach staging system: L/N/S/C3:
  - Location, Number, Size, anatomic configuration, site of communication to urethral lumen, and continence status

EPIDEMIOLOGY
- Incidence 1–5% of general population
- No racial predilection
- Females > Males

RISK FACTORS
- Trauma from childbirth
- Urethral trauma from instrumentation
- Recurrent UTIs or urethral infections resulting in urethral gland dilation

PATHOPHYSIOLOGY
- Congenital
- Trauma:
  - Obstetric injuries, urethral instrumentation, vaginal surgery, intraurethral injections
- Infections:
  - Repeat infections lead to destruction of paraurethral glands and often abscess formation within the periurethral and urethral glands.
    - Obstructed glands can rupture into urethral lumen and remain as outpouchings off the urethra after they reepithelialize.

ASSOCIATED CONDITIONS
- UTIs
- Urethral calculus in diverticulum
- Urethral carcinoma in diverticulum
- Urinary incontinence:
  - Women with stress urinary incontinence have a 1.4% incidence of urethral diverticulum.
  - 60% of patients with urethral diverticulum have stress urinary incontinence.

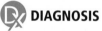 **DIAGNOSIS**

SIGNS AND SYMPTOMS
History
- Classic presentation of 3 Ds (dysuria, dribbling [post-void], and dyspareunia)
- Obstetric history (trauma during delivery)
- STD history
- Pain assessment and localization
- Urinary incontinence
- Urinary frequency and/or urgency
- Vaginal discharge (yellow or green and often with foul odor)
- Recurrent UTIs or persistent dysuria

Review of Systems
Any or all may be present:
- Pain: Urethral pain, pain with intercourse, pain during or after urination, and lower abdominal pain
- Urinary incontinence: Stress, urge, mixed
- Urinary retention or incomplete voiding
- Blood or pus in urine
- Awareness of vaginal or urethral mass

Physical Exam
Focused genitourinary exam with patient in lithotomy position:
- Half-speculum placed over posterior vaginal wall will help visualize the anterior vaginal wall
- Tender anterior vaginal mass on palpation
- Expression of pus through the urethral meatus
- Mass may be either midline or lateral (above and below urethra).
- Firmness or hardness may reflect presence of stone or neoplasm.
- Cough stress test and evaluation for urethral hypermobility help screen for urinary incontinence.

TESTS
- Tests should focus on patient symptoms and lead to a diagnosis based on clinical suspicion that narrows the differential diagnosis.
- PVR urine sample
- Screen for UTI (urine dipstick, urinalysis, urine culture).
- Culture if pus present
- Urine cytology if hematuria present
- Screen for STDs.
- Urodynamic testing should be performed if symptoms of urinary incontinence

Lab
- UA (bacteruria, hematuria, elevated leukocytes, and/or nitrites)
- Urine culture
- Urine cytology (if hematuria)
- PCR test or cervical culture for *Neisseria gonorrhea* and *Chlamydia trachomatis*
- Wet-mount or vaginitis culture (if abnormal vaginal discharge)

Imaging
- Proper imaging techniques should correctly diagnose urethral diverticula and aid surgical excision.
- Imaging should provide data regarding number, location, size, configuration, and communication to urethra:
  - Voiding cystourethrography (VCUG)
  - Positive-pressure urethrography (PPUG)
  - Cystourethroscopy (apply digital pressure to anterior vaginal wall to help express fluid through neck of sac)
  - MRI: Most sensitive for detecting urethral diverticula

DIFFERENTIAL DIAGNOSIS

Infection
- Urethral infections are believed to contribute to urethral diverticula formation.
- Most common infectious agents:
  – Escherichia coli
  – C. trachomatis
  – N. gonorrhea

Tumor/Malignancy
Malignancy in diverticula are rare:
- Adenocarcinoma, SCC, mesonephric carcinoma
- Treatment is surgical excision with or without radiation therapy.

Trauma
- Direct urethral trauma is believed to contribute to urethral diverticula formation.
- Obstetric trauma
- Direct urethral instrumentation or iatrogenic trauma

Other/Miscellaneous
- Urethrocele
- Urethritis
- Urethral caruncle
- Ectopic ureterocele
- Skene gland abscess
- Vaginal wall inclusion cyst
- Anterior vaginal cysts of embryologic origin (Gartner duct cyst)
- Urethral carcinoma
- Vaginal carcinoma
- Vaginal leiomyoma or leiomyosarcoma

 TREATMENT

GENERAL MEASURES
- Urethral diverticula can be managed conservatively or by surgery.
- Women with a diverticular abscess or symptomatic infection should be treated before any management path is chosen.
- Image mass before surgical excision.

SPECIAL THERAPY
Complementary and Alternative Therapies
Work best with small asymptomatic urethral diverticula.
- Observational management
- Post void digital decompression
- Aspiration of diverticulum
- Packing the diverticulum with cellulose
- Injection of diverticulum with Teflon

MEDICATION (DRUGS)
- Prophylactic antibiotics for recurrent UTIs
- Routine preoperative antibiotics
- Bladder antispasmodics such as opium suppositories or anticholinergics should be used both pre- and postoperatively if needed.

SURGERY
- Complete excision of urethral diverticula through a transvaginal approach using multiple-layer closure without overlapping suture lines is preferred technique.
- Surgical treatment best for persistent symptoms despite treatment of infections and for women with recurrent infections.
- Surgery requires resection of the sac and closure of the neck of the diverticulum.
- Distal urethral diverticula may be treated with incision and drainage alone or marsupialization.
- Foley or Tratner catheter should be placed preoperatively.
- Once the diverticulum is identified, a U-shaped vaginal incision is made and a vaginal flap is created.
- Next periurethral fascia flaps are dissected off the localized diverticular cavity.
- Circumferential dissection down to level of the abnormal communication is made and the diverticulum is excised.
- Urethra is then closed in a vertical fashion avoiding excessive tension.
- Periurethral fascia is closed as a 2nd layer in a horizontal fashion; if this tissue is poor or on a lot of tension a fat-pad interposition graft should be used (Martius graft).
- Autologous flap or xenografts may be used to reinforce large periurethral defects after excision of diverticula.
- Vaginal wall is then closed and a suprapubic catheter is left in place and vaginal packing used.
- If underlining stress incontinence is present, surgery may be combined with a pubovaginal sling or intraurethral injection.
- If stress incontinence develops postoperatively caution should be used in placing synthetic mesh devices and a more traditional autologous pubovaginal sling should be used.

 FOLLOW-UP

DISPOSITION
Issues for Referral
Early referral to physicians experienced in the management of urethral diverticula

PROGNOSIS
- Risk of recurrence: 12%
- Risk of postoperative stress incontinence: 8.5%
- Risk of urethrovaginal fistula: 4.2%
- Risk of urethral stricture: 2.1%

PATIENT MONITORING
- After surgery, drain bladder for 10–14 days.
- A postoperative voiding cystourethrogram should be performed to confirm closure.
- Pelvic rest for 6 weeks after surgery
- Follow up visits at 2 and 6 weeks

BIBLIOGRAPHY

Dmochowski R. Surgery for Vesicovaginal Fistula, Urethrovaginal Fistula, and Urethral Diverticulum. In: Walsh PC, ed. Campbell Urology, 8th ed. Philadelphia: W.B. Saunders; 2002:1195–1217.

Lee JW, et al. Female urethral diverticula. Best Pract Res Clin Obstet Gynaecol. 2005;19:875–893.

Vasavada SP. Urethral Diverticula. In: Walters MD, et al., eds. Urogynecology and Pelvic Reconstructive Surgery, 3rd ed. Philadelphia: Mosby; 2007: 461–471.

 MISCELLANEOUS

SYNONYM(S)
- Paraurethral cysts
- Periurethral microcysts
- Pseudo-diverticula
- Urethral diverticula

ABBREVIATIONS
- PCR—Polymerase chain reaction
- PVR—Postvoid residual
- SCC—Squamous cell carcinoma
- STD—Sexually transmitted disease
- UTI—Urinary tract infection

CODES
ICD9-CM
- 599.2 Urethral diverticulum
- 593.89 Urethral diverticulum (acquired)
- 594.0 Urethral diverticulum (with stone)
- 753.4 Urethral diverticulum (congenital)

 PATIENT TEACHING

PREGNANCY CONSIDERATIONS
Perform cesarean delivery if history of prior repair for urethral diverticulum.

URINARY TRACT INFECTION

Rocco A. Rossi, MD

 BASICS

DESCRIPTION
- A UTI is defined as the growth of a urinary tract pathogen.
- Bacteriuria is defined as:
  - 10^5 CFU in clean catch specimen
  - 10^2 CFU in a suprapubic catheter specimen
- Recurrent UTI: ≥ 2 infections in 6 months or 3 in 12 months
- Asymptomatic bacteriuria: Presence of a positive urine culture in an asymptomatic person
- Acute cystitis: Infection of the urinary bladder
- Pyelonephritis: Infection of the kidney and/or renal pelvis

Age-Related Factors
- Highest incidence occurs in the late teens and early 20s.
- Postmenopausal women are at risk due to atrophy of the vaginal epithelium.

EPIDEMIOLOGY
- 50–60% of women report having a UTI during their lifetime.
- Sexually active women have up to 0.5 episodes per year.
- Incidence reaches its peak during patient's early 20s.

RISK FACTORS
- Female
- Sexual activity
- Pregnancy
- Diabetes
- Obesity
- Postmenopausal
- Diaphragm use
- Vaginal spermicides
- Sickle cell trait
- Anatomic abnormalities
- Urinary tract calculi
- Neurologic disorders
- Catheterization

PATHOPHYSIOLOGY
- Periurethral and perineal colonization of the urinary tract
- Renal infection may also arise from bacteremia or lymphatic spread.
- Common pathogens:
  - *Escherichia coli*: 80–85% of cases
  - *Staphlococcus saprophyticus, Proteus mirabilis, Klebsiella, Enterococcus*, Group B Streptococcus

ASSOCIATED CONDITIONS
- Diabetes
- Obesity
- Sickle cell trait
- Urinary tract calculi
- Pregnancy
- Neurologic disease
- STDs

 DIAGNOSIS

SIGNS AND SYMPTOMS
The diagnosis or UTI and pyelonephritis in adults can be made from history and physical exam alone.

History
Dysuria, frequent voiding, urgency, hematuria

Review of Systems
Fevers and chills, nausea and vomiting, altered mental status (elderly), shortness of breath

Physical Exam
- Urethral discharge, suprapubic tenderness
- Pyelonephritis: Flank pain, CVA tenderness, and pulmonary sequelae in severe infection

TESTS
Lab
- UA:
  - Pyuria: ≥ 10 WBC
  - WBC casts indicative of upper UTI
  - Hematuria
- Urine dipsticks:
  - Leukocyte esterase: Detects pyuria
  - Nitrites: Detect Enterobacteriaceae
- Urine culture:
  - Not necessary for every patient, but may want to consider when:
    - Atypical symptoms, persistent symptoms or recurrence, complicated infection (i.e., pregnancy)

Imaging
As indicated when urinary tract calculi, anatomic abnormalities, or other complicating circumstances are suspected

DIFFERENTIAL DIAGNOSIS
Infection
Infection of other organ systems in proximity to the urinary tract:
- Vaginitis, STDs (chlamydial urethritis with sterile pyuria), PID, appendicitis, TOA

Hematologic
Sickle cell trait

Metabolic/Endocrine
Virulent or recurrent UTI may be a sign of diabetes.

Immunologic
Recurrent UTI warrants consideration of immunocompromised states.
- HIV, leukemia, etc.

Tumor/Malignancy
Tumors can lead to hematuria and pain along the urinary tract.

Trauma
Leading to pain and hematuria

Other/Miscellaneous
- Pregnancy-related pain
- Interstitial cystitis
- Other causes of urinary frequency:
  - Pelvic mass
  - DM
  - Overactive bladder

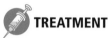 **TREATMENT**

GENERAL MEASURES
- Increased hydration
- Phenazopyridine t.i.d. provides symptomatic relief of dysuria, frequency, and urgency until UA or culture can be performed and antibiotics started.
  - Produces topical bladder analgesia
  - Available OTC
  - Turns urine bright orange
  - Does not treat infection

MEDICATION (DRUGS)
- Acute cystitis:
  - First line:
    - TMP/SMX 160/800 mg b.i.d. $\times$ 3 days
  - Second line:
    - Fluoroquinolones: Moxifloxacin cannot be used due to inadequate urinary concentrations
  - Nitrofurantoin 100 mg b.i.d. for 7days
- Pyelonephritis:
  - Uncomplicated
    - TMP/SMX or Fluoroquinolones orally as an outpatient for 14 days
  - Complicated (pregnancy, systemic toxicity): Inpatient treatment using parenteral antibiotics:
    - Fluoroquinolones or ampicillin/gentamicin are 1st-line therapy in nonpregnant patients.
    - Parenteral therapy is usually required for 48–72 hours followed by oral therapy to complete a 14-day course.
    - See "Pregnancy Considerations" for therapy recommendations in pregnant patients.

Pregnancy Considerations
- See chapter on UTI/pyelonephritis in pregnancy for more detailed background and therapy information.
- Acute cystitis:
  - Nitrofurantoin 100 mg b.i.d. for 3–7 days
  - Amoxicillin 500 mg b.i.d. for 3–7 days
  - Cephalexin 500 mg b.i.d. to q.i.d. for 3–7 days
  - No fluoroquinolones
  - Asymptomatic bacteriuria should be treated as acute cystitis when diagnosed in pregnancy.
- Recurrent UTI: ≥2 infections during the pregnancy:
  - Obtain urine culture with susceptibilities.
  - Treat with regimens for acute cystitis and then suppression with:
    - Nitrofurantoin 100 mg q.h.s.
    - Cephalexin 500 mg q.h.s.
- Pyelonephritis:
  - Inpatient parenteral therapy for a minimum of 48 hours; patient must be afebrile for 24 hours with symptomatic improvement:
    - IV cephazolin or IM ceftriaxone are first line.
    - Ampicillin/Gentamicin.
    - Suppression is given for the remainder of the pregnancy.
    - Monitor for sepsis and pulmonary sequelae.

SPECIAL THERAPY
Complementary and Alternative Therapies
Cranberry or lingonberry juice has been suggested to reduce recurrence risk, but well-designed RCT is lacking.

SURGERY
As indicated for urologic and neurologic disease processes

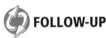 **FOLLOW-UP**

DISPOSITION
Issues for Referral
Reasons leading to UTI outside the scope of therapy that a gynecologist can offer:
- Urologic, neurologic, hematologic, immunologic state

Pediatric Considerations
- Extensive labial adhesions can predispose to urinary symptoms, including recurrent UTI and dribbling.
- Repeat episodes of UTI in girls should prompt referral to urology to rule out urinary tract abnormalities, including reflux, that may predispose to renal parenchymal scarring.

PROGNOSIS
Recurrent UTI

PATIENT MONITORING
- Pregnant patients should have a urine culture collected at their initial pregnancy visit and should have subsequent urine dip sticks at all pregnancy visits.
- Follow-up based on symptoms and complicating factors.

BIBLIOGRAPHY
Avorn J, et al. Reduction of bacteriuria and pyuria after ingestion of cranberry juice. *JAMA*. 1994; 271:751–754.

Finn SD. Clinical practice: Acute uncomplicated urinary tract infection in women. *N Engl J Med*. 2003:343:259–266.

Foxman B. Epidemiology of urinary tract infections: Incidence, morbidity, and economic costs. *Am J Med*. 2002;113(Suppl 1A):5S.

Hansson S, et al. The natural history of bacteriuria in childhood. *Infect Dis Clin North Am*. 1997;11:499.

Hooten TM, et al. Acute uncomplicated cystitis in an era of increasing antibiotic resistance: A proposed approach to empirical therapy. *Clin Infect Dis*. 2004;39:75.

Hooten TM, et al. A prospective study of risk factors for symptomatic urinary tract infection in young women. *N Engl J Med*. 1996;335:468.

Hooten TM. Recurrent urinary tract infection in women. *Int J Antimicrob Agents*. 2001;17:259–268.

Jepson RG, et al. Cranberries for treating urinary tract infections. Cochrane Renal Group. *Cochrane Database Syst Rev*. 2, 2007.

Nicolle LE, et al. Infectious Diseases Society of America guidelines for the diagnosis and treatment of asymptomatic bacteriuria in adults. *Clin Infect Dis*. 2005;40:643.

Pappas PG. Laboratory in the diagnosis and management of urinary tract infections. *Med Clin North Am*. 1991;75:313.

Sheffield JS, et al. Urinary tract infection in women. *Obstet Gynecol*. 2005;106:1085–1092.

Stamm WE. Measurement of pyuria and its relation to bacteriuria. *Am J Med*. 1983;75:53.

Vazquez JC, et al. Treatments for symptomatic urinary tract infections during pregnancy. *Cochrane Database Syst Rev*. 2000;CD002256.

Waren JW, et al. Guidelines for antimicrobial treatment of uncomplicated acute bacterial cystitis and acute pyelonephritis in women. *Clin Infect Dis*. 1999;29:745–758.

Wing DA, et al. A randomized trial of three antibiotic regimens for the treatment of pyelonephritis in pregnancy. *Obstet Gynecol*. 1998;92:249.

 MISCELLANEOUS

CLINICAL PEARLS
- A 3-day course of antibiotic therapy is the most efficacious and has the least side effects for those with uncomplicated cystitis.
- Pyelonephritis requires a 14-day course of therapy and, depending on circumstances, continuous suppression.
- Asymptomatic bacteriuria does not require therapy unless complicated by pregnancy.

ABBREVIATIONS
- CFU—Colony forming unit
- DM—Diabetes mellitus
- PID—Pelvic inflammatory disease
- RCT—Randomized controlled trial
- TMP/SMX—Trimethoprim/Sulfamethoxazole
- TOA—Tubo-ovarian abscess
- UTI—Urinary tract infection
- UTI—Urinary tract infection

CODES
ICD9-CM
- 595 Diseases of the urinary system:
  - 590–599

 PATIENT TEACHING

Encourage proper hygiene and emphasize the need to complete antibiotic therapy and/or maintain suppression medication.

PREVENTION
- Postcoital antibiotic prophylaxis
- Post voiding
- Daily continuous antibiotic prophylaxis
- Intermittent self-treatment

UTERINE FIBROIDS

Amber M. Shiflett, MD
Bryan D. Cowan, MD

 BASICS

DESCRIPTION
- Uterine myomas are benign, smooth muscle cell tumors, also called fibroids and leiomyomas.
- Described by location, although most myomas involve >1 layer of the uterus:
  - Subserosal: Projects into the pelvis, causing irregular uterine contour; may be pedunculated
  - Intramural: Within uterine wall
  - Submucosal: Projects into the uterine cavity
  - May arise from cervix or broad ligament
- Range from microscopic to easily palpable; size described in gestational weeks
- May be single or multiple
- Most common solid pelvic tumor in women
- Most common indication for hysterectomy

Age-Related Factors
Develop during hormonally active reproductive years; ~70% of women at age 45 demonstrate fibroids on sonography.

Staging
Based on the location of the fibroid:
- Submucous location: Type 0, I, II
- Intramural location (confused with Submucosal Type II)
- Subserous location

EPIDEMIOLOGY
- True incidence and prevalence are unknown because myomas are usually asymptomatic
- If symptomatic, typically in women between the ages of 30 and 40
- Black women are 2–3 times more likely to develop myomas than white women
- Black women tend to be younger at both time of diagnosis and hysterectomy, have higher uterine weights, and are more likely to be anemic

RISK FACTORS
- Nulliparity
- Obesity
- Black race

Genetics
- Family and twin studies suggest a genetic predisposition
- Associated with hereditary syndromes:
  - Reed syndrome: Uterine and subcutaneous myomas
  - Bannayan-Zoana syndrome: Uterine myomas, lipomas, hemangioma
  - Familial hereditary leiomyomas and renal cell carcinoma (linked to a genetic defect in the Krebs cycle [fumarate hydratase])

PATHOPHYSIOLOGY
- Abnormal uterine bleeding:
  - Increased vascularity and venous congestion
  - Increased surface area of uterine cavity
- Compression of pelvic structures
- Acute pelvic pain:
  - Torsion of pedunculated myoma
  - Protrusion of submucosal myoma through cervix
  - Infarction as myoma outgrows blood supply
- Impaired fertility:
  - Mechanical obstruction or distortion of uterine cavity may interfere with implantation or with ovum or sperm transport.

ASSOCIATED CONDITIONS
- Iron-deficiency anemia
- Endometritis
- Adenomyosis
- Impaired fertility

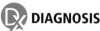 **DIAGNOSIS**

SIGNS AND SYMPTOMS
History
- Menstrual, sexual, obstetric histories
- Quantify blood loss during menses

Review of Systems
- Pelvic/Reproductive:
  - Heavy, prolonged, painful menses (submucosal myomas):
    - May be associated with fatigue, pallor, shortness of breath, palpitations
  - Pelvic pressure or fullness
- Acute pelvic pain
- GI:
  - Increased abdominal girth
  - Constipation, tenesmus (posterior myomas)
- Urinary:
  - Frequency, urgency (anterior myomas)

Physical Exam
- Enlarged, firm, irregular uterus
- Peritoneal signs (infarcted myoma)
- Conjunctival pallor, tachycardia

TESTS
Lab
hCG, CBC, type and cross before surgery

Imaging
- TVU to confirm diagnosis, evaluate for ovarian neoplasm
- Sonohysterogram to locate intramural lesions
- Abdominal plain films may show concentric calcifications
- MRI to visualize individual myomas
- Hysterosalpingography to define extent of submucous myomas before surgery or to evaluate uterine cavity and patency of fallopian tubes
- Renal US to evaluate for urinary obstruction

DIFFERENTIAL DIAGNOSIS
- Abnormal uterine bleeding:
  - Anovulation
  - Endometrial hyperplasia or malignancy
- Pelvic pain:
  - Endometriosis
  - Adenomyosis
  - Ectopic pregnancy
  - Torsion or rupture of ovarian cyst
  - PID
- Pelvic mass:
  - Pregnancy
  - Adenomyosis
  - Uterine polyp
  - Ovarian mass:
    - Functional cyst
    - Benign neoplasm
    - Malignancy
  - Leiomyosarcoma

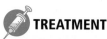 **TREATMENT**

GENERAL MEASURES
- Control severe bleeding and pain
- Treat iron-deficiency anemia

MEDICATION (DRUGS)
- Can reduce myoma size and uterine volume as well as bleeding
- Goal is to temporarily reduce symptoms and myoma size
- May be sufficient for women nearing menopause
- Side effects and expense limit long-term use
- None shown to improve fertility
- Myomas regain pretreatment size within 3–4 months after drug is stopped.
- OCPs may prevent but will not treat established myomas.
- 3 classes have demonstrated effective reduction of fibroids: GnRH-agonist, GnRH-antagonist, and progesterone antagonists.
- GnRH agonists:
  - Cause hypoestrogenic state:
    - Leuprolide: 3.75 mg IM monthly or 11.25 mg IM depot every 3 months
    - Nafarelin: 400 μg intranasally b.i.d. (alternate nostrils)
    - Goserelin: 3.6 mg implant SC every 28 days
  - Reduce uterine size by up to 65% and induce amenorrhea in most women
  - Maximum response achieved by 3 months
  - Associated with hot flushes, headaches, vaginal dryness, mood swings, joint and muscle stiffness, and reversible bone loss, although addition of HRT may reduce side effects
  - Not well studied beyond 6 months' use
- GnRH-antagonists are not FDA approved for treatment of myomas in the US.
- Mifepristone, selective estrogen response modifiers, and interferon-alfa may have benefit, but their use is largely investigational.

SURGERY

- Indications for surgery:
  - Contraindication to or intolerance of drug therapy
  - Failure of medical management to control abnormal bleeding or anemia
  - Concern for malignancy
  - Mass effect causing pain, pressure, or urinary or GI tract symptoms
  - Distortion of uterine cavity causing infertility or repeated pregnancy loss
- Carries risk of infection, bleeding, damage to adjacent organs, adhesion formation
- Hysterectomy:
  - Definitive treatment
  - Indicated for extensive disease, suspected malignancy, and myomas in association with other pelvic abnormalities
  - Significant improvement in symptoms, quality of life
  - Appropriate only if future pregnancy not desired
- Abdominal myomectomy:
  - Removal of myomas via laparotomy while preserving uterus
  - Indicated for multiple myomas or uterus larger than 16 weeks in size
  - Preferred in women desiring future pregnancy
  - Removal of multiple myomas may involve more time and greater blood loss than hysterectomy
- Considerations after myomectomy:
  - Adhesions may impair fertility
  - Postpone pregnancy for healing to occur
  - Cesarean delivery is probably preferable
- Laparoscopic myomectomy:
  - Removal of myomas via laparoscope while preserving uterus
  - Indicated for 1 or 2 easily accessible myomas <8 cm in diameter and uterine size <16 weeks
  - Risk of uterine rupture during pregnancy is controversial
- Hysteroscopic myomectomy:
  - Removal of submucosal myomas via transcervical operative endoscope
  - May be performed as same-day surgery with local anesthesia and sedation
  - More effective when combined with endometrial ablation, but ablation precludes future pregnancy
- Myolysis:
  - Coagulation/Freezing of myoma
  - May carry increased risk of adhesions and uterine rupture
- Uterine artery embolization:
  - Fluoroscopic guidance: Gel, beads, or coils are introduced through a catheter in the common femoral artery to the uterine artery
  - Disrupts blood supply, causing degeneration
  - Minimally invasive procedure under conscious sedation, with more rapid recovery
  - Usually requires overnight hospitalization for pain control
  - Resolution of bleeding symptoms in up to 90% at 6 months, but limited studies
  - Associated with significant pain and fever; sepsis and death have been reported
  - Disruption of blood supply to ovaries and endometrium causing permanent amenorrhea reported in up to 3% of women <40
  - Unknown effects on later fertility and pregnancy

- High-intensity focused ultrasound (HIFU):
  - Technique using HIFU in the MRI
  - This technique uses array focusing to generate heat in tissue areas of the fibroid.
  - No surgery is required.
  - Currently, patients are in the MRI unit for ~3–4 hours.
  - This technique is developmental.

ALERT

Rapid growth (increase in uterine size by 6 weeks in 1 year) in a nonpregnant woman, growth in a menopausal woman, or new pain suggest malignancy and should prompt surgical removal

 FOLLOW-UP

DISPOSITION

Issues for Referral

- Refer to fertility specialist if infertility
- Urology if ureteral obstruction
- Interventional radiologist for uterine artery embolization or HIFU

Pregnancy Considerations

- Most myomas do not grow in pregnancy; when they do, most of the growth is in the 1st trimester.
- Large myomas may be associated with pain and premature labor.
- Increased risk of abruption, preterm labor, and rupture of membranes if placenta overlies myoma.

PROGNOSIS

- Most symptomatic women require surgery
- May recur after myomectomy:
  - Risk increases with number of myomas
  - Up to 50% recurrence at 5 years
  - Up to 25% require 2nd surgery
- Regress during menopause
- HRT may stimulate growth

PATIENT MONITORING

- Serial exam or US every 6–12 months to determine growth pattern if asymptomatic:
  - Examine at same time in cycle to limit effects of hormonal stimulation on tumor size
- Watchful waiting may be appropriate for large, asymptomatic myomas in women approaching menopause if malignancy has been excluded.
- Annual bone mineral density studies if GnRH agonist are continued >6 months; consider calcium and bisphosphonate therapy

BIBLIOGRAPHY

ACOG Committee on Gynecologic Practice. Uterine artery embolization. *Obstet Gynecol* 2004;103: 403–404.

de Kroon CD, et al. Saline infusion sonography in women with abnormal uterine bleeding: An update of recent findings. *Curr Opin Obstet Gynecol* 2006;18(6):653–657.

Griffiths A, et al. Surgical treatment of fibroids for subfertility. *Cochrane Database Syst Rev*. 2006;3: CD003857.

Practice Committee of the American Society for Reproductive Medicine. Myomas and reproductive function. *Fertil Steril*. 2006 Nov;86(5 suppl): S194-4–9.

Speroff L, et al. *Clinical Gynecologic Endocrinology and Infertility*, 7th ed. Lippincott, Williams, & Wilkins 2005:136–140, 1043–1044.

Stewart EA, Morton CC. The genetics of uterine leiomyomata: What clinicians need to know. *Obstet Gynecol*. 2006;107(4):917–921.

Sudarshan S, et al. Mechanisms of disease: Hereditary leiomyomatosis and renal cell cancer—a distinct form of hereditary kidney cancer. *Nat Clin Pract Urol*. 2007;4(2):104–110.

Wallach EE, et al. Uterine myomas: An overview of development, clinical features, and management. *Obstet Gynecol*. 2004;104:393–406.

White AM, et al. Uterine fibroid embolization. *Tech Vasc Interv Radiol*. 2006;9(1):2–6.

 MISCELLANEOUS

SYNONYM(S)

- Fibroid
- Fibroleiomyoma
- Fibroma
- Fibromyoma
- Leiomyofibroma
- Myofibroma
- Myoma
- Leiomyoma

CLINICAL PEARLS

- Most women undergo hysterectomy to treat symptomatic uterine fibroids.
- Myomectomy is selected to preserve the uterus for women who wish future pregnancies, or women who desire retention of the uterus.
- Endoscopy is used to treat easily accessible uterine fibroids by laparoscopy, or pedunculated submucous fibroids (hysteroscopy).
- Less invasive treatments are now available, but must be considered "developmental"; include uterine artery embolization, HIFU, cryolysis, and radio frequency ablation.

ABBREVIATIONS

- GnRH—Gonadotropin-releasing hormone
- HCG—Human chorionic gonadotropin
- HIFU—High-intensity focused ultrasound
- HRT—Hormone replacement therapy
- OCP—Oral contraceptive pill
- PID—Pelvic inflammatory disease
- TVU—Transvaginal ultrasound

CODES

ICD9-CM

- 218.0 Submucous leiomyoma of uterus
- 218.1 Intramural leiomyoma of uterus
- 218.2 Subserous leiomyoma of uterus
- 218.9 Leiomyoma of uterus, unspecified

 PATIENT TEACHING

ACOG Patient Education Pamphlets: Uterine fibroids

UTERINE AND PELVIC ORGAN PROLAPSE

Christina Lewicky-Gaupp, MD
Dee E. Fenner, MD

ALERT

Geriatric Considerations
Pelvic organ prolapse and uterine prolapse are diseases associated with aging. Their incidence continues to rise as the median age of the population increases.

 BASICS

DESCRIPTION
- ACOG defines POP as the "protrusion of the pelvic organs into or out of the vaginal canal."
- Uterine prolapse occurs when the strength of the supporting connective tissue in the pelvis diminishes and the uterus descends into the vagina. Complete protrusion of the uterus with inversion of the vagina can occur in extreme cases (procidentia).
- The development and severity of prolapse are associated with a woman's vaginal parity, intrinsic risk factors, and aging.
- Collagen disorders, pelvic muscle and structural abnormalities, and chronic straining can predispose a woman to developing prolapse.

Age-Related Factors
With aging, the risk of prolapse increases. Prolapse itself worsens with increasing age.

Staging
Prolapse is staged according to the Pelvic Organ Quantification System (POP-Q):
- Stage 0: No prolapse
- Stage I: Most distal portion of prolapse is >1 cm above hymen
- Stage II: Most distal portion of prolapse is ≤1 cm proximal to or distal to hymen
- Stage III: Most distal portion of prolapse is >1 cm below hymen but is still less than total vaginal length (cm) minus 2
- Stage IV: Complete eversion of the genital tract; the distal portion of prolapse is at least equal to or more than total vaginal length (cm) minus 2

EPIDEMIOLOGY
- Only women develop pelvic organ prolapse
- Prolapse predominantly affects:
  - Peri- and postmenopausal women
  - Women that are vaginally parous
  - Caucasian women vs. Asian and African American women
- In a sub-analysis of the WHI trial, the overall annual incidence of uterine prolapse was 1.5 cases per 100 woman-years.

- According to the NIH definition of prolapse as "uterine descent to within 1 cm or lower of the hymen," 30–90% of women experience some degree of prolapse.
- However, only 3–5% of women have prolapse that extends beyond the introitus.
  - These are the women who have bothersome symptoms.
  - Up to 11% of women will have surgery in their lifetime for prolapse before the age of 80.

RISK FACTORS
- Vaginal childbirth
- Increased weight of vaginally delivered infants
- Increased BMI
- Advanced age
- Caucasian race
- Collagen-vascular disorders
- Neurogenic disorders
- Chronic increases in intra-abdominal pressure from abdominal and pelvic tumors, obesity and pulmonary diseases that cause chronic coughing
- Chronic constipation
- Occupations requiring heavy lifting
- Antecedent surgery to correct POP

Genetics
- Possibly linked to family history
- Increased incidence in patients with a history of other hernias

PATHOPHYSIOLOGY
- Aging and vaginal birth are the most important factors.
- Incidence of prolapse increases with number of vaginal deliveries; <2% of prolapse occurs in nulliparous women.
  - Labor and vaginal delivery can cause pudendal neuropathy and stretching or tearing of the levator ani muscles which ultimately lead to permanent neuropathy and muscle weakness.
- Connective tissue disorders (e.g., Marfan syndrome), neurogenic disorders (e.g., multiple sclerosis), cloacal agenesis, chronic constipation, pelvic tumors or ascites, and chronic coughing resulting from lung disease all increase risk.

ASSOCIATED CONDITIONS
- Rarely does the uterus prolapse alone.
- In nearly all cases, the anterior (cystocele) and posterior (rectocele and/or enterocele) vaginal walls descend along with the uterus.

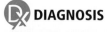 **DIAGNOSIS**

SIGNS AND SYMPTOMS
- Pelvic pressure
- Bulging sensation in vagina or at introitus
- Dyspareunia
- Incomplete bladder emptying
- Low back pain
- Difficulty with defecation, often requiring splinting or supporting the perineum with the hand
- Many patients with mild prolapse that does not extend outside of the hymen have no symptoms.

History
Obstetrical history including number of pregnancies, mode of deliveries, episiotomies, extent and repair of vaginal/perineal lacerations
- Previous pelvic surgery
- Congenital abnormalities
- Medical comorbidities

Review of Systems
Standard review of symptoms is appropriate, focusing on *when* and *how* prolapse was first discovered, *how long* the progression of prolapse was, and *how bothersome* the symptoms are.

Physical Exam
Formal evaluation requires performing the POP-Q:
- With straining, the cervix will descend toward or beyond the introitus.
- Supine and standing exam may be required to ensure full extent of prolapse is appreciated.
- Test Kegel strength (ability to squeeze the levator muscles or pelvic floor).
- Brief neurologic exam (e.g., test integrity of bulbocavernosis reflex).

TESTS
- If surgery is planned, urodynamic studies can be performed.
  - Prolapse can mask occult incontinence by kinking off the urethra which, after surgery, will become unkinked.
- If ulceration or bleeding is present, a PAP smear and vaginal/cervical/endometrial biopsies should be done to rule out malignancies.

Lab
- Basic metabolic panel to evaluate renal function
- Urinalysis to rule out UTI
- Postvoid residual to ensure adequate bladder emptying (should be <100 cc)

Imaging
- Consider intravenous pyelogram to rule out ureteral obstruction if prolapse is severe.
- Consider pelvic ultrasound or CT scan to rule out other pelvic pathology.

DIFFERENTIAL DIAGNOSIS
Infection
Hyperkeratosis of the cervical and vaginal tissues can occur if prolapse extends beyond the introitus.
- Chronic irritation and drying can result in bleeding and ulceration:
  - Must rule-out infectious causes of vaginal bleeding and ulceration such as STDs, candidiasis.

Tumor/Malignancy
- Ensure bulge through introitus is not a fibroid tumor or malignancy.
- If bleeding or erosion is present, vulvar or vaginal malignancy should be ruled out.
- Rarely, ascites can force the prolapse of the pelvic organs.

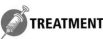 TREATMENT

GENERAL MEASURES
- Treatment of asymptomatic prolapse is unnecessary.
- First-line therapies include pessary placement and physical therapy with pelvic floor muscle exercises (see below).
  - Pessaries are indicated for women who are unfit for or don't desire surgery.
  - Proper pessary fitting and maintenance are required.
- Surgical therapy is indicated for women who are good candidates and desire definitive management or who fail conservative therapies.

SPECIAL THERAPY
Complementary and Alternative Therapies
Biofeedback and pelvic muscle training and exercises (Kegels) can be considered for mild, symptomatic prolapse.

MEDICATION (DRUGS)
- Estrogen can be prescribed for women using pessaries to prevent erosions or for women undergoing reconstructive pelvic surgery to aid in the healing process.
- Precautions: If the uterus is present, progesterone should be prescribed to offset the potential for endometrial carcinoma.

SURGERY
- Patients without additional pelvic pathology who no longer desire future fertility:
  - Vaginal, abdominal, laparoscopic or robot-assisted hysterectomy with vaginal vault suspension to uterosacral or sacrospinous ligaments or to sacrum
  - Concomitant repairs of anterior, posterior or paravaginal defects should be repaired and culdoplasty performed when necessary.

- Equal success rates of ~85% have been reported with vault suspensions via abdominal and vaginal routes.
- Uterine suspension is an option for patients who desire future reproductive function.
- Older women who are not sexually active and do not plan to be in the future can be treated with an obliterative procedure such as a colpocleisis.

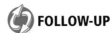 FOLLOW-UP

DISPOSITION
Postop follow-up within 4–6 weeks after surgery:
- Prior to discharge, voiding trial should be done:
  - If bladder is not adequately emptying, intermittently self-catheterization for 1–3 weeks or a Foley leg-bag for 3–7 days
  - With leg-bag, follow-up within 1 week for another trial of voiding

Issues for Referral
The option for nonsurgical treatment should be discussed with patients.
- If surgical treatment is warranted by symptoms or patient preference, the surgeon should be familiar with and have sufficient surgical experience with the treatment options. Referral to a urogynecologist may be warranted.

PROGNOSIS
- If left untreated, it is expected that the incidence/severity of prolapse will increase with age; however, natural progression of untreated symptomatic prolapse is not known.
- Pessary use may delay worsening.
- Surgical correction usually successful initially, but reoperation rate ~29%
- Bladder outlet/ureteral obstruction can lead to renal compromise in cases of severe prolapse that is left untreated.

PATIENT MONITORING
- Expectant management is appropriate.
- If a pessary is placed and the patient is unable to remove it herself, remove, clean, and replace every 3–6 months.

BIBLIOGRAPHY

American College of Obstetrics and Gynecologists. Pelvic Organ Prolapse. Practice Bulletin Number 79, February 2007.

Davis K, et al. Pelvic floor dysfunction: A conceptual framework for collaborative patient-centered care. *J Adv Nurs*. 2003;43(6):555–568.

Handa V, et al. Progression and remission of pelvic organ prolapse—a longitudinal study of menopausal women. *Am J Obstet Gynecol*. 2004;190(4).

MacLennan AH, et al. The prevalence of pelvic floor disorders and their relationship to gender, age, parity and mode of delivery. *Br J Obstet Gynaecol*. 2000;107:1460–1470.

Swift SE. Epidemiology of pelvic organ prolapse. In: Bent AS, et al., eds. *Ostergard's Urogynecology and Pelvic Floor Dysfunction*. 5th ed. Philadelphia, PA: Lippincott & Wilkins; 2003:35–41.

Swift SE, et al. Correlation of symptoms with degree of pelvic organ support in a general population of women: What is pelvic organ prolapse? *Am J Obstet Gynecol*. 2003;189(2):372–377.

 MISCELLANEOUS

SYNONYM(S)
- Genital prolapse
- Total or partial procidentia
- Uterine descensus

CLINICAL PEARLS
- Clinically symptomatic pelvic organ prolapse must be distinguished from asymptomatic prolapse. Therapy should address symptoms.
- Pelvic organ prolapse can be managed expectantly with annual monitoring, conservatively with a pessary or with definitive surgical treatment.
- How to manage prolapse is a decision that should be made between the patient and her physician and is individualized.
- 4 domains relate to pelvic organ prolapse:
  - Prolapse symptoms—pressure and bulge
  - Urinary tract function—incontinence and retention
  - Bowel function—fecal incontinence, constipation, difficult evacuation
  - Sexual function—pain, embarrassment, difficulty with penetration

ABBREVIATIONS
- POP—Pelvic organ prolapse
- POP-Q—Pelvic organ prolapse quantification system

CODES
ICD9-CM
- 618.2 Uterovaginal prolapse, incomplete
- 618.3 Uterovaginal prolapse, complete

 PATIENT TEACHING

- For at least 6 weeks after surgery, patients should
  - Avoid lifting >10 pounds and any strenuous or prolonged exercise.
  - Remain on pelvic rest with no intercourse, douching or tampon use.
- Stool softeners are helpful to maintain good bowel habits, especially postoperatively.
- Kegel exercises can be performed.
- American College of Obstetricians & Gynecologists (ACOG), 409 12th St., SW, Washington, DC 20024-2188; (800) 762-ACOG.
- American Urogynecologic Society: www.augs.org

PREVENTION
- Maintain healthy weight and bowel habits.
- Appropriately manage symptoms of other illnesses such as asthma and COPD.
- Protective effect of Cesarean section is uncertain.

UTEROVAGINAL ANOMALIES

Lesley L. Breech, MD

 BASICS

DESCRIPTION
- Uterovaginal anomalies include vaginal anomalies such as vaginal agenesis and longitudinal and transverse vaginal septa.
- Uterine abnormalities include:
  - Unicornuate
  - Bicornuate
  - Septate uterus
  - Arcuate uterus
  - Uterine didelphys

Age-Related Factors
- Obstructive anomalies tend to be diagnosed earlier, with the development of a mucocolpos in infancy or hematometrocolpos in adolescence.
- Nonobstructive anomalies of the uterus or vagina are not usually detected until potential sexual or obstetric issues develop.

Staging
The most commonly used classification system remains that proposed by the American Fertility Society, now the American Society of Reproductive Medicine, in 1988.

EPIDEMIOLOGY
- Actual incidence of Müllerian anomalies is unknown.
- Conditions are generally under-reported at birth and over-reported in the reproductive years.
- Uterine anomalies occur in:
  - ~3–4% of fertile and infertile women
  - ~5–10% of women with recurrent early pregnancy loss
  - Up to 25% of women with 2nd trimester loss or preterm delivery
- The septate uterus is considered the most common of the uterine anomalies, occurring in ~1% of the fertile population.

PATHOPHYSIOLOGY
- Uterovaginal anomalies are primarily caused by abnormalities in the development of the Müllerian system. The Müllerian system develops into the fallopian tubes, uterus, and upper vagina.
- The paired Müllerian ducts elongate caudally, cross the Wolffian ducts medially, and fuse in the midline to form the primitive uterovaginal canal.
- The caudal end of the uterovaginal canal fuses with the urogenital sinus.
- Finally, the Müllerian ducts canalize, and the midline septum resorbs in a caudal to cephalad manner.
- The main categories of defects are:
  - Agenesis and hypoplasia
  - Lateral fusion defects
  - Vertical fusion defects
  - DES-related exposure

- The unicornuate uterus occurs when 1 of the Müllerian ducts fails to develop (hypoplasia). Uterine didelphys results from failure of the 2 Müllerian ducts to fuse together (lateral fusion) creating 2 cervices and 2 endometrial cavities. A bicornuate uterus also results from failure of lateral fusion; however, a single cervix and 2 endometrial cavities result.
- A transverse septum may develop due to incomplete fusion between the Müllerian tubercle and the sinovaginal bulbs or canalization failure of the vaginal plate. The lower vagina and hymenal region develop from the urogenital sinus.

ASSOCIATED CONDITIONS
- Abnormalities in the kidneys and urologic system are often associated with uterovaginal anomalies.
- The unicornuate uterus is associated with a high incidence (40%) of renal abnormalities usually ipsilateral to the anomalous side.
- A longitudinal vaginal septum often occurs with uterine anomalies such as a septate uterus or a uterine didelphys.
- Skeletal anomalies have been reported in association with 12–30% of Müllerian anomalies.

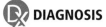 **DIAGNOSIS**

SIGNS AND SYMPTOMS
History
- Women may present with cyclic or noncyclic pain, dysmenorrhea suggestive of an obstructive phenomenon, retrograde menstruation, and endometriosis.
- Obstructive lesions tend to produce pain and discomfort due to the accumulation of mucous or menstrual products.
- Uterine anomalies are most commonly implicated in poor obstetric outcomes.
- Abnormalities of space, vascular supply, and local defects contribute to increased rates of recurrent pregnancy loss (21–33%), preterm delivery, and malpresentation.
- Women with unicornuate uteri have impaired pregnancy outcomes:
  - Spontaneous abortion rate: 36.5%
  - Preterm delivery rate: 44.6%
  - Live birth rate: 54.2%
- Women with a uterine didelphys have acceptable reproductive outcomes:
  - Spontaneous abortion rate: 32.2%
  - Preterm birth rate: 28.3%
  - Term delivery rate: 36.2%
  - Live birth rate: 55.9%

- Women with a bicornuate uterus may also experience obstetric complications:
  - Spontaneous abortion rate: 36%
  - Preterm birth rate: 23%
  - Term delivery rate: 40%
  - Live birth rate: 55.2%
  - ~1/3 of patients may experience cervical incompetence.
- The septate uterus is associated with the poorest obstetric outcomes. A compilation of studies of both partial and complete septa noted:
  - Pregnancy loss rates: 44.3%
  - Preterm delivery rate: 22.4%
  - Term delivery rate: 33.1%
  - Live birth rate: 50.1%
- A patient with an incomplete transverse vaginal septum may report light bleeding/spotting of dark blood between normal menstrual periods.
- Complaints associated with a longitudinal septum may include difficulty using tampons, dyspareunia, or in rare cases, obstructed labor.

Review of Systems
Inquiry regarding cyclic lower abdominal or pelvic pain would be pertinent when evaluating for a possible obstructive concern. Women with known urinary and renal anomaly can lead to suspicion of a possible uterovaginal anomaly.

Physical Exam
- A complete physical exam, including an external view of the perineum, is always important.
- Attention to spinal concerns, such as scoliosis or cervical spine abnormalities, and abnormalities in the digits are important.
- Bilateral labial traction and the use of a probe can assist in determining the vaginal length. Sometimes a longitudinal vaginal septum can be visualized in the office.
- If a patient is able to tolerate a speculum examination, visualization of the entire vagina with documentation of the cervical anatomy is appropriate.

TESTS
- Serum hormone levels are rarely beneficial.
- As described in cases of vaginal agenesis, elevated androgens would lead to determination of a serum karyotype to rule out forms of mixed gonadal dysgenesis.
- The mere presence of a uterovaginal anomaly does not mandate evaluation of a serum karyotype.

Imaging

- Abdominopelvic imaging is essential including evaluation of urogenital anatomy, including kidneys, ureters, and uterus/vagina.
- Hysterosalpingogram has historically been used to assess fallopian tube patency and the presence of complex communication with other systems.
  - This modality is not appropriate for use in an adolescent population, unless multidisciplinary evaluation under anesthesia is performed.
- US can be helpful in evaluating genitourinary anatomy, including kidneys, bladder, and uterus:
  - Allows assessment of internal and external uterine contour, a pelvic mass suggestive of a hematocolpos or hematometrocolpos, and kidneys
  - Inexpensive and, if a more complex anomaly is suspected, MRI can be requested
- MRI is gold standard in evaluating reproductive anomalies:
  - Distinguishes myometrial tissue from fibrous uterine communication and can differentiate a bicornuate uterus from a didelphys or a septate uterus, without the need for invasive surgery.

DIFFERENTIAL DIAGNOSIS

- Anomalies to consider include both uterine and vaginal abnormalities.
- Uterine anomalies include uterine didelphys, bicornuate uterus, septate uterus, and a unicornuate uterus, with a possible contralateral uterine remnant or horn.
- Vaginal anomalies include both transverse and longitudinal septa, and distal vaginal agenesis (see Vaginal Agenesis).

Infection

In obstructive conditions, attempts at drainage should be deferred until definitive treatment. Attempts at needle aspiration, with inadequate drainage and outflow of accumulated menstrual products, can introduce infection to a previously sterile collection.

Immunologic

In obstructive conditions, retrograde menstruation may lead to the development of endometriosis.

- Expert opinion supports the suggestion that the endometriosis resolves after relief of the obstruction.

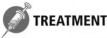

TREATMENT

GENERAL MEASURES

- Establishment of an adequate outflow tract is essential at puberty and menarche. Appropriate timing of surgery is important if postoperative dilation or serial exams are needed.

- In asymptomatic women or women with primary infertility, surgical treatment is controversial.
- In general, uterine anomalies do not prevent conception or implantation. Women can have normal reproductive outcomes.
- Surgery is indicated for women with pelvic pain, endometriosis, obstructive anomalies, and documented poor obstetric outcomes such as recurrent pregnancy loss or preterm deliveries.
- Menstrual suppression may be desirous in cases of suspected obstruction.
  - In cases requiring a more elaborate reconstruction, complete suppression with a GnRH agonist may be necessary preoperatively. Such treatment prevents continued accumulation of menstrual product, and therefore, allows stabilization of pain, to plan and schedule surgical intervention.

SURGERY

- The goals of surgery include treatment of pelvic pain, restoration of pelvic anatomy and uterine architecture, and preservation of fertility.
- The unicornuate uterus may be associated with a rudimentary horn on the contralateral side in 74% of cases:
  - In the majority of cases, the horn does not communicate with the unicornuate uterus.
  - If the horn contains active endometrium, it must be removed to prevent pain and obstruction.
- Surgical reconstruction does not improve pregnancy outcomes, but cervical cerclage may be beneficial in patients with a unicornuate uterus.
- The uterine didelphys has the best reproductive outcomes of all uterine anomalies, so it is only rarely necessary to consider a uterine unification procedure (metroplasty).
- Only after confirmed cases of recurrent pregnancy loss or severely preterm delivery is it appropriate to consider metroplasty of a bicornuate uterus. Exclusion of other causes of pregnancy loss should be performed 1st.
- For women with a septate uterus, hysteroscopic metroplasty has been demonstrated to significantly improve the live birth rate (80%) and miscarriage rates (15%).
  - This procedure is recommended when the uterine septum is implicated in recurrent pregnancy loss, 2nd trimester loss, malpresentation, or preterm delivery.

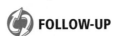

FOLLOW-UP

DISPOSITION

Issues for Referral

Uterovaginal reconstructive surgery often requires complex techniques, and patients may benefit from referral to a center with expertise in the procedures and long-term experience with reproductive outcomes.

BIBLIOGRAPHY

Acien P. Incidence of müllerian defects in fertile and infertile women. *Hum Reprod*. 1997;12:1372–1376.

American Fertility Society. Classifications of adnexal adhesions, distal tubal occlusion secondary to tubal ligation, tubal pregnancies, müllerian anomalies and intrauterine adhesions. *Fertil Steril*. 1988;49: 944–955.

Grimbizis GF, et al. Clinical implications of uterine malformations and hysteroscopic treatment results. *Hum Reprod Update*. 2001;7:161–174.

Lin PC, et al. Female genital anomalies affecting reproduction. *Fertil Steril*. 2002;78:899–915.

Nahum GG. Uterine anomalies; how common are they, and what is their distribution among subtypes? *J Reprod Med*. 1998;43:877–887.

Raga F, et al. Reproductive impact of congenital Müllerian anomalies. *Hum Reprod*. 1997;12: 2277–2281.

 MISCELLANEOUS

CLINICAL PEARLS

- A special circumstance of uterine didelphys occurs with a solitary kidney and an obstructing vaginal septum on the contralateral side.
  - Resection of the septum is necessary to allow menstrual flow after menarche. Adolescents often present with pain, primary amenorrhea, and a pelvic mass (hematocolpos within the obstructed hemivagina).

ABBREVIATION

GnRH—Gonadotropin-releasing hormone

CODES

ICD9-CM

- 752.2 Didelphys uterus, septate uterus
- 752.3 Uterine anomaly (bicornuate uterus, unicornuate uterus, uterine anomaly with only 1 functioning horn)
- 752.49 Septate vagina

 PATIENT TEACHING

- Patients with known urologic anomalies or renal agenesis should consult with a primary care physician regarding precautions to protect urinary health.
- Adult women should be counseled regarding obstetric prognosis, in order to seek appropriate reproductive medical support when indicated.
- Discussion of obstetric prognosis in adolescents should take into account the adolescent's cognitive and psychosocial development. Parents can be helpful in suggesting the appropriate timing of this discussion.

VAGINAL AGENESIS

Lesley L. Breech, MD

 BASICS

DESCRIPTION
- Vaginal agenesis describes the condition in which the vagina is absent or poorly developed. Some patients may have a small distal vaginal dimple.
- Most common cause is congenital absence of the uterus and vagina referred to as Müllerian aplasia, Müllerian agenesis, or Mayer-Rokitansky-Kuster-Hauser syndrome (MRKH).

Age-Related Factors
Most patients are diagnosed during adolescence with a chief complaint of primary amenorrhea.

Staging
- The American Society of Reproductive Medicine, previously the American Fertility Society, devised a classification system for uterovaginal anomalies in 1988.
- Vaginal agenesis is considered a Class I defect, dysgenesis of the Müllerian ducts.

EPIDEMIOLOGY
- 2nd most common cause of primary amenorrhea behind gonadal dysgenesis.
- Occurs in 1 of every 4,000–10,000 females:
  - Most patients will have rudimentary uterine remnants; however, in 2–7% of patients, active endometrium may be present, necessitating surgical management.

RISK FACTORS
Genetics
Multiple gene defects have been evaluated, without identification of a discrete inheritable defect.

PATHOPHYSIOLOGY
- Vaginal agenesis is caused by failure of embryologic growth of the müllerian ducts, with resultant anomalies of the müllerian structures.
- Variation can occur with the presence or absence of the uterus. A single midline uterus may be present, but more commonly uterine remnants, sometimes with an endometrial cavity, are present:
  - Due to the separate embryologic source, the ovaries are normal in structure and function.

ASSOCIATED CONDITIONS
- Associated congenital anomalies include urologic (25–50%) and skeletal abnormalities (10–30%).
- Skeletal abnormalities can include:
  - Scoliosis
  - Cervical spinal abnormalities
  - Digital abnormalities
- Auditory dysfunction and cardiac defects may also be present.

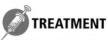 **DIAGNOSIS**

SIGNS AND SYMPTOMS
History
- Young women present with normal secondary sexual development and the absence of menses. Occasionally a diagnosis is made earlier due to evaluation for other conditions.
- If an endometrial lining is present in the uterine structure, patients may complain of cyclic abdominopelvic pain due to the accumulation of menstrual fluid in the uterus (hematometra).

Physical Exam
- Clinicians should perform a complete physical exam with attention to the presence of scoliosis, digital abnormalities.
- An exam of the external genitalia is mandatory.
- Bilateral labial traction is essential to assist in determining vaginal patency.
- Gentle insertion of a probe into the vagina is an atraumatic way to determine length.

TESTS
Chromosomal analysis may differentiate this condition from disorders of testosterone synthesis or receptor sensitivity in XY individuals—androgen insensitivity syndrome.

Lab
A normal, female range of serum testosterone can be useful to rule out androgen insensitivity.

Imaging
- A pelvic US is beneficial to confirm the presence of normally located and appearing ovaries. Additional imaging should also be performed to assess for possible renal anomalies.
- MRI is another useful modality to look at uterine remnants, which may remain somewhat high in the pelvis along the sidewall:
  - Considered the gold standard in the evaluation of reproductive anomalies.

DIFFERENTIAL DIAGNOSIS
Included in the differential diagnosis are:
- Congenital absence of the vagina
- Androgen insensitivity syndrome (see topic)
- 17-Hydroxylase deficiency
- Low transverse vaginal septum (See Uterovaginal Anomalies.)
- Imperforate hymen (see topic)

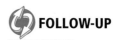 **TREATMENT**

GENERAL MEASURES
- Nonsurgical creation of a neovagina should be the first-line approach:
  - Success rates with this approach can be >90%.
- In the event of failure of this option or patient preference, there is no consensus regarding the best surgical therapy for vaginal agenesis.
- There is, however, agreement regarding waiting until at least mid to late adolescence to create a neovagina.
- It is not rare to see an individual with vaginal agenesis who, through repeated coital pressure, has developed a functional vaginal pouch.

SURGERY
- Surgery should be reserved for patients who fail an attempt at nonsurgical creation of a neovagina. Several procedures have been described with limited data regarding long-term outcomes, including sexual outcomes.
- Common surgical methods include the use of a split thickness skin graft, a bowel (most commonly the sigmoid colon) neovagina, or use of peritoneal lining.

FOLLOW-UP

DISPOSITION
Issues for Referral
- Because of the complex medical and psychological factors involved in managing this condition, patients often benefit from referral to a center experienced in the nonsurgical techniques of management.
- Patients who fail the nonsurgical approach or decide to proceed with surgical creation of a neovagina require referral to an experienced pelvic reconstructive surgeon:
  - Success is greatest on the 1st surgical attempt.

PATIENT MONITORING

The neovagina has the same risk as a native vagina for STIs. Examination for malignancies or other problems should occur on an annual basis. No data support the frequency of cytologic screening.

BIBLIOGRAPHY

American College of Obstetrics and Gynocologists. Committee Opinion No. 355: Vaginal agenesis: diagnosis, management, and routine care. *Obstet Gynecol*. 2006;108:1605–1609.

American Fertility Society. Classifications of adnexal adhesions, distal tubal occlusion secondary to tubal ligation, tubal pregnancies, müllerian anomalies and intrauterine adhesions. *Fertil Steril*. 1988; 49:944–955.

Evans TN, et al. Vaginal malformations. *Am J Obstet Gynecol*. 1981;141:910–912.

Oppelt P, et al. Clinical aspects of Mayer-Rokitansky-Kuster-Hauser syndrome: Recommendations for clinical diagnosis and staging. *Hum Reprod*. 2006;21:792–797.

Reindollar RH, et al. Delayed sexual development: A study of 252 patients. *Am J Obstet Gynecol*. 1981:140(4):371–380.

 MISCELLANEOUS

SYNONYM(S)

- Mayer-Rokitansky-Küster-Hauser syndrome (MRKH)
- Müllerian agenesis
- Müllerian aplasia
- Vaginal aplasia
- Vaginal agenesis
- Uterovaginal agenesis

ABBREVIATIONS

- MRKH—Mayer-Rokitansky-Küster-Houser
- STI—Sexually transmitted infection

CODES

ICD9-CM

- 752.40 Vaginal anomaly
- 752.49 Vaginal agenesis

 PATIENT TEACHING

Resources are available both for patients and parents through several sources. An especially good resource using "teen-friendly" terms is the Web site maintained by Boston Children's Hospital, www.youngwomeneshealth.org

VAGINAL INTRAEPITHELIAL NEOPLASIA (VAIN)

Jay E. Allard, MD
John Farley, MD
Cynthia Macri, MD

 BASICS

DESCRIPTION
- VAIN is defined as the presence of cytologic atypia of vaginal squamous cells without invasion.
- Increasing diagnosis over the last several years is likely the result of increased cytologic screening, heightened awareness, and liberal use of colposcopy.
- VAIN is much less common than cervical or vulvar intraepithelial neoplasia.
- The pathophysiology is extrapolated from information regarding CIN and VIN.

Age-Related Factors
The average patient is between 40 and 60 years old.

Staging
- Because VAIN is a premalignant lesion, it is not classically staged. However, it is classified into various categories, similar to those of CIN, according to the depth of epithelial involvement.
- VAIN I:
  – Lower 1/3 of the epithelium is involved with squamous cell atypia (the level closest to the basement membrane).
- VAIN II:
  – Lower 2/3 of the epithelium is involved with squamous cell atypia.
- VAIN III:
  – >2/3 of the epithelium is involved with squamous atypia.
  – Carcinoma in-situ, which encompasses the full thickness of the epithelium, is included under VAIN III.

EPIDEMIOLOGY
- True incidence unknown, estimated to be 0.2–0.3 cases per 100,000 women in the US
- Average age at diagnosis: 40–60

RISK FACTORS
- Most common: HPV infection
- Genetic and acquired immunosuppression (i.e., HIV infection)

Genetics
Intercalation of HPV DNA into the host genome, with expression causing the development of VAIN

PATHOPHYSIOLOGY
- 2 proposed etiologies:
  – Vaginal extension of unidentified cervical disease
  – Unlikely in most cases because VAIN is often multifocal, can occur several years after hysterectomy, is independent of the amount of vaginal cuff excised, often observed in the absence of cervical disease
- Common embryologic origin of vaginal epithelium with other lower genital tract epithelium may make all of these tissues more susceptible to similar carcinogenic stimuli. Exposure to HPV, in particular, has been shown to induce neoplasia in the vast majority of cervical epithelium.
  – More mature, stable squamous epithelium of the vagina (as opposed to the cervical transformation zone), may serve to be somewhat protective of the vaginal epithelium, thereby leading to a decreased incidence of VAIN as compared to CIN.
  – Women exposed to DES in utero have increased incidence of VAIN, possibly due to squamous metaplasia of vaginal epithelium.

ASSOCIATED CONDITIONS
Prior or concurrent neoplasia elsewhere in lower genital tract

 DIAGNOSIS

SIGNS AND SYMPTOMS
History
- Typically asymptomatic, however may present with:
  – Postcoital spotting
  – Vaginal discharge
- History of abnormal Pap smear in a patient who has had a hysterectomy or who does not have an identifiable cervical lesion on colposcopy should prompt evaluation for VAIN.

Physical Exam
- Digital palpation to assess vaginal wall thickening or irregularity
- Speculum examination with application of acetic acid:
  – Lesions appear raised or flat, white, granular
  – Sharply demarcated borders
  – May note vascular punctuation on colposcopy
- Majority of lesions are found in upper 1/3 of vagina

- Markedly irregular lesions or lesions with significant vascular abnormalities raise suspicion of an invasive process:
  – Perform excisional biopsy of this type of lesion
  – Schiller or Lugol iodine solution can improve visualization of border boundaries

TESTS
Colposcopy of suspicious lesions:
- Colposcopically directed biopsy taken from lesions

Lab
Biopsy for histologic diagnosis

Imaging
Not indicated

DIFFERENTIAL DIAGNOSIS
The differential diagnosis for VAIN includes CIN and VIN.

Infection
- Yeast vulvo-vaginitis can cause areas of aceto-whitening
- Other vulvo-vaginitis with discharge

Tumor/Malignancy
Melanoma

Trauma
Vulvar trauma with small abrasions from intercourse can appear aceto-white

Drugs
Topical vaginal medications or lubricants can be adherent to vaginal wall and simulate a lesion.

Geriatric Considerations
A postmenopausal patient may have atrophic vaginal mucosa causing abnormal findings on Pap smear:
- 4 weeks of topical estrogen treatment may accentuate visualization of a true abnormality and improve detection of VAIN.

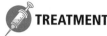 **TREATMENT**

GENERAL MEASURES
- A range of treatment options are available including:
  – Excision
  – Ablation
  – Topical chemotherapy
  – Radiation

- Therapy selection is based on:
  - Previous treatment failures
  - Presence of multifocal disease
  - Desire to preserve sexual function
  - Medical risks of surgery
  - Exclusion of invasive disease prior to therapeutic management

SPECIAL THERAPY

- Intracavitary radiation therapy:
  - Higher rates of morbidity than other therapies
  - Reserved for patients with:
    - Prior treatment failures
    - Medical risks precluding surgery
    - Extensive, multifocal disease
- Complications associated with intracavitary radiation therapy:
  - Vaginal atrophy
  - Vaginal stenosis
  - Vaginal shortening
  - Detrimental effects on bowel and bladder
  - Earlier menopause
  - Poor wound healing if subsequent surgery is required on irradiated tissue
- Complications can often interfere with sexual function and thorough colposcopic follow-up examination
- Must rule out invasion by thorough colposcopic examination and biopsy prior to treatment

MEDICATION (DRUGS)

- Chemotherapy
- Topical application of 5–FU:
  - Advantages:
    - Treats entire vaginal mucosa at 1 time
    - Incorporates coverage of multifocal disease
    - Treats disease in vaginal folds and invaginations
    - Relatively inexpensive
    - Administered in outpatient setting
  - Appropriate first-line treatment in patients with early lesions, multifocal disease, or in those who are poor surgical candidates
  - Disadvantages/Complications:
    - Vaginal irritation, burning, ulceration
    - Columnar metaplasia of the vaginal epithelium may develop
  - External application of petroleum jelly or zinc oxide cream may help prevent ulceration
  - Topical estrogen may reduce discomfort
  - Must rule out invasion by thorough colposcopic examination and biopsy prior to treating with 5–FU
  - Dosing:
    - Multiple dosing protocols with similar efficacy

SURGERY

- Surgical excision permits histologic diagnosis, an advantage over other treatments
- Multiple approaches including:
  - Local excision
  - Partial vaginectomy
  - Total vaginectomy
  - Electrosurgical loop excision
  - Laser vaginectomy
- Choice of approach is dictated by location of lesions, extensiveness of disease, and persistence of disease.
- Complications:
  - Vaginal shortening
  - Vaginal stenosis
  - Postoperative morbidity, especially if an abdominal approach is necessary
- Ablation:
  - CO_2 laser is preferred
  - ~1/3 of patients require additional treatments
  - Advantages:
    - Minimal sexual dysfunction
    - Well tolerated
    - Satisfactory healing
  - Complications:
    - Pain
    - Bleeding
  - Must be able to visualize entire area of abnormal epithelium
  - Must rule out invasion prior to ablation by thorough colposcopy and biopsy

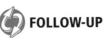 **FOLLOW-UP**

DISPOSITION

Issues for Referral

Patients should be referred to a specialist for persistent or recurrent disease, or when disease location is unable to be elucidated.

PROGNOSIS

5–FU, surgical excision, laser ablation, and intracavitary radiation are successful in ~80% of patients with VAIN; ~20% recurrence rate.

PATIENT MONITORING

Gynecologic exam and vaginal cytology performed at 3-month intervals for 1 year, followed by 6-month intervals for 1 year, then yearly screening.

BIBLIOGRAPHY

Berek JS, et al., eds. *Novak's Gynecology.* 12th ed. Baltimore: Williams & Wilkins; 1996.

Berek JS, et al., eds. *Practical Gynecologic Oncology.* 4th ed. Philadelphia: Lippincott Williams & Wilkins; 2005.

Holschneider CH, et al. Vaginal intraepithelial neoplasia. *UpToDate Online,* 2006; version 14.2.

Hoskins WJ, et al., eds. *Principles and Practice of Gynecologic Oncology.* 4th ed. Philadelphia: Lippincott Williams & Wilkins; 2005.

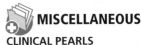 **MISCELLANEOUS**

CLINICAL PEARLS

Skin hooks may be used to gently evert vaginal recesses in patients who have had a hysterectomy, to improve visualization.

ABBREVIATIONS

- 5–FU—5–Fluorouracil
- AIS—Adenocarcinoma in situ
- CIN—Cervical intraepithelial neoplasia
- DES—Diethylstilbestrol
- HPV—Human papillomavirus
- VAIN—Vaginal intraepithelial neoplasia
- VIN—Vulvar intraepithelial neoplasia

CODES

ICD9-CM

- 623.0 Dysplasia of vagina
  - *Excludes:* Carcinoma in situ of vagina (233.3)

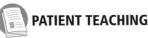 **PATIENT TEACHING**

- After treatment avoid:
  - Deep tub baths for 2 weeks
  - Strenuous exercise for 2 weeks
  - Intercourse for 6 weeks or during treatment with 5–FU
- Additionally, call your physician if you develop:
  - Worsening pain not relieved by pain medication
  - Persistent nausea or vomiting
  - Temperature >100.4°F (38°C)
  - Bleeding or abnormal drainage from your vagina
  - Worsening redness or swelling around your vulva

PREVENTION

- In 2006, the FDA approved a quadrivalent HPV vaccine for vaccination of females 9–26 years of age to prevent the following diseases caused by HPV Types 6, 11, 16, and 18:
  - Cervical cancer
  - Genital warts (condyloma acuminata)
  - The following precancerous or dysplastic lesions:
    - Cervical AIS
    - CIN grade 2 and grade 3
    - VIN grade 2 and grade 3
    - VAIN grade 2 and grade 3
    - CIN grade 1
- This vaccine is not intended to be used for treatment of cervical cancer, CIN, VIN, VAIN, or genital warts.
- The vaccine has not been shown to protect against diseases due to non-vaccine HPV types.

VAGINITIS, ATROPHIC

Thuong-Thuong Nguyen, MD

 BASICS

DESCRIPTION
- Vaginal epithelium thinning secondary to estrogen deficiency, resulting in vaginal dryness and inflammation

Age-Related Factors
- Atrophic vaginitis is most common in menopausal and postmenopausal women.
- May also be present postpartum in a woman who is breastfeeding

EPIDEMIOLOGY
10–40% of postmenopausal women have symptoms of atrophic vaginitis.

RISK FACTORS
- Menopause, either natural or surgical (oophorectomy): Decline in endogenous estrogen
- Premenopause:
  – Ovarian failure: Spontaneous or secondary to radiation or hemotherapy
  – Antiestrogenic medications: Tamoxifen, danazol, leuprolide, medroxyprogesterone
  – Postpartum loss of placental estrogen
  – Lactation: Prolactin, antiestrogenic effects
  – Immunologic disorder
  – Smoking
  – No vaginal delivery

PATHOPHYSIOLOGY
- Circulating estrogen, mainly estradiol, helps maintain vaginal epithelium elasticity and moistness by stimulating the production of collagen and hyaluronic acid, respectively.
- Estrogen stimulates nonkeratinized stratified squamous epithelium to thicken, form rugae, and fill with glycogen:
  – Glycogen from sloughed cells are converted into lactic acid by Döderlein's lactobacilli, creating an acidic environment (pH 3.5–5) that is protective against urogenital infections.
- Significant reduction in circulating estrogen after menopause results in:
  – Thin and less elastic vaginal epithelium, more susceptible to trauma and irritation
  – Shortened and less rugated vaginal canal
  – ~50% less vaginal secretions
  – Increased pH and predisposition to infection by *Staphylococcus, Streptococcus,* coliforms, and diphtheroids

ASSOCIATED CONDITIONS
The genital and urinary tract share a common embryologic origin. The urethral epithelium, bladder, pelvic muscle floor, and pelvic fascia are also estrogen dependent. Dysuria, hematuria, urinary frequency may occur.

 DIAGNOSIS

SIGNS AND SYMPTOMS
- The majority of women with mild to moderate vaginal atrophy are asymptomatic.
- Symptoms of atrophic vaginitis generally appear only after estrogen levels have been low for an extended period.
- Early on, women may notice a slight decrease in vaginal lubrication upon arousal, which is one of the 1st signs of estrogen insufficiency.
- Genital symptoms: Itching, dryness, burning, dyspareunia, yellow malodorous vaginal discharge, leukorrhea, pruritus, pressure sensation
- Urinary symptoms: Dysuria, hematuresis, urinary frequency, UTI, stress incontinence

History
- Menstrual history
- Last menstrual period or final menstrual period
- Symptoms of menopause: Hot flashes, age of mother's menopause
- Obstetric history, number of vaginal deliveries, number of weeks postpartum, lactation (breast-feeding or pumping; fully breastfeeding or supplementing)
- Sexual history: Dyspareunia, sexually active, use of lubricants, STIs
- Medications, chemotherapy, radiation
- PMH: Immunologic disorder
- Smoking
- Exogenous agents that may cause or further aggravate symptoms:
  – Perfumes, powders, soaps, deodorants, panty liners, spermicides, and lubricants may contain irritant compounds.
  – In addition, tight-fitting clothing and long-term use of perineal pads or synthetic materials

Review of Systems
Special attention to GU symptoms

Physical Exam
General:
- External genitalia: Loss of labial and vulvar fullness, sparsity of pubic hair, dryness of labia, vulvar lesions, vulvar dermatoses:
  – Areas of microtrauma or fissures at peri-introital area and posterior fourchette may be seen at colposcopy, if indicated
  – Signs suggesting lichen sclerosus:
    ○ Fusion of labia minora with majora (loss of architecture)
    ○ Introital stenosis
  – Signs suggesting vulvar vestibulitis:
    ○ Areas of focal erythema in hymenal sulcus

- Urethral:
  – Urethral caruncle, signifying eversion of urethral mucosa
  – Urethral polyps
  – Ecchymoses
- Vaginal:
  – Pallor of urethral and vaginal epithelium, decreased vaginal moisture
  – Smooth or shiny vaginal epithelium; superficial epithelium may be lost entirely
  – Loss of elasticity or turgor of skin and vaginal epithelium
  – Shortening and narrowing of the vaginal canal, with loss of distensibility
  – Lack of/flattening of rugae
  – Easily traumatized epithelium with areas of traumatic subepithelial or epithelial hemorrhage or petechiae
  – Pelvic organ prolapse
  – Rectocele
  – Cystocele

TESTS
Lab
- Serum hormone levels are generally not helpful to assess for menopause, as FSH can wax and wane during menopausal transition.
- A low level of circulating estradiol may be present, but is not clinically useful (≤25 pg/mL).
- Pap smear can confirm the presence of urogenital atrophy.
  – Maturation index: Cytologic examination of smears from the upper 1/3 of the vagina show an increased proportion of parabasal cells and a decreased percentage of superficial cells.
- An elevated pH level (postmenopausal pH levels >5), monitored by a pH strip in the middle 3rd of the vaginal vault, may also be a sign of vaginal atrophy.
- Microscopy: On microscopic evaluation, loss of superficial cells is obvious with atrophy, but there may also be evidence of infection with *Trichomonas, Candida,* or bacterial vaginitis.

Imaging
TVUS of the uterine lining that demonstrates a thin endometrium measuring between 4 and 5 mm signifies loss of adequate estrogenic stimulation.

DIFFERENTIAL DIAGNOSIS
Infection
- Candidiasis
- Bacterial vaginosis
- Trichomoniasis

Metabolic/Endocrine
POF (ovarian insufficiency)

Immunologic
Contact irritation or reaction to perfumes, powders, deodorants, panty liners, perineal pads, soaps, spermicides, lubricants, tight-fitting or synthetic clothing

Other/Miscellaneous
• Vulvar lichen sclerosus
• Vulvar vestibulitis

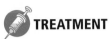 **TREATMENT**

GENERAL MEASURES
• Moisturizers and lubricants may be used in conjunction with estrogen therapy or as alternative treatment:
  – Women who choose not to take HRT, have medical contraindications, or experience hormonal side effects.
  – Daily moisturizer: Replens, a long acting polycarbophil-based, bioadhesive polymer, produces a moist film over the vagina:
    ○ Relieves vaginal dryness, normalizes pH
  – Water-based lubricants with intercourse: Astroglide, K-Y personal lubricant
• Sexual activity is a healthful prescription for postmenopausal women:
  – Vaginal intercourse encourages vaginal elasticity and pliability, and the lubricative response to sexual stimulation.
  – Fewer symptoms and less evidence of vaginal stenosis and shrinkage
  – Coital activity, including masturbation, associated with fewer symptoms

SPECIAL THERAPY
Complementary and Alternative Therapies
Insufficient evidence to support the use of DHEA-containing vaginal creams

MEDICATION (DRUGS)
• Estrogen replacement:
  – Restores normal pH levels; thickens and revascularizes the epithelium
  – Increases the number of superficial cells
  – May alleviate existing symptoms or even prevent development of urogenital symptoms if initiated at the time of menopause.
  – Contraindications to estrogen therapy include:
    ○ Estrogen-sensitive tumors
    ○ End-stage liver failure
    ○ Past history of venous thromboembolism
  – Adverse effects of estrogen therapy include:
    ○ Breast tenderness
    ○ Vaginal bleeding and a slight increase in the risk of an estrogen-dependent neoplasm
    ○ Venous thromboembolism
    ○ Increased risk of endometrial carcinoma and hyperplasia conclusively related to unopposed, estrogen intake
  – Routes of administration include oral, transdermal, and intravaginal.

  – Dose frequency may be continuous, cyclic, or as-needed for symptomatic relief.
  – The amount and duration required to eliminate symptoms depends on the degree of vaginal atrophy.
• Systemic administration of estrogen has been shown to have a therapeutic effect on symptoms of atrophic vaginitis. Additional advantages include a decrease in postmenopausal bone loss and alleviation of hot flashes.
  – Standard dosages of systemic estrogen, however, may not eliminate the symptoms of atrophic vaginitis in 10–25% of patients.
  – Systemic estrogen in higher dosages may be necessary to alleviate vaginal symptoms.
  – Some women require coadministration of a vaginal estrogen product applied locally.
• Low-dose local estrogen preferred:
  – Creams, pessaries, tablets, rings similarly effective in treatment of symptoms: Symptom relief with little endometrial proliferation
  – Vaginal rings, Estring or Phadia: Estradiol-impregnated silastic ring is inserted into the vagina and delivers 6–9 μg of estradiol daily for 3 months. Favored most for comfort and ease of use.
  – Creams, conjugated estrogens (Premarin): Daily for 3 weeks, then twice weekly for 12 weeks
  – Tablet, Vagifem: 25 μg estradiol twice a week
  – Higher-dose local estrogen treats atrophic vaginitis, hot flushes, and bone loss.
    ○ Vaginal ring, Femring: Releases 50–100 μg/d; replaced in 3 months.

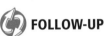 **FOLLOW-UP**

DISPOSITION
Issues for Referral
Urogynecology for urinary symptoms or pelvic organ prolapse

PROGNOSIS
• Most women get relief of symptoms with vaginal formulations of estrogen.
• Systemic estrogens may require the addition of vaginal estrogen formulations.
• Nonestrogen therapies are less effective for most women than estrogen.

PATIENT MONITORING
Assess compliance (frequency of use) and need for progestin therapy in women on estrogen therapy:
• TVUS may be helpful in assessing endometrial proliferation.

BIBLIOGRAPHY

Bachmann GA, et al. Diagnosis and treatment of atrophic vaginitis. *Am Fam Phys.* 2000;61:3090.

Ballagh SA. Vaginal hormone therapy for urogenital and menopausal symptoms. *Semin Reprod Med.* 2005;23(2):126–140.

Botsis D, et al. Transvaginal sonography in postmenopausal women treated with low-dose estrogens locally administered. *Maturitas.* 1996;23:41–45.

Cardozo L, et al. Meta-analysis of estrogen therapy in the management of urogenital atrophy in postmenopausal women: Second report of the Hormones and Urogenital Therapy Committee. *Obstet Gynecol.* 1998;92:722.

Castelo-Branco C, et al. Management of post-menopausal vaginal atrophy and atrophic vaginitis. *Maturitas.* 2005;52(Suppl 1):S46.

Leiblum S, et al. Vaginal atrophy in the postmenopausal woman: The importance of sexual activity and hormones. *JAMA.* 1983;249:2195.

Nyirjesy P. *Vaginitis.* Washington, DC: American College of Obstetrics and Gynecologists. Practice Bulletin, Number 72; May 2006.

Pandit L, et al. Postmenopausal vaginal atrophy and atrophic vaginitis. *Am J Med Sci.* 1997;314:228.

Santen RJ, et al. Treatment of urogenital atrophy with low-dose estradiol: Preliminary results. *Menopause.* 2002;9:179.

Suckling J, et al. Local oestrogen for vaginal atrophy in postmenopausal women. *Cochrane Database Syst Rev.* 2003;CD001500.

Willhite LA, et al. Urogenital atrophy: Prevention and treatment. *Pharmacotherapy.* 2001;21:464.

 MISCELLANEOUS

SYNONYM(S)
• Urogenital atrophy
• Senile vaginitis

CLINICAL PEARLS
• Women who are breastfeeding may be unaware of the possibility of atrophic vaginitis and can benefit from education and therapy.
• 75–80% of women with atrophic vaginitis do not inform their health care provider of their symptoms because they believe these are part of aging.

ABBREVIATIONS
• DHEA—Dehydroepiandrosterone
• FSH—Follicle-stimulating hormone
• HRT—Hormone replacement therapy
• PMH—Postmenopausal hormone
• POF—Premature ovarian failure
• TVUS—Transvaginal ultrasound

CODES

ICD9-CM
627.4 Postmenopausal or senile vaginitis

 PATIENT TEACHING

ACOG Patient Education Pamphlet: Vaginitis

PREVENTION
• Regular sexual activity including masturbation is associated with fewer symptoms of atrophic vaginitis, even without therapy.
• Initiation of estrogen therapy at time of menopause may alleviate and prevent symptoms of atrophic vaginitis.

VAGINITIS: BACTERIAL VAGINOSIS

Emily Boyd, MD
Jeffrey F. Peipert, MD, PhD

 BASICS

DESCRIPTION
- BV is a clinical syndrome caused by replacement of vaginal hydrogen peroxide–producing *Lactobacillus* species by a variety of anaerobic bacteria, *Gardnerella vaginalis*, and *Mycoplasma hominis*.

Age-Related Factors
- Estrogen is crucial for a healthy vaginal ecosystem.
- In the reproductive years, estrogen maintains a healthy vaginal epithelium, leading to larger numbers of lactobacilli.
- In prepubertal and postmenopausal years, the vaginal epithelium can be thin, and the pH of the vagina can be higher (≥4.7), which can lead to overgrowth of many organisms.

EPIDEMIOLOGY
- Most frequent causes of vaginal discharge:
  - Bacterial vaginosis: 22–50%
  - Vulvovaginal candidiasis: 17–39%
  - Trichomoniasis: 4–35%
- >50% of affected women are asymptomatic.

RISK FACTORS
- Generally not considered an STI, however a sexually associated infection
- Multiple sex partners
- New sex partner
- Douching
- Inherent lack of vaginal hydrogen peroxide–producing lactobacilli
- Exposure to other STIs
- Black race
- IUD use

PATHOPHYSIOLOGY
- Cause is not fully understood.
- Lactobacilli are the most prominent organism in the vagina:
  - Maintain acidic pH (3.8–4.2)
  - Acidic pH prevents growth of *G. vaginalis* and anaerobes
  - Lack of lactobacilli is characteristic of BV
  - Allows 100–1,000-fold increase in pathogenic bacteria
- Vaginosis versus vaginitis: In vaginosis there is notable lack of WBCs:
  - *Mobiluncus* and *Bacteroides* species produce succinic acid.
  - Succinic acid alters WBC migration.
  - Typically results in few WBCs on saline wet-mount

Pregnancy Considerations
- BV during pregnancy is associated with the following adverse outcomes:
  - Preterm delivery
  - Premature rupture of membranes
  - Preterm labor
  - Chorioamnionitis
  - Postpartum endometritis

ASSOCIATED CONDITIONS
- Postoperative infections (e.g., post abortion, post hysterectomy)
- Postpartum infections (e.g., endometritis)
- STIs

 DIAGNOSIS

SIGNS AND SYMPTOMS
History
- Include questions regarding sexual history, duration of symptoms, and location of symptoms.
- Also question history of treatment of symptoms including self-treatment.
- Thin white-gray vaginal discharge noted
- Malodor noticed after menses, intercourse
- May cause itching, burning, or irritation of vagina

Physical Exam
- Thin, homogenous discharge adherent to vulvar and vaginal epithelium
- Collect sample from anterior or lateral vaginal wall
- Saline wet prep:
  - Note lack of lactobacilli
  - Note clue cells (>20% of epithelial cells diagnostic)
  - Note lack of WBCs

TESTS
- Gram stain (gold standard):
  - Nugent scoring determines the relative concentration of lactobacilli, Gram-negative and Gram-variable rods and cocci, Gram-negative curved rods.
- Amsel's clinical criteria (3 of the following):
  - Homogenous, thin white or gray discharge
  - Clue cells on wet mount (>20% of epithelial cells)
  - Vaginal fluid pH >4.5
  - Positive whiff test (fishy odor produced) with or without addition of 10% KOH
- Amsel's criteria: Sensitivity 92% and specificity of 77%
- Similar sensitivity and specificity when combining any 2 of Amsel's clinical criteria

Labs

- A few tests are available commercially.
- Affirm: DNA probe–based test for high concentration *of G. vaginalis.*
- QuickVue Advance: Tests for elevated pH and trimethylamine
- Pip Activity TestCard: Tests for proline aminopeptidase
- Pap smear has limited clinical utility for diagnosis due to low sensitivity.

DIFFERENTIAL DIAGNOSIS

Infection

- Vaginitis:
  - Candidiasis (See Vaginitis; Vulvovaginal Candidiasis.)
  - Trichomonas vaginalis (See Sexually Transmitted Diseases [STDs]: Trichomonas.)
  - Inflammatory vaginitis (See Vaginal Signs and Symptoms: Vaginal Discharge.)
- Cervicitis:
  - *Neisseria gonorrhoeae* (See Sexually Transmitted Diseases [STDs]: Gonorrhea.)
  - *Chlamydia trachomatis* (See Sexually Transmitted Diseases [STDs]: Clamydia.)
  - HSV (See Sexually Transmitted Diseases [STDs]: Herpes Simplex Virus.)

Other/Miscellaneous

Atrophic vaginitis (See Vaginitis: Atrophic.)

 TREATMENT

GENERAL MEASURES

- General treatment goals:
  - Treat symptoms of vaginal infection.
  - Reduce risk of post procedure infection after hysterectomy or abortion:
    - ○ Some specialists recommend screening and treating high-risk women with BV.
    - ○ Some specialists recommend treatment and/or prophylaxis prior to procedures.
    - ○ Potential for reduction of other STIs
- Pregnancy treatment goals:
  - Treat symptoms of vaginal infection.
  - Possibly reduce preterm birth in high-risk women
  - Potentially reduce other STIs

MEDICATION (DRUGS)

- CDC recommended regimens (2006):
  - Metronidazole 500 mg PO b.i.d. for 7 days
  - Metronidazole gel 0.75% 1 applicator full (5 g) intravaginally for 5 days
  - Clindamycin cream 2% 1 applicator full (5 g) intravaginally for 7 days
- CDC alternative regimens (2006):
  - Clindamycin 300 mg PO b.i.d. for 7 days
  - Clindamycin ovules 100 g intravaginally once at bedtime for 3 days
- If Metronidazole allergy:
  - Clindamycin cream intravaginally is preferred
- Treatment of sexual partners:
  - Not shown to prevent recurrence
  - Not recommended
- Caution:
  - Use of alcohol should be avoided with metronidazole, which can cause disulfiram-like reactions.
  - Clindamycin is oil-based and can weaken condoms and diaphragms for up to 5 days.
- In pregnancy:
  - Metronidazole 500 mg PO b.i.d. for 7 days
  - Metronidazole 250 mg PO t.i.d. for 7 days
  - Clindamycin 300 mg PO b.i.d. for 7 days
  - Clindamycin topical should not be used in the 2nd half of pregnancy.

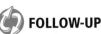 FOLLOW-UP

DISPOSITION

Issues for Referral

Multiple recurrences may warrant referral to specialist in vulvovaginal diseases/gyn infectious disease.

PROGNOSIS

Good

PATIENT MONITORING

- In nonpregnant patients:
  - No return visit is necessary.
  - Instruct patient to return for recurrence of symptoms.
  - Metronidazole gel 0.75% twice weekly for 6 months after completion of recommended therapy may be useful in preventing recurrence for up to 6 months.
- In pregnant patients:
  - Consider screening and treatment of women with high-risk pregnancy.
  - Consider follow-up 1 month after treatment completed.

BIBLIOGRAPHY

American College of Obstetricians and Gynecologists. Vaginitis. ACOG Practice Bulletin No. 72. *Obstet Gynecol.* 2006;107:1195–1206.

Centers for Disease Control and Prevention. Sexually Transmitted Disease Guidelines, 2006. *MMWR.* 2006;55(No. RR-11):50–52.

Gutman RE, et al. Evaluation of clinical methods for diagnosing bacterial vaginosis. *Obstet Gynecol.* 2005;105:551–556.

Landers DV, et al. Predictive value of the clinical diagnosis of lower genital tract infection in women. *Am J Obstet Gynecol.* 2004;190:1004–1010.

Sobel JD, et al. Suppressive antibacterial therapy with 0.75% metronidazole vaginal gel to prevent recurrent bacterial vaginosis. *Am J Obstet Gynecol.* 2006;194:1283–1289.

 MISCELLANEOUS

SYNONYM(S)

- Nonspecific vaginitis
- *Gardnerella* vaginitis

ABBREVIATIONS

- BV—Bacterial vaginosis
- HSV—Herpes simplex virus
- STI—Sexually transmitted infection

CODES

ICD9-CM

616.10 Vaginitis, bacterial

 PATIENT TEACHING

PREVENTION

- Good perineal hygiene
- Douching is not recommended for prevention or treatment.
- Nonperfumed soaps
- Safe sex practices with regular condom use

VAGINITIS: PREPUBERTAL VULVOVAGINITIS

Judith Lacy, MD

BASICS

DESCRIPTION
- Vulvovaginal inflammation is the most common gynecologic condition in the prepubertal age group and accounts for a majority of pediatric gynecologic clinic visits.
- In most circumstances, the vulva is inflamed and the vagina may be uninvolved or secondarily affected. Some of the more common etiologies of prepubertal vulvovaginitis include:
  - Nonspecific vulvovaginitis:
    - Poor vulvar hygiene practices
    - Chemical irritants
  - Foreign body:
    - Most common is toilet paper
  - Infectious vulvovaginitis:
    - Group A-hemolytic streptococcus
    - *Shigella flexneri*
    - *Enterobius vermicularis* (Pinworms)
    - Human papillomavirus
  - Dermatologic conditions:
    - Lichen sclerosus
    - Psoriasis
    - Eczema
    - Seborrhea

Age-Related Factors
- In girls <2 years or still in diapers, candidal infections are common.
- After a child is out of diapers, candidal infections are rarely seen in the unestrogenized prepubertal female.
- If a true candidal infection is diagnosed in the toilet-trained child, rule out diabetes mellitus and immunocompromised states.

EPIDEMIOLOGY
~70% of nonspecific vulvovaginitis in prepubertal girls is associated with coliform bacteria due to poor vulvar hygiene:
- Improved vulvar hygiene is the therapeutic approach, and antibiotics are not necessary.

RISK FACTORS
- Several factors predispose the *normal* prepubertal female to vulvovaginitis:
  - Structural factors:
    - Thin, atrophic epithelium
    - Lack of labial fat pads
    - Lack of pubic hair
    - Short perineal body
  - Chemical factors:
    - Lack of estrogenization
    - Neutral vaginal pH
    - Lack of lactobacilli
  - Hygiene-related factors:
    - Fecal contamination
    - Spread of respiratory pathogens
- Other factors increase the risk:
  - Foreign body
  - Sexual abuse, sexually transmitted organisms

PATHOPHYSIOLOGY
The hypoestrogenic state of the prepubertal female is a major contributing factor that increases susceptibility to vulvovaginal inflammation. The majority of cases involve primary irritation of the vulva with secondary involvement of the lower 3rd of the vagina. Consequently, once pubertal estrogen levels are attained, the incidence of vulvovaginitis decreases significantly.

ASSOCIATED CONDITIONS
Overweight and obesity predispose to difficulty attaining adequate hygiene.

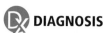

DIAGNOSIS

SIGNS AND SYMPTOMS
History
- Common complaints associated with prepubertal vulvovaginitis include:
  - Vaginal discharge
  - Vulvar erythema
  - Vulvar pruritus
  - Vulvovaginal discomfort
  - Vulvovaginal irritation
  - Abnormal odor
  - Urinary complaints
  - Vaginal bleeding
- Evaluation of vulvovaginal complaints in the prepubertal female involves obtaining a thorough history with the following elements:
  - Duration of symptoms
  - Pattern of symptoms
  - Prior evaluation and workup
  - Previous therapy and results:
    - Antifungals
    - Antibiotics
    - Steroid creams
  - Hygiene habits:
    - Wiping technique (front-back preferable)
    - Bathing habits (tub bath is preferable)
    - Laundry detergents
    - Soaps and bubble bath (cause chemical irritation)
    - Type of underwear (cotton is preferable)
  - Family and personal history of dermatologic disorders (eczema/lichen sclerosis)
  - Foreign body insertion in any orifice
  - Screening for sexual abuse

Physical Exam
- Tanner staging: Breasts
- Tanner staging: Pubic hair
- Genital examination:
  - Positioning:
    - Frog-leg
    - Knee-chest
    - Seated on mom's lap
  - Inspection:
    - Vulvar hygiene (presence of smegma or stool)
    - Labia/Vulva (color, inflammation)
    - Vaginal introitus and epithelium (estrogenized?)
    - Hymen (delicate margin vs. attenuated or scarred)
  - Assessment:
    - Discharge
    - Bleeding (See Bleeding, Abnormal Uterine: Prepubertal.)
    - Erythema
    - Hypo- or hyperpigmentation
    - Trauma (scarring)
    - Presence of foreign body visible at introitus
  - Rectal exam (palpation of foreign body, ovarian or vaginal mass)

TESTS
- Suspect infectious etiology:
  - Obtain vaginal sample with Calgiswab for culture, wet prep and Gram stain:
    - Bacterial: Typically mixed or "normal" flora, even with symptoms
    - Fungal: Rare
  - If abuse suspected, *culture:*
    - *Neisseria gonorrhea*
    - *Chlamydia trachomatis*
    - *Trichomonas*
- If foreign body suspected:
  - Copious saline irrigation of vagina

Imaging
- Rarely indicated
- If metal foreign body suspected:
  - Radiograph/Flat plate
- If bleeding and tumor suspected:
  - US
  - MRI

DIFFERENTIAL DIAGNOSIS
After obtaining a thorough history and appropriate physical examination, a differential diagnosis may include the following:

Infection
- Streptococcal
- *Shigella*
- Pinworms
- *Gonorrhea, Chlamydia,* or *Trichomonas:*
  - Strongly suggest abuse
  - Reporting and referral for abuse evaluation
- HPV:
  - Up to age 2–3 years, may have been perinatally acquired
  - >3 years of age, evaluate for sexual abuse

Tumor/Malignancy
Rare vaginal tumor (may present with bleeding):
- Sarcoma botryoides
- Other rare vaginal tumors

Trauma
- Foreign body
- Sexual abuse

Drugs
Chemical irritation from inappropriate topical medication

Other/Miscellaneous
- Nonspecific vulvovaginitis
- Lichen sclerosus (see topic)
- Eczema
- Seborrhea
- Psoriasis

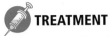 **TREATMENT**

GENERAL MEASURES

- Nonspecific vulvovaginitis is the most frequently diagnosed cause of prepubertal vulvovaginal inflammation. Therapy should consist of strict hygiene measures to include the following:
  - Sitz baths/daily tub baths
  - No soaps
  - No bubble bath
  - Mild laundry detergent
  - Cotton underwear
  - No underwear at bedtime
  - No tight fitting clothing
  - Thorough drying after bathing
  - Wiping front-to-back
- Foreign body:
  - Saline irrigation of vagina
  - Examination under anesthesia:
    ○ Vaginoscopy

MEDICATION (DRUGS)

- Lichen sclerosus (see topic)
- Specific Infectious etiology:
  - Streptococcal:
    ○ Amoxicillin 40 mg/kg divided t.i.d. for 10 days
  - Shigella:
    ○ TMP-SMX 6–10 mg/kg divided b.i.d. for 14 days
  - Pinworms:
    ○ Mebendazole 100 mg PO, then repeat in 14 days
  - Trichomonas:
    ○ Metronidazole 15 mg/kg divided t.i.d. for 7–10 days
  - Gonorrhea:
    ○ Ceftriaxone 125 mg IM single dose
  - *Chlamydia* (children >8 years):
    ○ Tetracycline 25–50 mg/kg divided q.i.d. for 7 days
- Persistent mixed bacterial/nonspecific vulvovaginitis:
  - Topical estrogen cream to labia b.i.d. for 7–14 days will increase cornification of vaginal epithelium, making it more resistant to inflammation:
    ○ Demonstrate to mother amount of cream
    ○ Demonstrate application site
    ○ Caution against PRN use

SURGERY

Pelvic examination under anesthesia with vaginoscopy may be required if symptoms are persistent (not recurrent), bleeding, examination in office is inadequate

 FOLLOW-UP

DISPOSITION

Issues for Referral

- Avoid traumatizing the child with an exam, as subsequent exams will be difficult or impossible:
  - If unable to perform an adequate exam or insufficient experience with pediatric gynecology, consider referral to a gynecologist with pediatric experience
- If sexual abuse is suspected, reporting is mandatory, and referral to clinician with experience in the evaluation of pediatric sexual abuse is indicated

PROGNOSIS

- Recurrent vulvovaginitis is common; hygiene measures typically lapse over time:
  - A follow-up visit immediately after treatment to assess resolution of symptoms and signs will help to differentiate persistent vs. recurrent infection.
- Persistent vulvovaginitis requires further evaluation. If a foreign body is suspected and vaginal irrigation is unsuccessful, examination under anesthesia with vaginoscopy is warranted.

BIBLIOGRAPHY

Emans SJ. Vulvovaginal Problems in the Prepubertal Child. In: Emans SJ, et al, *Pediatric and Adolescent Gynecology,* 5th ed. Philadelphia: Lippincott Williams & Wilkins; 2005:83–119.

Farrington PF. Pediatric vulvo-vaginitis. *Clin Obstet Gynecol.* 1997;40:135–140.

Kass-Wolff JH, et al. Pediatric gynecology: Assessment strategies and common problems. *Semin Reprod Med.* 2003;21:329–338.

Merkley K, et al. Vulvovaginitis and vaginal discharge in the pediatric patient. *J Emerg Nurs.* 2005;31: 400–402.

Rau FJ, et al. Vulvovaginitis in children and adolescents. In: Sanfilippo JS, et al. *Pediatric and Adolescent Gynecology*, 2nd ed. Philadelphia: W.B. Saunders; 2001:199–215.

 MISCELLANEOUS

CLINICAL PEARLS

- After toilet training, girls' desires for independence lead to less maternal supervision of toileting; mothers should be encouraged to monitor vulvar hygiene (avoiding hypervigilence).
- Daily baths are preferable to showers to facilitate vulvar hygiene.
- Girls should be shown how to gently wash between the labia using a clean washcloth to remove smegma.
- Ascertain child's terms for genital anatomy, but encourage use of anatomically correct terms.
- Be suspicious of abuse if vulvovaginal symptoms seem out of proportion to anatomic findings and/or the child is exhibiting inappropriately sexualized behavior or other behavioral disturbances.

CODES

ICD9-CM

- 041.0 Staphylococcal
- 041.1 Streptococcal
- 041.4 *E. coli*
- 098.0 Gonococcal vaginitis
- 127.4 Pinworm infection
- 131.01 Trichomonal vaginitis
- 616.10 Vaginitis and vulvovaginitis NOS:
- 623.5 Noninfective leukorrhea
- 701.0 Lichen sclerosis
- 939 Foreign body in genitourinary tract
- 995.53 Child sexual abuse

 PATIENT TEACHING

PREVENTION

With the implementation of strict vulvar hygiene measures, the majority of vulvovaginal disorders can be prevented:

- Sitz baths/daily tub bath
- No soaps
- No bubble bath
- Mild laundry detergent
- Cotton underwear
- No underwear at bedtime
- No tight fitting clothing
- Thorough drying after bathing
- Wiping front-to-back

VAGINITIS: VULVOVAGINAL CANDIDIASIS

J. D. Sobel, MD

 BASICS

DESCRIPTION
- Yeast vulvovaginitis usually presents as an acute inflammation of both vagina and vulva almost always caused by *Candida* species and rarely by non-*Candida* organisms
- Symptoms and signs vary from mild, moderate, to severe, with infrequent attacks in some women and recurrent attacks in others (≥4 attacks/per year).

Pediatric Considerations
Because *Candida* species depend on estrogen to alter vaginal epithelium and bacterial flora, VVC is extremely rare in prepubertal girls. Most episodes of vulvar pruritus and inflammation in children are NOT due to yeast.

Geriatric Considerations
Attacks of VVC likewise diminish in postmenopausal women not receiving HRT.

EPIDEMIOLOGY
~75% of women will develop at least 1 lifetime episode, 1/2 of whom subsequently have >1 attack.

PATHOPHYSIOLOGY
Microbiology
- Any *Candida* species may cause symptomatic vulvovaginitis, however >90% due to *C. albicans*.
- Non-*albicans* species (*C. glabrata, C. parapsilosis, C. tropicalis*) are less frequent pathogens and also less virulent, more likely to simply colonize vaginal secretions and serve as innocent bystanders.

Pathogenesis
Pathogenesis of VVC is complex and multifactorial in etiology.

RISK FACTORS
- Risk factors exist for colonization as well as for transformation from colonization to frank acute symptomatic vulvovaginitis.
- Risk factors for vaginal colonization include:
  - Genetic predisposition (only recently defined)
  - Behavioral factors (e.g., receptive oral sex, coital frequency, oral contraceptives)
  - Biologic factors (e.g., uncontrolled diabetes, pregnancy, antibiotic administration, HIV infection)
- Dermatologic conditions involving vulva (e.g., eczema, psoriasis, atopy, lichen sclerosus) also predispose to yeast colonization.
- Transformation to symptomatic vaginitis may occur for a variety of reasons but more often than not, no recognizable precipitating factor is evident. Known precipitating factors include:
  - Antibiotic administration, both systemic and local
  - Occasionally dietary factors are responsible (e.g., refined sugar excess)
  - Sexual activity including receptive oral sex
- Acute symptomatic VVC most frequently occurs in the week preceding menses.
- The attack rate of symptomatic VVC following antibiotics is 20–25%.

 DIAGNOSIS

SIGNS AND SYMPTOMS
History
- Vulvovaginal pruritus is almost invariably present
- Other manifestations of inflammation include:
  - Irritation
  - Soreness
  - Burning
  - Burning on micturition (See Urinary Symptoms: Dysuria.)
  - Dyspareunia (see topic)
  - Discharge: A variable white clumpy discharge, but often absent (See Vaginal Signs and Symptoms: Discharge.)

Physical Exam
- Signs include:
  - Vulva:
    - Erythema
    - Edema
    - Excoriation
    - Fissure formation
  - Vagina:
    - Erythema
    - Edema
    - Clumpy white adherent discharge of VVC but also may be milky.
- None of the symptoms and signs is specific and diagnosis cannot be made by exam alone.

TESTS
Lab
- pH: Normal 4.0–4.5:
  - All other forms of infectious vaginitis have pH ≥4.5
- Saline microscopy:
  - Yeast/Hyphae only found in 50% of women with VVC
  - No increase in PMNs
  - Normal flora or "rods" seen
- 10% KOH microscopy:
  - Yeast/Hyphae found in 60–70% of VVC
- Culture (delays diagnosis by 48 hours):
  - Always positive
  - Nonessential if microscopy positive
  - Essential for refractory vaginitis/clinically unresponsive to antimycotic therapy
  - Essential for recurrent *Candida* vaginitis
- Nonculture confirmation:
  - PCR (now commercially available)
  - Affirm DNA probe: Excellent, not inexpensive
  - No better than culture

DIFFERENTIAL DIAGNOSIS

- Easy to differentiate from other infectious causes of vaginitis (i.e., bacterial vaginosis, trichomoniasis, cervicitis), because all have increased pH (>4.5)
- Most important alternative diagnosis of normal pH vulvovaginitis is:
  - Contact dermatitis (chemical or hypersensitivity)
- In older women atrophic vaginitis always has increased pH (>4.5).

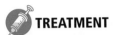

TREATMENT

GENERAL MEASURES

- Decide whether patient has uncomplicated or complicated *Candida* vaginitis. Most patients have uncomplicated VVC characterized by mild or moderate disease caused by *C. albicans,* with no tendency to a recurrent pattern, are immunocompetent.
  - Uncomplicated VVC requires short-course (including single-dose) therapy for clinical cure.
- In contrast, complicated VVC is characterized by severe disease, non-*albicans Candida*, recurrent infection, and immunocompromised host requires more prolonged therapy for 5–7 days.
- Recurrent VVC (>4 episodes/year):
  - Long-term maintenance regimen: Once weekly fluconazole 150 mg (long-term cures ~50%)

MEDICATION (DRUGS)

- Intravaginal agents:
  - Butoconazole 2% cream 5 g intravaginally for 3 days*
  - Butoconazole 2% cream 5 g (Butoconazole1– sustained release), single intravaginal application
  - Clotrimazole 1% cream 5 g intravaginally for 7–14 days*
  - Clotrimazole 100-mg vaginal tablet for 7 days
  - Clotrimazole 100-mg vaginal tablet, 2 tablets for 3 days
  - Miconazole 2% cream 5 g intravaginally for 7 days*
  - Miconazole 100-mg vaginal suppository, 1 suppository for 7 days*
  - Miconazole 200-mg vaginal suppository, 1 suppository for 3 days*
  - Miconazole 1,200-mg vaginal suppository, 1 suppository for 1 day*
  - Nystatin 100,000–unit vaginal tablet, 1 tablet for 14 days
  - Tioconazole 6.5% ointment 5 g intravaginally in a single application*
  - Terconazole 0.4% cream 5 g intravaginally for 7 days
  - Terconazole 0.8% cream 5 g intravaginally for 3 days
  - Terconazole 80-mg vaginal suppository, 1 suppository for 3 days
- Oral agent:
  - Fluconazole 150 mg PO tablet, 1 tablet in single dose

- Vaginitis due to *C. glabrata*:
  - High failure rate with azoles including fluconazole
  - Make sure treatment is indicated and that *C. glabrata* is not an innocent bystander.
  - Trial of boric acid vaginal capsules 600 mg/d (cure rates ~70%)
  - If symptoms and yeast persist, worth trying 3% amphotericin and 17% flucytosine cream made up by compounding pharmacy, 5 g daily for 14 days. Cure rates >90%, but expensive

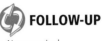 FOLLOW-UP

- None required
- HIV testing is not required.

BIBLIOGRAPHY

Centers for Disease Control and Prevention. Sexually transmitted disease treatment guidelines 2006. *MMWR Morb Mortal Weekly Rep.* 2006;(55).

Sobel JD. Vulvovaginal candidosis. *Lancet.* 2007;369:1961–1971.

 MISCELLANEOUS

SYNONYM(S)

- Candida vaginitis
- Fungal vaginitis
- Monilial vulvovaginitis
- Vaginal candidiasis
- Vulvovaginal candidosis
- Yeast vaginitis
- Yeast vulvitis

CLINICAL PEARLS

Ready access to over-the-counter antifungal agents is associated with wasted financial expenditures, unfulfilled expectations, and a delay in correct diagnosis.

ABBREVIATIONS

- HRT—Hormone replacement therapy
- PCR—Polymerase chain reaction
- PMN—Polymorphonuclear leukocytes
- VVC—Vulvovaginal candidiasis

CODES

ICD9-CM

112.1 Candidal vulvovaginitis

VESICO-VAGINAL FISTULA

Matthew A. Barker, MD
Mickey M. Karram, MD

 BASICS

DESCRIPTION
- Urogenital (genitourinary) fistulas are abnormal connections between the vagina and the urethra, bladder, or ureter.
- VVFs are the abnormal communications between the vagina and bladder. They are also the most common.
- VVF are congenital or acquired:
  - Developed countries: 75% of VVF caused by gynecologic or other pelvic surgery.
  - Developing countries: 90% of VVF are caused by obstetric trauma during normal obstructed labor.
  - Congenital VVF are extremely rare and associated with other urogenital malformations.

Pediatric Considerations
VVF in young nulliparous patients with no prior surgical history should be evaluated for congenital anomalies of the urinary tract.

Staging
Classification of VVF:
- Simple fistulas: Small size (<0.5 cm) and present as single nonradiated fistula
- Complex fistulas: Previously failed fistula repair, large size (>2.5 cm), or fistula present in irradiated tissue

EPIDEMIOLOGY
- The true incidence of VVF is unknown.
- In the US, the incidence of VVF after hysterectomy is 0.1–0.2%.
- In developing countries, VVF occur in ~2% obstructed labors.

RISK FACTORS
- Trauma to genitourinary tract greatest risk of VVF
- Pelvic surgery risks:
  - Prior cesarean section, endometriosis, prior pelvic irradiation
  - Radical hysterectomy
- Obstetric risks:
  - Obstructed labors, operative vaginal deliveries, cesarean deliveries, peripartum hysterectomies
- Other risk factors: Malignancy, gastrointestinal surgery, IBD, urinary tuberculosis, retained foreign bodies (e.g., pessaries)
- Conditions that interfere with wound healing increase the risk of VVF formation (e.g., infection, diabetes, smoking, peripheral vascular disease, chronic steroid use, and previous tissue injury)

PATHOPHYSIOLOGY
- Direct injury to the GU tract
- Fistulas that occur as a result of tissue ischemia, necrosis, or infection present later in postoperative course, usually 7–21 days.

ASSOCIATED CONDITIONS
- 10% of VVF are associated with a simultaneous ureteral component injury.
- Urodynamic studies showed that 47% of VVF are associated with stress urinary incontinence, 44% with detrusor overactivity, and 17% with poor bladder compliance.

DIAGNOSIS

SIGNS AND SYMPTOMS
History
Most common presenting symptom is continuous urinary drainage from vagina:
- Drainage may present immediately or more commonly several days to weeks after trauma or injury.
- Leakage may be continuous or intermittent, and can be confused with stress incontinence postoperatively.
- Foul-smelling or persistent vaginal discharge often precedes urinary leakage.
- Urine extravasation into abdominal cavity commonly presents as abdominal pain, nausea, vomiting, anorexia, abdominal distension, or ileus.
- Flank pain and/or fever may be sign of pyelonephritis or an ascending UTI.
- Vagina smells of urine.
- Patients void small amounts of urine because bladder never gets full.
- Complaints of intermittent, frequent episodes of urine leakage in varying amounts

Review of Systems
Any or all may be present:
- Leakage of urine from vagina
- Hematuria
- Vulvar irritation
- Recurrent urinary tract infections
- Persistent vaginal discharge
- Abdominal or flank pain
- Abnormal urine stream

Physical Exam
- Diagnosis demands leakage confirmed to be urinary and that an extraurethral source is identified.
- A complete physical exam should be part of initial evaluation of all patients with suspected VVF.
- Vaginal exam should focus on visualizing extraurethral leakage of urine:
  - Assess vaginal length and capacity, estrogen status of epithelial tissue, and examine for support.
  - Identify area of leaking and assess for induration or fibrosis around suspected fistula.
  - VVFs associated with hysterectomy are typically located near the vaginal apex.

TESTS
Office testing can often distinguish between fistulas involving bladders or ureters:
- Oral phenazopyridine with tampon in the vagina will diagnose fistula but not localize it.
- Retrograde bladder filling with methylene blue or sterile milk will help localize and diagnose VVF during vaginal exam:
  - The Moir test uses cotton swabs or sterile gauze placed in vagina; bladder is filled retrograde with methylene blue: Clear fluid is from ureter; changes color if from bladder

ALERT
IV methylene blue must be used with caution because of the risk of methemoglobinemia.

- Cystoscopy is indicated in most cases to demonstrate size, location, and proximity of VVF to ureteral orifices as well as to fully evaluate the bladder.
- Urodynamics may help evaluate bladder function and diagnose other urinary disorders.

Lab
- Measure urea concentration of vaginal fluid
- UA and culture
- CBC with differential
- BUN and serum creatinine
- Vaginal wet mount
- Vaginal and/or cervical culture

Imaging
- Always assess ureteral integrity with either intravenous urography or retrograde pyelography (best way to identify ureterovaginal fistula or combined uterovaginal fistula and VVF)
- Cystogram phase of IVP suggests VVF if early pooling of urine in vagina or urinary extravasation is seen.

- VCUG determines presence and location of a fistula and may also see vesicoureteral reflux, cystocele, or urethral diverticulum.
- Renal US may miss up to 20% of ureteral injuries.

DIFFERENTIAL DIAGNOSIS
Infection
Spontaneous vaginal discharge or vaginal infections
Tumor/Malignancy
- Radiation exposure to pelvis leads to VVF that typically appears 6–12 months after treatment.
- Always evaluate for recurrence of malignancy in patients with VVF and a history of irradiation.
Trauma
Birth trauma and gynecologic surgery account for most VVFs.
Other/Miscellaneous
- Persistent vaginal discharge from a peritoneal sinus tract, fallopian tube drainage, lymphatic fistula
- Urinary incontinence
- Bladder dysfunction (detrusor overactivity)
- Ectopic ureteral drainage or ureteral vaginal fistula

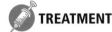

TREATMENT
GENERAL MEASURES
- Cystourethroscopy should be routinely performed during pelvic surgery to identify injuries.
- Small VVFs can be managed with continuous catheter drainage if they occur within 7 days of surgery. Repeat or perform VCUG to evaluate VVF. If not closed, surgery is indicated.
- If ureters are compromised or concern for an ureterovaginal fistula exists, then double-J stents should be placed. If unable to place stents, consider percutaneous nephrostomy tubes.
- Conservative management of ureterovaginal fistulas is warranted if:
  – There is minimal to no obstruction of the injured ureter
  – Only mild periureteral extravasation exists
  – There is improvement in associated upper tract obstruction on follow-up radiologic studies
- If spontaneous closure does NOT occur, then surgical repair with possible ureteroneocystostomy is indicated.

SPECIAL THERAPY
Complementary and Alternative Therapies
If surgery is delayed, sanitary protection and skin care will be needed, as well as close follow-up for emotional and psychological support.

MEDICATION (DRUGS)
- Conservative treatment may involve a trial of urethral catheter drainage and anticholinergic medicines.
- Occlusive techniques with endoscopic laser or fibrin glue products have been described (proceed to surgery if fails).
- Estrogen for atrophic vaginal tissues for at least 4–6 weeks in conjunction with other treatment modalities help tissue healing.

SURGERY
- Surgical results are improved when surgery is performed on mature fistula tract.
- Surgical repair can be either transvaginal, transabdominal, or through a transvesical approach.
- VVF identified in 1st 24–48 hours can be safely repaired immediately.
- Urethrovaginal fistulas are approached vaginally and are circumscribed and over-sewn rather than excised.
- Vaginal approach requires appropriate vaginal caliber and length for repair and creation of a vaginal flap. Closure of VVF is done with a 3 layer nonoverlapping suture lines over the excised fistula tract that is placed on little tension.
- Martius graft can be used to help separate suture lines, provide support, and introduce new blood supply to the anterior vagina.
- Latzko transvaginal technique involves excision of vaginal epithelium around fistula with partial colpocleisis and closure of vagina over VVF; allows vaginal tissue to reepithelialize as transitional epithelium.
- Abdominal approach can be used in all VVF repairs (especially complex cases) except those extending to the urethra.
- Urinary diversions utilizing small or large bowel can be used, especially in irradiated patients with small bladder capacities.
- Reconstructive techniques can be used: Fibrofatty labial interposition tissues, anterior/posterior bladder flaps, myocutaneous flaps, and gracilis muscles flaps, as well as combined myocutaneous flaps
- Surgical repair principles:
  – Adequate exposure of fistula tract
  – Watertight closure
  – Well-vascularized tissue used for repair
  – Multiple-layer closure
  – Tensionfree, nonoverlapping suture lines
  – Adequate urinary drainage early after repair
  – A VVF in an irradiated field may have difficulty healing; always rule out recurrence of malignancy before repair.

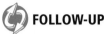

FOLLOW-UP
DISPOSITION
Issues for Referral
Early referral to physicians experienced in the management of VVF should be made.

PROGNOSIS
Success rates for surgical repair of VVF range from 84–100%.

PATIENT MONITORING
- After surgery, drain bladder for 10–14 days.
- A postoperative VCUG should be performed to confirm closure (stop anticholinergics 24–48 hours before test).
- Pelvic rest for 6 weeks after surgery.
- Follow-up visits at 2 and 6 weeks after surgery.

BIBLIOGRAPHY
Angioli R, et al. Guidelines of how to manage vesicovaginal fistula. *Crit Rev Oncol Hematol.* 2003;48:295–304.

Dmochowski R. Surgery for Vesicovaginal Fistula, Urethrovaginal Fistula, and Urethral Diverticulum. In: Walsh PC, ed. *Campbell's Urology.* 8th ed. Philadelphia: W.B. Saunders; 2002:1195–1217.

Hilton P. Vesico-vaginal fistula: New perspectives. *Curr Opin Obstet Gynecol.* 2001;13:513–520.

Karram MK. Lower urinary tract fistulas. In: Walters MD et al., eds. *Urogynecology and Pelvic Reconstructive Surgery.* 3rd ed. Philadelphia: Mosby; 2007:445–460.

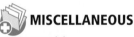

MISCELLANEOUS
SYNONYM(S)
- Ureterovaginal fistula
- Ureterouterine fistula
- Urethrovaginal fistula
- Urogenital or genitourinary fistula
- Vesicouterine fistula
- Vesicovaginal fistula

ABBREVIATIONS
- IVP—Intravenous pyelogram
- VCUG—Voiding cystourethrogram
- VVF—Vesico-vaginal fistula

CODES
ICD9-CM
- 593.83 Ureteral fistula
- 596.2 Vesical fistula, not elsewhere classified
- 599.1 Urethral fistula
- 619.0 Urinary-genital tract fistula

PATIENT TEACHING

Good general nutrition and adequate hydration

Pregnancy Considerations
- Access to prenatal care and appropriate obstetric facilities
- Perform cesarean delivery if history of prior repair for VVF

VULVAR ABSCESS, SKENE'S GLAND ABSCESS, BARTHOLIN'S ABSCESS

S. Paige Hertweck MD,

 BASICS

DESCRIPTION
Deep tissue infections of the vulva:

- Typically occur within confines of labia majora
- Bartholin's glands abscesses more common than primary labial abscesses
- Periclitoral abscesses similar to other vulvar abscesses except in location.
  - Lesions thought to be periclitoral abscesses must be differentiated from pilonidal cysts arising in periclitoral region that will require complete surgical excision instead of incision and drainage.
- Skene's gland (periurethral gland) abscesses are uncommon, periurethral in location and when very enlarged can cause labial enlargement

Age-Related Factors
Bartholin's abscess:

- Usually presents ages 20–29
- Rare after age 40, presence at that age suspicious for malignancy and requires biopsy and/or complete excision

EPIDEMIOLOGY
- Most infections are related to aerobic and anaerobic organisms commonly seen in the vaginal and cervical flora
- Community-acquired methicillin-resistant Staphylococcus aureus (MRSA) is an increasingly seen pathogen in labial abscesses especially in children
- Bartholin's abscesses typically have both anaerobic and aerobic organism on culture but also have association with gonorrhea and chlamydia.

RISK FACTORS
- Most cases occur without predisposing risks but predisposing factors include:
  - Diabetes
  - Pregnancy
  - Trauma (e.g., scratching, shaving)
  - Previous impetigo
- Community-acquired methicillin-resistant Staphylococcal aureus labial abscesses may be due to:
  - Shared athletic equipment
  - Shared razors
  - Family members with MRSA

Genetics
No genetic pattern

 DIAGNOSIS

SIGNS AND SYMPTOMS
History
- Localized edema, erythema and pain of the labia
- History of vulvar abrasion, injury or trauma
  - Not always elicited
- History of pre-existing epidermal inclusion cyst
- Possible fever

Review of Symptoms
Dermatologic conditions: Eczema or history of impetigo

Physical Exam
- +/− Fever
- Location of abscess:
  - True labial abscess:
    ○ Unilateral, tender, swollen, erythematous labia
  - Bartholin's abscess:
    ○ Cystic painful swelling of the posterior labia in the area of the Bartholin's gland (at 5:00 or 7:00 position of vagina introitus)
  - Skene's abscess:
    ○ Swelling at the anterior vagina just beneath the urethra

- Urinary symptoms:
  - Urgency
  - Frequency
  - Dysuria
  - Postmicturition dribbling
- Possible labial discharge if ruptured

TESTS
Bartholin's gland abscesses have been associated with chlamydia and gonorrhea infections

Lab
Test urine or endocervix for chlamydia and gonorrhea

Imaging
No imaging indicated

DIFFERENTIAL DIAGNOSIS
Infection
- Cellulitis
- Necrotizing fasciitis

Tumor/Malignancy
In women >40 years, consider biopsy for Bartholin's gland malignancy

Other/Miscellaneous
- Mesonephric cyst of the vagina
- Lipoma
- Fibroma
- Hernia
- Hydrocele
- Epidermal inclusion cyst
- Neurofibroma
- Aberrant breast tissue

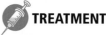 **TREATMENT**

GENERAL MEASURES
- Pain relief will occur with drainage of pus
  - Spontaneous
  - Surgical
- Women with abscesses already with a "point" or that rupture spontaneously may require only sitz baths, not antibiotics.
- Use warm sitz baths or hot packs to bring abscess to a "point" then proceed with incision and drainage if spontaneous rupture does not occur

MEDICATION (DRUGS)

- Treat with systemic antibiotics:
  - Cover both aerobic and anaerobic bacteria
  - Need staph aureus coverage based on local sensitivities—consider use of clindamycin as initial therapy
- If unruptured:
  - Initiate broad-spectrum antibiotics (1 dose Ceftriaxone 125 mg IM plus clindamycin 300 mg PO q.i.d. for 7 days) to cover skin bacterial flora, anaerobic bacteria and possibly gonorrhea and chlamydia (e.g., Ceftriaxone 125 mg plus clindamycin 300 mg q.i.d. for 7 days OR ofloxacin 400 mg BID and Flagyl 500 mg b.i.d. for 7 days)
  - Draw a line on the skin surrounding the abscess to delineate the furthest extent of inflammatory change. If margins progress—consider possibility of necrotizing fasciitis

SPECIAL THERAPY

Complementary and Alternative Therapies

- Give a single dose intraoperative clindamycin
- Then follow with incision, curettage and primary suture under general anesthesia.
  - Expose abscess cavity and curette lining,
  - Pass interrupted polypropylene sutures beneath but not through the cavity and close the defect.
  - Remove sutures on 6th postoperative day.
- Sclerotherapy:
  - After incision and drainage, place crystalloid silver nitrate stick 0.5 cm in length and diameter placed into cavity. Patient may experience mild burning.
    - Follow-up in 48 hours to clean wound.

SURGERY

- Bartholin's abscess—Treat in ED or office:
  - After infiltrating with local anesthetic, make stab incision over thinnest most medial aspect of abscess (preferably at or behind the hymenal ring):
    - Evacuate abscess cavity
    - Gently probe for loculations
    - Place Word catheter (a short catheter with an inflatable Foley balloon) into abscess cavity and fill bulb with saline
    - Tuck end of catheter inside vagina to minimize discomfort
    - Leave Word catheter in place for at least 2–4 weeks to promote formation of an epithelialized tract for drainage of glandular secretions.
  - Marsupialization with creation of larger opening than stab wound as alternative management
  - Excision of gland reserved for recurrent cases unresponsive to other treatment modalities
  - Skene's abscess
  - If spontaneous drainage does not occur or recurs, excision and correction of possible coexisting urethral diverticulum is required
- General anesthesia may be required:
  - In a child or adolescent
  - If pain precludes in office I&D

 FOLLOW-UP

DISPOSITION

Issues for Referral

Consultation or referral if necrotizing fasciitis suspected:

- High mortality rate
- Wide debridement and excision required

PROGNOSIS

- Recurrence of Bartholin's abscess not rare after initial gland abscess and damage of gland orifice
- Recurrence less likely with use of Word catheter than with simple incision and drainage, as epithelialized tract is established.

PATIENT MONITORING

Follow-up to monitor for spontaneous drainage or the need for surgical intervention and/or recurrence.

BIBLIOGRAPHY

Faro S. Pyogenic conditions of the vulva. In: Kaufman RH, et al., eds. *Benign Diseases of the Vulva and Vagina*. 5th ed. Philadelphia: Mosby; 2005: 264–266.

Larsen T, et al. Treatment of abscesses in the vulva. *Acta Obstet Gynecol Scand*. 1986;65:459–461.

Yuce K, et al. Outpatient management of Bartholin gland abscesses and cysts with silver nitrate. *Aust N Z J Obstet Gynaecol*. 1994;34:93.

 MISCELLANEOUS

CLINICAL PEARLS

- Labial abscesses that start initially as a papule and rapidly expand into a large abscess over 24 hours are highly suggestive of MRSA and require immediate antibiotic coverage and incision and drainage.
- Recurrent periclitoral abscesses require complete excision and biopsy.
  - May be secondary to presence of pilonidal cyst

ABBREVIATIONS

MRSA—Methicillin resistant staphylococcus aureus

CODES

ICD9-CM

- 597.0 Skene's gland abscess
- 616.3 Bartholin's gland abscess
- 616.4 Vulvar abscess

 PATIENT TEACHING

Need follow-up to monitor for spontaneous drainage or need for intervention for recurrence

PREVENTION

Reduce exposure to STDs and vulvar trauma (i.e., scratching, shaving)

VULVAR CANCER

Jessica Kassis, MD

 BASICS

DESCRIPTION

- 4th most common gynecologic cancer
- 5% of female genital tract malignancies
- Subtypes (most to least common):
  - Squamous cell (90%):
    - Occur on vestibule and labia
    - Keratinizing type associated with vulvar dystrophies in older women
    - Warty, Bowenoid type associated with HPV 6,18, and 33 found in younger women
    - Verrucous carcinoma usually locally destructive but rarely metastasizes:
      - Cauliflowerlike appearance
  - Melanoma (5%):
    - Most commonly women >65
    - May develop de novo or within existing nevus
    - Usually arise on clitoris or labia minora
    - Usually not due to sun exposure
  - Basal cell carcinoma (2%):
    - Most commonly women >65
    - Usually locally destructive but rarely metastasizes
    - Pearly lesion with rolled edges with central ulceration
    - Complete physical exam for concomitant malignancy
  - Extramammary Paget disease (<1%):
    - >65
    - Multifocal intraepithelial neoplasia
    - Pruritus is the most common symptom
    - Eczematoid; well-demarcated, slightly raised edges, red background, dotted with small, pale islands
    - May occur on the vulva, mons, perineum/perianal area, or inner thigh
    - Evaluate for coexisting malignancy in breast, cervix, ovary, urethra, rectum (20–30%)
  - Bartholin gland carcinoma (<2%):
    - Rare but most common cause of adenocarcinoma of the vulva
    - Median age 57
    - Cancer arising for Bartholin gland may be adenocarcinomas, squamous carcinomas, adenosquamous, transitional cell, or adenoid cystic carcinomas
    - Most often solid and deeply infiltrating into labia majora
    - Biopsy required of any enlargement in Bartholin gland in women >40
  - Sarcoma (1–2%):
    - Leiomyosarcoma is the most common
    - Enlarging painful masses in labia majora
    - Other histologic subtypes include malignant schwannomas, neurofibrosarcomas, liposarcomas, rhabdomyosarcomas, angiosarcomas, epithelioid sarcomas, and fibrosarcomas
  - Rare vulvar malignancies:
    - Endodermal sinus tumors
    - Merkel cell carcinoma
    - Lymphoma
    - Dermatofibrosarcoma protuberans

Age-Related Factors

- Elderly patients: High incidence of antecedent dystrophic lesions including lichen sclerosus adjacent to tumor (most common type).
- Premenopausal patients: Related to smoking and HPV, often with preexisting warty VIN

Staging

- Surgical:
  - T = Tumor:
    - T1 : Tumor $\leq$2 cm
    - T2: Tumor >2 cm
    - T3: Lower urethra or vagina involved
    - T4: Rectum, bladder, or upper urethra involved
  - N = Nodes:
    - N0: Node negative
    - N1: Unilateral positive node
    - N2: Bilateral positive nodes
  - M = Metastasis:
    - M0: No metastatic disease
    - M1: Positive pelvic nodes, distant metastasis
- FIGO:
  - Stage 0: Intraepithelial carcinoma (in-situ)
  - Stage I (T1, N0, M0): Lesions $\leq$2 cm in size, confined to vulva and/ or perineum. No nodal metastasis:
    - IA: Stromal invasion <1 mm.
    - IB: Stromal invasion >1 mm
  - Stage 2 (T2, N0, M0): Lesions >2 cm in size, confined to vulva and/or perineum. No nodal metastasis
  - Stage 3 (T1–3, N1, M0; T3, N0–1, M0): Tumor of any size with either spread to the lower urethra, vagina, anus, or unilateral regional lymph node metastasis
  - Stage 4A (T1–3, N2, M0): Tumor of any size invading either upper urethra, rectal or bladder mucosa, pelvic bones, or bilateral regional lymph node metastasis
  - Stage 4B (any T, any N, any M): Tumor of any size with distant lymph node metastasis including pelvic nodes

EPIDEMIOLOGY

- Predominantly disease of postmenopausal women >65, although the median age of diagnosis is declining
- Annual incidence of 1.5 cases per 100,000 women
- Incidence of VIN in younger women is on the rise:
  - Incidence of vulvar cancer has remained stable despite the rise in VIN, likely secondary to early detection
- 3,490 new cases annually in the US with 880 deaths

RISK FACTORS

- Smoking
- HPV
- Vulvar dystrophy (lichen sclerosus)
- Vulvar or cervical intraepithelial neoplasia
- History of cervical cancer
- Immunodeficiency syndromes

Genetics

Vulvar melanoma may be secondary to defects in oncogenes/tumor suppressor genes that have been linked to familial melanoma

PATHOPHYSIOLOGY

Vulvar cancer can spread via 3 routes:

- Hematologic: Cancer will arise in distant sites such as bone, lungs, liver
- Lymphatic: To regional nodes
- Direct: To anus, urethra, vagina

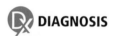 **DIAGNOSIS**

SIGNS AND SYMPTOMS

History

- <1% of women are symptomatic
- Vulvar lump or mass
- Vulvar pruritus
- Vulvar discharge or bleeding
- Dysuria

Review of Systems

Symptoms may be present if distant metastasis to bone, liver, lungs, or distant lymph nodes has occurred.

Physical Exam

- Unilateral vulvar raised plaque, ulcer, or mass on labia majora. May be fleshy, nodular, or warty
- Labia minora, mons, clitoris, and perineum less commonly involved
- +/– Groin lymphadenopathy
- 10% of cases too extensive to determine origin
- Should include pelvic exam, rectal exam

TESTS

- Biopsy of lesion:
  - Biopsy center and representative areas of lesion
  - Biopsy specimen should include underlying connective tissue and surrounding skin.
- Pap smear +/– colposcopy of cervix, vagina, and vulva
- +/– Cystoscopy, sigmoidoscopy if any concern of advanced disease

Lab

May be appropriate to evaluate for distant metastasis (bone, liver, etc.)

Imaging

- CXR to evaluate for lung metastasis
- CT chest/abdomen/pelvis to evaluate for intra-abdominal, intrathoracic, or lymphatic metastasis

DIFFERENTIAL DIAGNOSIS
- Epidermal inclusion cyst
- Lentigo
- Disorders of Bartholin gland
- Acrochordon
- Seborrheic keratosis
- Hidradenoma
- Lichen sclerosus
- Condyloma acuminata
- Syphilis
- Lymphogranuloma venereum
- Granuloma Inguinale

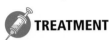 ## TREATMENT
SURGERY
- Should be individualized to patient, histologic type, and stage of disease. Most conservative approach to obtain remission is appropriate.
- Squamous cell vulvar carcinoma:
  - Stage 1A (<1 mm stromal invasion):
    o Radical local excision without lymph node dissection (groin lymph node metastases are rare).
    o Minimum 1 cm clear margin (ideally 2 cm)
  - Stage IB (>1 mm stromal invasion):
    o Radical wide local excision and ipsilateral inguinofemoral lymph node dissection (superficial and deep) for lateralized lesions
    o Bilateral lymph node dissections for central lesions.
    o Risk of groin node metastasis 8%
    o Minimum 1 cm clear margin (ideally 2 cm)
  - Stage II:
    o Modified radical vulvectomy and inguinofemoral lymphadenectomy
    o Unilateral lymphadenectomy if lesion is unilateral
    o Bilateral lymphadenectomy if lesion is bilateral or central.
    o Minimum 1 cm clear margin (ideally 2 cm)
    o Consider adjuvant radiation therapy in patients with high-risk primary lesions, 1–2 positive lymph nodes, and unclear margins
  - Stage III:
    o Preoperative radiation therapy: May decrease tumor size, allowing for less extensive surgical resection.
    o Chemoradiotherapy: Studies thus far have shown promise for 5-FU and cisplatin in conjunction with radiation therapy. RCTs not undertaken to date.
    o Neoadjuvant chemotherapy: Thus far inferior to chemoradiotherapy. Further studies necessary.
    o Radical vulvectomy and exenteration: Highly morbid procedure. Reserved for cases in which other options have been unsuccessful.

- Vulvar melanoma:
  - Wide local excision or radical vulvectomy if necessary
  - <1 mm thick: 1-cm skin margins
  - 1–4 cm thick: 2-cm margins
  - The depth should be at least 1 cm and extend to the muscular fascia below.
- Basal cell carcinoma:
  - Radical local excision without lymph node dissection. Rarely metastasize.
- Extramammary Paget disease:
  - Wide local excision or vulvectomy
  - Moh micrographic surgery (systematic excision, microscopically controlled)
  - Role of radio-/chemoradiotherapy not defined
- Bartholin-gland carcinoma:
  - Traditionally radical vulvectomy and bilateral groin dissection.
  - Recent good results with hemivulvectomy or radical local excision.
  - Postoperative irradiation decreases local recurrence.
- Sarcomas:
  - Wide local excision
  - Chemotherapy followed by surgery for rhabdomyosarcoma

 ## FOLLOW-UP
DISPOSITION
Issues for Referral
- Average delay from onset of symptoms to diagnosis approaches 1 year.
- Prompt diagnosis allows curative surgery.
- Because successful treatment often involves multimodality therapy, gynecologic oncologists are well suited to direct the care of women with vulvar cancer.

PROGNOSIS
- Prognostic factors:
  - Stage
  - Tumor size
  - Depth of invasion
  - Nodal Involvement
  - Older age
- Survival by stage:
  - Stage I: 90%
  - Stage II: 85%
  - Stage III: 70%
  - Stage IV A: 25%
  - Stage IV B: 5%

PATIENT MONITORING
- Long-term follow up is necessary as recurrence >5 years after diagnosis approaches 10%.
- Should include biannual routine gynecologic exams with palpation of inguinal nodes as well as visual inspection of vulva for at least 2 years following surgery

- Perineal recurrence can be cured with re-excision in ~75%, whereas inguinal recurrences are more difficult to cure.

BIBLIOGRAPHY

Al-Ghamdi A, et al. Vulvar squamous cell carcinoma in young women: A clinicopathologic study of 21 cases. *Gynecol Oncol*. 2002;84(1):94–101.

Berek, J, et al. *Practical Gynecologic Oncology*. Philadelphia: Lipincott Williams & Wilkins; 2005.

Homesley HD, et al. Radiation therapy versus pelvic node resection for carcinoma of the vulva with positive groin nodes. *Obstet Gynecol*. 1986;68(6): 733–740.

Jemal A, et al. Cancer statistics, 2007. *CA Cancer J Clin*. 2007;57(1):43–66.

Modifications in the staging for stage I vulvar and stage I cervical cancer. Report of the FIGO Committee on Gynecologic Oncology. International Federation of Gynecology and Obstetrics. *Int J Gynaecol Obstet*. 1995;50:215.

 ## MISCELLANEOUS
SYNONYM(S)
Bowen disease

ABBREVIATIONS
- FIGO—International Federation of Gynecology and Obstetrics
- HPV—Human papillomavirus
- RCT—Randomized controlled trial
- STI—Sexually transmitted infection
- VIN—Vulvar intraepithelial neoplasia

CODES
ICD9-CM
184.4 Malignant neoplasm of vulva, unspecified

 ## PATIENT TEACHING
PREVENTION
- Women with new-onset vulvar pruritus or mass should seek medical attention.
- Close attention including visualization of the vulva and necessary biopsies for any woman with new-onset vulvar pruritus or mass
- Close follow-up of those with VIN
- The recently available quadrivalent HPV vaccine is currently indicated for 9–26-year-olds for prevention of cervical cancer, cervical dysplasias, vulvar or vaginal cancer, and genital warts.
- Abstinence from sexual activity is the most effective way to avoid STIs, including HPV.
- Use of latex condoms reduces the likelihood of HPV acquisition.

Section II

VULVAR EPIDERMAL HYPERPLASIA

Paul D. DePriest, MD
Brook A. Saunders, MD

 BASICS

DESCRIPTION

- VEH is a benign disorder histologically characterized by variable hyperkeratosis, acanthosis without findings of atypia, inflammation, or other associated dermatoses.
- The only differentiating findings between VEH and lichen simplex chronicus is that in the latter there are histologic changes of dermal chronic inflammation and the presence of vertical collagen streaks in the papillary dermis.
- Historically this disorder was called vulvar dystrophy and squamous hyperplasia of the vulva.
- According to the ISSVD, VEH is categorized as a non-neoplastic epithelial disorder of the vulva.

Age-Related Factors

Very little is known about risk factors for the development of VEH, however the age of onset is usually between 30 and 60 years.

EPIDEMIOLOGY

- Vulvar pruritus is a common gynecologic symptom.
- Unfortunately, the incidence of VEH is unknown.

RISK FACTORS

There are no convincing risk factors for this disorder.

Genetics

- VEH and lichen sclerosis have been found to exhibit allelic imbalance similar to changes noted in differentiated VIN III.
- There is no known familial relationship in this disease.

ASSOCIATED CONDITIONS

VEH is frequently associated with other vulvar skin disturbances:

- Lichen sclerosis
- VIN

 DIAGNOSIS

SIGNS AND SYMPTOMS

History

- Women with VEH present with complaints of localized pruritus:
  - Frequently women presenting with these symptoms will be found to have associated lichen sclerosis.
- Any persistent or recurrent abnormalities should be biopsied to rule out neoplastic changes.

Physical Exam

- Any woman presenting with vulvar pruritus will require a thorough examination of the vulvar skin. Magnification with a hand lens or colposcope is useful.
- The exam should include a thorough visual inspection of the vulvar skin extending to the mons anteriorly, medial thigh creases laterally, hymenal ring internally, and to the perianal region posteriorly.
- The patient should be asked to point to the specific area of irritation.
- VEH is characterized by localized erythema or areas of thickened white skin.
- In patients with associated lichen sclerosis thinned, white vulvar skin changes may be the most prominent feature.

TESTS

A skin biopsy should be performed in any patient presenting with persistent complaints of focal pruritus or in those women who have a localized lesion (see Vulvar Biopsy).

- Biopsies are best performed after instillation of a small volume of 1% Lidocaine using a syringe and fine-bore needle.

- A 3–4 mm punch biopsy instrument is used to target and incise the lesion.
- The lesion is removed with fine scissors or a scalpel.
- Bleeding can be managed with local pressure and application of silver nitrate. Seldom is suturing required.
- Excisional biopsies should be performed if punch biopsies are insufficient.
- All biopsy material should be placed in formalin and sent for permanent histologic evaluation

Lab

- Thorough histopathologic evaluation of the biopsy material is necessary.
- Review by a dermatopathologist is sometimes helpful in differentiating VEH from other non-neoplastic vulvar disorders.

DIFFERENTIAL DIAGNOSIS

Infection

Vulvar infections:

- Candidiasis
- HPV
- HSV

Tumor/Malignancy

SCC of the vulva:

- VIN:
  - VIN I
  - VIN II
  - VIN III

Other

Dermatoses:

- Lichen sclerosis
- Lichen simplex chronicus
- Dermatitis:
  - Contact

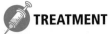

TREATMENT

GENERAL MEASURES

- Treatment of VEH consists of local application of topical corticosteroids.
- The relative potency of the corticosteroid cream/lotion/ointment should match the severity of the lesion and the symptom state of the patient.
- Depending on the specific compound chosen, corticosteroid cream/lotion/ointment should be applied by the patient 1–3 times daily for the 1st 2–4 weeks.
- The dose and potency of the corticosteroid cream/lotion/ointment should be tapered and stopped as soon as improvement is noted.
- Most patients will require intermittent retreatment.
- Every effort should be made to limit the treatment intensity and duration.
- Long-term high-potency corticosteroid use can cause marked skin atrophy and rebound dermatitis.

MEDICATION (DRUGS)

Corticosteroid options include (lowest to highest potency):

- Hydrocortisone
- Triamcinolone acetonide cream
- Betamethasone valerate
- Clobetasol propionate

SURGERY

On rare occasions, patients with a persistent, unresponsive lesion will require local excision of VEH.

FOLLOW-UP

DISPOSITION

Issues for Referral

- Persistent symptoms
- Enlarging lesion despite adequate treatment

PROGNOSIS

- VEH, like lichen sclerosis, appears to have an indolent course and only rarely is associated with vulvar dysplasia or cancer.
- Corticosteroid topical treatment of VEH has been shown to yield excellent response rates (>75%).

PATIENT MONITORING

- The indolent and chronic nature of VEH calls for vigilant long-term follow-up with examination of the vulva.
- Careful follow-up exams should be scheduled since a small proportion of women with VEH are at risk for the development of high-grade, differentiated VIN or invasive cancer.

BIBLIOGRAPHY

Ayhan A, et al. Vulvar dystrophy: An evaluation of 285 cases. *Eur J Gynaecol Oncol*. 1997;18(2):139–140.

Blanchard A. Benign Vulvar Diagnosis, Clinical Gynecology. Churchill Livingstone Elsevier; 2006:219–231.

Kagie MJ, et al. The relevance of various vulvar epithelial changes in the early detection of squamous cell carcinoma of the vulva. *Intern J Gynecol Cancer*. 1997;7:50–57.

Kerman R, ed. *Blaustein's Pathology of the Female Genital Tract*. New York: Springer; 2002.

Rouzier R, et al. Prognostic significance of epithelial disorders adjacent to invasive vulvar carcinomas. *Gynecol Oncol*. 2001;81:414–419.

MISCELLANEOUS

SYNONYM(S)

- Squamous cell hyperplasia of the vulva
- Vulvar dystrophy

CLINICAL PEARLS

- When treating VEH, start with an intermediate-strength corticosteroid cream such as 0.1% triamcinolone applied 3 t.i.d.
- After 1–2 weeks, decrease the application rate to b.i.d.
- At 1 month, decrease to 1 application per day.
- If symptoms are controlled for 2 weeks on this regimen, then decrease to every other day dosing.
- Finally, attempt to lower the potency of the cream or stop treatment altogether.

ABBREVIATIONS

- HPV—Human papillomavirus
- HSV—Herpes simplex virus
- ISSVD—International Society for the Study of Vulvovaginal Disease
- SCC—Squamous cell carcinoma
- VEH—Vulvar epithelial hyperplasia
- VIN—Vulvar intraepithelial neoplasia

CODES

ICD9-CM
624.3 Vulvar epidermal hyperplasia

PATIENT TEACHING

- Instruct the patient that careful follow-up will be necessary.
- Discuss the rare but important association between VEH and intraepithelial neoplasia and SCC.
- Teach the woman about the importance of self-examination and, if necessary, to utilize a hand mirror.
- Instruct the patient that prolonged corticosteroid application can actually worsen the symptoms.
- The patient should be made aware that the 1st treatments with corticosteroids may cause a burning sensation.

VULVAR INTRAEPITHELIAL NEOPLASIA

Paul D. DePriest, MD
Brook A. Saunders, MD

 BASICS

DESCRIPTION
- VIN is a lesion characterized histologically by disorientation of squamous epithelial cells limited by the basement membrane without extension to the underlying dermis.
- This epithelial disorientation shows a lack of normal cell maturation from the transition of replicating basal cells to the terminally differentiated superficial cell layer.
- In 1986, the ISSVD simplified the terminology for vulvar intraepithelial abnormalities and adopted a single term: VIN.
- VIN, usual type, is related most closely to HPV infections, smoking, and immunosuppression.
- VIN, differentiated type, occurs in older women and is related to lichen sclerosis and vulvar epithelial hyperplasia.
- Both forms of VIN possess oncogenic potential.
- VIN, differentiated type, is most frequently found adjacent to vulvar SCC and is largely unrelated to HPV infections.
- ~2/3 of vulvar cancers have no traceable linkage to prior HPV infections.
- In non-HPV related cases, SCC results from a chronic process of inflammation, impaired immunity, lichen sclerosis, or epithelial hyperplasia.

Age-Related Factors
- VIN, usual type, occurs in younger women, aged 20–50, and is highly associated with HPV infections.
- VIN, differentiated type, occurs in older women, aged 40–70, and is rarely associated with evidence of HPV infections.

Staging
- Historically, VIN was graded 1–3 from mild to severe intraepithelial neoplasia.
- In 2004, the ISSVD updated the classification system:
  - Usual type (VIN 1 warty type, VIN 2 basaloid type, VIN 3 mixed type)
  - Differentiated type

RISK FACTORS
- Primary:
  - HPV
  - Lichen sclerosis
  - Vulvar epithelial hyperplasia
- Secondary:
  - Smoking
  - Immunosuppression

PATHOPHYSIOLOGY
- The development of VIN is multistep and multifactorial.
- Usual type:
  - HPV infections with high risk subtypes
  - Persistence of infection (immunosuppression)
  - Virally mediated immortalization of squamous cells (enhance by tobacco use)
- Differentiated type:
  - Lichen sclerosis and vulvar epithelial hyperplasia
  - Chronic skin irritation and inflammation
  - Impaired immunity

ASSOCIATED CONDITIONS
- HPV infections
- Lichen sclerosis
- Vulvar epithelial hyperplasia

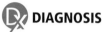 **DIAGNOSIS**

SIGNS AND SYMPTOMS
History
Women with VIN may be asymptomatic or may present with complaints of vulvar pruritus, burning, or irritation.

Physical Exam

> **ALERT**
> - It is imperative that the physician carefully inspect the external genitalia in *all* women presenting for gynecologic evaluation regardless of symptom complex:
>   - This exam should include inspection of the vulva from the mons anteriorly to the thigh creases bilaterally, to the hymenal ring internally, and to the perianal region posteriorly.

- Symptomatic patients should be asked to point out exactly the site of chronic irritation.
- VIN is extremely variable in appearance ranging from minimal erythema to dark brown raised nodules.
- Any lesion on the vulvar skin that exhibits abnormalities of color, surface contour, or thickness deserves magnified exam with a hand lens or colposcope.
- Magnified exam is utilized to identify the focality (discrete vs. multifocality), surface contour (flat, warty, erosive), and color of the lesion(s).
- Application of 3–5% acetic acid to the vulvar skin may help identify lesion margins. Aceto-white changes are highly variable in vulvar tissues depending on patient age, lesion type, and degree of local inflammation.

> **ALERT**
> - Any vulvar lesion that exhibits contour abnormalities and/or discoloration ranging from red, white, gray, or dark brown/black should be biopsied.
> - Any ulcerated or excoriated lesion should be biopsied.
> - If a vulvar lesion is noted, a thorough exam of the entirety of the vulvar skin, vagina, and cervix is required to rule out multicentric disease.

TESTS
- Biopsies are best performed after instillation of a small volume of 1% Lidocaine using a syringe and fine-bore needle.
- A 2–4 mm punch biopsy instrument is used to target and incise the lesion.
- The lesion is removed with fine scissors or a scalpel.
- In cases were a punch biopsy is considered inadequate due to lesion size, then an excisional biopsy should be performed.
- The biopsy material should be placed immediately into a fixative solution, such as formalin.
- Bleeding can be managed with local pressure and application of silver nitrate. Seldom is suturing required.
- The patient should use a lukewarm water sitz bath b.i.d. for 1 week to promote rapid healing.

Labs
- Careful histopathologic evaluation of the biopsy material is necessary.
- Gynecologic pathologist review of the biopsy material affords a reliable diagnosis.

DIFFERENTIAL DIAGNOSIS
The differential diagnosis in women with VIN includes infectious and neoplastic processes.

Infection
- Candidiasis (chronic)
- HSV
- HPV
- Syphilis

Immunologic
Immunocompromised women are at higher risk of VIN as well as vulvar cancer and vulvar infections:
- Women with HIV
- Medically immunosuppressed patients:
  - Transplant recipients on steroids

Tumor/Malignancy
Invasive vulvar cancer can be indistinguishable from VIN on physical exam:
- SCC
- Melanoma

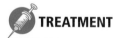 **TREATMENT**

GENERAL MEASURES
- Treatment of high-grade VIN consists of wide local excision or ablation followed by careful long-term follow-up.
- Young women with VIN, usual type, benefit from cautious excision in an effort to limit vulvar distortion and scarring.
- Take great care to avoid removing excess skin, thereby causing vulvar distortion, chronic pain, dyspareunia, and impaired self-image.
- Multiple repeat excisions may be needed over time.
- Every effort should be made to obtain negative margins, particularly in high-grade and in differentiated lesions.
- Any patient with recurrent vulvar symptoms or lesions deserves careful exam and re-biopsy.
- No treatment modality has been shown to be singularly curative.

- In choosing the appropriate treatment of VIN, take into account the severity of the lesion, focality of the lesion, patient's age, and potential negative impact of vulvar skin distortion.
- Laser ablation of VIN has been shown to be associated with more scarring than simple excision.

MEDICATION (DRUGS)

- More conservative medical treatments including α-interferon injections, imiquimod, and local 5–FU applications have been evaluated.
- Unfortunately to date, none of these treatment modalities has been shown to equal or exceed the cure rates of local excision/ablation.

SURGERY

Cold knife excision, laser excision, or laser ablation

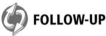

FOLLOW-UP

DISPOSITION

Issues for Referral

Women with recurrent or persistent VIN may benefit from specialty referral to:

- Gynecologic oncologist
- Plastic surgeon

PROGNOSIS

- Recurrence rates are highest in young women with HPV-related disease (20–35%).
- Recurrence rates are highest for VIN I–II, usual type.

PATIENT MONITORING

- Following excisional or ablative therapy, the patient should have vulvar exams using magnification at 3–4 month intervals for 1 year. Any recurrent abnormality should be biopsied and excised if necessary.
- The utilization of a colposcope with application of 3–5% acetic acid may facilitate differentiating VIN from other vulvar abnormalities.

BIBLIOGRAPHY

Cardosi R, et al. Diagnosis and management of vulvar and vaginal intraepithelial neoplasia. *Obstet Gynecol Clin N Am*. 2001;28:685–702.

Jones R. Vulvar intraepithelial neoplasia: Current perspectives. *Eur J Gynaecol Oncol*. 2001;22: 393–402.

Modesitt S, et al. Vulvar intraepithelial neoplasia III: Occult cancer and the impact of margin status on recurrence. *Obstet Gynecol*. 1998;92:962–966.

Preti M, et al. Squamous vulvar intraepithelial neoplasia. *Clin Obstet Gynecol*. 2005;48:845–861.

Sideri M, et al. Evaluation of CO(2) laser excision or vaporization for the treatment of vulvar intraepithelial neoplasia. *Gynecol Oncol*. 1999;75:277–281.

Sideri M, et al. Squamous vulvar intraepithelial neoplasia: 2004 Modified Terminology. ISSVD Vulvar Oncology Subcommittee. *J Reprod Med*. 2005;50: 807–810.

MISCELLANEOUS

SYNONYM(S)

- Vulvar carcinoma-in-situ
- Vulvar dysplasia

ABBREVIATIONS

- 5-FU—5-Fluorouracil
- HPV—Human papillomavirus
- HSV—Herpes simplex virus
- ISSD—International Society for the Study of Vulvovaginal Disease
- SCC—Squamous cell carcinoma
- STD—Sexually transmitted disease
- VIN—Vulvar intraepithelial neoplasia

CODES

ICD9-CM

184.4 Vulvar intraepithelial neoplasia

PATIENT TEACHING

- Women with VIN should be counseled concerning the possibility of recurrence and the need for vigilant follow-up.
- Women with VIN should understand the relationship between intraepithelial neoplasm and vulvar cancer.
- Encourage patients to avoid exposure to STDs that initiate this disorder (HPV).
- Teach women about the associated risks of smoking.
- Women should be taught self-exam of the vulvar skin and encouraged to seek assistance if any lesion is detected.

VULVAR LICHEN SCLEROSUS

Elisabeth H. Quint, MD
Meghan B. Oakes, MD

BASICS

DESCRIPTION
- LS is a chronic, lymphocyte-mediated skin disorder most commonly seen on the female genital skin.
- It is characterized by a thin, whitened, crinkled parchment-like appearance of the skin.
- Long-standing disease can lead to narrowing of the introitus, labial atrophy, and scarring.

Age-Related Factors
- This disease is most commonly seen in older women (50% >50), but happens across the lifespan.
- 7–12% occurs in premenarchal girls.

EPIDEMIOLOGY
- Little epidemiologic data are available; the true prevalence is unknown.
- Incidence is 1:300–1,000 in women who presented to a dermatologist.
- Extragenital LS found in 11% of women
- 5–100% of all vulvar cancer have been associated with LS.

RISK FACTORS
LS has been reported after repeated trauma and irritation (Koebner phenomenon).

Genetics
A genetic susceptibility is suggested by familial reports, but a clear pattern of inheritance has not been established.

PATHOPHYSIOLOGY
- The exact cause of LS is unknown.
- Autoimmune causes have been implicated:
  - 22% of women with LS have autoimmune disease, 42% have autoantibodies, and 60% have ≥1 autoimmune-related phenomena.
  - Studies have shown enhanced T-cell activity in LS.
- Sex hormones have been implicated:
  - LS is more common in low-estrogen states.
  - Decrease in local androgen receptors may be the cause.
- Infectious etiologies have been suggested, but never proved:
  - Conflicting results regarding *Borrelia burgdorferi*

ASSOCIATED CONDITIONS
A strong association with autoimmune disorders has been suggested.

DIAGNOSIS

SIGNS AND SYMPTOMS

History
- The most significant symptom of LS is intense itching.
- Ask about symptoms:
  - Pruritus (mild to severe)
  - Pain/Burning/Soreness
  - Dysuria
  - Dryness/Dyspareunia
  - Vaginal discharge
  - Genital/Anal bleeding (often due to excoriations from scratching, but may also result from "blood blisters") (see Bleeding, Abnormal Uterine: Prepubertal).
- Ask about timeline:
  - Length of symptoms
  - Continuous/Fluctuating
- Ask about previous treatments:
  - Steroids, progesterone, testosterone

Review of Systems
Other associated symptoms:
- Labial stenosis/fusion (late sequelae) and obliteration of normal anatomy
- Constipation or pain with defecation (girls are more likely than women to report urinary or bowel symptoms)

Physical Exam
- Diagnosis is often made on symptoms and vulvar appearance, especially in young girls.
- Vulvar exam:
  - Hypopigmentation
  - Parchmentlike crinkling of skin
  - Hourglass or figure-of-8 distribution around vulva and anus
  - Telangiectasias
  - Blisters/Bullae, may be hemorrhagic
  - Fissures
  - Edema (particularly of the clitoral hood)
  - Scratch effects: Excoriation, ulcers
  - Labial fusion or obliteration
  - Introital narrowing
  - Nongenital lesions are rare

TESTS

Lab
- In adults, a vulvar punch biopsy is often indicated to make the diagnosis. The edge of the lesion is the best place to take the biopsy (see Vulvar Biopsy).

- Direct immunofluorescence can be done on the biopsied skin to rule out pemphigoid as well as lichen planus.
- In children, history and physical exam are often adequate to make the diagnosis.
- Despite reports of autoantibodies in patients with LS, a workup for autoimmune disease is generally not warranted.

DIFFERENTIAL DIAGNOSIS

Infection
Postinflammatory hypo/hyperpigmentation

Metabolic/Endocrine
Postmenopausal atrophy (See Menopausal Symptoms.)

Immunologic
Vitiligo

Tumor/Malignancy
- VIN (See Vulvar Intraepithelial Neoplasia.)
- Squamous cell hyperplasia
- SCC (See Vulvar Cancer.)

Trauma
Sexual abuse (See Sexual Abuse and Vulvar and Vaginal Trauma.)

Drugs
Topical steroid overuse with atrophy

Other/Miscellaneous
Dermatologic conditions:
- Eczematous dermatitis
- Lichen planus
- Paget disease
- Psoriasis
- Labial adhesions (see topic)
- Scleroderma
- Pemphigus/Pemphigoid

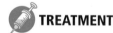

TREATMENT

GENERAL MEASURES
- Avoid strong soaps and detergents.
- Wear white, 100% cotton underwear.
- Defer undergarments at night.
- Panty liners may be avoided if they contribute to irritation.
- Use adequate lubrication with intercourse.
- Keep vulva clean and dry to prevent superinfection if ulcerations are present.
- Wear white cotton gloves at night to minimize scratching.

MEDICATION (DRUGS)

- Potent topical corticosteroids, followed by a lower potency taper, are the first-line treatment.
- Ultra-potent steroids (e.g., clobetasol propionate 0.05% ointment)
- Creams, gels, and liquid versions of these medications are not ultrapotent and should not be used.
- Many different treatment schedules have been proposed:
  – Use ultrapotent steroids b.i.d. for 1 month, then once daily for 2 months.
  – Apply thinly, not to exceed 30 g in 3 months.
- Follow this with mid-potency steroids for several months, followed by a low-potency steroid for long-term maintenance use.
  – Side effects include:
    ○ Burning
    ○ Irritation
    ○ Epithelial atrophy
    ○ Maceration
    ○ Hypopigmentation
- Nighttime sedation for severe itching may be used for severe pruritus.
- Patients may become irritated by the vehicle and may need steroids mixed in Aquaphor.
- Secondary infections are treated with antibiotics.
- If the patient is nonresponsive to steroid treatment, then biopsy and consider an alternative diagnosis.
- Occasionally, intralesional injection of corticosteroids are helpful in resistant disease.
- New research has shown promising, though early, results with the use of tacrolimus for LS.
- The use of testosterone in petrolatum has been advocated in the past, but is no longer recommended due to side effects and unclear benefit.
- Oral retinoids have been used with good results; however, the side effect profile precludes its use to only very severe refractory cases.

Pediatric Considerations

- This disease is seen in premenarchal girls (1:900, 7–12% of all cases of LS).
- Girls, more often than adults, present with constipation or pain with defecation.
- The vulvar appearance is similar to that of adults, with the addition of vesicles, bruising, and ulcers.
- No consistent data on the effect of puberty on the course of the disease.
- Treatment include ultrapotent steroids, but a shorter course: b.i.d. for 2 weeks, then once a day for 2 weeks, then taper to a midpotency steroid.

- Consider using emollient forms of the steroids.
- Nighttime sedative is recommended to prevent scratching.

Pregnancy Considerations

- Clobetasol is FDA pregnancy category C.
- Systemic absorption of clobetasol is low, but can be increased with prolonged use, occlusive dressings, and use over large surface areas.

SURGERY

- Surgery is rarely required and only to repair functional impairment caused by scarring.
- Indications include:
  – Narrowed introitus
  – Fused labia
  – Buried clitoris (smegmatic pseudocyst)

 ## FOLLOW-UP

DISPOSITION

Issues for Referral

Referral to gyn/oncology or dermatology if malignancy is diagnosed on biopsy

PROGNOSIS

- LS has no cure, but can be clinically controlled with symptom management.
- The symptoms often disappear, but the scars remain. Only in 20% of patients do skin changes revert. Further scarring can be prevented by maintenance therapy.
- 4–6% of treated LS is associated with malignancy.

PATIENT MONITORING

- Initially need frequent follow-up to assess response to therapy.
- For long-term follow-up, guidelines vary from every 3 months to annually.
- In adults, all suspicious areas should be biopsied, including thick plaques, ulcerations, nodules, and color changes.
- Biopsy in children, if required by suspicious areas or failure to improve, often requires general anesthesia.
- Patients should be instructed in self-examination.
- Sexual dysfunction is more common in women with LS and should be addressed in follow-up.

BIBLIOGRAPHY

Carlson JA, et al. Vulvar Lichen sclerosus and squamous cell carcinoma. *Hum Pathol.* 1998;29: 932–948.

Cooper SM, et al. Does treatment of vulvar lichensclerosus influence its prognosis? *Arch Dermatol.* 2004;140:702–706.

Kaufman RH, et al. Non-neoplastic Epithelial Disorders of the Vulvar Skin and Mucosa. In: *Benign Diseases of the Vulva and Vagina*, 5th ed. New York: Elsevier Mosby; 2005:274–290.

Luesley DM, et al. Topical tacrolimus in the management of lichen sclerosus. *Br J Obstet Gynaecol.* 2006;113:832–834.

Smith YR, et al. Vulvar Lichen sclerosus: Pathophysiology and treatment. *Am J Clin Dermatol.* 2004:5:105–125.

Val I, et al. An overview of lichen sclerosus. *Clin Obstet.* 2005;48:808–817.

 ## MISCELLANEOUS

SYNONYM(S)

- Until 1976, Lichen sclerosus et atrophicus (LSA)
- Kraurosis vulvae
- Leukoplakia
- Hypoplastic dystrophy
- Lichen planus sclerosus et atrophicus

CLINICAL PEARLS

- LS is a chronic skin condition, usually diagnosed in children by symptoms (pruritus) and visual inspection of the vulva.
- Biopsy to confirm the diagnosis is indicated in adults.
- Ultrapotent topical steroids are used to treat the symptoms, but do not cure the disease.
- Any change in appearance over time must be reevaluated by biopsy, due to a 5% increased risk for SCC of the vulva.

ABBREVIATIONS

- ISSVD—International Society for the Study of Vulvovaginal Diseases
- LS—Lichen sclerosus
- LSA—Lichen sclerosus et atrophicus
- SCC—Squamous cell carcinoma
- VIN—Vulvar intraepithelial neoplasia

ICD9-CM

701.0 Lichen sclerosus

PATIENT TEACHING

- Provide information about the condition.
- Explain, without alarm, the risk of malignancy and the need for monitoring and follow-up.
- Patients should be instructed in self-examination of the vulva:
  – Look for thick irregular white plaques, erosions, ulcers, nodules, or color changes.

PREVENTION

There are no known preventive measures.

VULVAR ULCERS/APHTHOSIS

Helen R. Deitch, MD
Jill S. Huppert, MD, MPH

 BASICS

DESCRIPTION

- Vulvar aphthae are painful, non–sexually transmitted ulcerations of the vulva that heal spontaneously.
- Because vulvar ulcerations are most commonly considered to be sexually transmitted, vulvar aphthae are often misdiagnosed as herpes.
- Aphthae have been described on the labia majora, minora, introitus, perineum, and in the vagina, and are often accompanied by systemic symptoms.
- 1st described in adolescent females by Lipshutz in 1913, they are similar in etiology to and often found in association with oral aphthae.
- Current gynecologic literature is limited to case reports. Case series describe findings in the pediatric population.

Age-Related Factors
Studies describing vulvar aphthosis across multiple age groups are lacking. Related oral aphthosis initially presents in adolescence and peaks in the 3rd and 4th decades.

Pediatric Considerations
- Vulvar aphthosis has a predilection for adolescent females.
- Their initial presentation is more common in pubertal females (Tanner stage 2–4 breast development) who are premenarchal or within the 1st year of menarche.

Staging
Gynecologic literature describing vulvar aphthosis is sparse. The following system is based on the description of oral aphthae from dermatologic literature.

- Classification by morphology:
  – Minor aphthae:
    ○ Single to few shallow ulcers <1 cm in diameter
    ○ Heal within 7–10 days
  – Major aphthae:
    ○ Single to few ulcers >1 cm
    ○ Heal in weeks to months
  – Herpetiform aphthae:
    ○ 10–100 small grouped ulcers (1–3 mm)
    ○ Heal in days to weeks

- Classification by disease type:
  – Simple aphthosis:
    ○ Recurrent attacks of minor, major or herpetiform aphthae with distinct ulcerfree periods
  – Complex aphthosis:
    ○ Constant presence of >3 oral aphthae OR
    ○ Recurrent oral and genital aphthae AND exclusion of Behçet's disease.
    ○ May be primary (idiopathic) aphthae or secondary to other systemic diseases
    ○ IBD is the most common

EPIDEMIOLOGY

Pediatric Considerations
- Most common in white adolescent females, but they have been described in Asian and African American patients.
- Hormone milieu of adolescence is thought to contribute to occurrence of ulcers.
- 50% will have a history of or develop oral ulcerations.
- 1/3 will have a recurrence of their vulvar lesion (complex aphthosis).
- No association has been made with the phase of the menstrual cycle.
- Outbreaks may be more common in the spring.

RISK FACTORS
- Adolescent white female
- Stress
- Viral infections associated but not likely causal:
  – EBV and CMV have been described in association with vulvar aphthosis.

PATHOPHYSIOLOGY
- Has not been delineated
- Viral or bacterial causes have not been identified.

ASSOCIATED CONDITIONS
- Vulvar aphthosis may be the initial presentation of Behçet's disease.
- Long-term monitoring for recurrent ulcers and other manifestations of Behçet's is important.
- Diagnostic criteria for Behçet's disease:
  – 3 recurrent episodes of oral aphthae within a year, plus 2 other findings including:
    ○ Recurrent genital aphthae
    ○ Ocular lesions
    ○ Skin lesions
    ○ Positive pathergy test

 DIAGNOSIS

SIGNS AND SYMPTOMS

History
- Vulvar pain or dysuria with vulvar swelling and presence of a vulvar scab prior to development of the ulceration.
- Systemic complaints such as fever, headache, and malaise are common.
- Other complaints may include gastrointestinal, upper respiratory, arthralgias, oral lesions, skin lesions.

Review of Systems
- Obtain a sexual history, asking about voluntary sexual activity and abuse.
- Focus on other symptoms of Behçet's disease:
  – Concurrent or a history of oral ulcerations
  – Visual changes
  – Skin lesions or rashes
- Inquire about symptoms of systemic inflammatory diseases:
  – Abdominal pain
  – Weight loss
  – Diarrhea

Physical Exam
- Ulcer appearance:
  – Shallow with sharply demarcated boarders that are often raised
  – May have an overlying gray exudate or hard gray-brown eschar
  – Associated cellulitis is common
- Location:
  – May occur on the labia minora, majora, perineum, and in the vagina
  – Medial aspect of the labium minus is most common
  – "Kissing" ulcers on opposing surfaces may occur
- Size:
  – Variable; lesions >1 cm are common
- Other physical findings:
  – Look for oral aphthae, skin nodules, rashes

TESTS
- Exclude STIs, especially HSV
- Other special testing depends on the patient's risk factors for STIs, and history that suggests other systemic illnesses.

Lab
- Minimal testing required for all patients:
  – Viral culture or PCR for HSV in all patients, regardless of reported sexual activity
  – RPR or VDRL for syphilis
- High-risk populations:
  – HIV
- Travel outside the US:
  – LGV:
    ○ Testing for *Chlamydia trachomatis* L 2–3 serovars
  – Chancroid:
    ○ Culture for *Haemophilus ducreyi*
- Biopsy may be indicated if recurrent lesions or severe case.

DIFFERENTIAL DIAGNOSIS
Vulvar aphthosis is a diagnosis of exclusion and requires excluding diseases primarily of the vulva and systemic illness that secondarily cause vulvar ulcerations (secondary complex aphthosis).

Infection
- Infectious etiologies can be divided into both sexually and non–sexually acquired infections:
  – Sexually acquired vulvar ulcerations:
    ○ HSV
    ○ Syphilis
    ○ HIV
    ○ LGV
    ○ Chancroid
- Non–sexually acquired systemic infections; evidence for a temporal but not necessarily causal association with:
  – EBV
  – CMV
- Local infections:
  – Folliculitis
  – Hidradenitis suppurativa

Hematologic
Cyclic neutropenia

Metabolic/Endocrine
Progesterone autoimmune dermatitis:
- Painful recurrent ulcerations that occur as an allergic reaction to endogenous progesterone

Immunologic
- Behçet's disease
- Crohn's disease:
  – Ulcerations usually described as "knifelike"
  – May precede GI symptoms
- Celiac disease
- Lichen sclerosus
- Lichen planus
- Pemphigus and pemphigoid:
  – Lesions are bullous

Tumor/Malignancy
- Paget disease of the vulva
- Vulvar SCC

Trauma
History is usually sufficient to rule out trauma.

Drugs
- Methotrexate and other chemotherapeutic agents
- Drug reactions: NSAIDs

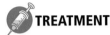

TREATMENT

GENERAL MEASURES
- Outpatient supportive therapy and pain control are usually all that is necessary.
- Frequent sitz baths help with discomfort and healing.
- Hospitalization may be necessary for uncontrolled pain or urinary retention.

MEDICATION (DRUGS)
- Oral or topical analgesics such as lidocaine jelly are helpful.
- Consider topical corticosteroids after infectious etiologies have been excluded (e.g., clobetasol topical ointment 0.5% b.i.d. for 1–2 weeks).
- In the oral aphthosis literature, amlexanox 5% oral paste, applied q.i.d. for 3–5 days, is safe and effective.
- Antibiotics may be needed to treat concurrent surrounding cellulitis if present.

SURGERY
Some patients may require general anesthesia to complete an adequate exam to establish the diagnosis, and biopsy may be performed, but resection of lesions is not recommended.

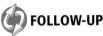

FOLLOW-UP

DISPOSITION
Issues for Referral
Subspecialty referral evaluation for suspected Behçet's disease or secondary aphthosis is indicated for:
- Patients with recurrent vulvar and oral aphthae or extra genital involvement:
  – Ophthalmologic examination for uveitis and iritis
  – Rheumatologic evaluation
  – Gastrointestinal evaluation

PROGNOSIS
- Vulvar aphthosis is a self-limited condition.
- Ulcerations heal spontaneously.
- Healing occurs within 3 weeks for 75% of patients
- ~1/3 can expect a recurrence:
  – Recurrences are usually shorter in duration with smaller, less painful ulcers.

PATIENT MONITORING
Long-term surveillance for evidence of Behçet's disease or secondary complex aphthosis is recommended.

BIBLIOGRAPHY

Complex aphthosis: A large case series with evaluation algorithm and therapeutic ladder from topicals to thalidomide. *J Am Acad Dermatol.* 2005;52(3 Pt 1):500–508.

Criteria for diagnosis of Behçet's disease. International Study Group for Behçet's Disease. *Lancet.* 1990; 5;335(8697):1078–1080.

Deitch HR, et al. Unusual vulvar ulcerations in young adolescent females. *J Pediatr Adolesc Gynecol.* 2004;17(1):13–16.

Huppert JS, et al. Vulvar ulcers in young females: A manifestation of aphthosis. *J Pediatr Adolesc Gynecol.* 2006;19(3):195–204.

MISCELLANEOUS

CLINICAL PEARLS
- Exclude HSV infection in all women presenting with vulvar ulcerations, regardless of age or sexual history.
- Patients with complex aphthosis need evaluation for secondary causes, especially IBD.
- Long-term monitoring for evidence of Behçet's disease is recommended.

ABBREVIATIONS
- CMV—Cytomegalovirus
- EBV—Epstein-Barr virus
- HSV—Herpes simplex virus
- IBD—Inflammatory bowel disease
- LGV—Lymphogranuloma venereum
- PCR—Polymerase chain reaction
- RPR—Rapid plasma reagin
- SCC—Squamous cell carcinoma
- STI—Sexually transmitted infection
- VDRL—Venereal Disease Research Laboratory

CODES
ICD9-CM
- 136.1 Behçet's syndrome
- 528.20 Oral aphthae
- 616.10 Vulvitis (includes aphthous)
- 616.51 Ulceration of vulva in diseases classified elsewhere

PATIENT TEACHING

Patients, especially young adolescents and their parents, must understand that these lesions are not sexually transmitted, heal spontaneously, and do not recur in most patients.

PREVENTION
Treatment of underlying conditions in secondary complex aphthosis

VULVAR VESTIBULITIS

Diane E. Elas, MSN, ENRC, ARNP
Rudolph P. Galask, MD, MS

BASICS

DESCRIPTION
- Vestibulitis is an inflammation of the vulvar vestibule.
- The vulvar vestibule is defined as the ringlike portion of the vaginal opening:
  - Anatomically, it is the area medial to the Hart line on the labia minora, extending to and including the hymenal ring.
  - It includes the Bartholin duct, lesser vestibular duct, and urethral meatus.
- 3 criteria have been established for the diagnosis of vulvar vestibulitis (Friedrich criteria):
  - Severe pain on vestibular touch or attempted vaginal entry
  - Tenderness to pressure localized within the vulvar vestibule
  - Physical findings of erythema of various degrees confined to the vestibule

Age-Related Factors
- May 1st be noticed with the onset of menses when attempts to insert or wear a tampon comfortably are unsuccessful.
- Otherwise, it is 1st noted with either onset of coital activity or may develop anytime after when the female is sexually active.

EPIDEMIOLOGY
The prevalence rate is unknown; possibly ≥16%.

RISK FACTORS
Genetics
No definitive genetic links at this time.

PATHOPHYSIOLOGY
Inflammation of the vulvar vestibulitis has been associated with:
- Exposure to contact irritants
- Recurrent vaginal infections (yeast and/or bacterial)
- HPV infection
- HSV infection
- Altered immune function
- In most cases the etiology is unknown.

ASSOCIATED CONDITIONS
- Decreased libido
- Decreased self-esteem
- Depression
- Marital discord

DIAGNOSIS

SIGNS AND SYMPTOMS
History
- Females with vulvar vestibulitis may experience vulvar burring and/or pain with day-to-day activities as well as with coital activity.
- Insertional pain:
  - Penis/Vibrators
  - Tampons
- Pain to touch:
  - Positional pain such as with sitting
  - Tight/Restrictive clothing
  - Wiping/Cleansing

Review of Systems
- Prior sexual abuse/trauma
- Prior/Current STD
- Urologic symptoms, without UTI
  - Dysuria
  - Urinary urgency/frequency

Physical Exam
- Exam of the vulva and vestibule for erythema limited to the vestibule.
- Pain with insertion of speculum or on bimanual examination.

TESTS
Pain on Q-tip touch test.

Lab
- Cultures as indicated:
  - *Chlamydia*
  - *Gonorrhea*
  - HSV
- Wet-prep of vaginal discharge:
  - Maturation index
  - Clue cells
  - *Lactobacillus*, present or absent
  - RBCs
  - Trichomonads
  - WBCs
  - Yeast: Buds or hyphae

DIFFERENTIAL DIAGNOSIS
Infection
- Bacterial vaginosis
- HSV
- HPV
- Yeast vulvovaginitis
- UTI

Immunologic
Possible underlying immunodeficiency

Tumor/Malignancy
VIN may also be present in patients with vestibulitis.

Trauma
- Female genital mutilation
- Genital trauma
- Sexual/Physical/Emotional abuse

Other/Miscellaneous
- Dermatologic:
  - Atrophic vaginitis
  - Contact dermatitis
  - Lichen sclerosus
  - Lichen planus
  - Sjögren syndrome
  - Genital ulcer:
    - Aphthous
    - Behçet's (rare)
    - HSV
- Other:
  - Interstitial cystitis/painful bladder syndrome
  - Pelvic floor muscle (levators) dysfunction

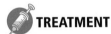

TREATMENT

GENERAL MEASURES
- No definitive therapy is available at this time. This is related to the fact that the etiology is not understood and, in many cases, is probably multifactorial in nature.
- Pelvic floor rehabilitation:
  - Pelvic floor relaxation exercises
  - Vaginal dilators for deconditioning
- Supportive/Protective:
  - Daily occlusive skin protectant to vestibule, such as olive oil or zinc oxide ointment.
  - Strict attention to vulvar skin care hygiene to eliminate exposure to contact irritants
  - Warm water soaks

SPECIAL THERAPY
Complementary and Alternative Therapies
Low oxalate diet with calcium citrate supplementation may or may not be helpful.

MEDICATION (DRUGS)
Multiple treatment strategies exist that include the following:
- Topical:
  - Low- to medium-potency steroid ointments
  - Anesthetics, specially prior to intercourse

- Systemic:
  - Amitriptyline
  - Gabapentin
- Other:
  - Anti-infectives/Antifungals to treat concomitant infections
  - Antidepressants to treat associated depression
  - Estrogen to treat concomitant atrophic vaginitis

SURGERY
Vestibulectomy

FOLLOW-UP

DISPOSITION
Issues for Referral
- Chronic pain clinic referral
- Health psychologist: Depression/marital problems
- Physical therapist: Pelvic floor dysfunction
- Vulvar disease specialist: For vestibulitis unresponsive to treatment

PROGNOSIS
Prognosis is variable. Condition may be acute, intermittent, or chronic.

PATIENT MONITORING
Frequent follow-up to assess response to treatment and evaluate for development of depressive or marital issues.

BIBLIOGRAPHY

Farage MA, et al. Vulvar vestibulitis syndrome: A review. *Eur J Obstet Gynecol Reprod Biol*. 2005;123:9–16.

Friedrich EG. Vulvar vestibulitis syndrome. *J Reprod Med*. 1987;32:110–114.

Nyirjesy P. Is it vulvar vestibulitis? *Contemporary OB/GYN*. 2007;January:64–74.

MISCELLANEOUS

SYNONYM(S)
- Vestibular adenitis
- Vestibulodynia
- Vulvar dysesthesia
- Vulvar vestibulitis syndrome
- Vulvodynia

ABBREVIATIONS
- HPV—Human papillomavirus
- HSV—Herpes simplex virus
- STD—Sexually transmitted disease
- UTI—Urinary tract infection
- VIN—Vulvar intraepithelial neoplasia

CODES

ICD9-CM
- 289.3 Vestibular adenitis
- 616.10 Vestibulodynia
- 616.10 Vulvar vestibulitis
- 625.9 Vulvodynia
- 782.0 Vulvar dysesthesia

PATIENT TEACHING

Vulvar skin care hygiene:
- Daily skin protectant to vestibule to keep urine, vaginal discharge, and menstrual discharge from coming in contact with the inflamed area
- Decrease/Eliminate exposure to contact irritants
- Decrease mechanical irritation to the vulva/vestibule
- Use a nonirritating lubricant with coital activity, such as olive oil/vegetable oil.

Section II

Section III
Women's Health and Primary Care

ACOG GUIDELINES FOR SCREENING AND WELL-WOMAN CARE

Jennifer Lang, MD
Beth Y. Karlan, MD

 BASICS

DESCRIPTION
- The ob-gyn has an important role to play in the prevention and early diagnosis of many diseases that cause serious morbidity and mortality. There is a growing emphasis on the incorporation of primary and preventative health care into the field.
- The goal of primary and preventative health care should be to promote health and wellness in a way that is age-appropriate and tailored to a woman's individual risk factors.
- The focus of primary care medicine is:
  - Health maintenance
  - Preventative services
  - Early detection of disease
  - Continuity of care
- Principle of "screening": Testing healthy individuals with the goal of identifying those at increased risk for a disease or condition
- A screening test should be accurate, highly sensitive, and reasonably highly specific.

Age-Related Factors
ACOG makes guidelines for screening and well-woman care that are divided into different age groups: Ages 13–18, 19–39, 40–64, ≥65.

EPIDEMIOLOGY
Each woman should discuss a personal risk-profile with her physician, who will also note US epidemiologic trends:
- Heart disease is the #1 cause of death in women: ~1/3 of all deaths or 350,000 deaths/yr
- Cancer is the #2 cause of death in women. By disease site:
  - #1 Lung
  - #2 Breast
  - #3 Colorectal
- Stroke is the #3 cause of death in women, and a leading cause of disability.
- 18.5% of US women are current smokers.
- 30% of HS senior girls are current smokers.
- 49% of all pregnancies are unintended.
- 35% of US women will have an induced abortion by age 45.
- In 2000, 35 of 50 states had a prevalence of obesity of ≥20%.
- 70% of white women >80 have osteoporosis.

RISK FACTORS
Genetics
- Take a thorough family history
- Be observant of body habitus and other stigmata that may alert you to a genetic condition or predisposition to a particular disease:
  - Consider consultation with geneticist or genetics counselor if history is suspicious.

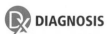 **DIAGNOSIS**

SIGNS AND SYMPTOMS
History
- History should be age-appropriate in content and style, and focus on age-group's specific risk factors and major causes of morbidity and mortality.

- Age 13–18:
  - Risk-taking behaviors: Sexual practices, reckless driving, alcohol and other drugs, screen for eating disorders
- Age 19–39:
  - Assess diet, nutrition, physical activity
  - Sexual practices: Contraceptive choices, pregnancy planning; don't assume heterosexual orientation
  - Depression
  - Intimate partner violence
  - Alcohol/Tobacco/Recreational drug use
  - Breast cancer risk assessment
- Age 40–64:
  - Menopausal symptoms, sexual function, incontinence of urine or stool, family history
- ≥65:
  - Nutrition, ADLs, home environment, abuse or neglect

Interacting with the Health System
- Use every opportunity to identify women at risk and direct them to appropriate resources:
- ~5% of ED visits for women related to intimate partner violence.
- Assuming heterosexuality may alienate some and cause avoidance of future health care interactions.

DIFFERENTIAL DIAGNOSIS
Infection
- HIV and AIDS is a growing problem for women.
  - 30% of 40,000 new HIV diagnoses in US are women.
  - >2/3 of these are in African American women.
  - Primary risk is high-risk heterosexual contact.
- Screening recommended at each check-up, even women who consider themselves low-risk
- Annual testing: High-risk sex, or IV drug user
- Cervical cancer is an AIDS-defining illness.

Hematologic
Iron-deficiency anemia is a common morbidity:
- Investigate heavy bleeding and offer treatment
- Multivitamins recommended in all women; iron supplementation in pregnancy and if iron-deficient

Metabolic/Endocrine
- Obesity in US is epidemic and a major cause of morbidity and mortality (see Diet:Obesity).
  - Calculate BMI
  - Advise about healthy diet and exercise.
  - Reducing obesity will have the health benefits of reducing risk for:
    - Type 2 DM, CAD, some cancers, osteoarthritis, sleep apnea, hypertension
- Diabetes mellitus increasing rates due to obesity:
  - No recommended screening Type 1 DM
  - Type 2 DM can be diagnosed in 1 of 3 ways:
    - Random glucose >200 mg/dL with symptoms of hyperglycemia
    - Fasting serum glucose ≥126 mg/dL
    - 2–hour 75 g OGTT glucose >200 mg/dL
  - Screening for Type 2 DM is recommended for:
    - All adults age ≥45; if normal, every 3 years
    - Adults with hypertension or hyperlipidemia
    - Overweight individuals, BMI ≥25
    - Women with PCOS
    - History of GDM, or baby >4 kg birthweight
    - 1st-degree relative with Type 2 DM

- Menopause is defined as 12 months of amenorrhea (see topics):
  - Median age is 51
  - Perimenopause is the 3–5 years before menopause.
  - The menopausal symptom complex includes vasomotor, urogenital, and psychologic symptoms:
    - Hot flushes, night sweats, sleep disturbances, vaginal dryness, mood changes
  - HRT is the most effective treatment for vasomotor symptoms, but also has health risks associated with its use.
    - Assess risk/benefit analysis for each individual before it is prescribed or denied.
- Hypothyroidism affects many women, causing low energy, depressed mood, other health risks:
  - ACOG recommends screening for with TSH levels every 5 years after age 40.
- Osteopenia and osteoporosis are a major cause of morbidity and mortality for women:
  - Bone density decreases roughly 1% per year after menopause.
  - Osteopenia: Bone density 1–2.5 SD below the mean for reference population-healthy women
  - Osteoporosis: ≥2.5 SD below this mean
  - Encourage adequate dietary calcium and Vitamin D; most women require supplements to achieve the recommended daily intake.
  - Pharmacologic therapy with a bisphosphonate, SERMs, or hormonal therapy may be required.

Tumor/Malignancy
- Breast cancer affects 1 in 8 women during their lifetimes.
  - 2nd leading cause of cancer-related deaths in the US
  - Age is the most important risk factor. Family history is 2nd most important. Others include: Early menarche, nulliparity, 1st child at age >30, late menopause, alcohol use, high fat diet, obesity, exposure to ionizing radiation, biopsy-confirmed atypical hyperplasia
  - Mammography is less sensitive in women <50 years old, using HRT, or with dense breasts.
  - For average-risk women, ACOG recommends mammograms every 1–2 years after age 40; annually after 50.
- Colorectal cancers are the 3rd leading cause of cancer-related deaths:
  - Screening should begin by age 50 in average-risk women, using 1 of the following 5 methods:
    - Yearly patient-collected fecal occult blood test
    - Flexible sigmoidoscopy every 5 years
    - Yearly patient-collected fecal occult blood test + flexible sigmoidoscopy every 5 years
    - Double-contrast barium enema every 5 years
    - Colonoscopy every 10 years
- Skin cancer:
  - No formal screening recommendation for women of average risk.
  - Consider yearly dermatologic exams for "high-risk":
    - Fair-skinned women, age ≥65, atypical moles, >50 moles, increased recreational or occupational exposure to sunlight, family history of skin cancer, evidence of precursor lesions

Drugs

Alcohol, tobacco, and illicit drug use is associated with high-risk behaviors, particularly in adolescents.

- These include motor vehicle accidents, unprotected intercourse, fires, falls

PSYCHOSOCIAL CONSIDERATIONS

- Major depressive disorder: Women are at a higher lifetime risk than are men; women have a 20% lifetime chance of major depressive disorder.
- Screen for depression by asking about feeling "down, depressed, or hopeless" or having decreased interest or pleasure in doing things.
  - In the elderly, may masquerade as dementia; it should be recognized and treated

PREGNANCY

- 50% of all pregnancies are unintended.
  - Preconception counseling can help prevent unintended pregnancies, and improve the health and wellness of women and fetuses once pregnancy occurs.
- Identify medical issues or conditions that could affect future pregnancies.
- Provide counseling regarding healthy diet with folate supplementation of 0.4 mg/d.
- Assess a woman's risk for genetic disorders, with referral to counseling or testing as needed:
  - Counsel women to abstain from alcohol, tobacco, and recreational drug use

SPECIAL GROUPS

Adolescents

- It is essential to disclose federal and state laws when caring for adolescents that may affect confidentiality or require mandatory reporting.
- In the sexual history, ask about coerced or nonconsensual sex that may include violence, abuse, incest.
- The pelvic exam should begin when the patient becomes sexually active (though no later than age 21), with annual testing for *Chlamydia trachomatis* and *Gonorrhea*:
  - The PAP test should begin 3 years after 1st intercourse, but no later than age 21.
- Assess Tanner stage during the physical exam, and investigate patients who fall outside the norms for their age and racial background (see Puberty).

Women with Chronic Illness

- Many women suffer from chronic illness and disease such as multiple sclerosis, HIV, lupus, and rheumatoid arthritis.
- Consider immunocompromised states as risk factors for persistent HPV infection, and subsequent cervical, vaginal, and vulvar dysplasia.
- Steroid use is also a risk factor for diabetes and osteoporosis.
- Women with a chronic illness still need primary care.

Older Women

- Life expectancy is increasing, and thus so is the population of women >65. Primary care issues include vision, hearing, musculoskeletal system, ADLs, continence of urine and feces, nutrition, mental status, depression, home environment, social support network.
- Issues of abuse or neglect in elders: Mistreatment may involve physical, psychological, financial, or neglect (most common form of elder mistreatment).

BIBLIOGRAPHY

Branson BM, et al. Revised recommendations for HIV testing of adults, adolescents, and pregnant women in health care settings. *MMWR Recomm Rep.* 2006 Sep 22;55(RR14):1–17.

Eaton DK, et al. Youth risk behavior surveillance-United States, 2005. Centers for disease control and prevention. *MMWR Surveill Summ.* 2006;55(5):1–108.

Human Papilloma Vaccination, ACOG Committee Opinion No 344. American College of Obstetricians and Gynecologists. *Obstet Gynecol.* 2006;108:699–705.

Jemal A, et al. Cancer Statistics, 2006. *CA Cancer J Clin.* 2006;56:106–130.

Nelson HD, et al. Screening women and elderly adults for family and intimate partner violence: A review of the evidence for the US Preventitive Services Task Force. *Ann Intern Med.* 2004;140:387–396.

Peipert JF, et al. *Clinical updates in women's health care: Primary and preventative care.* ACOG, April 2007; Vol. VI, No. 2.

Scholle SH, et al. Characteristics of patients seen and services provided in primary care visits in OB/GYN: Data from NAMCS and NHAMCS. *Am J Obstet Gynecol.* 2004;190:1119–1127.

Screening for osteoporosis in post menopausal women: Recommendations and rationale. US Preventive Services Task Force. *Ann Intern Med.* 2002;137:526–528.

Screening for thyroid disease: Recommendations statement. US Preventive Services Task Force. *Ann Intern Med.* 2004;140:125–127.

Siris ES, et al. Identification and fracture outcome of undiagnosed low bone marrow density in post-menopausal women: Results from the National Osteoporosis Risk Assessment. *JAMA.* 2001;286:2815–2822.

US Department of Health and Human Services, Healthy People 2010: Understanding and improving health, 2nd ed. Washington, DC: www.healthypeople.gov.

US Preventive Services Task force. Screening for depression: Recommendations and rationale. *Ann Intern Med.* 2002;136:760–764.

MISCELLANEOUS

CLINICAL PEARLS

- Below are screening and vaccination guidelines for average-risk women:
  - Annual PAP beginning 3 years after 1st intercourse, no later than age 21:
    - If age ≥30, HPV negative, with 3 consecutive normal PAP tests and no history of severe dysplasia or other high-risk feature, can perform Pap every 2–3 years.
  - HPV/Cervical cancer vaccine age 9–26 (most effective if given before onset of sexual activity)
  - Mammography every 1–2 years age 40–50, then annually
  - Lipid profile every 5 years ≥45 years
  - Fasting glucose every 3 years ≥45 years
  - TSH every 5 years ≥40
  - Colorectal screening as above, beginning age 50
  - Bone density beginning age 60, with DEXA scans no more frequently than every 2 years in absence of new risk factors.
  - Yearly dental exams

- BP at least every 2 years
- Annual influenza vaccine age ≥50
- Tetanus-diptheria-pertussis booster every 10 years
- Goals for health and wellness:
  - BP <120/80
  - Total cholesterol <200
  - LDL <100
  - Triglycerides <150
  - BMI between 18.5–24.9
  - Diet high in fiber, including fruits, vegetables, whole grains, and lean protein
  - Diet low in saturated fats
  - Moderate exercise at least 5 days a week for 30 minutes at a time
  - Vigorous exercise at least 3 days a week for 20 minutes at a time
  - Avoidance of tobacco and other drugs

ABBREVIATIONS

- ACOG—American College of Obstetricians and Gynecologists
- ADLs—Activities of daily living
- BP—Blood pressure
- CAD—Coronary artery disease
- DEXA—Dual-energy x-ray absorptiometry
- DM—Diabetes mellitus
- GDM—Gestational diabetes mellitus
- HDL—High-density lipoprotein
- HPV—Human papilloma virus
- HRT—Hormone replacement therapy
- LDL—Low-density lipoprotein
- OGTT—Oral glucose tolerance test
- PCOS—Polycystic ovarian syndrome
- SERM—Selective estrogen receptor modulator
- STI—Sexually transmitted infection
- TSH—Thyroid stimulating hormone

LEGAL ISSUES

The physician should be aware of and fully disclose to the patient any state or federal laws that may influence their ability to promise confidentiality or offer specific services. Many states have mandatory reporting laws that physicians must observe or face criminal charges. This is most relevant in the following areas:

- Abortion:
  - Parental notification laws
  - Gestational age restrictions
- Child abuse or neglect
- Intimate partner violence
- STIs
- Mental illness

PATIENT TEACHING

- Women should be active participants in their own health and wellness.
- Teach breast self-exam; encourage a woman to be familiar with the appearance, shape, and texture of her breasts so she can alert the physician to any changes.
- Helpful, educational web sites:
  - ACOG www.acog.org
  - American Heart Association www.americanheart.org
  - American Diabetic Association www.diabetes.org
  - American Cancer Society www.cancer.org
  - Center for Disease Control www.cdc.gov
  - Women's Cancer Network www.wcn.org

CANCER SCREENING: CERVICAL CYTOLOGY

Michelle Berlin, MD, MPH

BASICS

DESCRIPTION
- "Pap test" or "Pap smear" is entrenched in medical terminology and frequently is used to refer to cervical cytology regardless of actual method used to obtain or process the cytology, either by conventional slide or liquid based technology.
- Cervical cytology, using the Pap smear, is a screening test for premalignant cervical dysplasia and cervical cancer:
  - Designed to have high sensitivity (detection of cases)
  - Need for further evaluation determined by result
  - 2006 TBS guidelines current: www.asccp.org
- Cervical dysplasia:
  - CIN—cervical intraepithelial neoplasia
- ASCUS—atypical squamous cells of undetermined significance
- ASC-H—atypical squamous cells, cannot exclude HSIL
- LSIL—low-grade squamous intraepithelial lesion
- HSIL—high-grade squamous intraepithelial lesion

Age-Related Factors
- Differing recommendations
- USPSTF:
  - Begin 3 years after onset of sexual activity or age 21 (whichever comes 1st)
  - For well-screened women >65: Low yield with screening (see "ALERT")
  - No Pap screening needed for women who have undergone hysterectomy for benign indications (Must ensure that cervix has been removed by review of surgical report, speculum and/or bimanual exam. Standard hysterectomy, particularly cesarean hysterectomy or performed internationally, may NOT include removal of cervix.)
  - USPSTF recommendations evidence-based
- Recommendations of others (not all evidence-based):
  - ACS:
    - Annual screening beginning 3 years after onset of sexual activity or age 21
    - Until age 30: Annual or every 2-year screening
    - Age 30+: Women who have had 3 normal Pap test results in a row may get tested every 2–3 years with Pap
    - Women ≥70 can stop screening IF they have had 3 or more documented, consecutive, technically satisfactory normal/negative cervical cytology tests and no abnormal/positive cytology tests within the past 10 years.

- ACOG:
  - Annual screening 3 years after beginning of sexual activity but no later than age 21
  - <30: Annual screening
  - ≥30: May extend interval to 2–3 years if no history of CIN II or III, no DES exposure, not immunocompromised or have HIV
  - After hysterectomy for benign indications (and no prior history of CIN 2 or CIN 3): Routine screening may be discontinued

Pediatric Considerations
- See above recommendations for initiation of cervical cytology screening ~3 years after 1st vaginal intercourse or age 21.
- Guidelines are based on:
  - The high frequency of mild abnormalities on cervical cytology
  - High rates of spontaneous resolution and viral clearing over time
  - The time typically required for progression of low- to high-grade CIN
- The guidelines assume that adolescent reproductive health care with provisions of confidential screening and services is available to adolescents.

ALERT
Women at low risk of cervical cancer, who may consider Pap screening every 2–3 years (rather than annually) are:
- Well-screened: Had 3 or more documented, consecutive, technically satisfactory normal/negative cervical cytology tests, and no abnormal/positive cytology tests within the past 10 years
- No history of CIN 2 or 3
- Not immunocompromised, DES-exposed, or HIV-positive

EPIDEMIOLOGY
- Most cases of cervical cancer are found in women:
  - Who have never had Pap screening
  - Have not had Pap screening in the past 5 years
  - >55
- 11,500 new cases expected in 2007
- 3,670 deaths expected in 2007

RISK FACTORS
- HPV infection (HPV infection is common; most women with HPV will not develop cervical cancer.)
- Multiple sexual partners
- Early onset of sexual activity
- Smoking
- Immunosuppression and/or chronic steroid use

ASSOCIATED CONDITIONS
Immunosuppression; women with HIV, diabetes, conditions requiring chronic steroid use (e.g., severe asthma, rheumatoid arthritis) are at increased risk of cervical dysplasia and cervical carcinoma

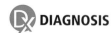

DIAGNOSIS

TESTS
Lab
Pap test (2 types):
- Conventional: Obtained with spatula + cytobrush or cervical broom; specimen smeared onto glass slide then fixative applied (spray or liquid)
- Liquid-based: Obtained with cervical broom; placed into liquid-filled container. Major advantages:
  - Ability to test for HPV, gonorrhea, and *Chlamydia* from liquid
  - Decreased amount of extraneous material in final slide
  - Greater sensitivity than conventional Pap test

DIFFERENTIAL DIAGNOSIS
Infection
- Presence of inflammatory debris with cervicitis or vaginitis may obscure or compromise the interpretation of cervical cytology, particularly with conventional Pap test.
- In patient with suspected cervical or vaginal infection, either:
  - Obtain Pap and treat infection simultaneously
  - Treat infection and obtain Pap after treatment
  - Pros/Cons: If Pap obtained during infection, may need to repeat Pap. If infection treated 1st, patient may not return for Pap later.

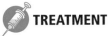 **TREATMENT**

GENERAL MEASURES
Geriatric Considerations
Postmenopausal women:

- Atrophy can mimic cervical cytologic abnormalities.
- If patient is postmenopausal (with no risk factors or prior history of abnormal Paps), consider short course of vaginal//oral/transdermal patch estrogen and repeat Pap.

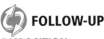 **FOLLOW-UP**

DISPOSITION
Issues for Referral
- Results of Pap dictate follow-up.
- No abnormalities: Regular screening
- ASCUS, LSIL, HSIL: See ASCCP and other recommendations for follow-up and treatment

PROGNOSIS
The widespread adoption of cervical cytology screening in the US resulted in a 74% reduction in deaths from cervical cancer from 1955–1992.

BIBLIOGRAPHY

American Cancer Society. Detailed Guide: Can Cervical Cancer Be Prevented? http://www.cancer.org/docroot/CRI/content/CRI_2_4_2X_Can_cervical_cancer_be_prevented_8.asp?sitearea=. Accessed 09/06/07.

American College of Obstetricians and Gynecologists. Cervical Cytology Screening. ACOG Practice Bulletin No. 45. *Obstet Gynecol*. 2003;102:417–427.

American Society for Colposcopy and Cervical Pathology (ASCCP 2001 Bethesda Consensus Guideline), http://www.asccp.org/consensus.shtml.

U.S. Preventive Services Task Force. Screening for Cervical Cancer: Recommendations and Rationale. AHRQ Publication No. 03-515A. January 2003. Rockville MD: Agency for Healthcare Research and Quality, http://www.ahrq.gov/clinic/3rduspstf/cervcan/cervcanrr.htm.

 MISCELLANEOUS

ABBREVIATIONS
- ACOG—American College of Obstetricians & Gynecologists
- ACS—American Cancer Society
- ASC-H—Atypical squamous cells, cannot exclude HSIL
- ASCUS—Atypical squamous cells of undetermined significance
- CIN—Cervical intraepithelial neoplasia
- DES—Diethylstilbestrol
- HPV—Human papillomavirus
- HSIL—High-grade squamous intraepithelial lesion
- LSIL—Low-grade squamous intraepithelial lesion
- TBS—Bethesda system
- USPSTF—US Preventive Services Task Force

 PATIENT TEACHING

- Regular Pap smears are important.
- Pap smear frequency depends on history, risk factors, patient and provider preference
- End of child-bearing does not mean end of need for Pap screening
- Even women who receive HPV vaccine needs Pap screening

PREVENTION
ALERT
- HPV vaccine will prevent up to 70% of cervical cancer cases.
- Even women who receive the HPV vaccine must continue to undergo regular Pap screening.

Section III

CANCER SCREENING: COLORECTAL CANCER

Jennifer Lang, MD
Beth Y. Karlan, MD

 BASICS

DESCRIPTION

- Colorectal cancers are by definition cancers that develop in the colon or the rectum.
- The colon is divided into 4 parts: Ascending, transverse, descending, and rectosigmoid colon.
- Most cancers develop slowly, over years.
- Adenomatous polyps have the potential to become cancer.
- Hyperplastic and inflammatory polyps are not precancerous, but may reflect a greater likelihood of developing colorectal cancers.
- Dysplasia is a precancerous condition, usually found in patients with ulcerative colitis or Crohn's disease.
- 95% of colorectal cancers are adenocarcinomas. Less common types are:
  - Carcinoid tumors
  - GI stromal tumors
  - Lymphomas

Age-Related Factors

- Risk of colorectal cancers increases dramatically >50 years.
- >90% of colorectal cancers are diagnosed in patients >50.

EPIDEMIOLOGY

- Colorectal cancers are the 3rd most common cancers, and the 2nd leading cause of cancer-related deaths in the US.
- 75,810 new cases were diagnosed in US women in 2006.
- 27,300 women died from colorectal cancer in 2006.
- A woman's lifetime risk of developing colorectal cancer is 1:18.
- Her lifetime risk of dying from colorectal cancer is 1:45.

RISK FACTORS

- Age >50
- Personal history of colorectal cancer
- History of polyps
- History of ulcerative colitis or Crohn's disease
- Family history of colorectal cancer
- African American race
- Diet high in fats, especially from animal sources
- Obesity
- Smoking
- Heavy use of alcohol
- Diabetes

Genetics

- 15% of colorectal cancers are considered hereditary, or "familial."
- 3–5% have a known inherited genetic susceptibility
- HNPCC or Lynch syndrome (3–4%):
  - Autosomal dominant inheritance pattern
  - Genetic defect involves microsatellite instability and mutations in DNA mismatch repair gene families MLH 1 and MSH 2.

ALERT

- Also at increased risk for endometrial, ovarian, gastric, small bowel, pancreatic, renal, ureteral and biliary carcinomas
- Many women with HNPCC will originally present with abnormal vaginal bleeding and endometrial cancer.
- FAP:
  - Develop hundreds of polyps in the colon and rectum
  - Polyps become cancerous beginning age 20, almost 100% of patients will develop cancer by age 40 if no surgical prophylaxis

PATHOPHYSIOLOGY

Colon polyps can be premalignant and develop into cancer if left undetected and untreated.

ASSOCIATED CONDITIONS

Endometrial and ovarian malignancies

 DIAGNOSIS

SIGNS AND SYMPTOMS

History

- Take a detailed medical history.
- Age
- Past medical history:
  - IBD
  - Colonic polyps: Precancerous or cancerous
  - Other cancers (may suggest syndrome, such as Lynch)
  - Diabetes
- Compliance with recommended screening tests:
  - Last fecal occult blood test
  - Last flexible sigmoidoscopy or colonoscopy
- Medications:
  - Multivitamin containing folate
  - Use of HRT
- Family history:
  - Relatives with known cancers or precancerous lesions
  - Their age at time of diagnosis
- Social history:
  - Diet
  - Exercise habits
  - Smoking
- Review of systems with special attention to GI system:
  - Weight loss, weight gain
  - Abdominal pain, bloating, early satiety
  - Bowel movements: Frequency, change in caliber, blood in stool
- Special attention to GU system:
  - Abnormal menses
  - Postmenopausal bleeding

Physical Exam

Digital rectal exam

TESTS

ALERT

- Begin screening for colorectal cancer in average-risk individuals at age 50.
- Utilize 1 of the following options:
  - Yearly patient-collected fecal occult blood testing
  - Flexible sigmoidoscopy every 5 years
  - Yearly patient-collected fecal occult blood testing plus flexible sigmoidoscopy every 5 years
  - Double contrast barium enema every 5 years
  - Colonoscopy every 10 years
- All positive tests should be followed-up by colonoscopy
- Virtual colonoscopy, another acceptable screening method, is more sensitive and specific than barium enema, but less so than colonoscopy.
- Single-sample FOBT done at the time of annual exam should not be used for screening because of extremely low specificity

SPECIFIC DISEASES

Drugs

Some medications have been associated with both increased and decreased risks of colorectal cancers:

- 5–ASA, used to treat IBD, may decrease colorectal cancers.
- HRT use reduces the risk of colorectal cancer and may improve survival after diagnosis of colorectal cancer.

SPECIAL GROUPS

Adolescents

- Colorectal cancer is extremely rare in childhood.
- An inherited predisposition should be excluded based on family history and/or genetic testing.
- These patients are at risk for developing secondary GI and extraintestinal malignancies.

Women with Chronic Illness

- Women with IBD (ulcerative colitis or Crohn's disease) should have regular screening for colorectal cancers.
- Many may benefit from 5–ASA to treat their disease and decrease risk of colon cancer.

Geriatric Considerations

- Decisions to stop colorectal cancer screening should be made individually based on several guidelines:
  - Individuals with a life-expectancy of <5 years should not be screened.
  - Individuals who, after extensive counseling, would decline treatment should not be screened
- Decisions to continue or discontinue screening in the elderly should be based on:
  - Health status
  - Benefits and potential harms of the test
  - Preferences of the patient
  - Should NOT be based solely on age

BIBLIOGRAPHY

Cheng X, et al. Subsite-specific incidence and stage of disease in colorectal cancer by race, gender and age group in the United States 1992–1997. *Cancer*. 2001;92(10):2547–2554.

Cotton PB, et al. Computer tomographic colonography (virtual colonoscopy): A multicenter comparison with standard colonoscopy for detection of colorectal neoplasia. *JAMA*. 2004;291:1713–1719.

Durno C, et al. Family history and molecular features of children, adolescents and young adults with colorectal carcinoma. *Gut*. 2005;54:1146–1150.

Gross CP, et al. Relation between Medicare screening reimbursement and stage at diagnosis for older patients with colon cancer. *JAMA*. 2006; 296(23):2815–2822.

Harewood GC, et al. A prospective controlled assessment of factors influencing acceptance of screening colonoscopy. *Am J Gastroenterol*. 2002; 97(12):3186–3194.

Jemal A, et al. Cancer Statistics 2006. *CA Cancer J Clin*. 2006;56:106–130.

Kinney AY, et al. Colorectal cancer surveillance behaviors among members of typical and attenuate FAP families. *Am J Gastroenterol*. 2007;102(1): 153–162.

Luciani MG, et al. 5-5-ASA affects cell cycle progression in colorectal cells by reversibly activating a replication checkpoint. *Gastroenterology* 2007;132(1):221–235.

Lynch HT, et al. Lynch syndrome: Genetics, natural history, genetic counseling, and prevention. *J Clin Oncol*. 2000;18(21 Suppl):19S–31S.

Mandelson MT, et al. Hormone replacement therapy in relation to survival in women diagnosed with colon cancer. *Cancer Causes Control*. 2003;14(10): 979–984.

Reddy BS, et al. Prevention of colon cancer by low doses of celecoxib, a cyclooxygenase inhibitor, administered in diet rich in omega-3 polyunsaturated fatty acids. *Cancer Res*. 2005;65(17):8022–8027.

Schroy PC 3rd, et al. Family history and colorectal cancer screening: A survey of physician knowledge and practice patterns. *Am J Gastroenterol*. 2002;97(4):1031–1036.

Smith RA, et al. American Cancer Society guidelines for the early detection of cancer: Update of early detection guidelines for prostate, colorectal and endometrial cancers. *CA Cancer J Clin*. 2001; 51:150.

Walter LC, et al. Screening for colorectal, breast and cervical cancer in the elderly: A review of the evidence. *Am J Med*. 2005;118(10):1078–1086.

MISCELLANEOUS

ACCESS ISSUES

- Most insurance plans cover routine cancer screening, including colorectal cancer.
- Underinsured patients may avoid screening programs for fear of medical expenses.
- Changes in Medicare reimbursement for screening colonoscopy and greater public awareness have led to increased use of colonoscopy and increased probability of being diagnosed at an early stage.

CLINICAL PEARLS

- Begin colorectal cancer screening in average-risk individuals at age 50 by 1 of the following options:
  - Yearly patient-collected fecal occult blood testing
  - Flexible sigmoidoscopy every 5 years
  - Yearly patient-collected fecal occult blood testing plus flexible sigmoidoscopy every 5 years
  - Double-contrast barium enema every 5 years
  - Colonoscopy every 10 years
- All positive tests should be followed up by colonoscopy
- High-risk factors:
  - Colorectal cancer or adenomatous polyps in a 1st-degree relative <60 or 2 1st-degree relatives of any ages
  - Family history of FAP or HNPCC
  - Personal history of colorectal cancer, adenomatous polyps, ulcerative colitis, Crohn's disease
- Screen high-risk individuals earlier:
  - FAP: Start screening in teen years
  - HNPCC: Start screening in 20s, annual colonoscopy should begin by age 40
  - Women from HNPCC families should be screened for endometrial cancer
- Sigmoidoscopy alone will miss 50% of colon cancers

ABBREVIATIONS

- CRC—Colorectal cancer
- FAP—Familial adenomatous polyposis
- FOBT—Fecal occult blood test
- GI—Gastrointestinal
- HNPCC—Hereditary non-polyposis colon cancer
- HRT—Hormone replacement therapy
- IBD—Inflammatory bowel disease

CODES

ICD9-CM

- 45.23 Colonoscopy
- 45.24 Sigmoidoscopy (flexible)
- 45.25 Colonoscopy with biopsy
- 45.42 Colonoscopy with polypectomy
- 88.01 Virtual colonoscopy
- 153.9 Malignant neoplasm of the colon, unspecified
- 211.3 Benign polyps of the colon
- 558.9 Inflammatory bowel disease

PATIENT TEACHING

- Encourage an active lifestyle, diet low in saturated fats from animal sources and high in fruits, vegetables, and whole grain foods.
- Encourage compliance with screening protocols. Colorectal cancers are preventable if precancerous polyps are identified and removed.
- Teach patients to recognize signs and symptoms that may indicate colorectal cancer and to seek contact with a healthcare provider if they experience any of these signs or symptoms.
- American Cancer Society Web site www.cancer.org
- American Society of Colon & Rectal Surgeons (ASCRS) www.fascrs.org
- National Cancer Institute www.cancer.gov
- Colon Cancer Foundation www.coloncancerfoundation.org

CANCER SCREENING: LUNG CANCER

Jennifer B. Hillman, MD
Corinne Lehmann, MD

 BASICS

DESCRIPTION

There are 4 major histologic types of lung cancer:

- Adenocarcinoma: 30–40%
- Squamous cell carcinoma: 20–30%
- Large cell carcinoma: 10%
- Small cell carcinoma: 20%

Age-Related Factors

- More women than men have a diagnosis of lung cancer before age 50 years.
- Highest incidence of lung cancer at ages 55–65

Staging

- See "Revised International Staging System, 1997"; tumor (T), nodal involvement (N), metastasis (M):
- Stage is based on TNM status:
  - Stage IA: T1N0M0
  - Stage IB: T2N0M0
  - Stage IIA: T1N1M0
  - Stage IIB: T2N1M0, T3N1M0
  - Stage IIIA: T3N1M0, T1N2M0, T2N2M0, T3N2M0
  - Stage IIIB: T4N0M0, T4N1M0, T4N2M0, T1N3M0, T2N3M0, T3N3M0, T4N3M0
  - Stage IV: Any T, any N, M1

EPIDEMIOLOGY

- Lung cancer is the leading cause of cancer mortality in men and women worldwide.
- Lung cancer mortality among women has dramatically increased since the 1960s:
  - Surpassed breast cancer in 1987
  - 2 times as many women in the US are expected to die from lung vs. breast cancer

RISK FACTORS

- Cigarette smoking:
  - Estimated to account for 80–90% of cases:
    - RR for development of lung cancer in smokers vs. nonsmokers 10–30
    - RR of 1.5 among those exposed to long-term 2nd-hand smoke
    - Magnitude of risk increases with duration and total exposure level.
- Female gender:
  - Women have a higher RR per given exposure to cigarette smoking than men.
  - Women with lung cancer are more likely than men to never have smoked.

Genetics

Family history of lung cancer is a risk factor:

- Significant interaction with smoking

PATHOPHYSIOLOGY

- Carcinogens and tumor promoters ingested via cigarette smoking.
- Molecular genetic studies of lung cancer cells reveals activation of dominant oncogenes and inactivation of tumor suppressor genes

ASSOCIATED CONDITIONS

Paraneoplastic syndromes are common:

- Hypercalcemia
- SIADH
- Eaton-Lambert syndrome (disorder of neuromuscular junction transmission, manifesting as muscle weakness)

 DIAGNOSIS

SIGNS AND SYMPTOMS

History

- Majority of patients are symptomatic at time of presentation:
  - Symptoms may be related to primary lung mass:
    - Cough: 45–75% of all cases
    - Hemoptysis: 27–57%
    - Chest pain: 25–50%
    - Dysphagia
    - Hoarseness
    - Dyspnea
    - Horner syndrome (see below)
  - Symptoms related to local or distant metastatic lesions:
    - Pleural effusion
    - SVC syndrome
    - Bone pain
    - Neurologic symptoms due to brain metastasis: Seizures, nausea, confusion
  - Other symptoms:
    - Weight loss
    - Venous thrombosis
- 10% of patients are asymptomatic at time of diagnosis
  - Diagnosed by routine CXR

Review of Systems

Virtually every organ system may be affected

Physical Exam

- Examination may be completely normal.
- Some findings on exam may include the following:
  - Cachexia
  - Focal neurologic examination
  - Digital clubbing
  - Lung examination abnormalities:
    - Unilateral wheezing, crackles, dullness to percussion
    - Asymmetrically decreased breath sounds due to elevated hemidiaphragm
  - Findings of SVC syndrome:
    - Facial or upper extremity swelling
    - Plethora
    - Dilated neck veins
  - Findings of Horner' syndrome: Exophthalmos, ptosis, miosis, ipsilateral loss of sweating

TESTS

> **ALERT**
> - Currently no recommended screening guidelines for lung cancer
> - Previous studies have evaluated targeted use of sputum cytology, CXR:
>   - Studies only included men
>   - No survival difference in the screened vs. nonscreened groups
> - Use of low-dose spiral CT scan of the chest more recently evaluated as screening measure:
>   - Screened at-risk men and women
>   - No convincing evidence to recommend widespread screening with chest CT yet

Labs

Staging laboratory testing after diagnosis of lung cancer includes:

- CBC
- Serum electrolytes, including phosphorous, calcium, and magnesium
- Liver function testing
- Glucose
- EKG
- Tuberculosis skin testing
- Pulmonary function testing (respiratory insufficiency)
- Arterial blood gas (respiratory insufficiency)

Imaging

Additional staging should include:

- CXR
- Radiograph of suspicious bony lesions
- CT scan chest, abdomen, and pelvis
- CT scan head if suspicious for brain metastasis
- Consider MRI of brain if locally advanced or metastatic disease
- PET scan
- Barium swallow exam (esophageal symptoms)
- Radionuclide scan of bone if suspected metastasis, PET scan not available

DIFFERENTIAL DIAGNOSIS

- Finding a primary lung mass on CT or CXR as the 1st sign of lung cancer is rare but does occur.
- SPNs are usually 1–6 cm densities seen on CXR, surrounded by normal lung tissue, with circumscribed margins, of any shape:
  - 35% of SPNs in adults are malignant.
  - <1% are malignant in nonsmokers <35 years of age

Infection

- Some types of pneumonia may appear round and mass-like:
  - Consider postobstructive pneumonia:
    - Patients with exposure to tobacco or asbestos
- Pulmonary tuberculosis
- Fungal infections: Histoplasmosis, coccidiosis

Tumor/Malignancy

Breast cancer:

- Metastatic lesions to lungs are common.
- Breast mass may appear to be intrathoracic on CXR.

TREATMENT

GENERAL MEASURES
- Primary prevention of tobacco use and cigarette smoking is critical.
- Secondary prevention through smoking cessation programs reduces risk of lung cancer.
- Treatment is based on categorization as small cell verses non–small cell, and stage.
- Non–small cell lung cancer:
  - Surgical resection for stages IA, IB, IIA, IIB and some IIIA can be curative:
    - Discussion of potential risks/benefits of adjuvant chemotherapy
    - Curative potential with radiation therapy for "nonoperable" patients
  - Stage IIIA:
    - Surgical resection with complete mediastinal lymph node resection and consideration of preoperative chemotherapy
  - Stage IIIB:
    - Chemotherapy combined with radiation therapy
  - Stage IV:
    - Radiation therapy to symptomatic local sites
    - 2-agent chemotherapy for ambulatory patients
- Small cell lung cancer:
  - Limited stage:
    - Combination chemotherapy and radiation therapy
    - Consider prophylactic cranial radiation therapy for chemo responders
  - Extensive stage:
    - Combination chemotherapy

SPECIAL THERAPY
Complementary and Alternative Therapies
- Smoking cessation is critical to the reduction of risk for lung cancer:
  - Support groups and other smoking cessation programs can be helpful.
- Chemoprevention among smokers has not been proven to be a useful intervention:
  - Vitamin E and β-carotene actually increase the risk of lung cancer in heavy smokers.

MEDICATION (DRUGS)
- Use of bupropion, nicotine replacement, and the combination of bupropion and nicotine replacement greatly increases likelihood and duration of smoking cessation.
- Zyban or bupropion SR:
  - Patient should plan to quit after 5–7 days of treatment
  - Begin 150 mg/d for 3 days
  - Increase to 150 mg PO b.i.d. for 7–12 weeks

- Nicotine replacement has various forms and doses:
  - Nicotine transdermal patch:
    - Smoking cessation should begin with onset of nicotine replacement therapy
    - Start 21 mg/24 hr patch if smoking >10 cigarettes/d
    - Decrease to 14 mg/24 hr patch after 6 weeks
    - Decrease to 7 mg/24 hr patch after 2 weeks
    - Discontinue patch after 2 weeks
  - Nicotine gum, >25 cigarettes/d:
    - Start 4-mg piece gum q1–2h for 6 weeks
    - Decrease to 1 piece q2–4h for 3 weeks
    - Decrease to 1 piece q4–8h for 3 weeks, then discontinue
    - Maximum: 20 pieces/d
  - Nicotine gum, <25 cigarettes/d:
    - Start with 2-mg piece gum q1–2h for 6 weeks
    - Follow taper outlined above
  - Nicotine replacement is also available as lozenges, nasal spray, and inhaler.
- New medication varenicline (Chantrix) was FDA approved for use in smoking cessation 2006:
  - Partial nicotine agonist helping to reduce cravings for nicotine
  - Appears to be equally or more efficacious than bupropion SR
  - Patient should plan to quit after 7 days of treatment:
    - Start 0.5 mg PO daily for 3 days
    - Increase to 0.5 mg PO b.i.d. for 4 days
    - Titrate to 1 mg PO b.i.d. for 12 weeks

SURGERY
See "General Measures."

FOLLOW-UP

DISPOSITION
Issues for Referral
- Diagnosis or concern for lung cancer should prompt referral to a trained specialist and may involve referral to multidisciplinary team that includes medical oncologist, radiation oncologist, pulmonary specialist, and thoracic surgeon.
- OB/GYN may recommend follow-up with primary clinician for smoking cessation, including medication and/or nicotine replacement.

PROGNOSIS
- Prognosis for smoking cessation:
  - Relapse is common:
    - On average takes 2 to 3 attempts
    - Those who quit for ≥ 3 months are more likely to remain cigarettefree for life.
  - 10–15 years after quitting, the risk of premature death approaches that of someone who has never smoked.
  - Women who stop smoking before becoming pregnant or within the 1st 3 months of pregnancy can reverse the risks of low birth weight and other pregnancy-related risks.
- Overall prognosis of lung cancer is poor:
  - 5–year survival rate is 14%

- Patients with stage I or II non–small cell lung cancer treated with surgery have a 50–85% 5-year survival rate.
- Long-term survivors are at risk for a 2nd primary lung cancer: 3–5%/yr

PATIENT MONITORING
Continued follow-up with multidisciplinary team is recommended.

BIBLIOGRAPHY

Baldini EH. Women and Lung Cancer. Up To Date, 2006.

Kasper DL, et al. *Harrison's Principles of Internal Medicine*, 16th Ed. New York: McGraw-Hill; 2006.

Lancaster T, et al. Physician advice for smoking cessation. *Cochrane Database Syst Rev* 2004; 4:CD000165. DOI: 10.1002/14651858. CD000165.pub2

Mountain CL. Revisions in the international system for staging lung cancer. *Chest*. 1997;111:1710–1717.

Strauss GM. Overview and Clinical Manifestations of Lung Cancer. Up To Date, 2006.

The International Early Lung Cancer Action Program Investigators. Survival of patients with stage I lung cancer detected on CT screening. *N Engl J Med*. 2006;355:1763–1771.

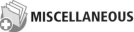

MISCELLANEOUS

ABBREVIATIONS
- RR—Relative risk
- SIADH—Syndrome of inappropriate antidiuretic hormone
- SPN—Solitary pulmonary nodule
- SVC—Superior vena cava

CODES
ICD9-CM
231.0–231.9 Malignant neoplasm of respiratory and intrathoracic organs

PATIENT TEACHING

- Resources from the American Lung Association at http://www.lungusa.org
- National Cancer Institute (NCI) http://www.cancer.gov/cancertopics/smoking
- Information for patients trying to quit smoking http://smokefree.gov/
- Office on Smoking and Health of the Centers for Disease Control and Prevention http://www.cdc.gov/tobacco/

PREVENTION
- Primary prevention of tobacco use and cigarette smoking is critical:
  - Discourage smoking at routine visits, particularly among adolescents and young adults.
- Secondary prevention through smoking cessation programs reduces risk of lung cancer:
  - Assess readiness for smoking cessation during any encounter with a current smoker.

CANCER SCREENING: MAMMOGRAPHY

Carolyn D. Runowicz, MD
Merieme Klobocista, MD

 BASICS

DESCRIPTION
- A screening mammogram is used to detect breast cancer in asymptomatic women.
- Low-dose x-ray that allows visualization of the internal structures of the breast:
  - Film screen or digital mammography:
    - The DMIST trial showed the 2 techniques overall are equal in screening.
    - Digital mammography detects breast cancer better in women: <50 years, women with heterogeneously dense or extremely dense breast on mammography, and pre- or perimenopausal women.
- Single most effective method of early detection:
  - Mammography detects 80–90% of breast cancer in asymptomatic women.
- Although women should be informed about the benefits and limitations of screening and the possibility of harms associated with false-positive findings, mammography saves lives through the early detection of breast cancer.

Age-Related Factors
- The incidence and mortality rates from breast cancer increase with age:
  - 95% of new cases occurred in women >40 in 1998–2002.
  - 97% of breast cancer deaths occurred in women >40 in 1998–2002.
  - For women <45, the 5-year relative survival rates are slightly lower than for women >45.

EPIDEMIOLOGY
- Breast cancer is the most common malignancy diagnosed in women, and it is the 2nd leading cause of death from cancer in women.
- 1 in 8 lifetime risk of developing breast cancer
- Decline in mortality is attributed to improvements in early detection, therapy, and awareness.

RISK FACTORS
- The most important risk factors for breast cancer are age and sex.
- Nonmodifiable risk factors:
  - Family history (5–10% result from inherited mutations, mostly BRCA1 and BRCA2)
  - Age at 1st birth
  - Age at menarche (<12)
  - Age at menopause
  - Dense breasts
- Modifiable:
  - Postmenopausal obesity
  - Use of hormone therapy
  - Alcohol consumption
  - Physical inactivity
- The Gail model has been used to assess short-term and lifetime risk of breast cancer. Because it utilizes limited family history, it should not be used if the patient's family history is the primary source of risk:
  - Risk is based on age of menarche, age at birth of 1st child, number of breast biopsies, the presence of atypical hyperplasia, and limited family history.
- BRCAPRO model is used to determine the likelihood of BRCA1/2 mutations and to estimate the lifetime risk of breast cancer.
- The Claus model can be used to estimate either short-term or lifetime risk of breast cancer. It is useful for women with affected 1st- and 2nd-degree relatives:
  - Risk is based on family history and age of cancer onset.
- Additional risk factors include previous chest irradiation, a personal history of breast cancer, or a family history of diseases associated with breast cancer such as Li-Fraumeni or Cowden syndromes.
- Chemoprevention:
  - Tamoxifen has been shown to reduce the risk of breast cancer (invasive and ductal carcinoma in situ).
  - Raloxifene has been shown to reduce the risk of invasive breast cancer with a safer risk profile than tamoxifen.
- Surgical prevention:
  - Prophylactic mastectomy

Genetics
- After controlling for age and sex, the greatest increase in risk for breast cancer has been a strong family history, especially BRCA1 and BRCA2 carriers.
  - These genes are associated with an increased risk of breast cancer and ovarian cancer.
  - However, only 5–10% of breast cancer is due to inherited mutations.
- Risk factors associated with genetic mutations:
  - History of >2 relatives with breast or ovarian cancer
  - Breast cancer before age 50 in a relative or in the patient
  - Relatives with both breast and ovarian cancer
  - >1 relatives with 2 cancers (breast/ovary)
  - Male relatives with breast cancer
  - A family history of breast or ovarian cancer and Ashkenazi Jewish heritage
- Risk can be inherited from maternal and paternal side. When risk is inherited from the paternal side, there may be no history of an affected 1st-degree relative.

PATHOPHYSIOLOGY
- During the introduction of mammography from 1980–1987, incidence rates of smaller tumors (<2 cm) more than doubled.
- From 1988–1999, the trend continued and stabilized after 1999.
- Most cases of ductal carcinoma in situ are detectable only through mammography.

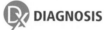 **DIAGNOSIS**

SIGNS AND SYMPTOMS
History
Breast surgery, family history of breast or ovarian cancer, previous hx atypical hyperplasia or LCIS on bx

Physical Exam
- Recommendations for CBE:
  - For average-risk asymptomatic women:
    - Age 20–40: Part of periodic health exam, at least every 3 years
    - >40: Part of a periodic health exam annually
- Recommendations for BSE:
  - Women should be educated about benefits and limitations of BSE beginning in their 20s.

Imaging
- Screening mammography (Screen-film or full-field digital):
  - Average risk patient: Annual, begin at age 40.
- High risk patient: Options to consider are:
  - Begin at age 30 or earlier if clinically indicated and/or
  - Shorter mammography screening intervals (e.g., every 6 months) and/or
  - Addition of MRI screening and/or
  - Addition of US screening
- Older women: Take into consideration current health status and estimated life expectancy:
  - If a woman is in good health and is a candidate for treatment, then screening should be continued.
  - If a woman has a limited life expectancy (e.g., <3–5 years), functional limitations, and/or multiple or severe comorbidities, cessation of screening can be considered.
- Risks of mammography:
  - Missed cancers (10–20%)
  - False-positives that may result in anxiety, repeat radiologic studies, needle aspiration or biopsy. ~5–10% of women have their mammograms interpreted as abnormal or inconclusive until further tests are done.
- US:
  - Diagnostic adjunct to mammography
  - Image-guided biopsy of a mass
- MRI:
  - Diagnostic adjunct to mammography and breast US
  - Used for screening in high-risk women (e.g., BRCA mutations)

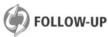 **FOLLOW-UP**

DISPOSITION
Issues for Referral
A persistent palpable breast mass requires evaluation: A normal mammography alone is not always sufficient to rule out malignancy.

BIBLIOGRAPHY

Breast Cancer Facts & Figures 2005–2006. American Cancer Society, 2005.

Pisano ED, et al. Diagnostic performance of digital versus film mammography for breast-cancer screening. N Engl J Med. 2005;353:1773–1783.

Smith R, et al. American Cancer Society Guidelines for Breast Cancer Screening: Update 2003. CA Cancer J Clin. 2003;53:141–169.

Vogel VG, et al. Effects of tamoxifen vs raloxifene on the risk of developing invasive breast cancer and other disease outcomes: The NSABP Study of Tamoxifen and Raloxifene (STAR) P-2 Trial. JAMA. 2006;295:2727–2741.

Wender R, et al. Cancer screening. Prim Care Clin Office Pract. 2002;29:697–725.

 MISCELLANEOUS

ABBREVIATIONS
- BSE—Breast self-exam
- CBE—Clinical breast exam
- LCIS—Lobular carcinoma in situ

American Cancer Society Guidelines for Early Breast Cancer Detection, 2003

Women at Average Risk   Begin mammography at age 40.

For women in their 20s and 30s, it is recommended that clinical breast examination be part of a periodic health examination, preferably at least every 3 years. Asymptomatic women aged 40 and older should continue to receive a clinical breast examination as part of a periodic health examination, preferably annually.

Beginning in their 20s, women should be told about the benefits and limitations of breast self-examination (BSE). The importance of prompt reporting of any new breast symptoms to a health professional should be emphasized. Women who choose to do BSE should receive instructions and have their technique reviewed on the occasion of a periodic health examination. It is acceptable for women to choose not to do BSE or to do BSE irregularly.

Women should have an opportunity to become informed about the benefits, limitations, and potential harms associated with regular screening.

Older Women   Screening decisions in older women should be individualized by considering the potential benefits and risks of mammography in the context of current health status and estimated life expectancy. As long as a woman is in reasonably good health and would be a candidate for treatment, she should continue to be screened with mammography.

Women at Increased Risk   Women at increased risk of breast cancer might benefit from additional screening strategies beyond those offered to women of average risk, such as earlier initiation of screening, shorter screening intervals, or the addition of screening modalities other than mammography and physical examination, such as ultrasound or magnetic resonance imaging. However, the evidence currently available is insufficient to justify recommendations for any screening approaches.

Section III

CONTRACEPTION, BARRIER: MALE CONDOMS

Susan M. Coupey, MD
Dominic Hollman, MD

BASICS

DESCRIPTION
- The male condom is a common, well-known form of barrier contraception. It is placed over the penis, covering the glans and shaft, and mechanically prevents semen from reaching the female reproductive system.
- History:
  - Described as early as 1564 by Italian anatomist Gabriello Fallopio
  - Casanova referred to them in his memoirs (18th century)
  - Originally made from animal intestine (sheep, calves, goats)
  - Vulcanized rubber developed by Hancock & Goodyear (1840s) led to less expensive production
  - Development of latex in 1930s led to condoms of greater tensile strength, longer shelf life
  - Increased popularity in 1980s due to recommendation of condom use for prevention of AIDS
- Characteristics:
  - Made from latex, polyurethane, synthetic elastomers (Tactylon), or natural membrane (lambskin)
  - Thickness ranges from 0.03–0.1 mm
  - Reservoir tip available for collection of semen
  - Manufactured in a range of sizes
  - Available with or without lubricant
  - Available with or without spermicide (i.e., nonoxynol-9)
  - Variety of textures, colors, or flavors

Age-Related Factors
- Recommended for use by sexually active males without age restriction
- Higher failure rate observed in adolescents, likely due to improper use

EPIDEMIOLOGY
- Condoms are the 3rd most common method of birth control for all US women: 9 million women and their partners.
- Condoms are the most common method of birth control used at 1st intercourse.
- 11% of all women age 15–44 report condoms as their current method of contraception.
- Of women who have had sex, 90% report using a condom at least once.
- Recent evidence shows adolescents are more likely to use condoms with a "casual" partner than with a "serious" partner.

MECHANISMS OF ACTION
Mechanically prevents semen from reaching female genital tract, thus preventing fertilization.

EFFICACY
- With perfect use, the pregnancy rate is 2–3% per year. Typical use results in 5–15% pregnancy rate per year.
  - Consistent, concurrent use of male condom and female condom provides efficacy approaching that of hormonal contraceptives.
- No increase in efficacy with spermicide-lubricated condoms
- Rate of breakage: 0–7%
- Rate of slippage: 0–6%
  - Rates of breakage and slippage increased in polyurethane as compared to latex condoms
  - Increased breakage, no difference of slippage rate in Tactylon as compared to latex

DIAGNOSIS

HISTORY
Medical history:
- Condom purchase does not require a medical history or a doctor visit.

Physical Exam
Not indicated

TESTS
Lab
Not indicated

Imaging
Not indicated

TREATMENT

MEDICATIONS/DRUG INTERACTIONS
- Latex condoms should not be used with oil-based lubricants:
  - Oil-based lubricants degrade latex in <60 seconds.
  - Avoid petroleum-based products, body oils, and lotions.
  - Oil-based lubricants may be used with nonlatex condoms.
- Intravaginal antifungals can cause degradation of latex:
  - Condom efficacy is decreased when used concurrently with these medications.
- Latex condoms should not be used by latex-allergic individuals

PATIENT SELECTION
All sexually active males

Indications
- Prevention of pregnancy
- Prevention of STIs

Contraindications
Latex allergy

Informed Consent
Available without prescription. Patient should be informed about proper condom use.

Patient Education
Efforts to educate the US population occur in clinical, community, and school settings:
- Clinical: Many organizations have provided guidelines for patient education including:
  - American Academy of Pediatrics
  - American Medical Association
  - American Academy of Family Physicians
  - US Department of Health and Human Services
- Community:
  - Youth development programs
  - Community-based HIV prevention programs
  - Television advertising remains controversial; many stations are resistant
- School programs take various forms:
  - Abstinence-only programs
  - Pregnancy prevention programs: Have resulted in increased condom use
  - HIV prevention programs: Have resulted in increased condom use

Risks
- Minimal risk exists with condom use:
  - Latex allergy
  - Improper use may result in decreased prevention of pregnancy or disease transmission
- Factors which may lead to nonuse:
  - Reduced spontaneity
  - Decreased sensation for some partners (improved sensation reported with polyurethane condoms)
  - Difficulty maintaining erection
  - Genital irritation

Benefits, Including Noncontraceptive
- Condoms are effective in preventing STIs:
  - Reduction in STI transmission is well-documented with latex condoms; evidence is less available for polyurethane or Tactylon.
  - Natural-membrane condoms do not prevent HIV or other STIs due to relatively large pores, which do not prevent viral passage.
- Condoms reduce the rate of transmission of the following:
  - HIV
  - *Neisseria gonorrhoeae*
  - *Chlamydia trachomatis*
  - *Treponema pallidum*
  - HSV-2
  - Hepatitis B virus
  - *Trichomonas vaginalis*
  - HPV:
    - ○ Condom usage promotes regression of CIN and enhances the clearance of HPV
    - ○ Skin-to-skin transmission of infections (HSV, HPV) may still occur by contact of skin not covered by condom.
- Additional benefits:
  - Accessibility (no prescription required and widely available)
  - Low cost
  - Easy to use
  - No systemic effects
  - Reversibility
  - May prolong intercourse
  - Involves the male in preventive health decisions

Alternatives
- Multiple other contraceptive methods are available.
- Combined estrogen/progestin hormonal methods:
  - OCP
  - Contraceptive patch
  - Vaginal ring
- Progestin-only hormonal methods:
  - DMPA injection
  - POP
  - Mirena IUD
- IUDs:
  - Mirena IUD
  - Copper IUD
- Nonhormonal methods:
  - Diaphragm
  - Cervical cap
  - Sponge
  - Spermicidal jelly, foam, cream
  - Female condom

SPECIAL GROUPS
Mentally Retarded/Developmentally Delayed
Limited only by ability to properly use condoms

Adolescents
- Adolescents are a key demographic target for condom education and use. Multiple factors make condoms an ideal form of contraception (with or without a 2nd method) in this age group:

- Prevents STI transmission as well as pregnancy
- Easily accessible without a prescription; may be available in schools
- Inexpensive
- Inexperienced female partners may not be familiar with or have access to other forms of birth control.

Women with Chronic Illness
- Condoms are highly recommended for women who are unable to use hormonal contraception due to a chronic medical condition.
- Especially recommended for immune-suppressed individuals to decrease risk of STIs

 FOLLOW-UP

PATIENT MONITORING
Routine STI testing at regular intervals in sexually active patients

COMPLICATIONS
Latex allergy in 1–3% of US population:
- Health care workers and individuals with chronic illness are particularly susceptible to allergy.

BIBLIOGRAPHY

Hogewoning CJ, et al. Condom use promotes regression of cervical intraepithelial neoplasia and clearance of human papillomavirus: A randomized clinical trial. *Int J Cancer*. 2003;107:811–816.

Kaplan DW. Condom use by adolescents. *Pediatrics*. 2001;107(6):1463–1469.

McNaught J, et al. Barrier and spermicidal contraceptives in adolescence. *Adolesc Med Clin*. 2005;16(3):495–515.

Mosher WD, et al. Use of contraception and use of family planning services in the United States, 1982–2002. Advance Data from Vital and Health Statistics; No. 350. Hyattsville, MD: National Center for Health Statistics, 2004.

 MISCELLANEOUS

SYNONYM(S)
Several slang terms for condom exist:
- Rubber
- Skin
- Raincoat
- Prophylactic

ABBREVIATIONS
- CIN—Cervical intraepithelial neoplasia
- HSV—Herpes simplex virus
- HPV—Human papillomavirus
- IUD—Intrauterine device
- OCP—Oral contraceptive pill
- DMPA—Depot medroxyprogesterone acetate (Depo-Provera)
- POP—Progestin-only pill
- STI—Sexually transmitted infection

LEGAL ISSUES
Age/Consent or Notification for Minors
There are no age restrictions on purchase of condoms.

Emergency Contraception
EC should be used in the event of condom breakage, slippage, or nonuse.

ACCESS ISSUES
Condoms are relatively easy to obtain:
- Condoms are readily available at pharmacies, convenience stores, and many other locations.
- Many schools provide condoms to students.
- Health care facilities often will provide condoms to patients.

CODES
ICD9-CM
V25.49 Other contraceptive method

 PATIENT TEACHING

Proper use is essential for optimal prevention of pregnancy and STI transmission. Recommendations include the following:
- Store condoms in cool, dry place prior to use.
- Use a new condom for each act of intercourse (vaginal, oral, anal).
- Remove carefully from package.
- Place condom before any genital contact.
- Space should be left at tip of condom by gently squeezing the end of it as it is unrolled to allow for semen collection.
- Withdraw penis while still erect (to prevent leakage).
- Remove condom a safe distance from female genitalia.
- Use a secondary contraceptive method (plan B, spermicide) if condom breaks or leaks.
- Spermicide-containing condoms are no longer recommended:
  - Spermicide may cause vaginal irritation, leading to ulcers and increased risk of HIV transmission.
- Condom use along with hormonal contraception is ideal ("belt and suspenders" approach).
- Never reuse a condom.

Section III

Anita L. Nelson, MD
Monica Hau Hien Le, MD

BASICS

DESCRIPTION
- Barrier methods for contraceptive management that allow more female control include the female condom, diaphragm, sponge, Lea's shield, and cervical cap.
  - Female condom: Single-use polyurethane sheath 7.8 cm in diameter and 17 cm in length between 2 flexible support rings with 8 hours of maximal wear time.
  - Diaphragm: Dome-shaped rubber cup with flexible rim, used with spermicide, must be left in place 6 hours after intercourse and may be worn up to 24 hours. Diaphragm must be fitted and prescribed by physician.
  - Contraceptive sponge: Single use, pillow-shaped polyurethane sponge containing 1 g of nonoxynol-9 spermicide that must be left in place 6 hours after coitus and may be worn for up to 24 hours of protection, available OTC.
  - Lea's shield: Oval device of medical-grade silicone rubber that fits over cervix with spermicide in the dome; left in place for 8 hours after coitus and worn for up to 48 hours.
  - FemCap: A hat-shaped silicone rubber cap placed over the cervix with a brim that is applied to the vaginal fornices; used with spermicide. 2 sizes, available only by prescription; left in place for 8 hours after coitus and worn for up to 48 hours.
  - Cervical cap (no longer available in US): Soft rubber cap fit snugly around cervix, used with spermicide, worn for up to 48 hours.
- Vaginal spermicides are used with most of these barrier methods. Nonoxynol-9 (N9) is the spermicide generally used in the US.

Age-Related Factors
- Parity affects the efficacy of the sponge.
- Fitting for the diaphragm requires assessment of vaginal muscle tone which may be affected by age and parity.

EPIDEMIOLOGY
- Effectiveness of each method is heavily based on correct and consistent use and parity.
- 1/2 of those who became pregnant while using vaginal barrier method report imperfect use.

MECHANISM OF ACTION
- Physical barrier to sperm passage.
- If spermicide is used, it will immobilize sperm in vagina.

EFFICACY
Rates of unintended pregnancy during the 1st year of typical use and the 1st year of correct and consistent ("perfect") use:

	Typical use	Perfect use
Female condom	21%	5%
Diaphragm	16%	6%
Contraceptive sponge		
Parous women	32%	20%
Nulliparous women	16%	9%
Lea's Shield	*	9%
FemCap	*	14%
Spermicide	29%	

*No data are available.

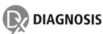

DIAGNOSIS

HISTORY
- Medical history:
  - Beware if history of latex allergy or TSS.
- Family history:
  - Not applicable.

Physical Exam
- Rule out significant pelvic relaxation if planning to use diaphragm or considering early precoital placement of other methods that may be dislodged by Valsalva.
- Diaphragms, Lea's shield, and FemCap are less effective with markedly anteverted or retroverted uterus.
- Fitting a diaphragm: Insert index and middle fingers into the vagina until the middle finger touches the posterior wall of the vagina.
  - Mark with your thumb the point at which your index finger touches the pubic bone.
  - Place the diaphragm rim on the tip of your middle finger. The opposite rim should lie just in front of your thumb. The distance between the middle finger and the thumb equals diaphragm diameter (in millimeters).
  - A properly fit diaphragm should cover the cervix completely, rest behind the symphysis pubis and against the vaginal walls.
  - Place largest size that patient cannot feel and that fits correctly without buckling around edges.

- FemCap sizing: Nulliparous and parous sizes
- Ensure that patient is able to place and remove method in the office.

TESTS
Ensure that patient is able to successfully place and remove method.

Labs
- No lab tests required prior to initiation or needed to follow-up women using barriers.
- As with intercourse, use of barrier may cause abnormal inflammatory changes on Pap smear if used within 48 hours.
- No routine screening tests are necessary:
  - STI, UTI, and pregnancy checks as indicated by age and clinical history.

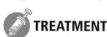

TREATMENT

MEDICATIONS
Antifungal medications applied topically reduce the effectiveness of barrier methods.

PATIENT SELECTION
Indications
Women who desire to use nonhormonal, female-controlled barrier method and who are willing to accept higher failure rates

Contraindications
- History of TSS
- Latex allergy (cap and diaphragm)
- N9 allergy

Informed Consent
- As indicated in Title X clinics
- Provide patient education including risks, benefits, alternatives, and side effects; document that this was provided

Patient Education
- Ensure patient can successfully insert and remove device prior to relying on it as a contraceptive method.
  - Have patient demonstrate placement/removal in office using samples.
  - Carefully instruct patient on timing of insertion and removal of vaginal barrier method and need for spermicide.
  - Each barrier may be placed early, but must be placed prior to intromission.

- Female condom: Compress ring within the condom. Use leading edge of ring to guide condom through introitus and advance through vagina. Once in place at the top of the vault, rotate inner ring 90° to stabilize condom at top of vault. Patient or partner should place penis inside condom and stabilize outer ring against introitus/vulva. Partner should avoid excessive friction against condom. Condom should be removed carefully after ejaculation to avoid spillage. Dispose of condom and its contents in solid-waste receptacle. If noise apparent prior to or with use, additional lubricant/spermicide may be added.
- Diaphragm: Use with spermicidal gel in dome. Leave in place for at least 6 hours after ejaculation. Add additional spermicide (any type) into vagina without removing device prior to each additional act of intercourse. Use diaphragm for a maximum of 24 hours.
- Contraceptive sponge: Add liquid to sponge to activate foam prior to insertion. Leave in place for 6 hours after ejaculation. Remove sponge and replace with fresh one prior to each subsequent act of intercourse. Use handle on sponge to remove it.
- Lea's shield: Dome should be filled with spermicidal gel prior to insertion. Handle should tuck behind symphysis pubis. May be worn for up to 48 hours, but must be left in place for at least 8 hours following ejaculation. Additional spermicide may be added to the vagina for subsequent acts of intercourse if desired. Use handle to guide removal.
- FemCap: Dome should be filled with spermicidal gel prior to insertion. Broad brim should be placed against posterior vaginal wall for stabilization. Ensure cap covers cervix. May be used for up to 48 hours, but must be left in place for at least 8 hours following ejaculation. Use handle to facilitate removal.
- Discuss cleansing and storage of devices:
  - Diaphragms, Lea's shield and FemCap should be washed with mild soap and water, dried, and stored in cool dry place.
  - Diaphragms should be inspected for any signs of cracking or rim inflexibility.
  - If device becomes malodorous, soaking in nondestructive antiseptic solution (mouthwash) may freshen device.
- Advise patient not to use latex barrier (diaphragm or cap) with any vaginal antifungal agent or other petroleum-based medication (clindamycin cream) or lubricant (Vaseline, baby oil, vegetable oil).
- Discuss early return to office and use of alternative method in case of vaginal barrier method problems.
- Prescribe EC and encourage use of EC should barrier not be used or if it becomes dislodged or is prematurely removed.

Risks
- The spermicide N9, used with barrier methods, can cause vulvovaginal disruption, theoretically increasing susceptibility to HIV, and provides no protection against other STIs.
- Use of diaphragm and spermicide increases vaginal *Escherichia coli* colonization and possible risk of bacterial vaginosis (and possibly ascending infection) and UTIs.
- Latex allergy (varies from local skin irritation to possible anaphylaxis) with use of diaphragm or cap

- TSS is a rare disorder caused by toxin release from *Staphylococcus aureus*. Absolute risk is 3 for every 100,000 women using vaginal barrier methods.

Benefits, Including Noncontraceptive
- Female condoms theoretically provide STI protection equivalent to male condoms with correct usage, although limited studies to support that data.
- The diaphragm may reduce cervical dysplasia.
- The diaphragm and sponge may reduce STI risk but should NOT be routinely recommended as a primary method for STI prevention.

Alternatives
Male barrier method (male condom), hormonal methods (pills, patch, ring, injection, implant), IUDs, withdrawal, natural family planning.

SPECIAL GROUPS
Mentally Retarded/Developmentally Delayed
- Consider the woman's manual dexterity and understanding of timing needed for insertion/removal.
- May be challenging to use correctly and consistently.

Adolescents
- Consider STI risk and the understanding of timing considerations for use of each method.
- Consider STI protection in choosing barrier method.
- Evaluate if adolescent is able to place the barrier method at the time of coitus and later remove it.

Women with Chronic Illness
- While no harm in use, may not provide adequate contraceptive protection for women with serious medical conditions.
- In patients with arthritis, consider the manual dexterity required for insertion and removal.

 FOLLOW-UP

DISPOSITION
Issues for Referral
Send to emergency room for symptoms of TSS.

CONTINUATION
- Assess patient and partner level of comfort and consistent usage of barrier method at each visit.
- Treatment based on symptomatology.
- Assess for allergy to N9.
- Assess for partner penile pain or patient cramps, bladder pain, or rectal pain when wearing a diaphragm or cap; fitting adjustment may help alleviate symptoms.
- Assess for symptoms of UTI, yeast infection, and bacterial vaginosis.

PATIENT MONITORING
- Diaphragm must be refitted annually, after weight change >10 pounds, and after each pregnancy.
- If diaphragm user experiences frequent UTIs, consider reevaluating size of device.
- Recurrent vaginal irritation without evidence of infection may indicate an allergy to spermicide or latex.

COMPLICATIONS
- Diaphragms and Lea's shields may cause cervical or vaginal erosions.
- TSS reported with diaphragm and sponge use, but potential exists with any female barrier method.
- Allergic reactions possible with latex devices and with use of spermicide.

- Increased risk of UTIs associated with increased number of gram-negative rods in vagina resulting from barrier use.

BIBLIOGRAPHY
Hatcher RA, et al. *Contraceptive Technology,* 18th ed. New York: Ardent Media; 2004.

Roddy RE, et al. A controlled trial of nonoxynol 9 film to reduce male-to-female transmission of sexually transmitted diseases. *N Engl J Med.* 1998;339(8):504–510.

Speroff L, et al. *A Clinical Guide for Contraception.* Philadelphia: Lippincott Williams and Wilkins; 2005.

Vijayakumar G, et al. A review of female-condom effectiveness: Patterns of use and impact on protected sex acts and STI incidence. *Int J STD AIDS.* 2006;17(10):652–659.

 MISCELLANEOUS

CLINICAL PEARLS
- The diaphragm, sponge, shield, and FemCap may be combined with the male condom to increase protection against pregnancy and STIs.
- Diaphragm, shield, and cap are routinely used with spermicide. Spermicide may also be used with the female condom.
- The female condom should NOT be used in combination with the male latex condom.

ABBREVIATIONS
- EC—Emergency contraception
- N9—Nonoxynol-9
- STI—Sexually transmitted infection
- TSS—Toxic shock syndrome
- UTI—Urinary tract infection

LEGAL ISSUES
Age/Consent or Notification for Minors
- Parental consent as required by state law.
- Formal consent not required except in Title X clinics.

Emergency Contraception
- Prescribe routinely and prophylactically with instructions regarding use for method problems.

ACCESS ISSUES
- Cervical cap no longer available in US.
- FemCap available online only.
- Clinician fitting and prescription are necessary for all barriers except the female condom.

 CODES

ICD9-CM
- V25.02 Fitting of diaphragm; prescription of foams, creams, or other agents
- V25.4 Surveillance of previously prescribed contraceptive methods

PATIENT TEACHING

PREVENTION
- Discuss early return to office and use of alternative method in case of vaginal barrier method problems.
- Routinely prescribe EC and instructions for use in the event of method failure.

CONTRACEPTION: COUNSELING

Eve Espey, MD, MPH

 BASICS

DESCRIPTION
- Contraceptive counseling is paramount to help assist a woman in choosing a method that fits her personal lifestyle and offers a/n:
  - High degree of effectiveness
  - Acceptable side effect profile
- Determination of a woman's likelihood of consistent and continuing use of a given method will help avoid unintended pregnancy.
- Contraceptive counseling includes counseling about emergency contraception, a postcoital method.

Age-Related Factors
- Adolescents have the highest rates of unintended pregnancy of any age group.
- Adolescents have the highest rates of discontinuation of common contraceptives like DMPA and birth control pills.
- Married women are more likely to use contraceptives consistently and correctly.

EPIDEMIOLOGY
- ~50% of all pregnancies in the US are unintended.
- ~50% of the unintended pregnancies in the US come from the 7% of women who use no contraceptive method.
- The other half of unintended pregnancies in the US come from the 93% of women who use a method inconsistently, incorrectly, or use a method with a high failure rate.
- The most common contraceptive methods used in the US are sterilization, birth control pills, and condoms:
  - The 2 top reversible methods (birth control pills and condoms) are highly user-dependent.
  - Top-tier contraceptive methods do not require continuing compliance on the part of the woman:
    ○ Intrauterine contraception
    ○ Hormonal implants
- Improved use of emergency contraception could reduce unintended pregnancy by 1/2.
- 20% of reproductive aged women were uninsured in 2003. They rely on a number of underfunded family-planning programs for contraception.
- 26 states have mandated coverage of contraceptives for insurance plans that offer prescription benefits. These laws have improved access to contraception.

RISK FACTORS
- All sexually active women of reproductive age are at risk for unintended pregnancy.
- Young, unmarried, poor women of color are at higher risk for unintended pregnancy.
- Adolescents are at higher risk of contraceptive failure.

Genetics
Women with unusual genetic and/or medical conditions such as hypercoagulable disorders, rheumatologic disease, or seizure disorders need more personalized counseling about methods that are safe and effective.

 DIAGNOSIS

SIGNS AND SYMPTOMS
History
- The majority of serious adverse events that occur as a result of hormonal contraceptives may be determined by taking a detailed medical history.
- Estrogen-containing contraceptives are contraindicated (the risks outweigh the benefits) for women with a history of:
  - Migraines with aura
  - History of thromboembolism (DVT, PE)
  - Uncontrolled HTN
  - Stroke
  - MI
  - Smoking (>15 cigarettes/d for women >35 years)
- A sexual and contraceptive history are helpful in assisting a woman choose an appropriate method:
  - A 17-year-old G2P2 who has used pills as her only method of birth control in the past should consider another method.
  - A 37-year-old G1P1 who has relied on condoms should not be discouraged from continuing to use them.

Physical Exam
- A pelvic exam is rarely necessary to initiate contraceptives and may be a deterrent for certain populations, like adolescents.
- In the absence of medical contraindications, an exam should not be required to counsel about and initiate most contraceptives.
- Blood pressure and weight should be measured.

TESTS
- Testing to rule out pregnancy and STIs is appropriate depending on the patient's age, history, and willingness.
- Urine pregnancy testing
- Cervical or urine gonorrhea and *Chlamydia* testing
- Pap smear as indicated. Although cervical cytology testing is not mandatory prior to initiating contraception, regular testing is indicated for preventive health maintenance. Initiation of contraception should not be dependent on Pap testing.

Imaging
Imaging is not required for initiation of contraceptive methods.

 TREATMENT

GENERAL MEASURES
- Counseling should stress:
  - Thorough review of all contraceptive options
  - Nonjudgmental but realistic expectations about difficulty of adhering to a given method:
    ○ Adolescents who must "hide" contraceptives may have more difficulty adhering to a daily pill regimen.
    ○ Uninsured women may have difficulty continuing DMPA injections.
  - Nuisance side effects:
    ○ Anticipatory guidance may improve ability to adhere.
  - Guidance on missed pills, patch, shot, etc.
  - The method's ability to protect against STIs and the need for a dual method (i.e., pills and condoms) for women at risk of unintended pregnancy and STIs
- Studies indicate that women have negative misperceptions about various contraceptive methods:
  - Identify specific negative perceptions
  - Respectfully give accurate information
- Noncontraceptive benefits of certain hormonal contraceptives are generally underappreciated:
  - Cycle control
  - Reduction in dysmenorrhea
  - Reduction in acne
  - Reduction in uterine and ovarian cancer

- Postpartum women and women who have undergone termination of pregnancy may be particularly motivated to use contraceptives and should be counseled thoroughly about the variety of options.
- Breast-feeding women may have concerns about the impact of hormonal contraception on lactation and should be counseled according to available evidence.

CONTRACEPTIVE CHOICES
- Most effective:
  – Sterilization
  – Intrauterine contraception
  – Hormonal implants
- Very effective:
  – DMPA
- Effective:
  – Birth control pills
  – The patch
  – The vaginal ring
- Less effective:
  – Condoms
  – Diaphragm
  – Spermicidal foams, films, jelly

SURGERY
Sterilization/Permanent contraception should be offered as an option. It may be performed by:
- Mini-laparotomy is most commonly performed for bilateral tubal ligation in the immediate postpartum period.
- Laparoscopy is used for the majority of interval procedures, most commonly with inert metal clips or cautery.
- Hysteroscopy; the Essure sterilization system places coils hysteroscopically into both tubal ostia.
- Vasectomy, male sterilization, is accomplished by interrupting the vas deferens.

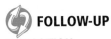 **FOLLOW-UP**

DISPOSITION
Issues for Referral
Women with complicated medical problems may be referred to family-planning experts for specific advice regarding contraceptive choices.

PROGNOSIS
Pediatric Considerations
- States vary in their laws about parental notification or consent for contraceptives.
- It is important to be aware of relevant state laws regarding consent for contraceptives.

COMPLICATIONS
- True medical complications of hormonal contraceptives are rare in healthy young women.
- Risks of morbidity and mortality are typically greater with pregnancy than with contraceptive methods.
- Contraindications to estrogen-containing hormonal contraceptives include migraine with aura; history of DVT, MI, or stroke; HTN; and smoking >35 years of age.

BIBLIOGRAPHY

Mosher WD, et al. Use of contraception and use of family planning services in the United States, 1982–2002. *Adv Data*. 2004;350:1–35.

Santelli JS, et al. Contraceptive use and pregnancy risk among U.S. high school students 1991–2003. *Perspect Sex Reprod Health*. 2006;38(2):106–111.

Sonfield A, et al. U.S. Insurance coverage of contraceptives and the impact of contraceptive coverage mandates, 2002. *Perspect Sex Reprod Health*. 2004;36(2):72–79.

WHO Department of Reproductive Health and Research. *Selected Practice Recommendations for Contraceptive Use*, 2nd ed. Geneva: World Health Organization; 2004.

 MISCELLANEOUS

SYNONYM(S)
- Birth control
- Contraception
- Family planning

CLINICAL PEARLS
- Many women request birth control pills because that is the method they are familiar with.
- Even if a woman requests a specific contraceptive method, review other options with her to assure that she is aware of available options.

- Avoid scaring women about rare medical complications and instead focus on the nuisance side effects that are more likely to lead to discontinuation.
- Consider discussing intrauterine contraception and implants with all women who desire reversible contraception. Even if they choose another method, you have given them education about methods they may be unfamiliar with and could use in the future.
- Remember to discuss emergency contraception with all women, even if they have decided on a method.

ABBREVIATIONS
- DMPA—Depot medroxyprogesterone acetate/ Depo-Provera
- DVT—Deep vein thrombosis
- MI—Myocardial infarction
- PE—Pulmonary embolism
- STI—Sexually transmitted infection

 CODES
ICD9-CM
V25 Encounter for contraceptive management

 PATIENT TEACHING

- Discuss the full range of contraceptive options.
- Encourage long-term methods with the highest effectiveness.
- Give anticipatory guidance about nuisance side effects.
- Speak in lay language, explaining concepts in simple terms.
- Give information without making judgments.
- Ask open-ended questions:
  – "What problems do you anticipate in using this method?"
  – "What have you heard about this method, either positive or negative?"
- Validate the woman's feelings.
- Maintain confidentiality.
- Educate patients about the noncontraceptive benefits of different contraceptive methods.

Section III

CONTRACEPTION, EMERGENCY

Patricia A. Lohr, MD, MPH
Beatrice A. Chen, MD

 BASICS

DESCRIPTION

EC is birth control used up to 120 hours after unprotected vaginal intercourse to prevent pregnancy. Options for EC in the US are:

- ECPs:
  - Combined estrogen and progestin
  - Progestin-only (Plan B)
- Copper T IUD

> **ALERT**
> ECPs are not the same as mifepristone (RU-486) and do not cause an abortion. ECPs are not effective if a woman is already pregnant and will not adversely affect an established pregnancy.

Age-Related Factors

EC is indicated for women of any age at risk of unintended pregnancy.

EPIDEMIOLOGY

Widespread use of EC could prevent as many as 1.5 million unintended pregnancies annually:

- 90% of pregnancies following rape could be prevented if all women had access to EC after a sexual assault.
- An estimated 51,000 abortions were avoided due to EC use in 2000.
- Most women seeking EC use a regular form of contraception, usually condoms.
- Up to 50% of clients request EC after a condom break/slip.

MECHANISM OF ACTION

- ECPs:
  - Primary mechanism: Inhibition or delay in ovarian follicular development or maturation
  - Other possible mechanisms if taken after ovulation:
    - Interference with corpus luteum function
    - Thickening of cervical mucus that impedes sperm transport or function
    - Alteration of fallopian tube transport of sperm, egg, or fertilized ovum
    - Impairment of endometrial receptivity to implantation
- Copper T IUD:
  - Prevents fertilization of ovum
  - May prevent implantation of a fertilized egg

> **ALERT**
> EC is not considered abortifacient because it does not interrupt an established pregnancy, which is defined by the FDA, NIH, and ACOG as beginning with implantation.

EFFICACY

- The point in the menstrual cycle when unprotected intercourse occurs and how quickly EC is used impact effectiveness. EC is more effective when used as soon as possible after unprotected sex.
- ECPs:
  - Progestin-only (Plan B):
    - 89% reduction in pregnancy risk
  - Combined estrogen and progestin:
    - 75% reduction in pregnancy risk
- Copper T IUD:
  - >99% reduction in pregnancy risk

 DIAGNOSIS

HISTORY

Medical history:

- Ensure that patient does not want to get pregnant.
- Ascertain whether she may already be pregnant or if a pregnancy test is indicated:
  - Obtain date of last menstrual period and whether it was normal.
  - Establish whether time of 1st episode of unprotected intercourse was >1 week prior to presentation.
- Determine time of most recent episode of unprotected intercourse.
- Inquire about a regular method of birth control.

Physical Exam

- A physical exam is not necessary prior to ECP administration in an asymptomatic patient.
- Before IUD insertion, perform a pelvic examination to assess uterine size and position and to exclude pelvic infection.

TESTS

None required

Labs

If there is a high suspicion of pregnancy, perform a urine pregnancy test:

- If the test is positive, EC is not indicated.
- If the test is negative, it does not mean that EC is not necessary.

Imaging

None required

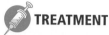 **TREATMENT**

MEDICATIONS

- No data are available about the interactions of ECPs with other drugs.
- Medications that reduce the efficacy of OCPs may also reduce the efficacy of ECPs. These include but are not limited to:
  - Rifampin
  - Griseofulvin
  - Phenytoin
  - St. John's wort
  - Some antiretroviral agents
- Copper IUD effectiveness is not affected by any medications.

PATIENT SELECTION

- Routine counseling and advance supply of EC is recommended by ACOG.
- ECPs:
  - Progestin-only (Plan B):
    - Within 120 hours of unprotected intercourse
    - 2 tablets of levonorgestrel 0.75 mg PO as single dose
  - Combined estrogen-progestin:
    - Within 72 hours of unprotected intercourse
    - 2 doses of EE (100–120 μg) and a progestin, typically levonorgestrel, (0.5–0.6 mg) PO 12 hours apart
- Copper T IUD:
  - Within 120 hours of unprotected intercourse
  - IUD is inserted in usual fashion

Indications

Unprotected vaginal intercourse in a woman not desiring pregnancy. This may be due to, but is not limited to, any of the following scenarios:

- Lack of contraceptive use
- Rape
- Contraceptive failure such as a condom slip/break, IUD expulsion, dislodged cervical shield, or errors in practicing coitus interruptus, periodic abstinence, or abstinence
- Failure to use a back-up method when:
  - ≥2 combined OCPs are missed
  - 1 POP is missed or taken ≥3 hours late
  - ≥2 days have elapsed from the start date of a new vaginal ring or contraceptive patch
  - ≥14 days have passed from the due date of Depo-Provera injection

Contraindications

- ECPs:
  - Pregnancy
  - Hypersensitivity to any component of ECPs
  - Undiagnosed abnormal genital bleeding

- Copper T IUD:
  – Pregnancy
  – Wilson disease
  – Allergy to any component of the IUD
  – Uterine cavity distortion precluding proper insertion
  – Undiagnosed abnormal genital bleeding
  – Endometrial or cervical cancer
  – PID (current or within 3 months)
  – Cervicitis (current or within 3 months)
  – Puerperal or post-abortion sepsis (current or within 3 months)

Informed Consent
Women should be aware of efficacy, benefits, risks, alternatives of EC.

Patient Education
- EC will decrease but not completely exclude risk of pregnancy.
- The sooner EC is used after unprotected intercourse, the better it works.
- If ECPs do not work, the pregnancy will be unharmed. Pregnancy risk following IUD insertion is extremely low, but is at increased risk of miscarriage or septic abortion. The IUD may require removal.
- ECPs will not prevent pregnancy due to unprotected intercourse following treatment.
- The next menstrual period may be early, on time, or delayed. Failure to have a menstrual period within 3 weeks of EC use requires a urine pregnancy test.
- Progestin-only ECPs have a low risk of side effects. Nausea and/or vomiting is the most common (18%/4%). Combined pills are more likely than progestin-only to cause nausea and vomiting (43%/16%).
- EC does not protect from STIs, including HIV.

Risks
No deaths or serious complications have been causally linked to ECPs. Use of EC has not been shown to increase frequency of unprotected intercourse or decrease the use of regular forms of contraception.

Benefits, Including Noncontraceptive
- ECPs:
  – Reduced risk of unintended pregnancy
- Copper T IUD:
  – Marked reduction in risk of unintended pregnancy
  – Can be used as ongoing contraception for up to 12 years

SPECIAL GROUPS
Mentally Retarded/Developmentally Delayed
- No medical contraindications to use of EC in this group.
- If long-term contraception is indicated, IUD is preferable.

Adolescents
Plan B ECPs are available at pharmacies in the US without a prescription for women and men ≥18 years. Persons ≤17 cannot obtain Plan B without a prescription.

Women with Chronic Illness
- There are no known medical situations in which the risks of ECPs outweigh the benefits.
- Progestin-only ECPs or an IUD may be preferable in women with thromboembolic disease, heart disease, acute focal migraine, or severe liver disease, however this has not been tested in formal trials.

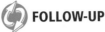 ## FOLLOW-UP

DISPOSITION
Issues for Referral
Refusal to provide EC by pharmacies, individual pharmacists, or physicians is an issue of political and legislative debate. If refusal is allowed by law, it should be accompanied by referral to provide access.

CONTINUATION
- ECPs are not recommended for routine use because they are less effective than regular contraception.
- Using an IUD for EC is highly effective and can be left in place for long-term contraception.
- Ongoing methods of contraception can be initiated after completing treatment with ECPs.

PATIENT MONITORING
- No scheduled follow-up is necessary. However, if menses do not occur within 3 weeks of use a pregnancy test is indicated.
- Symptoms suggestive of an ectopic pregnancy, such as persistent irregular bleeding or lower abdominal pain, require immediate evaluation.

COMPLICATIONS
- Side effects of ECPs include nausea, vomiting, breast tenderness, headache, dizziness, fatigue, and abdominal pain. Most side effects resolve in 24 hours.
- Progestin-only ECPs (Plan B) are more effective and have fewer side effects than combined ECPs, making them preferable.
- If vomiting of ECPs occurs within 2 hours of administration, repeat the dose.
- Meclizine 50 mg PO 1 hour prior to dosing combined ECPs lowers the risk of nausea and vomiting.

BIBLIOGRAPHY

Blanchard K, et al. Differences between emergency contraception users in the United States and the United Kingdom. *J Am Med Womens Assoc.* 2002;57(4):200–203, 214.

Croxatto HB, et al. Mechanism of action of hormonal preparations used for emergency contraception: A review of the literature. *Contraception.* 2001; 63(3):111–121.

Emergency contraception. ACOG Practice Bulletin No. 69. American College of Obstetricians and Gynecologists. *Obstet Gynecol.* 2005;106: 1443–1452.

Jones RK, et al. Contraceptive use among U.S. women having abortions in 2000–2001. *Perspect Sex Reprod Health.* 2002;34:294–303.

Ngai SW, et al. A randomized trial to compare 24h versus 12h double dose regimen of levonorgestrel for emergency contraception. *Hum Reprod.* 2004;20:307–311.

Stewart F, et al. Emergency Contraception. In: Hatcher RA, et al., eds. *Contraceptive Technology*, 18th revised ed. New York: Ardent Media; 2004.

Stewart FH, et al. Prevention of pregnancy resulting from rape: A neglected preventive health measure. *Am J Prev Med.* 2000;19:228–229.

Trussell J, et al. Emergency contraception: A cost effective approach to preventing unintended pregnancy. Available at: http://ec.princeton.edu/questions/ec-review.pdf. Accessed December 28, 2006.

von Hertzen H, et al. Low dose mifepristone and two regimens of levonorgestrel for emergency contraception: A WHO multicentre randomized trial. *Lancet.* 2002;360:1803–1810.

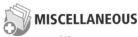 ## MISCELLANEOUS

SYNONYM(S)
- "Morning after pill" or "day after pill"
- Emergency birth control
- Post-coital emergency contraception
- EC or ECPs

CLINICAL PEARLS
- Taking both Plan B tablets at the same time is as effective as taking them 12 hours apart.
- Taking the Plan B tablets 24 hours apart is as effective as taking them 12 hours apart.
- IUDs and progestin-only ECPs can be used up to 120 hours after unprotected intercourse.
- Combined estrogen-progestin ECPs are only used up to 72 hours postcoitus.
- EC can be used more than once, even within the same menstrual cycle, if indicated.
- There are no recommendations in the US for use of ECPs when client is taking medications that might reduce ECP efficacy. The Faculty for Sexual and Reproductive Health Care Clinical Effectiveness Unit in the UK recommend using double the dose of progestin-only ECPs.

ABBREVIATIONS
- EC—Emergency contraception
- ECP—Emergency contraceptive pill
- EE—Ethinyl estradiol
- IUD—Intrauterine device
- OCP—Oral contraceptive pill
- POP—Progestin-only pill
- STI—Sexually transmitted infection

LEGAL ISSUES
Age/Consent or Notification for Minors
- Persons ≤17 must have a prescription to obtain Plan B from a pharmacy.
- Parental notification or consent is not necessary to obtain EC.

ACCESS ISSUES
- Plan B is available at pharmacies without a prescription for persons ≥18.
- Access is limited for adolescents <18 who must have a prescription to obtain Plan B from a pharmacy.
- In some states, EC can be obtained directly from a pharmacist.

CODES
ICD9-CM
V25.03 Encounter for emergency contraceptive counseling and prescription

 ## PATIENT TEACHING

- Routine counseling about the use, availability, and safety of EC should be offered to all persons.
- Additional patient education can be obtained at http://ec.princeton.edu/

PREVENTION
Obtaining EC in advance improves access to EC.

CONTRACEPTION, HORMONAL: COMBINATION ORAL CONTRACEPTIVES

Bliss Kaneshiro, MD
Alison Edelman, MD, MPH

BASICS

DESCRIPTION

- COCs contain an estrogen (EE) and a progestin (norgestimate, desogestrel, gestodene, levonorgestrel, cytoproterone acetate, ethynodiol diacetate, or drospirenone)
- Decreases in estrogen and progestin content and appropriate selection criteria have led to a decrease in side effects and complications.
- Packaging formulation:
  - In 21- or 28-day cycles, the last 2–7 pills in a 28-day pack are placebo pills.
  - 21/7 (hormonally active/placebo)
  - 21/2/5 (hormonally active/placebo/EE)
  - 24/4 (hormonally active/placebo)
  - Chewable formulation is available.
  - Monophasic pills contain the same dose of EE and progestin for all hormonally active days.
  - Multiphasic preparations use varying levels of EE or progestin:
    - Developed to lower the total steroid dose administered
    - No proven clinical advantage over monophasic pills
- Extended regimens delay or skip the placebo week:
  - 84/7 with 7 placebo and 84/7 with EE
  - 28/0 for 365 days and ongoing

Age-Related Factors

Successful use and efficacy are dependent on daily use:

- Young adolescent may find this more difficult.

EPIDEMIOLOGY

- Popular method of contraception in the US since the 1960s
- 80% of US women will use this form of birth control during their lifetimes.

MECHANISM OF ACTION

- Acts on pituitary and hypothalamus to inhibit gonadotropin secretion, thereby preventing ovulation:
  - Progestin suppresses LH secretion, eliminating LH surge.
  - Estrogen suppresses FSH secretion, decreasing follicular maturation.
- Progestational agent also thickens cervical mucus, decreases peristalsis in fallopian tube, and makes endometrium unreceptive to implantation.
- Estrogen stabilizes the endometrium to prevent irregular bleeding.

EFFICACY

- Perfect use failure rate: 0.1%
- Typical use failure rate: 7.6%
- Suggestion that obese women may have a higher failure rate; results not consistent

DIAGNOSIS

HISTORY

- Medical history:
  - Medical, surgical, and menstrual history
  - Current medications
  - Contraceptive history including past methods and contraceptive failures
  - Last act of intercourse and what contraceptive method was used
- Family history:
  - Review family history for close relatives with VTE; if a hypercoagulable trait is suspected, an evaluation is warranted before starting COCs.

Physical Exam

- BP
- Women can be prescribed COCs without a clinical breast and pelvic exam.

TESTS

Lab

- No lab studies are mandatory prior to use
- Cervical cytology as health maintenance, but not prerequisite to COC use

TREATMENT

MEDICATIONS

- Accelerated metabolism of COCs in women taking medications that increase liver microsomal activity (phenobarbital, phenytoin, griseofulvin, rifampin, carbamazepine, barbiturates, primidone, topiramate, oxcarbazepine)
- Women who take these medications may use COCs if they cannot use other methods and understand that there is decreased contraceptive efficacy.

PATIENT SELECTION

- Patients should be able to comply with daily pill taking; COCs may be more difficult to adhere to than other methods of contraception.
- Can be initiated on any day of the menstrual cycle:
  - "Quick Start" method with initiation on the day patient is given the prescription improves compliance and does not increase breakthrough bleeding.
  - Use a backup method for 7–10 days.

Indications

- Reversible contraception
- Hyperandrogenism:
  - Useful in idiopathic hirsutism and PCOS
- Dysmenorrhea
- Menorrhagia, abnormal uterine bleeding

Contraindications

- Conditions in which risks outweigh benefits:
  - Previous thromboembolic or ischemic event
  - Complicated valvular heart disease
  - Known hereditary thrombophilias
  - History of an estrogen-dependent tumor:
    - Known or suspected breast cancer
  - Markedly impaired liver function, acute or chronic cholestatic liver disease
  - Undiagnosed abnormal uterine bleeding
  - Hypertriglyceridemia
  - Multiple risk factors for arterial cardiovascular disease such as age >35 and smoking
  - Migraine with aura
  - Uncontrolled HTN
  - Known or suspected pregnancy
  - Major surgery with prolonged immobilization
  - Smoking >15 cigarettes a day in woman >35 years
- Conditions requiring clinical judgment (see evidence based Guidelines from WHO):
  - Seizure disorders requiring anticonvulsants
  - History of obstructive jaundice in pregnancy
  - Smoking
  - Major surgery without prolonged immobilization
  - HTN
  - Uterine leiomyoma
  - Diabetes
  - Hepatic disease
  - Sickle cell disease
  - Gallbladder disease
  - Uncomplicated valvular heart disease

Informed Consent

- Patients should understand the risks and benefits of COCs.
- All contraceptive options should be reviewed with the patient before they choose the contraceptive option that is best for them.
- It should be emphasized that use of COCs is safer than pregnancy in terms of health risk.

Patient Education

- Missed pills are cause of contraceptive failure:
  - A back-up method should be used if ≥2 pills are missed.
- Patients should not delay starting their next pill pack; pregnancies usually occur because of a failure to initiate the next pill cycle on time.
- Even if no pills have been missed, patients may consider using a back-up method after an episode of gastroenteritis.

Risks
- Side effects can include nausea and breast discomfort; in most cases these resolve in the 1st few months of use.
- Estrogen increases production of clotting factors:
  – Increased risk of venous thromboembolism (12–20 events per 100,000 per year)
  – Low-dose COCs do not increase the risk of MI or stroke in healthy, nonsmoking women regardless of age.
- Increase in BP through activation of renin-angiotensin system:
  – Oral contraceptive–induced HTN occurs in 5% of high-dose COC users.
  – Small increases in BP can be observed with low-dose COCs although clinically significant HTN has not been reported.
- Major depression is rarely associated with low-dose COCs.
- May be an increased risk of benign hepatic adenomas, no increased risk of liver cancer
- No differences in weight gain compared to placebo
- Conflicting data regarding increased risk of cervical cancer in COC users; difficult to control for confounding and enhanced screening in COC users
- No effect of past COC use or duration of use on the risk of breast cancer; COC use does not increase breast cancer risk in women with a family history of breast cancer.
- No increase in infertility or miscarriage rates

Benefits, Including Noncontraceptive
- Decreased risk of ectopic pregnancy
- Reduction in menstrual blood flow, decrease in iron-deficiency anemia in women with menorrhagia
- Decreased incidence of benign breast disease
- Decreased incidence of ovarian cysts
- Lowered risk of ovarian cancer, including BRCA1/BRCA2-associated ovarian cancer
- Lowered risk of endometrial cancer
- Treatment of hyperandrogenism
- Improves acne
- COCs decrease transmission of certain STIs by thickening cervical mucus.

Alternatives (See chapters on Contraception)
- Other estrogen containing contraceptives:
  – Transdermal contraceptive patch
  – Contraceptive vaginal ring
- Contraceptives that contain only progestin:
  – POPs or "mini-pill"
  – Progestin injection (IM or SC)
  – Implantable contraceptive rods
  – Progestin-secreting IUD
- Nonhormonal contraceptives:
  – Copper IUD
  – Barrier methods (male and female condoms, diaphragm, cervical cap, sponge)
  – Spermicides
  – Fertility awareness–based methods
- Permanent methods, including female sterilization and vasectomy

SPECIAL GROUPS
Pregnancy Considerations
- Inadvertent use during pregnancy does not increase the risk of congenital anomalies.
- COCs can diminish the quantity and quality of lactation; progestin-only methods may be preferable in breast-feeding women.
- COCs should not be used in women who are <6 weeks postpartum due to an increased risk of thromboembolism.
- COCs may be used immediately following a 1st or 2nd trimester pregnancy termination.

Mentally Retarded/Developmentally Delayed
No specific contraindication, although methods that do not require daily pill taking may be easier to comply with.

Adolescents
- There is no evidence that COC use impairs the growth and development of adolescents.
- Compliance may be a concern in this population; methods that are easier to adhere to may be preferable.

Women with Chronic Illness
- No effect on insulin requirement is expected with low-dose COCs in women with diabetes:
  – Insulin and glucose changes with low-dose COCs are minimal and rarely clinically significant.
- COCs can be used in women with well-controlled HTN although BP should be periodically monitored and, if other comorbidities exist, alternative contraception should be considered.

 FOLLOW-UP

CONTINUATION
Unscheduled bleeding in the 1st few months of use can lead to dissatisfaction and discontinuation, as can other side effects.

PATIENT MONITORING
- Patients should be seen in 3–6 months to determine satisfaction with contraceptive choice and review BP.
- Women who are satisfied with their contraceptive method should be seen for yearly health-maintenance screening, including exclusion of problems by history, measurement of blood pressure, palpation of the liver, and breast and pelvic exam.

COMPLICATIONS
- Women who develop a serious complication should discontinue the COC.
- Women who experience contraceptive failure or unplanned pregnancy should receive counseling about pregnancy options and discontinue COC.

BIBLIOGRAPHY

Holt VL, et al. Body mass index, weight and oral contraceptive failure risk. *Obstet Gynecol.* 2005;105:46–52.

Rosenberg MJ, et al. Compliance and oral contraceptives: A review. *Contraception.* 1995;52:137–141.

Speroff L, et al. *A Clinical Guide for Contraception.* Philadelphia: Lippincott Williams & Wilkins; 2005.

Trussell J. Contraceptive failure in the United States. *Contraception.* 2004;70:89.

Westoff C, et al. Quick start: A novel oral contraceptive initiation method. *Contraception.* 2002;66:141–145.

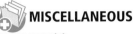 **MISCELLANEOUS**

SYNONYM(S)
- Birth control pills (BCPs)
- Oral contraceptives (OCs)
- Oral contraceptive pills (OCPs)
- "The pill"

CLINICAL PEARLS
Continuous COC regimens (only active hormone pills are taken and no placebo pills are taken) and extended COC regimens (placebo pills taken every 3–6 months) are safe and effective methods of contraception:
- Can be used to treat endometriosis, dysmenorrhea, PMDD
- Minimizing frequency of menses is more convenient for many women.
- Breakthrough bleeding is a common problem with continuous and extended COC use.

ABBREVIATIONS
- BP—Blood pressure
- COC—Combined oral contraceptive
- EE—Ethinyl estradiol
- FSH—Follicle-stimulating hormone
- HTN—Hypertension
- LH—Luteinizing hormone
- MI—Myocardial infarction
- PCOS—Polycystic ovarian syndrome
- PMDD—Premenstrual dysmorphic disorder
- STI—Sexually transmitted infection
- VTE—Venous thromboembolism
- WHO—World Health Organization

LEGAL ISSUES
Age/Consent or Notification for Minors
The ability of minors to obtain contraceptive services without parental notification varies by state.

Emergency Contraception
- Yuzpe method utilizes COCs:
  – 100 mg EE and 0.50 mg levonorgestrel taken within 72 hours of intercourse and repeated 12 hours later
- Levonorgestrel as 0.75 mg, repeated in 12 hours or combined as a single dose is more efficacious and better tolerated.

CODES

ICD9-CM
V25.01 Oral contraceptive initiation or counseling

 PATIENT TEACHING

ACOG Education Pamphlet: Birth Control Pills, AP159

Section III

CONTRACEPTION, HORMONAL: IMPLANTABLE

Carrie Cwiak, MD, MPH
Melissa Kottke, MD

 BASICS

DESCRIPTION
- Implanon is the only subdermal contraceptive implant currently available in the US:
  - A single 4 cm x 2 mm flexible rod:
    - Contains 68 mg of the synthetic progestin, etonogestrel (the active metabolite of desogestrel), in an ethylene vinyl acetate core
    - Provides up to 3 years of contraception
- Norplant™, a 6-rod implant system, was available in the US until 2000. It released the synthetic progestin levonorgestrel and was effective for 5 years.
  - Implanon is similar to Norplant except:
    - Implanon is easier to insert and remove
    - With Implanon, bleeding patterns do not improve over time
- Etonogestrel implant
- Implanon
- Subdermal contraceptive implant

Age-Related Factors
WHO category 1 for women ages 18–45 years regardless of smoking history:
- Category 1: No restriction on use
- All women who smoke should be encouraged to stop.

Pediatric Considerations
- Implanon has only been studied in women >18 years of age.
- Safety and efficacy after menarche expected to be the same in teens as in adult women.

Geriatric Considerations
Implanon has not been studied in postmenopausal women and is not indicated in this population.

EPIDEMIOLOGY
Since 1998, 2.5 million women in >30 countries have used Implanon™.

MECHANISMS OF ACTION
- Implanon prevents pregnancy primarily by inhibiting ovulation:
  - 0% ovulation in users in the 1st 2 years and <1% in the 3rd year
- Also increases the thickness of cervical mucus
- Thins the endometrial lining

EFFICACY
- In clinical studies, the cumulative Pearl index is 0.38 pregnancies/100 women-years of use.
- Efficacy may be reduced in patients taking hepatic enzyme–inducing medications.

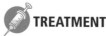 **DIAGNOSIS**

HISTORY
- Medical history:
  - A complete patient history should be elicited, including:
    - Future plans for pregnancy
    - Past experience with contraceptive methods
    - Current medications
    - Sexual history
  - LMP and current use of contraception or last episode of unprotected sex can help determine if a urine pregnancy test is needed before implant placement.
- Family history:
  - Women may use Implanon™ regardless of family history.

Physical Exam
- Examine site (inner upper arm on patient's nondominant side) before placement of implant.
- A breast or pelvic exam is not required before implant placement.

TESTS
A Pap smear or cervical cultures are not required before implant placement.

Labs
No laboratory tests are required before implant placement.

Imaging
- A nonpalpable Implanon rod can be located with US using a high-frequency transducer (10 MHz), or by MRI.
- Implanon is not radio-opaque and will not be seen with X-ray or CT.

TREATMENT

ALERT
Clinicians must attend and complete an Organon USA, Inc. sponsored training program before inserting or removing Implanon.

MEDICATIONS
- Hepatic enzyme–inducing medications that may decrease the efficacy of Implanon include:
  - Rifampicin
  - Phenytoin
  - Carbamazepine
  - Oxcarbazepine
  - Primidone
  - Topiramate
  - Barbiturates
- A back-up contraceptive method, like condoms, should be used with these listed medications.

PATIENT SELECTION
- Safe in recently postpartum women
- Does not decrease milk quality or production in lactating women
- Good for those who cannot use estrogen due to contraindications or side effects
- Safe for many women with medical conditions in whom pregnancy may be dangerous

Indications
- Any reproductive-age woman seeking highly effective, long-term, reversible contraception
- Recommended timing of insertion:
  - Between days 1–5 of menstrual cycle
  - When switching from combined hormonal contraception within 7 days of last dose
  - When switching from progestin-only method within last day of pill, on day of removal of implant or IUS, or when next injection due
  - Within 5 days of 1st trimester miscarriage or abortion
  - Within 21–28 days following delivery (after 28 days if exclusively breastfeeding) or 2nd trimester abortion
- If placed according to this recommended timing, no back-up contraception is needed.
- If placed at other times when pregnancy can be ruled out, back-up contraception or abstinence is necessary for the 1st 7 days.

Contraindications
Contraindications to Implanon™ include:
- Active thromboembolism
- Pregnancy
- Hepatic tumors or active liver disease
- Undiagnosed abnormal vaginal bleeding
- Current or recent personal history of breast cancer
- Hypersensitivity to any component of Implanon

Pregnancy Considerations
Current pregnancy is a contraindication to insertion of a contraceptive implant. If a woman who has an Implanon in place is pregnant and plans to continue the pregnancy, the implant should be removed.

Informed Consent
- Review all other appropriate contraceptive methods.
- Review risks, benefits, and side effects of Implanon™.
- Review insertion and removal procedure in detail.
- Have patient sign a written consent for the placement of a contraceptive implant.

Patient Education
- A change in menstrual bleeding pattern should be expected.
- No protection from HIV or STIs

- Must be inserted and removed by trained clinician
- May be removed in the office at any time at the request of the patient

Risks
- Irregular and unpredictable bleeding changes
- Possible pain, infection, bleeding or bruising, paresthesias, or scar formation at insertion site with insertion and/or removal
- Ovarian cysts, which often resolve spontaneously
- Ectopic pregnancy.
  – Although overall risk of pregnancy is low with Implanon, if a person becomes pregnant with an Implanon in place, it may be more likely to be ectopic.
- Rare adverse reactions include: Weight increase, headache, acne, emotional lability, breast pain, abdominal pain, and depression.
- No HIV or STI protection

Benefits, Including Noncontraceptive
- Long-term, highly effective contraception
- High continuation rate in clinical trials
- Total amount of menstrual bleeding decreased:
  – 20% amenorrhea rate
- Menstrual and ovulatory pain decreased by as much as 88% in 1 trial
- No loss of BMD
- No action needing at time of intercourse, allowing for spontaneity
- Easy to insert and remove
- Rapidly reversible, with immediate return to fertility
  – >90% of users ovulate within 3 months of removal

Alternatives
- A woman may choose any other hormonal or nonhormonal reversible contraceptive method suitable to her.
- A woman may choose permanent sterilization for herself or vasectomy for her male partner.
- All women not seeking contraception should be encouraged to take folic acid.

SPECIAL GROUPS
Mentally Retarded/Developmentally Delayed
- Involve the patient in the decision as much as possible.
- Ensure that parent or guardian consent is obtained and in the patient's best interest.

Adolescents
- May be ideal for adolescents who have trouble remembering to take pills or return for injections.
- See Pediatric Considerations.

Women with Chronic Illness
- Good for those who cannot use estrogen due to contraindications or side effects
- Safe for many women with medical conditions in whom pregnancy may be dangerous:
  – Smokers >35
  – Women with HTN or CVD
  – Women with diabetes or obesity

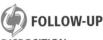

FOLLOW-UP

DISPOSITION
Issues for Referral
- Refer to only properly trained clinicians for implant insertion and removal:
  – For an available trained clinician, contact Organon USA Inc. at 1-877-IMPLANON.

- Nonpalpable rods require localization, which may need to be performed by a radiologist:
  – Nonpalpable Implanon™ rods should 1st be located with US using a high-frequency transducer (10 MHz) or by MRI before any attempt at removal.
  – Removal may be performed in consultation with a radiologist.

CONTINUATION
- High (68%) continuation rate at 1 year
- Current data shows efficacy for up to 3 years of use

PATIENT MONITORING
- Follow-up visit after implant insertion to check site
- Thereafter, observe recommended follow-up for other screening exams and tests
- Removal of Implanon™ recommended after 3 years

COMPLICATIONS
- Pregnancy:
  – Occurs rarely and typically is the result of an unrecognized early pregnancy at time of insertion
  – Provide options counseling and refer for termination if desired.
  – Remove implant if patient plans to continue the pregnancy.
- Local skin reactions:
  – Infection is very rare and can be treated with oral antibiotics.
  – Very rarely will the implant need to be removed secondary to infection not responding to antibiotics.
- Hematomas are rare but can occur:
  – Risk may be reduced by use of pressure bandage and ice postinsertion
- Pain postinsertion is often mild and can be managed with oral analgesics.
- Inability to palpate implant in patient's arm:
  – Patient should use nonhormonal back-up method until implant is localized.
  – Locate with 10-MHz US or MRI
  – Implant is not radio-opaque and will not be seen with X-ray or CT.

BIBLIOGRAPHY

Funk S, et al. Safety and efficacy of Implanon™, a single-rod implantable contraceptive containing etonogestrel. *Contraception*. 2005;71:319–326.

Hatcher RA, et al. Tiger, GA: Bridging the Gap Foundation, 2005.

Implanon TM™ [package insert]. Roseland, NJ: Organon USA Inc.; 2006.

Medical Eligibility Criteria for Contraceptive Use, 3rd ed. Geneva: World Health Organization; 2004.

Selected Practice Recommendations for Contraceptive Use, 2nd ed. Geneva: World Health Organization; 2005.

 MISCELLANEOUS

See "Subdermal Contraceptive Implant Insertion."

SYNONYM(S)
- Subdermal contraceptive implant
- Etonogestrel implant, Implanon™

CLINICAL PEARLS
- Likely not an ideal method for a woman who desires pregnancy within the next year

- Structured patient counseling on expected bleeding changes *before* implant insertion increases user satisfaction and continuation of progestin-only contraceptive methods:
  – Use supplemental estrogen to treat unacceptable bleeding patterns.

ABBREVIATIONS
- BMD—Bone mineral density
- CVD—Cardiovascular disease
- EC—Emergency contraception
- IUS—Intrauterine system
- LMP—Last menstrual period
- STI—Sexually transmitted infection
- WHO—World Health Organization

LEGAL ISSUES
Age/Consent or Notification for Minors
Observe state laws concerning minors' ability to consent for contraception.

Emergency Contraception
Use EC as back-up for 1st 7 days if deviating from the recommended timing of insertion (see Indications, above).

ACCESS ISSUES
- For an available trained clinician, or to receive training in insertion or removal of Implanon, contact Organon USA Inc. at 1-877-IMPLANON.
- Insurance coverage may limit access.

 CODES

ICD9-CM
- V25.5 Encounter for contraceptive management, insertion of implantable subdermal contraceptive
- V25.43 Encounter for contraceptive management, surveillance of previously prescribed contraceptive methods (checking, reinsertion, or removal of contraceptive device), implantable subdermal contraceptive
- V45.52 Other postprocedural states, presence of contraceptive device, subdermal contraceptive implant

PATIENT TEACHING

- Counsel patient on expected bleeding changes before insertion.
- After insertion:
  – Complete User Card and give to patient as a reminder to have implant removed after 3 years
  – May be removed at any time pregnancy is desired prior to 3 years
  – Male condoms are recommended every time HIV and STI is a possibility

PREVENTION
- After insertion:
  – Keep the pressure bandage on for 24 hours to minimize bruising
  – Return if fever, or pus or significant swelling, bleeding, or pain at insertion site
  – Return if signs of pregnancy or positive pregnancy test
  – Return if bleeding pattern or side effects are unacceptable
- Follow other recommendations for follow-up (Pap smears, exams, etc.)
- Return in 3 years for removal or when pregnancy desired

CONTRACEPTION, HORMONAL: INJECTABLE

Alexandra Emery-Cohen, MD
Andrew M. Kaunitz, MD

 BASICS

DESCRIPTION
- DMPA (Depo-Provera) was approved for the treatment of endometriosis in 1960, and approved as a contraceptive in 80 countries around the world by 1980.
- It was not approved by the FDA for use as a contraceptive in the US until 1992.
- DMPA is given as 150-mg IM injection at 12-week intervals.
- With consistent, well-timed injections, its annual failure rate is well under 1%; in actual practice, however, a "typical" failure rate is ~3%.
- A new subcutaneous DMPA is available "Depo-subQ-Provera 104" with a 30% lower total dose than the IM form:
  - The SC version is also effective for 12 weeks, with studies showing no pregnancies reported in 16,000 women cycles.

Age-Related Factors
Since its approval, DMPA has become an increasingly popular form of birth control and has been deemed responsible for the decreasing rates of teen pregnancy in the US.

EPIDEMIOLOGY
- DMPA is currently used by over 2 million women in the US.
- Over 400,000 adolescents in the US currently use DMPA.

MECHANISMS OF ACTION
- Inhibits ovulation and causes changes in the endometrial and cervical mucous resulting in decreased sperm transport and implantation.
- In spontaneously menstruating women initiating DMPA, ideally the 1st DMPA injection should be given 5 days after the onset of the menstrual cycle (with the 1st day of menses considered day 1) and repeated at 12-week or 3-month intervals.
- Ovulation is suppressed for at least 14 weeks, allowing a 2-week "grace period" for women presenting later than 12 weeks following their previous injection:
  - If women present for their next injection >14 weeks (98 days) following their previous injection, pregnancy should be excluded prior to proceeding with the next contraceptive injection.
- Fertility usually returns in 6–9 months after the next injection would have been given.

ALERT
- It may take as long as 18–22 months for fertility to return.
- Thus, another contraceptive option may be a better choice than DMPA for a woman wanting to conceive in the next year or so.

EFFICACY
- When used correctly (injections given every 12 weeks, no later than 14 weeks), DMPA has an annual failure rate of <1%.
- With typical use (delay between injections, etc.), the annual failure rate is ~3%.

 DIAGNOSIS

HISTORY
- Medical history:
  - DMPA, a progestin-only method, may be appropriate for women with contraindications to the use of estrogen, such as a history of:
    ○ Migraines with aura
    ○ Smoking >15 cigarettes/d in women >35 years
    ○ Thromboembolism: DVT or PE
    ○ HTN
- Family history:
  - DMPA does not increase the risk of breast, endometrial, or ovarian cancer.
  - Thus, while a family history of these conditions is important to a woman's overall future health and risk assessment, DMPA is not contraindicated, and in fact, may represent a good contraceptive choice.

Physical Exam
- A pelvic examination is not required prior to the initiation of DMPA, as it may be a deterrent to contraceptive care, particularly in adolescents.
- Routine screening exams should be encouraged for women seeking contraception.

TESTS
Lab
- A urine pregnancy test may be indicated prior to initiation, as appropriate.
- Pap testing/cervical cytology testing should be performed per screening guidelines, but is not required prior to initiation of DMPA.

- STD screening/testing is appropriate, as indicated, particularly in young women and adolescents in whom annual screening is appropriate. STD testing is not required prior to DMPA initiation.
- Cervical or urine screening may be appropriate

Imaging
No imaging is necessary prior to the initiation of DMPA.

TREATMENT

PATIENT SELECTION
- Because use of DMPA is associated with high contraceptive efficacy due to its prolonged duration of ovulation suppression, and the lack of need for daily contraceptive actions, DMPA represents a sound choice for women who may find consistent use of oral contraception challenging.
- Women are most likely to be successful in using a contraceptive method that they have chosen.
- Women should be informed of the contraceptive options, alternatives, benefits, and side effects of contraceptive methods.
- Clinicians should determine if there are any contraindications to use of the women's chosen method and, if not, use of this method should be encouraged.

Indications
Use of DMPA has not been found to be associated with increased incidence of stroke, MI, or venous thromboembolism, and can therefore be safely used by women who are not appropriate candidates for estrogen-progestin contraceptives.

Risks
- Common side effects include:
  - Initial irregular (unscheduled) bleeding/spotting
  - Long-term: Amenorrhea
- ~50% of users report no menstrual cycle by 1 year.
- Women often worry about weight gain with DMPA. Although observational studies have found use of DMPA to be associated with weight gain, this may reflect baseline differences between women who choose DMPA and those who choose other contraceptives.
  - The only randomized, blinded trial of DMPA vs. placebo found no impact on appetite or weight.

ALERT

- Use of DMPA lowers ovarian estradiol production, and BMD declines during DMPA use:
  - Although the FDA has recently put a black-box warning on the use of DMPA, indicating that skeletal health concerns should cause clinicians to review use of DMPA prior to continuing injections >2 years, existing studies indicate that BMD fully recovers in teens and adult women following DMPA discontinuation.
  - No increased incidence of fractures has been noted in >30 years of DMPA use worldwide.
  - For these reasons, the American College of Obstetricians and Gynecologists, the Society for Adolescent Medicine and the World Health Organization do not recommend routinely restricting use of DMPA contraception due to skeletal health concerns.
- Accordingly, skeletal health concerns should not prevent clinicians from initiating and continuing DMPA in their teen and adult patients.

Benefits, Including Noncontraceptive

DMPA has several noncontraceptive benefits including:

- Decreased risk of:
  - Endometrial cancer
  - Iron deficiency anemia
  - PID
  - Ectopic pregnancy
- Protection against symptomatic uterine leiomyomas
- Use of DMPA can provide effective treatment of pain in women with:
  - Endometriosis
  - Menorrhagia
  - Dysmenorrhea
  - PMS symptoms
  - Seizures refractory to conventional anticonvulsants
  - Hemoglobinopathy
  - Endometrial hyperplasia
  - Vasomotor symptoms in menopausal women
  - Metastatic endometrial cancer
- The subcutaneous formulation of DMPA has been approved for the treatment of endometriosis. This route appeals to women who prefer the smaller needle and the potential for injections away from a clinic setting.

Alternatives

- Use of other hormonal, nonhormonal, or progestin-only contraceptives
- For women with contraindications to estrogen use, other progestin-only methods which may be appropriate include:
  - POPs or "mini-pills"
  - Implants: Implanon
  - Levonorgestrel IUS

SPECIAL GROUPS

Mentally Retarded/Developmentally Delayed

- DMPA has been used extensively for menstrual suppression in individuals with developmental disabilities for whom menses present concerns related to:
  - Hygiene
  - Behavioral changes
  - Need for contraception
  - Medical concerns such as:
    ○ Catamenial seizures
    ○ Menstrual headaches
    ○ Other
- Families, patients, and caretakers should be advised that rates of amenorrhea are ~50% at 1 year, and that unscheduled bleeding is common prior to achieving amenorrhea.

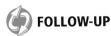 **FOLLOW-UP**

CONTINUATION

- Management of unscheduled bleeding should include:
  - Preventive guidance prior to initiation:
    ○ Women repeatedly expressing concerns regarding irregular bleeding should be examined and assessed for such conditions as cervicitis, uterine fibroids/adenomyosis, and endometrial polyps.
    ○ Women who may be unable to tolerate unscheduled bleeding may be better candidates for an alternative method of contraception.
- Although some clinicians treat persistent bleeding on DMPA with estrogen or NSAIDs, the efficacy of these strategies is uncertain.

PATIENT MONITORING

Women who are up to date with their periodic well-woman care returning for follow-up injections need only see the nursing personnel administering the injections (e.g., injection visit only); no clinician visit is needed in this setting.

BIBLIOGRAPHY

American College of Obstetricians and Gynecologists. Use of hormonal contraception in women with coexisting medical conditions. ACOG Practice Bulletin, Number 73. *Obstet Gynecol*. 2006;107: 1453–1472.

Kaunitz AM. Beyond the pill: New data and options in hormonal and intrauterine contraception. *Am J Obstet Gynecol*. 2005;192:998–1004.

Kaunitz AM. Depo-Provera's black box: Time to reconsider? *Contraception*. 2005;72:165–167.

Trussell J. Contraceptive failure in the United States. *Contraception*. 2004;70:89–96.

Westhoff C. Depot-medroxyprogesterone acetate injection (Depo-Provera): A highly effective contraceptive option with proven long-term safety. *Contraception*. 2003;68:75–87.

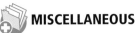 **MISCELLANEOUS**

SYNONYM(S)

- "Depo"
- DMPA
- Depo-Provera
- "The shot"

CLINICAL PEARLS

Women who receive proactive counseling regarding menstrual changes anticipated with DMPA use will be those most satisfied with their clinical care and those most likely to continue their contraception long-term.

ABBREVIATIONS

- BMD—Bone mineral density
- DMPA—Depot medroxyprogesterone acetate, Depo-Provera
- DVT—Deep venous thrombosis
- IUS—Intrauterine system
- PE—Pulmonary embolism
- PID—Pelvic inflammatory disease
- PMS—Premenstrual syndrome
- POP—Progestin-only pills
- STD—Sexually transmitted disease

LEGAL ISSUES

Emergency Contraception

All women should be advised of the availability of emergency contraception without a prescription (OTC) for women over 18 years old. Clinicians should consider the prophylactic prescription of emergency contraception for those younger than age 18.

CODES

ICD9-CM

- J1055 (to charge for the contraceptive itself)
- 90772 Therapeutic injection (to charge for the injection service)

 PATIENT TEACHING

ACOG Patient Education Pamphlet: *Hormonal Contraception—Injections, Implants, Rings, and Patches* (2007)

PREVENTION

~50% of all pregnancies in the U.S. are unintended, and among adolescents, 80–90% are unintended. The use of effective long-acting contraception including DMPA is 1 reason for declining adolescent pregnancy rates in the US.

CONTRACEPTION, HORMONAL: PROGESTIN-ONLY PILLS

Albert George Thomas, MD, MSc

 BASICS

DESCRIPTION
- Progestin-only pills (POPs) were 1st developed in 1973.
- Contains only progestin (P), not estrogen
- Consists of either:
  - Norethindrone (0.35 mg) or
  - Norgestrel (0.075 mg); no longer available in US
- Also known as the "mini-pill"
- Progestin dose 1/3 of that in COCs
- Serum P levels 1/4 of that seen with combination OCPs because of estrogen/progestin interactions
- 28 pills, all active hormone dose; no placebo
- Minipills

ALERT
There are few contraindications to use of POPs

Pregnancy Considerations
Non teratogenic, although FDA Category X

Age-Related Factors
- No age-related contraindications
- An option for any sexually active female at risk for pregnancy

EPIDEMIOLOGY
- Used < combination OCPs:
  - 4% of OCP market in Australia
  - 0.2% of OCP market in the US
- Niche product for:
  - Women with contraindications to the use of estrogen
  - Breast-feeding women after 6 weeks postpartum

MECHANISMS OF ACTION
- Progestin effects:
  - Thickened cervical mucus
  - Decreased tubal motility
  - Endometrial atrophy
- Inconsistent ovulation suppression

EFFICACY
- National survey data does not distinguish between COCs and POPs:
  - Thus, 1-year failure rate in typical use is cited as the same as COCs: 8%
  - Failure rate is likely higher with POPs.
  - POPs are often used in women who may be subfertile as a result of breast-feeding or older age.
- Back-up contraception is indicated if taken >3 hours late.

 DIAGNOSIS

HISTORY
- Medical history:
  - FDA-mandated labeling is for entire class of oral contraceptives, thus includes contraindications to COCs, because the safety of POPs has not been evaluated in women with these contraindications:
    - Known or suspected carcinoma of the breast
    - Undiagnosed abnormal genital bleeding
    - Hypersensitivity to any component of the product
    - Benign or malignant liver tumors
    - Acute liver disease
- Family history:
  - Family history of venous thromboembolism does not contraindicate POPs

Physical Exam
Annual gynecology exam as indicated for preventive health care, but not required prior to prescription of POPs:
- BP
- Breast exam
- Pelvic exam

TESTS
Risk-based screening as indicated for preventive health care, but not required prior to prescription of POPs:
- Breast cancer
- Cervical dysplasia
- STI

TREATMENT

MEDICATIONS
Drugs that increase metabolism of hormones
- Antitubercular drugs:
  - Rifampicin
- Anticonvulsants:
  - Phenytoin
  - Carbamazepine
  - Barbiturates
  - Primidone
  - Topiramate
  - Oxcarbazepine

PATIENT SELECTION
- Pregnancy risk
- Lactating 6 weeks postpartum
- Although contrary to package labeling, many experts believe that POPs are a reasonable contraceptive choice for women at high risk or for those known to have:
  - Coronary artery disease
  - Cerebrovascular disease
  - Venous thromboembolic disease
  - HTN
  - Other conditions in which use of estrogen is contraindicated

Indications
- Pregnancy risk
- Lactating 6 weeks postpartum
- Estrogen contraindication
- Desire low-progestin exposure

Contraindications
See "Medical History"

Informed Consent
Patients should be informed that the failure rate of POPs in young fertile women may be higher than that of COCs, and that it is essential that the pills be taken at the same time each day to maximize efficacy.

Patient Education
- Anticipatory counseling
- Address side effects:
  - BTB and spotting:
    - 23.1%: Irregular menses
    - 7.7%: Amenorrhea

Risks
1 study of lactating women with a history of gestational DM who used POPs had almost triple the risk of type 2 DM compared with use of COCs.

Benefits, Including Noncontraceptive
- Little impact on:
  - Coagulation factors
  - Blood pressure
  - Lipid levels
  - Carbohydrate metabolism
- Minimal hormone exposure
- Prevents pregnancy
- Prevents ectopic and intrauterine pregnancy, but if pregnancy does occur, the likelihood that the pregnancy is ectopic is higher in POP users than in noncontraceptors (5% vs. 2%)
- 1 study in breast-feeding women suggested that POP use protected against the reversible reduction in spinal BMD typically seen with breastfeeding.
- Protection against endometrial cancer

Alternatives

- For women without contraindications, COCs are an alternative.
- Progestin only alternatives:
  - Subdermal implant
  - Injectable: DMPA
  - Levonorgestrel IUS

SPECIAL GROUPS

Mentally Retarded/Developmentally Delayed

- Oral agents may be less useful:
  - Requires daily oral intake
  - Compliance may be a concern.

Adolescents

- May be less useful in adolescents, as POPs require consistent pill-taking at the same time and are quite unforgiving of missed pills.
- No protection from STIs

Women with Chronic Illness

May be useful for women with:

- HTN
- Sickle cell disease
- Heart disease
- DM
- Hyperlipidemia
- SLE
- History of DVT
- Thrombogenic mutations
- Stroke
- Migraine headache with aura
- AIDS on antiretrovirals
- Griseofulvin use
- Gallbladder disease
- Stable hepatitis carriers

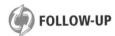 FOLLOW-UP

DISPOSITION

Issues for Referral

- May be dispensed by primary care
- Prescription required

CONTINUATION

- 1-year discontinuation rate
- 47.5% in 1 study secondary to irregular menses

PATIENT MONITORING

No specific monitoring required

COMPLICATIONS

Discontinue for idiosyncratic reactions

BIBLIOGRAPHY

Arowojolu AO, et al. Comparative evaluation of the effectiveness and safety of 2 regimens of levonorgestrel for emergency contraception in Nigerians. *Contraception*. 2002;66(4):269–273.

Broome M, et al. Clinical experience with the progestogen-only pill. *Contraception*. 1990;42(5):489–495.

Burkett AM, et al. Progestin only contraceptives and their use in adolescents: Clinical options and medical indications. *Adolesc Med Clin*. 2005;16(3):553–567.

Glasier A. Emergency postcoital contraception. *N Engl J Med*. 1997;337(15):1058–1064.

Graham S, et al. The progestogen-only mini-pill. *Contraception* 1982;26(4):373–388.

Hussain SF. Progestogen-only pills and high blood pressure: Is there an association? A literature review. *Contraception* 2004;69(2):89–97.

McCann MF, et al. Progestin-only oral contraception: A comprehensive review. *Contraception*. 1994;50(6 Suppl 1):S1–S195.

Perheentupa A, et al. Effect of progestin-only pill on pituitary-ovarian axis activity during lactation. *Contraception*. 2003;67(6):467–471.

Randomised controlled trial of levonorgestrel versus the Yuzpe regimen of combined oral contraceptives for emergency contraception. Task Force on Postovulatory Methods of Fertility Regulation. *Lancet*. 1998;352(9126):428–433.

Trussell J, et al. The role of emergency contraception. *Am J Obstet Gynecol*. 2004;190(4 Suppl 1):S30–S38.

Trussell J. Contraceptive failure in the United States. *Contraception*. 2004;70(2):89–96.

von Hertzen H, et al. Low dose mifepristone and two regimens of levonorgestrel for emergency contraception: A WHO multicentre randomised trial. *Lancet*. 2002;360(9348):1803–1810.

 MISCELLANEOUS

CLINICAL PEARLS

- Take POP at same time daily.
- Use condom backup for 1 week if:
  - Pill is missed or
  - Delayed for 3 hours
- Trial of POPs prior to progestin implant or injection has been suggested as an option that can be discontinued more easily than the implant or long-acting injection, although data are not available.
- Many experts suggest that POPs are an excellent choice for medical conditions such as HTN, diabetes, previous DVT.

ABBREVIATIONS

- BMD—Bone mineral density
- BTB—Breakthrough bleeding
- COCs—Combination oral contraceptives
- DM—Diabetes mellitus
- DVT—Deep venous thrombosis
- DMPA—Depo-medroxyprogesterone acetate
- EC—Emergency contraception
- IUS—Intrauterine system
- OCP—Oral contraceptive pill
- P—Progestin or progestogen
- POP—Progestin only pill
- SLE—Systemic lupus erythematosus
- STI—Sexually transmitted infection
- UCG—Urine chorionic gonadotropin

LEGAL ISSUES

Age/Consent or Notification for Minors

State-by-state differences:

- As of August 2006, nearly 1/2 of states explicitly allow all minors to consent to contraceptive services.
- A small number of states have no explicit policy.

Emergency Contraception

- Plan B, emergency contraceptive pill contains 2 doses of 0.75 mg levonorgestrel (See Contraception, Emergency).
- When norgestrel-containing POP was available, high-doses (20 pills) were sometimes used.

ACCESS ISSUES

Generic formulations:

- Less expensive
- Readily available

CODES

ICD9-CM

- V25.05 Oral contraceptive agent

 PATIENT TEACHING

- Quick start initiation:
  - Immediate start
  - UCG negative
  - Give EC PRN
- Dual usage: "Belt and suspenders" approach with concurrent condoms and POPs:
  - STI prevention
- Consistent daily pill usage; same time daily
- 28 active pills

PREVENTION

Dual method use to minimize risks of STIs

CONTRACEPTION, HORMONAL: TRANSDERMAL PATCH

Paula K. Braverman, MD

 BASICS

DESCRIPTION

- The hormonal patch, marketed in the US since 2002 under the trade name Ortho Evra, is a reversible combined hormonal method providing transdermal delivery of EE + norelgestromin:
  - 0.75 mg EE and 6 mg norelgestromin
  - 20 cm^2 matrix type patch with 3 layers:
    ○ Beige-colored polyethylene/polyester backing
    ○ Middle adhesive layer with hormones
    ○ Release liner, removed before application
- 3 patches each worn consecutively for 7 days followed by a patch-free week

Age-Related Factors

The patch is particularly appropriate for women who have difficulty taking daily COCs.

- Younger adolescents have more difficulty taking COCs than do adults and older women:
  - Compliance better with patch than with OCPs
- Older adolescents may do as well as adults with COCs, but may prefer patch's ease of use.

EPIDEMIOLOGY

- National data on usage patterns not available.
- Telephone, mail, and internet survey of 200,000 patch users through March 2003 showed:
  - No difference in use by marital or parenting status
  - Most (86%) had used another form of contraception prior to switching to the patch:
    ○ 2/3 had switched from OCPs.

MECHANISMS OF ACTION

- Mechanism of action is the same as with other combined hormonal contraceptives, with the primary mechanism being inhibition of ovulation.
- Suppression of gonadotropins
- Changes in cervical mucous that impair ability of sperm to access the uterus
- Changes in the endometrium that inhibit implantation
- Because of the transdermal delivery system, hormonal metabolism avoids 1st-pass liver effects:
  - Hormone levels plateau within 28 hours and reach steady state in 2 weeks.
  - Absorption at all recommended application sites (buttock, upper outer arm, abdomen, upper torso) is therapeutic and comparable.
  - Delivers daily dose of 150 μg norelgestromin and 20 μg EE
- Average concentration of EE is 60% higher than an OCP with 35 mg EE
- Hormonal levels are low or not measurable within 3 days of removal.

EFFICACY

- Overall Pearl index 0.88/100 women years
- Compliance is better than COCs in multiple studies in all age groups.
- Efficacy similar in various age and racial groups.
- Pregnancy rates higher if >198 lbs (90 kg):
  - Pearl index for <90 kg, 0.6/100 women years
- In women at high risk for unintended pregnancy or abortion with lower continuation rates:
  - Pearl index 14.84/100 women years

 DIAGNOSIS

HISTORY

- Medical history:
  - Chronic medical conditions
  - Current medications
  - Menstrual history
  - Previous contraceptive use
  - History of STIs
  - Pregnancy history and outcome(s)
  - Medical conditions that would be a contraindication for COCs
- Family history:
  - Family history should include a focus on potential inherited conditions that would contradict use of estrogen-containing hormonal contraceptives such as:
    ○ Hereditary thrombophilias
    ○ History of DVT or PE

Physical Exam

- Comprehensive physical exam including pelvic exam is an important part of routine health maintenance but not required prior to prescribing.
- BP and weight should be measured to determine if BP is within acceptable limits and if the weight >90 kg:
  - Can be prescribed if BP is controlled and stable
  - Counsel about potential decreased efficacy at higher weights, but the patch is not contraindicated, providing that the patient is appropriately informed

TESTS

No specific laboratory tests are needed.

Labs

- If family history shows DVT or PE in 1st-degree relative, consider evaluation for hypercoagulation disorder including factor V Leiden, protein C, protein S, antithrombin III deficiency, prothrombin mutation
- If known hyperlipidemia requiring medical treatment, consider retesting lipids after initiating:
  - Changes in lipids in patch users are not usually clinically significant.
  - However, patients with familial hypertriglyceridemia may have significant elevations in triglycerides.
- If history indicates liver dysfunction, perform liver function tests prior to use.
- If pregnancy suspected, do pregnancy test.
- If a hormonal abnormality such as PCOS or a hematologic disorder (eg, VWD) suspected, complete evaluation prior to prescribing, since hormonal contraceptives may alter test results and prevent diagnosis of the underlying condition.
- STI, HIV testing, and Pap smears should be performed at recommended intervals for health maintenance but are not required prior to prescribing.

 TREATMENT

MEDICATIONS

- Decreased efficacy may occur with:
  - Drugs that induce the hepatic microsomal P450 system:
    ○ Certain anticonvulsant medications
    ○ Anti-HIV protease inhibitors
    ○ Herbal products such as St. John's wort
  - Drugs that may increase hormone levels:
    ○ Atorvastatin
    ○ Ascorbic acid
    ○ Acetaminophen
    ○ Itraconazole
    ○ Ketoconazole
- Most antibiotics do not affect contraceptive efficacy of the patch:
  - Exception: Rifampin

PATIENT SELECTION

Patients who meet medical eligibility criteria, can use properly, weigh <90 kg, and who choose transdermal contraception are good candidates.

Indications

For contraception in postmenarchal women

Contraindications

Medical conditions in which the use of the patch represents an unacceptable health risk include:

- Thrombophlebitis, thromboembolic disorders
- History of DVT or thromboembolic disorders/ thrombogenic mutations
- Cerebrovascular or CAD, valvular heart disease with thrombogenic complications
- Uncontrolled HTN (≥160 systolic, ≥100 diastolic)
- Diabetes with vascular involvement
- Headaches with focal neurologic symptoms/aura
- Major surgery with prolonged immobilization
- Breast cancer (current)
- Acute or chronic liver disease with abnormal liver function
- Hepatic adenoma or carcinoma
- Breast-feeding <6 weeks postpartum
- Women >35 who smoke ≥ 15 cigarettes a day:
  - Women >35 who smoke are at increased risk of serious cardiovascular side effects.

Informed Consent

Clinicians should inform patients of potential complications from the patch.

Patient Education

- Review prior to use
- 1st patch cycle should begin on day 1 of menses or the Sunday after 1st day of menses
- Attach patch to clean dry skin free of creams, lotions, powders:
  - Buttock, abdomen, upper outer arm, or upper torso (but not near the breast)
- Press patch firmly and be sure it is completely attached.
- If patch partially or totally detaches, it must be replaced with a new patch (e.g., not reapplied if it is not sticky):
  - Provide a prescription for replacement patches.
  - Pregnancy protection is maintained if patch is off <24 hours. However, if patch has been off >24 hrs, start a new 4-week cycle.

- Apply new patch weekly to a new skin location on same day of the week for 3 weeks.
- During the 4th week of the cycle, no patch is worn. A new patch cycle is started on the patch change day 1 week later.
- Up to 48 hours of extra hormone protection is provided in each patch; if the duration of use exceeds 7 days, the patch change day can remain the same as long as it is changed within 48 hours of the scheduled change day.
- A new patch cycle must be started 7 days after the last patch is removed to ensure contraceptive efficacy (e.g., hormone-free period cannot exceed 7 days).

Risks
- Serious adverse events that have been associated with COCs and are presumed to be similar for the patch include thrombophlebitis, venous thrombosis, arterial thromboembolism, PE, MI, cerebral hemorrhage, cerebral thrombosis, HTN, gall bladder disease, hepatic adenomas, benign liver tumors, and retinal thrombosis.
- Conflicting data about whether there is a greater risk of VTE than with COCs:
  - 1 study comparing patch to OCPs with 35 μg EE + norgestimate showed no greater risk of nonfatal VTE.
  - Another study showed a 2-fold greater risk of VTE compared to same OCP.
  - Current labeling describes the increased levels of EE and possible greater risk of VTE.

Benefits, Including Noncontraceptive
- Ability to use the method on a weekly rather than a daily basis
- Androgen levels have been shown to decline in patch users, thus providing benefit with PCOS.
- It is presumed, but not yet proven, that the patch has the same noncontraceptive benefits as OCPs for acne and menstrual disorders such as dysfunctional uterine bleeding, PCOS, and dysmenorrhea. No studies evaluate the affects on bone density or cancer prevention.

Alternatives
- Reversible contraceptive alternatives include other forms of hormonal contraception, barrier method contraception, and the IUD.
- Permanent sterilization (male or female)

SPECIAL GROUPS
Mentally Retarded/Developmentally Delayed
Use for contraception or menstrual regulation may be helpful in girls with developmental delay, although some girls will "pick" at skin lesions or the patch, causing the patch to be dislodged.

Adolescents
- Only a few small studies to date on the use of the patch in adolescents
- Overall, these studies indicated satisfaction with the method and good short-term compliance.
- 1 study showed that up to 1/3 experienced detachments, which is higher than that reported in adults. Another study showed poor condom use among patch users:
  - Review instructions and emphasize the need to also use condoms for STI protection.

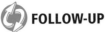 **FOLLOW-UP**

CONTINUATION
Except for the previously mentioned study in an adolescent high-risk population, compliance in general has been good with the patch and better than OCPs in many studies.

PATIENT MONITORING
Patient follow-up within the 1st 3 patch cycles is useful to review compliance, side effects, and to check weight and BP. Follow-up visit in 6–12 months depending on whether or not close monitoring of side effects or compliance is needed.

COMPLICATIONS
Most adverse reactions observed in studies resolved by the 3rd patch cycle:
- Breast tenderness
- Nausea
- Headache
- BTB
- Patch detachment:
  - Only 4.7% of 70,000 patches worn for 6–13 cycles detached partially or totally.
  - Have been demonstrated to stay in place under various conditions of physical activity, temperature, humidity, and water immersion
- Application site reaction/rash or pruritus
- Dysmenorrhea
- Possible increased risk of VTE

BIBLIOGRAPHY

Abrams LS, et al. Pharmacokinetics of norelgestromin and ethinyl estradiol delivered by a contraceptive patch (Ortho Evra™/ Evra™) under conditions of heat, humidity, and exercise. *J Clin Pharmacol.* 2001;41:1301–1309.

Bakhru A, et al. Performance of contraceptive patch compared with oral contraceptive pill in a high-risk population. *Obstet Gynecol.* 2006;108:378–386.

Burkman RT. The transdermal contraceptive system. *Am J Obstet Gynecol.* 2004;190:S49–S53.

Cole JA, et al. Venous thromboembolism, myocardial infarction, and stroke among transdermal contraceptive users. *Obstet Gynecol.* 2007; 109:339–346.

Harel Z, et al. Adolescents' experience with the combined estrogen and progestin transdermal contraceptive method Ortho Evra. *J Pediatr Adolesc Gynecol.* 2005;18:85–90.

Jick SS, et al. Risk of nonfatal venous thromboembolism in women using a contraceptive transdermal patch and oral contraceptives containing norgestimate and 35 μg of ethinyl estradiol. *Contraception.* 2006;73:223–228.

Rubinstein ML, et al. An evaluation of the use of the transdermal contraceptive patch in adolescents. *J Adolesc Health.* 2004;34:395–401.

Zieman M, et al. Contraceptive efficacy and cycle control with the Ortho Evra™/Evra™ transdermal system: The analysis of pooled data. *Fertil Steril.* 2002;77(Suppl 2):S13–S18.

 MISCELLANEOUS

SYNONYM(S)
- Contraceptive patch
- OrthoEvra, Evra
- "The patch"
- Transdermal contraceptive system

CLINICAL PEARLS
- The patch is a well-tolerated form of combined hormonal contraception that may have better patient compliance than OCPs.
- Conflicting data are currently available about the risk of VTE events compared to COCs.

ABBREVIATIONS
- BP—Blood pressure
- BTB—Breakthrough bleeding
- CAD—Coronary artery disease
- COC—Combination oral contraceptive
- DVT—Deep vein thrombosis
- EE—Ethinyl estradiol
- MI—Myocardial infarction
- OCP—Oral contraceptive pill
- PCOS—Polycystic ovary syndrome
- PE—Pulmonary embolism
- STI—Sexually transmitted infection
- VTE—Venous thromboembolism
- VWD—von Willebrand disease

LEGAL ISSUES
Age/Consent or Notification for Minors
Adolescents may request confidential contraceptive services. For minors < age 18:
- The clinician should determine if the adolescent is a mature minor who can understand the risks and benefits of the patch.
- Parental consent is not needed for sites receiving federal Title X funding:
  - Review state laws for non-Title X sites.
  - If no law is applicable, clinical judgment of the minor's ability to give informed consent should be used.

ACCESS ISSUES
Check insurance coverage for use as an initial contraceptive choice. Some will only cover after evidence that the patient has tried and failed another method, such as OCPs.

CODES
ICD9-CM
There is no specific ICD9 code for the patch:
- V25.02 Contraception, prescription, specified agent NEC
- V25.49 Contraception, prescription, repeat

PATIENT TEACHING

PREVENTION
For individuals at risk for acquiring STIs, discuss and encourage concurrent condom use.

Section III

CONTRACEPTION, HORMONAL: VAGINAL RING

Susan A. Ballagh, MD

BASICS

DESCRIPTION
- NuvaRing is the only contraceptive ring currently available in the US.
- It provides:
  - 0.015 mg of EE
  - 0.120 mg of etonogestrel (progestin)
- The hormones are released gradually by placing the ring in the vagina. It is worn for 21 days, then removed and discarded. A withdrawal bleeding occurs, and a new ring is placed into the vagina within 7 days to begin the next cycle.

Age-Related Factors
- WHO category 1 for women ages 18–39
- WHO category 2 for women >40
- All women using estrogen-containing contraceptives should be advised to reduce or preferably quit smoking.

Pediatric Considerations
NuvaRing has been studied in sexually active teens and appears to be safe for this age group. It is not intended for use prior to normal menarche.

Geriatric Considerations
NuvaRing has not been studied in menopausal women and is not indicated for them. Other ring products are available for hormone therapy in that population (Femring for vasomotor and vaginal symptoms and Estring for urogenital symptoms).

ALERT
Smokers >35 should not use the ring; they should switch to estrogen-free birth control.

EPIDEMIOLOGY
In developed countries (where average desired family size is small), of the 28 million pregnancies occurring every year, an estimated 49% are unplanned, and nearly half of these end in abortion.

MECHANISMS OF ACTION
- The ring inhibits ovulation by blocking pituitary output of LH and FSH.
- It also thickens cervical mucus and thins the endometrium predominantly due to the progestin.
- EE stabilizes the endometrial lining to minimize bleeding.
- The ring can sit in any location within the vagina for hormone release.

EFFICACY
The ring prevents pregnancy in 98 of 100 couples who use it for 1 year (Pearl index):
- Efficacy is reduced when women take hepatic enzyme–inducing medications.
- There is no evidence that the vaginal route of delivery alters contraceptive safety or effect.

Pregnancy Considerations
- Current pregnancy is a contraindication.
- If a woman becomes pregnant while using the ring she should remove it.
- No documented increase in risk of ectopic pregnancy
- In event of exposure, there is no need to recommend pregnancy termination based on teratogenicity concerns.

DIAGNOSIS

HISTORY
- Medical history:
  - Personal or family history of conditions that would contraindicate use of combination hormonal contraception
  - Last menses is used to determine if NuvaRing can be started immediately.
- Family history:
- Women with a family history of unexplained thrombosis are at increased risk with estrogen-containing products.
- No need to test for familial thrombotic tendencies in women with a family history of thrombosis as these tests do not predict risk of thrombosis well.

Physical Exam
- Annual breast examination and/or mammogram recommended in women >40 prior to use.
- Record BP and weight

TESTS
- Pap smear or cervical cultures are not required.
- No pelvic exam is needed.
- Women should be encouraged to seek routine health screening.

Lab
- No laboratory tests are required before use.
- A urine pregnancy test may be clinically indicated in certain circumstances.

TREATMENT

MEDICATIONS
Medications that may alter the efficacy of NuvaRing include:
- Anticonvulsants may decrease effect:
  - Phenytoin
  - Carbamazepine
  - Barbiturates
  - Primidone
- Only a few anti-infectives decrease effect:
  - Rifampicin
  - Griseofulvin
  - Streptomycin:
    - Most antibiotics do not interact
    - Vaginal antifungals and nonoxynol-9 spermicide do NOT reduce serum levels.
    - Significant interactions reported with ARV therapy: Contraceptive steroid levels may be reduced or elevated, and ARV efficacy may be compromised.

PATIENT SELECTION
- Safe option for women who are candidates for combination contraceptives.
- More acceptable in women who have been sexually active
- Useful for women who forget to take pills daily

Indications
- Reproductive-age women who desire an easily applied, reversible contraceptive that they can control

- Backup contraception not needed if ring initiated:
  - Day 1–5 of the menstrual cycle
  - Anytime during proper use of another contraceptive
  - Within 5 days of a 1st trimester miscarriage or termination
  - Within 21–28 days after a 2nd trimester termination or a birth
- If pregnancy is ruled out, may start at other times with backup contraceptive for the 1st 7 days.

Contraindications
- Women should not use NuvaRing if they have:
  - Personal history of thromboembolism
  - Hepatic tumors or liver disease, including active viral hepatitis
  - Undiagnosed, abnormal vaginal bleeding
  - Suspicion or personal history of a hormone-sensitive cancer like breast or endometrial.
  - Sensitivity to Evatane or sex steroids
  - Current pregnancy
  - Migraine with aura
  - Multiple risk factors for arterial CVD:
    - Diabetes
    - HTN
    - Hyperlipidemia
  - Active cholelithiasis, or prior history of biliary tract disease on COCs
  - Plans for major surgery followed by prolonged immobilization
  - Personal history of ischemic CVD or stroke
  - Complicated valvular heart disease (pulmonary HTN, risk of atrial fibrillation, SBE)
  - Known vascular disease associated with diabetes or other conditions
  - Smokers >35
- Most women who desire hormonal contraception but have contraindications above will be more appropriate candidates for progestin only oral, injected, or intrauterine contraception.

Informed Consent
- Review all appropriate contraceptive methods.
- Review risks, side effects *and* benefits.

Patient Education
- Remind patients that NuvaRing does not provide protection from STIs
  - Barriers should be used to reduce STI risk.
- Ring placed like a tampon: Any comfortable position is acceptable, no "fit" is required.
- Ring may be left in place for intercourse. If it interferes with intimacy, remove prior to sex but replace it within 3 hours to maintain efficacy.
- The ring may accidentally come out with straining, tampon removal, or intercourse. Rinse with water and replace ring within 3 hours.
- Rarely rings have broken, causing discomfort or expulsion. Discard and replace with a new ring.
- If ring is left in place >35 days or is out over 7 days, offer EC if recently exposed to pregnancy, immediately begin a new cycle and use backup contraception.
- If no withdrawal bleeding after removing NuvaRing, review use and bleeding during the cycle and rule out pregnancy if indicated.

- Consider skipping the ring-free week if improper use is noted during a cycle.
- Dispose of the ring in a solid waste container.

Risks

- Limited data; thus risks listed are based on oral contraceptive experience:
  - Use of combination contraception increases the risk of thromboembolism compared to nonusers, up to 2 additional cases per 10,000 women per year. Risk is only while using drug.
  - Mortality from circulatory and CVD increases when estrogen-containing contraceptives are combined with cigarettes.
  - Risk of thrombotic and hemorrhagic stroke is increased, particularly in hypertensive women who smoke. This risk further increases with age.
  - The risk of breast cancer may be slightly increased among current or recent users. The risk disappears 10 years after discontinuation.
  - Risk of benign hepatic adenomas is increased by 3.3 cases per 100,000 women years and increases further with use beyond 4 years.
    - Liver cancer risk may be increased but is too rare to provide a reliable risk estimate.
  - Rare case reports of retinal thrombosis. Discontinue NuvaRing if there is vision loss, visual or retinal changes, or papilledema.
  - Gall bladder disease may develop or accelerate with use of estrogen-containing contraceptives.
  - Rare women will develop hypertriglyceridemia using estrogen-containing contraceptives.
  - Prediabetic or diabetic women may have decreased glucose tolerance with NuvaRing.
  - BP may increase in women using a combination contraceptive, especially if older, with prolonged use of the contraceptive.
  - Onset or exacerbation of migraine symptoms or persistent, recurrent, or severe new headaches
  - Identification of these problems warrants immediate discontinuation of NuvaRing.
- Common nuisance side effects:
  - Reported by 1–5% of NuvaRing users:
    - Vaginal infection
    - Vaginal irritation
    - Increased vaginal secretions
    - Headache or migraine
    - Weight gain/fluid retention
    - Nausea
  - Reported with other combined contraceptives:
    - Vomiting
    - Change in appetite
    - Abdominal cramps/bloating
    - Breast tenderness of enlargement
    - Irregular vaginal bleeding/spotting
    - Melasma, may persist after use
    - Rash
    - Depressed mood
    - Vaginal candidiasis
    - Intolerance of contact lenses

Benefits, Including Noncontraceptive

- Effective pregnancy prevention without daily attention
- Patient-controlled insertion and removal with rapid return to fertility once ring is discontinued.
- Benefits of combination contraceptives are assumed to apply to NuvaRing:
  - Reduced menstrual blood loss
  - Reduced risk of endometrial or ovarian cancer
  - Reduced infection in the upper genital tract
  - May alleviate symptoms of endometriosis
  - Reduced vaginal dryness

Alternatives

- Nonhormonal alternatives are less effective than NuvaRing or other combined contraceptive products except for copper IUD or sterilization.
- Only implants or injections are more efficacious hormonal methods than NuvaRing in typical use.
- When infection prevention is needed, may be combined with barrier methods to reduce STIs.

SPECIAL GROUPS
Mentally Retarded/Developmentally Delayed

- May aid caretakers in providing contraception to dependents since application and ring removal are all that is needed per cycle.
- Since NuvaRing is fully reversible, it does not require legal action to provide to women who are unable to consent to surgery or procedures.

Adolescents

May be helpful for sexually active teens who have difficulty taking pills, particularly if living in multiple locations, since the ring stays with them.

Women with Chronic Illness

- May be indicated to reduce the risk of pregnancy in women in whom pregnancy may be dangerous or life-threatening.
- Should be avoided in women with vascular disease or other risk factors that would increase the risk of estrogen use.

SURGERY

- Should be discontinued before major surgery that will require prolonged immobilization due to the increased risk of thromboembolism.
- No need to discontinue drug prior to a brief interval sterilization procedure

 ## FOLLOW-UP

CONTINUATION

In a comparative study, 88% continued ring use at 1 year compared to 74% of pill users.

PATIENT MONITORING

- Assess blood pressure and weight, regardless of side effects reported at office visit.
- No need for special monitoring.
- Annual prescription for low-risk, healthy, normotensive users.
- At initialization of new contraception, early follow-up visit may allow identification of incorrect use or side effects.
- Women with risk factors for vascular disease, diabetes, or HTN may benefit from early reassessment of their response to therapy.
- Smokers <35 should be offered smoking cessation therapy at least annually.

COMPLICATIONS

- Ectopic pregnancy is no more likely than intrauterine pregnancy with method failure.
- TSS has been reported in conjunction with tampon use. It has not been attributed to the ring alone.

BIBLIOGRAPHY

Furlong LA. Ectopic pregnancy risk when contraception fails. A review. *J Reprod Med*. 2002;47(11):881–885.

Guttmacher Institute: Sharing Responsibility Women, Society and Abortion Worldwide, 1999. Page 42. Accessed 03/19/07 at http://www.guttmacher. org/pubs/sharing.pdf.

Marinez-Frias ML, et al. Prenatal exposure to sex hormones: A case-control study. *Teratology*. 1998;57(1):8–12.

Medical Eligibility for Contraceptive Use: Low-Dose Combined Oral Contraceptives, 3rd ed. Geneva: WHO, 13.

NuvaRing® Physician's Insert 75137. Roseland, NJ: OrganonUSA Inc., 2005. Accessed 03/01/07 at http://www.nuvaring.com/Authfiles/ Images/ 309_103003.pdf

Sabatini R, et al. Comparison profiles of cycle control, side effects and sexual satisfaction of three hormonal contraceptives. *Contraception*. 2006; 74:220–223.

 ## MISCELLANEOUS

SYNONYM(S)

- Etonogestrel/Ethinyl Estradiol ring
- NuvaRing
- Vaginal hormonal contraceptive
- Vaginal ring

CLINICAL PEARLS

- Women rarely feel the ring once it is placed, but must experience the lack of sensation to believe it. Use samples if available.
- BTB is low from the 1st month of use.
- St. John's Wort (herbal) may reduce efficacy.

ABBREVIATIONS

- ARV—Antiretroviral therapy
- BTB—Breakthrough bleeding
- CVD—Cardiovascular disease
- EC—Emergency contraception
- EE—Ethinyl estradiol
- FSH—Follicle-stimulating hormone
- LH—Luteinizing hormone
- SBE—Subacute bacterial endocarditis
- STI—Sexually transmitted infection
- TSS—Toxic shock syndrome
- WHO—World Health Organization

LEGAL ISSUES
Age/Consent or Notification for Minors

Observe your state laws concerning minor's ability to consent for contraception.

Emergency Contraception

- Consider if the ring has been in place for >35 days, out for >7 days, or used inconsistently *and* patient has recently had sexual intercourse.
- NOT an emergency contraceptive

CODES

ICD9-CM

- V25.02 Prescription of contraceptive
- V25.09 General contraceptive counseling
- V25.49 Repeat prescription for contraceptive
- V25.9 Contraceptive management

CONTRACEPTION: INTRAUTERINE CONTRACEPTIVES (IUCs)

DeShawn L. Taylor, MD, MSc
Raquel D. Arias, MD

 BASICS

DESCRIPTION

- ParaGard T 380A intrauterine copper contraceptive and Mirena LNG-releasing IUS are the 2 IUCs available in US.
- Both frames contain barium sulfate for detection by radiograph.
- Monofilament polyethylene removal threads are attached at base of vertical stems.
- ParaGard T 380A Copper IUC:
  - T-shaped intrauterine contraceptive with polyethylene frame
  - Copper wound around stem and transverse arms to create total surface area of 380 mm^2
- Mirena LNG-IUS:
  - T-shaped polyethylene IUS with reservoir that contains 52 mg LNG
  - Sustained release of LNG directly into uterine cavity at an initial rate of 20 μg/d

EPIDEMIOLOGY

- IUC prevalence 1% in US
- IUC prevalence is 3–26 times higher in other developed countries:
  - Canada (3%)
  - United Kingdom (6%)
  - France (20%)
  - Finland (26%)

MECHANISMS OF ACTION

- IUCs produce a sterile foreign-body reaction within uterine cavity impeding sperm transport, fertilization, and implantation.
- Copper ions released from the copper IUC enhance inflammatory response.
- High local concentrations of LNG from the LNG-IUS render the endometrium inactive and cervical mucous impenetrable.
- IUCs are NOT abortifacients

EFFICACY

- ParaGard T 380A Copper IUC:
  - Device approved for 10 years of contraceptive use, but effective for 12 years
  - Typical use failure rate at 1 year: 0.8%
- Mirena LNG-IUS:
  - Device approved for 5 years of contraceptive use, but effective for 7 years
  - Typical use failure rate at 1 year: 0.1%

 DIAGNOSIS

HISTORY

Medical history:

- Note last menstrual period.
- Evaluate abnormal vaginal bleeding if present.
- Uterine fibroids or other acquired or congenital uterine anomalies may be incompatible with IUC insertion and proper placement.
- Previous PID, gonorrhea, or chlamydial infections not contraindications to IUC use, but women at high risk for STI acquisition may not be optimal candidates for IUC.
- Note chronic medical conditions.

Physical Exam

Perform speculum and bimanual examination:

- Exclude active pelvic infection
- Identify position of uterus
- Unrecognized retroflexed uterus may increase risk of perforation at time of IUC insertion.

TESTS

Urine pregnancy test

Lab

STI screen if indicated by physical exam/age

Imaging

- Not routinely indicated
- Pelvic sonography may be indicated to rule out distortion of uterine cavity if uterine fibroids or suspected congenital uterine anomaly.

TREATMENT

MEDICATIONS

Agents that induce hepatic enzymes have potential but unknown risk of decreased efficacy for LNG-IUS:

- Some antiepileptics
- Rifampin
- St. John's wort

PATIENT SELECTION

- Desire or necessity to avoid estrogen-containing contraceptives
- Age and parity not critical factors:
  - Nulliparous women can safely use IUCs.
- Language regarding monogamous relationships removed from ParaGard labeling:
  - There is no evidence to support upholding similar restrictions for Mirena users.

Indications

Women desiring highly effective, long-acting, reversible intrauterine contraception

Contraindications

- Pregnancy
- Puerperal sepsis (postpartum endometritis)
- Immediate post septic abortion
- Undiagnosed abnormal vaginal bleeding
- Malignant gestational trophoblastic disease
- Uterine or cervical malignancy
- Breast carcinoma (LNG-IUS):
  - Theoretical risk
- Distorted uterine cavity due to congenital or acquired conditions
- Current PID, purulent cervicitis, gonorrhea, or chlamydial infections
- Pelvic tuberculosis
- Contraindication specific to copper IUC:
  - Wilson disease and copper allergy

Informed Consent

- Discuss benefits, risks, and alternatives prior to IUC insertion.
- Signed consent forms are recommended.

Patient Education

- Protection against pregnancy begins immediately after insertion.
- Changes in menstrual patterns may occur and are expected.
- Use condoms to protect against STIs.
- Transient increased risk of pelvic infection in the 1st few weeks after insertion
- IUC can be spontaneously expelled.

Risks

- Changes in menstrual bleeding patterns
- Cramping and pain at time of IUC insertion
- Expulsion 2–10% in 1st year, then declines over time
- Perforation 1/1,000 insertions:
  - Occurs at the time of insertion
- PID risk greatest in 1st 20 days after insertion due to contamination of endometrial cavity at time of insertion:
  - Antibiotic prophylaxis should not be used routinely before IUC insertion

Benefits, Including Noncontraceptive

- Advantages of IUCs:
  - Highly effective
  - Long acting
  - Protective against ectopic pregnancy
  - Rapid return to fertility after discontinuation
- Noncontraceptive benefits:
  - LNG-IUS:
    - Reduces menstrual blood loss and improves levels of hemoglobin, hematocrit, and serum ferritin in women with menorrhagia
    - As effective as endometrial resection and ablation

○ Cost effective alternative to hysterectomy
○ Reduces menstrual bleeding and pain in women with uterine fibroids and adenomyosis
○ Reduces pain in women with endometriosis
○ Suppression of endometrium expected to decrease risk of endometrial cancer
– Copper IUC:
○ Reduces risk of endometrial cancer
○ May reduce risk of cervical cancer

Alternatives
Injectables and implants are other highly effective, long-acting, reversible contraceptive methods.

SPECIAL GROUPS
Mentally Retarded/Developmentally Delayed
• Common concerns are menstrual hygiene, premenstrual symptoms, and pregnancy
• LNG-IUS provides menstrual hygiene benefits
• May need to insert in operating room under general anesthesia

Adolescents
• Highly effective, long-term, reversible contraception is the goal.
• Given appropriate screening, counseling, and care, the IUC is a contraceptive option for adolescents.

Women with Chronic Illness
• IUC use safe in the following conditions:
– Cardiovascular and cerebrovascular disease
– HTN
– DVT and PE
– Epilepsy
– Migraine headaches with and without aura
– DM
– HIV-infection and AIDS, clinically well on antiretrovirals
– Valvular heart disease
• Antibiotics NOT recommended solely for bacterial endocarditis prophylaxis for GU procedures (2007 guidelines)

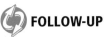 FOLLOW-UP

DISPOSITION
Issues for Referral
• Embedded or perforated IUC
• Pregnancy with IUC in situ

PATIENT MONITORING
• Follow up in 2–3 months after insertion to evaluate for pelvic infection and expulsion
• Patient should return sooner if she experiences any problems
• Inquire about risks for STI.
• Ask if patient can feel IUC strings and if they've changed in length.
• Inquire about bleeding patterns and offer reassurance.
• Evaluate and treat genital tract infections.

COMPLICATIONS
• Excessive bleeding:
– Bleeding due to copper IUC can be treated with NSAIDs.
– Provide iron supplementation if hemoglobin declines.
– Persistent abnormal bleeding requires clinical evaluation.

• Expulsion:
– Suspect if following symptoms present:
○ Unusual vaginal discharge
○ Cramping or pain
○ Intermenstrual or postcoital spotting
○ Dyspareunia (male or female)
○ Absence or lengthening of IUC strings
○ Visualization of IUC at cervical os or in vagina
• Uterine perforation:
– Copper induces adhesion formation in the peritoneal cavity that may involve adnexal, omentum, and bowel
– Prompt, preferably laparoscopic, removal recommended
• PID:
– No need to remove IUC during treatment
• Pregnancy:
– IUC should be removed at time pregnancy is diagnosed if strings are visible, regardless of patient's plan for the pregnancy
– 40–50% risk of spontaneous abortion if IUC left in place
– 30% risk of spontaneous abortion after IUC removed

BIBLIOGRAPHY

Guttmacher Institute. *State policies in brief; an overview of minors' consent law*. New York: Guttmacher Institute; January 1, 2007.

Hatcher RA, et al. *Contraceptive Technology*, 18th ed. New York: Ardent Media, Inc.; 2004.

Jensen JT. Contraceptive and therapeutic effects of the levonorgestrel intrauterine system: An overview. *Obstet Gynecol Surv*. 2005;60(9):604–612.

Kaunitz AM. Beyond the pill: New data and options in hormonal and intrauterine contraception. *Am J Obstet Gynecol*. 2005;192:998–1004.

Ora I, et al. Management of menstrual problems and contraception in adolescents with mental retardation: A medical, legal, and ethical review with new suggested guidelines. *J Pediat Adolesc Gynecol*. 2003;16(4):223–235.

Ortiz ME, et al. Mechanisms of action of intrauterine devices. *Obstet Gynecol Surv*. 1996;51(12 Suppl): S42–S51.

Speroff L, et al. *A Clinical Guide for Contraception*, 3rd ed. Philadelphia: Lippincott Williams & Wilkins, 2001.

United Nations Population Division. World Contraceptive Use 2005. Available at: www.un.org/esa/population/publications/contraceptive2005/2005_World_Contraceptive files/WallChart_WCU2005.pdf.

World Health Organization. Improving Access to Quality Care in Family Planning. *Medical Eligibility Criteria for Contraceptive Use*, 3rd ed. Geneva, Switzerland: World Health Organization; 2004

 MISCELLANEOUS

• Timing of IUC insertion:
– IUC may be inserted at any time in the cycle as long as evidence exists that patient is not pregnant.
– IUC insertion immediately after abortion or delivery is safe:
○ Expulsion rates are higher immediately after delivery and 2nd trimester abortions.

○ Balance higher expulsion rate with likelihood that patient will not return for delayed insertion.
– IUC insertion in breastfeeding women does not increase risk of perforation.
• *Actinomyces*-like organisms on Pap smear:
– *Actinomyces* species are normal inhabitants of the female genital tract.
– Found in Pap smears of up to 30% of plastic IUC wearers when cytologist looks for organism
– If patient asymptomatic, antibiotics and/or removal of IUC not necessary
– No evidence to support removing IUC and replacing after repeat Pap is negative:
○ If evidence of active infection, remove IUC and prescribe course of oral antibiotics
○ IUC must be removed during treatment because *Actinomyces* species preferentially grow on foreign bodies.

SYNONYM(S)
Intrauterine device (IUD)

ABBREVIATIONS
• DM—Diabetes mellitus
• DVT—Deep venous thrombosis
• IUC—Intrauterine contraceptive
• LNG-IUS—Levonorgestrel-releasing intrauterine system
• PE—Pulmonary embolism
• PID—Pelvic inflammatory disease
• STI—Sexually transmitted infection

LEGAL ISSUES
Age/Consent or Notification for Minors
• All minors ($\geq$12) may consent to contraceptive services in 25 states and District of Columbia.
• Certain categories of minors may consent to contraceptive services in 21 states:
– Married, pregnant, mature, health issues, etc.
• 4 states have no policy.

Emergency Contraception
• Copper IUC inserted within 120 hours of unprotected intercourse is 98% effective in preventing pregnancy.
• Good choice for women who want to continue copper IUC as long-term method of contraception

ACCESS ISSUES
Lack of medical insurance or insurance coverage for IUC limit access

CODES
ICD9-CM
• 69.7 Insertion of intrauterine contraceptive device
• 97.71 Removal of intrauterine contraceptive

PATIENT TEACHING

• Check to feel the string after menses.
• Call for fever, lower abdominal pain, or discharge suggesting PID.

PREVENTION
• LNG-IUS may help to prevent a hysterectomy for heavy uterine bleeding.
• IUC efficacy comparable to sterilization, and thus may prevent surgical sterilization.

Section III

CONTRACEPTION: SPERMICIDES

Susan A. Ballagh, MD

 BASICS

DESCRIPTION
- Spermicidal products, sold separately in the US, are intended for use alone, with condoms, or with vaginal or cervical barrier devices.
- Those products intended for use alone or with condoms contain 4% nonoxynol-9 (N-9) and are free of petroleum products.
- Products designed for use with cervico-vaginal barriers contain 2% N-9 or octoxynol-9.
- To be effective, spermicides must be placed in the vagina before intercourse within 1 hour after insertion and retained for 6 hours afterward. If spermicide is used alone, it should be reapplied before each ejaculation.
- Nonoxynol (N-9)-containing gels, inserts, creams, and film
- Octoxynol-9 containing creams

Age-Related Factors
WHO category 1 for all women. Not recommended for use by women who are not at risk for pregnancy.

EPIDEMIOLOGY
- Used throughout the world.
- Available in the US without a prescription.
- Current products have been marketed since the 1950s.

MECHANISM OF ACTION
- Nonoxynol-9 or octoxynol-9, the active ingredients, are detergents that damage membranes and inhibit or kill sperm. They must be present in the vagina before intercourse to be effective.
- Spermicides do not prevent STIs.

EFFICACY
- In a multicenter US clinical trial, the 6-month cumulative pregnancy rate for spermicide alone varied by dose:
  - 52.5 mg gel: 22% (range 16–28%)
  - 100 mg gel: 14% (range 9–19%)
  - 150 mg gel: 12% (range 7–17%)
- Method failure rate was higher for film than for gel or insert formulations.

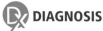 **DIAGNOSIS**

HISTORY
- Medical history:
  - Women with allergy to nonoxynol-9, octoxynol-9, or product excipients should avoid exposure.
  - Women with medical conditions or medication use that make pregnancy inadvisable should be encouraged to consider more efficacious contraceptive methods.
- Family history: Not pertinent with regard to method use.

TESTS
- None required prior to use.
- Women should be encouraged to seek appropriate preventive health care.

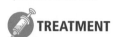 **TREATMENT**

MEDICATIONS
- None reported
- Spermicides with a petroleum base should not be used with latex condoms as they may damage or weaken the latex.

PATIENT SELECTION
- Safe in recently postpartum or breast-feeding women.
- Does not contain hormones.
- Particularly appropriate for women with infrequent coitus or those using contraceptives to space their children.

Indications
Spermicides are indicated for women who want a user-controlled method and accept a moderate risk of contraceptive failure.

Contraindications
- Women should not use spermicides if they have:
  - Hypersensitivity to nonoxynol-9, octoxynol-9, or other component in the product. The most common product additives are:
    - Methylparaben
    - Sorbic acid
    - Cellulose gum
    - Lactic acid
    - Povidone
    - Propylene glycol
    - Sorbitol
- Frequent use may increase the risk of acquiring HIV infection if exposed to the virus. Spermicide should not be used in the rectum.

Informed Consent
Not required. Available OTC.

Patient Education
- No prevention of STIs when used alone.
- Frequent use may increase the risk of HIV transmission.
- Avoid douching after placement of spermicide until 6 hours after the last ejaculation.
- Apply spermicide for each act of intercourse.

Risks
- Frequent use may increase the risk of HIV transmission.
- Dose-dependent increase in anaerobic gram-negative rods, peroxidase-negative lactobacilli, and bacterial vaginosis.

Pregnancy Considerations
No clear epidemiologic data links prenatal spermicide exposure to birth defects.

Common Nuisance Side Effects
- Vulvovaginal irritation noted by 1/5 of users
- Urinary symptoms noted by 15% or less

Benefits, Including Noncontraceptive
- Hormone-free
- User-controlled
- Available OTC
- Safe to use, no apparent teratogenic effects

Alternatives
For women seeking a reversible hormone-free method, consider the copper IUD for greater efficacy.

SPECIAL GROUPS
Pediatric Considerations
- Lower compliance with coitus-dependent products compared to oral contraceptives
- While some adolescents may have difficulty using a coitally based contraceptive consistently, others will choose spermicides due to availability without a prescription.

Women with Chronic Illness
- Women with prior hormone-dependent neoplasia may need hormone-free methods if their tumors express estrogen or progesterone receptors.
- Other methods with increased efficacy may be more appropriate if pregnancy is not advised.
- More effective methods should be used by women taking teratogenic medications. At least condoms should be used with spermicide in these cases.

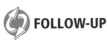 **FOLLOW-UP**

CONTINUATION
In a multicenter clinical trial, only 57% of women were still using spermicide at 6 months.

PATIENT MONITORING
None required

COMPLICATIONS
- If used improperly or not used at all, EC should be considered to decrease the risk of unplanned pregnancy.
- Minor vulvovaginal and urinary tract irritation is noted by up to 1/5 of women users.

BIBLIOGRAPHY

Bracken MB. Spermicidal contraceptives and poor reproductive outcomes: The epidemiologic evidence against an association. *Am J Obstet Gynecol*. 1985;151(5):552–556.

Grimes DA, et al. Spermicide used alone for contraception. *Cochrane Database Syst Rev*. 2005;(4):CD005218.

Louik C, et al. Maternal exposure to spermicides in relation to certain birth defects. *N Engl J Med*. 1987;317(8):474–478.

Raymond EG, et al. Contraceptive effectiveness and safety of five Nonoxynol-9 spermicides: A randomized trial. *Obstet Gynecol*. 2004;103: 430–439.

Richardson BA, et al. Evaluation of a low-dose nonoxynol-9 gel for the prevention of sexually transmitted diseases: A randomized clinical trial. *Sex Transm Dis*. 2001;28(7):394–400.

Roddy RE, et al. A controlled trial of nonoxynol-9 film to reduce male-to-female transmission of sexually transmitted diseases. *N Engl J Med*. 1998;339(8): 504–510.

Schreiber CA, et al. Effects of long-term use of Nonoxynol-9 on vaginal flora. *Obstet Gynecol*. 2006;107(1):136–143.

Van Damme L, et al. Effectiveness of COL-1492, a Nonoxynol-9 vaginal gel, on HIV-1 transmission in female sex workers: A randomized controlled trial. *Lancet*. 2002;360(9338):971–977.

 MISCELLANEOUS

CLINICAL PEARLS
Spermicides may be combined with periodic abstinence or withdrawal to improve efficacy.

ABBREVIATIONS
- EC—Emergency contraception
- STIs—Sexually transmitted infections
- N-9—Nonoxynol-9

LEGAL ISSUES
Age/Consent or Notification for Minors
Observe your state laws concerning minor's ability to consent for contraception.

Emergency Contraception
- Consider advance prescription of EC to cover nonuse for teens.
- Instruct all patients in EC as backup method available OTC for those >18.

 CODES

ICD9-CM
- V25.09 General contraceptive counseling
- V25.9 Contraceptive management

PATIENT TEACHING

- Use consistently 5–15 minutes before each coital act, as described in package labeling.
- Condoms are recommended to reduce exposure to HIV or STI. Spermicide has not been definitively shown to protect against STIs.
- Spermicides do not prevent STIs when used alone.
- Frequent use may increase the risk of HIV transmission.
- Avoid douching after spermicide use until 6 hours after the last ejaculation.
- Apply spermicide for each act of intercourse.
- Make sure fingers are dry before handling film. Place it on the cervical face.
- When spermicide is chosen as the contraceptive, provide information or an advance prescription for EC at that visit.

Section III

CONTRACEPTION: STERILIZATION, FEMALE

Ronald T. Burkman, MD

BASICS

DESCRIPTION
Voluntary female sterilization has become one of the most widely used family planning methods in the US and the world. 2 approaches most frequently used:

- Transabdominal: Interval or postpartum
- Transvaginal via hysteroscopy

Age-Related Factors
Majority of women selecting this approach are >30 and state they have completed their family.

EPIDEMIOLOGY
- Most common contraceptive method in the US.
- Data from the 1995 National Survey of Family Growth indicates:
  - 39% of women rely on female or male sterilization for contraception; 72% of these rely on tubal sterilization.
  - 700,000 tubal sterilizations are performed annually; >11 million women as of 1995 had had the procedure performed.
  - ~1/3 of tubal sterilizations are performed on unmarried women.

DIAGNOSIS

SIGNS AND SYMPTOMS
History
- Women electing female sterilization should undergo a history to screen for conditions that might contraindicate surgery:
  - Relative contraindications to transabdominal approaches include morbid obesity, multiple prior laparotomies, severe cardiovascular or pulmonary conditions, and other contraindications to surgery in general.
  - Contraindications specific to hysteroscopic sterilization include prior tubal surgery, hydrosalpinx, recent salpingitis, nickel or contrast media allergy.

Physical Exam
Physical exam as indicated for surgical procedures

TESTS
Minimal testing is required prior to female sterilizations procedures for healthy women

Lab
Testing specifically related to the procedure may include:

- Pregnancy test
- Other testing dependent on general medical status and risks associated with anesthesia

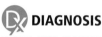

TREATMENT

GENERAL MEASURES
Female sterilization is a surgical procedure which can be accomplished transabdominally or via hysteroscopy.

PATIENT SELECTION
Informed Consent
The primary informed consent issue for sterilization is the concept that the procedure is intended to be permanent.

- At best, 50% of cautery and 85% of ring procedures can be reversed.
- Insurance rarely covers reversal.

Patient Education
Patient should be informed of the benefits, failure rates, risks, alternatives, and short- and long-term complications.

Benefits
- Contraceptive efficacy:
  - Data from CREST study indicates that over 10 years, risk of failure rate is roughly the same each year; data does not include hysteroscopic procedures.
  - 10-year cumulative failure rate (CREST study) for mechanical methods was 1.8% for rings and 3.7% for Hulka clip (similar data for other clips not available).
  - 10-year cumulative failure rates (CREST study) was 0.8% for postpartum tubal resection, 2% for interval tubal excision, and 2.5% for bipolar cauterization.

- Failure rate for hysteroscopic method <1% if both ostia occluded and 3 month HSG doesn't show patency; should note that bilateral placement fails in 6–12% of cases; no long-term data available.
- Noncontraceptive benefits:
  - Protection against ovarian cancer
  - Possible protection against acute salpingitis

Risks
- ~1/3 of pregnancies after non-hysteroscopic procedures are ectopic; higher rate with cautery procedures
- Mortality low, 4–6 per 100,000 procedures with most deaths related to anesthesia
- For nonhysteroscopic procedures, morbidity surgically relates to surgical problems, e.g. bleeding, adhesion occurring in 2–3% of cases and minor problems (e.g., pain) in 1.4%
- With hysteroscopic procedures, risks include: Expulsion of device (3%), tubal perforation (1%), minor complaints (e.g., back pain, dysmenorrhea) (7%)
- No strong evidence for a "posttubal sterilization syndrome, e.g., abnormal bleeding, dysmenorrhea, but some evidence for increased rates of hysterectomy after female sterilization though no biologic basis apparent

Alternatives
- Use of other long-acting contraceptive methods such as the IUD or DMPA provide similar efficacy and are non-permanent.
- Male sterilization—vasectomy (see chapter)

Medical
- IUD—medicated or nonmedicated
- DMPA

SURGERY
There are several approaches to accomplish female sterilization:

- Techniques:
  - Interval: Usually via laparoscopy, occasionally via minilaparotomy; involves bipolar cauterization of tubal segments or mechanical occlusion with clips or rings.
  - Postpartum: Accomplished at cesarean section or through minilaparotomy; usually involves resection of a segment of tube (Pomeroy) or division and ligation of the tube with burying of the proximal segment into the uterine myometrium (Irving)
  - Hysteroscopic method (Essure) involves placement of a microinsert device in the proximal tubal ostia to produce fibrosis; can be performed as an office procedure under local anesthesia.

ALERT

Women <30 years of age, regardless of parity, 2–3 times more likely to experience regret regarding sterilization. Careful counseling or use of equally efficacious long-acting methods like the copper IUD should be considered.

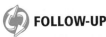 FOLLOW-UP

PATIENT MONITORING

Monitoring varies according to which approach chosen:

- With transabdominal approaches, patient needs to be aware that pregnancies occur at the same rate each year following the procedure but if ectopic, the highest rates are in the 1st 2–3 years postoperatively
- With hysteroscopic sterilization:
  - Backup contraception required until tubal blockage confirmed with HSG, usually 3 months
  - However, tubal patency still noted in 4–8% of women when HSG performed at 3 months postoperatively

BIBLIOGRAPHY

Piccinino LJ, et al. Trends in contraceptive use in the United States: 1982–1995. *Fam Plann Perspect*. 1998;30:4–10.

Peterson HB, et al. The risk of pregnancy after tubal sterilization: findings from the US Collaborative Review of Sterilization. *Am J Obstet Gynecol*. 1996;174:1161–1168.

Cooper JM, et al. Microinsert nonincisional hysteroscopic sterilization. *Obstet Gynecol*. 2003; 102:59–67.

Hillis SD, et al. Higher hysterectomy risk for sterilized than nonsterilized women: Findings from the US Collaborative Review of Sterilization. *Obstet Gynecol*. 1998;91:241–246.

Hillis SD, et al. Poststerilization regret: Findings from the United States Collaborative Review of Sterilization. *Obstet Gynecol*. 1999;93:889–895.

 MISCELLANEOUS

SYNONYM(S)

- Bilateral tubal ligation (BTL)
- Colloquial:
  - Having "a Tubal"
  - Having your "tubes tied"

ABBREVIATIONS

- BTL—Bilateral tubal ligation
- CREST—Collaborative Review of Sterilization
- DMPA—Depot medroxyprogesterone acetate
- HSG—Hysterosalpingogram

LEGAL ISSUES

Age/Consent

- Federal Medicaid guidelines do not allow payment for female sterilization until age 21.
- Federal Medicaid guidelines mandate a 30 day waiting period after female sterilization consent form is signed.
  - The mandatory waiting period may limit access for low-income women.
- Other state laws may preclude sterilization of other groups of women.
  - Women in a mental institution
- Spousal consent, age, number of children are not criteria for sterilization and nulliparity does not preclude sterilization.

CODES

ICD9-CM

- V25.2 Diagnostic code for female sterilization; modifier 66.32 if done postpartum as in-patient
- CPT codes for procedures
  - CPT 58670 Fulgeration (cautery) of fallopian tube
  - CPT 58671 Occlusion of fallopian tubes with rings or clips
  - CPT 58605 Postpartum procedure
  - CPT 58611 Procedure concurrent with cesarean section
  - CPT 58565 Hysteroscopic implants for sterilization; modifier 50 for bilateral placement

 PATIENT TEACHING

- Confirm that the decision is appropriate and ramifications have been considered; avoid making decision and proceeding with procedure after "significant" events (e.g., recent delivery, miscarriage, or pregnancy termination, divorce)
- Consider procedure irreversible; reversal of sterilization, while sometimes possible, is not a simple matter of "untying the tubes"
- Counsel that pregnancy risk, although low, exists for years after the procedure.
- With hysteroscopic sterilization, must use backup contraception until tubal occlusion confirmed by HSG
- Counsel on alternative reversible contraceptive approaches if any doubt exists.

Section III

CONTRACEPTION: STERILIZATION, MALE

Amy E. Pollack, MD
Mark A. Barone, DVM, MS

 BASICS

DESCRIPTION

- Male sterilization, also known as vasectomy, is one of the safest and most effective family planning methods and is one of the few contraceptive options for men. Vasectomy is a simple, minor surgical procedure that involves blocking each vas deferens so that sperm can no longer pass out of the body in the ejaculate. The vast majority of vasectomies are performed using local anesthesia.
- The procedure includes exposing and delivering the vas, occluding the vas, and separating the cut ends of the vas.
- Exposing and delivering the vas:
  - Conventional vasectomy (also known as traditional or incisional vasectomy):
    - Generally only the area around the skin entry site is anesthetized.
    - Either 1 midline incision or 2 incisions (1 overlying each vas) are made in the scrotal skin using a scalpel.
    - The incision(s) are closed with sutures.
  - NSV:
    - A deep injection of anesthesia alongside each vas is used in addition to anesthetizing the skin entry site.
    - 2 specialized instruments (a ringed clamp and dissecting forceps) replace the scalpel.
    - Both vasa are reached through the same small midline puncture in the scrotum.
    - Skin sutures are not necessary.
- Occluding the vas:
  - Division (cutting) and ligation with sutures:
    - The cut ends of the vas are tied off with absorbable or nonabsorbable sutures.
  - Cautery (electrosurgical or thermal):
    - A needle electrode or a cautery device is inserted into the vas lumen, and the luminal mucosa desiccated to create a firm scar that will occlude the vas.
  - Application of clips:
    - Clips are applied to the vas to compress a narrow segment, blocking passage of sperm.
    - After the vas is cut, a clip is applied to both of the cut ends.
  - Combinations of the above occlusions techniques are also used.
- Separating the cut ends of the vas:
  - Excision of a segment of the vas:
    - Common when division and ligation is used.
    - Sometimes no piece of vas is removed when clips or cautery are used.
  - Folding back:
    - 1 (or both) end of the cut vas is folded back upon itself and secured with a ligature or clip.
  - Fascial interposition:
    - Places a tissue barrier between the cut ends of the vas

- The thin layer of tissue that surrounds the vas is sutured (or secured with a clip) over 1 of the cut ends of the vas.
    - It can be used with any of the occlusion methods described above.
  - Combinations of the above are also used.

Age-Related Factors

Vasectomy is performed in men of reproductive age.

EPIDEMIOLOGY

- An estimated 526,501 vasectomies were performed in the US in 2002 (the most recent year for which data are available) for a rate of 10.2/1,000 men 25–49 years old.
- Although estimated numbers of vasectomies have increased over the past decade, the incidence rate remains unchanged.

 TREATMENT

PATIENT SELECTION

Indications

- Vasectomy is ideal for men and couples who are certain they do not want any more children.
- There is no medical reason to absolutely restrict a man's eligibility for vasectomy.
- Some conditions and circumstances indicate that precautions should be taken or that the procedure should be delayed, including:
  - Localized problems that make vasectomy more difficult to perform (e.g., inguinal hernia, large hydrocele or varicocele, and cryptorchidism).
  - Conditions that may increase the likelihood of complications (e.g., diabetes or coagulation disorders).

Informed Consent

The permanence of vasectomy is a significant consideration with respect to counseling and informed consent. Men who make informed decisions about vasectomy are more likely to be satisfied with their decision and less likely to experience regret. The key points that men should know to give truly informed consent are that:

- Highly effective, long-acting and temporary methods of contraception are available for women.
- Vasectomy involves surgery (details need to be explained before consent is given).
- The procedure involves risks in addition to the benefits (both of which need to be explained).
- If the procedure is successful, the man will not be able to have any more children.
- Vasectomy is permanent, although there is a small risk of failure.
- Vasectomy does not provide any protection against HIV or other STIs.

Patient Education

- Vasectomy should be considered a permanent end to fertility:
  - Although vasectomy reversal or assisted-reproductive technologies may allow a previously vasectomized man to father offspring, they are expensive, require technically demanding procedures, and results cannot be guaranteed.
- The contraceptive effect of vasectomy is not immediate because all sperm must 1st be cleared from the reproductive tract.
  - Another contraceptive should be used until success has been confirmed by semen analysis.
- Vasectomy provides no protection against transmission of HIV or other STIs. Men who are at risk should use condoms.
- Although vasectomy is highly effective, it is not 100% successful. Failure does occur, even years after the procedure was performed.

Risks

- Intraoperative complications such as vasovagal reaction, lidocaine toxicity, and excessive bleeding, are unusual and can generally be prevented if appropriate procedures are followed.
- Regret for having had a vasectomy can be high among some men (e.g., being in an unstable marriage at the time of sterilization, being <31, having no children or very young children, or making the decision to be sterilized during a time of financial crisis or for reasons related to a pregnancy). Good counseling reduces the risk of regret.

Benefits

- No worries about contraception
- Permanent and highly effective
- Most cost effective contraceptive method
- Removes burden for contraceptive from the woman

Alternatives

- The only other contraceptive option currently available to men is the condom.
- A wide range of contraceptive options are available to women.
- Vasectomy is simpler, safer, less expensive, and as effective as female sterilization.

 FOLLOW-UP

- Routine postprocedure follow-up visits are not necessary with NSV because no skin sutures are placed, or if absorbable sutures are used to close the skin incision when conventional vasectomy is used.
- It is generally recommended that men have semen analysis to confirm vasectomy success. Recommendations on when men should return in terms of time and/or number of ejaculations after vasectomy vary widely.

PROGNOSIS

- Men can resume normal activities after 2 or 3 days, although strenuous physical exercise should be avoided for ~1 week.
- Vasectomy is highly effective and 1 of the most reliable contraceptive methods.
- Although rare, failure does occur, sometimes long after the vasectomy procedure.
- The 1st-year failure rate in the US is estimated to be 0.15%, with a range of 0–0.5%.
- In general, vasectomy failure rates are believed to be similar to those for tubal ligation and lower than those for reversible methods.
- Vasectomy failure can result from spontaneous recanalization of the vas, occlusion of the wrong structure during surgery, and rarely, a congenital duplication of the vas that went unnoticed during the procedure.

COMPLICATIONS

- Vasectomy appears to be largely safe, with risks no greater than those found with any of the contraceptive options for women.
- Postoperative complications such as bleeding or infection as well as failure, although infrequent, do occur:
  - Most postoperative complications are minor and subside within 1 or 2 weeks.
  - The most frequent complaints after surgery are swelling of the scrotum, bruising, pain, and minor bleeding under the skin.
  - A scrotal support, mild pain medication, and local application of ice are usually sufficient for treatment.
  - More significant complications such as heavy bleeding, hematoma, or infection are quite rare.
  - Careful surgical technique, practicing aseptic technique, early recognition of a problem, and proper postoperative care and follow-up greatly reduce the risks of both minor and major complications after vasectomy.
- Chronic testicular pain (also known as postvasectomy pain syndrome):
  - Chronic testicular pain or discomfort is reported by some men after vasectomy.
  - While up to 1/3 to 1/2 of men have reported occasional testicular discomfort following vasectomy, only a small percentage of all vasectomized men (~2–3%) said the pain had negatively impacted their life or that they regretted having had the vasectomy.
  - Data for comparison on chronic testicular pain in the general population are limited.
- Potential physiological and mental health effects, as well as long-term sequelae of vasectomy, have been researched extensively over the past 3 decades. No significant long-term negative physical or mental health effects have been found:
  - Results of numerous well-designed studies have consistently shown no adverse effects of vasectomy in terms of heart disease, prostate or testicular cancer, immune complex disorders, and a variety of other conditions.

- Sexual function remains unaffected and vasectomy does not lead to impotence or other sexual difficulties, nor any reduction in the amount of semen ejaculated.
- Vasectomy has been reported to have no negative effects on sexuality, with some studies demonstrating a positive effect, perhaps because of the reduced worry about unintended pregnancy.

BIBLIOGRAPHY

EngenderHealth. *No-scalpel vasectomy: An illustrated guide for surgeons*, 3rd ed. New York: EngenderHealth; 2003.

Pollack AP, et al. In: Sciarra J, ed. *Gynecology and Obstetrics, Vol. 6: Fertility Regulation, Psychosomatic Problems, and Human Sexuality*, revised ed. Philadelphia: Lippincott Williams & Wilkins; 2000.

Sokal D, et al. A comparison of vas occlusion techniques: Cautery more effective than ligation and excision with fascial interposition. *Biomed Central Urology*. 2004;4:12. Available at http://www.biomedcentral.com/1471-1-2490/4/12.

 MISCELLANEOUS

- Despite the diversity of the US population, those men choosing vasectomy are a homogeneous group. They are primarily non-Hispanic white, well-educated, relatively affluent, and privately insured.
- Sperm production continues after vasectomy. Sperm are either destroyed/broken down by cells of the immune system or they degenerate.
- Antisperm antibodies are found in 50–80% of men following vasectomy, compared to 8–21% of men in the general population:
  - There is no evidence of any disease related to antisperm antibodies after vasectomy.
  - They may play a role in decreased fertility after vasectomy reversal, although conflicting results have been reported.

SYNONYM(S)

- No-scalpel vasectomy: Although technically a specific type of vasectomy
- Vasectomy

CLINICAL PEARLS

- Men should be told to clip the hair from around the scrotum and penis prior to the procedure as opposed to shaving. Shaving the scrotum is no longer recommended because it significantly increases the chance of a surgical-site infection.
- The NSV approach has a number of advantages over incisional vasectomy including fewer complications (e.g. infection, hematoma), less pain during and after the procedure, and earlier resumption of sexual activity.
- The same techniques are used to occlude the vas whether using conventional or NSV to expose the vas.

- Results from a number of recent studies suggest that there are some differences in effectiveness among different occlusion techniques:
  - Several studies found higher than expected failure rates for vasectomy by ligation (with suture or clips) and excision.
  - Results of an RCT demonstrated that use of fascial interposition with ligation and excision significantly improved the effectiveness of vasectomy.
  - Ligation and excision without fascial interposition should no longer be recommended.
  - Cautery has been shown to be highly effective and was found to significantly reduce failures compared to ligation and excision with fascial interposition:
    - Data on use of fascial interposition with cautery, differences in the effectiveness of thermal and electrocautery, and the importance of removing a segment of the vas when cautery occlusion is used are lacking.
- Open-ended vasectomy, in which the testicular end of the vas is left open, is a modification performed by some surgeons. In theory, success rates for reversal could be higher with open-ended vasectomy, but no studies have been reported in the literature.

ABBREVIATIONS

- NSV—No-scalpel vasectomy
- STI—Sexually transmitted infection

CODES

ICD9-CM

- 63.7 Vasectomy and ligation of vas deferens:
  - 63.70 Male sterilization procedure, not otherwise specified
  - 63.71 Ligation of vas deferens
  - 63.72 Ligation of spermatic cord
  - 63.73 Vasectomy

 PATIENT TEACHING

- After vasectomy, men should receive clear instructions about:
  - Postoperative care
  - Anticipated side effects
  - Actions to take if complications occur
  - Sites where they can access emergency care
  - Need for postoperative semen analysis
  - Importance of using alternate contraception until their semen is free of sperm
  - Reducing their risk of HIV and other sexually transmitted infections given that vasectomy provides no protection
  - Time and place for a follow-up visit
- ACOG Patient Information Pamphlet: Sterilization for women and for men. Available at http://www.acog.org/publications/patient_education/bp011.cfm
- Information from EngenderHealth available at: http://www.engenderhealth.org/wh/fp/cvas2.html

Section III

DIET

Seppideh Sami, MS, RD, LDN

 BASICS

DESCRIPTION

A healthy diet is a cornerstone for good health. Women's changing needs throughout stages of their life cycle, along with the corresponding specific nutrient needs from adolescence to reproductive years, pregnancy and postmenopause, will place them at risk for nutrition-related complications. Chronic diseases with a nutrition-related component will influence women's well-being. Nutrition screening and assessment, during a routine office visit or exam, may be used to identify patients with poor nutritional status or those at risk. A diagnosis of malnutrition will then need to be identified as caused by undernutrition, overnutrition, or impaired nutrient metabolism due to disease or trauma. The latter identification will help the timely and appropriate initiation of treatment, which may include interventions in addition to nutrition.

Age-Related Factors

Adolescence (Ages 11–19 years)
Needs for all nutrients are greater at this stage than at any other stage of life, except for pregnancy and lactation:

- Rapid growth and development: Bone development and increased body mass; protein, calcium and vitamin D needs increase
- Recommended intakes:
  - Protein = 0.85–0.95 g/kg body weight
  - Calcium = 1,300 mg/d = ~4.5 servings of calcium-rich foods
  - Vitamin D = 5–10 μg/d (200–400 IU)
  - Zinc = 8–9 mg/d
- Onset of puberty and menstruation
  - Iron needs increased due to menstruation
- Recommended intake:
  - 8–15 mg/d

Reproductive years
- Recommended intakes:
  - Protein = 0.8 g/kg body weight
  - Calcium = 1,000 mg/d
  - Vitamin D = 5 μg/day (200 IU)
  - Folate = 400 μg/d (max = 1 mg/d)

Pregnancy (See "Nutrition in Pregnancy")

Postmenopause
- Recommended intakes:
  - Protein = 0.8 g/kg body weight
  - Calcium = 1,000 mg/d
  - Vitamin D = 10 μg/d (400 IU) for 51–70 years and 15 μg/d for >70 years
- See Appendix IX for list of "Food Sources of Selected Nutrients"

EPIDEMIOLOGY

- Usual eating habits higher in fruits, vegetables, whole grains, legumes, low-fat dairy, and very lean meats associated with lower risk of chronic disease and related mortality
- Consumption of total fat, total energy, and refined carbohydrates has increased significantly.
- 27% of all foods consumed away from home
- Although healthier foods are more readily available, not always chosen
- Portion sizes of foods and beverages sold and consumed at and away from home have increased, leading to excess kcal intake and > risk of obesity and related chronic diseases.
- US women:
  - 75% have inadequate intakes of calcium
  - 90% have inadequate intakes of folate and vitamin E
  - ~8.9% have DM

Adolescents (11–19 years):
- 14% overweight; doubled since 1970
- Only 17% drink the recommended 3 servings milk per day
- Increased consumption of soft drinks, as primary beverage lead to less intake of calcium rich foods.
- 25% daily kcal intake from snacks
- In pregnancy, nutrient needs nearly double.

Older adults:
- Kcal needs decrease as age increases
- ~18% eat no vegetables

RISK FACTORS

General
- Adults are at nutritional risk if:
  - Weight loss >10% of UBW within last 6 months or >5% of UBW in 1 month, or a weight of 20% under or over IBW
  - Unable to adhere to usual eating pattern or consume adequate nutrition due to illness, surgery, swallowing difficulty, and malabsorption for >7 days

Adolescents:
- Typical eating habits: ↑ tendency to skip meals, eat / snack on nutrient-poor foods and beverages such as fast foods, or adopt fad diets
- Inappropriate dieting and 85% of eating disorders begin at this stage.
- At risk for deficiencies in vitamins A, B_6 & D, folate, calcium, magnesium, iodine, and zinc
- During pregnancy, at risk for deficiencies in vitamins A & C, niacin, chromium, and iron

Menstruating women:
- US women are not meeting their nutrient needs through their usual food intakes and are at risk for poor nutritional status and the sequelae of related chronic disorders.
- At risk for iron deficiency anemia and osteoporosis
- Eating away from home may increase risk of unhealthy eating patterns since such meals typically greater kcal, fat, cholesterol, and sodium while providing fewer amounts of fiber and vitamins.
- Abdominal obesity and higher fat diets lead to >LDL, <HDL, very high CVD risk.
- Alcohol intake positively correlated with increased breast cancer risk
- Women who have had 1 infant with neural tube defect are at high risk for a repeat incidence and need to take 4 mg of folate starting 1 month before pregnancy and at least throughout the 1st trimester.

Older adults:
In addition to risk factors listed above, at greater risk for:
- Dehydration
- Deficiency in calcium, vitamin D and Zinc; iron due to inadequate food intake
- Poor nutritional status due to poor chewing and swallowing, inability to shop and prepare meals

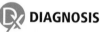 **DIAGNOSIS**

SIGNS AND SYMPTOMS

History

Diet History
- Diet history obtained to assess nutritional status, and to develop a treatment plan if necessary. Information must be obtained from patients with a diagnosis of or a family history of alcoholism, cancer, cardiovascular disease, DM, eating disorders, GI disorders, high blood pressure, lipid disorders, obesity, osteoporosis, renal disease, undernutrition.
- Information about specific dietary patterns must be obtained:
  - Vegetarian, or cultural practices
  - Use of supplements: Vitamins, minerals, herbs, protein, antioxidants
  - Use of laxatives, diuretics, etc.
  - Food allergies or intolerances

Social History
- Demographics, socioeconomic status, education, working conditions, living circumstances, and coping skills
- Culture, traditions, beliefs about foods and ethnicity
- Use of tobacco, illicit drugs, and alcohol

Physical Exam

Includes vital signs, height, weight, BMI, waist circumference, composition of fat and lean body mass, and physical appearance (hair, eyes, skin, mouth, nails, temporal muscles on head, skeletal muscles of arms and legs, subcutaneous fat stores)

TESTS
Lab
- Anemia:
  - CBC, serum Fe, Ferritin, TIBC, transferrin Saturation, MCV, RBC folate, serum vitamin B$_{12}$, reticulocyte count
- Fluids, electrolytes, calcium, phosphorus, magnesium, and serum glucose
- Tests of renal and hepatic function malabsorption:
  - Fecal fat, reducing substances in stool, fat soluble vitamins: A, D, E, K
- Tests for DM and hyperlipidemia

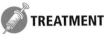 **TREATMENT**

GENERAL MEASURES
- Iron-deficiency anemia
  - Consumption of iron rich foods; ways to enhance absorption of non-heme iron (e.g., consumption of vitamin C-rich foods within the same meal)
- Overweight and obesity
  - ↓fat, ↑fiber, portion controlled meals; primarily whole foods
  - Plant-based regimens have been shown to be very effective.
- Cancer:
  - Healthful eating to prevent obesity
  - Plant-based regimen, minimally processed, primarily whole foods, ↓fat, ↑fiber
- CVD:
  - Plant-based regimen including cardio-protective foods rich in folic acid and soluble fiber, fish, nuts and seeds (rich in n-3 fatty acids), greens (rich in magnesium and potassium), whole grains (rich in micronutrients and lower glycemic load), soy and foods rich in monounsaturated fats such as olives, avocados, almonds provide strong evidence-based benefits.
- Diabetes:
  - Nutrition habits that allow lower kcal, lower fat intakes and weight loss
  - Lower fat, higher fiber plant-based regimens have been effective in improving blood glucose control.
- Osteoporosis:
  - Daily intake of foods rich in calcium, magnesium, and vitamin D
  - Supplementation is beneficial when baseline intakes are low to moderate.
  - Avoiding/Minimizing intake of nutrients and substances that interfere with absorption of calcium (e.g., caffeine, oxalates, excess animal protein, phosphoric acid and phosphates in processed foods, excess sodium, excess intake of wheat bran)
- Menopause:
  - Healthful eating habits that promote weight loss/prevent weight gain
  - Lower fat, higher fiber, whole foods (fruits, vegetables, legumes and whole grains)

- Postmenopause and old age:
  - Guidance on special supplementation if overall food and fluid intake is suboptimal (See Appendix X, Sample of Menu Planning Guides.)

SPECIAL THERAPY
Complementary and Alternative Therapies
Refer to:
- www.cmbm.org
- www.ncam.org

Supplements
- Calcium supplements:
  - If foods rich in calcium not regularly consumed 600 mg/d of calcium is recommended.
  - Form: Calcium carbonate, calcium citrate, calcium phosphate
  - Possible supplement vs. drug interaction to be discussed with patient
- Vitamin D supplements:
  - For patients with osteoporosis: 10 μg/d (400 IU)
- Folic acid:
  - Supplementaion before and during pregnancy
  - Lowers risk of neonatal NTD. Should start before conception and continue through the 4th week of pregnancy, until closure of neural tube.
  - 600–1200 μg/d folic acid throughout pregnancy, with max 1,000 μg/d.
  - With hx of child born with NTD up to 4,000 μg/d under physician supervision may be permitted.

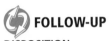 **FOLLOW-UP**

DISPOSITION
Issues for Referral
Referral to a registered dietitian:
- For further education and counseling to:
  - Provide further detailed education on issues listed in section "Education" and "Treatment & Prevention"
  - Assist and guide the patient to correctly fine tune their eating habits and help women learn ways through which they can achieve and maintain healthful eating habits and health-promoting practices.
  - Certified to work with patients diagnosed with eating disorders

PATIENT MONITORING
- Typical food intake
- Weight, BMI, waist circumference, body fat, and lean tissue composition
- Lab assays

BIBLIOGRAPHY

Arab L, et al. Ethnic differences in the nutrient intake adequacy of premenopausal United States women: Results from the 3rd National Health Examination Survey. *J Am Diet Assoc*. 2003;103:1008–1014.

Littleton LY, et al. In: *Neonatal, and Women's Health Nursing. Unit II: Health Care of Women. Chapter 8: Nutrition for Women Across the Life Span*. Delmar Thomson Learning; 2002:187–207.

Nutrition and Women's Health: Position of the American Dietetic Association and Dietitians of Canada. *Can J Diet Prac Res*. 2004;65:85–89.

Kleinman RE, ed. *Pediatric Nutrition Handbook. American Academy of Pediatrics*. 5th edition, 2004.

Russel MK, et al. The A.S.P.E.N. Nutrition Support Core Curriculum. Chapter 9. Nutrition Screening and Asessment. Available at www.nutritioncare.org. Accessed July 2007.

ABBREVIATIONS
- BMI—Body mass index
- CVD—Cardiovascular disease
- IBW—Ideal body weight
- UBW—Usual body weight

 PATIENT TEACHING

When a patient is diagnosed with malnutrition or at risk for it, treatment will include education. Referral to a registered dietitian for education and counseling is a component of effective therapy and treatment.

General Adult
- Anemia
- Nutrition-related deficiencies in Fe, vitamins: B$_{12}$, E, and folate
  - Education on rich sources of the respective nutrients as well as factors that enhance/hamper the absorption of the nutrients (e.g., vitamin C increases absorption of nonheme iron in plant foods)
  - Education on options for supplements
- Cancer:
  - Low-fat, high-fiber, whole foods
- CVD:
  - diet low cholesterol, low saturated fat, low total fat, and high fiber
  - Education on other food substances that decrease LDL cholesterol and atherosclerosis (e.g., garlic)
- Obesity:
  - Portion controlled, low fat, high fiber diet
- Osteoporosis:
  - Adequate calcium intake and review of nutrients that affect calcium balance (vitamin D, protein, sodium, oxalate, phosphorus, caffeine, fiber)
- Information on and referral to resources for food sources of nutrients of concern: (See Appendix IX, Food Sources of Selected Nutrients.)
- Vegetarian:
  - Education on appropriate food choices and supplementation (B$_{12}$ and calcium in some cases)
  - Referral to registered dietician for education and counseling
  - Referral to reliable resources such as www.vrg.org and www.nutritionMD.org.

DIET, EATING DISORDERS: ANOREXIA NERVOSA

Laurie A. P. Mitan, MD

 BASICS

DESCRIPTION
- Mental health illness with potentially grave medical complications
- Must meet following 4 criteria:
  - Refusal to maintain weight appropriate for height and age
  - Fear of gaining weight or being fat
  - Disturbed body image or denial of seriousness of current low weight or undue influence of shape on self-esteem
  - Amenorrhea
- Divided into restricting or binge-purge subtypes

Age-Related Factors
- Onset generally in early adolescence or young adulthood
- Relapse may occur at any age

EPIDEMIOLOGY
- Prevalence roughly 1% in US
- Female:Male is 10:1
- All socioeconomic classes affected equally

RISK FACTORS
- Female gender
- Residence in industrialized country
- Age <19 years
- Obsessive compulsive personality traits
- 1st-degree relative with eating disorder
- Any dieting in pediatric age group

Genetics
Susceptibility locus on chromosome 1 is an area of active research.

PATHOPHYSIOLOGY
Combination of genetic susceptibility, psychological factors, and environment

ASSOCIATED CONDITIONS
- Major depressive disorder
- Obsessive–compulsive personality disorder
- Substance abuse

 DIAGNOSIS

SIGNS AND SYMPTOMS
History
- Weight loss
- Fatigue
- Syncope or dizziness
- Cold intolerance
- Abdominal pain
- Constipation
- Amenorrhea
- Decreased concentration
- Measuring food
- Daily self-weighing practices
- Counting calories
- Excessive exercise
- Purging

Physical Exam
- Often normal early in disease process
- Vitals: Hypothermia, bradycardia, orthostatic pulse changes, hypotension
- BMI <18 or the 15th percentile in teens
- Skin: Dry, lanugo
- Cardiac: Poor peripheral pulses, arrhythmia
- Regression of breast tissue
- Vaginal dryness, hypoestrogenemia effects
- Delayed puberty and/or short stature in pediatric patients

TESTS
- EKG only if ill enough to hospitalize or hypokalemic
- DEXA if amenorrheic >6 months

Pediatric Considerations
Caution: Need appropriate software to calculate BMD Z-score in pediatric patients

Labs
To evaluate potential organ damage and monitor for refeeding syndrome:
- Renal panel
- Glucose, calcium, magnesium, phosphorous
- Liver function tests
- CBC
- TSH
- UA
- If diagnosis is unclear, consider additional tests for IBD, celiac disease, endocrinopathies, malignancy, CNS tumor.

Imaging
- Not routinely indicated
- MRI of brain, if obtained for other purposes, may reveal lateral ventricular enlargement, large cortical sulci, and decreased gray and white matter.
- Cardiac echo will reveal reversible mitral valve prolapse in 30% of patients.

DIFFERENTIAL DIAGNOSIS
- Female athlete triad
- Major depression with loss of appetite
- OCD with focus on counting (calories), germ fears (on food), or excessive exercise
- Substance abuse
- Anxiety disorder
- Globus hystericus
- PTSD: Sexual abuse, physical abuse
- Schizophrenia (adolescence is common age of onset)

Infection
PANDAS

Hematologic
Leukemia

Metabolic/Endocrine
- Hyperthyroidism
- Addison disease
- DM

Immunologic
Autoimmune disease (scleroderma or SLE)

Tumor/Malignancy
- CNS tumor
- Lymphoma

Drugs
Weight loss is common side-effect of many prescription and illicit drugs. However, body image will remain normal.

Other/Miscellaneous
- IBD
- Celiac disease

Geriatric Considerations
Anorexia nervosa may be misinterpreted as depression or loss of appetite from a medical condition in the elderly. Evaluation by mental health specialist may be helpful.

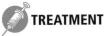

TREATMENT

GENERAL MEASURES

- All patients require multidisciplinary treatment to include:
  - Experienced mental health providers
  - Registered dietitian
  - Medical physician
- Initial evaluation should determine appropriate treatment setting (outpatient, intensive day treatment, inpatient, or residential)
- Consider inpatient medical hospitalization in an adult when:
  - Weight is <85% of ideal body weight
  - Heart rate <40 bpm
  - Blood pressure <90/60 mm Hg
  - Temperature <97°F
  - Electrolyte imbalance, potassium <3 mEq/L, dehydration, or glucose <60 mg/dL
  - Medical complication (e.g., poorly controlled diabetes, acute organ impairment)
- Consider acute psychiatric hospitalization if suicidal. Discuss all other psychiatric level of care options with experienced mental health provider.

Pediatric Considerations

- Admission criteria differ from adult criteria. Referral to pediatric specialists recommended.
- Consider medical hospitalization when:
  - Weight <85% of healthy body weight for age, height, and gender.
  - Acute food refusal with any weight loss
  - Heart rate in low 40 bpm range (must be taken when supine and at rest; recognize that vitals decrease further while asleep)
  - BP <80/50 mm Hg
  - Orthostatic changes (increase in pulse of >20 bpm or drop in BP of >10–20 mm Hg/min from supine to standing)
  - Any electrolyte abnormality

Pregnancy Considerations

- Treat as high risk. Patients with active anorexia have increased risk of low birth weight infant, increased rate of cesarean delivery, and higher rates of postpartum depression.
- Changes to body shape and weight may trigger relapse in patient with past history of anorexia nervosa.
- Recommend more attention to psychological needs during routine visits.

SPECIAL THERAPY

Complementary and Alternative Therapies

No evidence-based studies demonstrating effectiveness, however, stress-reducing therapies (e.g., yoga, meditation) may be of individual benefit.

MEDICATION (DRUGS)

- OCPs found to be of no benefit in protecting against or treating osteoporosis in adolescents and the majority of premenopausal women with anorexia nervosa
- Use of OCPs in premenopausal women with current weight <75% of ideal body weight may decrease rate of bone loss.
- Use of antidepressants or psychotropics should be reserved only for patients with coexistent mental health diagnosis (e.g., OCD).
- Defer making psychiatric medication decisions until weight restored, when possible.
- Calcium supplementation, 1,200 mg/d
- Vitamin D supplementation, 400–600 IU/d

SURGERY

Disturbed body image does not respond to cosmetic surgery in patients with a diagnosis of mental illness and is not recommended.

FOLLOW-UP

DISPOSITION

Issues for Referral

All preteens or prepubertal adolescents should be followed by providers experienced in growth and development.

PROGNOSIS

Recovery rates worse if:

- Onset of disease as adult
- Premorbid family dysfunction
- Dual diagnosis
- Treatment delayed >3 years

PATIENT MONITORING

- Frequency of visits determined by severity of illness and stage of illness.
- Weekly or twice-monthly appointment for medical stabilization in moderate to severe disease.
- Weight gain expectations of 1/2–1 lb/wk (200–500 g/wk) are safe as an outpatient.
- Restriction of physical activity is indicated early in treatment with gradual reintroduction as weight gain occurs.
- Coordination of care with mental health providers, dietitian, and family members is essential.
- Monitor for medical as well as mental health complications including refeeding syndrome, organ damage, gastroparesis, and suicidality.
- Monitor effect on social parameters including interpersonal relationships, school or job performance, behavior problems, substance abuse, domestic violence.

BIBLIOGRAPHY

American Psychiatric Association. Practice guideline for the treatment of patients with eating disorders, 3rd ed. Am J Psychiatry. 2006;163(7 Suppl):4–54.

Golden NH, et al. Eating disorders in adolescents: Position paper of the Society for Adolescent Medicine. J Adolesc Health. 2003;33:496–503.

National Collaborating Centre for Mental Health. Eating disorders: Core interventions in the treatment and management of anorexia nervosa, bulimia nervosa and related eating disorders. London: National Institute for Clinical Excellence; 2004.

Walsh TB, et al. Part IV: Eating Disorders. In: Evans DL, et al., eds. Treating and Preventing Adolescent Mental Health Disorders. What We Know and What We Don't Know. A Research Agenda for Improving the Mental Health of Our Youth. New York: Oxford University Press; 2005;257–334.

MISCELLANEOUS

ABBREVIATIONS

- BMD—Bone mineral density
- DEXA—Dual energy X-ray analysis
- DM—Diabetes mellitus
- IBD—Inflammatory bowel disease
- OCD—Obsessive compulsive disorder
- OCP—Oral contraceptive pill
- PANDA—Pediatric autoimmune neuropsychiatric disorders associated with streptococcal infection
- PTSD—Post-traumatic stress disorder
- SLE—Systemic lupus erythematosus
- TSH—Thyroid-stimulating hormone

CODES

ICD9-CM
307.1 Anorexia nervosa

PATIENT TEACHING

- www.ANAD.org
- http://www.aafp.org/afp/20040401/1729ph.html

PREVENTION

- Current area of research
- Primary prevention
- Several programs available for purchase geared at educators:
  - Encourage acceptance of all body shapes.
  - Promote high self-esteem in children and adolescents.
  - Role model healthy stress relieving techniques.
  - Focus on healthy behavior and not weight.
- Secondary prevention:
  - Never encourage an obese child or teen to engage in a weight loss plan without regular medical supervision.
  - Refer early any patients with symptoms suspicious for an eating disorder.

DIET, EATING DISORDERS: BINGE EATING DISORDER

Pauline Chang, MD

 BASICS

DESCRIPTION
- Recurrent binge eating episodes:
  - Duration of at least 2 days a week over a period of 6 months
  - Absence of compensatory behaviors (e.g., purging, fasting, excessive exercise) as seen in anorexia and bulimia
  - Lacks overconcern with body weight and shape
- Eating disorder NOS

ALERT
DSM-IV lists binge eating disorder as an EDNOS, but research criteria are suggested.

Age-Related Factors
- Studies suggest age of onset later than anorexia and bulimia, ~25 years
- Earlier age of obesity onset in obese patient with vs. without binge eating disorder

EPIDEMIOLOGY
- Lifetime prevalence: 2.8%
- Binge eating disorder present in 30% of patients seeking medical care for obesity
- Female > male (65% vs. 35%):
  - More equal in gender ratio than other eating disorders

RISK FACTORS
- Depression, negative self-esteem
- Adverse childhood events, including physical and sexual abuse
- Childhood obesity

Genetics
- Genetic predisposition shown in eating disorders and obesity:
  - Studies suggest a genetic component for binge eating disorder, but more research is needed

PATHOPHYSIOLOGY
- Pathophysiology of binge eating disorder is unknown.
- Hypotheses include the imbalance of serotonin and ghrelin
- Studies comparing obese patient with vs. without binge eating disorder show no significant differences in blood serum levels of glucose, insulin, lipids, or thyroid hormones.
- Negative emotional states and stress may play a role in triggering binge eating episodes.

ASSOCIATED CONDITIONS
- Overweight and obesity
- Depression
- Studies suggest binge eating disorder associated with increased risk of:
  - Mood disorders
  - Anxiety disorders
  - Impulse-control disorders
  - Personality disorders
  - Substance abuse

 DIAGNOSIS

SIGNS AND SYMPTOMS
- Binge eating is defined as eating large amounts of food in a discrete period of time:
  - More food than most people would eat under similar circumstances
  - Lack of control over eating during the episode
- Binge eating episode: Binge eating associated with 3 of the following symptoms:
  - Eating more rapidly than usual
  - Eating until feeling uncomfortably full
  - Eating when not feeling physically hungry
  - Eating alone because embarrassed about the amount of food consumed
  - Feeling disgusted with oneself, depressed, or very guilty after binge eating

ALERT
Obesity is not one of the criteria of binge eating disorder.

History
- Food diary, history of compensatory behaviors (e.g., purging, fasting, excessive exercise, laxative use)
- GI: Abdominal pain, bloating, constipation
- Reproductive: Menstrual history
- Past medical history:
  - Chronic medical conditions
  - Medications
  - Substance abuse
  - Learning difficulties
- Psychiatric history:
  - Signs/Symptoms of depression
  - Hypersexuality
  - Hypersomnia
  - Oral or tactile exploratory behavior
- Family history:
  - Eating disorders

Physical Exam
- General:
  - Appearance
  - VS
  - Weight, BMI
- HEENT:
  - Dental
  - Parotid gland
  - Thyroid
- Cardiovascular
- Abdominal:
  - Masses
  - Tenderness
- Mental status exam
- Neurologic exam

TESTS
EKG, if abnormalities in VS or cardiovascular exam

Labs
- CBC
- Basic metabolic panel
- Thyroid function tests
- Lipid panel

Imaging
Brain imaging if indicated by finding on neurologic exam

DIFFERENTIAL DIAGNOSIS
- Bulimia nervosa (See Diet, Eating Disorders: Bulimia Nervosa.)
- Anorexia nervosa (See Diet, Eating Disorders: Anorexia Nervosa.)
- EDNOS

Metabolic/Endocrine
- Hypothyroidism
- Cushing disease

Tumor/Malignancy
CNS tumor

Drugs
- Steroid-induced hyperphagia
- Medication-related hyperphagia

Other/Miscellaneous
- Klüver-Bucy syndrome
- Kleine-Levin syndrome
- Prader-Willi syndrome
- Major depressive disorder (See Mood Disorders: Depression.)

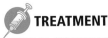 **TREATMENT**

GENERAL MEASURES
- CBT and interpersonal psychotherapy are main treatments for binge eating disorder.
- Most patients seek medical care for weight loss treatment:
  - Important to treat eating disorder before treating obesity

SPECIAL THERAPY
Complementary and Alternative Therapies
- CBT and interpersonal psychotherapy to reduce binge eating episodes:
  - Goals in therapy:
    - Focus on eating behaviors
    - Normalizing food intake
    - Alter dysfunctional thinking about food, shape, and weight
    - Development of coping skills not related to food

MEDICATION (DRUGS)
- Trial use of antidepressants, mainly SSRIs:
  - Shown to reduce frequency, but less so than CBT and psychotherapy
  - Withdraw of antidepressant therapy frequently leads to immediate relapse.
  - Other 2nd-generation antidepressants and TCAs also studied
- Studies with topiramate, an anticonvulsant associated with weight loss, shows potential in treating binge eating disorder.

SURGERY
Further studies are needed on the impact of binge and other eating disorders on the short- and long-term outcomes of bariatric surgery.

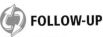 **FOLLOW-UP**

DISPOSITION
Issues for Referral
- Mental health specialists for CBT or interpersonal psychotherapy
- In morbid obesity, weight loss options include bariatric surgery:
  - Not shown to exacerbate binge eating episodes

PROGNOSIS
- Mean duration of binge eating disorder: 8.1–14.4 years
- May develop comorbidities of obesity (e.g., diabetes type II, cardiovascular risks), if obesity is present
- More research needed on prognosis of binge eating disorder

PATIENT MONITORING
- Monitor for signs of depression.
- Monitor for compensatory behaviors (e.g., purging, fasting, excessive exercise, laxative use) and development of other eating disorders.
- Monitor for comorbidities of obesity.

BIBLIOGRAPHY

American Psychiatric Association Task Force on DSM-IV. *Diagnostic and Statistical Manual of Mental Disorders*, 4th ed. Washington, DC: American Psychiatric Association; 1999.

Brownley KA, et al. Binge eating disorder treatment: A systematic review of randomized controlled trials. *Int J Eat Disord*. 2007;40(4):337–348.

de Zwaan M. Binge eating disorder and obesity. *Int J Obes Relat Metab Disord*. 2001;5(Suppl 1): S51–S55.

Halmi KA. Eating Disorder. In: Sadock BJ, et al, eds. *Comprehensive Textbook of Psychiatry*, vol. 2, 7th ed. Philadelphia: Lippincott Williams & Wilkins; 2000;1668–1669.

Hudson JI, et al. The prevalence and correlates of eating disorders in the national comorbidity survey replication. *Biol Psychiatry*. 2007;61(3):348–358.

Pope HG Jr., et al. Binge eating disorder: A stable syndrome. *Am J Psychiatry*. 2006;163(12): 2181–2183.

Steiger H, et al. Phenotypes, endophenotypes, and genotypes in bulimia spectrum eating disorders. *Can J Psychiatry*. 2007;52(4):220–227.

 MISCELLANEOUS

CLINICAL PEARLS
Binge eating disorder is defined as an EDNOS.
- Obesity is not one of the criteria for binge eating disorder.
- CBT and interpersonal psychotherapy are main treatments for binge eating disorder.
- In obese patients, treat the eating disorder before treating obesity.

ABBREVIATIONS
- CBT—Cognitive behavioral therapy
- EDNOS—Eating disorder not otherwise specified
- HEENT—Head, eyes, ears, nose, throat
- SSRI—Selective serotonin reuptake inhibitors
- TCA—Tricyclic antidepressant

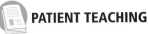 **CODES**

ICD9-CM
307.50 Eating disorder, Not Otherwise Specified

PATIENT TEACHING

- Promote awareness of stressors that trigger binge eating episodes.
- Development of non–food related coping skills.
- Educate about comorbidities of obesity and other eating disorders (e.g., bulimia, anorexia).
- ACOG Patient Education Pamphlet: Eating Disorders

PREVENTION
- Primary: Not well established
- Secondary: Treatment compliance, weight loss

Section III

DIET, EATING DISORDERS: BULIMIA NERVOSA

Michael G. Spigarelli, MD, PhD

 BASICS

DESCRIPTION
- Binge eating (eating a large amount of food in an uncontrolled manner) followed by inappropriate compensatory behaviors to prevent weight gain.

Age-Related Factors
- Predominant age: Adolescents and young adults
- Increasingly seen in older women

EPIDEMIOLOGY
- Incidence:
  – 1–2% in women 16–35 years of age
- Mean age of onset: 18–19
- Female > male (10–20:1)
- Prevalence:
  – 28.8 women, 0.8 men per 100,000 per year

RISK FACTORS
- Female gender
- Personal and family history of obesity and dieting
- Poor body image
- Unrealistic family expectations regarding weight, body shape, or eating
- Severe life stressor; achievement pressure; competition stressors
- Low self-esteem:
  – Perceived pressure to be thin
  – Perfectionistic or obsessional thinking
- History of anorexia nervosa
- Environment that stresses thinness or physical fitness (e.g., military, ballet, cheerleading, gymnastics, dancing, skating, or modeling).
- Family history of substance abuse, affective disorders, eating disorder, or obesity
- Diabetes
- Poor impulse control, substance or alcohol abuse

Genetics
The incidence of bulimia has been shown to be increased in identical twins, suggesting an underlying genetic basis.

PATHOPHYSIOLOGY
Bulimia nervosa has been linked to low serotonin levels:
- Low serotonin levels are further decreased by nutritional deficiencies, which further worsen the disease.
- These low levels of serotonin persist despite weight and behavioral recovery.

ASSOCIATED CONDITIONS
- Major depressive disorder and dysthymia
- Anxiety disorders
- Substance abuse/dependence
- Bipolar disorder
- OCD
- Schizophrenia
- Borderline personality disorder

DIAGNOSIS
SIGNS AND SYMPTOMS
History
Diagnostic criteria (must meet all criteria):
- Recurrent episodes of binge eating (eating in a discrete period of time > most people would typically eat) coupled with a perceived lack of control during binge
- Recurrent inappropriate compensatory behavior to prevent weight gain such as:
  – Self induced vomiting
  – Misuse of laxatives, diuretics, enemas, or other medications
  – Fasting
  – Excessive exercise
- The binge eating and inappropriate compensatory behaviors both occur, on average, at least twice per week for 3 months.
- Self-evaluation is unduly influenced by body shape and weight.
- The disturbance does not occur exclusively during episodes of anorexia nervosa.
- 2 recognized subtypes:
  – Purging type: Regularly engages in self-induced vomiting or the misuse of laxatives, diuretics, or enemas
  – Nonpurging type: Uses other inappropriate behaviors, such as fasting or excessive exercise, but does not regularly engage in self-induced vomiting or the misuse of laxatives, diuretics, or enemas

Physical Exam
Typically without findings (benign exam):
- Eroded tooth enamel (long-standing disease)
- Asymptomatic, parotid gland enlargement
- Calluses, abrasions, bruising on dominant hand or thumb
- Peripheral edema

TESTS
Psychological self-report screening:
- Eating Attitudes Test
- Eating Disorder Inventory
- Eating Disorder Screen for Primary Care
- Bulimia Test-Revised
- Bulimia Investigatory Test Edinburgh
- SCOFF Questionnaire:
  – Do you make yourself Sick (induce vomiting) because you feel uncomfortably full?
  – Do you worry that you have lost Control over how much you eat?
  – Have you recently lost >1 stone (14 lb) in a 3-month period?
  – Do you think you are too Fat, even though others say you are too thin?
  – Would you say that Food dominates your life?
  – A score ≥2 indicates a likely eating disorder.

Lab
- All laboratory results may be within normal limits (not necessary for diagnosis)
- If abnormal present, typically present with:
  – Hypokalemia
  – Hypochloremia
  – Hypomagnesemia
  – Hyponatremia
  – Hypocalcemia
  – Hypophosphatasemia
  – Alkalosis
  – Leukopenia
  – Elevated BUN
  – Elevated basal serum prolactin
  – Elevated serum amylase (mild)

Imaging
- Typically no need for imaging, except in long-standing disease.
- DEXA scan as screen for osteoporosis; related to long-standing malnutrition

DIFFERENTIAL DIAGNOSIS
- Anorexia, binge eating/purging type
- Major depressive disorder
- Psychogenic vomiting
- Hypothalamic brain tumor
- Epileptic equivalent seizures
- Klein-Levin syndrome
- Body dysmorphic disorder
- Borderline personality disorder

Infection
Malnourishment can lead to impaired ability to fight infection.

Hematologic
Malnourishment can lead to anemia.

Metabolic/Endocrine
Malnourishment can lead to irregular menses.

Immunologic
Malnourishment can lead to impaired ability to fight infection.

Trauma
Attempts to induce vomiting (particularly with foreign objects) can lead to damage to the airway, oropharynx, or esophagus.

Drugs
- Ipecac, although less readily available at present, can be used to increase purging.
- Laxative, diuretics, and enemas can be frequently used (abused).

TREATMENT

GENERAL MEASURES
- Most individuals are treated as outpatients.
- Treatment best accomplished by treatment team: Medical, nutritional, therapist).
- Outpatient:
  - Build trust, increase motivation for change
  - Assess psychological and nutritional status
  - Establish prescribed eating plan to develop regular eating habits; realistic weight goal
  - Involve patient in establishing target goals
  - Educate about ineffectiveness of purging for weight control and adverse outcomes
  - Address calories, weight, and purging ruminations
  - Challenge fear of loss of control
  - Develop plan to cope with triggers
  - CBT is effective
  - Establish relapse prevention plan
  - Gradual laxative withdrawal, if necessary
  - Nutritional education, relaxation techniques
  - After vomiting, avoid brushing teeth and consider using nonacidic mouthwash
  - Limiting acidic foods, beverages to meal time
- Inpatient:
  - If possible, admit to eating disorders unit
  - Supervised meals and bathroom privileges
  - Monitor weight and physical activity
  - Monitor electrolytes
  - Return control to patient as able
  - Balanced diet, normal eating pattern
  - Introduce challenge foods
  - Monitor excess activity
  - Encourage enjoyable activities

SPECIAL THERAPY
Complementary and Alternative Therapies
- When outpatient and/or inpatient therapy are ineffective or short lived, residential programs (6–12 weeks at treatment center) may be necessary.
- Emerging data demonstrating yoga as complementary therapy

MEDICATION (DRUGS)
- SSRIs, particularly fluoxetine, typically at higher doses than the typical antidepressant range (60–80 mg/d) have been shown to be effective in reducing symptoms with relatively few side effects.
- Augmentation of SSRIs with atypical antipsychotic medications (risperidone or quetiapine) or buspirone (BuSpar) have been suggested by some although definitive placebo-controlled, double-blind studies have not been done.
- Antidepressant medication should be continued at full therapeutic dose for at least 1 year beyond resolution of symptoms.
- Contraindications:
  - Hypersensitivity

- Precautions:
  - Serious toxicity following overdose is relatively uncommon.
  - Patients may vomit medication, need to have plan to take medication when less likely to purge following the medications
- Significant interactions:
  - MAOIs should not be combined with SSRI or TCAs.
- Additional medications:
  - Polyglycol preparations (such as MiraLax) with sufficient water, can prevent constipation during laxative withdrawal.
  - PPIs can help to decrease some of the metabolic sequela by decreasing loss of gastric acid.

FOLLOW-UP

DISPOSITION
Issues for Referral
- Bulimia nervosa is a chronic disease that typically requires treatment from a team of individuals (physician, nutritionist, and therapist) capable and comfortable treating individuals with this condition.
- Low threshold for referral
- Close follow-up to assure patient has sought treatment

PROGNOSIS
- With effective treatment:
  - 50% asymptomatic after 2–10 years
  - 30% remissions, relapses, or subclinical behaviors
  - 20% no significant change
- Without treatment:
  - Likely to remain chronic/relapsing problem
  - Greater weight fluctuations, other impulsive behaviors, and personality disorder diagnoses may predict poor prognosis.

PATIENT MONITORING
Weight and electrolyte monitoring is important:
- Large weight fluctuations associated with worsening disease
- Hypokalemia can be severe and may require magnesium replacement to restore total body stores to normal levels.

BIBLIOGRAPHY

American Psychiatric Association. *Diagnostic and Statistical Manual of Mental Disorders*, 4th ed. Washington, DC: American Psychiatric Association: 1994.

Fisher M. Treatment of eating disorders in children, adolescents, and young adults. *Pediatr Rev*. 2006; 27(1):5–16.

Kreipe RE, et al. The Role of the Primary Care Practitioner in the Treatment of Eating Disorders. In: Fisher M, et al., eds. *The Spectrum of Disordered Eating: Anorexia Nervosa, Bulimia Nervosa, and Obesity. Adolesc Med State of the Art Rev.* 2003;14(1):133–147.

le Grange D, et al. Bulimia nervosa in adolescents: A disorder in evolution? *Arch Pediatr Adolesc Med.* 2004;158(5):478–482.

Mehler PS. Clinical Practice. Bulimia nervosa. *N Engl J Med*. 2003;349(9):875–881.

MISCELLANEOUS

SYNONYM(S)
- Binge/Purge syndrome
- Eating disorder—bulimia

CLINICAL PEARLS
- Despite clinical evidence, many individuals, including those with bulimia nervosa, view this disease as a personal choice. This mistaken attribution delays and hinders treatment.
- Experience dictates that the intense loss of control an individual experiences during bingeing is intensely unsettling.
- Discussing the possibility of someday gaining control can provide the therapeutic opportunity for a medical provider to make a difference.
- Ask patients what they think about their weight and what they do to control their weight.
- Discuss weight-control pressure that each patient experiences.
- When a patient discloses bingeing and/or purging behavior, reassure them that treatments can help them gain control of their eating and weight.
- As a provider, seek treatment for any personal eating disorder issues.

ABBREVIATIONS
- CBT — Cognitive behavioral therapy
- DEXA — Dual-energy X-ray absorptiometry
- MAOI — Monoamine oxidase inhibitor
- OCD — Obsessive-compulsive disorder
- PPI — Proton pump inhibitor
- SSRI — Selective serotonin reuptake inhibitor
- TCA — Tricyclic antidepressant

CODES
ICD9-CM
307.51 Bulimia nervosa

PATIENT TEACHING

Helpful information for patients can be found at:
- http://www.nationaleatingdisorders.org/ nedaDir/files/documents/handouts/EdSurGde.pdf
- http://www.4women.gov/faq/Easyread/ bulnervosa-etr.htm

PREVENTION
Proven method prevents bulimia; however, early treatment has been shown to prevent worsening of the disease. For young individuals, particularly young women it is important to:
- Maintain a healthy body image.
- Improve self-esteem.
- Seek treatment for depression, anxiety, and other mental illnesses.

DIET: OBESITY

Sharon Phelan

 BASICS

DESCRIPTION
- An excess of adipose tissue that contributes to mortality and morbidity
- Associated with excessive caloric intake to the energy expenditures by activity
- BMI defined as weight in kilograms (kg) divided by height in meters (m) squared:
- – Overweight: BMI 25–29.9 kg/m^2
  Obesity: BMI 30 kg/m^2 or greater:
    - ◦ Type I: 30–34.9
    - ◦ Type II: 35–39.9
    - ◦ Type III/extreme obesity: >40
- Commonly a chronic condition and life-long issue
- BMI may not be accurate in very athletic individuals who have a high lean muscle mass or in the older woman who tends to have increased adipose-to-lean muscle ratio.

EPIDEMIOLOGY
- Female > Male (33% vs. 27%)
- Rapidly increasing nationally, with a 50% increase nationally in the past decade
- Being overweight during midlife increases risk of death by 20–40% even if otherwise healthy and nonsmoker
- Prevalence:
  – Overweight: 35%
  – Obesity: 31%
  – Ideal: 33%

Pediatric Considerations
- BMI cutoff is related to a patient being ≥95% for their age.
- High in minority children
- Increase risk of adult obesity, type 2 diabetes, HTN, metabolic syndrome, depression, self-esteem issues
- Adolescents:
  – Overweight: 17%

RISK FACTORS
- Overweight or obese in childhood
- Increase intake of refined carbohydrates
- Decreased fresh fruits and vegetables
- Decreased physical activity both at work and daily activities
- Lower socioeconomic status, Hispanic or African American ethnicity
- Obese parents
- Pregnancy, especially with excessive weight gain

Genetics
The human genome was developed in an environment of subsistence diet so there is no limit to the human body's ability to store calories as fat.

PATHOPHYSIOLOGY
- Increased adipose tissue leads to increased insulin resistance, increased tissue insulin levels, and chronic hyperinsulinemia with resultant secondary HTN and hyperlipidemia.
- Leptin, insulin adiponectin, and other neurohormonal factors interact to influence food intake and energy expenditure.
- Estrogen has been found to interact with leptin and its role in the relation of eating behavior and fat distribution.
  – In states of increased estrogen influence the fat distribution is more over thighs and buttocks (gynecoid).
  – In situations of great androgen influence, the fat distribution is more abdominal or central (android) and has a greater associated morbidity.
- Other endocrine dysfunctions (e.g., hypothyroidism, hypothalamic disorders, Cushing syndrome) have been associated with obesity.
- Certain medications (e.g., steroids, Depo-Provera, certain neuroleptic drugs) will cause weight gain but not typically to the obese level.

ASSOCIATED CONDITIONS
- HTN
- Dyslipidemia
- Type 2 diabetes
- CHD
- Depression
- Increased surgical risks
- Stroke
- Gallbladder disease
- Osteoarthritis
- Sleep apnea
- Cancers (breast, endometrial and colon)
- Infertility
- Menstrual problems

 DIAGNOSIS

SIGNS AND SYMPTOMS
History
- Full medical history indicated with particular emphasis on:
  – Weight during key times in life: Adolescence, prepregnancy,
  – Rate of weight gain; sudden weight gain concerning of medical problem
  – Screening for comorbidities associated with obesity
  – Medications that might contribute to weight gain
  – ROS to check for any undiagnosed condition (although rarely is obesity due to hypothyroidism despite patient's statements)
- Assess interest in changing behavior or initiating weight loss activities.
  – Dietary patterns; food diary
  – Stressors that provoke/trigger eating

Physical Exam
- Height and weight to calculate BMI
- Waist-hip ratio if BMI <35; if >35 inches strongly associated with medical conditions with a more android distribution
- BP
- Clinical signs of hypothyroidism, metabolic syndrome (Syndrome X), or Cushing syndrome

TESTS
Labs
If signs of underlying endocrine dysfunction, test fasting lipids, glucose levels

Imaging
None indicated

DIFFERENTIAL DIAGNOSIS
- Most patients do not have a secondary cause for obesity.
- Secondary causes that can be related to obesity etiology include:
  – Hypothyroidism (See Thyroid Disease.)
  – PCOS, metabolic syndrome or Syndrome X (See Polycystic Ovarian Syndrome and Metabolic Syndrome.)
  – Congenital adrenal hyperplasia (See Congenital Adrenal Hyperplasia.)
  – Cushing syndrome
  – Perimenopause (See Menopause.)
  – Hypothalamic lesions
  – Medications

TREATMENT

Prevention is the best management. Assess weight annually and alert patient as she is gaining weight so she can modify habits prior to becoming overweight or obese. This is key because most interventions do not work well over the long term.

GENERAL MEASURES
- Assess willingness to start on a major behavioral lifestyle modification. If not interested, let patient know you are willing to help once she does want to lose weight.
- Most successful weight-loss programs are multidisciplinary and combine diet modification, increased activity, and occasionally medication.
- Target goal is 1–2-pound loss a week over 6 months.
  – Maintain weight for a period, then resume goal of losing 1–2 lb/wk if appropriate
- A 10–15% body weight loss in an obese person can positively impact other comorbidities even if the patient remains obese.

SPECIAL THERAPY

Complementary and Alternative Therapies

- Diet:
  - Recommend special diet to overweight patients, or to those with increasing weight gain, as a general preventive measure.
  - Behavioral aspects to diet:
    - This should be seen as a modification of life-long eating and not a short-term "punishment."
    - Encourage structured meals; no snacking and fast foods.
    - Eat slowly.
    - Decrease portion size, avoid all-you-can-eat restaurants and sugary drinks.
  - Low-fat, high complex-carbohydrate, and high-fiber diets are the most compatible with long-term acceptance and are the basis for many of the commercial programs such as Weight Watchers.
  - Low-carbohydrate diets (e.g., Atkins, South Beach Diet) are currently very popular but are less compatible with long-term dietary change.
  - Bottom line is the amount of calorie restriction relative to activity. (No-fat baked goods made with corn syrup will result in a patient on the Atkins diet gaining weight while remaining "fat free.")
  - A deficit of 500 kcal/d results in ~1 pound lost per week.
  - Very low-calorie diets under medical supervision can result in a greater initial loss but overall long-term success is poor with much of the weight regained.
- Activity:
  - Activity alone will not generally result in significant weight loss but if integrated into daily activity will improve long-term maintenance of loss.
  - Exercise for 30–60 minutes daily for 5+ d/wk. Start with activities that the patient can tolerate and sustain. Brisk walking is the best overall activity initially. Eventually, weight training and aerobic combination is best.
  - Use of pedometers to document walking at work and home may help document activity.

MEDICATION (DRUGS)

- Medications help over placebo but generally only by 5–10 pounds over the course of a year. Also, once stopped, weight tends to return quickly.
- Categories of medications:
  - Appetite suppressants (e.g., antihistamines [OTC], amphetamines, sibutramine): These are centrally mediated, plateau at 4–6 months, and work for people who eat because they are hungry.
  - Antidepressants (SSRIs): Work by decreasing appetite and potentially helping with underlying depression that may motivate women to overeat.
  - Lipase inhibitors (e.g., Orlistat [OTC]): Prevents fat absorption through intestine and helps patients follow a low-fat diet due to side effect.

SURGERY

- Bariatric surgery has the best success with patients with BMI >40, or >35 with comorbidities.
  - Significant morbidity and mortality (1–2%), so other modes of weight loss should be tried 1st.
  - Long-term consequences are a better maintenance of lower BMI but also malabsorption of key vitamins.

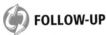 FOLLOW-UP

DISPOSITION

Issues for Referral

- If comorbidities of HTN, diabetes, etc. are present, encourage the patient to seek professional help from a nutritionist, internist with interest in weight loss, or surgeon if a candidate for bariatric surgery.
- If patient is not motivated to address the problem, let the patient know you are there to help once she is ready and be sure the patient understands the medical risks of continued obesity.

PROGNOSIS

- Long-term maintenance of weight loss is difficult. Patients tend to yo-yo, often gaining more weight than originally lost.
- If patient is not motivated to lose weight, attempts will not be successful.
- Complications of obesity:
  - HTN
  - Diabetes
  - Hyperlipidemia
  - Gall bladder disease; may be worse with rapid weight loss
  - Osteoarthritis
  - Gout
  - Thromboembolism
  - Sleep apnea
  - Cancer: Colon, breast, endometrial
  - Poor self-esteem
  - Occupational discrimination

PATIENT MONITORING

- Patients who weigh themselves daily or at least weekly are more likely to maintain weight loss.
- If patient is not motivated or is unsuccessful in weight loss, monitor annually for the development of comorbidities associated with obesity.

BIBLIOGRAPHY

CDC. Department of Health and Human Services. Overweight and obesity. Available at: www.cdc.gov/nccdphp/dnpa/obesity/index.htm.

Gardner CD, et al. Comparison of the Atkins, Zone, Ornish, and LEaRN diets for change in weight and related risk factors among overweight premenopausal women. *JAMA*. 2007;297:969–977.

Christakis NA, and Fowler JH. Spread of Obesity in a Large Social Network over 32 years. *N Engl J Med*. 2007;357:370–379.

U.S. Department of Health and Human Services. Dietary Guidelines for Americans 2005. Available at: www.health.gov/dietary guidelines.

 MISCELLANEOUS

CLINICAL PEARLS

Once patient is motivated, the key to success is to set reasonable goals:

- Dietary modification as life-long improvement in eating habits
- 10% weight loss will cause improvement in many comorbidities:
  - Activity should be something relatively easy and do-able, build up to more advanced exercises:
    - Simply walking more is a start.
  - Get a family member to be a partner in the process.
  - Let the patient know there will be challenges and set-backs, but these are not failures.

ABBREVIATIONS

- BMI—Body mass index
- CHD—Coronary heart disease
- HTN—Hypertension
- PCOS—Polycystic ovary syndrome
- ROS—Review of Systems
- SSRI—Selective serotonin reuptake inhibitor

CODES

ICD9-CM

278.0 Obesity and overweight:

- 278.00 Obesity
- 278.01 Morbid obesity
- 278.02 Overweight

PATIENT TEACHING

- Maintaining a healthy weight involves changes in behavior and choices for a lifetime, not just during a diet.
- There are no quick ways of losing weight that will maintain weight loss; no magic pill.
- The more steadily and slowly (1–2 lb/wk) the weight comes off, the more likely it will stay off.
- Diet and exercise/activity go hand in hand.

PREVENTION

- Encourage patients to weigh themselves regularly and modify eating habits if gaining weight.
- At physician visits, weigh the patient and alert her to changes in weight, especially excessive gains.
- Watch during times of risk for excessive weight gain, such as pregnancy and menopause.

DOMESTIC VIOLENCE

Jill Powell, MD
Linda R. Chambliss, MD, MPH

 BASICS

DESCRIPTION
- The CDC uses the term "intimate partner violence" or IPV to describe physical, sexual, or psychological harm by a current or former partner or spouse:
  - IPV can occur among heterosexual or same-sex couples, and does not require sexual intimacy.
  - IPV, interpersonal violence, and DV, domestic violence, are interchangeable terms:
    - Previously used terms include wife abuse, spouse abuse
- May lead to "battered woman syndrome"
- Includes actual or threatened violence that leads to fear and emotional or physical injury including:
  - Physical abuse:
    - Pushing, kicking, biting, hair pulling, choking, slapping, hitting, beating, suffocating
    - Threats to use any form of weapon or actual use of a weapon
  - Sexual abuse:
    - Sexual assault including any nonconsensual sexual act
    - Sabotage of birth control methods
    - Refusal to follow safer sex practices
  - Emotional abuse:
    - Name calling, threats, harassment
    - Social isolation from family, friends, work
    - Control of food, money, transportation, medications, access to health care
    - Destruction of personal property
    - Pet abuse
    - Stalking
  - Financial abuse

EPIDEMIOLOGY
- Incidence:
  - ~2 million US women experience partner violence annually. IPV accounts for:
    - 22% of all violent crimes against women
    - ~1/3 of female homicides (compared to 1/20 male homicides)
- 0.9–21% of pregnant women experience partner violence
- Prevalence:
  - ~16% of random women selected from voter lists reported ongoing physical abuse.

RISK FACTORS
- Only consistent risk factor is being female.
- No typical "battered" woman
- Any woman can be a victim, regardless of socioeconomic status, religion, age, marital status, education level, or sexual orientation.
- Pregnancy and the postpartum period often initiates or exacerbates partner violence.

Genetics
- IPV/DV is seen in increased frequency in multiple family generations but stems from learned/modeled behaviors on both the part of the perpetrators and victims:
  - Because violence can occur in multiple generations, clinicians should be aware of family violence that includes child abuse and elder abuse as well

PATHOPHYSIOLOGY
- Perpetrators aim to achieve power and control over victims.
- Violence occurs repetitively but unpredictably.
- Typical cycle of violence described:
  - Tension-building phase fueled by anger, blaming, arguing, jealousy
  - Battering phase
  - Honeymoon phase including denial, excuses, blame, apologies, gifts, and/or promises that it will not occur again

ASSOCIATED CONDITIONS
- Medical conditions:
  - Headaches, backaches, chest or abdominal pain
  - Functional gastrointestinal disorders
  - Chronic pelvic pain
  - Sexual dysfunction
  - Exacerbation of pre-existing conditions/non-compliance
- Psychiatric conditions:
  - "Battered woman syndrome" leading to low self-esteem, chronic somatization, "doctor-shopping," polypharmacy, polysurgery
  - PTSD
  - Depression/Mood disorders
  - Sleep and eating disorders
  - Alcohol/Substance abuse

DIAGNOSIS

SIGNS AND SYMPTOMS
History
- Patients will rarely disclose without being asked.
- Even when asked, barriers exist to patient's disclosure including:
  - Fear of retaliation by the abuser
  - Fear of police/court involvement
  - Fear of loss of children
  - Embarrassment and shame
  - Not trusting the health care provider
  - Fear of deportation if the patient is an immigrant
  - Confidentiality concerns
  - Belief that physicians lack time or interest to discuss

- May present with acute injury, chronic somatic symptoms, or psychiatric issues
- Depression: Prior to widespread clinician awareness of and screening for IPV, studies documented that women referred for evaluation of depression and/or anxiety were frequently victims of domestic violence.

Physical Exam
- Poor eye contact
- Evasiveness
- Ecchymoses
- Fractures/Previous fractures by imaging
- Bite marks
- Marks from objects such as cords, ropes, cigarette burns
- Neck or tracheal signs of attempted strangulation
- Genital or anal injuries
- Difficult pelvic exam including unexplained crying, clenching knees and buttocks, inability to assume or maintain lithotomy position
- Recurrent/Refractory vaginitis/STD
- Unintended pregnancy
- Placental abruption/vaginal bleeding
- Direct fetal injury
- Uterine rupture
- Pelvic fractures
- Spontaneous abortion/intrauterine fetal demise
- Fetal growth restriction

TESTS
Periodic, universal screening by primary care, specialty, and acute-care providers is essential:
- Can be included on patient intake questionnaires or asked during the history-taking
- Must be asked when patient is alone, as perpetrator often will accompany patient
- Must avoid using family members as interpreters when screening if at all possible
- Question about specific behaviors, as many victims will not recognize that what they are experiencing is violence/abuse:
  - Has anyone threatened or hurt you verbally or physically?
  - Are you safe at home?
  - Are you afraid of anyone?

Labs
If petechiae or ecchymoses are present, CBC, coags, and consideration of testing for bleeding disorder may be indicated.

Imaging
Lab evaluation can rule out thrombocytopenia or other pathophysiology causing petechiae or ecchymoses.

DIFFERENTIAL DIAGNOSIS

- IPV should be considered and screened for in the evaluation of injury, vague, recurrent somatic complaints with no findings, chronic pelvic pain and sexual dysfunction, mood disorder/psychiatric illness, and substance abuse.
- Rarely, a patient may exhibit self-mutilating behaviors or Munchausen syndrome, but these should be diagnoses of exclusion.

Hematologic
- Petechiae, ecchymoses could be from physical abuse or from an acquired bleeding disorder.
- Lab evaluation as above

Trauma
- Types of injury should match any "accident" the patient reports (e.g., walking into a door should not bruise the front and back).
- Injuries (fractures, bruises, etc.) in varied states of healing are suspicious for abuse rather than accidental trauma/accidents.

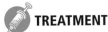 ## TREATMENT

GENERAL MEASURES
- Universal screening will elicit histories of previous and ongoing abuse in many women. Providers must be ready to:
  - Provide emotional support and validation that what the patient is experiencing is abuse.
  - Assess patient's and her family's immediate safety.
  - Provide information about community resources available for acute and chronic intervention when patient is ready.
  - Be familiar with whether mandatory reporting is required by your state.
  - If children in immediate danger or disclosure of any child abuse, notify appropriate authorities.
- Assist patient with developing a safety plan including:
  - Hide house and car keys outside to be able to leave quickly if necessary.
  - Pack an emergency bag to leave elsewhere with items for patient and children including:
    - Cash
    - Credit cards
    - Health insurance cards
    - Extra clothes
    - Favorite toy or stuffed animal
    - Medicines and necessities
  - Take original or pre-made copies of important papers including:
    - Birth certificates
    - Social security cards
    - Court papers
    - Titles or deeds
    - Pay stubs
    - Extra checks

- Clinicians should document all disclosure details and any physical findings:
  - Use patients, exact descriptions of abuse in quotation marks when possible
  - Document any other diagnostic findings (STD tests, imaging, etc.)
  - Photograph any physical findings if feasible:
    - Obtain and document consent from the patient
    - Label any photograph with patient's name, date/time, name of photographer
    - Use either instant imaging or 35 mm film cameras

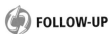 ## FOLLOW-UP

DISPOSITION
Issues for Referral
- Be familiar with community resources for various issues related to previous or ongoing partner violence including information about shelters, legal resources, crisis phone lines, etc.
- Offer materials to patients to take home but do not put information into her bag or pocket without her permission as many perpetrators will search these regularly.
- Patient can put information such as a crisis line phone number in hidden areas such as inside a shoe if she is concerned about taking it home otherwise.
- Have information displayed in private areas, such as the restroom, so that patients may take it without their partner knowing.

PROGNOSIS
IPV is not a rare cause of morbidity and mortality. Screening and identification can be lifesaving.

PATIENT MONITORING
Schedule periodic interval follow-up to reassess safety, coping, medical conditions, or allow opportunities for patient disclosure when ready.

BIBLIOGRAPHY

American College of Obstetricians and Gynecologists. Intimate Partner Violence and Domestic Violence. In: *Special Issues in Women's Health*. Washington, D.C: ACOG, 2005;169–188.

Chambliss L. Domestic violence: A public health crisis. *Clin Obstet Gynecol*. 1997;40:630–638.

MacMillan HL, et al. Approaches to screening for intimate partner violence in health care settings: A randomized trial. *JAMA*. 2006;296:530–536.

 ## MISCELLANEOUS

- National Coalition Against Domestic Violence (NCADV):
- 1–303–839–1852, www.ncadv.org

SYNONYM(S)
- Domestic violence
- Elder abuse
- Interpersonal violence
- Intimate partner violence
- Physical abuse
- Spouse abuse
- Wife abuse

CLINICAL PEARLS
Universal screening is paramount to improving patients' health and potentially saving lives.

ABBREVIATIONS
- DV—Domestic violence
- IPV—Intimate partner violence
- PTSD—Post-traumatic stress disorder
- STD—Sexually transmitted disease

CODES
ICD9-CM
- 995.81 Adult physical abuse
- 995.82 Adult emotional/psychological abuse
- 995.83 Adult sexual abuse
- V61.21 Counsel spousal abuse victim
- V15.41 History of physical abuse
- V15.42 History of emotional abuse

 ## PATIENT TEACHING

National Domestic Violence Toll Free Hotline Phone Numbers:
- 1–800–799–SAFE (7233)
- 1–800–787–3224 (TDD)

PREVENTION
Children who experience violence in their homes have higher rates of being victims (females) or perpetrators (males) as adults and need counseling and therapy to help break the cycle of violence in the family. Innovative programs geared toward educating adolescents about healthy dating relationships and partner violence may help to break the cycle of many before it begins.

FIBROMYALGIA

Tracy V. Ting, MD
T. Brent Graham, MD

 BASICS

DESCRIPTION
Chronic pain syndrome often identified by widespread musculoskeletal pain and common "tender points."

Pediatric Considerations
Uncommon, although can be seen particularly in adolescent females

Geriatric Considerations
Common; polypharmacy may play a role

EPIDEMIOLOGY
- Most commonly affects women from adolescence to elderly.
- Prevalence in US: 2%:
  - Incidence increases with age
  - Chronic pain affects 10–11% of general population.

RISK FACTORS
Risk factors typically associated with poor sleep hygiene, decreased activity +/− cognitive dysfunction or impaired mood:
- Severe fatigue
- Nonrestorative sleep (i.e., sleep apnea, irregular sleep patterns)
- Sudden change/decrease in physical activity
- Cognitive disturbance
- Mood disorders (symptoms of anxiety and/or depression):
  - 30% of patients have a coexisting mood disorder.

Genetics
- Increased risk in 1st-degree relatives:
  - Familial aggregation
  - Aggregation with mood disorders
- Genetic polymorphisms:
  - Serotonin

PATHOPHYSIOLOGY
Unknown etiology:
- Often triggered by physical and emotional stressors
- Disorder of pain regulation
- Hypothalamic-pituitary-axis dysfunction
- Elevation of substance P in CSF

ASSOCIATED CONDITIONS
These conditions often fall under the category of chronic pain syndromes:
- IBS
- Restless leg syndrome
- Chronic headaches

DIAGNOSIS

SIGNS AND SYMPTOMS
History
Often marked by change in lifestyle:
- Decreased physical activity
- Poor sleep patterns
- Stress or trauma

Physical Exam
- Widespread musculoskeletal pain
- Often display pain with pressure to at least 11 of 18 "trigger points":
  - Insertion of suboccipital muscle
  - Anterior cervical (C5–C7)
  - Mid-point of trapezius muscle (superior)
  - 2nd costochondral junction
  - Origin of supraspinatus muscle
  - 2 cm distal to lateral epicondyle
  - Just posterior to greater trochanter
  - Gluteal (upper outer quadrant)
  - Medial fat pad of the knee

TESTS
- No diagnostic test confirms diagnosis. Initial screening studies may be useful to rule out other diseases.
- A sleep study may be necessary to rule out sleep apnea.

Lab
- Normal CBC, renal and liver profiles
- Normal ESR
- Normal TSH
- Normal creatinine phosphokinase and aldolase

Imaging
Not useful

DIFFERENTIAL DIAGNOSIS
Infection
Epstein-Barr virus

Hematologic
Anemia

Metabolic/Endocrine
Hypothyroidism

Other/Miscellaneous
- Muscle strain/joint sprain
- Myositis
- Polymyalgia rheumatica
- Temporomandibular joint disease
- Chronic fatigue syndrome
- Chronic headaches/migraines
- Mood disorders

TREATMENT

GENERAL MEASURES
Optimal treatment involves a multidisciplinary approach:
- Rigorous physical therapy/aerobic exercise
- Improved sleep hygiene
- Stress management
- Educational intervention

Pregnancy Considerations
Therapeutic approach often limited to physical and psychosocial therapy

SPECIAL THERAPY
Complementary and Alternative Therapies
- CBT
- Biofeedback
- Hypnotherapy
- Heat therapy:
  - Hot packs, US

MEDICATION (DRUGS)

ALERT
There are risks of potential long-term abuse with specific medications.

- NSAIDs and glucocorticoids no more effective than placebo.
- Acetaminophen (Tylenol): Intermittently for symptomatic relief
- Tramadol (Ultram): Intermittently for symptomatic relief
- Cyclobenzaprine (Flexeril): Start at 10 mg q.h.s.
- Amitriptyline (Elavil): Start at 10 mg q.h.s.
- Fluoxetine (Prozac): Start 20 mg/d; may need increased dose
- Duloxetine (Cymbalta): 60 mg/d PO or b.i.d.
- Pregabalin: 300–450 mg/d PO in 2 divided doses; initiate at 150 mg/d
- Tender point injections not very effective

SURGERY
Generally not indicated

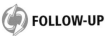 **FOLLOW-UP**

DISPOSITION
Issues for Referral
Referral often not warranted; however, some areas of involvement may require additional evaluation/therapy:

- Psychiatric counseling
- Neuropsychiatric testing
- Sleep disorders clinic

PROGNOSIS
- With resolution of sleep disturbance, may resolve totally
- Aggressive physical therapy is critical in those who do and particularly those who do not respond.
- ~5% of patients do not respond to any form of therapeutic intervention.
- Relapse is common.

PATIENT MONITORING
- For treatment efficacy at 6–8 weeks
- For medication side effects every 3–6 months

BIBLIOGRAPHY

Arnold LM, et al. A randomized, placebo-controlled, double-blind, flexible-dose study of fluoxetine in the treatment of women with fibromyalgia. *Am J Med*. 2002;112:191–197.

Arnold LM, et al. Family study of fibromyalgia. *Arthritis Rheum*. 2004;50:944–952.

Arnold LM, et al. A randomized, double-blind, placebo-controlled trial of duloxetine in the treatment of women with fibromyalgia with or without major depressive disorder. *Pain*. 2005; 119:5–15.

Busch A, et al. Exercise for treating fibromyalgia syndrome. *Cochrane Database Syst Rev*. 2002; 3:CD003786.

Crofford LJ, et al. Pregabalin for the treatment of fibromyalgia syndrome: Results of a randomized double-blind, placebo-controlled trial. *Arthritis Rheum*. 2005;52:1264–1273.

Fibromyalgia: New concepts of pathogenesis and treatment. *Intern J Immunopathol Pharmacol*. 2006;19:5–10.

Goldenberg DL, et al. Crofford management of fibromyalgia syndrome. *JAMA*. 2004;292: 2388–2395.

Gursoy S, et al. Significance of catechol-O-methyltransferase gene polymorphism in fibromyalgia syndrome. *Rheumatol Intern*. 2003; 23:104–107.

Lemstra M, et al. The effectiveness of multidisciplinary rehabilitation in the treatment of fibromyalgia: A randomized controlled trial. *Clin J Pain*. 2005; 21:166–174.

Lucas HJ, Brauch CM, Settas L, et al. Fibromyalgia: New concepts of pathogenesis and treatment. *Int J Immunopathol Pharmacol*. 2006;19(1):5–10.

McBeth J, et al. Hypothalamic-pituitary-adrenal stress axis function and the relationship with chronic widespread pain and its antecedents. *Arthritis Res Ther*. 2005;7:R992–R1000.

Mease P. Fibromyalgia syndrome: A review of clinical presentation, pathogenesis, outcome measures, and treatment. *J Rheumatol Suppl*. 2005;75:6–21.

Wolfe F, et al. The American College of Rheumatology 1990 criteria for the classification of fibromyalgia. Report of the multicenter criteria committee. *Arthritis Rheum*. 1990;33:160–172.

 MISCELLANEOUS

- Fibromyalgia is perhaps the most common cause of neck or back pain, and the most common rheumatologic problem in general.
- Associated with: "Chronic Fatigue Syndrome"; "Insomnia, Irritable Bowel Syndrome"; "Restless Leg Syndrome"

SYNONYM(S)
- Fibrositis
- Myofascial pain syndrome

CLINICAL PEARLS
Findings suggesting the diagnosis:
- Widespread musculoskeletal pain
- Exam significant for presence of tender points
- Otherwise unremarkable examination and laboratory studies

ABBREVIATIONS
- CBT—Cognitive behavioral therapy
- IBS—Irritable bowel syndrome
- TSH—Thyroid-stimulating hormone

 CODES

ICD9-CM
729.0 Fibrositis/Fibromyalgia

PATIENT TEACHING

- Resources: Fibromyalgia Network, National Fibromyalgia Research Association, The Arthritis Foundation, National Institute of Arthritis, Musculoskeletal and Skin Disease
- Education is crucial to rehabilitation:
  - Reinforce concept that disease is a benign disorder of pain dysregulation associated with poor sleep, fatigue, inactivity, and/or mood disorders.
  - Patients should be made aware of potential for relapse associated with emotional and/or physical stressors (including illness).

PREVENTION
- Good sleep hygiene
- Consistent aerobic exercise 30–45 minutes 3–5 times a week
- Treatment of underlying mood disorder
- Observe for medication side effects/abuse.

Section III

HEADACHES

Stephanie J. Nahas, MD, MSEd
Stephen D. Silberstein, MD

 BASICS

DESCRIPTION
- Primary headaches (diseases unto their own):
  - Tension-type headache
  - Migraine (with or without aura)
  - Cluster headache and other TACs
  - Others (stabbing, cough, exertional, coital, hypnic, thunderclap, trigeminal neuralgia)
- Secondary headaches (due to other causes):
  - Head and/or neck trauma
  - Cranial or cervical vascular disorder
  - Nonvascular intracranial disorder
  - Substance use or its withdrawal
  - Infection
  - Disorder of homeostasis
  - Disorder of cranial structures
  - Psychiatric

Age-Related Factors
- Prevalence of migraine and tension-type headaches highest for ages 35–45
- Migraine prevalence decreases with advanced age. Women with natural menopause may improve, whereas patients with surgical menopause often worsen.
- Cluster headache: Mean onset age 27–31
- Headache in older persons (>50) may be cause for concern.

EPIDEMIOLOGY
- Migraine and tension-type headaches are common.
  - Migraine has a 1-year prevalence of 18% in women, 6% in men.
  - Migraine usually presents in 1st 3 decades of life, but may present up to age 50.
  - Tension headache has a yearly prevalence of 38% in the general population.
- Cluster:
  - Incidence 15.6/100,000 person years (men) and 4.0/100,000 person-years (women)
  - Prevalence rate: ~0.4%
  - Male:female ratio: ~5.5:1 overall, 3:1 in blacks
- CDH (>15 d/mo):
  - Estimated at 4–5% worldwide
  - Chronic tension (leading cause), transformed migraine, new daily persistent headache, and hemicrania continua (rare)
- Other headaches are rare.
- Of note, CPH demonstrates female predominance of ~2:1
- Headache on the whole poses substantial burden on sufferers, families, and society:
  - Direct costs for migraine in US estimated at over $1 billion annually
  - Migraine costs US employers $13 billion annually (absenteeism, reduced function at work)

RISK FACTORS
- Tension, migraine, CPH: Female
- Cluster: Male, smoking, hazel eyes, head injury
- CDH: Obesity, medication overuse

Genetics
- As yet implicated in only 3 headache disorders:
  - Migraine and tension-type, see "Headaches During Pregnancy: Tension/Migraine"
  - Cluster: Autosomal dominant with incomplete penetrance
    - Less likely mitochondrial
    - No specific genes identified

PATHOPHYSIOLOGY
- Migraine involves activation of trigeminovascular system, which innervates large intracranial vessels and dura mater.
- Trigeminal nerve activation ensues, and neuropeptides are released resulting in leakage of plasma proteins.
- The trigeminal nucleus in the brainstem receives the afferents and may produce alterations of pain and sensory input, leading to nausea and sensory sensitivity.
- Aura results from "cortical spreading depression," which results in neuronal activation, then suppression
- Tension headache physiology is poorly understood but may be similar to migraine.
- Cluster headaches are mediated by trigeminal nociceptive pathways.
- Pathophysiology of most other headaches is poorly understood.

ASSOCIATED CONDITIONS
Most notable in migraine (See Headaches During Pregnancy: Tension/Migraine.)

 DIAGNOSIS

SIGNS AND SYMPTOMS
History
- History should allow you to classify headache:
  - Age at onset
  - Frequency, duration, and timing
  - Warning symptoms
  - Aura (See Headaches During Pregnancy: Tension/Migraine.)
  - Pain characteristics:
    - Intensity (mild, moderate, severe)
    - Constant or throbbing?
    - Dull or stabbing?
    - Unilateral or bilateral? Where?
    - Aggravated by activity?
  - Associated symptoms:
    - Nausea/Vomiting
    - Photophobia/Phonophobia
    - Restlessness
    - Autonomic features (conjunctival injection, lacrimation, rhinorrhea/congestion, eyelid/facial edema, ptosis and/or miosis)
  - Precipitating/Aggravating factors:
    - Stress (migraine and tension-type)
    - Hormonal changes (migraine)
    - Excessive stimuli (migraine > tension)
    - Alcohol (cluster > migraine)
    - Caffeine or its withdrawal (migraine)
    - Fasting (migraine and tension)
    - Exertion, coughing, sex (often benign)
    - Posture, neck movements (tension-type, cervicogenic)

- Talking/Chewing, touching face (trigeminal neuralgia)
  - Sleep changes (migraine)
  - Weather changes (migraine)
  - Relieving factors:
    - Rest?
    - Medication?
  - Prior treatment helps guide future treatment:
    - Medication or otherwise
    - Effective?
  - General and past health
  - Family history
  - Personal background
  - Emotional state
- Migraine and tension-type diagnostic criteria (See "Headaches During Pregnancy: Tension/Migraine.")
- Cluster headache diagnostic criteria:
  - 5 attacks lifetime
  - Severe unilateral orbital, supraorbital, and/or temporal pain lasting 15–180 minutes (untreated)
  - At least 1 of ipsilateral conjunctival injection and/or tearing, nasal congestion/rhinorrhea, eyelid edema, forehead/facial sweating, miosis/ptosis
  - Sense of restlessness or agitation
  - Frequency of 1 every other day to 8/d
  - Episodic: 2 attack periods for 7–365 days with pain-free interval at least 30 days
  - Chronic: Attacks recur for >1 year with remissions lasting <30 days, or no remissions
- PH, like cluster, but more frequent attacks throughout day and shorter lasting (2–30 min) with no restlessness
- Trigeminal neuralgia:
  - Facial pain, fraction of second to 2 minutes
  - Unilateral; face, jaw, ear; sharp/stabbing, severe; triggered by trivial stimuli including washing, shaving, smoking, talking, and/or brushing teeth, which activate "trigger zone" on face
- Exertional/Valsalva headaches tend to be triggered by specific activity, to be benign, and to respond to prophylactic NSAIDs, and particularly indomethacin

Physical Exam
- General exam excludes other medical contributors
- Comprehensive neurologic exam
- Funduscopic exam mandatory
- Special attention to head, jaw, neck

ALERT
Think of secondary causes when "red flags" are present, cued by the **"SNOOP"** mnemonic

- **S:** Systemic symptoms (fever, weight loss) or secondary risk factors (HIV, cancer)
- **N:** Neurologic symptoms/signs (altered consciousness, focal deficits)
- **O:** Onset: Sudden or split-second (think subarachnoid hemorrhage)
- **O:** Older: New or progressive >50 (think temporal arteritis)
- **P:** Prior history: 1st headache, different from usual headache, newly progressive headache

TESTS
Generally unnecessary, except in refractory cases or when secondary causes are suspected

Lab
- Routine to rule out disorders of homeostasis
- Drug screen
- ESR, C-reactive protein for temporal arteritis
- Other appropriate testing per history and exam

Imaging
- In refractory or suspected secondary cases:
  - CT, looking for:
    - Subarachnoid hemorrhage
    - Sinus disease
    - Mass lesion if papilledema seen
    - Blood or fracture in traumatic cases
- MRI: For what CT misses
- Myelogram/Cisternogram: CSF leak

DIFFERENTIAL DIAGNOSIS
Secondary causes may be present even in "typical" presentations; always keep in mind "Classic" worrisome headache patterns may have atypical or even benign etiology—Thunderclap headache, for example:
- Subarachnoid hemorrhage
- Arterial dissection
- Cerebral venous thrombosis
- Spontaneous CSF leak
- Pituitary apoplexy
- Unruptured aneurysm with rapid expansion
- Crash migraine (merely a sudden migraine)
- Idiopathic/Benign (the majority of cases!)

Infection
- Meningitis
- Lyme disease and others like it
- Sinusitis:
  - May present as any type of headache
  - True sinus headache is associated with documented sinus infection and resolves with antibiotics.
  - Most so-called "sinus headaches" are truly migraine with the autonomic feature of congestion/rhinorrhea.

Hematologic
- Cerebral venous thrombosis:
  - Risks include pregnancy, cancer, hypercoagulable state, dehydration in autoimmune disease, head trauma

Metabolic/Endocrine
Headache in these disorders is typically overshadowed by the other features of the disease.

Immunologic
- Giant cell (temporal) arteritis:
  - Older
  - Constitutional signs
  - Palpable, tender temporal artery
  - Blindness if untreated

Tumor/Malignancy
No reliable correlation exists between brain tumors and headache. It's a myth.

Trauma
Risk for subdural/epidural bleed, venous thrombosis, arterial dissection, CSF leak

Drugs
Cocaine, nitrites/nitrates, histamine, many other drugs with side effect of headache

Other/Miscellaneous
IIH (a.k.a. pseudotumor cerebri), with or without papilledema:
- Any kind of headache
- Young, overweight female
- LP diagnostic, pressure >200 mm CSF
- MRI may show small veins, slit-like ventricles
- Papilledema leads to vision loss if untreated

 TREATMENT

GENERAL MEASURES
- Acute home treatment must be effective, well tolerated.
- Emergency treatment must be aggressive yet safe.
- Prophylactic treatment is indicated when headaches are frequent (>1/week) or debilitating.
- Overuse of acute meds often worsens headache.
- Opioids should be *avoided* in most cases.
- Patients unable to function, in danger of losing employment should be hospitalized.

SPECIAL THERAPY
Complementary and Alternative Therapies
Most helpful in tension-type and migraine (See Headache During Pregnancy: Tension/Migraine)

MEDICATION (DRUGS)
- Migraine and tension-type (See Headache During Pregnancy: Tension/Migraine)
- Cluster: Acute and preventive treatment: Consider referral, as unusual in women
- PH: Indomethacin 50–300 mg/d, divided doses
- Trigeminal neuralgia: Carbamazepine (Tegretol) and other anticonvulsants
- IIH: Weight loss, drugs to reduce CSF production (acetazolamide, diuretics, topiramate)

SURGERY
- Occipital nerve stimulation: Migraine, cluster
- Deep brain stimulation: Cluster
- Microvascular decompression and ablative techniques: Trigeminal neuralgia
- Optic nerve sheath fenestration if vision threatened in IIH (but may not help headache)
- Shunts to be avoided in IIH if at all possible.

 FOLLOW-UP

DISPOSITION
Issues for Referral
Refer refractory cases to headache specialist early.

PROGNOSIS
Usually good; depends on comorbidities (especially psychiatric) and any underlying cause

PATIENT MONITORING
Drug specific. Recommend headache diary

BIBLIOGRAPHY

Headache Classification Subcommittee of the International Headache Society. *The International Classification of Headache Disorders*, 2nd ed. Cephalalgia 2004;24S1.

Lance JW, et al. *Mechanism and Management of Headache*. Philadelphia: Elsevier Butterworth Heinemann, 2005.

Silberstein SD, et al., eds. *Wolff's Headache and Other Head Pain*, 8th ed. New York: Oxford University Press; 2008.

 MISCELLANEOUS

CLINICAL PEARLS
- Most severe headaches are migraine
- Severe headaches with neck pain are usually migraine not tension.
- "Sick" headaches or "sinus headaches" are usually migraine.
- Beware of red flags:
  - Sudden onset
  - Older age of 1st onset
  - Systemic illness such as immunosuppression
  - Alteration of consciousness
  - Focal neurological deficits

ABBREVIATIONS
- CDH—Chronic daily headache
- CPH—Chronic paroxysmal hemicrania
- IIH—Idiopathic intracranial hypertension
- PH—Paroxysmal hemicrania
- TACs—Trigeminal autonomic cephalgias

CODES
ICD9-CM
- 346.20-346.21 Migraine variant:
  - Includes cluster, paroxysmal hemicrania,
  - 346.20 Episodic
  - 346.21 Chronic
- 350.1 Trigeminal neuralgia

PATIENT TEACHING

- Consider nonpharmacologic approaches such as biofeedback, relaxation, acupuncture, and physical therapy in selected patients.
- Develop strategies for managing acute attacks including options for moderate and severe attacks.
- Offer rescue therapy to prevent emergency room visits and increased disability.
- Encourage use of headache calendars for patients with frequent attacks.
- Preventative medications require an adequate trial of a few months to assess efficacy.

PREVENTION
- Avoidance of triggers when possible
- Regular sleep patterns
- Regular exercise
- Smoking cessation
- Avoiding overuse of acute attack medications
- Maintaining good general health
- Maintaining healthy weight

HEREDITARY THROMBOPHILIAS

Charles J. Lockwood, MD

BASICS

DESCRIPTION
- Inherited thrombophilias include a number of inherited conditions in which there is an increased risk of venous thrombosis and VTE. (See Table in Appendix; Deep Vein Thrombosis; Pulmonary Embolism; and Deep Vein Thrombosis/Pulmonary Embolus.)
- FVL is the most common heritable coagulopathy:
  - FVL results from a point mutation in the factor V gene that causes aPC resistance.
  - Heterozygous state is symptomatic.
  - Meta-analyses indicate that FVL is associated with fetal loss:
    - The risk of 1st trimester early pregnancy loss (<13 weeks) is modestly increased (OR, 2.01; 95% CI:1.13–3.58)
    - Stronger associated with late (>19 weeks) nonrecurrent fetal loss (OR 3.26;1.82–5.83)
    - Association with recurrent fetal losses >22 weeks (OR 7.83; 2.83–21.67)
  - Meta-analyses have found strong associations between placental abruption and both homozygosity and heterozygosity for the FVL mutation:
    - Homozygosity OR 16.9; 2.0–141.9
    - Heterozygosity OR 6.7; 2.0–21.6
  - The link between FVL and other adverse pregnancy events such as severe preeclampsia and IUGR is unproven and unlikely:
    - Similar conclusions regarding the other common thrombophilias including heterozygosity for the PGM, Protein C, S, and antithrombin deficiencies
- Other thrombophilias linked with VTE in pregnancy include:
  - Prothrombin G20201A promoter mutation (PGM)
  - Protein C deficiency
  - Protein S deficiency
  - Hyperhomocysteinemia:
    - May be responsive to folate therapy
  - Antithrombin deficiency

Age-Related Factors
Age >45 years is an independent risk factor for the occurrence of VTE.

EPIDEMIOLOGY
- FVL is present in 5% of European population.
- FVL accounts for >40% of VTE in women.
- Among pregnant women heterozygous for FVL:
  - The risk of thrombosis is only 0.2% without a personal or family history of VTE.
  - With a personal history or strong family history (1st-degree relative) with VTE, the risk is >10%.

RISK FACTORS
- The occurrence of VTE in a woman with an inherited thrombophilia is highly dependent on the presence of other predisposing factors including:
  - Pregnancy
  - Exogenous hormones
  - Obesity
  - Age >45 years
  - Immobilization
  - Concomitant thrombophilias
  - A personal or family history of VTE
  - Triggering factors:
    - Trauma
    - Surgery
    - Infection

Genetics
Homozygosity and heterozygosity for FLV or other specific thrombophilias

PATHOPHYSIOLOGY
- Factor V is a cofactor with factor X in the conversion of prothrombin to thrombin. Thrombin cleaves fibrinogen to fibrin, which polymerizes to comprise the majority of a clot.
- aPC is a natural anticoagulant that counterbalances and limits clotting by cleaving and degrading factor V.

- FVL is an autosomal dominant condition in which the coagulation factor cannot be inactivated by aPC.
  - The gene mutation prevents efficient inactivation of factor V by distorting the cleavage site.
  - Factor V remains active and facilitates overproduction of thrombin leading to excess fibrin generation and excess clotting.

ASSOCIATED CONDITIONS
- VTE (See Deep Vein Thrombosis)
- DVT (See Deep Vein Thrombosis/Pulmonary Embolus)
- PE (See Deep Vein Thrombosis/Pulmonary Embolus)
- Fetal loss (See Intrauterine Fetal Demise)
- Placental abruption (See Hemorrhage: Third Trimester)

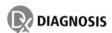

DIAGNOSIS

SIGNS AND SYMPTOMS
History
- Personal history of DVT/PE, fetal loss, abruption
- Family history of DVT/PE, fetal loss, abruption:
  - Attempt to obtain information about specific testing of the individual with VTE, although may have been prior to common testing for specific thrombophilias

TESTS
Labs
- aPTT as screening test
- If suspected on the basis of personal or family history, specific testing for the gene mutations of FVL and other thrombophilias may be indicated.

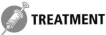 **TREATMENT**

MEDICATION (DRUGS)

- The presence of FVL, PGM, protein C or S deficiency, hyperhomocysteinemia unresponsive to folate therapy PLUS personal of strong family history of VTE warrant thromboprophylaxis during pregnancy and the puerperium.
- In the presence of these thrombophilias, but the ABSENCE of a personal or strong family history, thromboprophylaxis is only needed following a Cesarean delivery.
- In contrast, antithrombin deficiency, homozygosity for FVL, or PGM and compound heterozygosis for FVL and PGM carry higher risks for VTE and warrant antenatal and postpartum anticoagulation regardless of personal or family VTE history or mode of delivery.
- See Appendix for Table of Inherited Thrombophilias and Their Association with VTE in Pregnancy.

ALERT

Nonpregnant women with known thrombophilias should not receive exogenous hormones containing estrogen and are at increased risk of VTE following surgery or prolonged immobilization.

SURGERY

See Deep Vein Thrombosis/Pulmonary Embolus regarding prophylaxis at the time of surgery.

 FOLLOW-UP

DISPOSITION

Issues for Referral

- Consider consultation with hematologist for diagnosis.
- Consider consultation with maternal fetal medicine specialist for management issues in pregnancy or with recurrent pregnancy loss.

BIBLIOGRAPHY

Alfirevic Z, et al. How strong is the association between maternal thrombophilia and adverse pregnancy outcome? A systematic review. *Eur J Obstet Gynecol Reprod Biol*. 2002;101:6–14.

Friederich PW, et al. Frequency of pregnancy-related venous thromboembolism in anticoagulant factor-deficient women: Implications for prophylaxis. *Ann Intern Med*. 1996;125:955–960.

Gris JC, et al. Case-control study of the frequency of thrombophilic disorders in couples with late foetal loss and no thrombotic antecedent: The Nimes Obstetricians and Haematologists Study5 (NOHA5). *Thromb Haemost*. 1999;81:891–899.

Infante-Rivard C, et al. Absence of association of thrombophilia polymorphisms with intrauterine growth restriction. *N Engl J Med*. 20024;347:19–25.

Kosmas IP, et al. Association of Leiden mutation in factor V gene with hypertension in pregnancy and preeclampsia: A meta-analysis. *J Hypertens*. 2003;21:1221–1228.

Rey E, et al. Thrombophilic disorders and fetal loss: A meta-analysis. *Lancet* 2003;361:901–908.

Zotz RB, et al. Inherited thrombophilia and gestational venous thromboembolism. *Best Pract Res Clin Haematol*. 2003;16:243–259.

 MISCELLANEOUS

ABBREVIATIONS

- aPC—Activated protein C
- aPPT—Activated partial thromboplastin time
- CI—Confidence interval
- DVT—Deep venous thrombosis
- FVL—Factor V Leiden
- OR—Odds ratio
- PE—Pulmonary embolism
- PGM—Prothrombin gene mutation
- VTE—Venous thromboembolism

 CODES

ICD9-CM
289.81 Primary hypercoagulable state

PATIENT TEACHING

PREVENTION

- Identify candidates for prophylaxis with pregnancy or surgery.
- Avoid estrogen-containing contraceptives if known inherited thrombophilia.
- Avoid estrogen therapy for management of menopause if known inherited thrombophilia.

Section III

HYPERLIPIDEMIA

Paula J. Adams HIllard, MD

 BASICS

DESCRIPTION

- Abnormally high levels of plasma fats, including cholesterol, triglycerides, and lipoprotein, as defined by NCEP.
- The ATPIII focuses on primary prevention of CHD, particularly if multiple risk factors.
- Total cholesterol consists of VLDL, LDL, and HDL.
- Normal serum concentrations:
  - Total cholesterol:
    - <200: Desirable
    - 200–239: Borderline high
    - ≥240: High
  - LDL cholesterol:
    - <100: Optimal
    - 100–129: Near optimal/above optimal
    - 160–189: High
    - ≥190: Very high
  - HDL cholesterol:
    - <40: Low
    - ≥60: High
  - TG:
    - <150 mg: Normal
    - 150–199: Borderline-high
    - 200–499: High
    - ≥500: Very high
- Primary hypercholesterolemia: Elevated cholesterol as a result of an inherited disorder of lipid metabolism (familial hypercholesterolemia)
- Secondary hypercholesterolemia: Elevated cholesterol as a result of another disease process (i.e., nephrotic syndrome)
- Dyslipidemia
- Hypercholesterolemia
- Hypertriglyceridemia

Age-Related Factors

- In women, most CHD occurs after age 65.
- CHD is rare in women 20–45, except those with severe risk factors:
  - Elevated serum cholesterol in young adulthood predicts a higher rate of premature CHD in middle age
- Most CHD occurs in women with multiple risk factors and the metabolic syndrome.

EPIDEMIOLOGY

- Overall prevalence in women is ~29% and increases with age from 20% in 20–44 age group to 47.5% in >65 age group.
- CVD is the primary cause of death in American women, accounting for >500,000 deaths annually.
- Women become at increased risk for death from CHD ~10 years later than men.
- ~38% of women die within a year after a heart attack, compared to 25% of men.
- Within the 1st 6 years after a heart attack, 35% of women and 18% of men have a 2nd heart attack.

RISK FACTORS

- Factors that contribute to high risk for CHD and impact treatment goals:
  - Cigarette smoking
  - HTN (BP = 140/90 mm Hg or antihypertensive medications)
  - Low HDL cholesterol (<40 mg/dL)
  - Family history of premature CHD (male 1st-degree relative <55 years; CHD in female 1st-degree relative <65 years)
  - Age ≥55 years for women
  - DM
- CHD equivalents that also modify treatment goals:
  - Other atherosclerotic disease:
    - Peripheral arterial disease
    - Abdominal aortic aneurysm
    - Symptomatic carotid artery disease
  - Multiple risks factors that confer 10-year risk for CHD >20% (Framingham models for risk)
- Life habit risk factors: Obesity, physical inactivity, atherogenic diet
- Emerging risk factors: Homocysteine, prothrombotic and proinflammatory factors, impaired fasting glucose, subclinical atherosclerotic disease
- Metabolic syndrome:
  - Abdominal obesity (waist circumference >35 inches):
    - Atherogenic dyslipidemia: Elevated TG, small LDL particles, low HDL cholesterol
  - Elevated blood pressure
  - Insulin resistance
  - Prothrombotic and proinflammatory states
- Risk category establishes LDL treatment goal, lifestyle changes, and drug therapy

Genetics

- FHTG: Autosomal dominantly inherited disorder typically resulting from heterozygous mutations encoding the LDL receptor
- FCHL: Dominantly inherited lipid disorder

PATHOPHYSIOLOGY

- Primary FH: Defect of LDL receptor, resulting in the body's inability to properly use circulating LDL cholesterol, which accumulates within blood vessel walls, forming arterial plaques than can grow and occlude the lumen.
- FHTG: A severe elevation in serum triglycerides; can be associated with lipoprotein lipase deficiency or apolipoprotein C-II deficiency

ASSOCIATED CONDITIONS

- PCOS
- DM
- HTN
- Metabolic syndrome
- Overweight and obesity
- Peripheral arterial disease

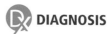 **DIAGNOSIS**

- Basic principle of prevention: Intensity of risk-reduction therapy adjusted to absolute risk
- 1st step is to assess risk status:
  - All adults ≥20 years, fasting lipoprotein profile once every 5 years
  - If nonfasting, total chol >200 mg/dL or HDL <40 mg/dL dictate fasting profile

SIGNS AND SYMPTOMS

History

- Family history of premature heart disease or occurrence of premature heart disease and hyperlipidemia in parents and grandparents:
  - Almost all cases of primary hyperlipidemia are of dominant inheritance.
- Lifestyle:
  - Smoking
  - Hormone therapy
  - Exercise
- 3-day diet history:
  - Evaluates dietary intake of calories and cholesterol with 3-day diet

Physical Exam

- Eye examination:
  - Arcus corneae: Deposits of cholesterol, resulting in a thin, white circular ring located on the outer edge of the iris
- Skin examination:
  - Tendon xanthomas: Thickened tissue surrounding the Achilles and extensor tendons
  - Xanthelasma: Yellowish deposits of cholesterol surrounding the eye
  - Palmar xanthomas: Pale lines in creases of palms
  - Eruptive xanthomas: Characteristic of hypertriglyceridemia; papular yellowish lesions with a red base that occur on the buttocks, elbows, and knees.

TESTS

Labs

- Lipid profile: Fasting serum lipoprotein levels:
  - Total cholesterol, HDL cholesterol, and TG
- Chemistry panel (ALT, AST, bilirubin, BUN, Crt, UA):
  - Screening test for liver and kidney disease
- Thyroid evaluation (T4, TSH):
  - Determines the presence of hypothyroidism

DIFFERENTIAL DIAGNOSIS

- Hypercholesterolemia:
  - Primary hypercholesterolemia (see above)
  - Hypothyroidism
  - Nephrotic syndrome
  - Liver disease (cholestatic)
  - Renal failure
  - Anorexia nervosa
  - Acute porphyria
  - Myelomatosis

- Medications (antihypertensives, estrogens, steroids, microsomal enzyme inducers, cyclosporine, diuretics)
- Pregnancy
- Dietary: Excessive dietary intake of fat, cholesterol, and/or calories
• Hypertriglyceridemia:
  - Primary hypertriglyceridemia
  - Acute hepatitis, nephritic syndrome, chronic renal failure, medications (diuretics, retinoids, COCs, DM, alcohol abuse, lipodystrophy, myelomatosis, glycogen storage disease, dietary [excess intake of fat and/or calories])

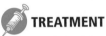 **TREATMENT**

GENERAL MEASURES
• Therapeutic lifestyle changes are indicated, and include:
  - Reduced intake of saturated fat (to <7% of total calories) and cholesterol (<200 mg/d)
  - Enhanced LDL lowering options such as plant stanol/sterols (2 g/d) and increased soluble fiber (10–25 g/d)
  - Weight reduction
  - Increased physical activity
• Diet nutrient composition
  - Saturated fat: <7% of total calories
  - Polyunsaturated fat: Up to 10% of total cal
  - Monounsaturated fat: Up to 20% of total calories
  - Total fat: 25–35% of total calories (keep trans fatty acids low)
  - Carbohydrates (especially complex carbohydrates like grains, fruits, and vegetables): 50–60% of total calories
  - Fiber: 20–30 g/d
  - Cholesterol: <200 mg/d
  - Total calories: Balance energy intake and expenditure to maintain desirable body weight/prevent weight gain
• Manage metabolic syndrome:
  - Weight management
  - Physical exercise

SPECIAL THERAPY
Complementary and Alternative Therapies
• RCT of 3 different garlic formulations did not show a beneficial effect on LDL cholesterol.
• Flaxseed preparations seem to have a beneficial effect of reducing total cholesterol and LDL, except little beneficial effect on LDL in postmenopausal women. Little effect on raising HDL.
• Oats, oat bran, and other soluble fibers can modestly reduce total and LDL cholesterol as part of a diet low in saturated fat.
• Other products, including red yeast, sitostanol, and β-sitosterol have been shown to lower total and LDL cholesterol.

MEDICATION (DRUGS)
• Individuals whose risk for CHD is high will require LDL-lowering drugs in addition to therapeutic lifestyle changes to reach LDL goals:
  - Addendum to NCEP ATP III guidelines recommend statins to reduce LDL to:
    ○ <70 for very high risk
    ○ <100 for moderately high risk

• Classes of drugs, effects:
  - Statins (HMG CoA reductase inhibitors):
    ○ 18–55% decrease LDL
    ○ 5–15% increase HDL
    ○ 7–30% decrease TG
  - Bile acid sequestrants:
    ○ 15–30% decrease LDL
    ○ 3–5% increase HDL
    ○ No change or increase TG
  - Nicotinic acid:
    ○ 5–25% decrease LDL
    ○ 15–35% increase HDL
    ○ 20–50% decrease TGPa
  - Fibric acids:
    ○ 5–20% decreases LDL (may be increased in patients with high TG)
    ○ 10–20% increase HDL
    ○ 20–50% decrease TG

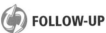 **FOLLOW-UP**

DISPOSITION
Issues for Referral
• Referral to dietician can be helpful.
• Internist or cardiologist may be indicated for active management of CHD risks.

PROGNOSIS
Risk of CHD based on Framingham risk tables

COMPLICATIONS
• Linked to premature coronary artery disease and vascular disease
• Severe hypertriglyceridemia can cause pancreatitis.
• Autopsy studies demonstrate that early coronary atherosclerosis or precursors of atherosclerosis often begin in childhood and adolescence and are related to high serum total cholesterol levels, high LDL cholesterol, plus high VLDL cholesterol levels and low HDL levels.
  - Significant atherosclerotic vessel disease can occur in the 1st decade of life in children with homozygous familial hypercholesterolemia.
• Hypercholesterolemia:
  - Premature heart disease
  - Stroke
  - Carotid artery disease
• Hypertriglyceridemia:
  - Pancreatitis

PATIENT MONITORING
• For patients with primary hyperlipidemia who are off medication, follow-up should be performed every 1–2 years with lipoprotein profile evaluation.
• For those patients on medication, follow-up should be conducted every 3 months.

BIBLIOGRAPHY

Grundy SM, et al. Implications of recent clinical trials for the National Cholesterol Education Program Adult Treatment Panel III guidelines. *Circulation* 2004;110(2):227–239.

National Heart, Lung, and Blood Institute, National Institutes of Health, US Department of Health and Human Services. *Third report of the National Cholesterol Education Program (NCEP) Expert Panel on Detection, Evaluation, and Treatment of High Blood Cholesterol in Adults (Adult Treatment Panel III)*. Bethesda MD: U.S. Department of Health and Human Services, Public Health Service, National Institutes of Health, National Heart, Lung and Blood Institute; 2001.

Natural Medicine Comprehensive Database—Flaxseed. At http://www.naturaldatabase.com. Accessed 09/27/07.

Trends in cholesterol screening and awareness of high blood cholesterol-United States, 1991-2003. *MMWR Morbidity Mortality Weekly Rep.* 2005; 54:865–870.

 MISCELLANEOUS

CLINICAL PEARLS
• Hyperlipidemia is 1 of the most important modifiable risk factors for CHD.
• LDL cholesterol is the major atherogenic lipoprotein and is the primary target of therapy.
• Aggressive lowering of LDL and early use of statins with therapeutic lifestyle changes can significantly reduce risk of CHD.
• COCs result in slight elevation of triglycerides; these elevations may be clinically significant in women with familial hypertriglyceridemia:
  - Periodic lipid screening is indicated for routine preventive healthcare, but is not required prior to initiating oral contraceptives in healthy women

ABBREVIATIONS
• ATPIII—Adult Treatment Panel III
• CHD—Coronary heart disease
• COC—Combination oral contraceptives
• DM—Diabetes Mellitus
• FCHL—Familial combined hyperlipidemia
• FH—Familial hypercholesterolemia
• FHTG—Familial hypertriglyceridemia
• HDL—High-density lipoprotein
• HTN—Hypertension
• LDL—Low-density lipoprotein
• NCEP—National Cholesterol Education Program
• PCOS—Polycystic ovary syndrome
• RCT—Randomized controlled trial
• TG—Triglycerides
• VLDL—Very low-density lipoprotein

CODES
ICD9-CM
• 272.1 Hypertriglyceridemia
• 272.2 Mixed hyperlipidemia
• 272.4 Hyperlipidemia
• 272.4 Combined hyperlipidemia

 PATIENT TEACHING

• Rosenson, RS. Patient information: High cholesterol and lipids (hyperlipidemia). Updodate.com at http://patients.uptodate.com/topic.asp?file=hrt_dis/7390 accessed 092707
• Patient information at http://www.NHLBI.nih.gov

PREVENTION
Primary prevention of CHD with lifestyle changes:
• Reduced intake of saturated fat and cholesterol
• Increased physical activity
• Weight control

HYPERTENSION

Max C. Reif, MD

BASICS

DESCRIPTION
- Normal BP <120/80 mm Hg
- Prehypertension 120–139/80–89 mm Hg
- HTN ≥140/90 mm Hg
- White coat HTN consists of elevated BP when measured at the office, with normal readings at home (present in 20% of patients with elevated in-office BP).
- Primary (essential) HTN accounts for 95% of all cases

Pediatric Considerations
Normal BP in the pediatric and adolescent age group is based on age and height percentile.

Age-Related Factors
- Women show progressive prevalence with age. In men, the prevalence is highest between ages 45 and 54.
- In patients >50, most of the cardiovascular risk is linked to the systolic BP.

EPIDEMIOLOGY
- Overall prevalence of HTN in US is 31.3%, translating into 65.2 million adults.
- African Americans have higher prevalence and greater risk of target-organ damage when compared to other ethnic groups.
- Incidence of renal artery stenosis is <1% in cases of mild HTN but as high as 10–40% in acute, severe, or refractory cases.

RISK FACTORS
- Family history
- Excess sodium intake
- Obesity
- Physical inactivity
- Mental stress
- Low birth weight
- Impaired glucose tolerance and metabolic syndrome increase risk for HTN, diabetes, and vascular disease
- Secondary HTN due to:
  – Combination oral contraceptives
  – Primary hyperaldosteronism
  – Renovascular disease
  – Rare causes:
    ○ Cushing' syndrome
    ○ Thyroid disorders
    ○ Pheochromocytoma
    ○ Acromegaly

Genetics
The cause of essential HTN is an even combination of genetic and environmental factors.

PATHOPHYSIOLOGY
- HTN causes arteriolosclerosis with increasing arterial stiffness, elevation of pulse pressure, and left ventricular hypertrophy.
- In more advanced stages, arteriolosclerosis leads to medial calcification of the arteries.
- Increased arterial stiffness leads to systolic HTN with large pulse pressure (difference between systolic and diastolic pressure).
- HTN is a major promoter of atherosclerosis, together with hyperlipidemia, diabetes, and cigarette smoking.
  – Atherosclerosis can lead to intimal arterial calcification.
  – The combination of left ventricular hypertrophy and coronary atherosclerosis causes a large increase in risk for chronic heart failure and sudden death.
- The renin-angiotensin system is a key regulator of BP and vascular function.
  – Inappropriate levels of angiotensin II not only cause HTN, but help promote inflammation, coagulation, excessive scarring, and arterial and left ventricular hypertrophy.
  – Angiotensin II has also been shown to accelerate atherosclerosis and increase the risk of developing diabetes.

ASSOCIATED CONDITIONS
- Diabetes
- Atherosclerosis
- Hyperlipidemia
- Metabolic syndrome
- PCOS

DIAGNOSIS

SIGNS AND SYMPTOMS
History
- Most patients with HTN are asymptomatic.
- Headache is present in ~20% of cases.
- Other symptoms are unusual, unless the patient develops target organ damage.
- Ask about:
  – Family history
  – Risk factors (smoking, diabetes, and hyperlipidemia)
  – Prior treatment of HTN
  – Dietary history
  – Sleep pattern
  – Drug intake
- Look for symptoms of target-organ damage:
  – Inquire about a h/o dyspnea
  – Edema
  – TIA
  – Stroke

Physical Exam
- Accurate measurement of BP:
  – Use the appropriate size cuff
  – Obtain at least 2 measurements with the patient sitting quietly for 5 minutes.
  – At initial visit, get both sitting and standing BP and check both arms.
- Determine BMI and waist circumference.
- Perform funduscopic exam.
- Palpate thyroid.
- Listen for carotid bruits.
- Look for signs of left ventricular hypertrophy and chronic heart failure.
- Listen for abdominal and peripheral bruits.
- Check pulses in all extremities.
- Obtain a neurologic exam, including cognitive function.

TESTS
Lab
- Essential:
  – Hematocrit
  – UA
  – Renal panel (BUN, creatinine, glucose, electrolytes)
  – Lipid profile
  – EKG
- Recommended:
  – Microalbumin test
  – GFR (by MDRD formula)
  – Serum uric acid
  – Serum calcium
- In some cases, 24-hour ABPM can refine the diagnosis, rule out white-coat HTN, and assess the effect of therapy.

> ### ALERT
> - Make sure to rule out metabolic syndrome. Any 3 of the following criteria are diagnostic:
>   – Abdominal girth >35 in (88 cm) in women
>   – HDL cholesterol <50 mg% in women
>   – Triglycerides >150 mg% (fasting)
>   – BP >130/85 mm Hg (untreated) or on antihypertensive medication
>   – Glucose >100 mg% (fasting)

Imaging
- If left ventricular hypertrophy or chronic heart failure is suspected, an EKG is indicated.
- If renal artery stenosis is suspected, renal arteriography may be indicated, although less invasive alternatives are MR angiography, CT angiography, duplex Doppler US

DIFFERENTIAL DIAGNOSIS
Causes of secondary HTN include:

Metabolic/Endocrine
- Primary hyperaldosteronism
- Cushing syndrome
- Acromegaly

Tumor/Malignancy
- Pheochromocytoma
- Cushing's disease (ACTH-producing pituitary tumor)

Drugs
OCPs

Other/Miscellaneous
Renal artery stenosis

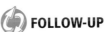

TREATMENT

GENERAL MEASURES

- Lifestyle changes and medication:
  - Recent data have shown that a delay of 6 mos in reaching goal BP increases risk for cardiovascular events.
  - Goal BP: Uncomplicated patients: <140/90 mm Hg
  - Patients with diabetes and/or renal disease: <130/80 mm Hg
- Goal blood BP may be more difficult to reach in patients with systolic HTN (especially older patients), and treatment goals must be weighed against the risk of hypotension and falling.
- Many experts recommend more aggressive BP lowering in patients at high risk (established vascular disease, chronic heart failure, decreased GFR [CKD stage 3 or higher] and proteinuria [>3 g/24 h]). Evidence for more aggressive BP lowering is circumstantial.
- Therapeutic lifestyle changes should be instituted in all patients:
  - Weight reduction (if indicated). Maintain normal BMI of 18.5–25 kg/m^2.
    - Weight loss of 10 kg can reduce BP by 5–20 mm Hg
  - Regular physical activity, such as brisk walking for 30 min, most days of the week.
  - Diet rich in fruits, vegetables, and low-fat dairy products. Reduce content saturated and total fat.
  - Reduce dietary sodium to 2.4 g/d (6 g of salt)
  - Limit consumption of alcohol to 1 standard drink per day for women

MEDICATION (DRUGS)

- Drug therapy should be initiated as soon as diagnosis of HTN is made.
- If lifestyle changes are effective, drugs can be reduced or discontinued.
- All major classes of antihypertensive drugs can be used as initial therapy.
- Many patients require >1 agent; if BP >20 mm Hg above goal, begin therapy with 2 drugs.
- Drugs should be up-titrated and added until BP reached.
- Thiazide diuretics. HCTZ and chlorthalidone are inexpensive and effective:
  - Use the lowest effective dose.
  - Can cause hypokalemia, hyponatremia, and hyperglycemia, especially at higher doses (>50 mg HCTZ or >25 mg chlorthalidone daily).
- ACE inhibitors:
  - Often combined with thiazide diuretic
  - Can improve symptoms of chronic heart failure, reduce proteinuria, slow progression of kidney disease, and reduce risk of developing diabetes.
  - Side effects include cough and angioedema (especially in black patients).
  - Available in generic form
  - Can cause hyperkalemia and acute rise in serum creatinine (usually benign).
- ARBs:
  - Similar to ACE inhibitors, but do not cause cough or angioedema (rare cases have been reported).
  - Recommended as 1st-line therapy in patients with diabetes type 2.

- Can be added to ACE inhibitors for further reduction in proteinuria and to improve symptoms and outcome in chronic heart failure.
  - Can cause hyperkalemia and acute rise in serum creatinine (usually benign).
- DRIs:
  - Recently approved. Similar to ARB
- β-Blockers:
  - Have differing effects on β_1 and β_2 receptors.
  - Lower heart rate and reduce sympathetic output.
  - Indicated for patients with chronic heart failure. Can cause hyperkalemia.
  - Many are available in generic form.
- CCBs:
  - Effective vasodilators
  - Dihydropyridines cause no change in heart rate.
  - Nondihydropyridines (verapamil and diltiazem) slow the pulse rate.
  - Useful in combination with ACE inhibitors and ARBs.
  - Do not combine β-blocker with nondihydropyridine CCB (risk of bradycardia).
  - CCBs are not indicated as 1st-line therapy in patients with kidney disease.
- Other antihypertensive agents include:
  - Loop diuretics (furosemide, bumetanide, torsemide)
  - Potassium-sparing diuretics (spironolactone, eplerenone, amiloride, triamterene)
  - Combined α- and β-blockers (labetalol and carvedilol)
  - Centrally acting α_2 agonists (clonidine)
  - Direct vasodilators (hydralazine, minoxidil)
  - Not recommended as initial therapy; can be added if standard therapy is inadequate.

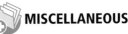

FOLLOW-UP

DISPOSITION

Issues for Referral

- Refractory HTN is defined as an inability to reach goal BP with 3 drugs, 1 of which is a diuretic.
- In that case, a workup for secondary HTN or referral to a specialist may be necessary.

PROGNOSIS

- Therapy is usually lifelong.
- Control of BP reduces the risk for:
  - Congestive heart failure by 40%
  - Risk for stroke by 30%
  - Risk for MI by 15%

PATIENT MONITORING

- Patients should be seen every month until goal BP is reached, and at 3–6-month intervals thereafter.
- Monitor serum urinalysis, creatinine, and potassium at least once a year, more often if medications are changed.

BIBLIOGRAPHY

Dickerson LM, et al. Management of hypertension in older persons. *Am Fam Physician.* 2005;71: 469–476.

Grundy SM, et al. Definition of metabolic syndrome: Report of the National Heart, Lung, and Blood Institute/ American Heart Association Conference on Scientific Issues Related to Definition. *Circulation.* 2004;109:433–438.

Neutel JM. The role of combination therapy in the management of hypertension. *Nephrol Dial Transplant.* 2006;21:1469–1474.

Pediatric/adolescent blood pressure tables. At http://www.nhlbi.nih.gov/guidelines/hypertensionHTN/child¯tbl.pdf.

The Seventh Report of the Joint National Committee on Prevention, Detection, Evaluation, and Treatment of High Blood Pressure (JNC 7). *JAMA.* 2003;289:2560–2572.

www.americanheart.org

www.nhlbi.nih.gov/guidelines/hypertension

MISCELLANEOUS

SYNONYM(S)

High blood pressure

CLINICAL PEARLS

- Some useful combinations of drugs: ACE inhibitor + thiazide, ARB + thiazide, β-blocker + thiazide, β-blocker + dihydropyridine CCB, ACE inhibitor + CCB, ARB + CCB.
- In patients with diabetes and/or kidney disease, initial therapy should include an ACE inhibitor or an ARB.
- Thiazide diuretics are ineffective if serum creatinine >2 mg%; substitute loop diuretics.

ALERT

ACE inhibitors, ARBs, and DRI are contraindicated in pregnancy.

ABBREVIATIONS

- ABPM—Ambulatory blood pressure monitoring
- ACE—Angiotensin-converting enzyme
- ACTH—Adrenocorticotropic hormone
- ARB—Angiotensin receptor blocker
- BMI—Body mass index
- BP—Blood pressure
- CCB—Calcium-channel blocker
- CKD—Chronic kidney disease
- DRI—Direct renin inhibitor
- EKG—Echocardiogram
- GFR—Glomerular filtration rate
- HCTZ—Hydrochlorothiazide
- MDRD—Modification of diet in renal disease
- MI—Myocardial infarction
- OCP—Oral contraceptive pill
- PCOS—Polycystic ovary syndrome
- TIA—Transient ischemic attack

CODES

ICD9-CM

- 277.7 Metabolic syndrome
- 401.9 Essential HTN
- 405 Secondary HTN

PATIENT TEACHING

NHLBI patient information at: http://www.nhlbi.nih.gov/health/dci/Diseases/Hbp/HBP¯WhatIs.html

PREVENTION

Maintenance of normal weight, regular exercise, and low-sodium diet may lower risk for developing HTN and target-organ damage.

IRRITABLE BOWEL SYNDROME

Paula J. Adams Hillard, MD

 BASICS

DESCRIPTION

IBS is a functional bowel disorder characterized by symptoms of abdominal pain or discomfort that is associated with disturbed defecation:

- Associated with:
  - Emotional distress
  - Impaired HRQL
  - Disability
  - High health care costs
- Rome III diagnostic criteria for IBS:
  - Recurrent abdominal pain or discomfort at least 3 days a month in past 3 months associated with 2 or more of:
    ○ Improvement with defecation
    ○ Onset associated with change in frequency of stool
    ○ Onset associated with change in form (appearance) of stool

Geriatric Considerations
- Reported less frequently among older individuals
- 1st presentation typically 30–50 years

EPIDEMIOLOGY
- Affects 4–22% of population
- Female > Male (1/5–3 times)
  - Similar prevalence white and black; possibly lower in Hispanics
- In US, up to 70% with IBS symptoms do not seek medical attention.
- In Australia, with better access to medical care, the consulting rate is 73%.

RISK FACTORS
Female

Genetics
Not established

PATHOPHYSIOLOGY
- Symptoms may occur in response to disruption of GI function from:
  - Infection
  - Dietary indiscretions:
    ○ Increased fat intake
    ○ Increased alcohol
  - Lifestyle changes:
    ○ Traveling
    ○ Vigorous exercise
  - Psychologic stress
- Quantitative differences between healthy controls and IBS patients in:
  - Motility of stomach, small intestine, colon, rectum:
    ○ These "abnormalities" occur in 25–75% of IBS patients.
  - In ileum, colon, and rectum, exaggerated response to meals, distension, stress, cholecystokinin, neostigmine, and corticotropin-releasing hormone

- Motility abnormalities may interact with low sensory thresholds:
  ○ Pain at lower volumes and pressures
  ○ Enhanced perception of visceral events (visceral hypersensitivity)
  - Possible role of altered gut immune function
  - Abnormalities in extrinsic autonomic innervation of the viscera
  - CNS stimulation of motility, secretion, immune function, blood flow
- Psychosocial factors:
  - Psychologic stress exacerbates GI symptoms.
  - Psychological and psychiatric comorbidity is common:
    ○ Prevalence of psychiatric disorder 40–90%
    ○ Psychological factors affect health status and clinical outcome: History of emotional, sexual, or physical abuse; stressful life events; chronic social stress or anxiety disorder; maladaptive coping style.
    ○ Psychologic factors influence which patients consult physicians.

ASSOCIATED CONDITIONS
- Women with IBS are 3 times more likely to have a hysterectomy than those without.
- Chronic pelvic pain
- Fibromyalgia

 DIAGNOSIS

SIGNS AND SYMPTOMS

History
- Symptoms that cumulatively support diagnosis:
  - Abnormal stool frequency (defined for research as >3/d or <3/wk)
  - Abnormal stool form (lumpy/hard or loose/watery)
  - Abnormal stool passage (straining, urgency, feeling of incomplete evacuation)
  - Passage of mucus
  - Bloating or feeling of abdominal distension
- Other GI symptoms occur commonly in individuals with IBS:
  - GERD
  - Dysphagia
  - Early satiety
  - Intermittent dyspepsia
  - Nausea
  - Noncardiac chest pain
- Factors suggesting that other diseases should be excluded before diagnosing IBS:
  - Age >50
  - Documented weight loss
  - Nocturnal symptoms
  - Family history of colon cancer
  - Rectal bleeding
  - Recent antibiotic use
- GI symptoms NOT commonly associated with IBS and suggesting other diagnoses:
  - Large volume diarrhea
  - Bloody stools
  - Nocturnal diarrhea
  - Greasy stools
- When symptoms occur, they occur frequently; over years, however, the symptoms wax and wane.

Physical Exam
- General physical exam, looking for signs NOT consistent with IBS:
  - Enlarged liver, abdominal mass, etc.
- Pelvic exam
- Rectal exam
- Assess pelvic floor muscle function

TESTS
- In general, if diagnostic criteria are fulfilled, there are no warning signs, and recent screening studies are normal, no further testing is required.
- If short duration of symptoms, worsening severity, family history of colon cancer or IBD, consider screening:
  - CBC
  - Fecal occult blood testing
  - Sedimentation rate
  - Serum chemistries
  - TSH
  - Colonoscopy if >50 years old or other features suggest

DIFFERENTIAL DIAGNOSIS

Infection
Parasitic, bacterial, viral, and opportunistic infections

Endocrine
- Diabetes
- Thyroid disease
- Addison disease
- Gastrinoma
- Carcinoid

GI
- Colon cancer
- Inflammatory bowel disease
- Celiac disease
- Gastroenteritis
- Pancreatic insufficiency

Immunologic
IBD

Tumor/Malignancy
- Ovarian cancer
- Ovarian benign neoplasm
- Colon cancer

Drugs
Side effects from medications

Other/Miscellaneous
- Chronic pelvic pain
- Fibromyalgia
- Somatization
- Depression
- History of abuse
- Lactose intolerance
- Depression
- Anxiety

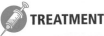 TREATMENT

GENERAL MEASURES
Determine concerns and explain symptoms:
- Diet:
  - Discuss diet and correct any obvious excesses.
  - Consider trial of wheat or dairy exclusion.
- Psychological treatments:
  - Treat anxiety or depression.
  - CBT and psychodynamic interpersonal therapy to improve coping.
  - Hypnotherapy may have long-lasting benefit.

SPECIAL THERAPY
Complementary and Alternative Therapies
Probiotics:
- Live micro-organisms, which, when administered in adequate amounts, confer a health benefit on the host
- Trials are ongoing on the use of probiotics for IBS:
  - Consuming a specific bifidobacteria strain significantly reduced symptoms of abdominal pain and bloating and bowel movement difficulty, but did not change bowel movement frequency or quality.

MEDICATION (DRUGS)
May target therapy based on subtypes:
- Antispasmodics may help pain.
- Soluble fiber for pain and bowel habits
- Serotonin type 3 (5HT3) antagonists improve global symptoms, diarrhea, and pain.
- 5HT4 agonists improve global symptoms, constipation, and bloating.
- SSRIs improve global symptoms without altering bowel habits.
- TCAs might benefit pain, especially with diarrhea.
- For constipation: Fiber or osmotic laxative
- For diarrhea: loperamide or diphenoxylate-atropine; possibly cholestyramine
- For pain/gas/bloating: Anticholinergic or antidepressants or psychological treatment

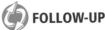 FOLLOW-UP

DISPOSITION
Issues for Referral
- In the presence of features suggesting an alternative diagnosis, referral to a gastroenterologist should be considered.
- Persistent, severe, worsening, or disabling symptoms should warrant referral.

PROGNOSIS
Although symptoms typically wax and wane over many years, IBS does not cause serious long-term health risks. <5% of individuals diagnosed with IBS will be diagnosed with another GI condition.

PATIENT MONITORING
Routine care and screening

BIBLIOGRAPHY
Drossman DA, et al. AGA technical review on irritable bowel syndrome. *Gastroenterology*. 2002;123(6): 2108–2131.

Holten KB, et al. Diagnosing the patient with abdominal pain and altered bowel habits: Is it irritable bowel syndrome? *Am Fam Physician*. 2003;67:2157–2162.

Spiller R. Clinical update: Irritable bowel syndrome. *Lancet*. 2007;369(9573):1586–1588.

 MISCELLANEOUS

SYNONYM(S)
- "Colitis"
- Irritable colon
- Spastic colon

CLINICAL PEARLS
Symptoms of IBS often worsen premenstrually, and may be a component of what the patient defines as PMS.

ABBREVIATIONS
- CBT—Cognitive behavioral therapy
- HRQL—Health-related quality of life
- IBD—Inflammatory bowel disease
- IBS—Irritable bowel syndrome
- SSRI—Selective serotonin reuptake inhibitor
- TCA—Tricyclic antidepressant
- TSH—Thyroid-stimulating hormone

CODES
ICD9-CM
564.1 Irritable bowel syndrome

 PATIENT TEACHING

- Irritable bowel syndrome at http://digestive.niddk. nih.gov/ddiseases/pubs/ibs/
- Irritable bowel syndrome tutorial at http://www.nlm. gov/medlineplus/tutorials/irritablebowelsyndrome/ htm/index.htm

PREVENTION
Some individuals find benefit in avoiding foods that are problematic for their bowel symptoms.

Section III

LESBIAN HEALTH

Susan R. Johnson, MD, MS

 BASICS

DESCRIPTION

- A lesbian is a woman who self-defines as having her primary emotional and sexual relationships with women.
- Other sexual minorities include bisexual, transgendered, and transsexual women.
- Sexual behaviors:
  - May be celibate, sexually active only with women, or with both men and women
  - ~75% of lesbians have had heterosexual sex at some time in their lives.
  - The most common sexual behaviors practiced are oral sex, vaginal penetration with fingers, and mutual masturbation.
  - Sex toys (with vaginal penetration) may also be used.

ALERT

Women currently having sex with both men and women are at high risk for unsafe sex (and STDs), alcohol and drug use, and eating disorders.

EPIDEMIOLOGY

- Prevalence between 1% and 5%
- An estimated 2.3 million women living in the US identify themselves as lesbian.
- The 2000 US Census reported a total of 293,000 households headed by female same-sex partners:
  - Likely an underestimate

RISK FACTORS

- More common compared to heterosexual women:
  - Alcohol use:
    - Everyday use more common
    - Heavy drinking more common
    - College-age lesbians 10 times more likely to drink
  - Tobacco use:
    - 2 times risk of current smoking
    - Increased risk begins in early adolescence
    - Risk 4-fold among college-age lesbians
  - Overweight and obesity rates higher
- Less common compared to heterosexual women:
  - Oral contraceptive use
  - Pregnancy (30% among lifetime lesbians, 70% if past heterosexual history)
- This risk profile could lead to higher rates of CVD, tobacco-related cancer, and ovarian, endometrial, and breast cancer, although reliable incidence data not available

Cancer

- Cervical cancer:
  - Risk depends on personal history of past and current heterosexual intercourse or abuse.
  - Risk of cervical cancer is highest in lesbians who:
    - Have been treated for abnormal Pap in the past or have a history of HPV
    - Have had sex with men (between 50% and 80% of lesbians report heterosexual intercourse at some point in their lives)

- Abnormal Pap smears and cervical cancer are uncommon but have been reported among lifelong lesbians.
  - Not all at-risk lesbians get appropriate Pap smear screening.
- Breast cancer:
  - WHI study found higher rate of breast cancer among older lesbians.
  - Mammogram screening rates are lower among lesbians in some studies.
- Ovarian cancer:
  - Lesbians may be at higher risk because of a lower likelihood of getting pregnant or using OCPs for a prolonged period of time.
  - Lesbians with a family history of ovarian cancer may want to consider the potential benefits of using OCPs to reduce their risk.

Cardiovascular Disease

WHI data showed higher rate of MI but not stroke or HTN among lesbians.

Mental Health Diagnoses

- Depression:
  - 2–3-fold higher rate
  - Suicidal ideation, plans increased
  - Discrimination stress may plan a role
- Anxiety disorders:
  - GAD 2–4-fold higher rate
  - PTSD, panic, phobia increased
- Multiple diagnoses: 3 times risk
- Alcohol abuse:
  - Alcohol abuse 2 times increase
  - Bar culture
  - Treatment issues: Regular AA may not be comfortable

STIs

- Bacterial vaginosis:
  - Rate higher than heterosexuals
  - Risk increases with more female partners and smoking
- *Candida* vaginitis:
  - As common as among heterosexuals
- *Chlamydia*:
  - Never reported if sex only with women
- Gonorrhea:
  - Never reported if sex only with women
- Hepatitis B:
  - Case report of transmission between women
- Herpes:
  - May be transmitted between women
- HPV:
  - May be transmitted from woman to woman
- HIV:
  - Transmission between women uncertain
  - IV drug abuse and bisexual practices increase risk
- Syphilis:
  - Case report of transmission between women
- *Trichomonas*:
  - Rare; usually only if history of recent sex with men
  - May be transmitted between women

STI Screening and Prevention Recommendations

- Screen based on woman's history
- Encourage safer sex practices:
  - Avoid menstrual blood
  - Dental dams for oral sex
  - Condoms on sex toys
  - Latex/Vinyl gloves for manual sex

Sexual and Physical Abuse

- Sexual abuse history:
  - 38% childhood sexual abuse survivors
  - 40% sexual assault as adults
- Intimate partner violence:
  - 10% rate, 1/2 that of heterosexual women
  - Less likely to be reported
- Targets for antigay verbal abuse, threats, violence

Parenthood

- Desire for children is common:
  - 30% children from past heterosexual relationship
  - Adoption
  - ART/DI:
    - Some clinics will not serve lesbians
- Psychosocial development of children of lesbians:
  - Similar to children of heterosexuals
  - Presence of partner matters

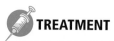 **TREATMENT**

GENERAL MEASURES

- Ask about sexual orientation:
  - <1/3 of physicians ask
  - Most lesbians do respond if asked
  - Revealing orientation is associated with regular care
- Language free of heterosexual assumptions (gender-neutral language):
  - "Are you in need of birth control?"
  - "Who is at home?"
  - "Are you having sex with men, women, or both?"
- Don't assume sex is/has been exclusively with women:
  - Discuss current birth control needs
  - Screen for STI based on history
- Respect the partner:
  - Treat her as the spouse.
  - Assure access if partner hospitalized.
  - Suggest durable power of attorney, as same-sex partners may not be legally recognized by the state.
- Employ the same screening guidelines and lifestyle advice for lesbians as for heterosexual women (i.e., appropriate Pap smear, mammogram, and colonoscopy screening, exercise, diet, and alcohol moderation)

BIBLIOGRAPHY

Bailey JV, et al. Lesbians and cervical screening. *Br J Gen Pract*. 2000;50:481–482.

Bailey JV, et al. Sexual behaviour of lesbians and bisexual women. *Sex Transm Infect*. 2003;79(2): 147–150.

Bailey JV, et al. Bacterial vaginosis in lesbians and bisexual women. *Sex Transm Dis*. 2004;31(11): 691–694.

Bailey JV, et al. Sexually transmitted infections in women who have sex with women. *Sex Transm Infect*. 2004;80(3):244–246.

Carroll NM. Optimal gynecologic and obstetric care for lesbians. *Obstet Gynecol*. 1999;93:611–613.

Case P, et al. Sexual orientation, health risk factors, and physical functioning in the Nurses' Health study II. *J Womens Health*. 2004;13(9):1033–1047.

Cochran SD, et al. Cancer-related risk indicators and preventive screening behaviors among lesbians and bisexual women. *Am J Public Health*. 2001;91:591–597.

Cochran SD, et al. Prevalence of mental disorders, psychological distress, and mental health services use among lesbian, gay, and bisexual adults in the United States. *J Consult Clin Psychol*. 2003;71(1): 53–61.

Dibble SL, et al. Comparing breast cancer risk between lesbians and their heterosexual sisters. *Womens Health Issues*. 2004;14:60–68.

Gruskin EP, et al. Gay/Lesbian sexual orientation increases risk for cigarette smoking and heavy drinking among members of a large Northern California health plan. *BMC Public Health*. 2006; 6:241. Available at http://www.biomedcentral. com/1471-2458/6/241

King M, et al. The health of people classified as lesbian, gay and bisexual attending family practitioners in London: A controlled study. *BMC Public Health*. 2006;6:127.

Makadon HJ. Improving health care for the lesbian and gay communities. *N Engl J Med*. 2006;354(9): 895–897.

Marrazzo JM, et al. Reproductive health history of lesbians: Implications for care. *Am J Obstet Gynecol*. 2004;190:1298–1304.

Marrazzo JM, et al. Sexual practices, risk perception and knowledge of sexually transmitted disease risk among lesbian and bisexual women. *Perspect Sex Reprod Health*. 2005;37(1):6–12.

Mercer CH, et al. Women who report having sex with women: British national probability data on prevalence, sexual behaviors, and health outcomes. *Am J Public Health*. 2007;97(6):1126–1133.

Mravcak SA. Primary care for lesbians and bisexual women. *Am Fam Physician*. 2006;74(2):279–286.

Ross LE, et al. Lesbian and bisexual women's recommendations for improving the provision of assisted reproductive technology services. *Fertil Steril*. 2006;86(3):735–738.

Remafedi G. Lesbian, gay, bisexual, and transgender youths: Who smokes, and why? *Nicotine Tobacco Res*. 2007;9:1,S65–S71.

Ridner SL, et al. Health information and risk behaviors among lesbian, gay, and bisexual college students. *J Am Acad Nurse Pract*. 2006;18(8):374–378.

Steele LS, et al. Regular health care use by lesbians: A path analysis of predictive factors. *Fam Pract*. 2006;23(6):631–636.

Valanis BG, et al. Sexual orientation and health: Comparisons in the Women's Health Initiative sample. *Arch Fam Med*. 2000;9:843–853.

Wilton T, et al. Lesbian mothers' experiences of maternity care in the UK. *Midwifery*. 2001;17: 203–211.

MISCELLANEOUS

LEGAL ISSUES

In most states, lesbians in committed relationships are not granted the same legal and financial protection that US laws confer to heterosexual couples:

- Civil marriage contracts are uncommon.
- Civil unions exist in only a small number of states.
- Many states have passed laws to prohibit recognition of same sex marriages.
- Some states have prevented recognition of any other state's domestic partnerships or civil unions.
- Without legal recognition, same-sex partners are not entitled to many state and >1,100 federal laws that protect married couples.

- Despite legally sanctioned inequality:
  - ~75% of Americans support laws to protect lesbians from prejudice and discrimination in employment and housing and to provide them with employment benefits, inheritance rights, employer-provided health insurance, and social security benefits.
  - The Kaiser Foundation survey found that 66% of Americans believe that homosexual behavior is a normal part of an individual's sexuality.

CLINICAL PEARLS

- www.glma.org: A gay and lesbian medical association/organization for health care professionals providing information about lesbian and gay health research, public policy, advocacy, and patient information.
- See Appendix on Developing a Patient-Friendly Office Environment

ABBREVIATIONS

- AA—Alcoholics Anonymous
- ART—Assisted reproductive technologies
- CVD—Cardiovascular disease
- DI—Donor insemination
- GAD—Generalized anxiety disorder
- HPV—Human papillovirus
- MI—Myocardial infarction
- OCP—Oral contraceptive pill
- PTSD—Post-traumatic stress disorder
- STD—Sexually transmitted disease
- WHI—Women's Health Initiative

PATIENT TEACHING

Patient resources available through the Gay and Lesbian Medical Association:

- http://www.glma.org/index.cfm?fuseaction= Page.viewPage&pageID=533

MENOPAUSE

Margery L. S. Gass, MD

 BASICS

DESCRIPTION
- Menopause is the permanent cessation of menses resulting from markedly decreased function of the ovaries or removal of the ovaries:
  - Spontaneous: Naturally occurring and defined as 1 year of no menses.
  - Induced: The result of bilateral salpingo-oophorectomy or noxious exposure (e.g., chemotherapy, radiation)
- Perimenopause includes the year following the last menses as well as the 3–5 years before the last menses, during which time menstrual irregularity is occurring.

Age-Related Factors
- Normal age range for menopause is 41–55
- Mean age is 51.4 years
- POF is characterized by amenorrhea, hypoestrogenism, and elevated gonadotropins in women <40 (See Ovarian Insufficiency [Premature Ovarian Failure])

EPIDEMIOLOGY
- ~1% of women have premature menopause.
- Smokers have an earlier menopause by ~1.5 years.
- Women living at high altitudes may have an earlier menopause.
- Women with severe malnutrition may have an earlier menopause.

RISK FACTORS
In addition to the items above, some autoimmune disorders have been associated with early menopause.

Genetics
- FMR1 premutation is associated with POF.
- Down syndrome is associated with early menopause (mean age in mid-40s).
- Turner syndrome mosaicism is associated with early or premature menopause:
  - Karyotype indicated in women with POF
- Some studies suggest an association between mother's age at menopause and daughter's age at menopause.

PATHOPHYSIOLOGY
- Menopause involves the depletion of the majority of ovarian follicles accompanied by a decline in inhibin B, followed by a decline in inhibin A, with a subsequent increase in FSH.
- The number of anovulatory cycles increase just prior to menopause, resulting in a relative progesterone deficiency and periods of unopposed estrogen.
- Estrogen levels can be erratic during perimenopause.
- The pathophysiology of vasomotor symptoms is not fully understood but appears to involve narrowing of the thermal comfort zone such that, when the core body temperature rises above the new upper limit, a hot flash is triggered.

ASSOCIATED CONDITIONS
- Many postmenopausal women have vaginal atrophy, often asymptomatic. Some experience dryness, irritation, dyspareunia. A small percentage may develop recurrent UTIs.
- Some women experience a transient disruption in sleep.
- A few women experience an increase in joint pain.

 DIAGNOSIS

SIGNS AND SYMPTOMS
History
- Cessation of menses, usually preceded by notably irregular cycles the previous year and mildly irregular (7 days early or late) the several years before that.
- Vasomotor symptoms:
  - Vasomotor symptoms (hot flashes and night sweats) are experienced in varying intensity by ~75% of women for unpredictable lengths of time:
    - 25% of symptomatic women have severe symptoms.
    - A small percentage has occasional hot flashes indefinitely.
- Vaginal dryness
- Dyspareunia
- Sleep disruption
- PMS type symptoms: Moodiness, irritability, breast tenderness, difficulty concentrating, anxiety

Physical Exam
- Thyroid palpation: Goiter, nodules
- Breast exam: Galactorrhea, nodules
- Pelvic exam: Decreased pubic hair and adipose tissue in the genitalia, vulvovaginal dryness, pallor of the mucosa, fewer rugae

TESTS
Labs
- Pregnancy test if indicated
- Prolactin level if galactorrhea is present or history is not convincingly menopausal
- TSH if history is not convincingly menopausal or if suspicious for thyroid disease
- Lipid profile if considering hormone therapy or per current guidelines
- FSH (>40 IU/mL) and estradiol (<20 pg/mL) only when diagnosis is in doubt:
  - It is desirable to have ≥2 elevated FSH levels since they are highly variable and change from day to day.

Imaging
- Mammogram per current guidelines or if considering HT
- Pelvic US if questionable pelvic exam, abnormal uterine bleeding, pelvic pain, or high risk for ovarian cancer
- BMD if age ≥65 or if <65 and postmenopausal with significant risk factors for osteoporosis

DIFFERENTIAL DIAGNOSIS
Infection
Vaginitis and vulvar dermatitis from various causes may produce symptoms that can be confused with symptoms of vaginal atrophy.

Metabolic/Endocrine
- Pregnancy
- Pituitary tumor, hyperprolactinemia
- Hypogonadotropic hypogonadism (low secretion of GnRH, low estradiol, low to normal GnRH, LH)
- Hyper-, hypothyroidism

Immunologic
Autoimmune disorders

Tumor/Malignancy
- Uterine pathology: Fibroids, polyps, hyperplasia, cancer can all cause irregular bleeding
- Cervical pathology: Polyps or cancer
- Carcinoid

Trauma
- Asherman syndrome: Amenorrhea secondary to intrauterine adhesions

Drugs
- Some psychiatric medications can result in amenorrhea (e.g., antidepressants).
- Chemotherapy may cause early menopause as a result of toxic effect on ovaries.

Other/Miscellaneous
- Vaginal pathology: Vaginitis, lichen sclerosis, vulvar vestibulitis, vulvodynia
- Psychological disorder: Depression, anxiety, panic attacks

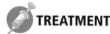 **TREATMENT**

GENERAL MEASURES
- Maintain healthy weight
- Nutritious variety of foods in moderate portions
- Exercise, stay fit, keep muscle tone (Kegel exercises, posture exercises)
- Regular sexual activity if important to patient
- Moisturizers and lubricants as needed for vaginal and sexual comfort. Avoid soap. Avoid fabric softener and anti-cling products on underwear.
- Calcium 500–600 mg b.i.d., and vitamin D 400 IU/d, 600 IU/d if >70 years old.
- Layered clothing allows accommodation to changes in ambient temperature for hot-flash control
- Avoid identified hot-flash triggers: Down comforters, thermal blankets, hot spicy foods, alcohol, emotional and stressful situations, bright lights
- Good sleep hygiene: Consistent sleep hours every day; avoid caffeine, alcohol, chocolate, getting too warm at night

SPECIAL THERAPY
Complementary and Alternative Therapies
- Paced respirations: Some evidence for decreasing hot flashes
- Black cohosh: Study results vary; Remifemin most well known 20 mg b.i.d. Minimal data beyond 6 months of use
- Isoflavones: Soy, red clover; most studies found no significant difference in number of hot flashes
- Acupuncture: Study results vary on effectiveness
- Cranberry juice or tablets may reduce frequency of recurrent UTIs.
- Valerian may help sleep latency
- Glucosamine may help joint pain

 ## MEDICATION (DRUGS)
- Hot flashes, vaginal atrophy (See Menopausal Symptoms; Vaginitis, Atrophic):
  - HRT is most effective therapy for menopausal symptoms. Use lowest effective dose for the shortest amount of time because of the small increased risk of venous thrombosis, stroke, breast cancer (especially with combined estrogen/progestogen) and dementia:
    o Estrogen alone if patient has had hysterectomy
    o Estrogen plus progestogen if patient still has uterus, either continuous progestogen daily, cyclic 12–14 days/month, or intrauterine progestin IUS (minimal data). Use continuous if trying to eliminate withdrawal bleeding and menstrual-type migraines.
    o Vaginal estrogen in very low doses if atrophic vagina is the only complaint; Vagifem and Estring should not raise the serum estradiol level above the menopausal level. Intermittent progestogen may be necessary for endometrial safety. Long-term safety data lacking.
    o Transdermal estrogen has less adverse effect on triglycerides, possibly lower rate of venous thrombosis; no head-to-head trials
    o Progestogens alone have also been demonstrated to reduce hot flashes
    o No data suggest that bioidentical or compounded hormones are any safer or any more effective than FDA-approved hormone therapy.
  - SSRIs, SNRIs appear to alleviate menopausal symptoms (venlafaxine 37.5–75 mg/d, paroxetine CR 12.5–25 mg/d, fluoxetine 10–20 mg/d):
    o Studies have reported a decrease in hot flashes as well as a decrease in moodiness, breast tenderness, and bloating.
  - SERMs vary in effects; some under investigation may provide mild improvement in vaginal atrophy along with a bone density benefit
  - Gabapentin 100–300 mg t.i.d.
  - Clonidine 0.2–0.3 mg patch or 0.1–0.2 mg/d PO daily or b.i.d

- Irregular perimenopausal bleeding (See Bleeding, Abnormal Uterine: Postmenopausal and Menopausal):
  - Cyclic progestogen (MPA 10 mg/d or micronized progesterone 200 mg/d 17–28 of the cycle, or day 14–25 if there is a short cycle) for anovulatory cycles
  - Low-dose OCPs if no contraindications can provide cycle control as well as contraception
  - A progestin-containing IUS has been approved for menopausal use in England
  - GnRH agonists can be used to create a medical menopause if severe anemia has occurred.

SURGERY
Hysteroscopy, D&C, endometrial ablation, or hysterectomy may be necessary in the case of failed medical management of menorrhagia.

 ## FOLLOW-UP
DISPOSITION
Issues for Referral
- Significant psychological symptoms
- Significant sexual dysfunction

PROGNOSIS
- Most of the symptoms associated with the acute phase of menopause subside with time. Vaginal atrophy, however, may not improve, but if the woman is not symptomatic, she does not have to be treated.
- For the woman with concomitant dyspareunia, a concerted effort may be required to achieve comfort again.

PATIENT MONITORING
- Annual examination:
  - Vital signs
  - Height, preferably with stadiometer
  - Thyroid palpation
  - Breast examination
  - Pelvic examination with Pap per guidelines
  - Mammogram
  - Stool guaiac $\geq$50 years old
  - Triglycerides if using hormone therapy
- Evaluate more frequently during symptomatic phase
- Additional pelvic exam for unscheduled uterine bleeding plus either endometrial biopsy or US to assess endometrial thickness (<5 mm reassuring)

BIBLIOGRAPHY

http://www.menopause.org/edumaterials/hormoneprimer.htm. Click on HT News for complete listing of hormone therapy products in the US and Canada.

Liu J, et al. *Management of the Perimenopause (Practical Pathways in Obstetrics & Gynecology Series)*. New York: McGraw-Hill; 2006.

Lobo RA. *Treatment of the Postmenopausal Woman*. San Diego: Elsevier. In Press.

Menopause Practice: A Clinician's Guide. www.menopause.org Website of the North American Menopause Society.

National Institutes of Health State-of-the-Science Conference statement: Management of menopause-related symptoms. *Ann Intern Med*. 2005;142(12 Pt 1):1003–1013.

Soules MR, et al. Executive summary: Stages of Reproductive Aging Workshop (STRAW). *Menopause*. 2001;8:402–407.

 ## MISCELLANEOUS
SYNONYM(S)
- Climacteric
- The Change

CLINICAL PEARLS
- Menopause is a normal, natural phase in a woman's life. Most symptomatic women feel better with time.
- ~50% of women with hot flashes who use HT will have some recurrence of hot flashes when they discontinue HT.

ABBREVIATIONS
- BMD—Bone mineral density
- FSH—Follicle-stimulating hormone
- GnRH—Gonadotropin-releasing hormone
- HT—Hormone therapy
- IUS—Intrauterine system
- LH—Luteinizing hormone
- MPA—Medroxyprogesterone acetate
- OCP—Oral contraceptive pill
- PMS—Premenstrual syndrome
- POF—Premature ovarian failure
- SERM—Selective estrogen receptor modulator
- SNRI—Selective norepinephrine reuptake inhibitors
- SSRI—Selective serotonin reuptake inhibitors
- TSH—Thyroid stimulating hormone
- UTI—Urinary tract infection

CODES
ICD9-CM
- 625.0 Dyspareunia
- 626.2 Excessive or frequent menstruation
- 627.1 Postmenopausal bleeding
- 627.2 Menopausal state, symptomatic
- 627.3 Vaginitis, postmenopausal atrophic
- 627.8 Other specified menopausal and postmenopausal disorders

 ## PATIENT TEACHING

- Our Bodies, Ourselves: Menopause. The Boston Women's Health Book Collective. New York: Touchstone. Simon and Schuster; 2006.
- Manson JE. Hot Flashes, Hormones & Your Health. New York: McGraw-Hill; 2006.
- Menopause Guidebook. www.menopause.org Website of the North American Menopause Society.

METABOLIC SYNDROME

Dana Rochester, MD
Nanette Santoro, MD

 BASICS

DESCRIPTION

- A cluster of metabolic factors that are thought to predict atherosclerotic cardiovascular risk and the development of diabetes.
- The metabolic disturbances include:
  - Central obesity
  - Insulin resistance
  - Glucose intolerance (type 2 diabetes, impaired glucose tolerance, or impaired fasting glycemia)
  - Dyslipidemia
  - Hypertension
- Recent literature has questioned whether the metabolic syndrome predicts cardiovascular risk beyond the risk associated with its individual components.

Age-Related Factors
The metabolic syndrome increases in incidence with aging.

EPIDEMIOLOGY
Due to varying definitions, prevalence is difficult to assess:

- Age-dependence is clear.
- ~25% of the US population are identified as having the metabolic syndrome.

RISK FACTORS
- Advancing age
- Abdominal obesity
- Family history of type 2 diabetes or atherosclerotic cardiovascular disease
- Sedentary lifestyle
- Atherogenic diet
- Ethnicity: Excess prevalence has been observed in Hispanic/Latin populations, reduced prevalence has been observed in Chinese/Japanese women compared to Caucasian women.

Genetics
Genetics may play a role in the expression of each metabolic risk factor.

PATHOPHYSIOLOGY
Although not completely understood, the pathogenesis is thought to be related to insulin resistance:

- Abnormal fat distribution (central obesity) with excess release of free fatty acids plays a role.
- A proinflammatory state also likely contributes.

ASSOCIATED CONDITIONS
- Obstructive sleep apnea
- PCOS
- Nonalcoholic fatty liver disease and/or nonalcoholic steatohepatitis
- Cholesterol gallstones
- Lipodystrophies
- Type 2 DM

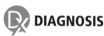 **DIAGNOSIS**

- Various groups that have proposed diagnostic criteria include the WHO, NCEP:ATP III, EGIR, and AACE.
- Essential components (see description) are the same, but differ in detail and criteria.
- The IDF and the NHBLI and AHA jointly are currently attempting to establish a unified definition.
- NCEP:ATP III definition is felt to be most clinically useful.
- ATP III Criteria 2001 include 3 or more of the following:
  - Central obesity: Waist circumference >102 cm (male), >88 cm (female Caucasian and African American; for Asian women use 80 cm as waist cutoff)
  - Hypertriglyceridemia: TG >150 mg/dL
  - Low HDL cholesterol: <40 mg/dL in men or <50 mg/dL in women
  - Hypertension: BP ≥130/85 mm Hg or on medication
  - Fasting plasma glucose: >100 mg/dL (includes diabetes)

Pregnancy Considerations
The metabolic syndrome cannot be diagnosed in pregnant women.

SIGNS AND SYMPTOMS

History
- Full cardiovascular risk assessment
- Family history of CVD or type 2 DM

Physical Exam
See ATP III diagnostic criteria above

TESTS

Lab
- Fasting lipids and glucose as stated in above ATP III criteria
- Other related metabolic parameters:
  - Atherogenic dyslipidemia: Apo B, small LDL particles
  - Dysglycemia: OGTT
  - Insulin resistance: Fasting insulin levels, HOMA-IR, elevated free fatty acids, M-value from insulin clamp
  - Vascular dysregulation: Endothelial dysfunction measurements, microalbuminuria
  - Proinflammatory state: Elevated CRP, inflammatory cytokines, decreased adiponectin levels
  - Prothrombotic state: Elevated fibrinogen, PAI-I

Imaging
- Not required for diagnosis of metabolic syndrome
- May demonstrate abnormal body fat distribution with:
  - DEXA (general body fat distribution)
  - CT/MRI (central fat distribution)
  - MRS (liver fat content)

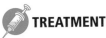 **TREATMENT**

GENERAL MEASURES

- 1st-line therapy targets lifestyle modification:
  - Moderate caloric restriction (to achieve 5–10% weight loss in 1st year)
  - Moderate increases in physical activity
  - Dietary changes to reduce saturated and trans fats, cholesterol, and if needed, salt intake; increase fiber intake
  - Smoking cessation
- Patients with high 10-year cardiovascular risk may be treated with drug therapy initially as well.

MEDICATION (DRUGS)

- Medical treatment is directed at individual components of the syndrome:
  - Obesity: Weight loss drugs not found to be very effective in treatment of obesity in US
  - Dyslipidemia: Statins for LDL and non-HDL cholesterol goals, fibrates for atherogenic dyslipidemia once LDL and non–HDL-C goal attained
  - Abnormal glucose tolerance: Some evidence that therapy with metformin, thiazolidinediones, or acarbose may prevent progression to type 2 diabetes but they are not recommended solely for the prevention of diabetes.
  - Elevated BP: Some investigators believe that ACE-inhibitors or ARBs are preferable for patients with the metabolic syndrome, but others believe the benefit is from BP reduction per se.
- For those at high cardiovascular risk, low-dose ASA is recommended.

SURGERY

Bariatric surgery is effective for severe obesity.

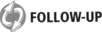 **FOLLOW-UP**

DISPOSITION

Issues for Referral

Patients may require referral to an endocrinologist or cardiologist.

PROGNOSIS

- Increased risk of developing CVD and type 2 diabetes:
  - Risk of developing diabetes is increased 5-fold.
- Both cardiovascular and all-cause mortality are increased.

PATIENT MONITORING

Long-term follow-up and management are indicated for all patients:

- Full cardiovascular risk assessment including Framingham 10-year risk scoring for CHD
- For impaired fasting glucose and possibly euglycemic patients, an annual OGTT should be performed to identify impaired glucose tolerance or diabetes.
- Maintenance of weight loss

BIBLIOGRAPHY

Alberti KGMM, et al. Metabolic syndrome- a new world-wide definition. A consensus statement from the International Diabetes Federation. *Diabetic Med*. 2006;23:469–480.

Eckel R, et al. The metabolic syndrome. *Lancet*. 2005;365:1415–1428.

Kain R, et al. The metabolic syndrome: Time for a critical appraisal. *Diabetes Care*. 2005;28: 2289–2304.

Grundy S, et al. AHA/NHBLI Scientific Statement: Diagnosis and management of the metabolic syndrome. *Circulation*. 2005;112:2735–2752.

 MISCELLANEOUS

SYNONYM(S)

- Insulin resistance syndrome
- Syndrome X
- The deadly quartet

Pregnancy Considerations

The metabolic syndrome cannot be diagnosed in pregnant women.

ABBREVIATIONS

- AACE—American Association of Clinical Endocrinologists
- ACE—Angiotensin-converting enzyme
- AHA—American Heart Association
- ARB—Angiotensin receptor blocker
- ASA—Acetyl salicylic acid—Aspirin
- CHD—Coronary heart disease
- CRP—Coronary-reactive protein
- CVD—Cardiovascular disease
- DEXA—Dual-energy X-ray absorptiometry
- DM—Diabetes mellitus
- EGIR—European Group for the Study of Insulin Resistance
- HDL—High-density lipoprotein
- HOMA-IR—Homeostasis model of assessment-insulin resistance
- IDF—International Diabetes Foundation
- LDL—Low-density lipoprotein
- MRS—Magnetic resonance spectroscopy
- NCEP ATPIII—3rd Report on the National Cholesterol Education Program's Adult Treatment Panel
- NHLBI—National Heart, Lung, and Blood Institute
- OGTT—Oral glucose tolerance test
- PAI-I—Plasminogen activator inhibitor
- PCOS—Polycystic ovary syndrome
- TG—Triglycerides
- WHO—World Health Organization

CODES

ICD9-CM

277.7 Metabolic syndrome

 PATIENT TEACHING

Lifestyle modification

PREVENTION

Target lifestyle risk factors to prevent CVD and type 2 DM.

MOOD DISORDERS: ANXIETY DISORDERS

Sharon B. Stanford, MD
Lesley M. Arnold, MD

 BASICS

DESCRIPTION
- Anxiety disorders are a cluster of diagnoses sharing anxiety as common theme.
- Panic disorder is characterized by recurrent, unexpected panic attacks followed by a month or more of worry or avoidant behavior. Panic disorder can occur with or without agoraphobia.
- Agoraphobia involves anxiety about being in a situation from which escape would be difficult or help might not be available.
- Specific phobia is characterized by an excessive fear of a particular object or situation that is avoided or endured with marked distress.
- Social phobia (social anxiety disorder) is an irrational fear of negative social evaluation, such as scrutiny by unfamiliar people or performance in unfamiliar situations.
- OCD is characterized by obsessions (persistent, intrusive, uncontrollable, anxiety provoking thoughts) or compulsions (repetitive behaviors performed in order to prevent or reduce distress).
- PTSD is a reaction to a traumatic experience lasting >1 month that involves reexperiencing the trauma through nightmares and flashbacks. The reaction includes increased arousal, emotional numbing, and efforts to avoid reminders of the event.
- Acute stress disorder involves similar symptoms to PTSD, but lasts <4 weeks.
- GAD involves persistent and excessive worry pertaining to multiple events or domains that continues for ≥6 months. Physical symptoms of GAD include feelings of restlessness, tiring easily, muscle tension, and sleep disturbance.

Age-Related Factors
Onset of most anxiety disorders is mid-adolescence to early 20s.
- Without treatment, symptoms tend to be chronic and intermittent throughout life.

EPIDEMIOLOGY
- Anxiety disorders are the most common cluster of mental disorders.
- Anxiety disorders are more common in women with a female:male ratio of 2:1.
- Specific phobia is the most common mental disorder among women in the US.

RISK FACTORS
- Family history of anxiety disorders
- Temperamental factors such as behavioral inhibition
- Environmental stressors, including emotional and physical abuse

Genetics
Anxiety disorders aggregate in families with heritability of 30–40% across the disorders:
- Risk of any anxiety disorder is 4–6 times greater in 1st-degree relatives compared to the general population.

PATHOPHYSIOLOGY
- Implicated neurotransmitters include norepinephrine, serotonin, dopamine, γ-aminobutyric acid (GABA), and glutamate.
- Dysregulation of the hypothalamic-pituitary-adrenal axis in PTSD

ASSOCIATED CONDITIONS
In a primary care setting, anxiety and depressive disorders present more commonly together than in isolation:
- Panic disorder and GAD are the anxiety disorders most associated with depression:
  - Up to 70% of patients with panic disorder present with comorbid depression.

 DIAGNOSIS

SIGNS AND SYMPTOMS
History
- Hypervigilance
- Frequent worry
- Panic attacks:
  - Discrete periods of intense physical symptoms that peak and resolve within a short time
  - Patients will often present to emergency care settings during or following panic attacks.
- Social withdrawal
- Physical symptoms of anxiety and panic including increased heart rate, muscle tension, difficulty sleeping, nausea, chest pain, and difficulty breathing
- Common obsessions include cleanliness, order, completeness, and fear of aggression.
- Common compulsions include handwashing, ordering, and checking, particularly for safety:
  - Examples include door locks and stoves.

Physical Exam
- Overall physical exam should be performed.
- Mental status exam:
  - Screen for depression and mania.
  - Specifically evaluate for history of substance use disorders.
- Appropriate evaluation of any abnormalities

TESTS
Labs
- Rule out other causes:
  - Screen for drugs of abuse
  - Check TSH
  - Complete metabolic panel:
    - Liver function for alcohol abuse/dependence
- CBC

DIFFERENTIAL DIAGNOSIS
- Rule out other medical conditions (cardiac, pulmonary, endocrine, and GI abnormalities) that may share anxiety symptoms
- Other psychiatric disorders associated with anxiety:

  - Substance intoxication and withdrawal
  - Tourette disorder:
    - Up to 2/3 with comorbid OCD
  - Other mental disorders including mood disorders, body dysmorphic disorder, hypochondriasis, and personality disorders.

Drugs
Common drugs that may worsen anxiety symptoms:
- Caffeine
- Sympathomimetics (i.e., pseudoephedrine)
- Stimulants (weight loss, ADHD drugs)
- Drugs of abuse:
  - Cocaine
  - Methamphetamine
  - Ecstasy
  - Opiate withdrawal
  - Alcohol withdrawal

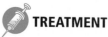 **TREATMENT**

GENERAL MEASURES
- CBT:
  - Relaxation techniques
  - Desensitization
  - Exposure and response prevention
  - Cognitive restructuring
  - Patient education
- Group or individual psychodynamic therapy:
  - Particularly useful with PTSD

SPECIAL THERAPY
Complementary and Alternative Therapies
Herbals often used for anxiety symptoms:
- Limited safety and efficacy data for Valerian, passion flower, St. John's wort

MEDICATION (DRUGS)
- Antidepressants treat anxiety disorders even in the absence of depressive symptoms.
- Exposure and response prevention, not medication, most effective for specific phobia.
- Important to assess mood frequently when starting an antidepressant due to possible increased risk of suicidal ideation

First Line
- SSRIs or SNRIs: For all anxiety disorders except specific phobia:
  - Side effects of SSRIs include headache, agitation, GI distress, and fatigue.
  - Side effects of SNRIs include nausea, dry mouth, constipation, fatigue, somnolence, increased sweating, and decreased appetite.
  - Sexual dysfunction may occur with SSRIs and SNRIs.
  - Indications for each drug listed in parentheses:
    - Fluoxetine (OCD, Panic: start 10 mg PO every morning, usual dose 20–60 mg/d, up to 80 mg daily for OCD)
    - Paroxetine (GAD, OCD, Panic, PTSD, Social Phobia: start 10 mg PO every morning, usual dose 20–50 mg/d)
    - Sertraline (OCD, Panic, PTSD, Social Phobia; start 25 mg PO daily, usual dose 50–200 mg/d)
    - Escitalopram (GAD: start 5 mg/d, usual dose 10–20 mg/d)
    - Fluvoxamine (OCD: start 50 mg PO qhs, usual dose 100–300 mg/d divided b.i.d.)

- SNRIs:
  - Venlafaxine (GAD, Social Phobia; start 37.5 PO daily; usual dose 75–150 mg/d)
    - Small dose-related risk of hypertension
  - Duloxetine (GAD; start 30 mg PO daily for a week; usual dose 60–120 mg/d)
- Taper antidepressants to avoid discontinuation syndromes (headache, dizziness, paresthesias, nausea for SSRIs and SNRIs).

Second Line
- Buspirone (GAD: Initial dose 5–10 mg PO b.i.d., usual dose range 15–40 mg in divided doses)
- Hydroxyzine (anxiety: initial dose 25 mg q6h p.r.n., usual range 50–100 q6h PRN)
- TCAs and MAOI: Considered 2nd- or 3rd-line drugs due to greater side-effect burden and concerns regarding toxicity
- Other drugs including citalopram, mirtazapine, anticonvulsants, and atypical antipsychotics have some evidence of efficacy for anxiety disorders.
- Benzodiazepines: Effective, but risk of dependence and withdrawal should limit use.

Pediatric Considerations
Black-box warning on all antidepressants for risk of suicidality in pediatric population and young adults up to age 24 when starting antidepressants or changing dose.

ALERT
- Screen for history of mania or hypomania before starting any antidepressant.
- Consider risk of serotonin syndrome when using SSRIs or SNRIs with triptan medications.

Pregnancy Considerations
- Pregnancy and the postpartum period are particularly vulnerable times for the development and worsening of anxiety symptoms.
- Pregnancy concerns:
  - Most women continue to have clinically significant anxiety symptoms during pregnancy.
  - In vulnerable women, OCD can develop or worsen during pregnancy.
  - Pharmacotherapy during pregnancy:
    - Consider psychotherapy (CBT) as 1st-line treatment during pregnancy
    - Avoid medication during 1st 12 wks gestation and near delivery if possible.
    - Lowest effective doses should be used.
    - Possible prematurity and low birth weight with SSRIs and TCAs.
    - SSRIs late in pregnancy may result in withdrawal syndrome in neonate.
    - Neonates exposed to SSRIs and SNRIs late in the 3rd trimester have developed complications requiring prolonged hospitalization, respiratory support, and tube feeding.
  - FDA MedWatch warnings:
    - Paroxetine exposure during 1st trimester associated with an increased risk of birth defects.
    - Reports of 6-fold increase in risk for persistent pulmonary hypertension in newborns with SSRI use after 20th week.

- Postpartum concerns:
  - Comorbid depressive symptoms are particularly common in postpartum period
  - GAD and social anxiety common in postpartum women
  - Postpartum women vulnerable to OCD:
    - Common obsession centers on fear of harming the baby
  - Pharmacotherapy in breast-feeding mothers:
    - All antidepressants have been shown to be present in breast milk.
    - Sertraline, paroxetine, and nortriptyline may be preferred due to undetectable drug levels in breast-fed infants.
    - Fluoxetine, citalopram, and doxepin should be avoided in breast-feeding.
    - Avoid benzodiazepines in breast-feeding.

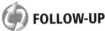

FOLLOW-UP

DISPOSITION
Issues for Referral
- Refer to a psychiatrist for complex, comorbid, severe, or treatment-refractory cases.
- Consider hospitalization for patients with suicidality or extreme difficulty functioning.
- Refer to psychotherapist (psychiatrist, psychologist, social worker, or other licensed psychotherapist) according to patient preference and ability to participate in therapy.

PROGNOSIS
- With the exception of specific childhood phobias that often remit spontaneously with age, untreated anxiety disorders are chronic and often worsen with time.
- Treatment of OCD is complicated both by potential relapse and incomplete response.
- PTSD is often chronic; up to 1/3 of patients are still symptomatic 10 years after diagnosis.
  - Despite this, prognosis for most anxiety disorders with appropriate treatment is good.
  - Psychotherapy and pharmacotherapy may be more effective than either treatment alone
- Length of treatment:
  - Treatment response is comparable for both psychotherapy and pharmacotherapy; may take 6–12 weeks
  - Maintenance therapy recommended for ≥12–18 months

PATIENT MONITORING
- Insomnia
- Suicidality common when a comorbid depressive disorder is present.

BIBLIOGRAPHY

American Psychiatric Association: Diagnostic and Statistical Manual of Mental Disorders, 4th ed., Text Revision. Washington, DC: American Psychiatric Association; 2000.

Baldwin DS, et al. Evidence-based guidelines for the pharmacological treatment of anxiety disorders: Recommendations from the British Association for Psychopharmacology. *J Psychopharmacol*. 2005; 19(6):567–596.

Eberhard-Gran M, et al. Use of psychotropic medications in treating mood disorders during lactation: Practical recommendations. *CNS Drugs*. 2006;20(3):187–198.

Hettema JM, et al. A Review and meta-analysis of the genetic epidemiology of anxiety disorders. *Am J Psychiatry*. 2001;158:1568–1578.

Rubinchik SM, et al. Medications for panic disorder and generalized anxiety disorder during pregnancy. *Prim Care Companion J Clin Psychiatry*. 2005; 7(3):100–105.

Wenzel A, et al. Anxiety symptoms and disorders at eight weeks postpartum. *Anxiety Dis*. 2005;19: 295–311.

MISCELLANEOUS

ABBREVIATIONS
- ADHD—Attention deficit disorder
- CBT—Cognitive behavioral therapy
- GAD—Generalized anxiety disorder
- MAOI—Monoamine oxidase inhibitor
- OCD—Obsessive compulsive disorder
- PTSD—Post-traumatic stress disorder
- RCT—Randomized controlled trial
- SNRI—Selective norepinephrine reuptake inhibitor
- SSRI—Selective serotonin reuptake inhibitor
- TCA—Tricyclic antidepressant
- TSH—Thyroid-stimulating hormone

CODES
ICD9-CM
- 300.01 Panic disorder without agoraphobia
- 300.21 Panic disorder with agoraphobia
- 300.22 Agoraphobia
- 300.29 Specific phobia
- 300.23 Social anxiety disorder
- 300.3 Obsessive compulsive disorder (OCD)
- 309.81 Posttraumatic stress disorder (PTSD)
- 300.02 Generalized anxiety disorder (GAD)

PATIENT TEACHING

- http://www.nimh.nih.gov/publicat/anxiety.cfm
- http://www.athealth.com/Consumer/disorders/nih_anxiety.html
- http://www.athealth.com/Consumer/disorders/nih_panic.html

PREVENTION
Some evidence with RCT that CBT and family-based group intervention can reduce the rate of anxiety disorders and prevent new onset in children.

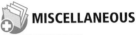

Section III

MOOD DISORDERS: BIPOLAR DISORDER

Pauline Chang, MD

BASICS

DESCRIPTION
- Illness characterized by periods of mood elevation
- Divided into 2 subtypes: Bipolar I and Bipolar II.
  - Bipolar I disorder:
    - At least 1 manic or mixed episode, with or without major depressive episodes
  - Bipolar II disorder:
    - At least 1 major depressive episode and 1 hypomanic episode
- Cyclothymia and bipolar disorder NOS also included in spectrum of bipolar disorders
  - Cyclothymia:
    - Chronic fluctuating mood disturbance, numerous periods of hypomanic and depressive symptoms
    - Duration of 2 years (1 year in adolescents and children)
  - Bipolar disorder NOS:
    - Bipolar features that do not meet criteria for any bipolar disorder

Age-Related Factors
The age of onset for bipolar disorder is generally between 15 and 24 years. If symptoms present after 60 years, condition may be secondary to other medical conditions.

EPIDEMIOLOGY
- Lifetime incidence:
  - Bipolar I: 0.8% (0.4–1.6%)
  - Bipolar II: 0.5%
  - Cyclothymia: 0.4–1.0%
  - Underdiagnosed: Patients typically present with depressive episode, history of mania symptoms not explored.
- Gender:
  - Bipolar I: Male = Female
  - Bipolar II: Female > Male
- No variation in race or ethnicity
- Socioeconomic status:
  - Bipolar I: Increased in low SES
  - Bipolar II: Increased in high SES

RISK FACTORS
- Family history of bipolar disorder, other mood disorders, or schizophrenia
- Negative stressful life events

Genetics
Studies of families and twins suggest a genetic component for bipolar disorder:
- Estimated 40–80% lifetime risk for monozygotic twins; 10–20% in dizygotic twins
- Non-Mendelian pattern, polygenic inheritance

PATHOPHYSIOLOGY
- Pathophysiology of bipolar disorder is unknown
- Hypotheses include the imbalance of neurotransmitters such as norepinephrine, dopamine, and serotonin and deficit in membrane sodium potassium-ATPase
- Environmental stress and abnormal sleep patterns also play a role in triggering manic or depressive episodes.

ASSOCIATED CONDITIONS
- Alcohol dependence
- Substance-related disorders
- Increased suicidal behavior

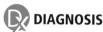

DIAGNOSIS

SIGNS AND SYMPTOMS
- Major depression: Depressive episode for a period of 2 weeks during which depressed mood or loss of interest or pleasure occurs (DSM-IV):
  - 5 of the following symptoms:
    - Depressed mood (most of the day, nearly every day)
    - Loss of interest or pleasure
    - Weight changes
    - Sleep pattern changes
    - Psychomotor agitation or retardation
    - Loss of energy
    - Feeling of guilt
    - Decreased concentration
    - Suicidal ideations
- Manic episode: Period of 1 week of abnormally, persistently elevated, expansive or irritable mood (DSM-IV):
  - Any duration if hospitalization required
  - Marked impairment in functioning, +/− psychotic features
  - 3 of the following symptoms (4 if only irritable mood):
    - Inflated self-esteem or grandiosity
    - Decreased need for sleep
    - Pressured speech
    - Distractibility
    - Increased goal-directed activity
    - Increased involvement in pleasurable activity with potential for painful consequences
- Hypomanic episode: Episode lasting for 4 days with same criteria as mania:
  - Not severe enough to cause functional impairment
  - No psychotic features

History
- Past medical history:
  - Hospitalizations
  - Chronic medical conditions
  - Medications
  - Substance abuse
- Psychiatric history:
  - Psychiatric hospitalizations
  - Assessment of risk taking behavior and psychotic features
  - Assessment for risk of suicide, homicide, and grave disability
  - Past suicide attempts
- Family history:
  - History of psychiatric disorders and suicides

Physical Exam
- General:
  - Appearance/Skin
  - VS
  - BP
- Thyroid exam
- Mental status exam
- Neurologic exam

TESTS
Labs
- CBC, basic metabolic panel
- Thyroid function tests
- Urine toxicology
- HIV, RPR (high-risk population)

Imaging
EEG or brain imaging if indicated by finding on neurologic exam

DIFFERENTIAL DIAGNOSIS
Differential diagnosis depends on presentation (depression vs. mania)

Infection
- HIV (See Sexually Transmitted Diseases: HIV/AIDS.)
- Tertiary syphilis (See Sexually Transmitted Diseases: Syphilis.)
- Influenza
- Infectious mononucleosis (depression)

Metabolic/Endocrine
- Hyperthyroidism/Hypothyroidism (See Thyroid Disease.)
- Cushing disease
- Addison disease
- Hyperparathyroidism (depression)
- Hypopituitarism (depression)
- Pernicious anemia

Immunologic
SLE (depression)

Tumor/Malignancy
- Cerebral malignancies
- Abdominal malignancies (depression)

Trauma
Head trauma

Drugs
- Steroid-induced (mania)
- Substance abuse
- Medication-related

Other/Miscellaneous
- Psychiatric:
  - Major depressive disorder (See Mood Disorders: Depression.)
  - Schizophrenia (mania)
  - Schizoaffective disorder
  - PTSD (mania)
  - Personality disorder: Narcissistic, histrionic, borderline (mania)
  - ADHD, conduct disorder (in children)
- Neurologic:
  - Head trauma
  - Neoplasm
  - MS
  - Epilepsy/Complex partial seizures
  - Cerebrovascular disorder
  - Huntington disease (mania)
  - Parkinson disease (depression)

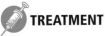

TREATMENT

GENERAL MEASURES
- Establish and maintain therapeutic alliance with patient to promote treatment compliance.
- Regulate sleep patterns and reduce stress.

ALERT
If bipolar disorder is misdiagnosed as unipolar depression, treatment with antidepressants may precipitate manic episode

SPECIAL THERAPY
Complementary and Alternative Therapies
Psychotherapy, CBT, and support groups as adjunct to pharmacologic treatment

MEDICATION (DRUGS)
- Acute mania:
  – Severe: Lithium or valproate plus atypical antipsychotic, hospitalization
  – Mild-moderate: Lithium, valproate, or olanzapine plus benzodiazepine
  – Second line: Carbamazepine or oxcarbazepine
- Acute depression:
  – Lithium or lamotrigine
  – If severe: Plus antidepressant
  – If refractory or pregnant: ECT
  – Second line: Bupropion or paroxetine
- Maintenance therapy:
  – At least 6 months of therapy because of high risk of relapse
  – Consider long-term/life-long therapy if 1–2 manic episodes or single severe episode
  – Lithium or valproate
  – Second line: Lamotrigine, carbamazepine, or oxcarbazepine
- Dosing:
  – Lithium: Start at 300 mg t.i.d., therapeutic level 0.5–1.2 mEq/L (0.6–0.8 mEq/L for maintenance)
  – Valproate: Start at 20–30 mg/kg/d, therapeutic level at 50–125 μg/mL
  – Carbamazepine: Start at 200–600 mg in t.i.d.-q.i.d. dosing, therapeutic level at 4–12 μg/mL

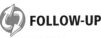

FOLLOW-UP

DISPOSITION
Issues for Referral
- Refer to mental health specialist for immediate stabilization.
- Therapeutic management if out of physician's scope of practice

PROGNOSIS
- Suicide: ~50% have at least 1 suicide attempt, 10–15% have completed suicide.
- High risk of recurrence: 80–90% will relapse after single manic episode.
- Rapid cycling ($\geq$4 mood episodes in 12 months) or mixed episode (meets both depressive and manic criteria) have worse outcome.
- Bipolar I with no history of major depressive episode has better outcome than with major depressive episode.

PATIENT MONITORING
- Monitor for suicidal or homicidal ideation and alcohol/substance abuse.
- Monitor for therapeutic levels after each dose increase and before next dose increase.
- Routine labs to monitor adverse effects of medications:
  – Lithium: Baseline BUN, Crt, and TSH and pregnancy test before initiating treatment:
    ○ BUN and Crt q2–3mo and TSH 1–2 times for 1st 6 months, then BUN, Crt, and TSH q6–12mo
    ○ TSH if breakthrough depression
  – Valproate: CBC and LFT every 6 months (minimum)
  – Carbamazepine: CBC and LFT q2wk for 2 months, then q3mo

ALERT
Pregnancy Considerations
- Treatment of bipolar disorder with Lithium associated with increase risk of birth defects:
  – Effective contraception strategy must be discussed
  – Carbamazepine decreases efficacy of OCP
- If pregnancy desired, discuss with mental health professional and obstetrician treatment options during pregnancy (e.g., off maintenance therapy during pregnancy)
- If continuing medication during pregnancy:
  – Monitor for NT defects, heart defects (Ebstein anomaly with lithium)
  – Close monitoring of therapeutic levels
  – High rate of relapse postpartum (>50%)
  – No breastfeeding on lithium (40% dose in breast milk)
  – Breastfeeding with valproate therapy not well studied

BIBLIOGRAPHY

American Psychiatric Association Task Force on DSM-IV. *Diagnostic and Statistical Manual of Mental Disorders: DSM-IV.* Washington, DC: American Psychiatric Association; 1999.

Belmaker RH. Bipolar disorder. *N Engl J Med.* 2004;351(5):476–486.

Blazer D. Mood Disorders. In: Sadock BJ, et al., eds. *Comprehensive Textbook of Psychiatry,* Vol. 1, 7th ed. Philadelphia: Lippincott Williams & Wilkins; 2000:1300–1306, 1369.

Hilty DM, et al. A review of bipolar disorder among adults. *Psychiatr Serv.* 1999;50(2):201–213.

Hirshfield R. *Practice guideline for the treatment of patients with bipolar disorder,* 2nd ed. In: American Psychiatric Association. Practice Guideline for the Treatment of Psychiatric Disorder: Compendium 2004. Arlington: American Psychiatric Publishing; 2004:525–586.

Muller-Oerlinghausen B, et al. Bipolar disorder. *Lancet.* 2002;359:241–247.

Muzina DJ, et al. Differentiating bipolar disorder from depression in primary care. *Cleve Clin J Med.* 2007;74(2):89–105.

MISCELLANEOUS

SYNONYM(S)
- Bipolar affective disorder
- Manic-depressive disorder
- Mood disorder

CLINICAL PEARLS
- Bipolar disorder is a spectrum of mood symptoms.
- If patient presenting with episode of major depression, evaluate for history of manic episode(s).
- If bipolar disorder is undiagnosed, starting antidepressant may precipitate mania.
- Monitor for suicidal ideations, 50% of patients will have at least 1 suicide attempt.

ABBREVIATIONS
- ADHD—Attention deficit/hyperactivity disorder
- CBT—Cognitive behavioral therapy
- DSM-IV—Diagnostic and Statistical Manual, 4th ed.
- ECT—Electroconvulsive therapy
- MS—Multiple sclerosis
- NOS—Not otherwise specified
- NT—Neural tube
- OCP—Oral contraceptive pill
- PTSD—Post-traumatic stress disorder
- RPR—Rapid plasmin reagent
- SES—Socioeconomic status
- SLE—Systemic lupus erythematosus
- TSH—Thyroid-stimulating hormone

CODES
ICD9-CM
- 296.4 Bipolar disorder, manic
- 296.5 Bipolar disorder, depressed
- 296.6 Bipolar disorder, mixed
- 296.7 Bipolar disorder, unspecified
- 296.8 Bipolar disorder, psychosis, other, and unspecified

PATIENT TEACHING

- Patients must adapt to idea that they have an illness that needs long-term therapy.
- Education and feedback regarding illness for patient and family
- Promote awareness of stressors, regular sleep patterns, and early signs of relapse.

PREVENTION
- Primary: Not well established
- Secondary: Treatment compliance

MOOD DISORDERS: DEPRESSION

Nada L. Stotland, MD, MPH

BASICS

DESCRIPTION
Disorder of mood, occurring chronically or in discrete episodes, and highly recurrent:
- 50% recurrence after single episode
- 75% after 2 episodes
- 90+% after 3 episodes
- Note confusion between "depression" as a normal, passing mood, and "depression" as a medical illness
- Bipolar disorder = manic-depression

Age-Related Factors
- Occurs at all ages
  - Peaks in reproductive years and in late life
- Female:Male ratio of 2:1 begins at puberty.

Pediatric Considerations
- Very young children can develop depression.
- Evidence that antidepressants are associated with suicidality in children is questionable.
- Depressed children should be evaluated by a child psychiatrist before medication is prescribed, and should be monitored closely.

Geriatric Considerations
- When medicating geriatric patients, "start low, go slow."
- Geriatric patients are at increased risk of suicide.
- Primary affect may be irritability rather than depressed mood.

EPIDEMIOLOGY
- Point prevalence for females 4–9%
- Lifetime prevalence for females up to 25%

Pregnancy Considerations
- All patients should be screened for depression.
- Media reports of adverse effects of maternal antidepressants on the newborn have frightened patients. This area is highly controversial.
- Mild-to-moderate cases can be treated with psychotherapy.
- The possible dangers of medication must be weighed against the known adverse effects of untreated depression, including premature birth.

RISK FACTORS
- Previous episode(s)
- History of abuse
- Family history
- Chronic illness
- Lack of social supports

Genetics
Clear family loading.

PATHOPHYSIOLOGY
- Multifactorial
- Environmental stress
- Effects of past or current abuse
- Changes in neurotransmitters and receptors:
  - Serotonin
  - Norepinephrine

ASSOCIATED CONDITIONS
- Anxiety disorders
- Alcohol and substance abuse
- Personality disorders
- Somatoform disorders

DIAGNOSIS

SIGNS AND SYMPTOMS
History
- Every day, most of the day, for 2 weeks:
  - Depressed or irritable mood
  - Inability to enjoy things (anhedonia)
  - Changes in sleep
  - Changes in appetite
  - Decreased energy
  - Decreased concentration
  - Guilt
  - Helplessness/Hopelessness
- Rule out bipolar disorder: Episodes of heightened mood/energy/confidence?

Physical Exam
Psychomotor retardation or agitation

TESTS
No specific diagnostic tests

Lab
Thyroid screen if clinically indicated (other signs and symptoms of hypothyroidism)

Imaging
Brain imaging differences between normal and depressed, but not diagnostic as of yet

DIFFERENTIAL DIAGNOSIS
Hematologic
Anemia

Metabolic/Endocrine
- Hypothyroidism
- Other metabolic conditions:
  - May exacerbate diabetes

Immunologic
Autoimmune disorders

Tumor/Malignancy
Most commonly associated with lung cancer

Trauma
Psychological trauma/posttraumatic stress

Drugs
- Frequently associated with alcohol/substance abuse
- Many prescribed general medical drugs have effects on mood

Other/Miscellaneous
Psychiatric conditions:
- Bipolar disorder:
  - Patients tend to present in depressed phase
  - Ask every patient about episodes of abnormally heightened mood/energy
- Anxiety disorders
- Personality disorders
- Psychotic disorders

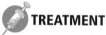

TREATMENT

GENERAL MEASURES
- Psychotherapy and medication equally efficacious for mild-to-moderate cases:
  - Cognitive-behavioral and interpersonal therapies have most empirical evidence
- Medication indicated for moderate-severe
- Combination medication/psychotherapy most effective
- Deep brain, magnetic, vagal nerve stimulation are expensive and controversial.
- ECT is safe and effective:
  - Unipolar electrodes, use of anesthesia and muscle relaxant
  - Possibility of memory loss:
    - Usually mild and short-term
  - Patients and families require reassurance because of stigma/old methods
  - Can be life-saving in extreme cases

PREGNANCY-SPECIFIC ISSUES
ECT ("shock treatment") is safe and effective in general and during pregnancy.

By Trimester
- Most postpartum depression is a continuation of depression during pregnancy.
- Patient may choose to decrease or discontinue antidepressant during 1st and end of 3rd trimester.

Risks for Mother
Discontinuing antidepressant has 65% risk of relapse.

Risks for Fetus
- Some reports of neonatal jitteriness with fluoxetine
- Some reports of pulmonary hypertension with paroxetine
- All studies are observational:
  - Impossible to completely control for severity of maternal depression

SPECIAL THERAPY
Complementary and Alternative Therapies
- St. John's wort:
  - Doses vary among preparations
  - German reports positive; US reports negative
- Light therapy: For seasonal depression
- Exercise is beneficial

MEDICATION (DRUGS)
- All antidepressants have similar efficacy as compared with placebo, but patients often need trials of up to 3 before finding 1 that works for them.
- Start at lowest dose, titrate up as tolerated.
- Choices are made on the basis of convenience, safety, cost, and side effects:
  - Tricyclic, but not SSRI, overdose can be fatal.
  - Side effects of activation or sedation can be useful.
  - Most antidepressants have antianxiety effects as well.
- SSRIs:
  - Fluoxetine 20–60 mg/d:
    - Once-a-week preparation available
  - Sertraline 50–200 mg/d
  - Paroxetine 20–50 mg/d
  - Escitalopram 20–40 mg/d
- Tricyclics/Heterocyclics:
  - Amitriptyline 150–300 mg/d, divided doses
  - Desipramine 150–300 mg/d, divided doses
- MAOIs: Not for primary care
- Other antidepressants:
  - Bupropion extended-release 150–300 mg/d:
    - Dopaminergic/Noradrenergic
    - Activating
    - Less weight gain
    - Fewer sexual side effects
    - Also prescribed for smoking cessation: Do not double-prescribe
  - Venlafaxine extended-release 150 mg/d:
    - Serotonin/Norepinephrine reuptake inhibitor
  - Duloxetine 60–120 mg/d:
    - Also appears useful for comorbid urinary stress incontinence, physical pain

SURGERY
No surgical approaches

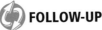 **FOLLOW-UP**

DISPOSITION
Issues for Referral
- Reassure patient she is not "crazy" or lazy
- Refer for:
  - Symptoms unimproved or worse
  - Inability to function in daily life
  - Comorbidity
  - Suicidality
- Make follow-up appointment to reassure patient of continued interest

PROGNOSIS
- 65% of patients respond to adequate therapy/medication.
- Up to 3 medication trials may be necessary before therapeutic response.
- If no improvement after 6–8 weeks:
  - Switch medications.
  - Increase dose to recommended limit.
  - Augment with thyroid, lithium, another antidepressant
- Recurrence (see "Description")

COMPLICATIONS
- Precipitation of manic episode
- Suicide
- Failure to adhere to regimens for other medical disorders

PATIENT MONITORING
- Close follow-up is essential.
- Have patient call after referral to report her satisfaction with mental health professional.
- When prescribing antidepressant, have patient:
  - Call 2–3 days after starting meds to report tolerability of side effects.
  - Return weekly until treatment response.
  - Return monthly to monitor continued response.
- Treat until premorbid mood achieved.
- Treat at least 9 months to avoid relapse.

BIBLIOGRAPHY

American Psychiatric Association: Diagnostic and Statistical Manual of Mental Disorders, 4th ed, Text Revision. Washington DC: APA; 2000.

Mellow AM, et al. Depression and Anxiety in Late Life. In: Mellow AM, ed. *Geriatric Psychiatry*. Washington DC: APPI, 2003; 1–34.

Schatzberg AF, et al. *Manual of Clinical Psychopharmacology*, 5th ed. Washington DC: APPI; 2005;33–148.

Wright JH. Computer-Assisted Cognitive-Behavior Therapy. In: Wright JH, ed. *Cognitive-Behavior Therapy*. Washington DC: APPI; 2004;55–82.

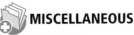 **MISCELLANEOUS**

CLINICAL PEARLS
- Screen every patient for depression.
- Diagnostic criteria are sound and treatment works.

ABBREVIATIONS
- ECT—Electroconvulsive therapy
- MAOI—Monoamine oxidase inhibitor
- SSRI—Selective serotonin reuptake inhibitor

 CODES

ICD9-CM
- 296.2 Major depressive disorder, single episode
- 296.3 Major depressive disorder, recurrent

PATIENT TEACHING

Psychiatric diagnoses and treatments still carry considerable stigma:
- Reassure patient that she is neither "crazy" nor lazy; depression is a disease like any other.
- Reassure patient that treatment works.
- Prepare patient for side effects and reassure that most will abate in days.
- Provide written materials for patient to take home.
- Determine whether family members are supportive, and offer to meet with and educate those who are not.
- Warn patient that abrupt discontinuation can produce withdrawal symptoms.
- Reading for patients: Solomon A. The Noonday Demon: An Atlas of Depression. New York: Simon & Schuster, 2001.
- Informational web sites:
  - www.mentalhealthamerica.org
  - www.nimh.gov
  - www.healthyminds.com

PREVENTION
Continued medication or psychotherapy decreases risk of recurrence.

Section III

PALLIATIVE CARE

Aaron Goldberg, MD
Weldon Chafe, MD

 BASICS

DESCRIPTION

Palliative care uses a multidisciplinary approach to relieve suffering and improve the quality of life in patients with advanced/terminal diseases. The approach focuses on pain relief and management of other symptoms, as well as open communication with both patients and their families. This includes treatment, goal setting, and various forms of psychosocial support.

EPIDEMIOLOGY

As the US population ages, the number of people living with advanced end-stage diseases will grow accordingly, resulting in a dramatic increase in the need for palliative care services.

RISK FACTORS

Patients treated by Ob/Gyn's most likely to require palliative care evaluation include patients with end-stage:
- Gynecologic cancer
- Breast cancer
- Lung cancer
- Colon cancer

Genetics

Refer to sections specific to underlying disease process.

PATHOPHYSIOLOGY

Refer to sections specific to underlying disease process.

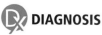 **DIAGNOSIS**

SIGNS AND SYMPTOMS
History
- Pain
- Anorexia
- Incontinence
- Nausea/Vomiting
- Dyspnea/Cough
- Skin ulceration/breakdown
- Level of function
- Treatment side effects
- Psychological distress (depression/anxiety/delirium)

Physical Exam
- Vital signs
- Urine output
- Weight loss
- Anemia
- Cachexia
- Weakness
- Delirium

TESTS

Measurement of performance status may be measured using the Gynecologic Oncology Group's scale:
- 0—Fully active (Karnofsky scale 90–100)
- 1—Restricted strenuous physical activity, but ambulatory (70–80)
- 2—Ambulatory; self care, unable to work up to 50% of waking hours (50–60)
- 3—Limited self care; bed or chair-bound up to 50% of waking hours (30–40)
- 4—Completely disabled, no self care (10–20)
- Further testing decisions must be evaluated based on expected benefits and impact on symptom relief.

Lab

Although lab tests are indicated in certain circumstances, in the palliative-care setting, patient evaluation and treatment typically is based on history and physical exam findings. Utility of laboratory tests must be weighed against potential for relief of suffering and prolongation of life.

Imaging

As for lab testing, noninvasive radiologic studies such as radiographs and CT scans may be considered to evaluate disease progression and emergence of acute illness; their utility must be weighed against the potential for relief of suffering and prolongation of life.

 TREATMENT

GENERAL MEASURES
- Pain management using medical therapy as described below:
  – Acute vs. chronic
  – Caused by disease process and/or its treatment
  – May be considered to have 4 steps (Berek):
    ○ Decrease painful stimuli: NSAIDs and acetaminophen are effective; muscle relaxants and massage for muscle spasms.

○ Increase pain threshold: Treat depression and anxiety appropriately and maintain compassionate and clear communication; massage and meditation may be helpful.
○ Use appropriate and effective dose of opioid analgesics: Employ regular dosing intervals and titrate dose to successful pain control.
○ Identify and treat neurogenic pain correctly: Consider TCAs, anticonvulsants, or corticosteroids as adjuncts to opioid analgesics.
- Nausea: Medical therapy as described below
- Anorexia/Cachexia: Medical therapy as described below
- Bowel obstruction:
  – Nasogastric tube placement, antiemetics, intravenous fluids and NPO
  – Surgical treatment decisions rest on prognosis, patient wishes, and likelihood of success at symptom relief
- Constipation: Rule out obstruction, medical therapy as described below.
- Dyspnea:
  – Nebulized fentanyl has been shown by research to be effective at relieving symptoms associated with end-of-life dyspnea.
  – Supplemental oxygen
- Anxiety/Depression: Appropriate anxiolytic and antidepressant therapy

SPECIAL THERAPY
Complementary and Alternative Therapies

Implantable devices that deliver pain medication intrathecally have been shown effective at improving pain control for those refractory to medical management.

MEDICATION (DRUGS)
- Pain control:
  – NSAIDs (avoid in renal failure and bleeding disorders)
  – Acetaminophen
  – Opioid analgesics: Dose equivalents (duration of action):
    ○ Morphine PO: 15 mg q4h (3–4 hours)
    ○ Morphine IV: 5 mg q4h (3–4)
    ○ Morphine SR: 45 mg q12h (12)
    ○ Oxycodone PO: 15 mg q12h (3–4)

- ○ OxyContin PO: 40 mg q12h (12)
- ○ Hydrocodone PO: 20 mg q4h (3–4)
- ○ Hydromorphone PO: 2–4 mg q4h (3–4)
- ○ Hydromorphone IV: 1 mg q4h (3–4)
- ○ Methadone PO: 5 mg q8h (6–8)
- ○ Fentanyl patch: 50 μg/hr q72h (72)
- ○ Fentanyl IV: 50 μg q1h (1)
- – Common side effects of opioids include:
  - ○ Constipation
  - ○ Nausea/Vomiting
  - ○ Respiratory depression
  - ○ Delirium
  - ○ Tolerance
  - ○ Pruritus
- – Use caution with morphine use in patients with renal insufficiency. Consider dose reduction or alternatives such as fentanyl, which is not renally cleared.
- Nausea:
  - – Metoclopramide IV: 10–20 mg q4h (avoid in bowel obstruction)
  - – Perchlorperazine PO/PR: 5–25 mg b.i.d./t.i.d.
  - – Ondansetron IV/PO: 4–8 mg q4h (24 mg dose common for chemotherapy related nausea; can cause constipation)
  - – Promethazine IV/PO: 12.5–25 mg (may cause sedation)
- Constipation (if obstruction ruled out)
  - – Docusate PO: 100 mg/d b.i.d.
  - – Lactulose PO: 15–30 mL(10 g/15 ml)
  - – Bisacodyl PO: 10–15 mg/d (also available as suppository)
  - – Magnesium citrate PO: 120–240 mL (max 300 mL)
  - – Castor oil PO: 15–60 mL once
- Anorexia/Cachexia:
  - – Megestrol acetate PO: 10–20 mL/d (40 mg/mL)
  - – Dronabinol PO: 2.5 mg b.i.d. (may cause hallucinations or agitation)
  - – Dexamethasone IV/PO/IM: 5 mg/d

SURGERY

- Depending on the life expectancy, patient wishes, and likelihood of success, surgical therapy most commonly is considered for bowel obstruction.
- For SBO due to metastatic disease, PEG tube placement offers a minimally invasive means of long-term bowel decompression and symptomatic relief.

 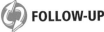

FOLLOW-UP

DISPOSITION
Issues for Referral
Palliative care referral is appropriate when benefits of further treatment outweigh the costs. Decisions should be made by balancing the clinician's knowledge, prior treatment response, treatment side effects, and the patient's values and wishes.

PROGNOSIS
Avoid providing specific timeframes, but offering a general range of expected survival in order to provide time for planning and to establish the finite nature of the disease process is appropriate.

PATIENT MONITORING
- Once in palliative care, care settings include inpatient palliative care units, nursing home facilities, and home hospice. Arrangements vary by medical condition, patient/family preferences and financial considerations.
- Typical monitoring includes (but not limited to):
  - – Vital signs
  - – Mental status
  - – Pain control
  - – Bowel function
  - – Nutritional status

BIBLIOGRAPHY

Berek JS, et al. *Practical Gynecologic Oncology*, 4th ed. Philadelphia: Lippincott Williams & Wilkins; 2005.

Coyne PF, et al. Nebulized fentanyl citrate improves patients' perception of breathing, respiratory rate, and oxygen saturation in dyspnea. *J Pain Symptom Manage*. 2002;23(2)157–160.

Meyer L, et al. Decompressive percutaneous gastrostomy tube use in gynecologic malignancies. *Curr Treat Options Oncol*. 2006;7(2):111–120.

Morrison RS, et al. Palliative care. *N Engl J Med*. 2004;350:2582–2590.

Santoso JT, et al. *Handbook of Gyn Oncology*. New York: McGraw-Hill; 2001.

Smith TJ, et al. Implantable drug delivery systems (IDDS) after failure of comprehensive medical management (CMM) can palliate symptoms in the most refractory cancer pain patients. *J Palliat Med*. 2005;8(4):736–742.

White KR, et al. Nonclinical outcomes of hospital based palliative care. *J Healthc Manage*. 2006;51(4): 260–273.

MISCELLANEOUS

- Decisions regarding end-of-life care, including advance directives and living wills, are necessary prior to initiation of palliative care. Complete documentation in the medical record must be maintained.
- Evidence suggests that inpatient palliative care units provide cost-effective care compared to other hospital settings.

CLINICAL PEARLS
- Patients receiving large doses of opioids should be placed on a bowel regimen.
- Patients with long-acting narcotic pain medication should be prescribed short-acting narcotics for breakthrough pain.

ABBREVIATIONS
- LBO—Large bowel obstruction
- PEG—Percutaneous endoscopic gastrostomy tube
- SBO—Small bowel obstruction
- TCA—Tricyclic antidepressant

CODES

ICD9-CM
Z51.5 Palliative care

PATIENT TEACHING

Patients and families should be counseled regarding expectations for prognosis (as noted above) and signs/symptoms associated with disease progression.

PREVENTION
Refer to sections on specific gynecologic and other malignancies for information regarding prevention.

Section III

PRECONCEPTION CARE

Merry K. Moos, BSN, FNP, MPH

BASICS

DESCRIPTION
- Many poor pregnancy outcomes are determined before prenatal care begins; prevention must be initiated before conception (preconception).
- For the majority, this goal is achievable during routine well-woman care.
- CDC-recommended activities before pregnancy include identifying and modifying biomedical, behavioral, and social risks to a woman's health or pregnancy outcome through prevention and management.
- Preconception care is part of a larger health model that impacts the health of women (before, between, and after pregnancy), infants, and families.

Age-Related Factors
Preconception focus is important in the care of all women of childbearing potential, regardless of childbearing intent.

EPIDEMIOLOGY
- Congenital anomalies are a leading cause infant mortality in US:
  - Structural anomalies occur 17–56 days following conception.
- Leading contributors to morbidity and mortality in women are also leading contributors morbidity and mortality in perinatal outcomes:
  - Obesity
  - Tobacco use
  - Alcohol use
- Risk factors for poor pregnancy outcome often are present before the start prenatal care:
  - Unintended conception (49% of all conceptions)
  - Chronic disease
  - Teratogenic exposures
  - Abnormal placentation

RISK FACTORS
- Chronic diseases
- Infectious diseases
- Previous poor reproductive outcomes
- Family history for genetic/inherited conditions
- Teratogenic exposures
- Nutrition status
- Personal health habits

Genetics
Exploring genetic risks before conception allows a woman or couple to become informed about the risks to potential offspring.

PATHOPHYSIOLOGY
- Most structural anomalies occur 17–56 days after conception.
- Day 17 is 3 days after the 1st missed menstrual period.
- Most congenital anomalies result from an interplay of the embryo's genetic predisposition and environmental insults during embryogenesis delivered via mother.

DIAGNOSIS

HISTORY
- Complete a well-woman history including special attention to:
  - Chronic diseases:
    ○ Diabetes
    ○ Hypertension
    ○ Thyroid disease
    ○ Autoimmune disease
    ○ Metabolic disorders
    ○ Hematologic disorders
    ○ Kidney disease
    ○ Mental health disorders including depression and anxiety
    ○ Other
  - Infectious diseases:
    ○ Vaccine-preventable diseases: Rubella, hepatitis b, varicella, influenza, tetanus
    ○ HIV/AIDS
    ○ Syphilis
    ○ *Chlamydia*, gonorrhea
    ○ Periodontal disease
    ○ Toxoplasmosis, CMV
- Reproductive profile:
  - Desires and timing for future pregnancy
  - Contraceptive options/choices
  - Previous pregnancies:
    ○ Intended or unintended
    ○ Maternal complications
    ○ Fetal/Neonatal/Infant outcomes
- Genetic/Inherited conditions:
  - Autosomal recessive diseases:
    ○ Sickle cell
    ○ Thalassemia
    ○ Cystic fibrosis
    ○ Tay-Sachs
  - Fragile X syndrome
  - Down syndrome
  - Other mental retardation
  - Muscular dystrophy
  - Familial hearing or vision loss
  - Diabetes

- Medications:
  - Teratogenic drugs:
    ○ Antiepileptic
    ○ Oral anticoagulants
    ○ Isotretinoin (Accutane)
    ○ Other category X drugs
- Other drugs or herbals known to adversely impact pregnancy outcome
- Nutrition status:
  - BMI <19 or >29
  - Folic acid supplementation
  - Other supplements
- Personal exposures:
  - Tobacco use/exposure
  - Alcohol use/exposure
  - Illicit drug use/exposure
  - Perception of safety at home and work
  - Exposure home or work to infections, environmental toxins
  - Social support

Review of Systems
Special attention to any positive findings and potential significance should the woman conceive

Physical Exam
- Routine well-woman exam with special attention to:
  - BMI
  - BP
  - Thyroid disorders
  - Lymphadenopathy
- Cardiovascular:
  - Murmurs/Bruits
  - Varicosities
- Breast
- Abdomen
- Pelvis:
  - Speculum exam with cervical testing for STDs, cervical cancer
  - Bimanual

TESTS
Lab
Based on risk status:
- Rubella titer, if not previously proven immune
- Varicella titer, if not known immune
- Hepatitis B surface antigen
- Anti-HCV antibody
- HIV
- RPR
- Chlamydia and gonorrhea

- Glucose (particularly if obese, strong family history or history of glucose intolerance of pregnancy)
- TSH
- CBC
- Hemoglobin electrophoresis
- Cystic fibrosis screening
- Tay-Sachs screening
- Other

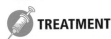
TREATMENT

GENERAL MEASURES
- Educate about the importance of planning when to conceive, for both medical and social reasons.
- Provide contraception based on patient desires regarding conception and health profile.
- Discuss decreasing fertility with age.
- Recommend beginning/continuing over-the-counter multivitamin with 400 μg of folic acid every day for rest of reproductive life, irrespective of desires regarding pregnancy.
- Discuss BMI and implications regarding own health, potential impact on conception and pregnancy; instruct/refer if interventions needed
- For all smokers, recommend smoking cessation using the 5A counseling approach:
  – Ask
  – Advise
  – Assess
  – Assist
  – Arrange
- If the patient has a chronic medical condition (e.g., diabetes, HTN, phenylketonuria, epilepsy) and desires or is at risk for pregnancy, refer to or consult with internist/specialist managing the condition to discuss disease/medication management before/during pregnancy.
- If genetic risks are present, refer for counseling regarding more specific risk calculations and options for testing, minimizing risks, etc.

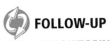
FOLLOW-UP

PATIENT MONITORING
As indicated by desire for planned or risk for unplanned pregnancy and identified risk factors

BIBLIOGRAPHY

American Academy of Pediatrics, Committee on Genetics. Maternal phenylketonuria. *Pediatrics.* 2001;107:427–428.

American College of Obstetricians and Gynecologists Committee on Practice Bulletins. Neural tube defects. Committee Opinion number 44. *Obstet Gynecol.* 2003;102:203–213.

American College of Obstetricians and Gynecologists, Committee on Obstetric Practice. Smoking cessation during pregnancy. Committee Opinion number 316. *Obstet Gynecol.* 2005;106:883–888.

American College of Obstetricians and Gynecologists, Preconception Work Group. The importance of preconception care in the continuum of women's health care. Committee Opinion number 313. *Obstet Gynecol.* 2005;106:665–666.

American College of Obstetricians and Gynecologists. *Guidelines for Women's Health Care,* 2nd ed. Washington, DC: ACOG; 2002.

American Diabetes Association. Preconceptional care of women with diabetes. *Diabetes Care.* 2004;27(Suppl):S76–S78.

Atrash HK, et al. Preconception care for improving perinatal outcomes: The time to act. *Maternal Child Health J.* 2006;10:S3–S11.

Barrett C, et al. Epilepsy and pregnancy: Report of an Epilepsy Research Foundation Workshop. *Epilepsy Res.* 2003;52:147–187.

CDC. Alcohol consumption among women who are pregnant or who might become pregnant-United States, 2002. *MMWR Morb Mortal Week Rep.* 2004;53(50):1178–1180.

Cefalo RC, et al. *Preconceptional Health Care: A Practical Guide,* 2nd ed. St. Louis: Mosby;1995.

Jack BW, et al. Preconception care: Risk reduction and health promotion in preparation for pregnancy. *JAMA.* 1990;264:1147–1149.

Korenbrot CC, et al. Preconception care: A systematic review. *Maternal Child Health J.* 2002;6:75–88.

MISCELLANEOUS

SYNONYM(S)
- Well woman care
- Interconceptional care

ABBREVIATIONS
- RPR—Rapid plasma reagin
- STD—Sexually transmitted disease
- TSH—Thyroid-stimulating hormone

CODES

ICD9-CM/ICD9
- 99385 Preventive Medicine Codes (new)
- 99385
- 99386 (established)
- 99395
- 99396
- v72.31 (annual visit with Pap) and/or v26.49 (Procreative management) and/or code for specific risk condition

PATIENT TEACHING

- ACOG Patient Education pamphlet available at http://www.acog.org
- March of Dimes Patient Education Information at http://www.modimes.org

RAPE/SEXUAL ASSAULT

Kathi Makoroff, MD
Megan McGraw, MD

 BASICS

DESCRIPTION
The legal definition varies from state to state:
- Typically defined as any sexual contact performed by 1 person on another without consent.
- Can involve threats or force.
- Also applies to a person who is unable to give consent.

EPIDEMIOLOGY
- >300,000 women and >90,000 men report being raped yearly.
- 1 in 3–4 women will be the victim of sexual assault in her lifetime.
- ~40% of sexual assaults are reported to law enforcement yearly, making sexual assault one of the most underreported crimes.
- 20–25% of college women report attempted rape or rape.
- The majority of female rape victims were raped at <18 years (54%), with 22% <12.

RISK FACTORS
- Risk factors do not imply causation of sexual assault; rather they are contributing factors to sexual violence.
- In 8 out of 10 cases of sexual assault, the victim knows the perpetrator.
- Victims are often raped again:
  - Among victims of sexual assault, women experienced 2.9 rapes and men 1.2 rapes in the previous year.
- The majority of perpetrators are male.

DIAGNOSIS

SIGNS AND SYMPTOMS
History
- The history should focus on the details of the events and injuries and should be thoroughly documented for forensic purposes.
- Key elements of the history include:
  - Date, time, place of assault
  - Description of perpetrators
  - Any use of force, threats, weapons, or drugs/alcohol
  - Any history of loss of consciousness or memory loss
  - Specific type of contact, penetration, ejaculation, and/or condom use
  - Types of bodily fluid contact
  - Bleeding, injury
  - Time of last voluntary intercourse
  - Last menstrual period
  - Medications including contraception
  - Last tetanus immunization
  - Patient's activity since assault:
    - Voiding, defecation
    - Changed clothes
    - Bathing or douching
    - Brushed teeth, eating or drinking
    - Tampon use

Physical Exam
- Evidence collection kit:
  - See local authorities for standardized evidence collection kit.
  - Perform if assault was ≤72 hours with a history of contact with perpetrator's genitalia, semen, blood, or saliva.
  - Maintain chain of evidence:
    - Since item collection can be used in court, it is crucial that potential evidence be handled carefully with documentation of those handling it.
    - Once evidence is collected, it should stay with you or designated SANE until secured by security/law enforcement per hospital policy.
  - Best evidence collection is a thorough collection that is expanded, not limited, by the patient's history. For many reasons patients may not disclose all details of the assault.
  - SANE or PSANE should perform the evidence collection, if possible.
  - All packaging should be made of paper/cardboard to preserve evidence.
- Complete physical exam:
  - Perform complete physical exam with emphasis on the following:
    - Abrasions
    - Lacerations
    - Bites
    - Foreign bodies
    - Bruising
    - Dried bodily fluid patches
  - Document all trauma or unusual marks.
  - Obtain photographs of injuries if possible.
- GU exam:
  - Use labial traction technique to visualize hymenal area.
  - Look for injury to the GU area:
    - Colposcopic exam permits better visualization.
    - Injuries may include bruising/abrasions, tears, active bleeding.
  - Examine perianal area for injury.
  - Perform speculum exam as indicated by injuries.
  - Obtain photographs of injuries if possible.
- A normal exam is common and can be consistent with a history of sexual assault.

Pediatric Considerations
- Avoid direct contact to the hymen if possible:
  - The prepubertal hymen is sensitive.
- An internal vaginal exam including speculum exam should only be considered in the prepubertal patient if the patient has internal (vaginal) bleeding or trauma.

ALERT
The internal vaginal exam/speculum exam should be performed under anesthesia in the prepubertal patient.

TESTS
Lab
- Pregnancy test
- Consider testing for *Neisseria gonorrhoeae*, *Chlamydia trachomatis*, and *Trichomonas vaginalis* based on history.
- Baseline hepatitis B, hepatitis C, HIV, and syphilis.
- Drug testing per drug-facilitated rape protocol if indicated by history:
  - Drug-facilitated rape protocol includes testing not only for routine drugs of abuse/alcohol but also for "date rape" drugs such as GHB, ketamine, Rohypnol (flunitrazepam).
  - Check with your local lab regarding availability of testing for specific drugs.
- Other testing as indicated by history and/or injuries.

Pediatric Considerations
Obtain *cultures* for *N. gonorrhoeae* and *C. trachomatis* in prepubertal children as legally admissible evidence:
- Urine or vaginal DNA- or RNA-based tests (NAAT) may be used to screen for *N. gonorrhoeae* and *C. trachomatis* but positive results must be confirmed by culture before treatment is initiated.

Imaging
As indicated by history and/or injuries

 TREATMENT

GENERAL MEASURES
- Treatment requires sensitivity and privacy:
  - Have support personnel available if possible.
  - Consider prompt mental health evaluation.
  - If possible, patient should be prioritized.
- Report to appropriate law enforcement agency and, when applicable, to child protection agencies.
- SANE or PSANE should perform the evidence collection and exam, if possible.

MEDICATION (DRUGS)
- Postpubertal and adult patients should be offered prophylaxis against STIs and pregnancy (for prepubertal patients, see Pediatric Considerations below):
  - *N. gonorrhoeae*:
    - Ceftriaxone 125 mg IM in a single dose OR
    - Cefixime 400 mg PO in a single dose OR
  - *C. trachomatis*:
    - Azithromycin 20 mg/kg (maximum 1 g) PO in a single dose OR
    - Doxycycline 100 mg b.i.d. for 7 days (if at least 8 years of age) OR
    - Erythromycin base 50 mg/kg/d q.i.d. for 14 days
  - *T. vaginalis*:
    - Metronidazole 2 g PO in a single dose
    - Consider administering metronidazole 24 hours later to decrease nausea.

- Hepatitis B:
  - If the hepatitis B status of the perpetrator is unknown and the patient is unimmunized or inadequately immunized, begin the hepatitis B vaccine series immediately:
    - Follow-up doses of hepatitis B vaccine are given at 1 and 6 months after the 1st dose.
  - If the perpetrator is known to be hepatitis B positive and the patient is unimmunized or inadequately immunized, administer:
    - HBIG (0.06 mL/kg) AND
    - Begin the hepatitis B vaccine series.
    - Follow-up doses of hepatitis B vaccine are given at 1 and 6 months after the 1st dose.
- HIV PEP:
  - There is little data concerning the risk of acquiring HIV from an unknown assailant.
  - The risk may be increased if any of the following are present:
    - Sexual assault occurs in a region with a high prevalence of HIV infection.
    - Multiple assailants
    - Assailant is known to have a risk factor for acquiring HIV such as IV drug use.
    - Anal penetration
    - The assailant was bleeding or the patient has bleeding or genital/anal injury
  - Antiretroviral drugs must be started no later than 72 hours following the assault and preferably within 4 hours.
  - The patients must remain on the antiretroviral regimen for 28 days.
  - Consult with a specialist familiar with HIV and HIV PEP for specific drug regimen and also for patient follow-up.
- Consider tetanus immunization.
- Pregnancy risk:
  - EC should be offered to all postpubertal and adult patients regardless of the timing of their menstrual cycle and assuming the patient is not already pregnant.
  - Plan B (levonorgestrel 0.75 mg), 2 tablets at the same time, can be administered up to 120 hours postassault.
  - It is more effective the earlier it is administered.
  - Few if any side effects from Plan B; antiemetics are generally not needed.

Pediatric Considerations
- Prophylactic treatments for STIs (excluding HIV and hepatitis B) and pregnancy usually are not indicated for the prepubertal patient.
- Testing for STIs should be considered; these may have forensic implications.

SURGERY
As indicated by history and/or injuries

FOLLOW-UP

DISPOSITION
- Admission as warranted by patient's injury
- Safety planning:
  - Medical staff should ask patient if she feels comfortable returning to place of residence.
  - If necessary, contact child protection agencies for safety planning for pediatric patients.

Issues for Referral
- Offer referrals for mental health counseling.
- Consider referral for follow-up for patients with injuries.
- Pediatric patients should be referred to a CAC if possible.

PROGNOSIS
- Well-documented, immediate and long-tem psychiatric issues follow assaults, including PTSD.
- Refer for mental health counseling.

PATIENT MONITORING
Follow-up testing:
- HIV, syphilis and hepatitis at 6 weeks, 3 months, and 6 months.
- Pregnancy testing in 2–3 weeks even if patient received EC.
- Testing for *N. gonorrhoeae*, *C. trachomatis,* and *T. vaginalis* in 1–2 weeks for patients who did not receive prophylaxis treatment or who have symptoms.

BIBLIOGRAPHY
Kellogg N. The evaluation of sexual abuse in children. *Pediatrics.* 2005;116:506–512.
MMWR Recommendations and Reports 55(RR11);1–94. Available at: http://www.cdc.gov/mmwr/preview/mmwrhtml/rr5511a1.htm.
National Center for Injury Prevention and Control. Sexual Violence: Fact Sheet. Available at: www.cdc.gov/ncipc.
Pickering LK, et al, eds. *Red Book: 2006 Report of the Committee on Infectious Diseases,* 27th ed. Elk Grove Village: American Academy of Pediatrics; 2006.

MISCELLANEOUS

CLINICAL PEARLS
A normal exam is common and consistent with a history of sexual assault.

ABBREVIATIONS
- CAC—Child advocacy center
- EC—Emergency contraception
- GHB—Gamma hydroxy butyrate
- NAAT—Nucleic acid amplification technology
- PEP—Postexposure prophylaxis
- PSANE—Pediatric sexual assault nurse examiner
- PTSD—Post-traumatic stress disorder
- SANE—Sexual assault nurse examiner
- STI—Sexually transmitted infection

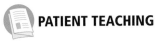

ICD9-CM
- V71.5 Rape
- 959.14 Genital trauma
- 995.53 Child sexual abuse

PATIENT TEACHING

- Refer patients to local rape crisis centers.
- Centers for Disease Control web site: www.cdc.gov
- National Institute of Mental Health web site: www.nimh.nih.gov

SEXUAL ABUSE

Daniel M. Lindberg, MD
Robert A. Shapiro, MD

 BASICS

DESCRIPTION
- Sexual abuse occurs when a child is engaged in sexual activities that he or she cannot comprehend, for which he or she is developmentally unprepared and cannot give consent, and/or that violate the laws or social taboos of society.
- Differentiate abuse from sexual play by considering developmental asymmetry and coercion:
  - Genital contact
  - Exhibitionism
  - Voyeurism
  - Involvement in pornography

Age-Related Factors
- Children of all ages are victims of sexual abuse. Differences in reporting patterns will influence reported rates by age. Most recent national statistics are from 2005:
  - 7% of victims were 0–3 years
  - 23% of victims were 4–7 years
  - 23% of victims were 8–11 years
  - 37% of victims were 12–15 years
  - 11% of victims were over 16 years
- Legal age of consent varies by state.

EPIDEMIOLOGY
By the age of 18, 12–36% of women and 4–9% of men report having an unwanted sexual experience although reports may underestimate prevalence.

RISK FACTORS
- Girls are more commonly affected than boys.
- Homes with single parents, marital discord or stepfathers increase risk to girls.
- Disabilities that impair ability to report abuse increase risk:
  - Blindness
  - Deafness
  - Mental retardation
- Race, ethnicity, and socioeconomic status have not been shown to increase risk for sexual abuse although reporting bias may exist.

ASSOCIATED CONDITIONS
- STIs are not common but screening should be considered.
- Behavioral changes:
  - Nightmares
  - Acting out
  - Toileting difficulties
- Long-term emotional distress:
  - PTSD
  - Major depression
  - Substance use disorders
  - Eating disorders
  - Somatization

DIAGNOSIS

SIGNS AND SYMPTOMS
History
- Although the history is usually the most important factor in determining whether sexual abuse has occurred, children may minimize or deny sexual abuse even in cases of proven abuse.
- When available, history obtained by a trained forensic interviewer is optimal. When the physician is the 1st point of contact, care should be taken to obtain a history that is not leading but is appropriate to the developmental abilities of the child:
  - If at all possible, the child should be interviewed separately from caregivers.
  - Use open-ended, nonleading questions.
  - Determine and then use the child's own terms for body parts.
  - Maintain neutral affect.
  - Generally, children <8–10 years are less developmentally capable of answering questions with "When?" and "How many?" Consider "Where?" and "Once or more than once?"
- Special questions (if possible):
  - Time of last episode of abuse
  - Once or more than once
  - Type of contact, if any
  - Coercion/Threats
  - Identity of perpetrator
  - Presence of ejaculation
  - Menstrual history
  - Prior episodes or allegations of abuse
  - History of pain, bleeding, dysuria, discharge, behavioral changes, nightmares, or toileting difficulties

Physical Exam
Physical findings indicative of sexual abuse are uncommon in both boys (<1%) and girls (<5%).

ALERT
- A normal physical exam cannot exclude even penetrating abuse. The physical exam cannot discriminate consensual from nonconsensual sexual activity in adolescents.

- Sufficient time to reassure the child is necessary. An exam should never be forced on an anxious child. If the alleged episode occurred >72 hours ago, and the child has no acute complaints or need for medical care, the physical exam can safely be deferred if the child's mood or the exam environment is not optimal.
- In the prepubertal child, the frog-leg exam, either on an examination table or trusted adult's lap, is usually sufficient for a full exam. Traction should be applied inferiorly and towards the examiner.

ALERT
- Speculum exam is contraindicated in prepubertal patients.

- The extragenital exam should specifically document any bruising or evidence of other trauma.
- The oropharyngeal exam can show signs of genital-oral contact:
  - Soft palate bruising or petechia
  - Torn frenulum
- Most children will not tolerate contact with the prepubertal hymen, which is extremely sensitive.
- There are few physical findings considered very concerning for sexual abuse:
  - Deep notch or transection of the posterior hymen (from 3–9 o'clock)
  - Unexplained acute bruising or laceration of the genitalia or rectum.
  - Absence of posterior hymen
- Several findings once thought to be concerning for sexual abuse have failed to demonstrate a convincing evidence and should not be used in diagnosis of sexual abuse without further evidence:
  - Labial adhesions
  - Size of the hymenal orifice
  - Venous pooling about the rectum
  - Generalized erythema or increased vascularity of the genitalia
  - Hymenal bands, bumps, or tags
  - Rectal tone. Note: A digital rectal exam is usually unnecessary in the evaluation of alleged child sexual abuse.

TESTS
Labs
Determining which children should be screened for STIs is controversial. While NAAT for gonorrhea and *Chlamydia* may have false-positives compared to culture, they are also likely to have increased sensitivity. While most practitioners do not use these tests to determine treatment or testimony in prepubertal children, one approach is to screen children by NAAT and follow positive tests with culture before treatment.
- Strong indications to test for STIs:
  - Symptoms of an STI including discharge, dysuria, or lower abdominal pain
  - Known STI in the perpetrator or high-risk characteristics
  - Sibling or household contact with an STI
  - Multiple assailants
- Other indications to test for STIs:
  - Patient or parental concern
  - Evidence of ejaculation or penetration

- Consider culture of vagina, rectum, and/or pharynx based on history of abuse.
  - The prepubertal hymen is extremely sensitive. In prepubertal patients, vaginal cultures can be obtained from the vulvar mucosa without penetrating the hymen.
  - Avoid any direct contact with the hymen to minimize patient discomfort.
- Positive cultures for gonorrhea should undergo confirmatory testing to exclude other *Neisseria* species. *Chlamydia* culture should be confirmed using fluorescein-labeled antibodies.
- Urethral sampling by swab is rarely necessary. Urine NAAT can be obtained or material from the tip of the urethra can be cultured.
- The diagnostic significance of STIs for sexual abuse varies with the disease.
  - While *Chlamydia*, gonorrhea, syphilis, and HIV are thought to be virtually diagnostic, trichomoniasis is slightly less specific and herpes, pediculosis, and condyloma are much less conclusive.
  - *Gardnerella* is not concerning for sexual abuse.
- Perinatal and rare nonsexual transmission of STIs should be considered or excluded if the STI is an important part of the diagnosis of sexual abuse.
- The decision to test for HIV, hepatitis, or syphilis should consider the circumstances of abuse, community prevalence of disease, patient or parent concern, and perpetrator characteristics.
  - Follow-up testing for HIV should be repeated at 6 weeks, 3 months, and 6 months. Syphilis testing should be repeated at 6 weeks.
- Forensic evidence collection ("rape kit") should be collected from a willing patient if the alleged abuse may include secretion of blood, saliva, or semen and the abuse may have occurred within 72 hours (120 hours in some states). Beyond 24 hours, useful evidence is most likely to come from the patient's clothes or underwear.

Imaging
Photodocumentation of genital and anal exams and any significant physical findings with a digital camera or colposcopy is useful.

DIFFERENTIAL DIAGNOSIS
- Vaginal discharge can result from several infectious or inflammatory causes in children (see chapter "Vaginitis Prepubertal Vulvovaginitis"):
  - *Streptococcus*
  - *Staphylococcus*
  - *E. coli*
  - *Enterococcus*
  - *Shigella*
  - *Salmonella*
  - Anaerobic infection
  - *Candida albicans*
  - *Gardnerella*
  - Poor hygiene
  - Foreign bodies (including toilet paper)
- Several conditions can mimic genital bleeding, bruising or lesions:
  - Lichen sclerosis
  - EBV, CMV, other viral infections
  - Aphthosis
  - Henoch-Schönlein purpura
  - Straddle injury
  - Anal fissures
  - Toilet seat injury
  - Hair tourniquet
  - Diaper dermatitis
  - Pinworms

- Foreign bodies (including toilet paper)
- Vulvovaginitis
- *Trichomonas hominis*
- Urethral prolapse
- UTI
- Hemolytic-uremic syndrome

 TREATMENT
GENERAL MEASURES

> **ALERT**
> Physicians are mandated reporters of child sexual abuse if they have a reasonable suspicion that abuse has occurred. The specific legal requirements differ by state. Reports must be made to the county child protection agency and/or law enforcement immediately. Upon agreement and when available, a hospital child protection team may assume this reporting requirement.

MEDICATION (DRUGS)
- Urgent treatment of presumptive STI is rarely needed in prepubertal children. Unlike in adolescents and adults, STIs are far less likely to ascend or cause more systemic complications.
- Confirmatory testing to identify false positives has legal importance, and false-positive test results are more common in this population given low disease prevalence.
- Confirmation of positive tests should be done using gold-standard tests or tests with high specificity.
- Treat proven STIs as usual.
- Prophylactic treatment for STIs is appropriate in postpubertal victims.
- EC should be offered as appropriate.
- While PEP for HIV after sexual assault has not been proven in adults or children, it should be considered for children who could start the regimen <72 hours after assault.
  - Consider local prevalence of disease, characteristics of assault, ability to strictly adhere to prophylaxis regimen, and perpetrator characteristics if known.
  - If PEP is considered, consult with a professional with experience treating HIV-infected children.

SURGERY
- Rarely, therapeutic procedures under anesthesia will be necessary:
  - Repair of severe perineal lacerations
  - Removal of foreign bodies
- In rare cases of acute assault requiring exam in an unwilling child, exam under anesthesia may be necessary.

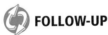 **FOLLOW-UP**
DISPOSITION
Issues for Referral
- Mental health follow-up:
  - Parents or caregivers should be alerted to potential behavioral or psychological symptoms. Children or adolescents with these symptoms should be referred for appropriate counseling.
    - Eating/Feeding disorders
    - Sleep disorders
    - Increased startle response
    - Suicidal/Homicidal ideation

- Medical follow-up:
  - Consider follow-up exam in 7–21 days for children with positive or questionable findings on physical exam.

PROGNOSIS
Poor prognostic signs:
- Closer relationship to perpetrator
- Failure of nonoffending caregiver to support child's disclosure
- More intrusive abuse
- Longer duration of abuse
- Violent or penetrating assault
- Abuse begins at a younger age

PATIENT MONITORING
- Victims of sexual abuse rarely require hospital admission in the absence of associated physical abuse, if a safe environment for discharge can be identified.
- Caregivers may supervise play with other children more closely for persistent sexual behavior.

BIBLIOGRAPHY

Adams J, et al. Guidelines for medical care of children who may have been sexually abused. *J Ped Adolesc Gynecol*. 2007;(20):163–172.

Berenson AB, et al. A case-control study of anatomic changes resulting from sexual abuse. *Am J Obstet Gynecol*. 2000;182:820–834.

Heger A, et al. Children referred for possible sexual abuse: Medical findings in 2384 children. *Child Abuse Neglect*. 2002;26:645–659.

Kellogg N, AAP Committee on Child Abuse and Neglect. The evaluation of sexual abuse in children. *Pediatrics*. 2005;116:506–512.

Putnam FW. Ten-year research update review: Child sexual abuse. *J Am Acad Child Adolesc Psychiatry*. 2003;42:269–278.

US Department of Health and Human Services, Administration on Children, Youth and Families. *Child maltreatment 2004*. Washington, DC: US Government Printing Office; 2006.

ABBREVIATIONS
- CMV—Cytomegalovirus
- EBV—Epstein-Barr virus
- EC—Emergency contraception
- NAAT—Nucleic acid amplification testing
- PEP—Post-exposure prophylaxis
- PTSD—Post-traumatic stress disorder
- STI—Sexually transmitted infection
- UTI—Urinary tract infection

CODES
ICD9-CM
- 995.53 Child sexual abuse
- 995.59 Other child abuse & neglect, multiple forms of abuse

 PATIENT TEACHING

PREVENTION
Programs that attempt to prevent child sexual abuse have not been proven to be effective. While children's knowledge increases with these programs, it is unclear whether they lead to a decreased rate of victimization or an increase in reporting by children.

SEXUAL DYSFUNCTION

Leah S. Millheiser, MD

 BASICS

DESCRIPTION

The evaluation and treatment of female sexual dysfunction combines the disciplines of physical and mental health; therefore, addressing it in the office setting can be an intimidating experience for both the clinician and the patient. However, it has been shown that a patient's report of a sexual health complaint increases by 41% when directly questioned by her clinician.

- 4 types of female sexual dysfunction:
  - Hypoactive sexual desire disorder: Persistent or recurring deficiency (or absence) of sexual fantasies/thoughts, and/or receptivity to, sexual activity.
  - Female sexual arousal disorder: Persistent or recurrent inability to attain, or maintain, sufficient sexual excitement
  - Female orgasmic disorder: Persistent or recurrent difficulty, delay in, or absence of attaining orgasm following sufficient sexual stimulation and arousal:
    - Primary: Never achieved orgasm
    - Secondary: Able to achieve orgasm at 1 point in time, but now no longer able
  - Sexual pain disorders:
    - Vaginismus: Recurrent or persistent involuntary spasm of the pubococcygeus muscles and the musculature of the outer 3rd of the vagina that interferes with vaginal penetration
    - Dyspareunia: Recurrent or persistent genital pain associated with sexual intercourse
- A woman must experience personal distress associated with her complaint to meet the criteria for female sexual dysfunction.

Age-Related Factors
- Sexual dysfunction affects women of all ages.
- Prospective research trials show worsening of most aspects of sexual function after menopause.

EPIDEMIOLOGY
- In the US, 43% of women (compared to 31% of men) suffer from a sexual complaint
- The frequency of sexual complaints in women of all ages is:
  - Desire: 17–55%
  - Arousal: 8–28%
  - Orgasm: 25%
  - Dyspareunia: 2–20%
  - Vaginismus: 6%

RISK FACTORS
- Physiologic:
  - Hormonal changes:
    - Menopause
    - Postpartum
  - Medications:
    - Antidepressants (SSRI, TCA)
    - Anxiolytics
    - Anticonvulsants
    - Antihypertensives (β-Blockers, diuretics)
    - Anticholinergics
    - Anti-androgenics
    - Hormones: OCPs, menopausal hormone therapy
    - GnRH agonists
    - SERMs
    - H_2 receptor blockers
  - Urogenital:
    - Genital atrophy

- Genital surgery
- Pelvic organ prolapse
- STI/PID
- Pelvic masses
- Chronic Illness:
  - Autoimmune disorders
- Neurologic disease
  - MS
  - Spinal cord injury
  - Stroke
- CVD:
  - Peripheral vascular disease
- Endocrine disorders:
  - DM
  - Hyperprolactinemia
- Fatigue
- Psychological:
  - Depression
  - Anxiety disorder
  - Stress
  - Substance abuse
  - Emotional, physical, sexual abuse
  - Body image problems
- Interpersonal:
  - Relationship conflict
  - Partner sexual dysfunction
  - Lack of privacy
  - Lack of partner
- Socio-cultural:
  - Societal taboos
  - Personal and family values
  - Conflict with religion
  - Cultural conflict
  - Lack of early sexual education

Genetics
Currently, no evidence exists for a genetic link in female sexual dysfunction.

PATHOPHYSIOLOGY
Based on both the psychological and physiologic dysfunction that may occur at any point during the sexual response cycles:
- Desire:
  - Sexual thoughts, feelings, fantasies
- Excitement:
  - Genital vasocongestion
  - Vaginal lubrication
- Plateau:
  - Expansion of inner 2/3 of vagina
  - Retraction of clitoris under hood
  - Full elevation of uterus
- Orgasm:
  - Rhythmic contraction of pelvic floor, vaginal, uterine, anal sphincter muscles
- Resolution:
  - Gradual return to pre-excitement state

ASSOCIATED CONDITIONS
See "Risk Factors"

 DIAGNOSIS

SIGNS AND SYMPTOMS
- Diminished or absent sexual libido
- Pain with attempted vaginal penetration
- Pain with noncoital stimulation of the genitals
- Decreased or absent vaginal lubrication during sexual situations

- Decreased or absent genital sensation to stimulation
- Difficulty achieving orgasm
- Diminished intensity of orgasm
- Lack of orgasm with sufficient stimulation

History
- The patient should be completely dressed during the history portion of the visit.
- Medical:
  - Past medical history/medications
  - Gynecologic: STI, PID, Endometriosis, Fibroids, Trauma, OB laceration, Pelvic surgery
- Social:
  - Alcohol/Drug/Tobacco use
  - Relationship issues
  - Life stressors
  - Body image problems
  - History of sexual, physical, emotional abuse
- Sexual:
  - Introductory question: "Ms. X, women may experience difficulties with sexual activity at any stage of life. Is there anything about your sex life that has been concerning to you?"
    - When did problem start
    - Did problem occur with other partners
    - Partner sexual dysfunction
    - Is problem situational
    - Is there desire mismatch
    - Age of 1st sexual experience
    - Number of lifetime sexual partners
    - Is sexual activity being forced upon patient
    - Masturbation
- Validated questionnaires useful in diagnosis and post-treatment: FSFI, FSDS, BDI

Physical Exam
- External female genitalia:
  - Ingrown hairs, lesions, infection, vulvar erythema, labial or clitoral hood fusion, vulvar atrophy, sensory deficits
- Vagina:
  - Atrophy
  - Lesions
  - Pelvic organ prolapse
  - Abnormal discharge
  - Contracted pelvic floor and/or thigh and abdominal muscles during attempted or actual exam of the vagina
- Cervix: Erythema, abnormal discharge, lesions
- Uterus: Enlargement, fibroids, cervical motion tenderness, mobility
- Adnexa: Masses, tenderness

TESTS
- Vestibulitis: Q-tip test
- Vaginal pH: Normal 3.5–5.0
- Wet mount
- Cervical cultures: GC/CT
- Pap smear

Lab
- Most patients do not require lab tests. Testing should be based purely on a patient's clinical presentation or obtained as a baseline prior to initiating certain types of therapies:
  - Free and total testosterone, SHBG, estradiol, TSH, prolactin, fasting glucose, hepatic panel, lipid panel

Imaging
Pelvic imaging, such as US, MRI, or CT, may be necessary to rule out underlying structural anomalies.

DIFFERENTIAL DIAGNOSIS
- Hypoactive sexual desire disorder:
  – Sexual aversion disorder
- Female sexual arousal disorder
- Female orgasmic disorder
- Sexual pain disorders
- See Risk Factors for conditions that may cause sexual dysfunction.

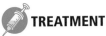 **TREATMENT**

GENERAL MEASURES
- No medications are FDA-approved for the treatment of female sexual dysfunction.
- Treatment of female sexual dysfunction is multidisciplinary.
- Discontinue medications associated with sexual dysfunction, if safe to do so.
- Use bupropion in premenopausal patients with antidepressant-related sexual dysfunction in the absence of anxiety.
- If OCPs are felt to be contributing to sexual dysfunction and are discontinued, provide alternate birth control.

SPECIAL THERAPY
Complementary and Alternative Therapies
- Pelvic floor physical therapy
- Sex therapy
- Psychology/Psychiatry
- Herbal therapy for hypoactive sexual desire disorder:
  – ArginMax: L-Arginine, ginseng, ginkgo biloba (pre- and postmenopausal)
- Herbal therapy for sexual arousal disorder:
  – Zestra (topical evening primrose oil, borage seed oil)

MEDICATION (DRUGS)
- Hypoactive sexual desire disorder:
  – Off-label:
    ○ Testosterone: Gel with concomitant estrogen use in postmenopausal women. Use of testosterone in healthy premenopausal women is not advised.
    ○ Bupropion
- Sexual arousal disorder:
  – Pharmacotherapy:
    ○ Vaginal estrogen
  – Off-label:
    ○ Sildenafil
    ○ Testosterone: Gel
  – Devices:
    ○ EROS clitoral therapy device
    ○ Vibrator therapy (self/partner exploration)
  – Replens vaginal moisturizer
  – Lubricants:
    ○ Water-based or Silicone-based
    ○ Women who are prone to yeast infections should use water or silicone-based lubricants that are glycerin-free.
    ○ Petroleum and oil-based lubricants should be avoided as they interfere with latex-containing items. Petroleum lubricants promote vaginal inflammation and yeast infections.

- Orgasmic disorder:
  – Off-label: Sildenafil; Interstim
  – Devices: Vibrator therapy; Vaginal weights
  – Kegel exercises
- Pain disorders:
  – Dyspareunia:
    ○ Treat underlying etiology
    ○ Pelvic floor physical therapy
  – Vaginismus:
    ○ Vaginal dilator therapy
    ○ Pelvic floor physical therapy

SURGERY
- Surgery has a limited role in the treatment of female sexual dysfunction, except as it pertains to sexual pain disorders.
- Pelvic masses, endometriosis, and vulvovaginal structural anomalies (septums, incompletely perforated hymens) may cause dyspareunia and often require surgical management.
- Medical and physical therapy should be the initial course of treatment, when possible.

 FOLLOW-UP

DISPOSITION
- Once a sexual complaint has been identified, bring the patient back for a thorough history and exam.
- Have a referral pool of clinicians in your area who treat female sexual dysfunction.

Issues for Referral
- Pelvic floor physical therapy: Vaginismus, dyspareunia
- Sex therapy:
  – Relationship difficulty in the setting of sexual dysfunction
  – Patient requires sex education
  – Multiple sexual dysfunctions
  – Lack of response to medical therapy
- Psychotherapy:
  – Depression
  – Anxiety disorder
  – History of abuse
  – Lack of response to medical therapy

PROGNOSIS
Treatment of female sexual dysfunction is most effective when the patient is compliant with clinician visits and therapy and has a supportive partner, if applicable. Patients and clinicians should not anticipate immediate partial or complete resolution of any type of female sexual dysfunction.

PATIENT MONITORING
Women placed on testosterone therapy should have their testosterone levels and hepatic panel checked every 3 months.

- If testosterone levels are supraphysiologic for an extended period, the patient may experience the rare and irreversible side effects of clitoromegaly, hoarseness of the voice, and male-pattern baldness.
- 3–8% of women on testosterone therapy experience acne and/or hirsutism.
- Lipid levels should be checked every 6 months.

BIBLIOGRAPHY

Basson, et al. Revised definitions of women's sexual dysfunction. *J Sex Med*. 2004;1(1):40–48.
Dennerstein L, et al. *Fertil Steril*. 2001;76:456–460.

Laumann, et al. Sexual dysfunction in the United States: Prevalence and predictors. *JAMA*. 1999; 281(6):537–544.
Montejo, et al. Sexual dysfunction secondary to SSRIs. A comparative analysis in 308 patients. *Actas Luso Esp Neurol Psiquiatr Cienc Afines*. 1996;24: 311–321.

 MISCELLANEOUS

In 2003, the American Foundation of Urologic Disease convened an international committee to revise the current classification of female sexual dysfunction. The proposed classification takes into account psychological, physiologic, and contextual factors that affect female sexual function. Until the new classification is officially adopted, the 1998 classification described continues to apply.

CLINICAL PEARLS
- Attempt to treat underlying medical condition prior to initiating medical or surgical therapy.
- Never assume heterosexuality or monogamy.
- Always refer to the patient's significant other as a "partner."

ABBREVIATIONS
- BDI—Beck Depression Inventory
- CVD—Cardiovascular disease
- FOD—Female orgasmic disorder
- FSAD—Female sexual arousal disorder
- FSD—Female sexual dysfunction
- FSDS—Female Sexual Distress Scale
- FSFI—Female Sexual Function Index
- GnRH—Gonadotrophin-releasing hormone
- HSDD—Hypoactive sexual desire disorder
- OCP—Oral contraceptive pill
- SERM—Selective estrogen receptor modulator
- SSRI—Selective serotonin reuptake inhibitor
- STI—Sexually transmitted infection
- TCA—Tricyclic antidepressant

CODES
ICD9-CM
- 302.72 Female sexual arousal disorder
- 302.73 Female orgasmic disorder
- 302.79 Sexual aversion disorder
- 625.1 Vaginismus
- 625.0 Dyspareunia
- 799.81 Decreased libido

 PATIENT TEACHING

- Educate patient (and partner) on the sexual response cycle.
- Inform patient that treatment may take an extended period and that the dysfunction may not completely resolve after treatment.
- Safe sexual practices

PREVENTION
- Educate clinicians on the topic of female sexual dysfunction.
- Ask all female patients, regardless of partner status and sexual orientation, about their sexual function at every annual visit.

SLEEP DISORDERS

Victoria Surdulescu, MD

 BASICS

DESCRIPTION

- Insomnia: Repeated difficulty with sleep initiation, duration, maintenance, or quality that occurs despite adequate opportunity for sleep, resulting in daytime impairment.
- SDB: Repetitive episodes of complete (apnea) or partial (hypopnea) upper airway obstruction during sleep:
  - Often result in decreased oxyhemoglobin saturation level and usually terminate in brief arousals, with sleep fragmentation and distorted sleep architecture.
- RLS: Sensorimotor disorder characterized by a strong, nearly irresistible urge to move the legs, worse at rest and during evening:
  - Circadian rhythm to RLS symptoms (worse in evenings and almost never upon awakening).
  - Sleep onset disruption and increased rates of depression reported with moderate-to-severe RLS
  - 80–90% RLS patients also report PLMS; may decrease sleep efficiency.
- SRLC: The most frequent type of leg complaint in pregnancy:
  - Unknown etiology
- PLMD: Repetitive, highly stereotyped periodic limb movements that occur during sleep (PLMS), with clinical sleep disturbance:
  - PLMS in up to 34% of people of age >60 years.
- Sleep in women may vary across their lifespan due to women's additional biologic states that may affect sleep (menstrual cycle, pregnancy, menopause).
  - Menstrual cycle:
    - Self-reported data indicates that ~70% women report sleep disturbances due to menstrual symptoms for an average of 2.5 days per month.
    - Dysmenorrhea: Reduced subjective sleep quality, sleep efficiency, and REM sleep (with possibly mood-worsening and pain threshold–reducing effects of sleep loss)
  - Menopause:
    - Multiple factors can disrupt sleep: Hot flashes, insomnia, mood changes, vaginal dryness, weight gain, nocturia, SDB

Pregnancy Considerations

- RLS, nocturnal heartburn, and snoring may worsen; significant maternal sleep disruption occurs mostly 2–4 months postpartum
- Snoring: ~20% women report onset of snoring during pregnancy
- RLS: 19–23% of pregnant women by the 3rd trimester
- Postpartum depression: 10–20% incidence of a major depressive episode during this period; difficult to differentiate between depression and symptoms of chronic sleep loss

Age-Related Factors

- Increased incidence of SDB in postmenopause (protective role of estrogen?), approaching male prevalence (4%, compared to 1.5–2% premenopause)
- Increased incidence of RLS, PLMD, and insomnia (with or without association with major depression) in older women

EPIDEMIOLOGY

- Insomnia:
  - Prevalence: Women > Men and younger adults
  - Prevalence varies according to the type of populations studied (healthy adults, chronically ill, psychiatric disorders, etc).
- SDB:
  - Wisconsin Sleep Cohort Study: 9% women (24% men) with SDB (defined as AHI ≥5/hr); 2% women (4% men) prevalence if sleepiness is included in definition of SDB
  - Sleep apnea: Postmenopausal prevalence up to 9.7% (from 3.2% premenopausal) for mild SDB (AHI 0–15/hr and moderate or severe snoring)
  - Association between SDB and hypertension, metabolic syndrome, and various other cardiovascular diseases (recurrent atrial fibrillation, stroke, congestive heart failure, nocturnal cardiac arrhythmias)
- Nocturnal leg cramps:
  - 8–10% outside pregnancy, up to 75% during the 3rd trimester
- Nonrestorative sleep associated with FM reported in 76% FM patients:
  - FM prevalence: ~3% of population, with 75% FM patients being women.
  - RLS possibly more frequent in FM patients.
  - Pain associated with FM may disrupt sleep, which in turn causes a lower pain threshold due to the chronic partial sleep deprivation.

RISK FACTORS

Genetics

- RLS: Possible genetic component
- SDB: Familial component of its pathogenesis.
  - The apparent familial aggregation of SDB may be due to a true genetic component or phenotype sharing of such traits as body fat distribution or size of airway, etc.

PATHOPHYSIOLOGY

- Insomnia:
  - Alteration of circadian cycle, depression, sleep interruption (i.e., from breast-feeding), hot flashes, inadequate sleep hygiene, environmental, medical, or neurologic disorders
- SDB:
  - Weight gain (distribution of visceral adiposity, loss of "protective" estrogen effect postmenopause)
  - Craniofacial and upper airway abnormalities
    - Micrognathia
    - Macroglossia
    - Nasal septal deviation, polyps, tonsillar hypertrophy

- PLMD:
  - Unknown association with SRLC; pregnant women carrying twins or triplets have higher incidence of PLMD than singleton mothers.
- RLS:
  - Low total body iron stores (ferritin level <50 ng/mL), and low folic acid levels, probably worsened during pregnancy:
    - Pregnant women should receive multivitamins with both iron AND folic acid throughout pregnancy.
  - Renal failure
  - Familial
  - Idiopathic

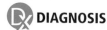 **DIAGNOSIS**

SIGNS AND SYMPTOMS

History

- Insomnia:
  - Careful sleep history, with attention to onset of symptoms, sleep duration and quality, relationship with various environments (e.g., sleep better away from home than in own bedroom may indicate psychophysiological insomnia), sleep hygiene, impact on daytime functioning, medication list and other illnesses.
  - Sleep diary kept for at least 2 weeks, as well as actigraphy, may be useful.
- SDB:
  - Snoring, waking up gasping for air, daytime sleepiness, morning headaches, mood disturbances, witnessed sleep apnea, and nocturia can be associated with SDB.
- RLS:
  - Characteristic "creepy crawly" (or "Pepsi in veins") sensation in legs and/or arms, with the urge to move the limbs and immediate relief from activity
- PLMS:
  - Usually reported by collateral history (bed partner) but occasionally associated with sleep fragmentation and daytime symptoms
- Depression:
  - Loss of interest in activities once perceived as pleasurable, flat affect, poor sleep quality or hypersomnia, easily crying and/or sad. Watch for it in postpartum period ("baby blues").
- FM:
  - 11 of 18 tender points (bilateral, above and below waist, include axial sites, widespread distribution and occurring for >3 months)
  - Sleep disturbance is major complaint in FM.

Physical Exam

- May be significant in SDB: Crowded posterior oropharyngeal examination (high Mallampati class), obesity, micrognathia, macroglossia, or other upper airway abnormalities.
- Positive for tender points in FM patients (see above)

TESTS

- Insomnia:
  - PSG evaluation is indicated only if another diagnosis (such as SDB or PLMD) is suspected.
  - Actigraphy may be helpful.
- RLS:
  - Ferritin and iron studies
  - Renal panel if suspect renal failure
- SDB:
  - NPSG
  - Thyroid function testing (subclinical hypothyroidism may contribute to the pathophysiology of SDB)

Imaging
When craniofacial abnormalities are suspected as the major contributing etiologic factor to the presence of SDB, x-ray cephalometry, CT, or MRI of the upper airway may be useful, especially if corrective surgery is contemplated.

 ## TREATMENT
GENERAL MEASURES

- Insomnia:
  - Psychological and behavioral interventions are effective and recommended in the treatment of both primary and secondary insomnia, in older adults as well in chronic hypnotic users.
  - Stimulus control therapy training of the patient to reassociate the bed and bedroom with sleep is recommended.
  - Relaxation training is recommended for chronic insomnia.
  - CBT is recommended for chronic insomnia.
- SDB:
  - Lifestyle modifications, including weight loss, avoiding alcohol and sedatives at bedtime, smoking cessation, nasal decongestion, and regular sleep-wake cycles
  - Positional therapy (avoiding sleep in supine position by sleeping in a nightshirt with a tennis ball inside a pocket sewn along mid-thoracic spine) for strictly positional SDB.
  - CPAP: 1st-line therapy for the treatment of SDB:
    - Usually initiated in the sleep laboratory, during a calibration night when the sleep technologist adjusts the pressure delivered to abolish apneas, hypopneas, respiratory effort-related arousals, oxyhemoglobin desaturations, and snoring.
  - Oral appliances for management of:
    - Primary snoring (i.e., snoring without polysomnographic evidence of SDB)
    - Mild-to-moderate sleep apnea
- RLS and PLMD:
  - Behavioral therapy for mild cases (physical activity, mental distractions, hot baths)
  - Discontinuing use of potential exacerbators, (caffeine, alcohol, nicotine, SSRIs, metoclopramide, dopamine antagonists, diphenhydramine)

MEDICATION (DRUGS)

- Insomnia:
  - Pharmacologic options: Hypnotics of various classes (benzodiazepines and benzodiazepine-receptor agonists, melatonin receptor agonists, OTC antihistamines)
- RLS/PLMD:
  - Iron supplementation to a ferritin level above 50 ng/mL
  - Dopaminergic agents (such as levodopa, ropinirole, pramipexole)
  - Opiates (good second-line agents)
  - Gabapentin
  - BRAs such as clonazepam, zaleplon, zolpidem)
- SDB:
  - No medication has been recommended for the treatment of SDB in the recent AASM Practice Parameters for the Medical Therapy of Obstructive Sleep Apnea.
  - Modafinil, a wakefulness-promoting agent, is indicated for the treatment of residual excessive daytime sleepiness in SDB patients who have sleepiness despite effective CPAP therapy and who lack other identifiable causes for their sleepiness.

SURGERY

- Of these disorders, surgical management plays a role only in the treatment of SDB.
- Upper airway surgical procedures:
  - Tracheostomy
  - UPPP
  - Nasal procedures (septoplasty, turbinectomy)
  - Genioglossus advancement and hyoid myotomy and suspension
  - Maxillo-mandibular advancement

 ## FOLLOW-UP
DISPOSITION
Issues for Referral

- Insomnia:
  - Referral to psychiatrist/psychologist for help with cognitive and behavior interventions, as well as for the management of major mood disorders
- SDB:
  - Referral to the sleep disorders center for testing and/or management
  - Referral to a dentist with expertise in the fitting and management of oral appliances
  - Referral to a center with expertise in the surgical options, as appropriate (patient declines or cannot tolerate CPAP therapy, or obvious craniofacial or upper airway abnormalities preclude successful CPAP use)
- FM:
  - Treatment is often difficult, costly, and of limited success.
  - Comprehensive, multidisciplinary approach, with individualized flexible strategies
  - Antidepressants, analgesics, muscle relaxants
  - Intermittent use of zolpidem or zaleplon for management of acute insomnia

- Nonpharmacologic therapies:
  - CBT
  - Exercise
  - Biofeedback
  - Hypnotherapy
  - Acupuncture

BIBLIOGRAPHY

Earley CJ. Clinical practice. Restless legs syndrome. *N Engl J Med*. 2003;348(21):2103–2109.

Morgenthaler T, et al. Practice parameters for the psychological and behavioral treatment of insomnia: An update. An American Academy of Sleep Medicine Report. *Sleep*. 2006;29(11):1415–1419.

Pien GW, et al. Sleep disorders during pregnancy. *Sleep*. 2004;27(7):1405–1417.

Young T, et al. The occurrence of sleep-disordered breathing among middle-aged adults. *N Engl J Med*. 1993;328(17):1230–1235.

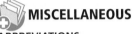 ## MISCELLANEOUS
ABBREVIATIONS

- AASM—American Academy of Sleep Medicine
- AHI—Apnea-hypopnea index
- BRA—Benzodiazepine receptor agonist
- CBT—Cognitive behavioral therapy
- CPAP—Continuous positive airway pressure
- FM—Fibromyalgia
- NPSG—Nocturnal polysomnography
- PLMD—Periodic limb movement disorder
- PLMS—Periodic limb movements of sleep
- RLS—Restless leg syndrome
- SDB—Sleep disordered breathing
- SRLC—Sleep-related leg cramps
- SSRI—Selective serotonin reuptake inhibitor
- UPPP—Uvulopalatopharyngoplasty

CODES
ICD9-CM

- 307.42 Idiopathic insomnia
- 307.02 Insomnia due to mental disorder
- 327.23 Obstructive sleep apnea
- 333.99 Restless legs syndrome
- 327.52 Periodic limb movement disorder
- 327.53 Sleep related leg cramps

PATIENT TEACHING

PREVENTION

- Implementation of good sleep hygiene
- Regular exercise
- Maintain ideal body weight.
- Avoid substances that interfere with sleep onset or maintenance, or that may worsen SDB (alcohol, caffeine, nicotine).
- Balanced nutrition to avoid iron deficiency

SUBSTANCE ABUSE

Preeti Patel Matkins, MD

 BASICS

DESCRIPTION

- DSM-IV defines alcohol abuse as a maladaptive pattern of use leading to significant impairment or distress in work, home, or school; leading to hazardous conditions, interpersonal problems
- DSM-IV defines substance dependence as a pattern of use having at least 3 of the following within the last 12 months:
  - Tolerance
  - Withdrawal
  - Use of substance more frequently or in larger amounts than intended
  - Persistent desire or unsuccessful attempts to reduce use
  - Use of time to obtain substance
  - Social interference
  - Continued use despite knowledge of untoward effects of substance

Pediatric Considerations
2005 Youth Risk Behavior Survey of over 13,000 adolescents:

- 38.4% ever used marijuana; 20.2% used at least once in last 30 days
- 7.6% ever used cocaine; 3.4% at least once in last 30 days
- 2.1% have used injectable illegal substances
- 2.4% have used heroin
- 6.2% have used crystal methamphetamine

Pregnancy Considerations
- Pregnant women may fear legal repercussions if they disclose substance abuse.
- Fetal outcomes:
  - IUGR
  - Low birth weight
  - Placental abruption
  - Preterm delivery
  - Neonatal withdrawal syndrome
  - SIDS
  - Learning problems

Geriatric Considerations
Consider drug interactions and pain-relieving medications.

EPIDEMIOLOGY
5–10% of women who receive prescriptions for mood-altering drugs will develop a dependence or addiction:

- Medically appropriate use may result in physical dependence.
- Psychological dependence or abuse
- Addiction

RISK FACTORS
- Alcohol abuse
- Tobacco use
- Physical or sexual abuse
- Comorbid conditions: Anxiety disorders, mood disorders, PTSD, eating disorders, trading sex for drugs

Genetics
- Family, twin, and adoption studies of families of drug abusers suggest genetic component of drug abuse vulnerability.
- Mouse genetic studies support a genetic component.
- Studies suggest that common genetic factors are involved in drug and alcohol abuse and certain psychological disorders in men.

PATHOPHYSIOLOGY

ALERT
Pathophysiology differs widely and depends on specific substance of abuse.

ASSOCIATED CONDITIONS
- Depression and other mental health conditions
- Conditions associated with IV needle use such as hepatitis B and C, HIV
- Health conditions:
  - Malnutrition
  - CNS changes
  - Heart disease
  - Liver disease

 DIAGNOSIS

SIGNS AND SYMPTOMS
History
- Behavioral: Social changes, withdrawal, job/school failure; driving while impaired, violence
- Physical:
  - Weight loss, anorexia, poor hygiene, symptoms of associated conditions
  - Acute withdrawal: Hallucinations, nausea, emesis, palpitations, hypertension, blackouts, seizures
  - Cravings

Physical Exam
- Physical exam findings differ widely, depending on specific substance of abuse.
- Ascertaining substance may be difficult outside of self-reporting without performing screening tests.
- Routine discussion/verbal screening is recommended.
- In addition to alcohol, marijuana, and cocaine, also ask about benzodiazepines, sedatives, hypnotics, tranquilizers, and narcotics. Also consider ecstasy, γ-hydroxybutyrate, ketamine.
- DAST is a 28-item screen.
- CAGE-AID: 1 yes indicates risk for abuse and/or dependence; 2 or more indicates high likelihood:
  - Ever Cut down on drug use?
  - Have people Annoyed you about your drug use?
  - Ever felt Guilty about drug use?
  - Ever had an Eye-opener (drugs) in the morning?

TESTS
Lab
- Urine toxicology:
  - Immunoassay tests for amphetamines, cocaine, opioids, marijuana, although individual "drug screens" may differ.
  - Results may be affected by dose, route of administration, and metabolism.
  - Some substances, such as marijuana, remain positive for several weeks after last use in chronic users.
  - Confirm with thin-layer chromatography.
- Serum alcohol level
- Specific levels for specific substances of abuse

Imaging
- Use as indicated by exam, history
- CT/MRI of brain may show atrophy, cortical and basilar lesion
- Old fractures

DIFFERENTIAL DIAGNOSIS
Other/Miscellaneous
- Substance-induced psychiatric disorders
- Other mental illnesses:
  - Common comorbid disorders present in up to 50% of substance abusers:
    - Antisocial personality disorder
    - Schizophrenia
    - Anxiety disorders
    - Bipolar disorder
    - Major depression
    - Dysthymia
    - Pathologic gambling
- Individuals with identified mental illness have ~30% chance of comorbid substance abuse disorder.

TREATMENT
GENERAL MEASURES
- Treatment should be tailored for substance involved.
- Marijuana:
  - Cravings occur with diminished use.
  - Hypnotics may be helpful initially.
  - SSRIs and/or anxiolytics may be helpful.
- Opioids:
  - Consider use of methadone or buprenorphine and tapering
  - Use detoxification center with frequent evaluation
- Cocaine and other substances:
  - Use community resources and experts

SPECIAL THERAPY
Complementary and Alternative Therapies
- Complementary and alternative therapies are frequently used in different treatment settings, including detoxification, residential, outpatient, and methadone treatment. It has been suggested that these therapies add value across the range of conventional substance abuse treatments.
- Few data support the effectiveness of these therapies or explain how/why they may be effective.
  - Recreational therapy
  - Relaxation training
  - Acupuncture
  - Guided imagery
  - Nutrition/Vitamins
  - Sweat lodges
  - Meditation/Transcendental meditation
  - Music therapy
  - Biofeedback
  - Hypnosis
- A Cochrane review of AA and other 12-step approaches involving psychosocial behavioral change did not show these programs to reduce alcohol use or achieve abstinence compared with other treatments.

MEDICATION (DRUGS)
Medication use depends on the specific substance abused, but may include:
- Hypnotics
- SSRIs
- Anxiolytics
- Methadone
- Buprenorphine

 FOLLOW-UP

DISPOSITION
Issues for Referral
Consultation with or referral to a psychiatrist may be helpful in assessing comorbid psychiatric conditions.

Issues for Intervention
- Method of intervention and referral in outpatient setting:
  - State concerns
  - Discuss health related outcomes, including fetal outcomes
  - Discuss patient insight
  - Develop plan for treatment, intervention
  - Monitor for progress and relapse
  - Be aware of community resources
- SBIRT initiative: Screening, brief intervention, and referral for treatment of those at risk for substance use–related problems

PROGNOSIS
The prognosis for substance abuse is varied, and depends on the substance, the length of time of abuse, patient motivation, and support available.

BIBLIOGRAPHY

2005 Youth Risk Behavior Surveillance-United States, 2005. *MMWR Morbid Mortal Week Rep.* 2006; 55(SS-5):1–108.

American Psychiatric Association. *Diagnostic and Statistical Manual,* 4th text revision. Washington, DC: American Psychiatric Press, 2000.

Brown RL, et al. Conjoint screening questionnaires for alcohol and other drug abuse validity in a primary care practice. *Wis Med J.* 1995;94:135–140.

Ewing J. Detecting alcoholism: The CAGE questionnaire. *JAMA.*1984;252:1906–1907.

Ferri M, et al. Alcoholics Anonymous and other 12-step programmes for alcohol dependence. *Cochrane Database Syst Rev.* 2006; Jul 193. CD005032

Skinner HA. Drug abuse screening and testing. *Addictive Behavior Testing.* 1982;7:363–367.

 MISCELLANEOUS

ABBREVIATIONS
- AA—Alcoholics Anonymous
- DAST—Drug abuse screening test
- DSM-IV—Diagnostic and Statistical Manual, 4th edition
- IUGR—Intrauterine growth restriction
- PTSD—Post-traumatic stress disorder
- SIDS—Sudden infant death syndrome
- SSRI—Selective serotonin reuptake inhibitor

CODES
ICD9-CM
305 Abuse, drugs:
- 4th digit specific to substance of abuse
- 5th digit:
  - 0 unspecified
  - 1 continuous
  - 2 episodic
  - 3 in remission

 PATIENT TEACHING

PREVENTION
- Routine education of substance abuse effects on behavior and fetal development
- Be aware of community resources

Section III

SUBSTANCE ABUSE: ALCOHOL

Preeti Patel Matkins, MD

 BASICS

DESCRIPTION
- DSM-IV defines *alcohol abuse* as a maladaptive pattern of use leading to significant impairment or distress in work, home, or school; leading to hazardous conditions, interpersonal problems
- DSM-IV defines *alcohol dependence* as a pattern of use having at least 3 of the following within the last 12 months:
  - Tolerance
  - Withdrawal
  - Use of substance more frequently or in larger amounts than intended
  - Persistent desire or unsuccessful attempts to reduce use
  - Use of time to obtain substance
  - Social interference
  - Continued use despite knowledge of untoward effects of substance
- Women have a faster transition from use to dependency to abuse.
- Women more likely to have comorbidities of depression, interpersonal violence, abuse, PTSD, unplanned pregnancies
- Children of women who abuse alcohol are more likely to be abused or neglected.
- Women have higher risk than men to develop liver disease, hepatitis, other complications.

EPIDEMIOLOGY
- ~2/3 of adults in US drink alcohol at least occasionally.
- Estimates that 1 of every 13 adults abuse alcohol or are alcoholics

Pediatric Considerations
2005 Youth Risk Behavior Survey of over 13,000 adolescents:
- 9.9% drove while using alcohol
- 74.3% had at least 1 drink in lifetime
- 43% had at least 1 drink in the last 30 days
- 25.5% had at least 5 drinks in a row at least once in the last 30 days

Pregnancy Considerations
- 18% of pregnant women drank alcohol while pregnant (1991 National Institutes of Drug Abuse and Addiction).
- There is no safe level of alcohol use in pregnancy.
- Alcohol abuse in pregnancy is associated with miscarriage, fetal anomalies.
- Outcomes in infant may include but are not limited to FAS, learning problems, decreased IQ, other neurodevelopmental problems.

Geriatric Considerations
National Institutes of Alcohol Abuse and Alcoholism statistics:
- Incidence of alcohol dependence in women >65 years old is 0.13%
- Incidence of alcohol abuse in women >65 is 0.38%
- Consider drug interactions

RISK FACTORS
- Genetics
- Early initiation
- Interpersonal violence
- Physical or sexual abuse
- Comorbid conditions: Anxiety disorders, mood disorders, PTSD, eating disorders

Genetics
- Genetic component has been established by family, twin, and adoption studies.
- Native American and Alaskan Natives have higher rates of alcohol dependence and abuse than other ethnic groups.

PATHOPHYSIOLOGY
Alcohol is a CNS depressant:
- Blocks NDMA receptors
- Increases GABA inhibition

ASSOCIATED CONDITIONS
- Major organ systems:
  - Dilated cardiomyopathy
  - HTN
  - Liver disease: Cirrhosis, fatty liver, hepatitis
  - Cholelithiasis
  - Pancreatitis
  - Peptic ulcer disease
  - Upper GI malignancies
  - CNS abnormalities
- Malnutrition
- Gout
- Trauma
- Interpersonal violence, abuse

DIAGNOSIS

SIGNS AND SYMPTOMS
History
- Behavioral: Social changes, withdrawal, job/school failure; driving while impaired, violence
- Physical:
  - Weight loss, anorexia, poor hygiene, symptoms of associated conditions
  - Acute withdrawal: Hallucinations, nausea, emesis, palpitations, hypertension, blackouts, seizures

Physical Exam
- Clinician can use interviews and questionnaires.
- Moderate drinking is 3–7 drinks per week in women.
- At risk for abuse in women if >7 drinks/week or >3 drinks per occasion (National Institute on Alcohol Abuse and Alcoholism).
- CAGE: 1 yes indicates risk for abuse and/or dependence; 2 or more indicates high likelihood:
  - Ever Cut down on drinking?
  - Have people Annoyed you about your drinking?
  - Ever felt Guilty about drinking?
  - Ever had an Eye-opener in the morning?
- AUDIT is a 10-item questionnaire developed by World Health Association in 1992.

ALERT
T-ACE and TWEAK are for alcoholism in pregnant women.

Review of Systems
- CV: HTN, dilated cardiomyopathy
- Lungs: Aspiration pneumonia
- Abdomen: Hepatomegaly, varices, pancreatic abnormalities, pain from ulcer disease
- Musculoskeletal: Ecchymosis, old fracture
- Skin: Bruising, caput medusa, telangiectasias, jaundice
- Neurologic:
  - Amnesia, peripheral neuropathy
  - Wernicke- Korsakoff syndrome of Vitamin B_1 (thiamine) deficiency and amnesia:
    - Delirium tremens start 48–72 hours after last alcohol intake.
    - Seizures begin 48–72 hours after last alcohol intake.

TESTS
Lab
- Urine pregnancy test
- Blood alcohol level (mg/dL):
  - <100: Incoordination, personality changes
  - 110–199: Speech/Gait abnormalities
  - 200–299: Emesis, nausea, worsened ataxia
  - 300–399: Amnesia, hypothermia, severe dysarthria
  - >400: Coma, respiratory failure
- Other tests of acute use: Urine tests, breathalyzer
- CDT rises 1–2 weeks after heavy alcohol use
- Less sensitive and less specific:
  - γ-Glutaryl transferase >30 μg/L indicates use of >4 drinks/d for at least 4–8 weeks
  - MCV >100 μg/m^3 indicates 4–8 weeks of heavy drinking
  - Elevated AST, ALT, ALK: An AST:ALT ratio >2.0, uric acid, triglycerides, cholesterol
  - Decreased BUN, hemoglobin/hematocrit, WBC count, platelet

Imaging
- Use as indicated by exam, history
- CT/MRI of brain may show atrophy, cortical and basilar lesion
- Old fractures

DIFFERENTIAL DIAGNOSIS
Rule out medical conditions that cause symptoms similar to intoxication or withdrawal:
- Traumatic brain injury
- Hypoglycemia
- Electrolyte imbalance
- Diabetic ketoacidosis
- Meningitis
- Other neurologic conditions
- Altered mental status with sepsis
- Stroke
- Coexisting psychiatric conditions:
  - Depression
  - Anxiety disorders
  - Abuse of other intoxicants

TREATMENT
GENERAL MEASURES
- General principles:
  - Engage family, if supportive
  - Utilize 12-step programs (AA), community resources, women's groups, adolescent specialists, mental health community, residential settings
- Acute evaluation: Support airway, breathing, circulation.
  - CIWA scores may help with dosage of medications:
    - Scores 1–7 for level of nausea/vomiting, tremors, paroxysmal sweats, anxiety, agitation, tactile disturbance, auditory disturbance, visual disturbances, headaches
    - Scores 1–4 for sensorium changes
    - Score of ≥15 indicates higher risk for withdrawal; <10 usually will not need medication for withdrawal

SPECIAL THERAPY
Diet
- May be deficient in vitamins B_1, B_6, folate, magnesium, phosphate, zinc
- IV fluids
- Follow electrolyte abnormalities
- May need cardiac monitoring

Activity/Restrictions
Take precautions against fall, head injury

MEDICATION (DRUGS)
- Use clinical evaluation and/or CIWA to guide need for treatment
- Thiamine (Vitamin B_1):
  - 100–200 mg IV prior to glucose-containing fluids to avoid Wernicke encephalopathy
  - Consider long-term supplement 100 mg/d
  - Safe in pregnancy and lactation; Category A
- Benzodiazepines (dose depends on CIWA score):
  - Drug of choice in acute withdrawal
  - Efficacious in reducing delirium tremors and seizures
- Disulfiram (125–500 mg/d):
  - Blocks alcohol oxidation by blocking acetyl aldehyde dehydrogenase
  - If combined with alcohol, acetyl aldehyde levels in blood result in unpleasant side effects
  - Use in select patients
  - Use with caution in patients with DM, seizure disorders
  - Monitor CBC, LFT, chemistries
  - Not studied in pregnant women; Category C
  - Lactation risk L5:
    - Excreted in breast milk
    - Can cause long-lasting inhibition of alcohol dehydrogenase in infant
    - Stop breastfeeding if on this medication
- Naltrexone (25 mg 1st dose, then 50 mg/d for 4–6 weeks):
  - Opioid receptor antagonist that blunts pleasurable effects of alcohol. Also reduces cravings for alcohol.
  - Must be opioid free 7–10 days prior to initiation
  - Contraindicated in liver/renal failure
  - Caution: Depression, suicidal ideation
  - FDA black-box warning of hepatic injury
  - Monitor LFTs; may increase GGT.
  - Not studied in pregnant women; Category C
  - Lactation L1 studies show that at a dose of 50 mg/d, the infant receives a relative dose 0.06–1%.
- Acamprosate (666 mg t.i.d.):
  - Binds NDMA and GABA receptors
  - Reduces cravings
  - Check baseline Crt
  - Use with caution in elderly, depressed patients
  - Contraindicated in renal failure
  - Adjust dosing for hepatic and renal failure; Crt clearance <30
  - Not studied in pregnant or nursing women; Category C
- SSRIs:
  - May be helpful
  - FDA black-box warning of suicidality (thoughts or actions about suicide)
  - Pregnancy and nursing category C

BIBLIOGRAPHY
2005 Youth Risk Behavior Surveillance—United States, 2005. *MMWR Morbid Mortal Week Rep.* 2006;55(SS-5):1–108.

American Psychiatric Association. *Diagnostic and Statistical Manual,* 4th text rev. Washington, DC: American Psychiatric Press; 2000.

Ewing J. Detecting alcoholism: The CAGE questionnaire. *JAMA.* 1984;252:1906–1907.

National Institute for Alcohol Abuse and Alcoholism. Available at: www.niaaa.nih.gov.

National Institute on Drug Abuse. Available at: www.nida.nih.giv.

Russell M, et al. Screening for pregnancy risk drinking. *Alcoholism Clin Exp Res.* 1994;18:1156–1161.

Sokol RT. The T-ACE questions: Practical prenatal detection of risk drinking. *Am J Obstet Gynecol.* 1989;160:836–871.

Substance Abuse and Mental Health Services Administration. Available at: www.samhsa.gov.

MISCELLANEOUS
ABBREVIATIONS
- AA—Alcoholics Anonymous
- AUDIT—Alcohol Use Disorder Identification Test
- CDT—Carbohydrate deficient transferrin
- CIWA—Clinical Institute Withdrawal Assessment for Alcohol
- DSM-IV—Diagnostic and Statistical Manual, 4th ed.
- FAS—Fetal alcohol syndrome
- NMDA—N-methyl-D-aspartate
- PTSD—Post-traumatic stress disorder
- SSRI—Selective serotonin reuptake inhibitor

CODES
ICD9-CM
- 305.0* Acute alcohol intoxication
  - 303.0* With dependence
- 303.9* Alcohol dependence
- 305.00 Alcohol abuse
- Maternal addiction with suspected fetal damage
  - 655.4 *Affecting management of pregnancy
  - 760.71 Affecting fetus or newborn
- Use 5th digit code:
  - 0 Unspecified
  - 1 Continuous
  - 2 Episodic
  - 3 In remission

PATIENT TEACHING

- Effects of alcohol on women: http://ncadistore. samhsa.gov/catalog/productDetails.aspx?ProductID =17638
- Alcohol help resources: http://www. mentalhealthscreening.org/events/nasd/help_add. aspx
- Publications for the National Institute on Alcohol Abuse and Alcoholism (NIAAA): http://www.niaaa. nih.gov/Publications/PamphletsBrochuresPosters/ English/

PREVENTION
- Routine education of patients about risks of alcohol use on behavior, injuries
- Discuss effects of alcohol on fetus with all women of child-bearing age.
- Recognize genetic tendencies and discuss strategies.
- Be aware of community resources.

SUBSTANCE ABUSE: PRESCRIPTION DRUGS

Lisa L. Park, MD
Michael G. Spigarelli, MD, PhD

 BASICS

DESCRIPTION

Definitions:

- Abuse: Maladaptive pattern of using drugs that causes physical, psychological, economic, legal or social harm to individual user or to others affected by drug user's behavior
- Dependence: Physiologic state of adaptation to a drug, usually characterized by development of tolerance to drug effects and emergence of a withdrawal syndrome during prolonged abstinence

Age-Related Factors

Substance abuse can begin in early childhood, typically by experimenting and modeling behavior seen in adult relatives. This can rapidly progress to addiction and go unnoticed until the situation has gotten significantly worse.

EPIDEMIOLOGY

Incidence/Prevalence (National Survey on Drug Use and Health 2005–2006)

- 45.4% of individuals have used an illicit substance in their lifetime, 8.3% within the last month.
- Illicit drug use in 4% pregnant women, 10% nonpregnant women
- 12% pregnant women used alcohol in the past month, 4% report binge drinking (≥5 drinks at 1 occasion)
- 16.6% pregnant women and 29.6% nonpregnant women currently smoke.
- Increasing rates of nonmedical prescription drug use, 60% obtained for free from friend or relative, 16% from a doctor
- Obstetricians and gynecologists are in a unique position to screen for substance abuse; women are more likely to seek care through primary care provider (PCP) or mental health professionals rather than directly seek substance abuse treatment.

RISK FACTORS

- Family history of substance abuse, spouse or peer substance abuse
- Comorbid psychiatric disorders such as depression, ADHD, bipolar disorder, eating disorder
- History of physical or sexual abuse
- Personal factors such as poor coping skills, low self-esteem, risk-seeking behaviors

Genetics

- Substance abuse tends to run in families
- Exact genetics of addiction are unknown

ASSOCIATED CONDITIONS

- Alcohol: Women progress more rapidly to alcohol dependence than men, are more likely to die while driving drunk than men with the same blood alcohol concentration (BAC) level.
- Violence: Females who abuse drugs are more likely to be victims of violence and abuse. 50% victims of sexual assault had been drinking.
- Sexual activity: People who consumed ≥5 drinks in 1 sitting, or used marijuana were more likely to have >1 sexual partner, and less likely to use condoms.

Pregnancy Considerations

Reproductive consequences: Opiates, cocaine, marijuana, cigarette use can all increase the risk of preterm labor and preterm delivery. Placental abruption and previa have been associated with cocaine use. There are specific teratogenic effects of illicit drugs including low birth weight and neurodevelopmental delay in the child.

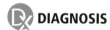 DIAGNOSIS

SIGNS AND SYMPTOMS

- Unless presenting in acute intoxication, symptoms can be vague.
- Symptoms may include: Allergic symptoms such as nose bleeds, nasal septal perforation (cocaine, inhalants), Antabuse types of reactions (intense feeling of unease with concomitant use of alcohol, for example with metronidazole, cephalosporins), behavioral changes, blackouts, chest pain, arrhythmias, bronchospasm, gastritis, constipation, headache, endocarditis, decreased attention, memory loss
- Gynecologic symptoms including menstrual dysfunction, galactorrhea, amenorrhea, or infertility may be seen.
- Thorough medical history, including obstetric/gynecologic history, is valuable for detecting substance abuse and its sequelae.
- Confidential interviewing, especially with adolescents, is crucial to obtaining an honest substance abuse history.
- Psychiatric history and current psychiatric status, including suicidal ideation or history of suicide attempts should be assessed.

Physical Exam

Complete physical exam including vital signs, assessment of mental status, breast and pelvic exam should be preformed.

- Physical signs include:
  - Tachycardia
  - Hypertension
  - Dilated or pinpoint pupils
  - Sluggish papillary response
  - Irritation of nasal mucosa
  - Cutaneous scars ("track marks")
  - SC fat necrosis from IV drug use
  - Tattoos in antecubital fossa
  - Skin abscesses and cellulitis
  - Hepatomegaly
  - Icterus

TESTS

Several screening tools are available:

- The CRAFFT screen has been validated in adolescents, can be used to screen for alcohol or other substance use, and gives a starting point for counseling patients.
  - C-Have you ridden in a car driven by someone who had been drinking or after you were drinking?
  - R- Do you use alcohol/drugs to relax, feel better, or fit in?
  - A- Do you drink/use drugs while alone?
  - F- Do you forget things while using drugs/alcohol?
  - F- Have family or friends told you that you need to cut down?
  - T- Have you gotten into trouble with the law, school, or work while using?
- The CAGE screen has been validated for screening for alcohol abuse.
  - C- Have you ever felt you should try to Cut down on your drinking?
  - A- Have people Annoyed you by criticizing your drinking?
  - G- Have you ever felt bad or Guilty about your drinking?
  - E- Have you ever had a drink first thing in the morning to steady your nerves or get rid of a hangover (Eye opener)?
- DAST is a 20 question test for drug abuse.

Lab

Actual components of laboratory tests may vary; verify with lab if concerned about specific drug(s) or substance(s) of abuse.

- Urine drug screens usually include:
  - Amphetamine
  - Barbiturates
  - Benzodiazepines
  - PCP
  - Marijuana
  - Cocaine
  - Opiates

- Urine toxicology screen is typically more comprehensive, and may include:
  - Phenothiazines
  - Antidepressants
  - Anticonvulsants
  - Analgesics
  - Synthetic narcotic analgesics
  - Sympathomimetic amines
  - Stimulants
  - Tranquilizers and psychotoxics hypnotics/sedatives
  - Miscellaneous agents
- Should obtain consent, even from minors, before obtaining drug screen
- Most likely to obtain positive drug screens: After the weekend (Monday), early morning, and during summer or following vacations

Imaging
Not typically indicated unless concern for acute intracranial bleed.

DIFFERENTIAL DIAGNOSIS
Infection
Main infectious risks result from a combination of poor judgement skills while intoxicated, coupled with high risk activities (sharing needles, incarceration, prostitution or poor choice of sexual partners) and malnutrition.

Hematologic
Anemia, particularly related to B_{12} and folate deficiency is common.

Immunologic
Impaired immunity can result from poor nutrition or infections, such as HIV.

Tumor/Malignancy
Addiction and chronic abuse of substances can lead to cancer, depending on the particular substance abused.

Trauma
- Intoxication can lead to decreased awareness which can lead to greater exposure to violence.
- Association with individuals who sell or use drugs can lead to greater exposure to violence.

Drugs
Virtually any chemical entity that can affect brain function can be addictive from medications (both prescription and over the counter), plants, solvents and cleaning chemicals as well as legal substances, such as alcohol and tobacco.

 TREATMENT
GENERAL MEASURES
- Acute treatment:
  - Stabilize patient if acutely intoxicated or in danger of withdrawal
  - Brief counseling intervention – 5 As
    - Assess: What, with whom, how, how much of the substance; stage of change (precontemplation, contemplation, preparation, action, relapse)
    - Advise: Educate patients about effects of drugs and alcohol, including effects on pregnancy, advise to reduce or stop use
    - Agree: On individual goals for reducing use or abstinence

- Assist: Patients with acquiring motivation, skills, support needed for behavioral change
- Arrange: Follow-up support, counseling, and referral to specialty treatment
- Long-term treatment
  - Work in conjunction with patient's primary care physician, therapist or psychiatrist
  - Criteria for inpatient or outpatient management dependent on acute intoxication, withdrawal potential, medical complications, emotional/psychiatric condition or complications, treatment acceptance, relapse potential, and recovery environment

SPECIAL THERAPY
Complementary and Alternative Therapies
No conclusive evidence exists documenting efficacy of alternate modalities.

MEDICATION (DRUGS)
Several agents are currently on the market.

- Antabuse, which when taken prior to alcohol ingestion, makes the individual violently ill, is not frequently used in clinical situation.
- Naltrexone has been used to treat opiate and alcohol addiction, long-acting injections are now available.
- Buprenorphine (a partial opiate receptor agonist) coupled with naloxone (Suboxone) prevents opiate withdrawal without the rush associated with addictive opiates.
- Methadone replacement therapy, using a long-acting opiate like methadone to prevent withdrawal from shorter acting opiates such as heroin has long been controversial and must be prescribed by an approved methadone clinic (not private offices).
- Bupropion, when coupled with nicotine replacement or Varenicline, has increased effectiveness of smoking cessation attempts.

 FOLLOW-UP
DISPOSITION
Issues for Referral
Any sign of severe, acute withdrawal or uncertainty regarding mental status changes should be referred to the nearest emergency department.

PROGNOSIS
Prognosis depends upon the desire of the individual to seek help, availability of a supportive environment and access to effective strategies and techniques.

PATIENT MONITORING
- Controlled substance prescriptions should be monitored, clearly documented, and if cause for concern, urine drug screens to ensure prescribed medication is present and other illicit agents are not present.
- Acute monitoring for severe withdrawal or confusion will allow appropriate treatment to be provided.

BIBLIOGRAPHY

American College of Obstetrics and Gynecology. Illicit Drug Abuse and Dependence in Women [presentation]. Available at: www.acog.org/departments/dept_notice.cfm?recno=18&bulletin=2207.

Dias PJ. Adolescent substance abuse. Assessment in the office. *Pediatr Clin North Am.* 2002;49(2):269–300.

Greenfield SF. Epidemiology of substance use disorders in women. *Obstet Gynecol Clin North Am.* 2003;30(3):413–446.

Kaul P, et al. Clinical evaluation of substance abuse. *Pediatr Rev.* 2002;23(3):85–94.

Kulig JW, American Academy of Pediatrics Committee on Substance Abuse. Tobacco, Alcohol, and other Drugs: The role of the pediatrician in prevention, identification and management of substance abuse. *Pediatrics.* 2005;115(3):816–821.

National Institute on Drug Abuse Web site. Available at: www.nida.nih.gov/.

National Survey on Drug Use and Health Web site. Available at: www.oas.samhsa.gov/nsduh.htm.

Substance Abuse and Mental health Treatment Locator Web site. Available at: http://findtreatment.samhsa.gov/

 MISCELLANEOUS
CLINICAL PEARLS
- Substance abuse is common and knows no socioeconomic bounds.
- It is important to build trust, provide support, and offer to be of assistance.
- Earlier intervention is more rapidly effective than delayed intervention.
- Failure to ask questions regarding substance abuse, particularly prescription abuse, can lead to prolonged difficulty and decreased chance for rehabilitation.

ABBREVIATIONS
- PCP—Primary care provider
- BAC—Blood alcohol concentration

CODES
ICD9-CM
- 303.XX Alcohol dependence
- 304.XX Drug dependence
- 305.XX Non dependent abuse of drugs

 PATIENT TEACHING

Fact sheets are available at:
- National Institute on Drug Abuse: http://www.nida.nih.gov/

PREVENTION
Information can be found at:
- www.csapdccc-csams.samhsa.gov/previnfo.aspx

SUBSTANCE ABUSE: TOBACCO

Vicki L. Seltzer, MD

 BASICS

DESCRIPTION

- Cigarette smoking is 1 of the 2 leading preventable contributors to premature death and disability in the US.
- The obstetrician-gynecologist can play a very important role in reducing morbidity and premature mortality in women by:
  - Advising their patients not to initiate smoking,
  - By advising smokers to quit, and
  - By assisting them in doing so.
- DSM IV substance dependence criteria nicotine dependence 305.10:
  - Tolerance
  - Withdrawal
  - The substance is often taken in larger amounts or over a longer period than was intended.
  - Persistent desire or unsuccessful attempts to cut down or control substance
  - Time spent in activities necessary to obtain/use the substance, and recover from its effects
  - Important social, occupational, or recreational activities given up or reduced because of use of the substance
  - Use is continued despite the knowledge of having a persistent or recurrent physical or psychological problem that is likely to have been caused or exacerbated by the substance
- Criteria for diagnosing nicotine withdrawal DSM IV 292.0:
  - Daily use of nicotine for at least several weeks
  - Abrupt cessation of nicotine use, or reduction in the amount of nicotine used, followed within 24 hours by 4 (or more) of the following signs:
    - Dysphoria or depressed mood
    - Insomnia
    - Irritability, frustration or anger
    - Anxiety
    - Difficulty concentrating
    - Restlessness
    - Decreased heart rate
    - Increased appetite or weight gain
  - The symptoms above cause clinically significant distress or impairment in social, occupational, or other important areas of functioning.

Age-Related Factors

- Adolescence is the most vulnerable time for the initiation of cigarette smoking:
  - >90% of adults who smoke had their 1st cigarette before they reached 20 years of age.
  - ~1/3 of girls in high school have smoked within the past month.
- ~29% of reproductive age women smoke.

EPIDEMIOLOGY

- Worldwide, >200 million women smoke cigarettes:
  - 100 million in developed countries and 100 million in developing countries
- Overall US statistics: 50% have never smoked, ~25% are current smokers, and 25% are ex-smokers
- ~3/4 of women who smoke indicate that they want to quit:
  - Only a small percentage of those who try to quit are successful with that specific attempt and remain abstinent; however, if a patient relapses she should be encouraged to try again.
- The mean number of cigarettes smoked per day is ~20.
- Between 8% and 15% of smokers are occasional or light smokers (<5 cigarettes/d).
- The prevalence of smoking has declined dramatically in the US; however, the prevalence of smoking has declined less in those who are younger, female, non-Caucasian, less educated, or poor and those with psychiatric or alcohol/drug problems.
- The mean age of initiation of smoking is 15.

RISK FACTORS

Psychiatric predictors of initiation of smoking include:

- Use and abuse of alcohol and other drugs, ADD, and depressive symptoms.

Genetics

Some evidence from twin and adoption studies that genetic factors (along with environmental factors) play a role in smoking initiation, use, and tobacco dependence.

PATHOPHYSIOLOGY

- Placental changes noted in smokers may include the types of findings seen with ischemia and chronic hypoxia.
- Dependence on tobacco refers to the compulsive use of this psychoactive drug in which tolerance and physiological dependence may also be present.
- The term physiological dependence has been used to refer more specifically to the physiological adaptation manifested by the emergence of withdrawal symptoms after cessation of use.
- The pathophysiological consequences of tobacco smoke exposure include tissue destruction contributing to lung disease, cellular changes contributing to cancer, and cellular and molecular reinforcing effects leading to dependence.

ASSOCIATED CONDITIONS

Cigarette smoking places women at increased risk for the following problems:

- Cancer (~90% of lung cancers and 30% of all cancers are associated with cigarette smoking):
  - Lung and bronchus:
    - US women's deaths from lung cancer have increased 600% since 1950.
    - In 1987, lung cancer surpassed breast cancer as the leading cause of cancer death in women.
  - Oropharynx
  - Esophagus
  - Pancreas
  - Bladder
  - Kidney
  - Cervix (preinvasive and invasive)
- Respiratory disorders:
  - Chronic sinusitis
  - More than tenfold increase in risk of dying from emphysema, bronchitis, and chronic airway obstruction
- Coronary artery disease:
  - ~55% of cardiovascular deaths in women under the age of 65 are associated with cigarette smoking.
- Cerebrovascular disease
- Peripheral vascular disease
- Fertility problems

Pregnancy Considerations

- Adverse pregnancy outcomes:
  - Spontaneous abortion
  - Ectopic pregnancy
  - IUGR
  - Perinatal loss
- Effects on infants:
  - May increase SIDS risk
  - Acute respiratory problems
  - Chronic respiratory problems

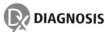 **DIAGNOSIS**

SIGNS AND SYMPTOMS

History

- Does the woman smoke now, and did she ever?
- When smoking was initiated
- Number of cigarettes smoked
- Times and situations in which desire to smoke is strongest
- Willingness to quit
- Prior quit attempts:
  - Methods used
  - Duration of abstinence
  - Triggers for failure

Physical Exam

Examine patient for any of the known morbidities associated with smoking (e.g., include problems listed in risk factors section and in the associated conditions section).

TESTS

Imaging

Studies are currently underway to evaluate benefits and risks of screening chest CTs in heavy smokers.

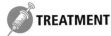 **TREATMENT**

GENERAL MEASURES

- U.S. Public Health Service: 5A's:
  - **A**sk about use:
    - Vital sign every visit
    - Current, former, never
  - **A**dvise the patient to quit:
    - Personalize the message to address risks that are most important to the patient.
  - **A**ssess patient's willingness to quit:
    - If yes, provide assistance and referral.
    - If no, conduct brief motivation intervention.
  - **A**id the patient in quitting: STAR plan:
    - **S**et date
    - **T**ell friends, family and co-workers
    - **A**nticipate challenges
    - **R**emove tobacco products
  - **A**rrange follow-up
- Counseling:
  - It has been demonstrated that the combination of counseling plus pharmacotherapy is most effective in achieving smoking cessation.
  - Counseling may be in group or individual.
  - For pregnant women it is usually preferable to focus on counseling and to avoid pharmacotherapy.

SPECIAL THERAPY

Complementary and Alternative Therapies

Little evidence of effectiveness:

- Hypnosis
- Acupuncture

MEDICATION (DRUGS)

- Preferable to avoid any medications during pregnancy unless necessary
- For women who are not pregnant, pharmacotherapy may include:
  - Nicotine replacement:
    - Nicotine patch, gum, nasal spray, lozenge, inhaler
  - Bupropion:
    - Contraindicated in patients with seizure disorders, a history of anorexia nervosa or bulimia, or patient taking MAO inhibitor in previous 14 days

 FOLLOW-UP

DISPOSITION

Issues for Referral

- Counseling plus pharmacotherapy improves abstinence results when compared with pharmacotherapy alone.
- Many health care facilities have smoking cessation programs available.

PROGNOSIS

- Most people who stop smoking will relapse at least once or more.
- If an individual relapses she should be encouraged to attempt to quit again.

PATIENT MONITORING

The 5th A in the 5 A's is **A**rrange for follow-up.

- Patients should communicate with their health care team at frequent intervals during the smoking cessation process.

BIBLIOGRAPHY

American College of Obstetricians and Gynecologists. ACOG Educational Bulletin: Smoking and women's health. American College of Obstetricians and Gynecologists. 1997;240:1–11.

A clinical practice guideline for treating tobacco use and dependence. A US public health service report. *J Am Med Assoc.* 2000;283:3244–3254.

Reichert VC, et al. Women and tobacco dependence. *Med Clin North Am.* 2004;88:1467–1481.

Seltzer V. Smoking as a risk factor in the health of women. *Int J Gynecol Obstet.* 2003;82:393–397.

 MISCELLANEOUS

CLINICAL PEARLS

To motivate women to stop smoking focus on the issues that are most important to them at their particular stage of life.

ABBREVIATIONS

- ADD—Attention deficit disorder
- DSM-IV—Diagnostic and Statistical Manual of Mental Disorders, 4th Edition
- IUGR—Intrauterine growth restriction
- MAO—Monamine oxidase
- SIDS—Sudden Infant death syndrome

CODES

ICD9-CM

305.1 Tobacco use disorder

 PATIENT TEACHING

- Counseling is an important component of successful smoking cessation and continued abstinence
- It has been demonstrated that when counseling is added to pharmacotherapy it achieves better success rates than pharmacotherapy alone
- http://www.surgeongeneral.gov/tobacco/
- http://www.smokefree.gov

PREVENTION

Because ~90% of women who smoke as adults began smoking prior to age 20, preventive efforts should be focused on children and adolescents.

TAMPONS AND MENSTRUAL HYGIENE PRODUCTS

Shibani Kanungo, MD, MPH
Hatim A. Omar, MD

 BASICS

DESCRIPTION

- Menstruation is a major stage of puberty in girls, usually starting at any age between the ages of 8 and 13.
- Women usually lose 1–4 Tbs (<80 mL) blood during normal menstrual period.
- A wide variety of menstrual hygiene products are available. They are available in 2 major categories:
  - Reusable
  - Disposable
- Menstrual hygiene products include:
  - Menstrual pads
  - Tampons
  - Menstrual cup
  - Padded panties
  - Sea sponges
  - Miniform
- Menstrual pads are used as a protective cover outside the vagina, to absorb menstrual flow; available in a wide variety of sizes, shapes, and brands.
- Maxi pads are for heavy days and mini pads or panty liners for light days:
  - With wings:
    ○ Pros: Keeps pads in place
    ○ Cons: Can abrade inner thigh
  - Without wings
  - Thong-shaped
  - Small, medium, large, hourglass shapes
  - Tube shape with straight sides
- Can be with:
  - Deodorant:
    ○ Pros: Smells good
    ○ Cons: Can cause local irritation
  - Nondeodorant:
    ○ Pros: Odor indicates vaginal infection and shouldn't be masked
    ○ Cons: No artificial smell

- Different sizes:
  - Regular maxis
  - Super maxis: Longer than standard pad for extra protection overnight or for heavy flow days
  - Thin maxis: Thinner than typical pad
  - Ultra-thin maxis: Even thinner than thin maxis; may have absorbent gel; useful for lighter-flow days
- Tampons are finger shaped devices used inside the vagina to absorb menstrual flow, are also available in a wide variety of sizes, shapes, and brands.
  - They are considered as medical devices by the FDA and require label with absorbency standards.
  - Pros:
    ○ More comfortable than pads,
    ○ Cosmetically appealing and can be worn during activities such as swimming and gymnastics
  - Cons:
    ○ Risk of TSS
    ○ Requires changing every 4–6 hours
    ○ Can cause irritation/discomfort/dryness
    ○ Learning curve for insertion and removal can cause clogging of sewer if flushed down the toilet.
    ○ Incidence of UTIs reported in 1 study to be significantly higher among tampon users than among pad users.
  - Available with a choice of applicators:
    ○ Plastic
    ○ Cardboard
    ○ Assembly required
    ○ None
  - Absorbencies as defined by FDA:
    ○ Light: ≤6 g of fluid
    ○ Regular: 6–9 g of fluid
    ○ Super: 9–12 g of fluid
    ○ Super Plus: 12–15 g of fluid
    ○ Ultra: 15–18 g of fluid

- FDA guidelines for decreasing the risk of contracting TSS:
    ○ Follow package directions for insertion
    ○ Choose the lowest absorbency for your flow
    ○ Change your tampon at least every 4–8 hours
    ○ Consider alternating pads with tampons
    ○ Don't use tampons between periods
    ○ Avoid tampon usage overnight when sleeping
    ○ Know the warning signs of TSS such as fever with chills, vomiting, diarrhea, dizziness
- Menstrual cup is a barrier, either inverted bell shape or diaphragmlike device, to collect menstrual fluid.
  - Pros:
    ○ Economical
    ○ Can be worn for 12 hours
    ○ Environmentally friendly
    ○ Comes in different sizes
  - Cons:
    ○ User must wash hands prior to use
    ○ Can be messy
    ○ Can leak
    ○ Needs proper cleaning and storage
    ○ Risk of TSS not well established, as product is not widely used
- Padded panties have washable absorbent pads, are economical, preferred alternative for allergies to synthetic materials used in disposable pads.
  - Not frequently used in US
- Sea sponges are ancient practical alternative to absorb menstrual flow
  - Pros:
    ○ Cost effective
    ○ Intravaginal absorbent
    ○ Environmentally friendly
    ○ Easy to use
  - Cons:
    ○ User needs to wash hands prior to use
    ○ Need to boil prior to use
    ○ Can leak and be messy
    ○ Risk of TSS not well established, as product is not widely used
    ○ Needs proper cleaning and storage

- Miniform is a small pad designed to fit between the labia minora.
  - Pros:
    - Small size
    - Discrete
    - For light days or tampon backup
    - Risk of TSS not well established, as product is not widely used
    - Company is exploring use for incontinence, and as a diagnostic testing mechanism for HPV
  - Cons:
    - Absorbs small amount of fluid
    - May be displaced during movement
    - Needs frequent changing
    - Costly
    - Not widely available

Pediatric Considerations

- Choice of menstrual hygiene products is a matter of personal preference, and many young adolescents choose to learn to use tampons even with the 1st menstrual period.
- For more information on TSS and or menstrual TSS see Septic Shock and Toxic Shock Syndrome.

BIBLIOGRAPHY

Omar HA, et al. Tampon use in young women. *J Pediat Adolesc Gynecol.* 1998;11(3):143–146.

The Museum of Menstruation and Women's Health. http://www.mum.org

The Tampon Safety and Research Act of 1999, H. R. 890, U.S.A. U.S. Food and Drug Administration. March-April 2000.

MISCELLANEOUS

ABBREVIATIONS

- FDA—U.S. Food and Drug Administration
- TSS—Toxic Shock Syndrome

PATIENT TEACHING

- Many girls are interested in using tampons from the onset of menarche.
- Mothers or other family may be concerned about tampons affecting virginity:
  - Reassurance
  - Assurances of normalcy

- Inability to use tampons:
  - Anxiety and vaginismus vs. hymenal abnormality
  - A guide to 1st tampon use at http://www.youngwomenshealth.org
  - Wikihow:
    - How to know when you're ready to star using a tampon at: http://www.wikihow.com/Know-when-You%27re-Ready-to-Start-Using-a-Tampon
    - How to use a tampon at: http://www.wikihow.com/Use-a-Tampon/

PREVENTION

- Imperforate hymen should be noted in delivery room or neonatal nursery.
- Hymenal variants and abnormalities should be detected by primary clinician in prepubertal years.

Section III

THYROID DISEASE

Adetokunbo Dawodu, MD
Susan R. Rose, MD

BASICS

DESCRIPTION
- Autoimmune thyroid disease:
  – Hashimoto thyroiditis
  – Graves disease
- Classification based on clinical effect:
  – Hypothyroidism:
    ○ Hashimoto thyroiditis
    ○ SAT
    ○ Postpartum thyroiditis; other thyroiditis
    ○ Postablative/post-thyroidectomy
    ○ Hypopituitarism or hypothalamic disease
    ○ Lithium
  – Thyrotoxicosis:
    ○ Graves disease
    ○ Toxic multinodular goiter
    ○ Thyrotoxicosis factitia
    ○ Gestational transient thyrotoxicosis
    ○ Thyrotoxicosis in trophoblastic disease
    ○ TSH-secreting pituitary adenoma
    ○ Pituitary resistance to thyroid hormone
    ○ Autonomous hyperfunctioning adenoma
    ○ Iodine induced thyrotoxicosis.
    ○ Struma ovarii
    ○ Amiodarone
  – Others:
    ○ Thyroid nodule
    ○ Thyroid carcinoma
    ○ Multinodular goiter
    ○ Sick euthyroid syndrome

Age-Related Factors
- Autoimmune thyroiditis:
  – Incidence increases with age
  – Mean age at diagnosis is 60 years.
  – 1.4–14 per 1,000/yr at ages 20–25 and 75–80 years.
- Graves disease:
  – Peak occurrence is in the 4th to 6th decade of life, also at puberty.
- SAT:
  – Common in women 40–50 years old.

Pediatric Considerations
- Maternal hypothyroidism in pregnancy may adversely affect neurologic development in fetus.
- Thyrotoxicosis in pregnancy is associated with preeclampsia and LBW.
- Neonatal hyperthyroidism is due to maternal transplacental transfer of TSH receptor-stimulating antibodies, not to maternal thyroid function.
- Hyperthyroidism may be initially misdiagnosed as ADHD. Check TFT when in doubt.

Pregnancy Considerations
- Poor control of underlying thyroid disease in pregnancy will lead to fetal complications.
- hCG is a weak thyroid stimulator, with thyrotoxicosis depending on hCG levels:
  – Subclinical hyperthyroidism in 10–20% of normal pregnant women
  – Hyperemesis gravidarum
  – Trophoblastic hyperthyroidism
- Hypothyroid pregnant patient may require 50% dose increment to maintain normal TSH

- Maternal complications of Graves disease:
  – Heart failure
  – Thyroid storm
  – Eclampsia

Geriatric Considerations
- Hyperthyroidism in the elderly may present with atrial fibrillation, confusion, dementia, agitation, anxiety, and congestive heart failure.
- Hypothyroidism is a significant cause of HTN in women >70 years.

EPIDEMIOLOGY
- Women are the highest risk population:
  – Prevalence of hypothyroidism is 0.8/100 population in the US with 95% being women
  – Autoimmune thyroiditis most common
  – Female > Male (5:1)
  – Mean incidence in women: 3.5/1,000 women/yr
  – 10% of 50-year-old women: Autoimmune thyroiditis
- Graves disease:
  – Female > Male (5–10 times)
  – Prevalence in US: 1.2/100, 88% are women
- SAT:
  – Female > Male (6:3)
- Thyroid neoplasia:
  – 0.4% of all cancer deaths
  – Thyroid cancer: 4–6.5% of all thyroid nodules.
- Postpartum thyroiditis:
  – 5–10% of pregnancies

RISK FACTORS
- Autoimmune thyroid disease:
  – Iodine and iodine-containing drugs
  – Age; prevalence increases with age
  – Irradiation
  – Exogenous cytokines given therapeutically (e.g., interferon alfa)
- Hypothyroidism:
  – Lithium therapy
  – Postpartum thyroiditis
  – Stress, post puberty, pregnancy
  – *Yersinia* infection
  – Smoking
- Thyroid neoplasm:
  – Hashimoto thyroiditis
- Subacute thyroiditis:
  – Infection
- Multinodular goiter:
  – Iodine deficiency
  – Hashimoto thyroiditis

Genetics
- Family history of autoimmune disease
- Association with HLA DR3 and CTLA4 gene in both Graves and Hashimoto disease.
- Postpartum thyroiditis has a weak association with HLA DR5.

PATHOPHYSIOLOGY
- Hashimoto disease: Infiltration of the thyroid by lymphocytes with destruction of thyroid follicular cells:
  – Hypothyroid
  – Euthyroid
  – Transient thyrotoxicosis in Hashitoxicosis

- Graves disease:
  – Stimulation of the thyroid by circulating antibodies to TSH receptor (TSHR-ab) mimicking TSH
  – Nonhomogeneous lymphocytic infiltration with hyperplasia and hypertrophy of follicles
  – Production of TSHR-ab leads to hyperthyroidism, goiter +/− orbitopathy

ASSOCIATED CONDITIONS
- Autoimmune thyroid disease may be seen in:
  – Insulin-dependent diabetes mellitus
  – ITP +/− pernicious anemia
  – Myasthenia gravis
  – Rheumatoid arthritis
  – Vitiligo
  – Autoimmune adrenal insufficiency
  – SLE
  – Autoimmune polyglandular syndrome type 2
  – Syndromes: Down, Turner, Noonan
- Medullary thyroid cancer:
  – Adrenal pheochromocytoma + parathyroid hyperplasia (MEN 2A), less often (MEN 2B)

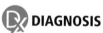

DIAGNOSIS

SIGNS AND SYMPTOMS
- Symptoms of hypothyroidism:
  – Fatigue, increased need for sleep, weight gain, hair loss, depression, cold intolerance, concentration decline, myalgia, new-onset constipation, muscle cramps, fatigue, irregular menses, galactorrhea, amenorrhea
  – May complain of neck swelling: Painless in Hashimoto or painful in subacute thyroiditis
- Symptoms of thyrotoxicosis:
  – Nervousness, fatigue, emotional lability, dyspnea, palpitation, increased appetite, diarrhea, weight loss, heat intolerance, sweating, oligomenorrhea, amenorrhea, infertility
  – Graves hyperthyroidism: Goiter, eye complaints (photophobia, tearing, retrobulbar pain)
- Neck swelling only:
  – Thyroid nodule
  – Multinodular goiter

History
- Fever, chills, or other systemic signs consistent with acute thyroiditis
- Medication history is important.
- History of autoimmunity in patient and family
- Recent pregnancy, exposure to iodine excess, recent thyroid surgery, or radioiodine treatments
- History of radiation exposure to head and neck in childhood, rapid growth, obstructive symptoms, dysphagia suggests malignancy
- Family history of cancers: Thyroid, pheochromocytoma

Physical Exam
- Hypothyroidism:
  – Skin is pale, yellowish, dry, and thick.
  – Hair is dull, coarse, and brittle.
  – Face may be edematous, eyelids puffy, supraclavicular fullness.
  – Nervous system: Decreased deep tendon reflexes with slow relaxation phase, Hashimoto encephalopathy
  – CVS: Bradycardia, diastolic hypertension, narrow pulse pressure

- Goiter:
  - Variable size
  - Firm, rubbery, with irregular surface; painless in Hashimoto
  - In SAT. goiter is painful
- Thyrotoxicosis:
  - Skin:
    - Warm, velvety, and moist.
    - Palmar erythema +/− nail changes in long-standing Graves.
    - Pretibial myxedema, thyroid acropachy
    - Hair is friable.
  - CVS:
    - Resting tachycardia, systolic murmur related to mitral valve prolapse, arrhythmias, signs of heart failure, A fib or flutter in elderly
  - Nervous system:
    - Fine distal tremor, brisk tendon reflex, shortened relaxation phase, clonus
    - Thyrotoxic neuropathy: Areflexic flaccid quadriparesis, acute psychosis
  - Variable thyroid enlargement:
    - Symmetrical, firm and rubbery, +/− bruit
  - Graves ophthalmopathy is variable: Exophthalmus, lid lag, lid retraction, chemosis.
  - Thyroid nodule: Note texture of lesion, fixation to structures, cord paralysis, enlarged lymph node

TESTS
Lab
- Thyrotoxicosis:
  - Low or undetectable TSH, Elevated FT4, T4, and T3
- TSHR ab is positive in Graves disease.
- Positive anti-TPO ab in Hashimoto
- Note elevated T4 seen in pregnancy, OCP, and chronic liver disease due to increased TBG
- Hypothyroidism:
  - Elevated TSH, low T4
- Normal thyroid function in multinodular goiter, thyroid nodule
- Subacute thyroiditis, postpartum thyroiditis may show biochemical hypothyroidism or hyperthyroidism
  - ESR is high in subacute thyroiditis

Imaging
- Radioactive iodine uptake to differentiate SAT, factitious thyrotoxicosis, amiodarone-induced thyrotoxicosis
- Thyroid US to evaluate thyroid nodules
- FNAB to be considered in multinodular goiter and thyroid nodules

DIFFERENTIAL DIAGNOSIS
- Thyroid disease can affect all organ systems.
- Depending on severity, may mimic unrelated disorder.

Infection
- Respiratory illness/COPD
- Conjunctivitis

Hematologic
- Thrombocytopenia
- Pernicious anemia

Metabolic/Endocrine
- CHF
- Prolactinoma
- Chronic renal insufficiency
- Nephrotic states

Tumor/Malignancy
Treatment of malignant tumors or hepatitis C or B with IL2 or interferon-α can lead to thyroid dysfunction.

Trauma
Trauma to neck may present as subacute thyroiditis.

Drugs
- Agents that inhibit thyroid hormone synthesis and secretion:
  - Lithium
  - Sulfonamides
  - Ethionamide
  - Ketoconazole
  - Sulfonylureas
  - Gabapentin
- Amiodarone-induced thyrotoxicosis

Other/Miscellaneous
- Parkinson disease
- Patients with neuropsychiatric illness may present with transient abnormalities in thyroid function.

 TREATMENT

SPECIAL THERAPY
Radioiodine therapy (Graves disease, multinodular goiter):
- Transient exacerbation of thyrotoxicosis post treatment
- Contraindicated in pregnant women
- Ophthalmopathy may develop and may require treatment with steroids

Complementary and Alternative Therapies
- Graves disease:
  - Iodine and iodine-containing compounds
  - Lugol's Iodine, SSKI is useful presurgery or in severe thyrotoxicosis
- Endemic goiter:
  - Iodine, or iodine plus thyroxine

MEDICATION (DRUGS)
- Graves disease +/− multinodular goiter if indicated:
  - Thioamides: Propylthiouracil, methimazole
  - β-Adrenergic antagonist drugs
- Hashimoto thyroiditis:
  - Thyroxine:
    - Start at a low dose and gradually increase for tolerance.
- Silent and postpartum thyroiditis:
  - Usually transient; hypo/hyperthyroid symptoms may require treatment.

SURGERY
Thyroidectomy:
- Thyrotoxicosis (Graves and other hot nodules)
- Establish diagnosis of mass after nonconclusive FNAB
- Treat benign/malignant tumors
- Remove large goiter
- Alleviate pressure
- Multinodular goiter if radioiodine not feasible
- MEN 2A

 FOLLOW-UP

DISPOSITION
Issues for Referral
- Graves ophthalmopathy
- Thyroid nodule

PROGNOSIS
- Postpartum thyroiditis: 70% recover but 30% develop permanent hypothyroidism.
- Graves disease: 30–40% have remission after medical therapy for 2 years.

- Hashimoto thyroiditis: 20% will have disappearance of antibodies.

PATIENT MONITORING
- Patients with subclinical autoimmune thyroiditis should be monitored yearly.
- During childhood, monitor at least every 6 months (infancy to 3 years, every 3 months)
- MEN 2A: Calcitonin and urinary catecholamine should be monitored.

BIBLIOGRAPHY

AACE. Medical guidelines for clinical practice for the evaluation and treatment of hyperthyroidism and hypothyroidism. *Endocr Pract.* 2002;8(6):457–469.

AACE and Associazione Medici Endocrinologi. Medical guidelines for clinical practice for the diagnosis and management of thyroid nodules. *Endocr Pract.* 2006;12(1):63–102.

Rose SR, et al. Update of newborn screening and therapy for congenital hypothyroidism. *Pediatrics.* 2006;117(6):2290–2303.

 MISCELLANEOUS

- Hypothyroid patient may need increased replacement if on certain medications:
  - Sucralfate, aluminum hydroxide, ferrous sulphate, Tegretol.
- Decrease dose in end-stage renal disease

CLINICAL PEARLS
In nonthyroidal illness, serum hormones are low but metabolism is normal:
- Low T4, low T3, TSH is normal/suppressed, RT3 is elevated.

ABBREVIATIONS
- CHF—Congestive heart failure
- SAT—Subacute thyroiditis
- TSH—Thyroid-stimulating hormone
- LBW—Low birth weight
- ADHD—Attention deficit-hyperactivity disorder
- TFT—Thyroid function tests
- hCG—Human chorionic gonadotropin
- ITP—Idiopathic thrombocytopenia
- SLE—Systemic lupus erythematosus
- T4/T3—Thyroxine/Triiodothyronine
- OCP—Oral contraceptive pill
- TBG—Thyroid binding globulin
- FNAB—Fine needle aspiration biopsy

CODES
ICD9-CM
- 193 Malignant neoplasm of thyroid gland
- 226 Benign neoplasm of thyroid glands
- 242.0 Toxic diffuse goiter, Graves disease
- 241 Nontoxic nodular goiter, thyroid nodule
- 243 Congenital hypothyroidism
- 245.2 Hashimoto thyroiditis
- 246.2 Cyst of thyroid
- 242.8 Thyrotoxicosis of other specified origin
- 246.9 Unspecified disorder of thyroid
- 648.1 Thyroid dysfunction
- V77.0 Thyroid disorders

Section IV
Common Pregnancy Signs and Systoms

ADVANCED MATERNAL AGE

Melissa Snyder Mancuso, MD
Marjorie Greenfield, MD

BASICS

DESCRIPTION
- No universal definition exists for advanced maternal age because many age-related risks, such as infertility, miscarriage, and chromosomal abnormalities, increase slowly starting at the youngest ages and continue to rise with time.
- 35 years was originally chosen as the maternal age at which to recommend genetic amniocentesis because at age 35 the chance of trisomy 21 (Down syndrome) was felt to equal the risk of the amniocentesis causing a miscarriage. The risks of miscarriage from amniocentesis are now lower than was previously believed.
- Most sources use 35 years as the definition of advanced maternal age.

EPIDEMIOLOGY
- The age-specific birth rate for women ages 35–39 was 45.4 per 1,000 in 2004.
- The percentage of all pregnancies represented by women >35 is ~14% and is expected to rise, given the increase in later marriage, 2nd marriage, availability of better contraception, and number of women delaying childbearing secondary to career or education.

PATHOPHYSIOLOGY
- The greatest risks to the older gravida are determined by coincident medical conditions.
- Karyotype analyses from pregnancies in women >35 show a higher incidence of aneuploidy compared with pregnancies in younger women. The age-related incidence of chromosomal nondisjunction during the 2nd phase of meiosis leads to a greater chance of abnormal chromosome number in the developing oocyte:
  - The chance of any major chromosomal abnormality for mothers at age 35 is 1 in 204 live births
  - At age 40, the risk increases to 1 in 65 live births.

ASSOCIATED CONDITIONS
Potential confounding factors to the relationship between advancing maternal age and obstetric outcomes include:
- Race
- Parity
- BMI
- Level of education
- Coexisting medical problems:
  - Diabetes
  - Cardiac disease
  - HTN
  - Renal compromise
  - Thyroid dysfunction

DIAGNOSIS

SIGNS AND SYMPTOMS
History
- For all women who at their expected delivery dates will be ≥35:
- Past medical history: Older women are more likely to have developed medical problems, including heart, kidney, and thyroid disease; obesity; HTN; and diabetes, which can complicate pregnancy and require more intense prenatal surveillance.
- Past gynecologic history: Fibroids, infertility treatment, and prior gynecologic surgery can affect pregnancy outcome.
- Past obstetric history: The best predictors of obstetric complications are prior obstetric events.
- Medications: Pay close attention to medications taken by these mothers. Some that are contraindicated in pregnancy include:
  - Lipid-lowering agents
  - Some psychotropic medications
  - Some antihypertensives

Physical Exam
The routine 1st prenatal physical exam is adequate for caring for the mature gravida.
- Pay close attention to blood pressure, given increased risk of hypertensive disorders at older ages.
- Fundal height/uterine size may be increased due to fibroids.

TESTS
- In addition to standard prenatal laboratory evaluation, routine 2nd trimester genetic amniocentesis should be offered to all women of advanced maternal age.
- Depending on risk assessment (see below), 1st trimester chorionic villus sampling may be suggested.
- Decisions about accepting genetic testing are personal, based on values, acceptance of risks, and what the parents would do if confronted with an abnormal result.
- Genetic counseling, if accessible, can help parents sort through the different available approaches.

Lab
Multiple markers screen for genetic abnormalities:
- 1st trimester:
  - Serum free hCG and PAPP-A can be used to estimate the risk of a chromosomal abnormality in the fetus. Some mothers found to be at increased risk choose to have 1st trimester chorionic villus sampling rather than wait for 2nd trimester amniocentesis.
- 2nd trimester:
  - Maternal serum AFP, hCG, uE3, and inhibin A can be used to estimate the risk of certain chromosomal abnormalities and NTDs after 15 completed weeks of gestation.
- Some protocols for screening include individual, sequential, or combined use of the 1st and 2nd trimester multiple marker tests.

Imaging
- If available, 1st trimester US evaluation of fetal nuchal translucency can be offered to refine the estimate of the risk of Down syndrome. Some mothers found to be at increased risk choose to have 1st trimester chorionic villus sampling rather than wait for 2nd trimester amniocentesis.
- 2nd trimester level 2 US can also help to detect anatomic evidence of chromosomal anomalies in mothers who decline routine amniocentesis.

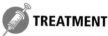

TREATMENT

GENERAL MEASURES
Women with singleton pregnancies who will be ≥35 at time of delivery should be offered prenatal diagnosis and formal genetic counseling.

PREGNANCY-SPECIFIC ISSUES
Risks for Mother
Women of advanced maternal age are at increased risk for a variety of maternal and pregnancy-related conditions when compared with younger women:
- Spontaneous abortion
- Ectopic pregnancy
- Hypertensive disorders
- Gestational DM
- Placental abruption
- Placenta previa
- Stillbirth
- Dysfunctional labor
- Cesarean delivery
- Maternal mortality

Risks for Fetus
Compared to offspring of younger mothers, the fetus of a mother >35 is at risk for:
- 1st and 2nd trimester miscarriage
- Chromosomal abnormalities
- Congenital malformations
- Perinatal morbidity and mortality

FOLLOW-UP

- Coincident medical problems and genetic risk assessment dictate whether follow-up needs to be different from routine prenatal care.
- The rise in perinatal morbidity and mortality in relation to maternal age cannot be fully explained by the increased frequency of medical problems at older ages.
- In the absence of medical problems or pregnancy complications, the recommended guidelines for fetal surveillance and induction of labor for older gravidas are no different than those for younger women.

DISPOSITION
Issues for Referral
Women with singleton pregnancies who will be ≥35 at delivery should be offered prenatal genetic diagnosis. These women should be referred for formal genetic counseling if available.

BIBLIOGRAPHY

Cleary-Goldman J, et al. Impact of maternal age on obstetric outcome. *Obstet Gynecol*. 2005;105: 983–990.

Gabbe S, et al., eds. *Obstetrics: Normal and Problem Pregnancies*, 4th ed. Philadelphia: Churchill Livingstone; 2002.

Jacobsson B, et al. Advanced maternal age and adverse perinatal outcome. *Obstet Gynecol*. 2004;104:727–733.

 MISCELLANEOUS

SYNONYM(S)
Elderly Primigravida or Multigravida

ABBREVIATIONS
- AFP—α-Fetoprotein
- hCG—Human chorionic gonadotropin
- NTD—Neural tube defect
- PAPP-A—Pregnancy-associated plasma protein A
- uE3—Unconjugated estriol
- US—Ultrasound

CODES
ICD9-CM
- 659.50 Elderly Primigravida
- 659.60 Elderly Multigravida

 PATIENT TEACHING

- Women who will be ≥35 at delivery may benefit from tracking fetal movement in the late 3rd trimester.

- Several approaches to fetal movement tracking have been validated:
  - Once daily method: The woman counts distinct fetal movements at a time of the day when her baby tends to be active. Perception of 10 distinct movements in a period of up to 2 hours is considered reassuring.
  - T.i.d. method: Women are instructed to count fetal movements for 1 hour 3 times per day. The count is considered reassuring if it equals or exceeds the woman's previously established baseline count. >5 movements is generally considered reassuring.
- If the fetal movements have not met criteria, the woman is instructed to call her doctor/midwife.

PREVENTION
- Women who are ≥35 should be offered contraception if desired. Hormonal contraceptives are generally acceptable for healthy, nonsmokers >35.
- Preconception counseling offers the opportunity to discuss individualized risks, as well as to perform testing such as cystic fibrosis screening. To decrease the risks of NTDs, preconception folate supplementation is indicated for all women who plan to or are at risk for becoming pregnant.

Section IV

ANEMIA IN PREGNANCY

Kellie Rath, MD

BASICS

DESCRIPTION
- Most commonly, anemia in pregnancy is physiologic.
- Reduction below normal in the mass of RBCs:
  - Measured by ≥ 1 of the major RBC components:
    - Hgb: Concentration of the major oxygen carrying component in whole blood
    - Hct: % volume of whole blood occupied by intact RBCs
  - RBC count: RBCs contained in a volume of whole blood
  - Adult nonpregnant female:
    - Hgb <12 g/dL or Hct <37%
  - Adult pregnant female:
    - 1st trimester Hgb <11 g/dL
    - 2nd trimester Hgb <10.5 g/dL
- Hgb/Hct depends on oxygen pressure:
  - Increased in neonates and people living above 4,000 feet
- Hgb, Hct, and RBC count are concentrations:
  - Dependent on RBC mass and plasma volume
  - Values decrease if RBC mass decreases or plasma volume increases

EPIDEMIOLOGY
Prevalence varies worldwide:
- 2–20% in developed countries
- 40–80% in developing countries

RISK FACTORS
- Socioeconomic factors:
  - Lower socioeconomic status
  - Young maternal age; prevalence of anemia decreases with increasing maternal age to 35
  - Race
  - Lower education
  - Unmarried
  - Late prenatal care
  - Substance use (alcohol, tobacco)
- Medical conditions:
  - Hemoglobinopathies
  - Cardiac
  - Renal
  - Pulmonary

PATHOPHYSIOLOGY
- Most commonly, anemia in pregnancy is physiologic:
  - Increased plasma volume exceeds the increase in red cell mass.
  - Total blood volume increases 40–50%.
  - Red cells mass increases 25%.
  - Plasma volume increases 50%.

- Iron deficiency:
  - Increased requirement in pregnancy to 1 g
  - 360 mg fetus and placenta
  - 450 mg RBC mass expansion
  - 200 mg vaginal delivery
  - 1 mg/d lactation
- Folate deficiency:
  - Increased folate requirement; $\sim$2 times the amount required in nonpregnant state
- Vitamin B_{12} deficiency:
  - Rare
  - Pernicious anemia, gastric bypass, colonic resection

DIAGNOSIS

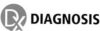

SIGNS AND SYMPTOMS
Physical Exam
- Depends on:
  - Rapidity of onset:
    - Hypovolemia if acute
    - Asymptomatic if mild and chronic
  - Underlying disease
  - Severity and type of anemia
- Decreased oxygen delivery to tissues:
  - Fatigue
  - Decreased exercise intolerance
  - Tachypnea
- Rectal exam can detect low-lying polyps:
  - Fecal occult blood testing; 3 times using take-home cards
  - In-office testing for occult blood is not recommended

Review of Systems
- Cardiovascular:
  - Dyspnea on exertion
  - Chest pain/angina
  - Syncope
  - Tachycardia, cardiomegaly, murmurs
  - Postural hypotension
- Dermatologic:
  - Skin:
    - Cool
    - Pallor
    - Jaundice
    - Purpura
    - Telangiectasia
  - Spoon-shaped nails (koilonychia)
- CNS:
  - Neuropathy
  - Altered mental status

TESTS
Labs
- CBC
- RBC indices:
  - MCV (normal: 80–100 μm^3)
  - MCH (normal: 27–34 pg/cell)
  - MCHC (normal: 33–36%)
- Iron studies
- Folate
- Hemoglobin electrophoresis
- Reticulocyte count:
  - Normal 0.5–1.5% (reticulocytes/1,000 RBCs)
  - Increased retic count: Increased erythropoietic response to continued blood loss or hemolysis
  - Stable anemia with low retic count: Impaired RBC production
  - Active hemolysis or blood loss with low retic count: Concurrent disorder
  - Low retic count with pancytopenia: Aplastic anemia
  - Low retic count with normal WBC and platelets: Pure RBC aplasia
- RI = reticulocyte count (%) $\times$ (patient Hct/normal Hct):
  - RI <2% implies inadequate RBC production
  - RI >2% implies increased RBC production with excessive RBC destruction or loss
- Stool for occult blood:
  - Fecal occult blood testing with take-home cards, testing on 3 samples
  - In-office testing is not recommended, as sensitivity of single stool sample is not adequate.
- Renal panel
- UA:
  - Hematuria
  - Hemoglobinuria in hemolytic anemia
- Specialized testing may be required to diagnose uncommon causes of anemia.

DIFFERENTIAL DIAGNOSIS
- Most common causes:
  - Physiologic anemia of pregnancy
  - Iron-deficiency anemia
- Less common or rare:
  - Megaloblastic:
    - Folic acid deficiency
    - Vitamin B_{12} deficiency
  - Chronic disease:
    - Chronic renal disuse (EPO deficiency)
    - Pyelonephritis
  - Hemoglobinopathies:
    - Sickle cell disease
    - Thalassemias
  - Hemolytic anemias:
    - Acquired (autoimmune, drug-induced, paroxysmal nocturnal hemoglobinuria)
    - Genetic (hereditary spherocytosis, red cell enzyme defects)

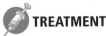

TREATMENT

GENERAL MEASURES
- Based on cause of anemia
- Balanced diet important to ensure proper nutrition, as common anemias of pregnancy are related to nutrition.
- No benefit to iron prophylaxis; only treat if truly anemic

PREGNANCY-SPECIFIC ISSUES
Risks for Fetus
- Untreated maternal iron deficiency anemia may lead to:
  - Preterm delivery
  - Low-birth-weight infant
- Untreated maternal anemia does not lead to fetal anemia.

MEDICATION (DRUGS)
- Iron deficiency:
  - $FeSO_4$ 300 mg PO t.i.d.
  - Investigate underlying cause
  - Increase Hgb expected in 2–3 weeks
- Folate deficiency:
  - Folic acid 1 mg/d PO
- Vitamin B_{12} deficiency:
  - B_{12} 1,000 μg/d IM for 1 week, then weekly for 1 month, then monthly
- Renal failure:
  - Endogenous erythropoietin is diminished.
  - Replace with recombinant erythropoietin
- Autoimmune hemolytic anemia:
  - Corticosteroids (prednisone 60 mg/d until response)
  - Immunosuppressive agents
  - Plasmapheresis
  - Splenectomy if splenic sequestration
- Drug-induced hemolytic anemia: Stop offending agent

- Anemia of chronic disease:
  - Treat underlying disease:
    - Hematologic parameters normalize within 2 months.
    - Neurologic symptoms present >6 months may be permanent.
- Aplastic anemia:
  - Antithymocyte globulin
  - Bone marrow transplantation
- Sickle cell anemia:
  - Supportive care with oxygen, rehydration, analgesia
  - Treat precipitating cause

FOLLOW-UP

DISPOSITION
Issues for Referral
- Underlying medical condition causing anemia
- Underlying hematologic condition causing anemia
- Concern of possible need for bone marrow biopsy to establish diagnosis
- Nutritional deficiency (dietary counseling)

Admission Criteria
- Unstable vital signs
- Ongoing blood loss
- Symptomatic anemia: Angina/Dyspnea/Syncope
- Pancytopenia
- Need for transfusion
- Need for aggressive evaluation

Discharge Criteria
Discharge vast majority of stable patients for outpatient workup.

PATIENT MONITORING
Mother
- Monitor for resolution of signs/symptoms of anemia after treatment
- Proper nutrition

Fetus
- May need to monitor fetal heart rate if viable fetus and severe symptomatic maternal anemia
- Growth scans

BIBLIOGRAPHY

Adebisi OY, et al. Anemia in pregnancy and race in the United States: Blacks at risk. *Fam Med.* 2005;37(9): 655–62.

Cunningham et al. *Williams Obstetrics,* 22nd ed. New York: McGraw-Hill; 2005.

Gabbe SG, et al. *Obstetrics: Normal and Problem Pregnancies,* 4th ed. Philadelphia: Churchill-Livingstone; 2002.

MISCELLANEOUS

CLINICAL PEARLS
- Pica has been associated with anemia.
- If patient is taking iron regularly, rectal exam will reveal dark stool.
- Regular iron use can be associated with constipation; thus, attention to dietary fiber and fluid intake is important.

ABBREVIATIONS
- Hct—Hemocrit
- Hgb—Hemoglobin
- MCH—Mean corpuscular hemoglobin
- MCHC—Mean corpuscular hemoglobin concentration
- MCV—Mean corpuscular volume
- RI—Reticulocyte index

CODES
ICD9-CM
648.2 Anemia

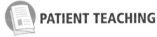

PATIENT TEACHING

- Encourage proper nutrition.
- Educate on risk factors for anemia.
- Educate on risk to fetus with untreated anemia.
- ACOG Patient Education Pamphlet: Nutrition During Pregnancy

Section IV

ANTEPARTUM FETAL TESTING

Barak M. Rosenn, MD

BASICS

DESCRIPTION
- The ultimate purpose of AFT is to prevent fetal demise. Additionally, AFT is utilized in an attempt to identify fetal compromise and allow intervention before it results in neonatal morbidity.
- There is, however, no compelling evidence from RCTs that such testing does indeed decrease the risk of fetal death.
- Nevertheless, AFT has been widely integrated into clinical practice throughout the world due to the wealth of observational and circumstantial evidence pointing to its association with improved pregnancy outcome.

Indications
Indications for AFT are not based on firm scientific evidence. Generally, AFT is employed when maternal or fetal circumstances are associated with an increased risk of fetal compromise and death. Some of the more common indications for AFT are:

- Maternal indications:
  - HTN
  - Diabetes
  - Autoimmune disease
  - Renal disease
  - Antiphospholipid syndrome
  - Poorly controlled thyroid disease
  - Hemoglobinopathy
  - Cyanotic heart disease
  - Advanced maternal age
- Fetal indications:
  - Poor fetal growth
  - Post term pregnancy
  - Decreased fetal movements
  - Oligohydramnios
  - Polyhydramnios
  - Multiple gestation
  - Fetal isoimmunization
  - Fetal cardiac anomaly
  - Fetal single umbilical artery

Concurrent Procedures
AFT may include >1 testing modality.

EPIDEMIOLOGY
- The percentage of pregnancies evaluated with AFT depends on the population—whether high-risk or routine obstetric—as well as the site and clinicians' clinical judgments.
- 1 report found that AFT occurred in <1% of pregnancies in the early 1970s, but had increased to 15% by the mid-1980s.

PATHOPHYSIOLOGY
Fetal hypoxemia and acidosis may result from extrinsic factors (placental dysfunction, maternal hypoxemia, etc.) or intrinsic factors (fetal cardiac failure, severe fetal anemia, etc.). Fetal hypoxia and acidosis may manifest in several ways that constitute the basis for AFT:

- Decreased fetal activity
- Redistribution of fetal blood flow resulting in decreased renal perfusion and oligohydramnios
- Loss of the normal autonomic regulation of fetal heart rate patterns
- Abnormal fetal heart rate patterns in response to uterine contractions

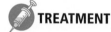

TREATMENT

PROCEDURE
AFT has several different modes:
- NST:
  - The patient is placed in the left lateral or semireclining position:
  - An external transducer is placed on the abdomen to register fetal heart beats and another transducer to register uterine contractions.
  - A reactive tracing is defined as:
    - Baseline 120–160 bpm
    - At least 2 accelerations that peak ≥15 bpm above baseline and last at least 15 seconds from baseline to baseline in a 20-minute period.
    - Absence of decelerations (except short sporadic variable decelerations lasting <30 seconds each)
    - The NST may need to be continued for a longer period due to the fetal sleep cycle.
    - Acoustic stimulation using an artificial larynx may be applied to wake the fetus and shorten the test time. A stimulus of 1–3 seconds is applied to the maternal abdomen up to 3 times.
    - A Cochrane review found that vibroacoustic stimulation offers benefits by decreasing the incidence of nonreactive antenatal cardiotocography tests and reducing the testing time.
    - The NPV of a reactive NST for fetal demise within 1 week is 99.8%.
  - If the NST does not meet criteria for reactivity, it is defined as a nonreactive NST:
    - The NST may be nonreactive in 50% of fetuses from 24–28 weeks.
    - The NST may be nonreactive in 15% of fetuses from 28–32 weeks.
    - Accelerations peaking at 10 bpm above baseline may be considered sufficient for determining reactivity in fetuses up to 34 weeks' gestation.
    - The PPV of a nonreactive NST for predicting fetal compromise is >30–40%.

- BPP:
  - The BPP is a physiologic assessment of the fetus that consists of 5 components:
    - NST
    - Amniotic fluid assessment (at least 1 vertical pocket of fluid measuring ≥2 cm)
    - Fetal breathing movements (≥1 episodes of breathing movements lasting at least 30 seconds within a 30-minute period)
    - Fetal movements (at least 3 body or limb movements within a 30-minute period)
    - Fetal tone (≥1 episodes of extension/flexion of an extremity or opening/closing of hand)
  - Each component receives 2 points if present or normal, 0 points if absent or abnormal.
    - A score of 8 or 10 is normal.
    - A score of 6 is equivocal.
    - A score of 4 or less is abnormal.
    - The BPP is abnormal if the largest vertical pocket of fluid is <2 cm.
    - The NPV of a normal BPP for stillbirth within 1 week is >99.9%.
  - The modified BPP consists of NST and AFI:
    - A reactive NST with an AFI of ≥5 cm constitute a normal modified BPP.
    - The NPV of a normal modified BPP is >99.9%.
  - A Cochrane review found insufficient evidence from RCTs to evaluate BPP as a test of fetal well-being.
- CST:
  - The CST documents fetal response to uterine contractions. During contractions, a transient decrease in uterine perfusion and fetal oxygenation occurs. Under this stress, the compromised fetus will have fetal heart pattern changes indicative of hypoxia.
    - The patient is placed in the left lateral or semireclining position.
    - A low-dose oxytocin drip is administered to achieve at least 3 contractions in a 10-minute period, each lasting at least 40 seconds.
    - Alternatively, maternal nipple stimulation can be used (the mother rubs the nipple for 2 minutes through her clothing) to attain uterine contractions.
    - The CST is negative when no late decelerations and no variable decelerations occur (excluding mild variable decelerations).
    - The CST is positive if late decelerations occur following ≥50% of the contractions.
    - The CST is equivocal when intermittent late decelerations or significant variable decelerations occur.
    - The CST is unsatisfactory when <3 contractions occur in a 10-minute period.
    - The NPV of a negative CST for stillbirth within 1 week is >99.9%.
    - A positive CST has a PPV of <35%.

- Doppler velocimetry:
  - Fetal arterial Doppler velocimetry measures flow in fetal vessels and is used to assess resistance downstream of the insonated vessel.
    - Umbilical artery velocimetry reflects resistance in the placenta.
    - Abnormal waveforms in the umbilical artery may reflect increased placental resistance, leading to placental dysfunction and fetal compromise.
    - Decreased diastolic flow in the umbilical artery, particularly AEDF or REDF, is associated with poor fetal outcome.
    - Fetal Doppler velocimetry is useful in situations of fetal growth restriction.
    - There is no benefit in using Doppler velocimetry in situations other than fetal growth restriction.
- Fetal movement monitoring:
  - Normal fetal movements are usually a sign of fetal health. A decrease in fetal movements or absent fetal movements will often occur in the compromised fetus prior to fetal demise. Therefore, maternal perception of fetal movements is a useful method of antenatal fetal surveillance.
  - There are various protocols of fetal movement monitoring:
    - The mother reclines or lies on her side and counts fetal movements. ≥10 movements in a period of up to 2 hours is considered reassuring.
    - The mother reclines or lies on her side and counts movements. If 4–5 movements are felt within <1 hour, the test is reassuring.
    - The mother counts movements for 1 hour 3 times a week. If the number of movements counted declines, further testing is warranted.
  - A Cochrane review found better compliance with the "count to 10" method, but concluded that more research was needed before incorporation in practice.

MANAGEMENT

- Initiation, timing, and frequency of AFT, as well as the response to abnormal test results, depend on many clinical factors:
  - Underlying maternal disease or fetal condition, gestational age, degree of abnormality of the test

- Extrinsic factors affecting test results (such as maternal medications, transient maternal hypoxia or acidosis)
- Given the high false-positive rates of all testing methods, abnormal AFT results should be interpreted within their clinical context, and an attempt should be made to establish their significance with additional testing.
- Timing and frequency:
  - Under most circumstances, AFT is started at 32–34 weeks.
  - In more extreme cases, AFT may begin as early as 26 weeks.
  - If there is no evidence of fetal compromise or significant maternal disease, AFT may be performed once a week.
  - Significant maternal disease or fetal compromise warrant AFT twice a week and daily surveillance of fetal movements.
  - In the postterm pregnancy, AFT should be performed twice a week and should include assessment of amniotic fluid volume.
- Abnormal AFT results:
  - A nonreactive NST should be followed by a BPP.
  - The BPP will be normal and the CST will be negative in up to 90% of patients following a nonreactive NST.
  - Decreased fetal movements should be followed by a NST or BPP.
  - An equivocal BPP (score of 6) in a term fetus is best followed by admission for delivery.
  - An equivocal BPP in a preterm infant should be repeated within 24 hours.
  - A BPP of ≤4 should prompt delivery.
  - AEDF or REDF on fetal Doppler velocimetry of the umbilical artery should prompt delivery or very close fetal surveillance.
  - Oligohydramnios requires either close fetal surveillance or, in the term fetus, initiation of delivery.

BIBLIOGRAPHY

ACOG Practice Bulletin 9. Antepartum fetal surveillance. October 1999.

Alfirevic. Biophysical profile for fetal assessment in high risk pregnancies. *Cochrane Database Sys Rev.* 2007.

Mangesi MMT. Fetal movement counting for assessment of fetal wellbeing. *Cochrane Database Sys Rev.* 2007.

 MISCELLANEOUS

SYNONYM(S)
Antipartum fetal surveillance

ABBREVIATIONS
- AEDF—Absent end diastolic flow
- AFI—Amniotic fluid index
- AFT—Antenatal fetal testing
- BPP—Biophysical profile
- CST—Contraction stress test
- HTN—Hypertension
- NPV—Negative predictive value
- NST—Non-stress test
- PPV—Positive predictive value
- RCT—Randomized clinical trials
- REDF—Reverse end diastolic flow

CODES

ICD9-CM
- 590.20 CST
- 590.25 NST
- 768.18 BPP with NST
- 768.19 BPP without NST
- 768.20 Doppler of fetal umbilical artery

Section IV

BACKACHE IN PREGNANCY
Donna Mazloomdoost, MD

 BASICS

DESCRIPTION
- Pain experienced in the back
- May be described as:
  - Cramps
  - Ache
  - Sharp pain
- Common musculoskeletal back and pelvic girdle pain increases with advancing pregnancy and can interfere with work, daily activities, and sleep.

EPIDEMIOLOGY
- 1/2 to perhaps >2/3 of all pregnant women will experience some back pain.
- Almost 1/5 experience pelvic girdle pain.

RISK FACTORS
Although discomfort in the back may be normal in pregnancy, several risk factors do exist:
- Prior back injury
- History of muscular disorder
- Improper posture
- Excess activity
- Obesity

Genetics
Although there may be some genetic component to chronic back pain, no definitive genetic predisposition to pregnancy-related back pain is known.

PATHOPHYSIOLOGY
Most back pain in pregnancy is related to 3 factors:
- Normal weight gain in pregnancy
- Exaggerated lordosis
- Hormonal changes in pregnancy with increasing joint laxity

ASSOCIATED CONDITIONS
Pelvic girdle pain including pubic symphysis

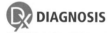 DIAGNOSIS

SIGNS AND SYMPTOMS
History
Elicit the following history:
- Onset:
  - Pre-existing prior to pregnancy
- Duration
- Severity
- Alleviating/Aggravating factors

Physical Exam
Important components of the physical exam:
- Check vital signs:
  - Particularly for fever
- Pulmonary/Cardiovascular exam
- Evaluate for costovertebral angle tenderness
- Musculoskeletal exam:
  - Palpate over the location of pain:
    ○ Common pregnancy musculoskeletal back pain is lumbar or sacroiliac in location.
- Neurologic exam
- Pelvic exam:
  - Concentrate on cervical exam

TESTS
Lab
Standard laboratory tests:
- UA:
  - Possible urine culture and sensitivity
- CBC:
  - Attention to WBC
- Consider ESR or CRP

Imaging
Imaging is typically avoided for the evaluation of back pain in pregnancy. If severe, may consider:
- US evaluation of kidneys
- MRI
- X-ray imaging provides little information with unnecessary radiation exposure to fetus and patient.

DIFFERENTIAL DIAGNOSIS
Infection
- Pyelonephritis
- Complicated UTI
- Meningitis
- Chorioamnionitis

Hematologic
Although very unlikely to be the cause, consider:
- Hemolytic uremic syndrome

Metabolic/Endocrine
- Vitamin D deficiency has been associated with chronic low back pain.
- In a diabetic patient, consider:
  - Diabetic ketoacidosis

Immunologic
Other rare causes of back pain:
- MS
- SLE

Tumor/Malignancy
Rare causes of back pain in pregnancy:
- Bone metastasis
- Leukemia/Lymphoma

Trauma
In a patient who may have suffered trauma such as motor vehicle accident, physical attack, or fall, consider:
- Placental abruption

Drugs
In a patient abusing illicit drugs, consider:
- Placental abruption in cocaine use
- Infection in IV drug use

Other/Miscellaneous
- Musculoskeletal:
  - Degenerative disk disease
  - Osteoarthritis
  - Tumor
- Obstetric:
  - Preterm or term labor
  - Placental abruption
- Neurologic:
  - Sciatica
  - Cauda equina syndrome
  - Tumor

Pediatric/Adolescent Considerations
- In adolescent populations, may need to consider:
  - Spondylolysis
  - Spondylolisthesis
  - Scoliosis
  - Osteomas
  - Sickle cell disease

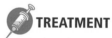 TREATMENT

GENERAL MEASURES
General treatment options for back pain include:
- Acetaminophen PRN (and sparingly)
- Heat therapy
- Physical therapy
- Exercise
- Activity modification
- Maternity back and abdominal support brace
- Physical therapy as indicated

- A Cochrane review found that for women with low-back pain, the following were beneficial in reducing pain intensity and back pain—related sick leave (although studies had moderate to high potential for bias):
  – Participating in strengthening exercises
  – Sitting pelvic tilt exercises
  – Water gymnastics
  – Acupuncture and stabilizing exercises relieved pelvic pain more than routine prenatal care.
  – Acupuncture showed better results compared to physiotherapy.

PREGNANCY-SPECIFIC ISSUES
In pregnancy, it is particularly important to:
- Avoid NSAIDs (especially 3rd trimester)
- Avoid heavy lifting
- Avoid high heel shoes, which increase the lumbar lordosis

By Trimester
- 1st trimester:
  – Consider miscarriage
- 2nd trimester:
  – Consider infectious causes
- 3rd trimester:
  – Consider preterm labor
  – Consider placental abruption

Risks for Mother
If no early intervention regarding activity, serious muscular and permanent injury may ensue.

Risks for Fetus
If preterm labor or abruption are not recognized, it may have significant consequences for fetus.

MEDICATION (DRUGS)
Avoid prescribing NSAIDs or narcotics. If patient requires more acetaminophen, consider referral to specialist in orthopedics or musculoskeletal medicine.

SURGERY
Surgery is reserved for extreme cases of disk disease, tumor, or neurologic problems. Should this be necessary, referral to a specialist is required.

 FOLLOW-UP

May need to have patient follow-up weekly if pain is severe to ensure a serious condition is not missed.

DISPOSITION
Issues for Referral
Referral to a specialist is necessary if:
- Pain is severe and not managed by conservative therapy
- Suspicion of malignancy or neurologic issue
- Consideration of physical therapy

PATIENT MONITORING
Patient monitoring is individualized and depends on diagnosis.

BIBLIOGRAPHY

Hayden JA, et al. Meta-analysis: Exercise therapy for nonspecific low back pain. *Ann Intern Med*. 2005;142:765.

Klutcher J, et al. Neurologic disorders complicating pregnancy. Available at: www.uptodate.com.

Nigrovic P, et al. Overview of the causes of back pain in children and adolescents. Available at: www.uptodate.com.

Pennick VE, et al. Interventions for preventing and treating pelvic and back pain in pregnancy. *Cochrane Database Syst Rev*. 2007;18(2):CD001139.

Runmarker B, et al. Pregnancy is associated with a lower risk of onset and a better prognosis in multiple sclerosis. *Brain*. 1995;118(Pt1):253.

Van der VG, et al. The effect of exercise on percentile rank aerobic capacity, pain, and self-rated disability in patients with chronic low-back pain: A retrospective chart review. *Arch Phys Med Rehabil*. 2000;81:1457.

Van Tulder MW, et al. Exercise therapy for low back pain. *Cochrane Database Syst Rev*. 2000; CD000335.

 MISCELLANEOUS

ABBREVIATIONS
- CBC—Complete blood count
- MS—Multiple sclerosis
- NSAIDs—Nonsteroidal anti-inflammatory drugs
- SLE—Systemic lupus erythematosus
- UA—Urinalysis
- UTI—Urinary tract infection

CODES
ICD9-CM
648 (requires 5th digit) Conditions complicating pregnancy

PATIENT TEACHING

Important to reassure patients that pain will improve and is unlikely to be associated with serious condition.

PREVENTION
While it has been suggested that back pain may be prevented with the following measures, a Cochrane review failed to find studies supporting these measures, although individuals may find them useful:
- Strength training prior to pregnancy
- Mild exercise (as deemed by the physician) early in pregnancy

Section IV

CONSTIPATION

Paula J. Adams Hillard, MD

 BASICS

DESCRIPTION
Constipation is defined for research as <3 bowel movements per week. Typically, stools are hard, small, and difficult to eliminate. It is a common symptom in pregnancy.

EPIDEMIOLOGY
Constipation occurs in ~1/3 of all pregnant women.

RISK FACTORS
Inadequate dietary fiber intake

PATHOPHYSIOLOGY
- Little change in GI secretion or absorption
- High levels of progesterone in pregnancy are likely responsible for decreased bowel motility.
- Decrease in small bowel transit time in 2nd and 3rd trimester compared with postpartum.
- Colonic transit times also slower:
  - Progesterone inhibits both amplitude and frequency of spontaneous colon muscle activity.
  - Decreased plasma concentration of motilin (a stimulatory GI hormone), possibly due to progesterone's inhibit of motilin release
- Gravid uterus may mechanically slow small bowel transit, particularly in 2nd and 3rd trimester.

ASSOCIATED CONDITIONS
Hemorrhoids, which may be symptomatic with itching, discomfort, or bleeding

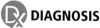 **DIAGNOSIS**

SIGNS AND SYMPTOMS
History
- Assess frequency, character of stools.
- Assess evacuation habits.
- Assess discomfort or pain.

Physical Exam
- Abdominal pain
- Rectal exam:
  - Presence of hemorrhoids

TESTS
Lab testing is not required.

DIFFERENTIAL DIAGNOSIS
- IBS (see chapter)
- Other conditions as listed in IBS

Metabolic/Endocrine
Hypothyroidism

Drugs
Iron, typically found in prenatal vitamins, is constipating for many women.

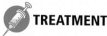 **TREATMENT**

GENERAL MEASURES
Dietary changes are most useful:
- Additional fiber, including fresh fruits and vegetables
- Hydration
- Avoidance of food typically described as constipating (e.g., cheese)
- Exercise has been recommended to prevent constipation, although in 1 study, there was no difference in rates of constipation between light, moderate, and vigorous physical activity.

PREGNANCY-SPECIFIC ISSUES
By Trimester
- Constipation may initially become bothersome in the 1st trimester:
  - Initiation of prenatal vitamins
  - High progesterone levels
- Constipation exacerbates hemorrhoids (occurring in 30–40%), particularly during the last trimester.

Risks for Mother
Discomfort, but not medically serious, and resolves postpartum

MEDICATION (DRUGS)

- Bulk-forming agents containing fiber (Metamucil) are the safest drugs to use; they are not absorbed systemically.
- Laxatives should be avoided if possible:
  - Anthraquinone laxatives are commonly reported to be contraindicated in pregnancy, although evidence for this lack of safety is not established.
  - Cassia senna (Senna) is frequently used in pregnancy and postpartum, and is Pregnancy Category C.
  - Castor oil is Pregnancy Category X; it may stimulate uterine contractions.
  - Milk of Magnesia can cause sodium retention.
  - Mineral oil can interfere with absorption of fat-soluble vitamins.
  - Stimulant laxatives, lactulose, sorbitol, and glycerine, if required

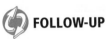 **FOLLOW-UP**

Typically, constipation resolves after delivery. This can be assessed at the postpartum visit.

DISPOSITION
Issues for Referral
If symptoms are severe, referral to a gastroenterologist may be indicated.

BIBLIOGRAPHY

Bianco A. Maternal gastrointestinal tract adaptation to pregnancy. Available at: UpToDate http://www.utdol.com. Accessed 09/23/07.

Derbyshire E, et al. Diet, physical inactivity and the prevalence of constipation throughout and after pregnancy. *Matern Child Nutr.* 2006;2(3):127–134.

 MISCELLANEOUS

CLINICAL PEARLS
Women presenting with constipation rarely have hypothyroidism as a cause, although women with hypothyroidism may present with constipation.

ABBREVIATION
IBS—Irritable bowel syndrome

 CODES
ICD9-CM
- 564.0 Constipation
- 648.8 Other specified complications of pregnancy

PATIENT TEACHING

- Up-To-Date Patient Information: Constipation in adults at http://patients.uptodate.com/topic.asp?file=digestiv/5719
- UK National Health Service patient information at http://cks.library.nhs.uk/patient˙information_leaflet/constipation

PREVENTION
- Attention to dietary fiber with bran, fruits, and vegetables
- Fiber supplement if needed
- Adequate fluid intake
- Adequate exercise

Section IV

DERMATOLOGIC CONCERNS OF PREGNANCY

Amy E. Derrow, MD
Debra Breneman, MD

 BASICS

- 2 conditions—PUPPP and PG—are unique to pregnancy. 1 is common, and will be seen by most obstetricians; the other is rare.
- PUPPP:
  - Polymorphic eruption of pregnancy
  - Toxic erythema of pregnancy
- PG:
  - Herpes gestationis
  - Gestational pemphigoid

DESCRIPTION

- PUPPP is the most common dermatosis of pregnancy. It is a benign, self-limited skin condition that poses no known risk to the mother or fetus.
- PG is a rare autoimmune blistering dermatosis of pregnancy. The clinical findings and course are variable and pose no known risk to the mother. Premature delivery and small-for-gestational-age infants have rarely been associated with PG.

EPIDEMIOLOGY

- PUPPP: Incidence is estimated to be between 1 in 130 and 1 in 300 pregnancies.
- PG: Incidence is estimated at 1 in 50,000 pregnancies.

RISK FACTORS

- PUPPP:
  - Primigravidas
  - Multiple gestation pregnancy (debated)
- PG:
  - A previous diagnosis of PG, since the condition frequently recurs with subsequent pregnancies and occasionally with re-onset of menses and the use of oral contraceptives.

Genetics

- Rare familial cases of PUPPP have been reported but no isolated identifiable genetic cause is known to date.
- With PG, an increased association with HLA-DR3 and DR4 is present.

PATHOPHYSIOLOGY

- PUPPP: The etiology is unknown but proposed hypotheses include:
  - Rapid abdominal wall distention causing connective tissue damage and triggering an inflammatory response
  - Dermal fibroblast proliferation secondary to unknown substance secreted by placenta in the 3rd trimester
- PG:
  - PG is caused by an IgG antibody that induces C3 complement deposition along the dermal–epidermal junction.
  - Activation of complement leads to chemoattraction of eosinophils and subsequent degranulation, leading to dissolution of the dermal–epidermal junction.

ASSOCIATED CONDITIONS

- PUPPP: None
- PG:
  - Hydatidiform mole
  - Choriocarcinoma
  - Grave's disease and other autoimmune diseases

 DIAGNOSIS

SIGNS AND SYMPTOMS

History

- PUPPP:
  - Pruritic, erythematous, papular eruption that classically begins in the abdominal striae and then spreads over a few days to involve the thighs, buttocks, breasts, and arms.
  - Onset is typically in the 3rd trimester (mean onset, 35 weeks) and resolves within 7–10 days of delivery. The mean duration is 6 weeks.
  - The condition rarely recurs with subsequent pregnancies.
- PG:
  - Sudden onset of intensely pruritic, erythematous papules and plaques that classically start on the trunk and rapidly progress to a generalized bullous eruption. The face, mucous membranes, palms, and soles are typically spared.
  - The eruption often begins in the 2nd or 3rd trimester (mean onset, 21 weeks). Lesions may resolve later in the course of pregnancy, but can frequently flare again at the time of delivery or immediately postpartum.
  - The eruption often clears within weeks to months of delivery.

Physical Exam

- PUPPP:
  - Polymorphous, erythematous, edematous papules and plaques with occasional vesicles, purpura, and polycyclic lesions distributed within the abdominal striae and on the breasts, buttocks, and proximal extremities
  - Classic sparing of the periumbilical region, face, palms, and soles
- PG:
  - Erythematous, edematous papules, plaques and tense vesicles and bullae predominantly involving the abdomen and periumbilical region, and extending to the flexural surfaces of extremities

TESTS

Skin biopsy:

- PUPPP:
  - Reveals nonspecific findings
  - Negative direct immunofluorescence studies on perilesional skin may be necessary to differentiate from the urticarial form of PG.
- PG:
  - Skin biopsy reveals a subepidermal vesicle with a perivascular infiltrate of lymphocytes and eosinophils.
  - Direct immunofluorescence studies on perilesional skin reveal C3 +/− IgG deposition along the basement membrane zone.

DIFFERENTIAL DIAGNOSIS

Infection

- PUPPP and PG:
  - Viral exanthem:
    - Evaluate for associated systemic symptoms such as fever, sore throat, congestion, etc.
- PG:
  - Herpes zoster:
    - Evaluate for lesions in a dermatomal pattern with associated dysesthesias and consider checking a viral culture to confirm diagnosis.
  - Varicella:
    - Evaluate for grouped vesicles on erythematous bases that are usually on the trunk and are associated with systemic symptoms such as fever, cough, congestion, etc. Consider checking a viral culture to confirm diagnosis.

Immunologic

- PUPPP:
  - Consider the urticarial form of PG, which can be differentiated by a perilesional skin biopsy for direct immunofluorescence (positive result indicates PG).
- PG:
  - Other autoimmune bullous dermatoses including:
    - Bullous pemphigoid, dermatitis herpetiformis, impetigo herpetiformis, and linear IgA bullous dermatosis
    - Differentiate by direct immunofluorescence studies

Trauma

Arthropod bites:

- Evaluate for history of recent mosquito bites, flea bites, scabies infestation, etc.

Drugs
Drug exanthem:
- Perform a thorough review of the patient's medications.

Other/Miscellaneous
- PUPPP and PG:
  - Urticaria:
    - Individual lesions are randomly distributed and last <24 hours.
- PG:
  - PUPPP:
    - Urticarial papules, plaques, and rarely vesicles typically begin in the abdominal striae and spare the periumbilical region. Direct immunofluorescence studies are negative.
  - Allergic contact dermatitis:
    - Evaluate for a history of allergen exposure in a pattern that is characteristic of that allergen.

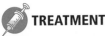 **TREATMENT**

GENERAL MEASURES
Given the benign, self-limited nature of these 2 conditions, treatment is aimed at supportive care for symptomatic relief.

PREGNANCY-SPECIFIC ISSUES
Risks for Mother and Fetus
Varies with treatment

MEDICATION (DRUGS)
- PUPPP and PG:
  - Topical doxepin
  - Topical corticosteroids
  - Oral antihistamines
  - Phototherapy (UVB)
  - Oral corticosteroids:
    - PUPPP for severe cases only
    - PG gold standard for treatment
- PG:
  - Steroid-sparing agents (note pregnancy category) such as:
    - Pregnancy Category A: Pyridoxine
    - Pregnancy Category C: Cyclosporine, dapsone

 ALERT
- Pregnancy Category D: Cyclophosphamide
- Pregnancy Category X: Methotrexate:
  - Plasmapheresis (may be added in severe cases if indicated)

 FOLLOW-UP

DISPOSITION
Issues for Referral
Dermatology: Refer for biopsy and immunofluorescence studies to distinguish PUPP from PG if necessary.

PATIENT MONITORING
Mother
PUPPP and PG: Varies with treatment

Fetus
- PUPPP: Varies with treatment
- PG: A milder, self-limited form of neonatal PG occurs in up to 10% of cases and rarely has been associated with prematurity and a tendency for small-for-gestational-age infants.

BIBLIOGRAPHY

Ambros-Rudolph, et al. The specific dermatoses of pregnancy revisited and reclassified: Results of a retrospective two-center study on 505 pregnant patients. *J Am Acad Dermatol*. 2006;54:395–404.

Aronson IK, et al. Pruritic urticarial papules and plaques of pregnancy: Clinical and immunopathologic observations in 57 patients. *J Am Acad Dermatol*. 1998;39:933–939.

Castro LA, et al. Clinical experience in pemphigoid gestationis: Report of 10 cases. *J Am Acad Dermatol*. 2006;55:823–828.

Engineer L, et al. Pemphigoid gestationis: A review. *Am J Obstet Gynecol*. 2000;183:483–491.

Kroumpouzos G, et al. Dermatoses of pregnancy. *J Am Acad Dermatol*. 2001;45:1–19.

 MISCELLANEOUS

CLINICAL PEARLS
- PUPPP:
  - Urticarial papules and plaques that initially develop in the abdominal striae during the 3rd trimester (sparing the periumbilical region).
  - Benign, self-limited course
- PG:
  - Autoimmune vesiculobullous eruption that initially develops on the abdomen and periumbilical region during the 2nd or 3rd trimester.
  - Diagnosis is confirmed by direct immunofluorescence studies.
  - Corticosteroids are the cornerstone of treatment.

ABBREVIATIONS
- PG—Pemphigoid gestationis
- PUPPP—Pruritic urticarial papules and plaques of pregnancy

CODES

ICD9-CM
646.8 Other specific complications of pregnancy

PATIENT TEACHING

PG patients should be educated about the potential risk of recurrence associated with subsequent pregnancies, re-onset of menses, and oral contraceptives.

PREVENTION
None

Section IV

ESTABLISHING ESTIMATED DATE OF DELIVERY (EDD)

Megan N. Beatty, MD

 BASICS

DEFINITION
- Duration of pregnancy is 40 weeks (280 days) from LMP or 266 days from fertilization.
- Establishing the fetus' GA is critical in managing pregnancy.
- Term pregnancy is 38–42 weeks from LMP.
- Pregnancy dating is based on the timing of earliest detection of:
  – β-Subunit of hCG, produced by the trophoblast and detectable in urine and serum after implantation, ~8–10 days after fertilization:
    ○ Current urine pregnancy tests are sensitive to 25 mIU/mL β-hCG.
    ○ Serum tests may detect 5 mIU/mL β-hCG.
  – TVUS reveals IUP with β-hCG ~1,500 mIU at ~5 wks from LMP.

EPIDEMIOLOGY
- >6 million women are diagnosed with pregnancy each year.
- Millions more seek diagnostic testing for pregnancy.

RISK FACTORS
- Unprotected intercourse
- Inconsistent/Incorrect use of contraception

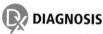 **DIAGNOSIS**

SIGNS AND SYMPTOMS
History
- Complete menstrual, sexual, contraception history
- Menstrual history:
  – LMP (NORMAL menstrual period—LNMP):
    ○ Bleeding in early pregnancy or implantation bleeding occurs in up to 20% of pregnancies.
  – Regularity of menstrual cycles
- Sexual history:
  – Number of partners
  – Recent episodes/dates of unprotected intercourse
  – Awareness of ovulation
- Contraception use:
  – Recent use of birth control or EC
  – Regularity of usage

Review of Systems
- Earliest signs and symptoms:
  – General:
    ○ Fatigue
  – Alterations in menstrual cycle:
    ○ Amenorrhea
    ○ Intermenstrual bleeding/spotting
    ○ Bleeding suddenly heavier/lighter than normal
  – GI system:
    ○ Nausea/Vomiting (especially 6–12 weeks' gestation)
    ○ Food cravings/aversions
    ○ Bloating/Constipation
    ○ Weight gain
  – GU system:
    ○ Urinary frequency/nocturia (secondary to enlarging uterus resting on the bladder)
    ○ Uterine cramping/pain
  – Musculoskeletal:
    ○ Low back pain
  – Breasts:
    ○ Tenderness
    ○ Enlargement/Heaviness
    ○ Darkening of skin around areola; 1st trimester
    ○ More prominent veins over surface

Physical Exam
- Presence of signs increases likelihood of pregnancy, but absence does not rule it out.
- Abdominal exam:
  – Uterus palpable above symphysis 12 weeks
  – At umbilicus 20 weeks
  – ~1 cm/week of gestation (e.g., 28 cm at 28 weeks)
- Vulva/Vagina:
  – Increased blood supply leads to blue-violet color of cervix (Chadwick sign) ~8–10 weeks.
- Uterus:
  – Softens (Hegar sign) ~6 weeks' gestation
  – Enlarged/Globular after 8 weeks' gestation
  – Increases by ~1 cm/wk after 4 weeks' gestation
  – Increased blood supply; uterine artery pulsation may be felt in lateral fornices on bimanual exam.
- Cervix:
  – Softens (Goodell sign) at 6 weeks' gestation
- Breasts:
  – Fullness
  – Tenderness
  – Darkening areolas
  – Increased venous patterns

TESTS
- Urine β-hCG:
  – Most common method used to confirm pregnancy
  – Identifies the β-subunit of hCG
  – Qualitative test (positive or negative)
  – Most home kits can detect hCG 25–50 mIU/mL
  – Depending on the brand, can detect 16–95% of pregnancies near the 1st day of the unexpected/missed menses
- Serum β-hCG:
  – Quantitative test (can be used to determine approximate GA in very early pregnancies)
  – Can detect as low as 5 mIU/mL
  – Sensitivity and specificity for pregnancy is between 97 and 100%.
  – False-positive occasionally seen with serum can be confirmed with urine testing.
  – Steep rise starts ~5 weeks' gestation, peaking by ~10 weeks' gestation
- Audible Doppler:
  – Can detect fetal cardiac activity audibly at 10–12 weeks' gestation

Imaging
- TVUS:
  – Can detect fetal cardiac activity as early as 5 weeks' gestation
  – Should see a gestational sac with β-hCG between 1,000 and 2,000 mIU/mL
- TAUS:
  – May detect a gestational sac by 4–5 weeks' gestation
  – Can detect fetal cardiac activity as early as 6 weeks' gestation
  – Up to 12 weeks' gestation, the crown-rump length is predictive of GA within 4 days.

DIFFERENTIAL DIAGNOSIS
- Many pregnancy symptoms are nonspecific and may be associated with a wide variety of other medical conditions.
- Amenorrhea (See Amenorrhea: Absence of Bleeding.)
- Nausea/Vomiting
- Breast symptoms (See Breast Signs and Symptoms: Breast Pain.)
- Fatigue
- Urinary frequency
- Weight gain

Infection
- Nausea/Vomiting:
  – Gastroenteritis
- Urinary frequency:
  – UTI

Metabolic/Endocrine
- Amenorrhea:
  – PCOS (See Polycystic Ovarian Syndrome.)
  – POF (See Ovarian Insufficiency (Premature Ovarian Failure).)
  – Hypo/Hyperthyroidism (See Thyroid Disease.)

Immunologic
- Amenorrhea (See Amenorrhea: Absence of Bleeding.)
- POF (See Ovarian Insufficiency (Premature Ovarian Failure).):
  – Hashimoto thyroiditis

Tumor/Malignancy
- Gestational trophoblastic disease (molar pregnancy)
- Fibroids:
  – Can be mistaken for enlarged pregnant uterus
- Ovarian mass

Drugs
- Amenorrhea (See Amenorrhea: Absence of Bleeding.):
  – Depo-Provera
  – Busulfan
  – Chlorambucil
  – Cyclophosphamide
  – Phenothiazines

Trauma
Asherman's syndrome (see topic)

Other/Miscellaneous
- Fatigue:
  - Thyroid disorders (See Thyroid Disease.)
  - Depression
  - Anemia
- Alterations in menstrual cycle:
  - PCOS
  - Thyroid/Pituitary abnormalities
  - Weight disorders (anorexia, obesity)
  - Outflow obstruction (cervical stenosis)
  - Excessive exercise
- Psychiatric disorders:
  - Pseudocyesis: Patient believes she is pregnant when she is not.
  - Anxiety can cause amenorrhea.
  - Depression can cause changes in appetite, fatigue, musculoskeletal pain.

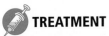 **TREATMENT**

PREGNANCY-SPECIFIC ISSUES
- Pregnancy dating is important for many reasons, including avoiding iatrogenic prematurity and appropriate management of pregnancy-related complications and conditions.
- Pregnancy dating should be based on a combination of factors from LMP and menstrual/sexual history, to physical exam, to correlation of quantitative β-hCG.
- Size > dates suggests:
  - Incorrect dating
  - Multiple pregnancy (see topic)
  - Molar pregnancy (see topic)
  - Hydramnios (see topic)
- Size < dates suggests:
  - Incorrect dating
  - IUGR (See Intrauterine Growth Restriction.)
  - Oligohydramnios (See Oligohydramnios.)
  - Intrauterine fetal demise (See Intrauterine Fetal Demise.)

By Trimester
- 1st trimester pregnancy dating is important:
  - The earlier the assessment of GA, the more accurate.
- 1st trimester issues include:
  - Ectopic pregnancy vs. spontaneous abortion

Risks for Mother
Ectopic pregnancy is the most common cause of maternal mortality in the 1st trimester. It is imperative to diagnose as quickly as possible. Discrepancies in expected rise of serum quantitative β-hCG over 48 hours aid in diagnosis (see Pregnancy-Related Conditions: Ectopic Pregnancy).

Risks for Fetus
Spontaneous abortion/miscarriage (See Pregnancy-Related Conditions: Spontaneous Abortion.)

MEDICATION (DRUGS)
Vitamins:
- Prenatal vitamins with 400 μg folic acid for all women of reproductive age
- Women with risk factors for NTDs (on seizure medications, history of precious pregnancy with NTDs) should take 4 mg/d folic acid.
- Iron sulfate supplementation for anemia

SURGERY
Planned cesarean delivery on maternal request:
- Requires accuracy of estimated GA and the calculated EDD:
  - Calculated EDD impacts the risk/benefit ratio of cesarean delivery on maternal request, as respiratory morbidity decreases in increasing GA.

 FOLLOW-UP

DISPOSITION
Issues for Referral
At the time of pregnancy diagnosis:
- Patients desiring to continue with their pregnancy should be counseled to seek prenatal care as soon as possible.
- Patients desiring to terminate their pregnancy should be referred to the proper center and counseled to seek this service as soon as possible, as the risks of abortion increase with increasing GA (see Unplanned Pregnancy and Options Counseling).

PATIENT MONITORING
- Prenatal care
- Initial evaluation:
  - Define the health status of the mother and fetus.
  - Estimate the GA of the fetus.
  - Initiate a plan for continuing obstetric care.
  - See topic on routine prenatal labs (see Prenatal Laboratory Testing, Routine).
- Measurement of fundal height with each prenatal visit correlates with appropriate fetal growth, and inappropriate growth should trigger fetal assessment.

BIBLIOGRAPHY
Bastion L, et al. Is this patient pregnant?: Can you reliably rule in or rule out early pregnancy by clinical examination? *JAMA*. 1997;278(7):586–591.

Cole L, et al. Accuracy of home pregnancy tests at the time of missed menses. *Am J Obstet Gynecol*. 2004; 190(1):100–105.

Cole LA, et al. Sensitivity of over-the counter pregnancy tests: Comparison of utility and marketing messages. *J Am Pharm Assoc*. 2005;45(5):608–615.

Cunningham F, et al, eds. *Williams Obstetrics*, 22nd ed. 2005.

Gardosi J, et al. Controlled trial of fundal height measurement plotted on customised antenatal growth charts. *Br J Obstet Gynaecol*. 1999;106(4): 309–317.

Kriebs J, et al. Ectopic pregnancy. *J Midwifery Womens Health*. 2006;51(6):431–439.

Patel M. "Rule out ectopic": Asking the right questions, getting the right answers. *Ultrasound*. 2006;22(2):87–100.

Ramoska E, et al. Reliability of patient history in determining the possibility of pregnancy. *Ann Emerg Med*. 1989;18:48–50.

Wilcox A, et al. Natural limits of pregnancy testing in relation to the expected menstrual period. *JAMA*. 2001;286(14):1759–1761.

 MISCELLANEOUS

SYNONYMS(S)
- Due date
- Estimated date of confinement (EDC)

CLINICAL PEARLS
Growth of fundal height measured from symphysis to fundus should be ~1 cm/wk of GA.

ABBREVIATIONS
- EC—Emergency contraception
- EDD—Estimated date of delivery
- GA—Gestational age
- hCG—Human chorionic gonadotropin
- IUP—Intrauterine pregnancy
- LMP—Last menstrual period
- NTD—Neural tube defect
- PCOS—Polycystic ovary syndrome
- POF—Premature ovarian failure
- TAUS—Transabdominal ultrasound
- TVUS—Transvaginal ultrasound
- UTI—Urinary tract infection

CODES
ICD9-CM
- V22 Normal Pregnancy
- V22.0 Supervision of normal 1st pregnancy
- V22.1 Supervision of other normal pregnancy
- V72.40 Pregnancy exam or test, pregnancy unconfirmed

 PATIENT TEACHING

Encourage women to record dates of menses.

PREVENTION
Prevention of unintended pregnancy and family planning:
- See topics on contraception in Section III, Women's Health and Primary Care.
- Patients should be informed that they can become pregnant during the menopausal transition, as ovulation can still occur.

EXERCISE IN NORMAL PREGNANCY

Thomas A. deHoop, MD

 BASICS

DESCRIPTION
More than ever, women are recognizing the benefits of regular exercise. The majority who continue exercise during pregnancy are motivated by the desire to achieve health benefits and maintain muscular and cardiovascular fitness. Risks and benefits to the mother and fetus should always be considered when exercise is continued in pregnancy.

EPIDEMIOLOGY
- Since Title IX legislation in 1972 (mandating equal funding of sports for males and females), participation of high school girls in after-school sports has increased 600%.
- In 1972, 1 out of 24 girls participated in high school sports; now, 1 out of 3.
- 1/4 of US women participate in regular exercise.

RISK FACTORS
Exercise in pregnancy is contraindicated for certain pregnancy conditions:
- Pregnancy-induced hypertension
- Preeclampsia
- Preterm labor
- Preterm rupture of membranes
- Incompetent cervix
- Utero-placental insufficiency
- Women at risk for IUGR
- Vaginal bleeding

PATHOPHYSIOLOGY
- Many changes occur in pregnancy and during exercise.
- Pregnancy-associated physiologic changes:
  - Increase in blood volume
  - Increase in plasma volume
  - Increase in red cell mass
  - Increase in cardiac output:
    ○ Begins at 5 weeks
    ○ Increases by 35% by week 12

- Exercise-associated physiologic changes:
  - Additional increase of 20% in blood volume and 40% in cardiac output over that associated with pregnancy alone
  - 40–50% decrease in splanchnic blood flow in nonpregnant women
  - Decrease in uterine blood flow:
    ○ Compensated by preferential shift of blood flow to the placenta
    ○ Compensated by increased oxygen extraction
    ○ Uterine blood flow decrease is 20–30% less in conditioned women.
  - Moderate exercise increases core temperature:
    ○ Theoretical concern in early pregnancy during organogenesis for possible increased risk of NTDs (seen in animal studies, not seen in humans)
    ○ By week 7, maximum maternal temperature with exercise falls by 0.3°.
    ○ Continues to fall by 0.1° per trimester
    ○ Increased blood flow improves heat dissipation.
    ○ Temperature at which sweating begins is lowered by week 7.
    ○ Increased maternal mass requires more heat to be generated to raise core temperature.
  - Fetal heart rate changes in healthy pregnancies:
    ○ Variable results
    ○ Rare episodes of bradycardia when exercising at *submaximal* levels (<70% of maximal anaerobic capacity)
    ○ Studies have demonstrated reactive fetal heart rate tracings 30 minutes after exercise.
    ○ Studies of selected (low-risk) patients have not shown a relationship to adverse fetal outcomes.
  - Miscarriage rates:
    ○ No studies confirm an increase in early pregnancy loss in women who continue to exercise during pregnancy.

ASSOCIATED CONDITIONS
- Fetal outcomes:
  - Impact on birth weight:
    ○ Inconsistent data; depends on level of prepregnancy fitness, intensity of exercise, and trimester when exercise occurred
    ○ Consistent evidence demonstrates no increase in the risk of IUGR in low-risk pregnancies.
  - Preterm labor:
    ○ No increase in preterm labor or delivery in women not already at risk
  - Apgar scores:
    ○ No negative impact identified
    ○ Some studies document improved scores.
- Maternal outcomes:
  - Fitness and well-being:
    ○ Improved in women who either start or continue exercise in pregnancy
    ○ Fewer symptoms of pregnancy such as anxiety, insomnia, somatic complaints, lowered self-image reported in regular exercisers.
  - Weight gain:
    ○ Conflicting data
  - Labor and delivery:
    ○ Conflicting data due to differences in prepregnancy fitness, exercise intensity, duration, and type
    ○ Trend toward less epidural use, shorter 2nd stage, fewer cesarean deliveries

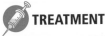 **TREATMENT**

PREGNANCY-SPECIFIC ISSUES

Risks for Mother

- Supine hypotension:
  - Compression of the vena cava in the supine position reduces venous return and therefore cardiac output.
  - Can lead to hypotension and syncope in times of increased cardiovascular demand
- Musculoskeletal injury:
  - Relative laxity of joints during pregnancy
  - Shift in center of gravity during pregnancy leads to increase risk of falls.

Risks for Fetus

Reduction in uterine blood flow

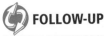 **FOLLOW-UP**

PATIENT MONITORING

Fetus

Women exercising near or above a submaximal threshold should consider antenatal testing of fetal well-being.

BIBLIOGRAPHY

Carpenter MW, et al. Fetal heart rate response to maternal exertion. *JAMA*. 1988;259:3006–3009.

Clapp JF. The changing thermal response to endurance exercise during pregnancy. *Am J Obstet Gynecol*. 1991;165:1684–1689.

Morris SN, et al. Exercise during pregnancy: A critical appraisal of the literature. *J Reprod Med*. 2005;50:181–188.

Pivarnik JM, et. al. Effects of chronic exercise on blood volume expansion and hematologic indices during pregnancy. *Obstet Gynecol*. 1994;83:265–269.

Sternfeld B, et. al. Exercise during pregnancy and pregnancy outcome. *Med Sci Sports Exercise*. 1995;27:634–640.

 MISCELLANEOUS

CLINICAL PEARLS

- Women who participate in non–weight bearing exercise are more likely to continue it longer.
- Doesn't guarantee an easier, shorter, or less painful delivery, but contributes to the overall feeling of well-being
- Women who maintain the same level of participation and diet after pregnancy as they did prior to pregnancy can expect to be near their prepregnancy weight in ~6 months.

ABBREVIATIONS

- ACOG—American College of Obstetricians and Gynecologists
- IUGR—Intrauterine growth restriction
- NTD—Neural tube defect

 PATIENT TEACHING

http://www.acog.org

PREVENTION

- Avoid activity that requires precise balance or an increased risk of falling.
- Walking is a good way for women who haven't been active to start an exercise program.
- Avoid lying flat on your back, instead elevate the right hip and tilt to the left.
- Hydrate frequently; avoid the feeling of thirst.
- Joint laxity may increase the risk of musculoskeletal injury.
- Don't try to maintain a specific level of fitness.
- Women who participate in non–weight bearing exercise (e.g., swimming) are better able to maintain that level of exercise longer into the pregnancy compared to women who participate in weight bearing exercise.
- ACOG suggests pregnant women avoid:
  - Downhill skiing
  - Contact sports
  - Scuba diving

Section IV

GENETIC SCREENING AND COUNSELING

Lee P. Shulman, MD

 BASICS

DESCRIPTION

- Perhaps no other field in obstetrics has undergone such profound changes as genetic counseling and screening.
- Initially performed to provide a numeric assessment of risk for a limited number of newborn abnormalities, genetic counseling and screening have now evolved into a process by which women and couples can choose from an array of screening and diagnostic options that empower them to learn about their pregnancy.
- The core principle of genetic counseling is nondirectiveness:
  – All counseling should be provided in a nondirective manner to ensure that the information provided to patients is free from bias and thus empowers women and couples to make decisions based on the available information and THEIR OWN moral and ethical beliefs, not those of the counselor.
  – This is a vital part of the counseling process, as the decisions made by the patient will greatly impact the patient and her family, as opposed to the counselor or other caregivers.

Pediatric Considerations
Counseling parents about the role of genetic testing to explain functional, organic, or developmental abnormalities in children is a seminal aspect of pediatric care for children with particular problems.

Geriatric Considerations
Genetic counseling and screening for inheritable cancer syndromes may be applicable to older family members to assess risk for cancer development in their offspring and family members.

RISK FACTORS
Genetics
- Counselors utilize a variety of communication and information-gathering techniques to gather information that will either determine actual risk or identify those genetic screening tests that would provide valuable information.
- Pregnancy screening tests:
  – Maternal serum screening (with and without US); hemoglobin electrophoresis for sickle cell disease and other hemoglobinopathies; cystic fibrosis; Jewish genetic disease screening
- Pregnancy genetic tests:
  – CVS, amniocentesis, PUBS
- Nonpregnancy genetic testing:
  – Inherited Thrombophilia Screening, BRCA testing for familial breast and ovarian cancer; HNPCC test for Lynch syndrome

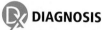 **DIAGNOSIS**

SIGNS AND SYMPTOMS
History
- A detailed history provides the foundation for all genetic counseling.
- This history should be augmented with written records whenever possible. Such records allow for arriving at a more accurate assessment of risk.
- All counseling should be done in a nondirective manner, to remove or minimize counselor-related bias from the process.
- A pedigree is usually drawn to provide a more visual tool for counselors and clinicians to review potential familial conditions. This pedigree should encompass at least 3 generations whenever possible.
- History taking also allows the counselor to communicate what tests and further information is needed from the patient to better assess the risk and determine what diagnostic testing would provide meaningful information to the patient.

Pregnancy Considerations
- Genetic counseling is a mainstay of prenatal care as it allows for the proper assessment of risk and provides invaluable information to women and couples concerning their options for prenatal detection of inherited and noninherited fetal abnormalities.
- With regard to pregnancy, genetic counseling is optimally performed prior to pregnancy to ensure that all risk assessment occurs prior to conception so that couple knows what screening and testing would be appropriate during the pregnancy.

Physical Exam
- Genetic counselors do not usually perform physical exams; however, genetics and other clinicians can examine patients to determine if physical signs are present that indicate that an individual has a particular condition or carries genes that would predispose the patient or offspring to genetic problems.
- This aspect of risk assessment is usually not a major component of prenatal counseling and screening, as the majority of these cases revolve around a risk for chromosome abnormality. However, a physical exam can provide invaluable information concerning the genetic assessment of pediatric and adult patients.

TESTS
- An increasingly important aspect of genetic counseling is the determination of appropriate genetic screening and diagnostic testing. This is becoming more challenging from the view of increasing complexity of the prenatal screening paradigms while trying to maintain the core principle of nondirective counseling.
- In many cases, several screens or tests exist to choose from; in such cases, the counselor's responsibilities lie in explaining the positive and negative aspects of the tests and encouraging the patient to choose which, if any, of the tests would best provide the information sought.
- Genetic maternal screening; most screens are offered on ethnic-specific conditions:
  – Sickle cell disease (African Americans)
  – Hemoglobin electrophoresis: Thalassemia (Mediterranean peoples), congenital hemoglobinopathies (Asia, Mediterranean, African)
  – Cystic fibrosis (Central-North Europeans)
  – Jewish genetic diseases
- Prenatal screening protocols:
  – Maternal serum screening:
    ○ Triple screen: 2nd trimester
    ○ Quad screen: 2nd trimester
    ○ Sequential screen: 1st and 2nd trimesters
  – Maternal screening:
    ○ 1st trimester: Serum analytes plus nuchal measurement
    ○ 1st and 2nd trimesters: Serum analytes plus nuchal measurement plus serum analytes in 2nd trimester
- Prenatal diagnostic testing:
  – CVS
  – Amniocentesis
  – Percutaneous umbilical sampling
- Genetic screening in gynecology/infertility:
  – Cystic fibrosis
  – Hereditary thrombophilia (e.g., factor V Leiden)
  – Genetic disease screening specific to each individual patient
- Cancer-specific testing (based on personal or family history of malignancy):
  – BRCA1/BRCA2: Breast/Ovarian cancer
  – HNPCC: Colon, breast, endometrial
  – Other testing specific to individual history of cancer

Lab

- Most genetic testing in children and adults involves obtaining a small blood sample from the patient or family member(s) to determine the presence or absence of specific gene sequences.
- Some genetic testing in cancer cases is best performed on malignant tissue.
- Lab involvement in prenatal cases can involve multiple tissue sources and more commonly evaluates chromosome complement rather than the presence or absence of gene mutations:
  - Maternal: Blood
  - Fetal: Blood (PUBS), amniotic fluid (amniocentesis), placenta (CVS)

Imaging

- US plays an increasingly important role in providing information leading to an accurate diagnosis in prenatal as well as pediatric and adult situations. Nonetheless, the application of US is not universal in non-prenatal genetic counseling and screening and is reserved for specific patients and conditions. Examples are:
  - Pediatric: Congenital renal abnormalities (Infantile polycystic kidney disease)
  - Adult: Ovarian cyst (ovarian cancer and BRCA mutations)
  - Prenatal: Pregnancy assessment

DIFFERENTIAL DIAGNOSIS

Genetic counseling and screening helps to formulate a differential diagnosis as well as to better assess the components of the differential diagnosis.

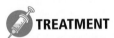 **TREATMENT**

GENERAL MEASURES

Once a diagnosis is made, genetic counseling serves to present treatment options available to the patient. In many cases, the counselor will help to facilitate further care by clinicians who can provide the medical or surgical interventions warranted.

- Pediatric: Medical, surgical, psychological, developmental (physical and occupational therapy)
- Adult: Cancer assessment, medical prevention, and intervention

PREGNANCY-SPECIFIC ISSUES

Prenatal: Medical, invasive diagnostic testing, fetal therapy, pregnancy termination

By Trimester

- 1st trimester: 1st trimester screening (nuchal translucency measurement with and without serum markers), ultrasound, CVS
- 2nd trimester: Triple screen, quad screen, sequential screening (1st and 2nd trimester), US, amniocentesis
- 3rd trimester: US

Risks for Mother

Based on particular genetic condition, although maternal risks above and beyond pregnancy are not common

Risks for Fetus

Based on particular genetic condition. Very small but finite increased risk for loss after CVS or amniocentesis.

MEDICATION (DRUGS)

Can be used in all pediatric, prenatal, and adult genetic situations to prevent or treat specific conditions. Most likely a component of pediatric and adult care.

SURGERY

Can be used in pediatric, prenatal, and adult genetic situations to prevent or treat specific conditions. Most likely a component of pediatric and adult care.

 FOLLOW-UP

- All genetic counseling sessions should be followed by a letter describing what was reviewed and what actions, if any, were taken. Frequently, a phone call will be placed to make sure that there are no further questions and to determine if the agreed-upon actions were, in fact, undertaken.
- All genetic screening results should be communicated to the referring clinician and to the patient. This is usually accomplished by a paper report, but is now increasingly accomplished by facsimile or e-mail notifications.

DISPOSITION

Issues for Referral

The detection of specific conditions may warrant referral to specialists for further evaluation, care, and intervention. Even the failure to detect a genetic abnormality may warrant referral for further evaluation and care in cases of abnormalities.

BIBLIOGRAPHY

ACOG Committee Opinion #298. Prenatal and preconceptional carrier screening for genetic disease in individuals of eastern European Jewish descent. August 2004.

ACOG Guidelines for Women's Health Care Edition 3.

ACOG Practice Bulletin #77. Screening for Fetal Chromosomal Abnormalities. January 2007.

ACOG Practice Bulletin #78. January 2007: Hemoglobinopathies in pregnancy

 MISCELLANEOUS

ABBREVIATIONS

- CVS—Chorionic villus sampling
- HNPCC—Hereditary nonpolyposis colon cancer
- PUBS—Percutaneous umbilical blood sampling

CODES
ICD9-CM

- 655.13 Known/Suspected chromosome abnormality
- 655.23 Hereditary disease history affecting fetus
- 659.53 Advanced maternal age
- V26.33 Genetic counseling

 PATIENT TEACHING

- National Society of Genetic Counselors Consumer information. Available at: www.nsgc.org
- American College of Medical Genetics. Available at: www.acmg.net
- American Society of Human Genetics. Available at: www.ashg.org

GESTATIONAL DIABETES: SCREENING AND MANAGEMENT

Barak M. Rosenn, MD

BASICS

DESCRIPTION
GDM is defined as carbohydrate intolerance that begins or is 1st recognized during pregnancy:
- GDM A1: GDM controlled with diet modification alone
- GDM A2: GDM requiring medical therapy

EPIDEMIOLOGY
- Prevalence: Varies between 2–5%
- No universal agreement on the criteria for defining GDM

RISK FACTORS
GDM parallel those for type 2 diabetes:
- Obesity
- Family history of diabetes
- Ethnicity (Hispanic, African-American, Asian)
- Advanced maternal age
- Prior GDM
- Prior LGA infant

PATHOPHYSIOLOGY
- GDM results from the physiologic increase in insulin resistance that occurs during the 2nd half of pregnancy:
  - Insulin resistance in pregnancy is believed to be due to the action of placental hormones.
  - When the maternal pancreas is incapable of producing sufficient insulin to overcome this resistance, the result is maternal hyperglycemia.
- Fetal glucose concentrations are directly related to maternal glucose concentrations.
- Maternal hyperglycemia results in fetal hyperglycemia.
- Fetal hyperglycemia leads to a variety of fetal, neonatal, and life-long complications.

ASSOCIATED CONDITIONS
- GDM is associated with maternal and fetal complications.
- Maternal complications:
  - Preeclampsia, infection, cesarean section, and birth trauma
  - At least 50% of women with GDM develop type 2 diabetes within 10–15 years.

- Fetal complications:
  - Stillbirth, excessive fetal growth, cardiac septal hypertrophy, and delayed lung maturation
- Neonatal complications:
  - Macrosomia, shoulder dystocia, hypoglycemia, hypocalcemia, hyperbilirubinemia, and hypomagnesemia:
    - For any given fetal weight, the risk of shoulder dystocia is about twice higher compared to infants of mothers without diabetes.
  - Long-term complications include an increased risk of childhood and adolescent obesity, as well as adult obesity and diabetes.

DIAGNOSIS

SIGNS AND SYMPTOMS
Physical Exam
No reliable physical findings aid in the diagnosis of GDM.

TESTS
Labs
- Glucosuria during pregnancy may be a normal finding and is not a reliable indicator of GDM.
- Screening for GDM:
  - There is considerable controversy worldwide regarding the optimal method for screening and diagnosing GDM.
  - In the US, most clinicians screen all pregnant women between 24–28 weeks' gestation.
  - GCT:
    - 50 g load of glucose
    - The GCT does not require the woman to be in the fasting state.
    - Maternal blood is drawn 1 hour after administering the GCT to determine plasma glucose concentration.
    - Using a cutoff value of 130 mg/dL plasma glucose concentration, this test has a sensitivity of 90% for identifying women with GDM.
- Diagnosis of GDM:
  - A diagnostic GTT is performed following a positive GCT.
  - The GTT consists of a 100 g glucose load administered after an overnight fast.

- Plasma glucose concentrations are determined in the fasting state and at 1, 2, and 3 hours.
- Cutoff levels are:
  - Fasting: 95 mg/dL
  - 1 hour: 180 mg/dL
  - 2 hours: 155 mg/dL
  - 3 hours: 140 mg/dL
- GDM is diagnosed when at least 2 values are at or above the cutoff levels.
- Some clinicians will establish the diagnosis of GDM when only 1 of the values is abnormal because clinical outcomes are similar to those in women with 2 abnormal values.

TREATMENT

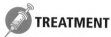

GENERAL MEASURES
- Management of women with GDM consists of frequent monitoring of blood glucose levels, modification of diet, medical therapy when necessary, monitoring of fetal growth and well-being, and planned delivery when necessary.
- Monitoring of glucose levels:
  - Self-monitoring of glucose levels by the patient is key to achieving normoglycemia:
    - Using a meter with memory, the patient should monitor herself before and 2 hours after each meal.
    - Goals of glycemic control are usually set at <95 mg/dL before meals and at <120 mg/dL 2 hours after meals with a mean glucose not exceeding 100–105 mg/dL.
  - Glucose levels should be reviewed every 1–2 weeks and modifications made in treatment if targets of control have not been achieved.
- Diet modification includes the following components:
  - Limiting the amount of carbohydrates in the diet to no more than 40% of total caloric intake (1 g of carbohydrate equals 4 Kcal)
  - Minimizing consumption of simple carbohydrates (sugars, fruit, sweets, etc.)
  - Choosing carbohydrates that are rich in fiber (whole-wheat instead of white bread, brown instead of white rice, etc.)

- Eating 3 small meals with 3 small snacks between meals and at bedtime
- Emphasizing the importance of consuming more protein and fat

PREGNANCY-SPECIFIC ISSUES
Risks for Mother
See "Associated Conditions."

Risks for Fetus
See "Associated Conditions."

MEDICATION (DRUGS)
- If the goals of glycemic control are not achieved with diet alone, the patient requires medical therapy.
- If the patient's fasting value on the GTT was abnormal, it is prudent to start medical therapy immediately in addition to diet modification.
- Oral hypoglycemic therapy:
  - Recently, the use of glyburide, a sulfonylurea oral hypoglycemic agent that does not cross the placenta, has been shown to be both efficacious and safe for use in pregnancy.
  - Providing the woman does not have an allergy to sulfa, treatment is started with 2.5 mg in the morning.
  - The dose is raised gradually every 3 days if glycemic control is not achieved: To 2.5 mg b.i.d., then 5 mg b.i.d., to a maximum of 10 mg b.i.d.
  - Modifications can be made based on the patient's individual response.
  - The importance of the snacks between meals should be emphasized in order to avoid hypoglycemia.
- Insulin therapy:
  - If glyburide is contraindicated or fails to achieve adequate control, insulin is used in split doses.
  - Several regimens are available for the administration of insulin:
    o The most commonly used regimen consists of a combination of regular (R) and intermediate acting NPH (N) insulins.
  - In the 3rd trimester, a total of 1 U insulin per kg maternal body weight is administered.

- 2/3 of the total dose is administered 1/2 hour before breakfast, consisting of 2/3 N and 1/3 R.
- The remaining 3rd of the total dose is administered in the evening: 1/2 of the evening dose administered as R insulin 1/2 hour before dinner, and the remaining 1/2 administered at bedtime as N insulin.
- The total dose should be raised by ~20% across the board every 3 days until the patient attains an adequate level of glycemic control.
- Modifications in this regimen should be made according to the patient's individual response.

 FOLLOW-UP

- Women with GDM should be tested 2–3 months postpartum to rule out abnormal glucose tolerance.
- Regular yearly follow-up should be continued to identify the development of abnormal glucose tolerance.
- Lifetime risk of DM for women with GDM is over 50%.
- Women with GDM have a 30–50% risk of developing GDM in subsequent pregnancies.

DISPOSITION
Issues for Referral
- Although many general obstetrician/gynecologists manage women with GDM, consultation with a maternal-fetal medicine specialist is advisable.
- Consultation with a nutritionist is a helpful adjunct in management.

PATIENT MONITORING
Mother
See above for glucose monitoring.

Fetus
- Sonographic evaluation of the fetus:
  - Fetal growth should be followed by US every few weeks to detect signs of diabetic fetopathy.
  - Sonographic signs of diabetic fetopathy include excessive fetal growth, excessive growth of the fetal abdomen, and septal hypertrophy.

- Most clinicians advocate antenatal fetal testing from 34 weeks onward, particularly in the presence of diabetic fetopathy.
- Poor glycemic control and diabetic fetopathy increase the risk of stillbirth.
- Timing of delivery:
  - Delivery should be timed to minimize the risks of stillbirth and shoulder dystocia while avoiding the complications of prematurity.
  - If the estimated fetal weight exceeds 4,000–4,500 g, elective caesarian delivery should be considered to avoid the risk of shoulder dystocia.
  - The newborn infant should be followed closely to detect the development of hypoglycemia and other metabolic complications.

BIBLIOGRAPHY
ACOG Practice Bulletin #30. Gestational Diabetes, 2001.

Diabetes Mellitus Complicating Pregnancy. In: Gabbe SG, et al., eds. *Obstetrics: Normal and Problem Pregnancies*, 5th ed. New York: Elsevier; 2007: 976–1010.

Langer O, ed. *The Diabetes in Pregnancy Dilemma.* University Press of America; 2006.

 MISCELLANEOUS

ABBREVIATIONS
- GCT—Glucose challenge test
- GDM—Gestational diabetes
- GTT—Glucose tolerance test
- LGA—Large for gestational age

CODES
ICD9-CM
648.83 Gestational diabetes

 PATIENT TEACHING

ACOG Patient Education Pamphlet: Diabetes and Pregnancy

PREVENTION
Weight management and exercise prior to and between pregnancies

LACTATION AND LACTATION SUPPRESSION
Ruth A. Lawrence, MD

 BASICS

DESCRIPTION
- Lactation is the production of milk by the mammary glands for the purpose of nourishing the infant from birth through weaning.
- Lactation suppression is carried out when the mother chooses not to breastfeed or the baby dies:
  - Termination of physiologic milk production
  - When a woman cannot or wishes not to breastfeed:
    - Medical contraindications to breastfeeding include HIV, HTLV, need to take radioactive compounds, or a few drugs.
    - Drugs of abuse
  - Management:
    - Firm brassiere or binder
    - Cold compresses for uncomfortable engorgement
    - Bromocriptine is not indicated.
    - The normal decline in prolactin postpartum in nonlactators occurs over 10–14 days.
    - Hormone treatment is ineffective.
    - Decreasing fluids is ineffective.

EPIDEMIOLOGY
Statistics from US CDC (2007 report from 2004 births) indicate:
- Ever breastfed: 73.8%
- Breastfed at 6 months: 41.5%
- Breastfed at 12 months: 20.9%
- Exclusive breastfeeding through 3 months: 30.5%
- Exclusive breastfeeding through 6 months: 11.3%

RISK FACTORS
- Family history of lactation failure
- Lack of family support for breastfeeding
- Lack of adequate support in the hospital
- Outside pressure in a bottle-feeding culture

Genetics
No known genetic link for lactation failure

PATHOPHYSIOLOGY
- Most women lactate spontaneously after a normal pregnancy.
- The breast responds to the hormones of pregnancy by proliferation of the ductal system and development of the alveoli, which become lined with cells that produce milk.
- The breasts increase in size, the nipples and areola become prominent.
- After 16 weeks' gestation, the breast will produce milk when the fetus and placenta are delivered.
- Breast development:
  - Asymmetric breasts
  - Tubular breasts
  - Other anatomic variations
- Postsurgical problems:
  - Augmentation
  - Reduction mammoplasty
  - Other surgical scarring

ASSOCIATED CONDITIONS
- Hormone failure
- Sheehan syndrome

 DIAGNOSIS

SIGNS AND SYMPTOMS
History
- Anatomic structure of breasts
- Presence of normal breast changes during pregnancy

Physical Exam
Observations during a feeding:
- Placement of infant at the breast: Facing mother abdomen to abdomen
- Attachment of baby to breast: Mother strokes lower lip with nipple

- Infant draws nipple and areola into mouth to form a teat.
- Infant compresses teat against hard palate.
- Peristolic motion of tongue stimulates let-down reflex.
- Let-down reflex stimulates pituitary to release oxytocin, which causes ducts to eject milk.
- Pituitary also releases prolactin to stimulate lacteal cells to continue to make milk.
- Infant swallows ejected milk.

TESTS
- Observation of milk release:
  - Swallowing of infant
  - Dripping of milk from opposite breast
- Measurement of adequate supply:
  - Weight gain (lose no >7% of birth weight)
  - Stooling at least 3 times daily in 1st month of life
  - Voiding at least 6 times daily in 1st month of life

Lab
Usually not indicated except in lactation failure

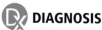 **TREATMENT**

GENERAL MEASURES
- During pregnancy:
  - Inspection of breasts to detect abnormal developments, inverted nipples
  - Breast should enlarge and nipples and areolae become more prominent.
  - No treatment is necessary, especially ointments, soaps, or exercises.
  - Inverted nipples can be everted with breast cups worn inside the brassiere the last 6 weeks of pregnancy.

- At delivery:
  – Infant should be put to breast soon after delivery (30–60 minutes) if infant is stable.
  – Breastfeeding should continue ~q2–3h.
  – Supportive care from knowledgeable staff
  – Assessment of milk production should be done prior to discharge:
    o Weight loss <7%
    o Stooling 3 times daily
    o Meconium gone by 72 hours
    o Voiding 6 times a day

PREGNANCY-SPECIFIC ISSUES
- Some women excrete a small amount of colostrum in the last few weeks of pregnancy.
- Breasts should not be massaged or pumped, as this may stimulate premature uterine contractions.

MEDICATION (DRUGS)
- When mother is medicated for concurrent conditions, consider secretion in breast milk.
- Most medications are safe, or their dosing can be modified to reduce amount that gets to the baby:
  – Information is available on common drugs.

SURGERY
Only emergency surgery should be performed on the breasts during pregnancy viz a breast abscess or a cancerous tumor.

BIBLIOGRAPHY

Breast-feeding Handbook for Physicians. American Academy of Pediatrics and the American College of Obstetricians and Gynecologists. 2006.

Hale TW. *Medications and Mothers' Milk,* 12th ed. Amarillo TX: Hale Publishing; 2006.

Lawrence RA and Lawrence RM. *Breast-feeding: A Guide for the Medical Profession,* 6th ed. Philadelphia: Elsevier-Mosby; 2005.

MISCELLANEOUS

CLINICAL PEARLS
Babies are born to breastfeed.

CODES
ICD9-CM
- V24.1 Lactating mother—supervision of lactation
- 676.4 Failure of lactation
- 676.5 Suppressed lactation
- 676.8 Other disorders of lactation—galactocele
- 676.9 Unspecified disorder of lactation

PATIENT TEACHING

- Breastfeeding Helpline. Available at: http://www.4woman.gov/Breast-feeding/index.cfm?page=ask
- Breastfeeding for Parents. Available at: La Leche League http://www.lalecheleague.org/nb.html
- ACOG Patient Education Pamphlet. Available at: http://www.acog.org/publications/patient_education/bp029.cfm
- New Mothers Guide to Breastfeeding: American Academy of Pediatrics, Joan Meek, ed., 2002.

Section IV

NUTRITION CONCERNS IN PREGNANCY

Seppideh Sami, MS, RD, LDN

 BASICS

DESCRIPTION

Pregnancy is marked by physiologic changes in the body causing symptoms that "only" occasionally warrant medical intervention. These symptoms can alter the energy and nutrient intake and needs of the pregnant woman. The most common symptoms include:

- Iron deficiency anemia (See Anemia in Pregnancy.)
- Morning sickness: Nausea and vomiting of pregnancy occurring any time during the day
- Leg cramps: Painful spasm of the calf
- Constipation: Hard stools, straining at defecation, sensation of incomplete evacuation ≥25% of the time, ≤2 bowel movements a week
- Heartburn: Irritation or burning sensation of the esophagus
- Hemorrhoids: Itching or painful mass of dilated veins in swollen anal tissue
  - Effects of iron supplements
- Pica: Abnormal craving or appetite leading to compulsive ingestion of nonfood substances

EPIDEMIOLOGY

- Iron deficiency anemia (See Anemia in Pregnancy.)
- Morning sickness:
  - 6th–12th wk gestation: ~75–80% report nausea; ~30–42% report vomiting
- Heartburn:
  - 2nd and 3rd trimesters >50% report symptoms
- Hemorrhoids:
  - Mainly during 3rd trimester, clears up after childbirth
- Leg cramps:
  - >50% occurs during 3rd trimester; ~45% report symptoms
- Constipation:
  - ~50% report symptoms
- Pica:
  - Ancient behavior
  - Regional practice; exists in some regions of southern US. Typically, observed in:
    - ○ Conjunction with poor diets due to poverty
    - ○ Women of lower socioeconomic levels
  - A deep-rooted cultural pattern, pica must be understood and treated with respect to improve chances of successful negotiation for appropriate change in behavior.

RISK FACTORS

- Any of the following factors, whether present before or during pregnancy indicate likely risk for poor nutritional status:
  - Poor eating habits/eating disorders leading to inadequate intake of fluid and essential nutrients
  - Avoidance of specific foods due to allergy or intolerance
  - Poor knowledge of good nutrition especially during pregnancy
  - Medications that interfere with nutrient absorption and metabolism
  - Nutrition-related chronic disease
  - Low hemoglobin and/or hematocrit
  - Excessive vomiting
  - Income at or below poverty level
- Note well: Symptoms listed under "Description", if not addressed/treated in a timely fashion, in conjunction with any of the factors listed above, can lead to inadequate intake and/or absorption of fluids and essential nutrients. This in turn will place the pregnant woman and her fetus at risk for specific nutrient deficiencies and poor birth outcomes.

PATHOPHYSIOLOGY

- Iron-deficiency anemia (See Anemia in Pregnancy.)
- Morning sickness:
  - Hormonal changes causing relaxation in GI muscle tone
- Leg cramps:
  - Possibly due to low serum calcium causing neuromuscular irritability
  - Magnesium deficiency has been linked to leg cramps, due to its close link to calcium metabolism
- Constipation:
  - Placental hormones relaxing the GI muscles
  - Growing uterus pressing on the intestines making elimination difficult
- Heartburn:
  - Hormonal changes causing relaxation of cardiac sphincter
  - The enlarging uterus places pressure on the diaphragm moving the gastric contents up into the esophagus and hence the burning sensation.
  - Full feeling due to gastric pressure, large meal, lack of normal space, or gas formation
- Hemorrhoids:
  - Increasing weight of the fetus and its downward pressure cause the enlargement of veins in the anus, often protruding through the anal sphincter.
  - Occasionally, these veins may rupture and bleed causing more pain and discomfort.

- Effects of iron supplements:
  - Ferrous sulfate may be given to counteract the physiologic dilution anemia of pregnancy due to the increased circulating blood volume.
- Pica:
  - Craving and consumption of nonfood substances (clay, dirt, ice, laundry starch)
  - May be indicative of iron deficiency anemia

ASSOCIATED CONDITIONS

- Iron deficiency anemia (See Anemia in Pregnancy.)
- Morning sickness:
  - Dehydration, carbohydrate depletion, metabolic disturbance, anemia
  - If untreated it may develop into hyperemesis gravidarum.
- Leg cramps:
  - Compromised sleep and ability to work
- Effects of iron supplements:
  - May cause gray/black stools, nausea, constipation or diarrhea
- Pica:
  - Inadequate nutrition due to substitution of non-food items for nutritious foods
  - Iron-deficiency anemia, zinc deficiency, constipation, lead poisoning
  - Fecal impaction due to clay ingestion

 DIAGNOSIS

SIGNS AND SYMPTOMS

History

- Typical daily food and liquid intake before pregnancy
- Past medical history review and inquiry about history of any specific condition of concern (anemia, pica, constipation, hemorrhoids, or heartburn with previous pregnancies)
- Prepregnancy weight and height
- History of herb/supplement use

Physical Exam

Typical physical observations associated with undernutrition:

- Fatigued with very low energy levels during pregnancy
- Abnormally high hair loss, dry, dull hair and eyes
- Dry, scaly skin, unhealthy color
- Cracked lips
- Poor dentition and discolored
- Swollen tongue and raw in appearance

TESTS
Anthropometrics: Current weight and weight trend during pregnancy

Labs
- Tests for iron deficiency and CBC
- Liver function tests and lipid panel
- Chemical panel 7
- Glucose test at the 3rd trimester
- Tests for pica:
  - Lymphocyte subset
  - Serum lead if lead poisoning is suspected

DIFFERENTIAL DIAGNOSIS
Hematologic
- Pica:
  - Tests for iron deficiency:
    ○ Serum: Iron, ferritin, transferrin

Other/Miscellaneous
- Current fluid and food intake
- Current meds/supplements including prenatal vitamins, additional iron, calcium, folic acid, herbal, and other supplement use

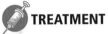 TREATMENT
GENERAL MEASURES
- Iron deficiency anemia (See Anemia in Pregnancy.)
- Morning sickness:
  - Eat dry crackers before getting out of bed.
  - Avoid high-fat foods.
  - Eat cold (vs. hot), small frequent meals, rich in fruits and complex carbohydrates.
  - Eat a high-protein bedtime snack.
  - Drink liquids between, not with, meals.
- Leg cramps:
  - Keep well hydrated.
  - Ensure adequate intakes of sodium, potassium, calcium, and magnesium; avoid foods rich in phosphorus (processed foods).
  - Magnesium lactate or magnesium citrate (with medical supervision)
- Constipation:
  - Adequate fluid intake (min 64 fl oz/d)
  - High-fiber diet (25–30 g/d using foods)
  - Regular exercise
- Heartburn:
  - Avoid spicy and acidic foods.
  - Eat small frequent meals.
  - Sit up for an hour after the meal.
- Hemorrhoids:
  - Adequate fluid intake (min 64 fl oz/d)
  - High-fiber diet (25–30 g/d using foods)
  - Regular exercise
  - Sufficient rest during the latter part of the day
- Effects of iron supplements:
  - Take iron supplement 1 hour before or 2 hours after a meal, with water or orange juice, but not with milk or tea. Iron absorption is enhanced by vitamin C-rich foods and reduced by dairy, eggs, tea, and whole-grain breads and cereal.

- Pica:
  - Appropriate eating pattern for healthy pregnancy with foods rich in iron, vitamin C, calcium, and zinc

PREGNANCY-SPECIFIC ISSUES
- Constipation:
  - Laxatives NOT recommended for treating constipation during pregnancy because they might stimulate uterine contractions and cause dehydration.
  - Mineral oils should NOT be used during pregnancy because there is an increased reduction in nutrient absorption.
- Heartburn:
  - OTC antacids not to be taken without medical supervision because some contain high levels of sodium (can cause fluid buildup in body tissues) and some may contain lead.

Risks for Mother
- General consequences of maternal malnutrition include fatigue, weakness, infections, anemia, increased risk of complications.
- Morning sickness:
  - Weight loss or inadequate weight gain
  - Complications due to dehydration and electrolyte imbalance
  - Increased risk for hospitalization
- Pica:
  - Inadequate nutrition due to substitution of nonfood items for nutritious foods
  - Iron-deficiency anemia, zinc deficiency, constipation, lead poisoning
  - Fecal impaction due to clay ingestion

Risks for Fetus
General consequences of maternal malnutrition:
- Increased risk of IUGR, prematurity and low birth weight
- Increased risk of fetal, neonatal, and infant death
- Increased risk of infection and birth defects
- Increased risk of brain damage and cretinism

 FOLLOW-UP
DISPOSITION
Issues for Referral
Refer to a registered dietitian for in-depth nutrition education and/or counseling.

PATIENT MONITORING
Mother
- General measures include food and fluid intake recall, current weight and trend, labs, physical signs
- For pica, monitor urine color (to be clear to pale yellow)

Fetus
Monitor growth and development.

BIBLIOGRAPHY
American Dietetic Association. Position of the American Dietetic Association: Nutrition and lifestyle for a healthy pregnancy outcome. *J Am Diet Assoc.* 2002;102(10):1479–1490.

American Pregnancy Association. Available at: www.americanpregnancy.org/pregnancyhealth/eatingfortwo.html. Accessed 06/01/07.

Centers for Disease Control and Prevention. Iron deficiency-United States, 1999–2000. *MMWR.* 2002;51:897–899.

Lutz C, et al. eds. Life Cycle Nutrition: Pregnancy and Lactation. In: *Nutrition & Diet Therapy: Evidence-Based Applications,* 4th ed. Philadelphia: F.A. Davis; 2006:211–212.

 MISCELLANEOUS
SYNONYM(S)
- Morning sickness:
  - Nausea, gravidarum; vomiting, emesis
- Constipation:
  - Lack of bowel movement, impaction
- Heartburn:
  - Gastric pressure or "a full feeling"
  - Acid indigestion
- Hemorrhoids:
  - Piles

ABBREVIATION
IUGR—Intrauterine growth restriction

CODES
ICD9-CM
- 648.2 Anemia
- 643.0 Morning sickness
- 729.82 Leg cramps
- 564.00 Constipation
- 787.1 Heartburn
- 671.8 Hemorrhoids
- 307.52 Pica

PATIENT TEACHING
General nutrition guidelines listed in "Treatment"

PREVENTION
- Generally appropriate eating plan for pregnancy with prenatal vitamins
- Guidelines for treatment apply to prevention also

POSTPARTUM FEVER

Cristiano Jodicke, MD

 BASICS

DESCRIPTION
- Postpartum fever or puerperal fever is defined as an oral temperature of 38°C (100.4°F) on 2 separate occasions at least 6 hours apart, or of >38.5°C (101.6°F) at any time.
- Postpartum fever is a sign that requires investigation to determine the specific etiology, which will then dictate treatment.
- Puerperal fever

EPIDEMIOLOGY
- A complication in 2–4% of vaginal deliveries
- 5–15% of scheduled cesarean deliveries
- 15–20% of unscheduled cesarean deliveries

RISK FACTORS
- Cesarean deliveries
- Membranes ruptured for >6 hours
- Multiple pelvic examinations
- Chorioamnionitis
- Increased duration of active labor
- Internal fetal monitoring
- Retained products of conception
- Multiparity
- Low socioeconomic status
- Urethral catheterization
- Previous UTI
- Operative vaginal delivery
- Obesity
- Chronic lung disease
- Smoking
- Intubation
- Nipple fissure
- Breast-feeding
- Breast engorgement
- DM
- Long operative duration
- Anemia
- Immunosuppressive therapy
- Immunodeficiency disorder
- Corticoid therapy
- Nutritional status

PATHOPHYSIOLOGY
- Pathophysiology depends on cause and site.
- Pelvic infections associated with vaginal pathogens that then lead to ascending genital tract infection
- Breast infections arise from skin flora (see Mastitis)
- Wound infections (see topics)

DIAGNOSIS

SIGNS AND SYMPTOMS
History
- Vaginal or cesarean delivery
- Premature rupture of membranes
- Pelvic pain
- Foul-smelling lochia
- Fever
- Chills
- Headache
- Malaise
- Anorexia
- Urinary system:
  - Flank pain
  - Dysuria
  - Urgency
  - Frequency
- Surgical incision/episiotomy:
  - Erythema
  - Induration
  - Drainage
  - Local pain
- Respiratory system:
  - Cough
  - Dyspnea
  - Pleuritic chest pain
- Breast:
  - Pain
  - Erythema
  - Engorgement

Physical Exam
- Vital signs:
  - Appearance; pallor
  - Temperature
  - Pulse
  - BP (with orthostatic assessment)
  - Pulse oximetry
- Pulmonary exam:
  - Rales
  - Rhonchi
  - Consolidation
- Back:
  - Costovertebral angle tenderness
- Breast (generally unilateral):
  - Erythema
  - Tenderness
  - Engorgement
- Abdomen:
  - Bowel sounds
  - Fundal tenderness
  - Generalized abdomen, lower abdomen, or suprapubic tenderness
  - Wound:
    - Erythema
    - Local tenderness
    - Induration
    - Discharge
- Pelvic exam:
  - Uterine tenderness
  - Adnexal/Parametrial tenderness
  - Foul-smelling lochia
  - Palpable mass
  - Palpable pelvic veins (rare)

TESTS
Lab
- CBC with differential
- UA with culture and sensitivity test
- Wound cultures
- Blood cultures:
  - Septicemia
  - Refractory to routine antibiotics
- Cervical or uterine cultures

Imaging
- Pelvic US
- CT
- MRI

DIFFERENTIAL DIAGNOSIS
Infection
- Endometritis
- UTI
- Mastitis
- Pneumonia
- Wound infection:
  - Abdominal (cesarean or postpartum sterilization) incision
  - Episiotomy
- Pelvic abscess
- Appendicitis

Hematologic
- Thrombophlebitis
- DVT
- PE
- Septic pelvic vein thrombosis

Metabolic/Endocrine
Thyroiditis

Drugs
Drug fever

Other/Miscellaneous
Atelectasis

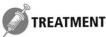 **TREATMENT**

GENERAL MEASURES
- Fluid management
- Cardiac monitoring
- Oxygen therapy, if necessary
- Assess for signs of septic shock or septicemia.
- Rule out intra-abdominal bleeding or wound hematoma.

PREGNANCY-SPECIFIC ISSUES
- Endometritis:
  - Parenteral broad-spectrum antibiotics: IV treatment until 24–48 hours afebrile. Continuing treatment with oral antibiotics is not necessary.
    o Clindamycin/Gentamicin (Ampicillin is added if enterococcal infection is suspected or if no improvement occurs by 48 hours.)
    o Clindamycin/Aztreonam
    o Metronidazole/Penicillin
    o Ampicillin/Gentamicin/Metronidazole
- Mastitis:
  - Local measures:
    o Ice packs
    o Analgesics
  - Antibiotics:
    o Dicloxacillin
    o Nafcillin
    o Vancomycin (penicillin allergy)
    o Surgical drainage (local abscesses)
- UTI:
  - Hydration
  - Antibiotic treatment
- Wound infection:
  - Drainage
  - Debridement
  - Irrigation
  - Broad-spectrum antibiotics
- Pneumonia:
  - Antibiotic treatment
  - Adequate oxygenation
  - Analgesia
- Atelectasis:
  - Adequate oxygenation
  - Reexpansion of the lung segments
  - Analgesia
  - Early ambulation
- Pelvic abscess:
  - Drainage
  - Broad-spectrum antibiotics
- Septic pelvic thrombophlebitis:
  - Broad-spectrum antibiotics
  - Anticoagulation

MEDICATION (DRUGS)
Choice of antibiotic therapy is dictated by source of infection and likely pathogenic organisms:
- Clindamycin 900 mg IV q8h
- Gentamicin 1.5 mg/Kg q8h or 5 mg/Kg q24h
- Ampicillin 2g IV q6h
- Metronidazole 500 mg PO/IV q6h
- Cefotetan 1–2 g IV q12h
- Cephalexin 500 mg PO q6h over 10–14 days
- Dicloxacillin 500 mg PO q6h
- Nafcillin 2g IV q4h
- Vancomycin 1g IV q12h

SURGERY
- Wound exploration and probing at bedside
- Wound infection/seroma/infected hematoma that result in open incision should be assessed for possible wound closure.
- If evidence of fascial dehiscence, surgical repair is required as emergency procedure (See Wound Dehiscence and Disruption.).

 FOLLOW-UP

All patients with a postpartum fever should undergo follow-up with an obstetrician/gynecologist, but ideally with the delivering obstetrician.

BIBLIOGRAPHY

Bonnar J. Venous thromboembolism and pregnancy. *Clin Obstet Gynecol*. 1981;8:455–473.

Chaim W, et al. Prevalence and clinical significance of postpartum endometritis and wound infection. *Infect Dis Obstet Gynecol*. 2000;8(2):77–82.

Cunningham FG, et al. Infections and disorders of the puerperium. In: *William's Obstetrics*, 20th ed. New York: McGraw-Hill; 1997:547–568.

Filker R, et al. The significance of temperature during the first 24 hours postpartum. *Obstet Gynecol*. 1979;53:358–361.

Gabbe SG. Puerperal endometritis, serious sequelae of puerperal infection. In: *Obstetrics: Normal and Problem Pregnancies*, 4th ed. 2002:1304–1308.

Gibbs RS. Clinical risk factors for puerperal infection. *Obstet Gynecol*. 1980;55(5 Suppl):178S–84S.

Gilstrap LC, et al. Postpartum endometritis. In: *Infections in Pregnancy*, 2nd ed. 1997:65–78.

Larsen JW. Guidelines for the diagnosis, treatment and prevention of postoperative infections. *Infect Dis Obstet Gynecol*. 2003;11:65–70.

Mead PB. Postpartum endometritis. *Contemp Ob Gyn*. 1990;35:29–34.

Seaward. International Multicentre Term Prelabor Rupture of Membranes Study: Evaluation of predictors of clinical chorioamnionitis and postpartum fever in patients with prelabor rupture of membranes at term. *Am J Obstet Gynecol*. 1997;177(5):1024–1029.

Suonio S.*Int J Gynaecol Obstet*. 1989;29(2):135–142.

Sweet RL, et al. Postpartum infection. In: *Infectious Diseases of the Female Genital Tract*, 3rd ed. 1995;578–600.

Yonekura ML. Treatment of postcesarean endomyometritis. *Clin Obstet Gynecol*. 1988;31:488–500.

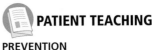 **MISCELLANEOUS**

CLINICAL PEARLS
The classic description of the temporal sequence of postpartum fever involves:
- Wind (lung—atelectasis, pneumonia)
- Water (urinary tract)
- Wound (infection)
- Wonder drugs (drug fever)

ABBREVIATIONS
- DM—Diabetes mellitus
- DVT—Deep venous thrombosis
- PE—Pulmonary embolism
- UTI—Urinary tract infection

CODES
ICD9-CM
- 672.02 (if delivered on current visit)
- 672.04 (if delivered during the previous episode of care)

PATIENT TEACHING

PREVENTION
- Antibiotic prophylaxis before cesarean
- Early ambulation
- Good hemostasis
- Excellent surgical technique
- Incentive spirometry
- Early urethral catheter removal

Section IV

PRENATAL LABORATORY TESTING, ROUTINE

Melissa Snyder Mancuso, MD
Marjorie Greenfield, MD

 BASICS

DESCRIPTION
- The goal of prenatal care is to ensure the health of both mother and fetus. This can be done by:
  - Identifying the patient at risk for complications.
  - Estimating the GA as accurately as possible.
  - Evaluating the health status of mother and fetus.
  - Encouraging and empowering the patient to do her part to care for herself and her baby-to-be.
- Routine and indicated laboratory testing are integral to good prenatal care.
- ACOG recommends specific laboratory tests to screen for treatable conditions and identify pregnancies that may need further workup or intervention.

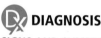 **DIAGNOSIS**

SIGNS AND SYMPTOMS
History
A complete medical and psychosocial history, including domestic violence screening, should be obtained at the initial visit and updated throughout the pregnancy.

Physical Exam
- A full physical exam should be performed at the 1st prenatal appointment.
- At each subsequent prenatal visit, the following should be recorded:
  - Weight
  - BP
  - UA for glucose and protein
  - Fundal height
  - Fetal heart rate and, in the late 3rd trimester, fetal position
  - Pelvic/Cervical exam if indicated

TESTS
A Pap smear should be obtained when indicated, regardless of gestation.

Lab
- 1st visit:
  - CBC
  - Blood type and antibody screen
  - Hemoglobin electrophoresis for patients at risk for sickle cell disease or thalassemia
  - Urine testing for glucose and protein
  - Urine culture
  - Rubella titer
  - Syphilis test
  - Gonorrhea/*Chlamydia* screening
  - Hepatitis B surface antigen
  - HIV testing (patient may opt out if chooses to decline)
  - Cystic fibrosis screening (information should be made available to all couples):
    - Cystic fibrosis carrier screening should be offered before conception or early in pregnancy when 1 partner is of Caucasian, European, or Ashkenazi Jewish descent.
    - Patients may elect to use either sequential or concurrent carrier screening; the latter option may be preferred if there are time constraints for decisions regarding prenatal diagnostic testing ortermination of the affected pregnancy.
    - It is reasonable to offer cystic fibrosis carrier screening to all couples regardless of race or ethnicity as an alternative to selective screening.
- 11–20 weeks:
  - Multiple markers screen should be offered:
    - Some centers are providing 1st trimester assessment of Down syndrome risk, which may include measurement of serum free hCG and PAPP-A.
    - 2nd trimester screening for Down syndrome, trisomy 18, and NTDs can be obtained after 15 completed weeks of gestation with maternal serum, hCG, uE3, and inhibin A

- 24–28 weeks:
  - Diabetes screening with a glucose challenge test (50 g oral glucose load with blood glucose testing 1 hour later):
    - If abnormal, may be followed by a 3-hour glucose tolerance test (100 g oral glucose load with blood drawn fasting, 1, 2, and 3 hours after ingestion of glucose). Specified cutoffs define gestational diabetes.
  - Hematocrit or hemoglobin
  - Repeat antibody screen in Rh-negative mothers prior to receiving prophylactic Rh immunoglobulin.
- 35–36 weeks:
  - Group B Streptococcus culture from vagina and rectum
  - High-risk patients should be screened again for *Gonorrhea, Chlamydia*, HIV, and syphilis.

Imaging
- US is optional but potentially helpful.
- 1st trimester US:
  - To confirm presence of viable IUP, evaluate a suspected ectopic or molar pregnancy, provide most accurate estimate of GA, assist with chorionic villus sampling, or evaluate pelvic masses
- 2nd trimester US:
  - Optimal timing for a single US evaluation in absence of specific indications is at 16–20 weeks, at which time dating can be confirmed and anatomy can be assessed.

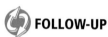 **FOLLOW-UP**

Further lab tests or imaging may be indicated on the basis of the results of the *screening* lab tests.

DISPOSITION
Issues for Referral
Abnormal screening labs or imaging may prompt referral to maternal-fetal medicine specialist or other medical specialist, as indicated.

PATIENT MONITORING

Prenatal charting should indicate performance and results of screening labs so that routine testing is offered at an appropriate time, and "catch-up" testing can be performed as indicated if prenatal labs are not obtained due to clinician or lab error, or patient nonadherence to recommendations.

BIBLIOGRAPHY

American College of Obstetricians and Gynecologists, American College of Medical Genetics. *Preconception and prenatal carrier screening for cystic fibrosis: clinical and laboratory guidelines.* Washington, DC: ACOG; Bethesda, MD: ACMG; 2001.

Cunningham F, et al., eds. *William's Obstetrics* 22nd ed. New York: McGraw-Hill; 2005.

MISCELLANEOUS

ABBREVIATIONS

- ACOG—American College of Obstetricians and Gynecologists
- AFP—α-Fetoprotein
- GA—Gestational age
- hCG—Human chorionic gonadotropin
- IUP—Intrauterine pregnancy
- NTD—Neural tube defect
- PAPP-A—Pregnancy-associated plasma protein A
- UE3—Unconjugated estriol

CODES

ICD9-CM

- V72.4 Pregnancy exam or test
- V77.6 Screening for cystic fibrosis
- 88.78 Ultrasound of the gravid uterus

PATIENT TEACHING

Patients should be made aware of the tests that are performed routinely, as well as other tests that might be elected (e.g., chorionic villus sampling or amniocentesis for advanced maternal age) as well as the choices that would be available if testing were abnormal (pregnancy termination, preparation for the birth of an infant with congenital anomalies, further testing).

PREVENTION

- Preconception counseling offers the opportunity to discuss individualized risks, as well as to perform testing such as cystic fibrosis screening.
- To decrease the risks of NTDs, preconception folate supplementation is indicated for all women who plan to or are at risk for becoming pregnant.

TERM LABOR

Jonathan A. Schaffir, MD

 BASICS

DESCRIPTION

- Labor: Regular uterine contractions causing cervical change.
- Term: GA between 37 and 42 weeks:
  - Average duration of singleton pregnancy is 280 days (40 weeks) from 1st day of LMP.
- Preterm: Occurring prior to 37 weeks' gestation (from LMP)
- Postterm: Pregnancy continuing beyond 42 weeks' gestation (from LMP)
- Stages of labor:
  - 1st stage is divided into latent and active phases:
    - Latent phase:
      - From onset of labor until increased rate of cervical dilation
      - Usually until 3–4 cm dilation
    - Active phase:
      - Increased rate of cervical dilation until complete dilation
  - 2nd stage:
    - From full cervical dilation until delivery of the infant
  - 3rd stage:
    - From delivery of infant until delivery of placenta

EPIDEMIOLOGY

GA at time of labor and delivery:

- 11% preterm
- 82% term
- 7% postterm

PATHOPHYSIOLOGY

- A multifactorial, incompletely elucidated mechanism for determining the onset of labor, the timing of which is largely under fetal control
- Removal of inhibitory effects on myometrium
- Activation of uterine tissues:
  - Increased prostaglandin synthesis
  - Increased gap junction formation
  - Upregulation of oxytocin receptors
- Increased myometrial activity coordinated by endocrine factors from fetoplacental unit

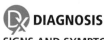 **DIAGNOSIS**

SIGNS AND SYMPTOMS

History

- Assess for symptoms of labor:
  - Onset and timing of contractions
  - Status of fetal membranes
  - Presence of mucoid vaginal bleeding ("show")
  - Amount of fetal movement
- Be sure to review prenatal information and risk factors.

Physical Exam

- Maternal assessment:
  - Vital signs
  - Cervical exam:
    - Dilation
    - Effacement
    - Station of presenting part
  - Adequacy of maternal pelvis
- Fetal assessment:
  - Abdominal palpation for size, presentation, and lie
  - Fetal heart monitoring to assure fetal well-being
  - Determine status of fetal membranes

TESTS

- External fetal heart rate monitor:
  - Ensure reassuring fetal status:
    - Normal baseline rate between 110 and 160
    - Adequate variability
    - Observe for decelerations in response to contractions

Lab

- CBC:
  - To assess preexisting degree of anemia
- Type and screen:
  - In case of need for peripartum blood transfusion
  - To rule out isoimmunization
- Group B streptococcus status should be noted:
  - Prophylactic antibiotics if known positive
- Other labs based on risk factors:
  - Preeclampsia labs if warranted by clinical signs
  - Coagulation studies if suspicion of abruption

Imaging

- When physical exam is questionable or limited, sonography can be used to confirm:
  - Presentation
  - Fetal size/GA
  - Presence of multiple gestation

DIFFERENTIAL DIAGNOSIS

- "False labor":
  - Contractions irregular and of less intensity
  - Lack of cervical change:
    - May need to observe 1–2 hours to assess change
- Preterm labor:
  - Be sure GA is accurate
  - Sonographic dating at term has 3-week range of error

 TREATMENT

GENERAL MEASURES

- Activity:
  - Walking may be allowed throughout labor in low-risk individuals:
    - Does not reduce labor duration or need for operative delivery
    - Contraindicated once narcotic analgesia or regional anesthesia provided

- Diet:
  - NPO during active labor:
    - Reduces risk of aspiration if emergent general anesthesia required
    - Frequent emesis in late active phase
    - Ice chips or lozenges permissible for oral comfort
- IV access:
  - To maintain adequate hydration
  - Allows access for medication delivery

Managing Labor

- Latent phase of 1st stage:
  - Variable duration, but averages 6.4 hours in nulliparae and rarely >20 hours
  - Hospital admission in this phase is discouraged unless there are concerns about fetal well-being or significant analgesia requirements
- Active phase of 1st stage:
  - Average rate of change is 3 cm/hr in nulliparae and 5.7 cm/hr in multiparae
  - Rates of change defined as normal are referred to as Friedman labor curves
  - <1.2 cm/hr change in nullipara or 1.5 cm/hr change in multipara is <5th percentile, and reason for lack of progress should be evaluated.
  - Cervical exams in this phase of labor should be frequent enough to document adequate progress (every 1–2 hours).
  - Amniotomy can be considered to shorten the active phase.
- 2nd stage of labor:
  - Usually involves active maternal expulsive efforts to achieve delivery
  - May require 2 hours in nulliparae and 1 hour in multiparae without regional anesthesia
  - Epidural anesthesia prolongs this stage.
  - Operative vaginal delivery may be considered:
    - Poor maternal expulsive efforts
    - Maternal contraindication to Valsalva
    - Suggestions of fetal compromise requiring expedited delivery
  - Routine episiotomy is not recommended:
    - Increased incidence of 3rd and 4th degree perineal lacerations
    - May be indicated to expedite delivery for fetal bradycardia or if shoulder dystocia anticipated

Active Management of Labor

- A system of educational and medical components to ensure labor progression and decrease dystocia
- Medical interventions:
  - Strict diagnosis of labor
  - Early amniotomy
  - Frequent examination for cervical change
  - High-dose oxytocin if dystocia diagnosed
- Efficacy:
  - Shortens labor
  - Reduces maternal and neonatal infection rates
  - Does not prevent cesarean delivery

MEDICATION (DRUGS)

- Pain management is individualized according to patient desires:
  - Narcotics:
    - Often used in latent phase of labor
    - Risk of neonatal depression if administered excessively or proximal to delivery
  - Regional anesthesia:
    - Epidural most common choice, provides continuous pain relief throughout labor
    - Risk of hypotension and decreased placental perfusion if mother inadequately hydrated
    - Pudendal or saddle block may be useful in 2nd stage to reduce perineal pain or assist with operative vaginal delivery
- Oxytocin:
  - Commonly used to augment or induce labor at term
  - Increases the frequency and intensity of contractions:
    - Generally reserved for protracted or arrested labor pattern
    - Rule out cephalopelvic disproportion or malpresentation prior to use.
  - Initiated at low dose (e.g., 2 mU/min) and gradually titrated upward until contractions adequate:
    - Excessive dose can cause hyperstimulation.

SURGERY

- Cesarean delivery:
  - Abdominal incision to deliver infant indicated when maternal or fetal health is jeopardized by labor:
    - Arrest of labor
    - Nonreassuring fetal assessment
    - Hemorrhagic complication
    - Malpresentation
    - Risk of infectious transmission (e.g., HSV)
- Cesarean on maternal demand with no medical indication is controversial.

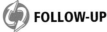 FOLLOW-UP

DISPOSITION

- Uncomplicated labor:
  - May deliver in any position, although lithotomy is most common
- Consider transfer to operative suite or larger delivery area if significant intervention may be anticipated:
  - Shoulder dystocia
  - Twin gestation
  - Breech presentation

Issues for Referral

- Perinatologist consultation:
  - Preferably obtained prior to presentation in labor
  - Major congenital anomaly
  - Severe maternal medical disease
- Referral to tertiary care center:
  - If institution is ill-equipped to handle complicated labor:
    - Level III nursery for premature infant or major anomaly
    - If intensive care might be needed for maternal medical disease

PATIENT MONITORING

Mother

- Monitor vital signs every 15–30 minutes:
  - More frequent following epidural anesthesia
- Temperature every 1–2 hours
- Assessment of pain experience
- Periodic assessment for bladder fullness:
  - May require bladder catheterization if loss of bladder sensation from regional anesthetic

Fetus

- Electronic fetal monitoring:
  - Performed on all women in labor in most hospitals
  - Assessment of fetal-well being
  - Monitoring regularity of uterine contractions
  - Never shown to significantly reduce overall perinatal mortality or cerebral palsy in low-risk parturients

- Intermittent auscultation:
  - Alternative monitoring in women at low risk of peripartum morbidity
  - Fetal heart auscultated during and following contraction:
    - Every 15–30 minutes in 1st stage of labor
    - Every 5–15 minutes in 2nd stage of labor
  - Requires 1-on-1 nursing

BIBLIOGRAPHY

American College of Obstetricians and Gynecologists. Intrapartum Fetal Heart Rate Monitoring. Practice Bulletin #70. Washington, DC: American College of Obstetricians and Gynecologists, 2005.

Liao JB, et al. Normal labor: Mechanism and duration. *Obstet Gynecol Clin N Am*. 2005;32:145–164.

Norwitz ER, et al. Labor and delivery. In: Gabbe SG, et al., eds. *Obstetrics: Normal and Problem Pregnancies*, 4th ed. New York: Churchill Livingstone; 2002:353–394.

Pates JA, et al. Active management of labor. *Obstet Gynecol Clin N Am*. 2005;32:221–230.

 MISCELLANEOUS

ABBREVIATIONS

- GA—Gestational age
- LMP—Last menstrual period

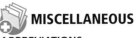

ICD9-CM
650 Normal labor and delivery

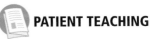 PATIENT TEACHING

- Childbirth education:
  - To decrease anxiety and familiarize patient with delivery plan
  - Different schools of thought:
    - Lamaze: Psychoprophylaxis to minimize pain associated with anxiety
    - Bradley: Emphasizes noninterventional approach
- Support person in labor:
  - May be professional "doula"
  - Benefits of having support person present:
    - Reduced analgesia requirements
    - Decreased intrapartum complications
    - Minimize postpartum emotional difficulties

THIRD STAGE OF LABOR

Jonathan A. Schaffir, MD

 BASICS

DESCRIPTION
3rd stage of labor refers to the interval from the delivery of the infant until the delivery of the placenta.

EPIDEMIOLOGY
- Mean length of time: 6 minutes
- 97th percentile: 30 minutes

RISK FACTORS
Prepare for possible placenta accreta if placenta does not separate after 30 minutes and risk factors present:
- Previous cesarean delivery
- Previous other uterine surgery
- History of endometrial infection
- Uterine leiomyomata
- Nonfundic implantation (cornu or lower segment)

PATHOPHYSIOLOGY
- Placental separation occurs as a result of uterine contractions.
- Influenced by oxytocin and prostaglandins
- Reduce area of placental bed
- Disrupt attachment in plane of spongiosa layer of decidua vera (Nitabuch layer)
- Compress and occlude myometrial arterioles to prevent postpartum hemorrhage.

ASSOCIATED CONDITIONS
- Postpartum hemorrhage:
  - May be immediate or delayed
  - See "Differential Diagnosis" below.
- Abnormal placentation:
  - Associated with above risk factors:
    - Placenta accreta: Attached directly to myometrium
    - Placenta increta: Invades myometrium
    - Placenta percreta: Penetrates uterine serosa; may invade to adjacent organs
- Uterine inversion:
  - Associated with grand multiparity, adherent placenta, and excessive cord traction

DIAGNOSIS

SIGNS AND SYMPTOMS
History
- Patient may present to hospital following extramural delivery.
- Obtain pregnancy history and description of delivery prior to arrival.

ALERT
Rule out twin gestation before managing 3rd stage!

Physical Exam
- Examine vagina and perineum:
  - Look for cervical or vaginal lacerations:
    - Particularly common after operative delivery
    - Exam may be performed after delivery of placenta as well.
- Examine umbilical cord:
  - Determine number of vessels:
    - Normal: 2 arteries and 1 vein
    - Single umbilical artery associated with other structural anomalies in 20% of cases
  - Determine length:
    - Average length 50–60 cm
    - Short cord poses risk of oligohydramnios, fetal distress, and adverse neonatal outcomes
- Examine placenta:
  - Abnormal cord insertion (marginal or velamentous):
    - Associated with risk of cord avulsion
  - Abnormalities in surface area
    - Infarction/Fibrosis
    - Calcifications
    - Abruption (appears as depressed area with adherent clot)
    - Associated with perfusion defects, growth restriction, fetal demise
  - Abnormalities of lobulation:
    - Missing cotyledon or accessory lobe
    - Associated with retained placental fragment and postpartum hemorrhage or infection
  - Abnormalities of disk interface:
    - Circumvallate or circummarginate placenta
    - Associated with growth restriction and fetal demise

TESTS
Lab
- Obtain cord blood for:
  - Type/Coombs test
  - Some states require cord blood screen for syphilis
  - Consider arterial and venous blood gases:
    - Delivery for fetal compromise
    - Low 5-minute Apgar score
    - Severe growth restriction
    - Abnormal fetal heart rate tracing
    - Maternal thyroid disease
    - Intrapartum fever
    - Multifetal gestations
  - Cord blood may also be collected for banking (see Patient Education below).
- Consider obtaining placental cultures in cases of intraamniotic infection:
  - Take swab from both maternal and fetal placental surfaces

Imaging
US may be useful to rule out retained placenta.
- Interrupted blood vessels along membrane surface suggest accessory lobe.
- Fragmented or absent cotyledons on placental inspection

DIFFERENTIAL DIAGNOSIS
Excessive bleeding in 3rd stage should prompt examination for causes of postpartum hemorrhage:
- Uterine atony
- Retained placental tissue
- Laceration of cervix, vagina or perineum
- Coagulopathy
- Uterine inversion
- Amniotic fluid embolism/anaphylactoid syndrome of pregnancy

Hematologic
Postpartum hemorrhage associated with abnormalities of clotting:
- Incidence of von Willebrand in general population ~1%

TREATMENT

GENERAL MEASURES

- Expectant versus active management
- Expectant: "Physiologic" or hands-off approach:
  - No clamping or cutting of cord until cessation of pulse:
    - Allows transfer of blood to infant up to 3 minutes after birth
    - May prevent neonatal anemia
  - Placental separation occurs without intervention. Signs of separation:
    - Lengthening of the umbilical cord
    - Gush of blood from vagina
    - Elevation and change in shape of uterine fundus
  - Placenta delivers spontaneously, aided by gravity or maternal expulsion.
- Active management:
  - Administration of uterotonic agent after delivery of infant:
    - Oxytocin most commonly administered
    - May be given either after delivery of the anterior shoulder, or on placental separation
  - Early cord clamping and cutting:
    - Draining the umbilical cord does not hasten delivery.
  - Controlled traction on umbilical cord to expedite separation:
    - Brandt-Andrews maneuver: Abdominal hand secures fundus above symphysis while cord is pulled downwards
    - Credé maneuver: Cord is held secure while abdominal hand pushes the fundus upward.
    - Excessive traction may result in avulsion of the cord or uterine inversion.
  - Advantages of active management:
    - Shorter 3rd stage of labor
    - Reduce incidence of postpartum hemorrhage
    - Reduce risk of anemia
    - Decrease need for postpartum blood transfusion

MEDICATION (DRUGS)

Uterotonics useful to prevent postpartum bleeding:

- Oxytocin:
  - May be given IV or intramuscular
  - Preferred agent for postpartum prophylaxis
  - IV bolus may cause hypotension
  - Usual effective dose: 10 units IM, or 20 units in 500 mL saline run IV
- Methylergonovine:
  - May be given PO or IM
  - Equally effective in preventing hemorrhage, but increased risk for manual removal of placenta

- Prostaglandins:
  - Tablets may be administered orally, rectally, or sublingually
  - Misoprostol demonstrated to be not as effective as injectable uterotonics in the prevention of postpartum hemorrhage.

SURGERY

- Manual or surgical exploration of the uterus may be required.
- Indications:
  - Suspected retained placenta
  - Excessive bleeding
  - Lack of separation after 30 minutes
  - May be considered after VBAC to determine if uterine scar intact
- Requires adequate anesthesia or sedation
- Prophylactic antibiotic should be considered to prevent postpartum endometritis.

FOLLOW-UP

Fundal assessment:

- Following delivery, fundal pressure applied:
  - Expresses clot remaining in uterus
  - Assess for adequate uterine contraction
  - Fundal height may be periodically assessed in postpartum period to assure adequate uterine tone.

BIBLIOGRAPHY

American College of Obstetricians and Gynecologists. Umbilical cord blood gas and acid-base analysis. Committee Opinion #348. Washington, DC: American College of Obstetricians and Gynecologists; 2006.

Magann EF, et al. 3rd stage of labor. *Obstet Gynecol Clin N Am*. 2005:32:323–332.

Maughan KL, et al. Preventing postpartum hemorrhage: Managing the 3rd stage of labor. *Am Fam Physician*. 2006;73:1025–1028.

Norwitz ER, et al. Labor and delivery. In: Gabbe SG, et al., eds. *Obstetrics: Normal and Problem Pregnancies*, 4th ed. New York: Churchill Livingstone; 2002:353–394.

MISCELLANEOUS

CLINICAL PEARLS

Avoid excessive traction: No matter your hurry; it leads to more worry!

ABBREVIATION

VBAC—Vaginal birth after cesarean

CODES

ICD9-CM

- 650 Normal labor and delivery
  - Includes placental delivery
- Retained placenta
  - 667.0 Without hemorrhage
  - 667.1 With hemorrhage

PATIENT TEACHING

- During pregnancy, discuss option of obtaining cord blood for private banking.
- Allows storage of cord blood for possible stem cell transfusion in future:
  - Explain that odds of needing such a transfusion (e.g., for leukemia or Fanconi anemia) is small unless there is a strong family history.
- Several private companies offer this service.
- Patient should make arrangements in advance and bring collection kit to delivery if banking is desired.
- Follow instructions in collection kit to maximize amount of cord blood collected.

PREVENTION

Avoid excessive traction on cord to prevent uterine inversion.

Section IV

UNPLANNED PREGNANCY AND OPTIONS COUNSELING

Suzanne T. Poppema, MD

BASICS

DESCRIPTION
- Nonvolitional occurrence of pregnancy
- Nondirective counseling to clarify options:
  – Pregnancy termination/abortion
  – Continued pregnancy with either:
    ○ Parenting
    ○ Placing baby for adoption
- Desire for pregnancy termination, abortion, elective abortion, therapeutic abortion

Age-Related Factors
- Adolescents have the highest rates of unintended pregnancy of any age group.
- Adolescents have the highest abortion ratio (abortions/1,000 live births) of any age group.
- Women in 40s have 2nd highest rates
- Abortion rates have declined in US since the 1990s.

EPIDEMIOLOGY
- 49% of US pregnancies unintended
- Rates of unintended pregnancy:
  – 51/1,000 among women age 15–44
- Frequency of unintended pregnancy (unplanned birth, abortion, or both):
  – 48% of women age 15–44
  – 60% of women by age 35–39
- Outcomes unintended pregnancies:
  – 48% end in abortion

RISK FACTORS
- All women of reproductive age
- Highest risk among women not using contraception
- Contraceptive failure contributes ~1/2 of unintended pregnancies

Genetics
Women with a desired but abnormal pregnancy (by amniocentesis, CVS, or US) may request options counseling.

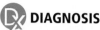 DIAGNOSIS

SIGNS AND SYMPTOMS
History
- Must confirm pregnancy
- Determine GA

Physical Exam
Exam corroborates history and US if indicated

TESTS
Testing to confirm pregnancy, presence of IUP, and/or GA:
- Urine pregnancy testing
- Quantitative β-hCG
- US

Imaging
- GA determines options
- Imaging not required if history and exam are consistent

TREATMENT

GENERAL MEASURES
- Prenatal care
- Options counseling:
  – Parenting
  – Adoption:
    ○ 1% of pregnancies
  – Abortion:
    ○ 48–54% of all pregnancies

MEDICATION (DRUGS)
Medical abortion is an option in early pregnancy.

SURGERY
Surgical abortion most commonly used in US

FOLLOW-UP

DISPOSITION
Issues for Referral
- Adoption agencies
- Abortion services
- Prenatal care services
- To another provider in a timely fashion if unable to give patient unbiased information
- To legal counsel if a minor requests abortion and judicial bypass in a state with mandatory parental notification or consent

PROGNOSIS
Pediatric Considerations
- Increased likelihood nonconsensual sex causing pregnancy
- Increased risks to fetus and adolescent patient with childbearing
- Be aware of laws governing adoption and abortion rights for adolescents:
  – Vary from state to state
- Know parental involvement requirements:
  – Vary from state to state
  – May mandate notification or consent

COMPLICATIONS
Risks of complications with both continued pregnancy and abortion should be addressed.
- Risks of morbidity and mortality greater with continued pregnancy than with pregnancy termination

BIBLIOGRAPHY

Henshaw S. Unintended Pregnancy in the United States. *Family Planning Perspect.* 1998;30(1): 24–29, 46.

Physicians for Reproductive Choice and Health. *Options Counseling.* Adolescent Reproductive Health Education Project Curriculum, New York: Physicians for Reproductive Choice. Oct. 2006.

Sonfield A. Preventing Unintended Pregnancy: The Need and the Means. The Guttmacher Report on Public Policy, New York: Guttmacher Institute. December 2003.

 MISCELLANEOUS

SYNONYM(S)
- Undesired pregnancy
- Unintended pregnancy
- Unplanned pregnancy

CLINICAL PEARLS
- Presentation with an unintended pregnancy is a critical entry point into medical system.
- Be prepared to provide options counseling.
- Feel comfortable with the emotions, biases, and uncertainties involved with pregnancy decision making.

ABBREVIATIONS
- CVS—Chorionic villus sampling
- GA—Gestational age
- hCG—Human chorionic gonadotropin
- IUP—Intrauterine pregnancy
- US—Ultrasound

CODES

ICD9-CM
V22 Normal pregnancy:
- May have other specified complications of pregnancy
- May have pregnancy with pre-existing medical conditions

 PATIENT TEACHING

- Do's:
  - Recognize personal biases.
  - Recognize patient ambivalence and stress.
  - Give information without making a judgment.
  - Ask open-ended questions:
    - "How do you feel about this pregnancy at this time?"
    - "How have you made difficult decisions in the past?"
  - Validate the woman's feelings:
    - "Many women in your situation are afraid, unsure, feeling guilty."
  - Recognize the woman's feelings of powerlessness.
  - Ask how the woman feels about pros and cons of this pregnancy.
  - Maintain confidentiality.
  - Assure the woman of your support regardless of her decision.
  - Be prepared to assist the woman in following through with whatever decision she makes.
- Don'ts:
  - Do not assume the diagnosis of a pregnancy is either good or bad.
  - Do not try to steer the woman to one decision over another.
  - Do not be judgmental.
  - Do not inject personal morality.
  - Do not rush the woman's decision.
  - Do not tell the woman how she should feel.
  - Do not try to "fix" or make the woman's feelings go away.

PREVENTION
Contraception:
- ~1/2 of unintended pregnancies result from the 7% women not using contraception

Section V
Pregnancy-Related Conditions

BREECH PRESENTATION AND OTHER ABNORMAL PRESENTATIONS

Inna V. Landres, MD

BASICS

DESCRIPTION
- Fetal presentation is the portion of the fetal body foremost within the birth canal or closest in proximity to the birth canal.
- In longitudinal lies, the presenting part is either cephalic or breech:
  - Cephalic: Vertex, sinciput (forehead), brow, face
  - Breech: Frank, complete, footling
- In transverse lies, the shoulder is the presenting part
- Abnormal lie

Age-Related Factors
GA related:
- Breech has decreasing prevalence with GA:
  - Term (37–40): 3–4% prevalence
  - 34 weeks: 5%
  - 32 weeks: 11%
  - 30 weeks: 17%
  - 28 weeks: 24%
  - Chance of spontaneous version after 36 weeks is 25%

EPIDEMIOLOGY
- Fetal presentation (from 68,097 singleton pregnancies at Parkland Hospital):
  - Cephalic (96.8%)
  - Breech (2.7%)
  - Transverse (0.3%)
  - Compound (0.1%)
  - Face (0.5%)
  - Brow (0.01%)
- Breech presentation:
  - Frank breech (50–70% of all breech): Both hips flexed and both knees extended
  - Complete breech (5–10% of all breech): Both hips and both knees flexed
  - Footling or incomplete breech (10–40% of all breech): 1 or both hips not flexed, 1 or both feet or knees present before the buttocks

RISK FACTORS
- Abnormal placental implantation:
  - Previa, low-lying placenta
- Uterine anomalies:
  - Septate uterus
  - Bicornuate uterus
  - Large leiomyomata
- Fetal anomalies
- Preterm delivery
- Abnormal amniotic fluid volume:
  - Oligohydramnios, polyhydramnios
- Multiple gestation
- Prior breech presentation

PATHOPHYSIOLOGY
Persistent breech presentation is associated with increased risk of:
- Perinatal morbidity from difficult delivery
- Prolapsed cord
- Uterine anomalies (septum, fibroids)
- Placenta previa
- Fetal, neonatal anomalies

ASSOCIATED CONDITIONS
Face
Mentum (chin) anterior or posterior:
- Management:
  - Usually successful vaginal delivery
  - Avoid fetal scalp electrodes
  - Avoid manual or forceps rotation

Brow
- Rarest!
- Usually converts to face or occiput:
  - Management:
    - If small fetus and large pelvis, try vaginal delivery.
    - If larger fetus, cesarean is usually required.

Transverse
Dorsosuperior (back up), or dorsoinferior (or back down)
- Management:
  - Attempt version after 39 weeks
  - If labor, delivery by cesarean only
- Delivery for transverse back-down presentation requires a vertical uterine incision or intra-abdominal version
- Prolonged labor risks include uterine rupture

Compound
An extremity presenting simultaneously with the presenting part:
- In vaginal delivery, the arm will typically retract with descent

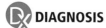

DIAGNOSIS

SIGNS AND SYMPTOMS
History
Consider risk factors predisposing to abnormal presentation (see above)

Physical Exam
- Leopold maneuvers
- Vaginal exam:
  - Face presentation is often confused for breech!

Imaging
- US to confirm suspected breech
- If considering vaginal delivery, evaluate for type of breech and degree of head flexion
- X-ray pelvimetry is not routinely used:
  - Clinical pelvimetry may be helpful if vaginal delivery is considered

DIFFERENTIAL DIAGNOSIS
- With frank breech, palpation of anus may suggest little cervical dilation
- Breech and face presentations may be confused
- Fetal anomalies may make determination difficult:
  - Breech with sacrococcygeal teratoma
  - Anencephaly

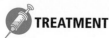

TREATMENT

GENERAL MEASURES
ACOG Committee Opinion July 2006 states that: "the decision regarding mode of delivery should depend on the experience of the health care provider."
ECV:
- Should be offered to all women near term with breech presentation (Level A evidence).
- Successful version translates into lower cesarean rates.
- Patient candidates for ECV:
  - Should have completed 36 weeks
  - Reassuring fetal heart tones by NST
  - ECV should not be attempted in labor or in patients with PROM
  - Assure availability of OR and anesthesia in case of emergency cesarean
  - Variable reported success rates: 35–85%
  - Transverse lie: 80–90% success for ECV
  - Success is more likely for parity, normal amniotic fluid, and an unengaged fetus.
  - Consider tocolysis for nulliparas.
  - Earlier gestation increases success rate but also increases rate of spontaneous reversion.
  - Complications:
    - Placental abruption
    - Uterine rupture
    - Preterm labor
    - Fetal distress
  - Isoimmunization: Always check Rh status and give Rhogam if indicated.

Cesarean Delivery

- A planned Cesarean delivery is the preferred mode for most patients due to lower neonatal morbidity and mortality as well as decreasing expertise of health care providers.
- The Term Breech Trial, a large, randomized, international multicenter trial demonstrated improved neonatal outcomes with a planned cesarean compared with a planned vaginal delivery (1.6% vs. 5% perinatal mortality, neonatal mortality, and serious morbidity)

Vaginal Delivery

- May be an option for select patients with an experienced provider
- Criteria for patient selection:
  - GA >37 weeks
  - Frank or complete breech presentation
  - Adequate maternal pelvis (prior term vaginal delivery preferred)
  - Detailed patient informed consent

SPECIAL THERAPY

Complementary and Alternative Therapies

- Nurse midwives and complementary medicine recommendations for converting near-term breech to cephalic presentation include:
  - Knee-chest position twice a day. Data for efficacy not available.
  - Lying head down on an ironing board positioned on a chair (creating angled surface). Data for efficacy not available
  - Moxibustion acupuncture (burning of moxa herbal preparation); benefit shown in 1 small RCT.
  - Hypnosis; benefit shown in 1 small RCT
  - Acoustic stimulation while performing ECV

SURGERY

See above for planned cesarean delivery.

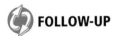 FOLLOW-UP

DISPOSITION

Issues for Referral

Referral to specialist with expertise in ECV could be considered.

PROGNOSIS

- Maternal:
  - Greater maternal morbidity due to high frequency of cesarean, emergency surgery, and failed ECV
  - Similar labor length with cephalic presentation for successful vaginal delivery
- Fetal:
  - Greater neonatal morbidity and mortality at every stage of gestation compared with cephalic presentation

COMPLICATIONS

Vaginal Delivery of Breech

- Head entrapment leading to hypoxia and acidemia
- Trauma from compression and traction
- Cord prolapse: More common with footling breech (15%)
- Entrapment of fetal arm behind neck
- Fractures of fetal humerus, clavicle
- Hyperextension of fetal head
- Preterm fetus: Incomplete cervical dilation
- Management of head entrapment:
  - Mauriceau maneuver: Flex head by suprapubic pressure and pressure on the maxilla
  - Piper forceps
  - Dührssen cervical incisions for incomplete cervical dilation

Cesarean Delivery

- Maternal morbidity due to surgery
- Longer hospital stay
- Increased blood loss

PATIENT MONITORING

- US to confirm suspected breech or abnormal presentation
- Avoid fetal scalp electrode for face presentation
- Continuous external fetal monitoring for footling breech due to high risk of cord prolapse
- NST before and after ECV

BIBLIOGRAPHY

ACOG Practice Bulletin No. 13. External Cephalic Version. Washington DC: ACOG; February 2000.

ACOG Practice Bulletin No. 340. Mode of Term Singleton Breech Delivery. Washington DC: ACOG; July 2006.

Cunnigham FG. *Williams Obstetrics*, 22nd ed. New York: McGraw-Hill; 2005

Hannah ME, et al. Planned cesarean section versus planned vaginal birth for breech presentation at term: A randomized multicentre trial. *Lancet*. 2000;356:1375.

 MISCELLANEOUS

CLINICAL PEARLS

- "A breech is not just a vertex upside down." (WE Brenner and CH Hendricks)
- Increased risk of structural and chromosomal anomalies

ABBREVIATIONS

- ECV—External cephalic version
- GA—Gestational age
- NST—Nonstress testing
- PROM—Premature rupture of membranes
- RCT—Randomized control trial

CODES

ICD9-CM

- 652.1 Breech or other malpresentation successfully converted to cephalic presentation
- 652.2 Breech presentation without mention of version
- 652.3 Transverse or oblique presentation
- 652.4 Face or brow presentation
- 669.6 Breech extraction, without mention of indication
- 761.7 Malpresentation before labor
- 763.0 Breech delivery and extraction
- 763.1 Other malpresentation, malposition, and disproportion during labor and delivery

 PATIENT TEACHING

ACOG Patient Education Pamphlet: If Your Baby Is Breech

CERVICAL INSUFFICIENCY

Mona Prasad, DO, MPH
Jay Iams, MD

 BASICS

DESCRIPTION
- Classic:
  - Painless cervical dilation leading to midtrimester loss, often repetitive:
    - Anatomically dysfunctional cervix
- Current:
  - Function of cervix not characterized by ability to maintain pregnancy alone:
    - Cervical function is a continuum.
    - Obstetric history and cervical length via ultrasound contribute

Age-Related Factors
Preterm delivery occurs more often at extremes of reproductive age. Cervical insufficiency does not specifically seem to be affected by age.

EPIDEMIOLOGY
- Incidence of cervical insufficiency is uncertain given lack of clear diagnostic criteria.
- Indirect estimate of cervical insufficiency determined by number of cerclages placed: 1/182–222 pregnancies

RISK FACTORS
- History of recurrent midtrimester pregnancy loss (≥2)
- Structural risk factors:
  - Congenital:
    - Congenitally short cervix
    - Müllerian duct abnormality
    - In utero DES exposure
  - Acquired:
    - Cervical lacerations following vaginal delivery
    - Prolonged 2nd stage of labor
    - Cervical injury at time of cesarean section
    - Surgical procedures to cervix (mechanical dilation or conization)
  - Uterine overdistention:
    - Multiple gestation
    - Polyhydramnios
- Biochemical risk factors:
  - Increased levels of relaxin
  - Deficiencies in cervical collagen
  - Infection:
    - Cervical or upper genital tract infection may lead to inflammation; cytokine and prostaglandin release may lead to cervical softening and effacement.

Genetics
Genetic defects in collagen synthesis may predispose to cervical insufficiency:
- Ehlers-Danlos syndrome

PATHOPHYSIOLOGY
4 pathways lead to a common outcome of cervical shortening and dilation:
- Congenital
- Loss of tissue
- Infection, inflammation
- Primary cervical disease

ASSOCIATED CONDITIONS
- Preterm delivery
- Chorioamnionitis
- Premature rupture of membranes

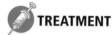 **DIAGNOSIS**

SIGNS AND SYMPTOMS
History
- Suspect if obstetric history of:
  - Short labors
  - Progressively earlier deliveries
  - Advanced dilation prior to labor
- Current history of:
  - Vaginal fullness or pressure
  - Vaginal spotting or bleeding
  - Increased volume of watery, mucousy or brown discharge
  - Vague low back pain, low abdominal pain

Physical Exam
- Vital signs, maternal temperature should be normal
- Absence of fundal tenderness or CVA tenderness
- Tocometry to evaluate presence of contractions
- Sterile speculum exam to:
  - Exclude ruptured membranes
  - Exclude vaginitis, cervicitis
  - Identify visual dilation of the cervix
  - Identify hourglassing membranes
- Sterile digital exam:
  - Evaluate cervical dilation and effacement

TESTS
No current tests are available for use in a nonpregnant female to predict cervical insufficiency in a future pregnancy.

Labs
- CBC
- UA
- Amniocentesis:
  - When clinical suspicion of intrauterine infection is high
  - Send fluid for Gram stain, culture, protein, and glucose

Imaging
- TAUS:
  - Evaluate viability of fetus
  - Evaluate estimated GA
  - Evaluate presence of fetal anomalies
  - Not good to assess cervix
- Cervical sonography:
  - Characteristics of cervical insufficiency:
    - Shortening to 20 mm or less
    - Dilation of internal os
    - Funneling of membranes into endocervical canal

DIFFERENTIAL DIAGNOSIS
- Infection:
  - UTI/Pyelonephritis
  - Vaginitis
  - Chorioamnionitis
- Preterm labor
- Premature rupture of membranes
- Placental abruption
- Musculoskeletal low back pain
- Round ligament pain

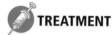 **TREATMENT**

GENERAL MEASURES
Optimal treatment for cervical insufficiency is not determined. Currently, no clinical evidence that any intervention proves to prolong pregnancy.

PREGNANCY-SPECIFIC ISSUES
Risks for Mother
If etiology of cervical insufficiency is intrauterine infection, mother is at risk for sepsis.

Risks for Fetus
If cervical insufficiency results in delivery, fetus has the attendant risks of prematurity. Extreme prematurity may result in neonatal death.

SPECIAL THERAPY
Complementary and Alternative Therapies
- Modified activity:
  - Bedrest
  - Pelvic rest
- Pessaries

MEDICATION (DRUGS)

17–Hydroxyprogesterone, 250 mg:

- Weekly IM injections weeks 16–36
- Prevents preterm birth in women with prior preterm birth; not studied in women with cervical insufficiency

SURGERY

Cerclage:

- Purse-string stitch around the cervix to reinforce the presumed weak cervix
- Multiple types:
  - MacDonald: Transvaginal approach
  - Shirodkar: Transvaginal approach
  - Abdominal: Requires laparotomy

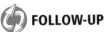 ## FOLLOW-UP

DISPOSITION

Issues for Referral

Once the diagnosis of cervical insufficiency is made, evaluation by a perinatologist is recommended. It may be necessary to obtain consultation in order to make the diagnosis.

PROGNOSIS

Prognosis is unpredictable. Depends upon degree of cervical insufficiency identified, possibility of underlying inflammation, and contributing obstetric history:

- In women with prior preterm birth, cervical length of <25 mm before 24 weeks has a positive predictive value for preterm delivery of 55%.
- Cervical cerclage has not been demonstrated to prolong pregnancy.
- Cervical cerclage placed in the presence of underlying inflammation may lead to increased risk of preterm delivery.

COMPLICATIONS

- Complications of cervical insufficiency:
  - Preterm delivery or midtrimester loss
- Complications of cervical cerclage:
  - Iatrogenic rupture of membranes
  - Chorioamnionitis
  - Suture displacement
  - Hemorrhage

PATIENT MONITORING

Mother

When diagnosis of cervical insufficiency is made:

- Activity modification:
  - Bedrest, pelvic rest
  - Inpatient or outpatient
- Serial US evaluation of cervix:
  - Every 2 weeks until 34 weeks
- Administration of corticosteroids to enhance fetal lung maturity:
  - When cervical length <25 mm
- Bowel regimen to prevent hard stools and excessive Valsalva
- If cerclage present and patient is candidate for vaginal delivery: Remove cerclage 35–36 weeks

Fetus

Routine fetal surveillance via US is not indicated with the diagnosis of cervical insufficiency.

BIBLIOGRAPHY

ACOG Practice Bulletin No. 48. Cervical Insufficiency. *Obstet Gynecol*. 2003;102:1091–1099.

Creasy RK, et al., eds. *Maternal-Fetal Medicine Principles and Practice*, 5th ed. Philadelphia: Saunders; 2004.

Johnson J, et al. Cervical Insufficiency. Available at: www.uptodate.com. Accessed 11/01/06.

Romero R, et al. The role of cervical cerclage in obstetric practice: Can the patient who could benefit from this procedure be identified? *Am J Obstet Gynecol*. 2006;194:19.

Sakai M, et al. Evaluation of effectiveness of prophylactic cerclage of a short cervix according to interleukin-8 in cervical mucus. *Am J Obstet Gynecol*. 2006;194:1419.

Vidaeff AC, et al. From concept to practice: The recent history of preterm delivery prevention. Part I: Cervical incompetence. *Am J Perinatol*. 2006;23:313.

 ## MISCELLANEOUS

ABBREVIATIONS

- CVA—Costovertebral angle
- DES—Diethylstilbestrol
- GA—Gestational age
- TAUS—Transabdominal ultrasound
- TVUS—Transvaginal ultrasound
- UTI—Urinary tract infection

 ## CODES

ICD9-CM

654.5 Cervical incompetence

PATIENT TEACHING

- Signs which may indicate cervical insufficiency:
  - Uterine contractions
  - Low, dull backache
  - Menstrual-like cramps
  - Pelvic pressure
  - Change in vaginal discharge
- Activity modification:
  - Level I:
    - 8–10 hours of sleep at night
    - 1 hour of rest, in the morning and afternoon
    - Light household chores
    - No exercise or strenuous activity
    - Short walks (2–3 blocks) if desired
    - Short shopping trips, to a movie, or out to dinner on occasion
    - Work limitation
  - Level II:
    - 8–10 hours of sleep at night
    - Rest most of the day
    - May get up to shower or use the restroom
    - Will need help with housekeeping, laundry, and grocery shopping
    - No walking, exercise, or sports
    - Work cessation
  - Level III:
    - 8–10 hours of sleep at night
    - Rest in bed all day
    - May get up to shower or use the restroom
    - No stairs
    - Will need help with all home chores
    - Meals in bed
    - Leave house only for doctor visits

Section V

CERVICAL RIPENING

Cecilia Gambala, MD, MSPH
Sarah Kilpatrick, MD, PhD

 BASICS

DESCRIPTION

Cervical maturation or cervical "ripening" refers to the use of either pharmacologic or nonpharmacologic methods to produce a more favorable cervix that is softer and more effaced. This effect will subsequently increase the likelihood of a successful induction of labor. The goal of preinduction cervical ripening is to decrease time to delivery and possibly lower the rate of cesarean delivery.

- Pharmacologic methods:
  - Hormonal methods:
    o Prostaglandins
  - Oxytocin
- Nonpharmacologic methods:
  - Membrane stripping
  - Mechanical dilators
  - Hygroscopic dilators
  - Balloon catheter (alone, with traction, with infusion)
  - Amniotomy

EPIDEMIOLOGY

Between 1990 and 2004, the rate of labor induction in the US increased from 9.5% to 21.2% of all births nationwide.

PATHOPHYSIOLOGY

- Pharmacologic methods:
  - PGEs:
    o 20 carbon bioactive lipid important for cervical maturation
    o E2: Dinoprostones (Cervidil, Prepidil)
    o E1: Misoprostol (Cytotec)
  - Oxytocin (Pitocin):
    o Potent endogenous uterotonic agent
    o Myometrial oxytocin receptor concentrations increase on average 100–200-fold during pregnancy, reaching a maximum during early labor.
- Nonpharmacologic methods:
  - Mechanical release of endogenous prostaglandins from the membranes and adjacent decidua, which may be involved in stimulating myometrial contractions and in the onset of labor
  - May trigger an autonomic neural reflex that promotes the release of oxytocin from the maternal posterior pituitary

 DIAGNOSIS

SIGNS AND SYMPTOMS
History

- Patients who require cervical ripening are those whose management plans include an induction of labor for either maternal or fetal indications.
- Induction refers to the initiation of uterine contractions before the spontaneous onset of labor for the purpose of delivery.
- Cervical ripening may be the 1st step to induction.
- Important obstetric history:
  - History of prior cesarean deliveries:
    o History of prior classical uterine incision contraindicated
- Other contraindications to induction of labor include but are not limited to:
  - Placenta or vasa previa
  - Transverse fetal lie
  - Active genital herpes infection
  - Allergies or adverse reactions to medications (i.e., prostaglandins, oxytocin, misoprostol)

ALERT
PGE1 use is contraindicated in patients with history of prior cesarean section or major uterine surgery.

Physical Exam

- Cervical exam with assessment of dilation, effacement, station, consistency, and cervical position
- Bishop score: If ≤6, then cervical ripening recommended for an increased likelihood for a successful induction of labor. Each parameter can score up to 3 points:
  - Dilation in centimeters
  - Closed, 0 points:
    o 1–2 cm, 1 point
    o 3–4 cm, 2 points
    o ≥5 cm, 3 points
  - Effacement %:
    o 0–30%, 0 points
    o 40–50%, 1 point
    o 60–70%, 2 points
    o ≥80%, 3 points
  - Station:
    o −3, 0 points
    o −2, 1 point
    o −1 or 0, 2 points
    o +1 or +2, 3 points

- Consistency:
  o Firm, 0 points
  o Medium, 1 point
  o Soft, 2 points
- Cervical position:
  o Posterior, 0 points
  o Midposition, 1 point
  o Anterior, 2 points
- Assess shape and adequacy of bony pelvis: Clinical pelvimetry
- Assess estimated fetal weight and presentation by Leopold maneuvers.

TESTS
- Routine labor and delivery admission testing
- NST to assess fetal well being
- Amniotic fluid assessment if indicated

Imaging
US to confirm vertex presentation if needed

TREATMENT

GENERAL MEASURES
- Document indications of induction of labor.
- Review history of any contraindications to labor and/or vaginal delivery.
- Confirm GA.
- Determine fetal position.
- Confirm fetal well being.
- Continuous fetal monitoring is necessary in appropriate situations.

PREGNANCY-SPECIFIC ISSUES
By Trimester
Doses of pharmacologic agents changes from 3rd trimester inductions to 2nd trimester inductions for termination. Oxytocin (Pitocin) is not as effective for induction of labor compared to other options available for 2nd trimester indications. Exact dosing considerations are listed in Medications section below.

Risks for Mother
- Failed induction
- Need for cesarean section
- Time
- Discomfort

Risks for Fetus
Intolerance to uterine contractions

SPECIAL THERAPY
Complementary and Alternative Therapies
Mechanical dilation using an intracervical catheter can be augmented with low-dose IV Pitocin.

MEDICATION (DRUGS)
- If a pharmacologic method is preferred for cervical ripening, the following drugs can be used. Consider changing induction method after 24 hours if no progress.
- Prostaglandin E2:
  - 3rd trimester:
    - Prepidil: 0.5 mg in 2.5-mL gel intracervical preparation q4–6h
    - Cervidil: 10 mg in timed-release intravaginal preparation q12h
    - PG gel: Dinoprostone in various concentrations (2–5 mg) in 10 mL gel
  - 2nd trimester:
    - Dinoprostone: 20 mg suppository q6h
- Prostaglandin E1, Misoprostol (Cytotec):
  - 3rd trimester:
    - 25–50 μg q4h intravaginally at external cervical os or posterior fornix
    - 50 μg PO q4h
  - 2nd trimester cervical ripening and induction for termination:
    - 100–200 μg intravaginally q3–4h
    - 400–800 μg intravaginally q6–12h
  - Tablets come in 100–200-μg forms
- Oxytocin 1–4 mIU/min, low-dose, continuous infusion

ALERT
- PGE1 use is contraindicated in patients with history of prior cesarean deliveries or major uterine surgery.

- Side effects: Tachysystole (more frequent with 50 μg) or hyperstimulation; nausea, diarrhea, and fever

SURGERY
- If a nonpharmacologic method is preferred, the following methods can be used. Keep in mind relative contraindications: Mucopurulent cervical discharge, ruptured membranes.

- Membrane stripping:
  - Digital separation of chorioamnionic membrane from the wall of the cervix and lower uterine segment
- Mechanical dilators, balloon catheters:
  - Intracervical Foley balloon catheter placed in the cervical canal at the lower uterine segment, latex or nonlatex in sizes 18–26 gauge.
  - The catheter balloon is then filled with 30 mL of sterile normal saline.
  - Traction is then applied by taping the catheter taut onto the patient's thigh.
  - Normal saline solution can also be infused through the catheter port at 30 mL/h (EASI; extra amniotic saline induction).
  - Can also use concomitantly with oxytocin
  - If not expelled spontaneously after 12 hours, remove and continue with another method.
- Hygroscopic dilators:
  - Absorbs water to swell and forcibly dilate the cervix
  - Laminaria: Desiccated seaweed
  - Dilapan polyacrylonitrile
  - Lamicel: Magnesium sulfate in polyvinyl alcohol
  - Placed into cervical canal at internal os after cleansing cervix with Betadine
  - Place gauze into vagina to keep dilators in place.
  - Remove 12–24 hours after placement and proceed with further ripening or induction.

ALERT
If latex allergy, balloon catheter is contraindicated.

 FOLLOW-UP

COMPLICATIONS
- Potential complications of PGE analogues:
  - Complications are dose related
  - Uterine hyperstimulation:
    - Intracervical PGE2 get (0.5 mg): 1%
    - Intravaginal PGE2 gel or vaginal insert: 5%
    - Subsequent FHR deceleration
    - Rarely, uterine rupture
    - Rarely, placental abruption
- Oxytocin:
  - Uterine rupture rare
  - Uterine hyperstimulation
  - Water intoxication with high concentration and hypotonic solutions
- Amniotomy:
  - Umbilical cord prolapse (rare)
  - Chorioamnionitis
  - Umbilical cord compression
  - Rupture of vasa previa

- Stripping the membranes:
  - Bleeding from undiagnosed placenta previa or low-lying placenta
  - Accidental amniotomy
- Mechanical dilators:
  - Risk of maternal or neonatal infection

PATIENT MONITORING
Mother
- With PG preparation:
  - Patient should remain recumbent for at least 30 minutes.
  - Record vital signs.
  - Uterine activity is monitored continuously for 30 minutes to 2 hours after administration of PGE2 gel.
  - If no increase in uterine activity and FHR unchanged, may transfer elsewhere
- With Misoprostol:
  - Uterine activity monitoring in hospital setting

Fetus
- With PGE2 vaginal insert:
  - Electronic fetal heart rate monitoring from placement of vaginal PGE2 until at least 15 min after removal.
- With misoprostol:
  - FHR monitoring in hospital setting

BIBLIOGRAPHY
ACOG Committee Opinion No. 342. Induction of Labor after Vaginal Birth after Cesarean Delivery. Washington, DC: ACOG; 2006.

Gabbe. *Obstetrics: Normal and problem pregnancies*, 4th ed. New York: Churchill Livingstone; 2002.

 MISCELLANEOUS

ABBREVIATIONS
- FHR—Fetal heart rate
- GA—Gestational age
- NST—Nonstress test
- PG—Prostaglandin

CHORIOAMNIONITIS

Yasser Y. El-Sayed, MD
Justin Collingham, MD

 BASICS

DESCRIPTION
- Chorioamnionitis is an infection of the amniotic fluid and its surrounding membranes.

EPIDEMIOLOGY
- Chorioamnionitis complicates .5–10% of deliveries.
- Frequency highest in preterm deliveries.
  - Up to 30% of preterm labor with intact membranes
  - 40% of PPROM with contractions
  - 75% of those who develop labor after admission for PPROM

RISK FACTORS
- Risks for term intrapartum chorioamnionitis:
  - Nulliparity
  - Prolonged labor or prolonged rupture of membranes (>24 hours associated with a 2–5-fold increase in risk)
  - Internal uterine or fetal monitoring
  - Multiple digital exams after ruptured membranes
  - Genital tract infections such as STDs, Group B streptococcus, bacterial vaginosis
- Risks for preterm chorioamnionitis:
  - Preterm labor or PROM (may also be a result of chorioamnionitis)
  - Obstetric procedures such as amniocentesis, emergent cerclage, or percutaneous umbilical cord sampling

PATHOPHYSIOLOGY
- The placenta and membranes act as mechanical and immunologic barriers to genital tract pathogens:
  - In term intrapartum chorioamnionitis after rupture of membranes and in PPROM, ascending infection is likely causative.
  - In preterm chorioamnionitis with intact membranes, a weakening of the membranes may provide a route for ascending infection.
- Most cases polymicrobial in nature:
  - *Bacteroides* sp.: 25%
  - *Gardnerella vaginalis*: 24%
  - Group B streptococcus: 12%
  - *Escherichia coli:* 10%
- Not associated with STIs

 DIAGNOSIS

SIGNS AND SYMPTOMS
History
A history of fevers with abdominal pain and foul-smelling discharge may be consistent with chorioamnionitis after ruptured membranes.

Physical Exam
Diagnosis of chorioamnionitis is typically made by documenting a maternal temperature of 38°C (100.4°F) with ≥1 of the following:
- Maternal tachycardia (>100 bpm)
- Fetal tachycardia (>160 bpm)
- Uterine tenderness
- Malodorous vaginal discharge

TESTS
Lab
- Leukocytosis of >15,000/mm^3 may be suggestive of infection.
- Subclinical chorioamnionitis may be detected by amniocentesis:
  - May be warranted with refractory preterm labor or when diagnosis of chorioamnionitis is uncertain
  - Culture remains gold standard, but following tests may be useful in supporting or refuting diagnosis of chorioamnionitis:
    - Gram stain for bacteria
    - Glucose (<15 mg/dL suggests infection)
    - WBC (>30 cells/mm^3 suggests infection)

DIFFERENTIAL DIAGNOSIS
Infection
Other maternal infections may present similarly, particularly in the nonlaboring patient, such as appendicitis or pyelonephritis.

Tumor/Malignancy
Degenerating uterine fibroids may present with abdominal pain, uterine tenderness, and a low-grade maternal temperature.

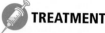 **TREATMENT**

GENERAL MEASURES
- Treatment for chorioamnionitis involves delivery of the fetus and maternal treatment with broad-spectrum antibiotics.
- If chorioamnionitis diagnosed intrapartum, augmentation of labor to expedite delivery is recommended.
- If chorioamnionitis diagnosed antepartum, delivery via induction or cesarean is warranted, with cesarean delivery reserved for usual obstetric indications.
- Early antibiotic treatment decreases both maternal and neonatal infectious morbidity.

PREGNANCY-SPECIFIC ISSUES
By Trimester
Diagnosis of chorioamnionitis before viability (23–24 weeks' gestation) typically warrants an induced previable delivery (termination).

Risks for Mother
- Common maternal complications in the developed world:
  - Bacteremia
  - Need for cesarean delivery
  - Postpartum hemorrhage secondary to atony
  - Wound infection after cesarean delivery
  - Endometritis
- Rare complications in the developed world but more common in the developing world:
  - Septic shock
  - DIC
  - ARDS

Risks for Fetus
- Risk of fetal infection with chorioamnionitis is 10–20%, with neonatal sepsis and pneumonia most common:
  - Infectious complications in preterm chorioamnionitis more common and severe
- Associations with increased risk of cerebral palsy and periventricular leukomalacia have been documented.

370

MEDICATION (DRUGS)

- Ampicillin 2 g IV q6h plus gentamicin 1.5 mg/kg q8h is the generally recommended regimen for intrapartum treatment of chorioamnionitis:
  - The addition of clindamycin 900 mg IV q8h after cesarean delivery is recommended to reduce anaerobic postsurgical infectious complications.
- Cefazolin 2 g IV and then 1 g IV q8h plus gentamicin is an alternative for those patients with a penicillin allergy and a low risk for anaphylaxis.
- Clindamycin 900 mg IV q8h plus gentamicin or vancomycin 1 g IV q12h are alternatives for those patients with a penicillin allergy and a risk for anaphylaxis.
- Continue antibiotics until patient is afebrile for 24–48 hours after cesarean delivery.
- Treatment options after vaginal delivery include:
  - Discontinuation of antibiotics
  - Treatment with additional dose after delivery
  - Treatment for 24–48 hours afebrile

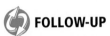 FOLLOW-UP

PATIENT MONITORING
Mother
Monitor for signs of endometritis after antibiotic treatment, such as maternal fever and fundal tenderness (or adult).

Fetus
Close observation of the infant after delivery is warranted, with empiric antibiotic therapy often initiated.

BIBLIOGRAPHY

Gibbs RS, et al. Quantitative bacteriology of amniotic fluid from patients with clinical intra-amniotic infection at term. *J Infect Dis*. 1982;145:1–8.

Gibbs RS, et al. A randomized trial of intrapartum versus immediate postpartum treatment of women with intra-amniotic infection. *Obstet Gynecol*. 1988;72:823–828.

Gibbs RS, et al. Progress in pathogenesis and management of clinical intra-amniotic infection. *Am J Obstet Gynecol*. 1991;164:1317–1326.

Yoon BH, et al. Clinical significance of intra-amniotic inflammation in patients with preterm labor and intact membranes. *Am J Obstet Gynecol*. 2001;185:1130–1136.

 MISCELLANEOUS

SYNONYM(S)
- Intra-amniotic infection
- Intrapartum fever

ABBREVIATIONS
- ARDS—Acute respiratory distress syndrome
- DIC—Disseminated intravascular coagulation
- PPROM—Preterm premature rupture of membranes
- PROM—Premature rupture of membranes
- STD/STI—Sexually transmitted disease/infection

CODES

ICD9-CM
762.7 Chorioamnionitis

 PATIENT TEACHING

Chorioamnionitis. Available at: http://www.clevelandclinic.org/health/health-info/docs/3800/3857.asp?index=12309

PREVENTION
Limiting unnecessary vaginal exams in labor

Section V

CORTICOSTEROID USE FOR FETAL LUNG MATURATION

Shirley L. Wang, MD

 BASICS

DESCRIPTION
- Antenatal glucocorticoids administered to women at risk for preterm delivery
- Reduces risk of RDS and IVH as well as overall perinatal morbidity and mortality by ~50% in premature infants
- GA: 24–34 weeks
- Single course of betamethasone 12 mg/d for 2 doses or dexamethasone 6 mg q12h for 4 doses.
- Clinical efficacy:
  - Reduction of RDS (9.0% vs. 25% in controls):
    - Max benefit in subgroup delivered 48 hours but <7 days after treatment (3.6% vs. 33.3%)
  - Meta-analysis shows reduction of IVH, necrotizing enterocolitis, neonatal mortality, systemic infection in the 1st 48 hours of life.

EPIDEMIOLOGY
~2% of all births in the US occur at 24–34 weeks, and thus would be candidates for antenatal glucocorticoids.

PATHOPHYSIOLOGY
Mechanism of action:
- Improves lung mechanics and gas exchange
- Maturational changes in lung architecture:
  - Accelerated morphologic development of type I and type II pneumocytes
- Biochemical maturation:
  - Regulates enzymes in type II pneumocytes
  - Stimulates phospholipid synthesis, subsequent release of surfactant

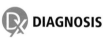 **DIAGNOSIS**

See Preterm Labor and Preterm Contractions.

 TREATMENT

GENERAL MEASURES
Gestational Age
- ACOG and NIH recommend administration at GA of 24–34 weeks.
- Prior to 24 weeks: Only a few primitive alveoli on which glucocorticoids can act
- After 34 weeks: No evidence of decreased RDS, IVH, neonatal mortality. Most likely because risk of such conditions low after 34 weeks.
- Antenatal Steroids For Term Caesarean Section (ASTCS) trial suggested the effectiveness of glucocorticoids in reducing respiratory distress from TTN after 37 weeks' gestation:
  - ACOG and NIH state that the use of glucocorticoids after 34 weeks can be considered if there is evidence of pulmonary immaturity.

PREGNANCY-SPECIFIC ISSUES
Risks for Mother
- Does not increase the risk of maternal death, chorioamnionitis, or puerperal sepsis
- Transient hyperglycemia:
  - Steroid effect begins ~2 hours after 1st dose, may last for 5 days.
  - In diabetic gravida, closely monitor and treat hyperglycemia.

Risks for Fetus
- Single course: Not associated with adverse neonatal events
- Can be associated with transient fetal heart rate changes that resolve 4–7 days after treatment:
  - Decrease in variability on days 2 and 3
  - Breathing and body movements commonly reduced
- Long-term studies of exposed fetuses have been reassuring.

MEDICATION (DRUGS)
- Betamethasone 12 mg IM q24h (2 doses)
- Dexamethasone 6 mg IM q12h (4 doses)
- Both regimens results in 75–80% occupancy of available glucocorticoid receptors.
- Higher or more frequent doses do not increase benefits.
- Hydrocortisone is extensively metabolized in the placenta; relatively little crosses into the fetal compartment and adequate fetal therapy *cannot be assured*.
- Use with PROM:
  - NIH consensus panel, 1994 recommendations:
    - Benefits of antenatal glucocorticoids outweigh the infection risk.
    - Antenatal glucocorticoid therapy is recommended for pregnancies complicated by PPROM at <30 to 32 weeks of gestation as long as there was no clinical evidence of chorioamnionitis.
    - Supported by meta-analysis of 15 trials, 2001

 FOLLOW-UP

Multiple courses of antenatal glucocorticoids are not recommended, as studies show they may result in harmful developmental effects on:
- Lung growth and organization
- Retinal development
- HPA axis
- Insulin resistance
- Renal glomerular number
- Somatic growth
- Head circumference
- Maturation of the CNS

DISPOSITION
Issues for Referral
Referral or transfer as necessary to provide appropriate level of neonatal care in the event of preterm delivery.

PATIENT MONITORING
Mother
For diabetic gravida, monitor and treat for possible transient hyperglycemia.

Fetus
Amniocentesis after administration of corticosteroids to assess for FLM is not predictive of RDS.

BIBLIOGRAPHY

ACOG Committee on Obstetric Practice. ACOG committee opinion: Antenatal corticosteroid therapy for fetal maturation. *Obstet Gynecol*. 2002;99(5 Pt 1):871–873.

Ballard PL, et al. Scientific basis and therapeutic regimens of use of antenatal glucocorticoids. *Am J Obstet Gynecol*. 1995;173(1):254–262.

Ballard PL. Hormones and lung maturation. In: *Monograms on Endocrinology*, vol. 28. Berlin: Springer-Verlag; 1986;1–345.

Harding JE, et al. Do antenatal corticosteroids help in the setting of preterm rupture of membranes? *Am J Obstet Gynecol*. 2001;184(2):131–139.

Liggins GC, et al. A controlled trial of antepartum glucosteroid treatment for prevention of respiratory distress syndrome in premature infants. *Pediatrics*. 1972;50:515.

Moore KL, et al. The respiratory system. In: *The Developing Human*, 5th ed. Philadelphia: W.B. Saunders; 1993;226.

Report on the Consensus Development Conference on the Effect of Corticosteroids for Fetal Maturation on Perinatal Outcomes. U.S. Department of Health and Human Services, Public Health Service, NIH Pub No. 95-5-3784, November 1994.

Roberts S, et al. Antenatal corticosteroids for accelerating fetal lung maturation for women at risk of preterm birth. *Cochrane Database Syst Rev*. 2006;3:CD004454.

Smolders-de Haas J, et al. Physical development and medical history of children who were treated antenatally with corticosteroids to prevent RDS: 10 to 12 year follow-up. *Pediatrics*. 1990;86(1):65–70.

Stutchfield P, et al. Antenatal betamethasone and incidence of neonatal respiratory distress after elective caesarean section: pragmatic randomised trial. *Br Med J*. 2005;331(7518):662. Epub 2005 Aug 22

MISCELLANEOUS
CLINICAL PEARLS

ALERT
NIH recommendations for use of antenatal corticosteroids:
- Benefits of antenatal administration of corticosteroids to fetuses at risk of PTD outweigh the potential risks:
  - Reduction in the risk of RDS
  - Reduction in mortality and IVH

- Candidates for antenatal treatment with corticosteroids: All fetuses between 24 and 34 weeks of gestation at risk of PTD.
- Decision to use antenatal corticosteroids should not be altered by fetal race or gender or by the availability of surfactant replacement therapy.
- Patients eligible for therapy with tocolytics should also be eligible for treatment with antenatal corticosteroids.
- Treatment:
  - 2 doses of 12 mg of betamethasone IM 24 hours apart
  - 4 doses of 6 mg of dexamethasone IM 12 hours apart
  - Optimal benefit begins 24 hours after initiation of therapy and lasts 7 days.
- In PPROM at <30–32 weeks of gestation in the absence of clinical chorioamnionitis, antenatal corticosteroid use is recommended.

ABBREVIATIONS
- ACOG—American College of Obstetricians and Gynecologists
- FLM—Fetal lung maturity
- GA—Gestational age
- HPA—Hypothalamic pituitary adrenal
- IVH—Intraventricular hemorrhage
- NIH—National Institutes of Health
- PPROM—Preterm premature rupture of membranes
- PROM—Premature rupture of membranes
- PTD—Preterm delivery
- RDS—Respiratory distress syndrome
- TTN—Transient tachypnea of the newborn

CODES
ICD9-CM
- 644.1 Other threatened labor
- 644.2 Early onset of labor
- 761.1 Premature rupture of membranes
- 769 Respiratory distress syndrome

PATIENT TEACHING

See "Preterm Labor" for teaching patients signs and symptoms of preterm labor.

PREVENTION
Antenatal corticosteroid use is preventive medicine for fetuses at risk for complications of prematurity.

Section V

DEEP VEIN THROMBOSIS AND PULMONARY EMBOLUS

Amy H. Picklesimer, MD, MSPH
Daniel Clarke-Pearson, MD

 BASICS

DESCRIPTION
Formation of blood clots of varying size within the deep veins, most commonly in the lower extremities or pelvis. These clots have the potential to embolize to the lung with potentially life-threatening consequences.

EPIDEMIOLOGY
- Incidence of DVT: 0.5–3:1,000 pregnancies
- Incidence of PE: 0.09–0.7:1,000 pregnancies
- Equally divided between antepartum and postpartum period
- Antenatally, equally divided among trimesters

RISK FACTORS
- Clinical risk factors:
  - Advanced maternal age
  - Increased parity
  - Multiple gestation
  - Trauma, especially orthopedic injuries
  - Surgery, including cesarean delivery
  - Prolonged immobility, as with bedrest
  - Indwelling central venous catheters
  - Travel (>4 hours)
  - Dehydration
  - Smoking
- Pathologic risk factors:
  - Inherited thrombophilia (see below)
  - Prior DVT or pulmonary embolism
  - Antiphospholipid antibodies
  - Lupus anticoagulant
  - Obesity
  - Malignancy
  - Nephrotic syndrome
  - Myeloproliferative disorders

Genetics
- 30% of patients with venous thromboembolism in pregnancy will be found to have an inherited thrombophilia.
- Plasma factors:
  - Factor V Leiden mutation
  - Prothrombin mutation (G20210A)
  - Protein C deficiency
  - Protein S deficiency
  - Antithrombin III deficiency
- Metabolic defects:
  - Hyperhomocysteinemia
  - MTHFR deficiency
- Impaired clot lysis (rare):
  - Dysfibrinogenemia
  - Plasminogen deficiency

PATHOPHYSIOLOGY
The classic triad is known as Virchow triad:
- Vessel wall injury:
  - Vessel damage caused during delivery
- Venous stasis:
  - Mechanical impedance of venous return caused by the gravid uterus
  - Increased vein distensibility caused by hormonal changes
- Changes in local clotting factors:
  - Normal pregnancy is characterized by progressive increases in clotting factors, a decrease in Protein S and resistance to activated Protein C.

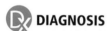 **DIAGNOSIS**

SIGNS AND SYMPTOMS
History
- DVT:
  - Often asymptomatic
  - Pain or tenderness
  - Limb swelling
- PE:
  - Tachypnea, dyspnea
  - Tachycardia
  - Pleuritic pain, cough, hemoptysis

Physical Exam
- Cannot reliably diagnose or exclude DVT
- Asymmetric limb swelling, >2 cm larger than opposite side
- Warmth or erythema of skin over area of thrombosis (rare)
- Homan sign: Calf pain with dorsiflexion of the foot, 50% sensitivity
- Lisker sign: Pain on percussion of medial tibia
- Bancroft or Moses sign: Pain on compression of calf against tibia in anteroposterior plane

TESTS
Labs
- Baseline labs: CBC, coagulation profile.
- D-dimer assay is not useful. Elevations are found in normal pregnancy.
- Arterial blood gasses may be misleading. Respiratory alkalosis is common in normal pregnancy.
- Evaluation for inherited thrombophilias in pregnancy:
  - Tests that are reliable in pregnancy:
    - Factor V Leiden (PCR tests)
    - Prothrombin Mutation (G20210A)
    - Antithrombin III
    - MTHFR deficiency
    - Protein C (2nd-generation tests)
    - Lupus anticoagulant
    - Anticardiolipin antibodies
  - Tests that are altered by pregnancy:
    - Protein S (levels reduced 40–60%)
    - Protein C (1st-generation tests only)
    - Hyperhomocysteinemia (levels reduced)

Imaging
- Doppler US of lower extremities:
  - Sensitivity and specificity >95%
  - Noninvasive, no fetal risk
  - Will not identify clots in pelvic veins or inferior vena cava
- MRI:
  - Can detect clots in pelvic veins
  - No adverse events in pregnancy reported, but safety remains unproven
- Contrast venography: not commonly used in pregnancy
- Spiral CT scanning:
  - High sensitivity and specificity for pulmonary embolism in experienced hands
  - Radiation exposure <V/Q scan
- V/Q scan:
  - Accuracy depends on pretest probability
  - Low (500 mrad) radiation exposure to fetus

DIFFERENTIAL DIAGNOSIS
- Physiologic changes of pregnancy
- Musculoskeletal pain
- Superficial venous thrombosis
- Cellulitis
- Compartment syndrome

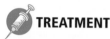 **TREATMENT**

GENERAL MEASURES
- Identifying candidates for prophylaxis:
  - Patients with a single previous episode of DVT associated with an identifiable, transient risk factor (excluding pregnancy and oral contraceptive use) do not require prophylaxis during pregnancy.
  - Patients with a single previous episode of DVT of uncertain etiology, and patients known to have inherited thrombophilias should receive prophylaxis during pregnancy and for at least 3 months postpartum.
  - Patients on long-term anticoagulation therapy due to multiple prior episodes of thrombosis or high-risk thrombophilias should continue to receive therapeutic does of either UFH or LMWH.
- DVT may be managed outpatient, but all patients with PE should be hospitalized. Anticoagulation is the primary therapy.
  - Precautions with anticoagulation:
    - Avoid IM injections
    - Monitor CBC, including platelets
    - Necrotic skin lesions may develop at injection sites

PREGNANCY-SPECIFIC ISSUES

By Trimester
- 1st trimester:
  - Warfarin is teratogenic, with a peak effect between 7–12 weeks gestation.
- 3rd trimester:
  - UFH is preferred in the late 3rd trimester as delivery approaches because it has a shorter half-life and its effects are more reliably reversed with protamine sulfate. Patients on LMWH should be switched to UFH no later than 37 weeks' gestation.

Risks for Mother
- Large PE may lead to cardiovascular instability or death.
- Anticoagulation carries additional risks for women who have preeclampsia, peptic ulcer disease, IBD, noncompliance and poor follow-up.
- Use of UFH for >7 weeks can increase the risk of osteoporosis.

Risks for Fetus
- Large PE may lead to maternal hypoxia and fetal distress.
- There is no increased risk for abruption for patients receiving anticoagulation.

MEDICATION (DRUGS)
- UFH:
  - Initial management: 80 U/kg IV bolus, followed by continuous infusion starting at 18 U/kg/h and adjusted to maintain aPTT of 1.5–2 times control.
  - Maintenance: Total number of units required over 24 hours of IV infusion given SC in 2 divided doses.
  - Due to variable dose-response relationships, particularly in pregnant women, requires frequent monitoring to maintain aPTT in therapeutic range
  - May be restarted 12 hours after cesarean delivery or 6 hours after uncomplicated vaginal delivery
- LMWH:
  - Either 1 mg/kg SC b.i.d. or 1.5 mg/kg/d SC
  - May be initiated in an outpatient setting
  - More predictable dose-response relationship. Factor XA levels should be measured 4 hours after dosing once each trimester, due to weight increases during pregnancy.
- Warfarin:
  - Does not cross into breast milk. May be safely used postpartum.
- Thrombolytic agents have been used with success in small series of pregnant women with life-threatening PE.

ALERT
LMWH should be held for 24 hours before administration of epidural or spinal anesthesia because of the risk for spinal hematoma. Patients receiving UFH may undergo spinal or epidural anesthesia once PTT normalizes.

SURGERY
- When anticoagulants and thrombolytics are contraindicated, filtering devices can be inserted into the vena cava to "trap" emboli before they reach the lungs.
- Very large clots can be surgically removed in certain circumstances.

 FOLLOW-UP

DISPOSITION
Issues for Referral
Vascular surgery or interventional radiology should be consulted for patient with large clots or cardiovascular instability.

PROGNOSIS
- 20% of untreated proximal (e.g., above the calf) DVTs progress to PE, and 10–20% of those are fatal. With aggressive anticoagulant therapy, mortality is decreased 5–10-fold.
- DVT confined to the infrapopliteal veins has a small risk of embolization, but these can propagate into the proximal system and therefore should be treated in pregnancy.

COMPLICATIONS
- PE (fatal in 10–20%)
- Arterial embolism (paradoxical embolization) with AV shunting
- Chronic venous insufficiency
- Postphlebitic syndrome (pain and swelling in affected limb without new clot formation)
- Treatment-induced hemorrhage
- Soft tissue ischemia associated with massive clot and high venous pressures: Phlegmasia cerulea dolens (rare but is a surgical emergency)

PATIENT MONITORING
Duration of treatment:
- All events during pregnancy should be treated with full anticoagulation for a minimum of 6 months. Low-risk patients may then be converted to prophylactic therapy for the remainder of pregnancy, through delivery, and for 6–12 weeks postpartum.
- High-risk conditions should be treated with full anticoagulation throughout pregnancy, delivery, and 6–12 weeks postpartum for a total treatment time of 6–18 months: Active cancer, continued immobilization, protein C/S deficiency, and elevated Factor VIII
- Very high-risk conditions should be continued indefinitely on anticoagulation: recurrent DVT, PE, or other thrombotic event, life-threatening event (large pulmonary embolism, limb-threatening DVT), cerebral or visceral vein thrombosis, antithrombin deficiency, homozygous Factor V Leiden, antiphospholipid antibodies with event, combined clotting disorders (Factor V Leiden with elevated homocysteine).

Mother
Investigate significant bleeding (hematuria or GI hemorrhage), because anticoagulant therapy may unmask a pre-existing lesion (e.g., cancer, peptic ulcer disease, arteriovenous malformation).

Fetus
No additional fetal monitoring is required.

BIBLIOGRAPHY
Bates SM. Treatment and prophylaxis of venous thromboembolism during pregnancy. *Thromb Res.* 2002;108(2-3):97–106.

Franchini M, et al. Inherited thrombophilia. *Crit Rev Clin Lab Sci.* 2006;43(3):249–290.

Nijkeuter M, et al. Diagnosis of deep vein thrombosis and pulmonary embolism in pregnancy: A systematic review. *J Thromb Haemost.* 2006;4(3):496–500.

 MISCELLANEOUS

See Hereditary Thrombophilias; Antithrombin Deficiency; Factor V Leiden; Protein C Deficiency; Protein S Deficiency; Prothrombin 20210 (Mutation); Pulmonary Embolism

ABBREVIATIONS
- aPTT—Activated partial thromboplastin time
- IBD—Irritable bowel disease
- LMWH—Low molecular weight heparin
- MTHFR—Methylene tetrahydrofolate reductase
- POP—Progestin-only pill
- PT—Prothrombin time
- UFH—Unfractionated heparin

CODES
ICD9-CM
- 671 Venous complications in pregnancy and the puerperium
- 671.93 Unspecified venous complication, antepartum condition or complication
- 671.94 Unspecified venous complication, postpartum condition or complication
- 673 Obstetrical pulmonary embolism
- 673.23 Obstetrical blood clot embolism, antepartum condition or complication
- 673.24 Obstetrical blood clot embolism, postpartum condition or complication

PATIENT TEACHING

Women with personal or family history of thrombosis should be offered screening for inherited or acquired thrombophilias (clotting disorders).

PREVENTION
Contraception is important in women with history of DVT/PE or with inherited thrombophilias because of increased risk with pregnancy, but estrogen-containing hormonal contraceptives are contraindicated because of potential additive risks:
- Increased risk of venous thromboembolism has not been demonstrated with progestin-only contraceptives:
  - Depot medroxyprogesterone acetate
  - POP
  - Subcutaneous implant
  - Levonorgestrel IUD

DOWN SYNDROME AND OTHER CHROMOSOMAL ABNORMALITIES

Lee P. Shulman, MD

 BASICS

DESCRIPTION

Normal female chromosome complement is 46,XX and for males is 46,XY. An alteration in the numeric complement or in the structure of any chromosome can lead to an unbalanced complement and result in functional and developmental problems.

- Numeric abnormalities:
  - Most common are nondisjunctional events, such as Down syndrome, trisomy 18, and trisomy 13
  - Some numeric abnormalities are the result of a loss of a chromosome, such as Turner syndrome (45,X).
- Structural abnormalities:
  - Any structural rearrangement including a duplication, deletion, or combination thereof can lead to an unbalanced complement.
  - Structural alterations can be de novo, spontaneous, or inherited from a parent. The detection of a structural chromosome abnormality in a fetus or child should lead to parental chromosome analyses.
- Mosaicism:
  - The existence of >1 cell line, usually with at least 1 normal cell line, in an individual. Affected individuals with abnormal mosaic complements are usually, but not always, less severely affected than individuals with nonmosaic abnormal complements.

ALERT

Chromosome abnormalities, including Down syndrome, are the most common reason that women choose to undergo prenatal diagnosis.

Age-Related Factors

- Survival usually depends on type of chromosome abnormality:
  - Numeric, non-sex chromosome: Few survive past childhood
  - Numeric, sex chromosome: Most with normal life expectancy
  - Structural non-sex chromosome: Usually not as lethal as numeric conditions, but usually associated with diminished life expectancy
  - Structural sex chromosome: Most with normal life expectancy
  - Mosaicism: If cell lines involve autosomes, usually diminished life expectancy. Sex chromosome abnormalities usually have no adverse effect on life expectancy.

Pediatric Considerations

- Most infants with non-sex chromosome (autosome) abnormalities show considerable developmental and functional abnormalities and many die in the 1st few years of life.
- Children with sex chromosome abnormalities usually show mild or no stigmata and are not usually characterized by severe developmental problems.

Pregnancy Considerations

- Men with Down syndrome are sterile, but women with Down syndrome can reproduce with only a slight increased risk of a similarly affected offspring.
- Most individuals with non-sex chromosome abnormalities do survive to reproduce, and those with sex chromosome abnormalities may have reduced fertility, frequently leading to the detection of the sex chromosome abnormality.

Geriatric Considerations

Affected individuals rarely survive to geriatric age.

EPIDEMIOLOGY

- Most autosomal abnormalities detected at birth or in early childhood.
- Sex chromosome abnormalities may not be detected until adulthood, commonly at the time of an evaluation for infertility or an abnormal pregnancy or child.

RISK FACTORS

- Risk for a fetus with numeric abnormalities like Down syndrome increase with maternal age.
- The risks for Down syndrome based on maternal age:
  - 20 years: 1/2,000
  - 35 years: 1/200
  - 37 years: 1/100
  - 45 years: 1/20
- Structural abnormalities not affected by parental age, but are rather associated with the presence of balanced parental chromosome rearrangements.

Genetics

- With regard to Down syndrome and other nondisjunctional events: An extra chromosome comes from the mother in >90% of the cases.
- Inheritance:
  - If child has trisomy 21, 1% risk for trisomy 21
  - 1–20% for parent with a balanced translocation; range depends on parent and type of rearrangement.
  - If the parental translocation is 21:21 (45,t [21:21]), the recurrence is 100%.
  - Increased inheritance in families with mosaic Down syndrome is not clear, but prenatal testing is recommended.

PATHOPHYSIOLOGY

Etiology of Down syndrome and other numeric abnormalities:

- Genetic: Nondisjunction or unequal chromosome division (95%)
- Genetic: Translocation (5%)

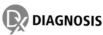 **DIAGNOSIS**

SIGNS AND SYMPTOMS

Down syndrome

- Infants and children:
  - Brachycephaly (100%)
  - Hypotonia (80%)
  - Posterior 3rd fontanel
  - Small ears, with or without superior ear folds, with or without low-set ears
  - Mongoloid slant, eyes (90%)
  - Epicanthic folds (90%)
  - Brushfield (speckled) spots of iris (50%)
  - Esotropia (50%)
  - Depressed nasal bridge
  - Enlarged tongue (75%)
  - Small chin
  - Short neck
  - Cardiac murmur (50%)
  - Abnormal dermatoglyphics, including single palmar crease, distal palmar triradius, and absence of plantar whorl (ball of foot)
  - Developmental delay, which may not be apparent in 1st year
  - Thyroid defects; low or high (5%)
  - Mild–moderate instability of neck at C1–C2
- Adults:
  - Most findings milder, but brachycephaly remains
  - Patients are retarded (IQ = 40–45) but usually personable and cooperative.
  - Most adults can care for their personal needs. Some have jobs, but all require a sheltered environment.
  - A small percentage of patients have some autistic features. A small percentage of patients are nonverbal.
  - A small percentage of patients have breathing problems and tracheomalacia.

TESTS

- The goal of prenatal screening and testing is a means of identifying affected pregnancies for those couples who wish to exercise reproductive choice.
- ACOG recommends that all women be offered invasive testing such as CVS or amniocentesis as well as screening using multiple markers, of which there are several types; some include US.
- Each testing strategy has different sensitivities and specificities.
- Serum prenatal testing:
  - 1st-trimester testing at 10–13 weeks' gestation: Uses sonographic determination of nuchal translucency combined with the serum PAPP-A and free β-hCG (or hCG itself)

– 2nd-trimester testing at 15–18 weeks gestation: Uses a combination of AFP, uE3, hCG, and inhibin A in maternal serum

– Integrated test: Uses a combination of both the 1st- and 2nd-trimester testing just described

– Serum integrated test: Uses the combination of 1st- and 2nd-trimester screening without US for nuchal translucency

– Sequential screening: Performing 2nd-trimester screening after 1st-trimester screening

• Prenatal invasive testing (chorionic villus biopsy at 10–13 weeks or amniocentesis at 14 weeks and beyond).

Lab
A chromosome test is definitive and should always be done because of the chance of translocation.

Imaging
Prenatal US will detect certain "soft signs" such as shortened femurs, clinodactyly (curved 5th finger), small external pinna, as well as cardiac defects, prominent nuchal translucency, and renal anomalies.

DIFFERENTIAL DIAGNOSIS
Minor familial anomalies such as Mongoloid slant, epicanthic folds, and depressed nasal bridge, particularly in a child with hypotonia

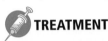

TREATMENT
GENERAL MEASURES
• Appropriate health care:
  – Genetic evaluation and counseling
  – Cardiac evaluation and ECG
  – Appropriate pediatric health care
  – Thyroid testing for any reasons (slowing of growth or weight gain, constipation) and thyroid treatment
• Parents can usually adapt to a special child.
• Most important is to address parental fears and treat the infant normally.
• Infant stimulation programs are recommended, but definitive proof of effectiveness is lacking.

PREGNANCY-SPECIFIC ISSUES
• Increased risk of fetal loss in all trimesters of pregnancy with autosomal abnormalities.
• No apparent increased risk for loss in cases of sex chromosome abnormalities, except for 45,X, which is most common chromosome finding in 1st-trimester losses.

By Trimester
Most chromosomally abnormal conceptuses are lost in the early 1st trimester, but pregnancies continue to show increased risk of loss in all 3 trimesters.

Risks for Mother
Usually no physical risk, but may have considerable adverse psychological impact

SPECIAL THERAPY
Physical Therapy
For those children with autosomal abnormalities, extensive physical and occupational therapy, along with special education, is required.

Complementary and Alternative Therapies
• Current enthusiasm for neural enhancers (e.g., piracetam, a GABA analog) not proven, but under study
• Experimental evidence that vitamin E prolongs the life of Down syndrome neurons in tissue culture

 FOLLOW-UP

DISPOSITION
Issues for Referral
Prenatal: Women at increased risk for Down syndrome and other chromosome abnormalities should be referred for genetic counseling and consideration of prenatal screening or diagnosis.

PROGNOSIS
• Autosomal abnormalities: Generally poor
• Sex chromosome abnormalities: Generally good, save for fertility
• Down syndrome children:
  – Development is normal in the 1st year in ~1/3 of cases and mildly delayed in the rest.
  – Development slows after age 1 y; language and cognition are moderately delayed.
  – The outcome and longevity may be dependent on congenital heart disease.
  – Some adult individuals can work in protected situations; a few are largely independent.
  – Intestinal complications and congenital heart disease may be of immediate concern.
  – Hypothyroid disease occurs after 6 months, and diminished growth is the principal sign.
  – Clinical Alzheimer disease in 1/3 of patients after age 35 years. Plaques in 100% of brains after age 20 years.
  – Premature aging: Most patients die at 50–60 years, earlier in presence of heart disease.

COMPLICATIONS
• Children with Down syndrome:
  – Bowel obstruction (fistula, intestinal anomalies [10%])
  – Hirschsprung disease (3%)
  – Thyroid disease (hypothyroidism and hyperthyroidism 5–8%)
  – Leukemia (1–20%)
  – Congenital heart disease (50%)
  – Alzheimer disease
  – Seizures (3–4%)
• Autosomal: Profound structural, functional, and development embarrassment, frequently necessitating medical and surgical intervention
• Sex chromosome: Most common complication is infertility, frequently, but not always requiring gamete donation or consideration of adoption

PATIENT MONITORING
Mother
Monitor pregnancy closely for continued pregnancy viability.

Fetus
• Monitor pregnancy closely for continued viability.
• Assess fetus for common structural abnormalities.
• Unable to predict outcome based on chromosome complement alone, including mosaic complements

BIBLIOGRAPHY
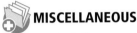
ACOG Practice Bulletin No. 77. Screening for Fetal Chromosomal Abnormalities. Washington DC: ACOG; January 2007.

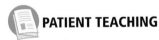 **MISCELLANEOUS**

CLINICAL PEARLS
• Older women, women with a history of a previous abnormal pregnancy, and women with abnormal US during pregnancy are at increased risk for child with Down syndrome and other chromosome abnormalities.
• Not all fetuses with chromosome abnormalities have detectable abnormalities on US.
• CVS and amniocentesis have been recently shown to be safe and reliable for detecting chromosome abnormalities.
  – Increased risk for miscarriage for either procedure is <1/1,000.

ABBREVIATIONS
• ACOG—American College of Obstetricians and Gynecologists
• AFP—α-Fetoprotein
• CVS—Chorionic villus sampling
• GABA—γ-Aminobutyric acid
• hCG—Human chorionic gonadotropin
• PAPP-A—Pregnancy-associated plasma protein A
• uE3—Unconjugated estriol

CODES
ICD9-CM
• 758.0 Down syndrome
• 655.13 Known or suspected chromosome abnormality
• 655.23 Hereditary disease history affecting fetus
• V82.4 Parental chromosome abnormality, not pregnant

PATIENT TEACHING
• National Down Syndrome Congress (800)–232–NDSC
• Down syndrome. Available at: Usenet Listserv at listserv@vm1.nodak.edu
• Down syndrome information and counseling. Available at: http://www.nas.com/downsyn
• Frank discussion of health issues, including piracetam. Available at: http://www.ds-health.com/

Section V

DYSTOCIA

Arin E. Ford, MD
James E. Ferguson, II, MD
Wendy F. Hansen, MD

BASICS

DESCRIPTION
- Dystocia simply means "difficult passage."
- Shoulder dystocia refers to impaction of a fetal shoulder behind the symphysis pubis.
- Fetopelvic disproportion usually (CPD): A disproportion between fetal size (head) relative to the maternal pelvis can lead to dystocia:
  - CPD is 1 cause of abnormal labor resulting in failure of progressive labor, which includes lack of progressive cervical dilation and/or lack of descent of the fetal head.
  - Dystocia is not diagnosed before an adequate trial of labor is achieved.
- Dystocia is defined as abnormal labor that results from abnormalities of:
  - Power (uterine contractions)
  - Passenger (fetal position, size, presentation)
  - Passage (maternal pelvis and soft tissues)

Age-Related Factors
- Possible connection between increasing maternal age, macrosomia, and increasing incidence of shoulder dystocia
- Nonprogression of 1st stage labor has been associated with increasing maternal age.

EPIDEMIOLOGY
- Shoulder dystocia incidence: 0.6–1.4% of vaginal births in the vertex presentation:
  - Neonatal morbidity: ~20%
  - ~50% of shoulder dystocias will occur in neonates <4,000 g.
  - Recurrence risk: ~14%
- CPD

RISK FACTORS
- Fetal macrosomia (≥4,000–4,500 g)
- Maternal diabetes
- Maternal obesity
- History of previous shoulder dystocia
- History of previous macrosomic fetus
- Postdate pregnancy (≥42 weeks)
- Prolonged active phase of labor
- Fetal anomalies
- Slow progress of labor associated with:
  - Inadequate uterine contractions
  - Chorioamnionitis
  - Pelvic contracture
- Longer duration of 2nd stage of labor associated with:
  - Occiput posterior position
  - Longer 1st stage of labor
  - Nulliparity
  - Short maternal stature
  - Birth weight
  - High station at complete dilation

Genetics
Dystocias are more likely with genetic conditions predisposing a fetus to anomalies that increase size.

ASSOCIATED CONDITIONS
- Fetal macrosomia
- Chorioamnionitis
- Maternal diabetes
- Maternal obesity
- Fetal anomalies
- Neonatal brachial plexus injury
- Neonatal hypoxic-ischemic encephalopathy
- Postpartum hemorrhage
- Maternal vaginal lacerations

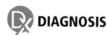

DIAGNOSIS

SIGNS AND SYMPTOMS
History
- Fetal macrosomia:
  - Recent US with EFW ≥4,500 g
  - History of previous macrosomic fetus
- Maternal diabetes
- History of previous shoulder dystocia
- Postdate pregnancy (≥42 weeks)
- Known fetal anomaly:
  - Cystic hygroma
  - Renal abnormalities
  - Hydrocephalus
  - Sacral teratoma
  - Hydrops

Physical Exam
- Leopold maneuver:
  - Palpation of maternal abdomen to assess fetal weight and lie
- Clinical pelvimetry to detect contracted maternal pelvic:
  - Measurement of various components of the female bony pelvis to assess for suspected CPD:
    ○ Pelvic inlet
    ○ Pelvic midcavity
    ○ Pelvic outlet
- "Turtle" sign:
  - Delivery of the fetal head with subsequent retraction of the head to the maternal perineum

TESTS
US:
- Assessment of EFW:
  - HC
  - BPD
  - AC
  - FL
- Subject to a high degree of error

Lab
Gestational diabetes evaluation (24–28 weeks):
- 1–hour GLT (50 g glucose load)
  - Abnormal 1-hour GLT: ≥140 mg/dL
  - Proceed with 3-hour GTT with 100 g glucose load

Imaging
Radiologic assessment of bony pelvis:
- X-ray pelvimetry
- CT pelvimetry
- Rarely used, not superior to clinical assessment regarding prediction

DIFFERENTIAL DIAGNOSIS
CPD
- Fetal size being too great for passage through relative maternal pelvis
- Affecting factors include:
  - Hereditary factors
  - Medical comorbidities (diabetes)
  - Pelvic structure
  - Abnormal fetal lie

Infection
Chorioamnionitis has been associated with dystocia as a *consequence* of prolonged labor.

Tumor/Malignancy
Uterine fibroids may cause dystocia.

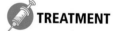

TREATMENT

GENERAL MEASURES
- See topic on shoulder dystocia for specific maneuvers to address.
- Oxytocin supplementation (See "Oxytocin Administration")
- Maternal hydration
- Ambulation

PREGNANCY-SPECIFIC ISSUES
Dystocias pose multiple risks to both mother and fetus/neonate.

Risks for Mother
- Postpartum hemorrhage: 11%
- 4th-degree vaginal lacerations: 3.8%
- Endomyometritis:
  - More common in cases involving Zavanelli maneuver, symphysiotomy, or hysterotomy for shoulder dystocia
- Rectal or urethral trauma

Risks for Fetus
- Shoulder dystocia:
  - Brachial plexus injury (4–40%, varies widely)
  - Erb-Duchenne palsy
  - Klumpke palsy
  - Neonatal fractures
  - Neonatal hypoxic-ischemic encephalopathy
  - Fetal or neonatal death
- Other dystocias/CPD

SPECIAL THERAPY
Complementary and Alternative Therapies
Role of continuous support in labor

MEDICATION (DRUGS)
Augmentation of labor is indicated if pelvic size is adequate. (See topic)

SURGERY
Cesarean delivery is indicated when dystocia unable to be resolved or when fetal well-being requires action.

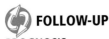 FOLLOW-UP

PROGNOSIS
Neonatal brachial plexus injury:
- <10% of all injuries are persistent.

COMPLICATIONS
- Maternal:
  - Postpartum hemorrhage
  - Severe vaginal lacerations
  - Sepsis
  - Rectal or urethral trauma
- Neonatal:
  - Brachial plexus injury
  - Fractures
  - Hypoxic-ischemic encephalopathy
  - Death

PATIENT MONITORING
Both mother and fetus/neonate require close intrapartum and postpartum monitoring.

Mother
- Intrapartum:
  - Vital signs
  - Bleeding
  - Pain control
- Postpartum:
  - Vital signs
  - Bleeding (hemoglobin/hematocrit)
  - Pain control
  - Infection or fever
  - Development of urinary or fecal incontinence or fistula due to lacerations

Fetus
- Intrapartum:
  - Fetal heart rate assessment:
    - Presence or absence of accelerations/decelerations
    - Presence or absence of variability
- Postpartum:
  - Cord gas assessment
  - APGAR scoring
  - Vital signs
  - Infection or fever
  - Imaging to rule out fractures
  - Pain control
  - Neurologic assessment

BIBLIOGRAPHY

ACOG Practice Bulletin No. 49. Dystocia and Augmentation of Labor. Washington DC: ACOG; 2003.

ACOG Practice Bulletin No 40. Shoulder Dystocia. Washington DC: ACOG; 2002.

ACOG Practice Bulletin No. 30. Gestational Diabetes. Washington DC: ACOG; 2001.

Lewis DF. *Am J Obstet Gynecol*. 1995;172:1369–1371.

Nocon JJ. Shoulder dystocia: An analysis of risks and obstetric maneuvers. *Am J Obstet Gynecol*. 1993; 168:1732–1739.

 MISCELLANEOUS

CLINICAL PEARLS
- Shoulder dystocia can not be accurately predicted or prevented.
- Shoulder dystocia is an obstetric emergency that requires anticipation and methodical efforts by an experienced clinician to achieve delivery with minimal morbidity to the mother or fetus.
- Few brachial plexus injuries (<10%) result in permanent damage to the neonate.

ABBREVIATIONS
- AC—Abdominal circumference
- BPD—Biparietal diameter
- CPD—Cephalopelvic disproportion
- EFW—Estimated fetal weight
- FL—Femur length
- GLT—Glucose loading test
- GTT—Glucose tolerance test
- HC—Head circumference

CODES
ICD9-CM
- 660.4 Shoulder (girdle) dystocia
- 660.9 Dystocia
- 763.1 Dystocia affecting newborn or fetus
- 763.1 Shoulder (girdle) dystocia affecting newborn or fetus
- 767.6 Brachial plexus palsy
- 767.6 Erb-Duchenne's palsy
- 767.6 Klumpke's palsy

PATIENT TEACHING

- Subsequent pregnancies:
  - Recurrence rate varies from 14%
  - Must consider multiple factors for mode of delivery:
    - DM
    - EFW compared with previous neonate
    - Severity of neonatal injury
    - Previous vaginal lacerations
- Brachial plexus injury:
  - <10% are persistent
  - Can occur without shoulder dystocia or at the time of cesarean delivery

PREVENTION
- Consider elective cesarean delivery:
  - Nondiabetic: EFW >5,000 g
  - Diabetic: EFW >4,500 g
- Continuous support in labor (nurses, midwives, doulas) has been associated with a reduction in cesarean and operative vaginal deliveries.
- The active management of labor has not been shown to lead to a reduction in cesarean deliveries.
- No recommendations exist to prevent shoulder dystocia.
- Always have a clear plan and practiced methodology to cope with the unexpected.
- Be prepared for a shoulder dystocia in *every* delivery.

Section V

ECTOPIC PREGNANCY

C. H. McCracken, III, MD

 BASICS

DESCRIPTION

Ectopic pregnancy is defined by the presence of the fertilized ovum outside the endometrial cavity. The ectopic pregnancy may be ruptured or unruptured. Hemorrhage from ectopic pregnancy is the leading cause of pregnancy-related maternal death in the 1st trimester.

Age-Related Factors

Women of reproductive age are at risk. Women >35 may be at higher risk than younger age groups.

EPIDEMIOLOGY

- Occur in ~2% of all US pregnancies
- The highest rate of ectopic pregnancy occurs in women aged 35–44 years.
- The highest incidence of ectopic pregnancy is in women aged 20–29.

RISK FACTORS

- Previous tubal surgery
- Previous ectopic pregnancy
- Tubal ligation
- Current IUD use
- Current use of progestin only contraceptive pills and implants
- In utero DES exposure
- History of PID
- Documented tubal abnormality
- History of infertility
- History of chlamydial or gonococcal cervicitis or PID:
  - >1/2 of ectopic pregnancies occur in women without risk factors.

Genetics

Primary ciliary dyskinesia (Kartagener syndrome) may be associated with an increased risk of ectopic pregnancy.

PATHOPHYSIOLOGY

Location:

- Most (97.7%) occur in the oviduct:
  - Ampullary: 81%
  - Isthmus: 12%
  - Fimbria: 5%
- Abdominal: 1.4%
- Interstitial or cornual: 2%
- Ovarian: 0.5%
- The incidence of heterotopic pregnancy is between 1:100 and 1:4,000.

ASSOCIATED CONDITIONS

Heterotopic pregnancy (concurrent ectopic pregnancy and intrauterine pregnancy):

- Rare condition, but may be increasing in frequency
- Heterotopic pregnancies may be more likely to occur after use of ART and IVF and embryo transfer.

 DIAGNOSIS

SIGNS AND SYMPTOMS

- Abdominal pain
- Amenorrhea
- Vaginal bleeding
- Dizziness, fainting
- Urge to defecate
- Pregnancy symptoms
- Passage of tissue
- Adnexal tenderness
- Abdominal tenderness
- Adnexal mass
- Uterine enlargement
- Orthostatic changes
- Fever

History

- Constitutional and symptoms of pregnancy:
  - Fatigue, nausea, breast symptoms, urinary frequency
- Menstrual:
  - Last menstrual period
  - Usual menstrual interval
  - Onset of unusual bleeding
- Reproductive:
  - Sexually active
  - Last intercourse
- Contraceptive:
  - Current form and usage:
    - Although IUDs very effectively prevent pregnancy, if a pregnancy occurs, it is more likely to be ectopic than if it occurred in the absence of IUD use.
    - Pregnancies occurring as a result of failure of POP OCPs or implants are more likely to be ectopic.
- Gynecologic:
  - Pelvic surgery
  - Infertility treatment
  - Upper reproductive tract infections
- Pain:
  - Onset
  - Duration
  - Location

Physical Exam

- A benign exam does not rule out an ectopic pregnancy.
- Vital signs:
  - Tachycardia
  - Orthostatic changes
  - Hypotension
- Abdominal exam:
  - Tenderness
  - Rebound and guarding
  - Cullen sign (periumbilical blue coloration is a sign of retroperitoneal hemorrhage)
  - Distention

- Pelvic exam:
  - Vaginal bleeding present
  - Adnexal mass
  - Fullness or pointing in the cul de sac on rectovaginal exam

ALERT

A soft and disproportionately large cervix with extrusion of dark tissue through the os is suggestive of a cervical pregnancy.

TESTS

- D&C:
  - The presence of trophoblasts with uterine curettage tissue will distinguish between an IUP and an ectopic pregnancy.
  - Disruptive to normal intrauterine pregnancies
- Culdocentesis:
  - Detects the presence of hemoperitoneum
  - Of little use with the availability of reliable TVUS

Lab

- Quantitative hCG:
  - Serial quantitative hCG evaluation, performed at 48-hour intervals, is useful if the diagnosis of ectopic pregnancy is not confirmed by exam and imaging studies.
  - A 66% or greater rise is expected in a normal pregnancy.
  - Falling levels are confirmatory of a nonviable pregnancy, but do not rule out an ectopic pregnancy.
- Serum progesterone:
  - Serum progesterone levels are less useful in confirming the diagnosis of ectopic pregnancy, but may be useful in distinguishing between a viable and a nonviable pregnancy.
  - In patients with a serum progesterone level <5 ng/mL, only 0.16% will have a viable pregnancy, 85% have spontaneous abortions, 14% have ectopic pregnancies.
- CBC
- Type and screen (especially if Rh status is unknown)

Imaging

- TVUS is the imaging modality of choice.
- A finding of an extrauterine gestational sac is diagnostic of an ectopic pregnancy.
- A negative pelvic ultrasound (absence of an adnexal mass or IUP) does not exclude the diagnosis of ectopic pregnancy.
- Normal US findings:
  - 4.5–5 weeks: Intrauterine gestational sac
  - 5–6 weeks: Yolk sac appears
  - 5.5–6 weeks: Double decidual sign
  - 5.5–6 weeks: Fetal pole with cardiac activity
- Presence of IUP does not exclude heterotopic pregnancy, but is typically reassuring, as heterotopic pregnancy is rare.

- US findings suggestive of ectopic pregnancy:
  - Complex adnexal mass
  - Fluid-filled adnexal mass surrounded by an echogenic ring (bagel sign)
  - Free fluid within the peritoneal cavity
  - A gestational sac or hyperechoic mass seen in the cornual area with myometrial thinning is suggestive of a interstitial pregnancy.
  - Intracervical location of a gestational sac with an echogenic rim is suggestive of a cervical pregnancy.
- Other modalities (not as useful as TVUS):
  - MRI
  - CT
  - Color Doppler flow Imaging

DIFFERENTIAL DIAGNOSIS

- Normal pregnancy
- Threatened abortion
- Missed abortion or blighted ovum
- Ruptured corpus luteum cyst
- Appendicitis
- Ovarian torsion
- Ovarian cyst

Infection

Antecedent pelvic infections increase the risk of ectopic pregnancy:

- *Chlamydia trachomatis*
- *Neisseria gonorrhoeae*

Metabolic/Endocrine

Elevated circulating levels of estrogen or progesterone can alter tubal contractility, thus increasing the risk of ectopic pregnancy.

Drugs

A history of in utero DES exposure confers a 4–5-fold risk of ectopic pregnancy.

TREATMENT

GENERAL MEASURES

Initial stabilization and volume resuscitation is necessary for the hemodynamically unstable patient, followed expeditiously by surgical management.

SPECIAL THERAPY

Complementary and Alternative Therapies

Expectant management:

- Limited use; must have careful patient selection
- Useful when hCG levels are low and declining
- Close follow-up is required.
- Methotrexate is often a better alternative to expectant management.

MEDICATION (DRUGS)

Methotrexate, a folic-acid antagonist, is the primary nonsurgical modality for treatment of ectopic pregnancy.

ALERT

Hemodynamic instability is a contraindication to medical management, and surgical intervention is required.

- Requirements for medical therapy:
  - Hemodynamically stable
  - No signs of hemoperitoneum or active bleeding
  - Patient is reliable and able to return for follow-up
  - No contraindications to methotrexate
- Relative indications:
  - Unruptured mass ≤3.5 cm
  - No fetal cardiac motion
  - hCG level <5,000
  - General anesthesia poses a significant risk
  - Nonlaparoscopic diagnosis
  - Desires future fertility
- Absolute contraindications:
  - Breastfeeding
  - Immunodeficiency
  - Alcoholism or alcoholic liver disease
  - Chronic liver disease
  - Preexisting blood dyscrasias
  - Known methotrexate sensitivity
  - Active pulmonary disease
  - Peptic ulcer disease
  - Hepatic, renal or hematologic dysfunction
- Relative contraindications:
  - Gestational sac ≥3.5 cm
  - Fetal cardiac motion

Regimens:

- Single dose:
  - Methotrexate 50 mg/m² IM injection on Day 0
  - No leucovorin rescue
  - 2nd dose if hCGs fail to decline 15% between days 4 and 7
- Multiple dose:
  - Methotrexate 1.0 mg/kg, days 0, 2, 4, and 6
  - Leucovorin 0.1 mg/kg, days 1, 3, 5, and 7
- Adverse drug effects: Nausea, vomiting, stomatitis, gastric distress, dizziness, severe neutropenia (rare), reversible alopecia (rare), pneumonitis
- Signs of treatment failure:
  - Significantly worsening abdominal pain
  - Hemodynamic instability
  - hCG levels that do not decline by at least 15% between day 4 and day 7
  - Increasing or plateauing hCG levels after the 1st week of treatment

SURGERY

- Laparoscopic or abdominal Incision
- Salpingectomy
- Salpingostomy
- Cornual resection for cornual or interstitial pregnancies
- Cervical pregnancy (see "Ectopic Pregnancy" in "Obstetric and Gynecologic Emergencies" section):
  - D&C

FOLLOW-UP

PROGNOSIS

- ~25% of conceptions after an ectopic pregnancy result in another ectopic.
- 1/3 of nulliparous women with an ectopic pregnancy will have a subsequent ectopic.

COMPLICATIONS

- Persistent ectopic pregnancy
- Tubal rupture
- Abdominal pregnancy

PATIENT MONITORING

- Weekly monitoring of hCG until the level is zero:
  - A decline of the hCG of <20% in 72 hours after surgical treatment is suggestive of incomplete treatment.
- Post treatment tubal patency may be assessed with a hysterosalpingogram.

BIBLIOGRAPHY

ACOG Practice Bulletin No. 3. Ory SJ, ed. *Medical Management of Tubal Pregnancy*. Washington, DC: ACOG; December 1998.

Mishell DR. Ectopic Pregnancy. In: Stenchever MA, et al., eds. *Comprehensive Gynecology*, 4th ed. St. Louis: Mosby; 2001:443–478.

Murray H, et al. Diagnosis and treatment of ectopic pregnancy. *Can Med Assoc J*. 2005;173(8): 905–912.

Seeber BE, et al. Suspected ectopic pregnancy. *Obstet Gynecol*. 2006;107:399–413.

Sowter MC, et al. Ectopic pregnancy: An update. *Curr Opin Obstet Gynecol*. 2004;16:289–293.

Stovall TG, et al. Single-dose methotrexate: An expanded trial. *Am J Obstet Gynecol*. 1993;168: 1759–1765.

MISCELLANEOUS

CLINICAL PEARLS

All Rh-negative unsensitized women should receive RhoGAM at the time of diagnosis.

ABBREVIATIONS

- ART—Assisted reproductive technologies
- DES—Diethylstilbestrol
- hCG—Human chorionic gonadotropin
- IUP—Intrauterine pregnancy
- IVF—In vitro fertilization
- OCP—Oral contraceptive pill
- PID—Pelvic inflammatory disease
- POP—Progestin-only pill
- STI—Sexually transmitted infection
- TVUS—Transvaginal ultrasound

CODES

ICD9-CM

See list for "Ectopic Pregnancy" in "Obstetric and Gynecologic Emergencies" section.

PATIENT TEACHING

- www.asrm.org/Patients/patientbooklets/ectopicpregnancy.pdf
- www.acog.org/publications/patient_education/bp155.cfm
- Methotrexate therapy:
  - Some abdominal pain, vaginal bleeding or spotting may occur.
  - Contact physician for sudden severe abdominal pain, heavy vaginal bleeding, dizziness, syncope, or tachycardia.
  - Avoid alcoholic beverages, folic acid–containing vitamins, NSAIDs, and sexual intercourse until the ectopic pregnancy has resolved.

PREVENTION

Prevention of STIs/PID; minimizing tubal surgery

FETAL ANATOMIC ABNORMALITIES

Christine Isaacs, MD
John W. Seeds, MD

 BASICS

DESCRIPTION

- Fetal anatomic abnormalities indicate a deviation from the expected normal anatomic architecture of a fetal organ or system.
- May be from intrinsic or extrinsic causes:
  - Fetal karyotype abnormalities
  - Single gene disorders
  - Multifactorial or polygenic disorders
  - Teratogenic or environmental factors
- May occur by chance, or be part of an identifiable syndrome
- May be single or multiple
- Major anomalies can impact survival/function.
- Minor anomalies may not affect normal life expectancy or lifestyle.

Age-Related Factors

Advanced maternal age (≥35 at time of delivery) can serve as an indication for consideration of invasive prenatal testing:

- Aneuploidy rates and associated fetal anomalies increase with increasing maternal age.

EPIDEMIOLOGY

- True incidence is difficult to determine given spontaneous miscarriage rates.
- ~ 3% risk for major congenital anomalies is generally accepted.
- With an aging obstetric population, chromosomal abnormalities may be increasing.

RISK FACTORS

- Chromosomal abnormalities risks:
  - Advanced maternal age, previous child with a chromosomal disorder
- Single gene defects risks:
  - Previous child with a gene disorder, heterozygous couples detected by screening programs
  - Ethnic background (e.g., Eastern European Jewish heritage increases risk of Tay-Sachs disease)
- Multifactorial disorders:
  - History of child with a multifactorial abnormality such as spina bifida or cleft lip increases risk in sibship
- Environmental factors:
  - Prenatal exposure to teratogenic drug such as alcohol or infectious agent such as toxoplasmosis

Genetics

As a general rule, 1 major organ anomaly, or 2 or more minor anatomic abnormalities correlates with a significant risk of aneuploidy. This should prompt referral for counseling and possible further testing.

PATHOPHYSIOLOGY

With teratogen exposure, timing of insult is critical:

- Very early exposures (up to 5 weeks GA) generally have an all-or-none effect: Abortion or normal.
- Exposure during organogenesis (5–10 weeks postmenstrual) can result in anatomic anomalies.

- Exposure beyond 10 weeks GA may cause variable functional disturbances (e.g., mental retardation) or growth abnormalities but not structural defects.

 DIAGNOSIS

SIGNS AND SYMPTOMS

History

Previous child or parental history of anatomic abnormalities or suspect ethnic origins

Physical Exam

- Maternal abdominal exam is of low yield in screening for fetal anatomic abnormalities.
- Major discrepancy in size of the uterus vs. expected GA, however, should prompt suspicion of possible polyhydramnios or oligohydramnios, which often are associated with anomalies and should prompt an early US evaluation.

TESTS

- Appropriate counseling and testing should be offered to patients at increased risk for fetal anatomic abnormalities.
- May be declined by patient

Labs

- 1st-trimester screening:
  - 10–14 weeks gestation
  - Measures nuchal translucency on US, maternal blood levels of free β-hCG, and pregnancy-associated PAPP-A.
    - Can lead to early detection of Down syndrome and associated fetal anomalies
  - CVS: 9–12 weeks gestation. Confirms abnormal karyotypes associated with fetal anomalies by obtaining chorionic villus cells under direct US guidance.
    - This early confirmation of genetic abnormalities allows for earlier pregnancy management options.
- 2nd-trimester serum screening:
  - 15–20 weeks' gestation
  - Tetra or quad screen measures maternal serum levels of AFP, hCG, uE3, and inhibin A and compares results to multiples of the (normal) median.
  - Abnormal serum screening tests are followed up with genetic counseling, a detailed/specialized US exam, and possible amniocentesis.
  - Amniocentesis ≥16 weeks:
    - Transabdominal needle aspiration of amniotic fluid under direct US guidance.
    - Desquamated fetal cells grown in tissue culture can provide karyotype or DNA analysis.
    - Pregnancy loss rate associated with amniocentesis ~0.6%.
    - As with CVS, amniocentesis provides prenatal diagnostic and prognostic information for direct management decisions regarding prenatal, postnatal or termination options.
- Screening tests have a high false-positive rate. Patients should be appropriately counseled.

Imaging

- 1st-trimester US:
  - Nuchal translucency:
    - Measurement of the hypoechoic subcutaneous layer behind the fetal neck in early pregnancy; when increased, can be associated with an increased incidence of Down syndrome, congenital heart disease, and other congenital anomalies.
    - Precise pathophysiology is unknown.
    - Follow-up testing for confirmation is essential.
- Standard US exam:
  - Performed during the 2nd or 3rd trimester, after ~16–20 weeks of gestation
  - Essential fetal elements include: Head and neck (cerebellum, choroid plexus, cisterna magna, midline falx, cavum septi pellucidi); chest; abdomen (stomach, kidneys, bladder, umbilical cord insertion site, umbilical cord vessel number); spine (cervical, thoracic, lumbar, sacral); extremities; sex; evaluation of multiple gestations)
- Specialized US exam:
  - Detailed anatomic exam of a suspected anomaly or of fetus. Components of exam are determined on an individual basis.
  - Specialized exams might include Doppler evaluation, fetal echocardiography, or additional fetal measurements. There is no universally agreed upon protocol.

DIFFERENTIAL DIAGNOSIS

>180 anomalies (both minor and major) can be identified by US, which may (or may not) suggest a definitive etiology or diagnosis. These include anomalies of the head and spine, heart and chest, abdomen and urinary tract, bowel, and limb abnormalities.

Infection

Common infections associated with fetal anatomic anomalies include:

- CMV
- Parvovirus
- Congenital syphilis
- Toxoplasmosis
- Rubella
- Varicella-Zoster virus

Hematologic

Severe fetal anemia

Immunologic

Rh isoimmunization can produce fetal anatomic abnormalities such as pericardial effusions and ascites.

Tumor/Malignancy

Fetal tumors, although rare, may present as abnormal masses on US:

- Teratoma
- Rhabdomyoma

Trauma

Fetal traumatic abnormalities have been rarely reported including gunshot wounds, blunt trauma, and rare suspected needle injuries.

Drugs

- Various drugs have been associated with fetal anatomic malformations, but few have been confirmed. Proven teratogens in common use include:
  - Antiseizure drugs (carbamazepine, phenytoin, valproic acid, phenobarbital)
  - Coumadin
  - Ethanol
  - Lithium
  - Retinoic acid
- Use of drugs associated with malformations should prompt timely referral to a MFM specialist.
- Preconception counseling should be provided when patients using such high-risk drugs are considering pregnancy.
- Contraceptive counseling should be provided to minimize the risks of unintended pregnancy.

Other/Miscellaneous

Lists of differential diagnoses for abnormal sonographic findings can be found in Sanders reference. MFM consultation will also provide the appropriate diagnostic support.

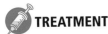

TREATMENT

GENERAL MEASURES

Findings suggestive of a fetal anomaly on maternal screening tests or on US, require prompt referral to MFM specialist. Subsequent collaboration may involve genetics specialists, pediatric cardiologists, pediatric surgeons, and neonatologists:

- Services often require tertiary care center facilities for delivery and management.

PREGNANCY-SPECIFIC ISSUES

Termination:

- Although many fetal anomalies may carry a favorable prognosis, certain anomalies (including lethal) may result in consideration of pregnancy termination.
- Parents should be informed of prognosis and options.
- State laws vary regarding pregnancy termination and legal limitations.
- Autopsy and genetic testing should be considered to confirm the diagnosis.
- Emotional support should be offered to the patient and family. Follow-up to assess patient's well being after hospital discharge is crucial.
- Counseling regarding early diagnostic interventions for subsequent pregnancies is imperative.

Risks for Mother

Special considerations for delivery may be required, including location, timing, induction, and mode (vaginal vs. cesarean). Risk and benefits must be reviewed to allow an informed decision.

Risks for Fetus

- Lethal fetal anomalies may result in death (IUFD) at any GA.
- Supportive care of the mother, including physical and emotional well-being is essential.
- Delivery of the dead fetus must be accomplished.
- A trained obstetric team with appropriate medical resources should manage delivery options.

SPECIAL THERAPY

Intrauterine transfusion may be lifesaving for severe fetal anemia.

MEDICATION (DRUGS)

Coordinated use of antiarrhythmic drugs may be indicated for specific fetal tachyarrhythmias.

SURGERY

In rare circumstances, fetal surgery in utero may be considered for certain fetal anomalies after weighing risks and benefits for both mother and fetus:

- Such interventions require referral to specialized centers.

FOLLOW-UP

DISPOSITION

Issues for Referral

- Referral to or consultation with a MFM specialist is the 1st step in an evaluation for suspected fetal anatomic abnormality.
- Fetal evaluation may be necessary throughout the pregnancy, most commonly with serial US exams. When fetal viability is reached, further assessment of fetal well-being may be necessary, and should be managed with obstetric specialists.

PROGNOSIS

Prognostic counseling must be individualized, based on the severity of the anatomic abnormality and the likely etiology.

- Major fetal anatomic anomalies may warrant corrective surgical intervention in the newborn period that may yield an optimistic prognosis.
- Specialized counseling and multidisciplinary medical decision making is often necessary.

COMPLICATIONS

Polyhydramnios or oligohydramnios associated directly with fetal malformations may cause severe morbidity in the mother.

PATIENT MONITORING

Close monitoring of maternal physiology as well as fetal well-being may be critical to an optimal outcome.

BIBLIOGRAPHY

ACOG Practice Bulletin No. 44. Neural Tube Defects. *Obstet Gynecol*. 2003;102(1):203–213.

ACOG Practice Bulletin No. 58. Ultrasonography in Pregnancy. *Obstet Gynecol*. 2004;104(6): 1449–1158.

ACOG Practice Bulletin No. 77. Sanders R, ed. Structural Fetal Screening for Fetal Chromosomal Abnormalities. *Obstet Gynecol*. 2007;109(1): 217–227.

Callen P, et al., eds. *Ultrasonography in Obstetrics and Gynecology*, 4th ed. Philadelphia: W.B. Saunders; 2000.

Fleischer A, et al., eds. *The Principles and Practice of Ultrasonography in Obstetrics and Gynecology*, 4th ed. East Norwalk, CT: Appleton & Lange; 1991.

MISCELLANEOUS

- Infants with congenital anomalies can impose significant economic and emotional stressors on families.
- The incidence of divorce and sibling maladjustment can be greater in such families and thus may require a multidisciplinary approach for support including social services, pastoral care, financial assistance, and support groups.

CLINICAL PEARLS

Worldwide, the most common major congenital fetal anomalies are cardiac malformations, followed by NTDs.

- NTDs are among the few birth anomalies for which primary prevention is possible via folic acid supplementation.
- Folic acid should be initiated *before* conception and maintained at least through the 1st 4 weeks of fetal development, as neural tube formation is nearly complete by the time of the 1st missed period and pregnancy test.
- All reproductive age women capable of pregnancy should take folic acid 400 μg/d.
- Women with a history of a child with a NTD should take folic acid 4 mg/d (prescription dosing).

ABBREVIATIONS

- AFP—α-Fetoprotein
- CMV—Cytomegalovirus
- CVS—Chorionic villus sampling
- GA—Gestational age
- hCG—Human chorionic gonadotropin
- IUFD—Intrauterine fetal demise
- MFM—Maternal-fetal medicine
- NTD—Neural tube defect
- PAPP-A—Pregnancy-associated plasma protein A
- uE3—Unconjugate estriol

CODES

ICD9-CM

- V28.3 Screening for malformation using ultrasonics
- 655.23 Hereditary disease in family possibly affecting fetus
- 655.33 Suspected damage to fetus from viral disease in the mother
- 655.43 Suspected damage to fetus from other disease in the mother
- 655.53 Suspected damage to fetus from drugs
- 655.83 Suspected or known fetal abnormality not elsewhere classified:
  - 5th-digit subclassification "3" indicates *antepartum* condition or complication

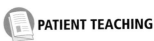

PATIENT TEACHING

PREVENTION

Folic acid supplementation preconceptionally

FETAL LUNG MATURITY

Gary Ventolini, MD

BASICS

DESCRIPTION
- The fetal pulmonary system is among the last organ system to become functionally mature; consequently, when a fetus reaches lung maturity, it is assumed that most organ systems are also prepared for neonatal self-sufficient existence.
- Fetal lung maturity is regarded as generally present by 39 weeks' gestation:
  - When an elective delivery is intended before 39 weeks' gestation ACOG recommends documenting confirmation of fetal lung maturity.
- The ability to test for fetal lung maturity represents 1 of the major achievements of modern obstetrics.
- Direct testing of fetal pulmonary function is not available antepartum. The assessment of lung maturity is inferred through the testing of surfactant, its function or turbidity, in the AF.
  - Surfactant is a complex lipoproteinic substance produced in the type II alveolar cells (pneumocytes) and packaged as lamellar bodies.
  - Surfactant's purpose is to prevent alveolar collapse by reducing surface tension, thus allowing reasonable pulmonary ventilation.
  - The presence of surfactant or its components in an adequate amount in the AF correlates with the likelihood of predicting pulmonary maturity.

Age-Related Factors
- Affects fetuses at 23–39 weeks' gestation
- Neonates
- Female neonates have less respiratory problems and better survival than males at equivalent GA.

EPIDEMIOLOGY
- The extended use of US in early pregnancy has contributed to more accurate gestational dating and has decreased iatrogenic premature births.
- The extent of lung disease in a premature neonate depends not only on the presence of surfactant but also on the stage of lung development:
  - The incidence of RDS in neonates delivered before 30 weeks' gestation is 70% and declines to ~20% in neonates' born between 32 and 37 weeks.

RISK FACTORS
Genetics
Fetal lung development and maturation, as any other fetal organ system is under genetic control, although its specific genetic pattern is still unknown.

PATHOPHYSIOLOGY
- Fetal lung development is conventionally divided into 4 stages:
  - Glandular sac stage: 5–16 weeks' gestation
  - Canalicular sac stage: 16–24 weeks' gestation
  - Terminal sac stage: 24 weeks' gestation until birth and childhood
  - Alveolar stage lasts from birth to 8 years of age.
- Fetal lung maturity is reached by 39 weeks' gestation, when enough surfactant is produced to assure neonatal self-sufficient respiratory function.

ASSOCIATED CONDITIONS
RDS:
- The presence of pulmonary maturity reduces the probability of a neonate developing RDS.

DIAGNOSIS

SIGNS AND SYMPTOMS
History
Establishment of GA supporting fetal lung maturity (See Establishing Estimated Date of Delivery.):
- Fetal heart tones documented for 20 weeks by fetoscope or for 30 weeks by Doppler
- At least 36 weeks since a valid positive pregnancy test performed
- US measurements at 6–11 weeks of crown-rump length confirms at least 39 weeks' gestation.
- US measurements at 12–20 weeks' gestation support a clinically determined GA of at least 39 weeks.

Physical Exam
- Maternal exam corroborates establishment of GA.
- *Neonatal* signs of fetal lung maturity at birth:
  - Normal APGAR scores at 1, 5, and 10 minutes
  - Absence of neonatal transient tachypnea
  - Absence of nasal flaring
  - Absence of subcostal and intercostals retractions
  - Absence of expiratory grunting
  - Absence of RDS

TESTS
- AF is obtained through amniocentesis.
- All tests of fetal lung maturity have high sensitivity and moderate specificity:
  - The positive predictive value of a result indicating fetal lung maturity is 95–98%.
- These test may be divided into 3 groups:
  - Quantification of surfactant or component with normal values:
    - L/S ratio: ≥ 2.5
    - PG: Present
    - TDX-FLMII: >55 mg/g
    - LBC: $\geq 50,000$
  - Measurements of surfactant function:
    - FSI
    - Shake test
  - Assessment of amniotic fluid turbidity

Lab
Immature and transitional values for quantitative tests:
- TDX-FLMII: Immature <40 mg/g and transitional between 40 mg/g and 55 mg/g
- LBC: Immature $<15,000$ and transitional between 15,000 and 50,000

ALERT
- Lab interference
- Contamination of AF by meconium or blood can cause the following interferences:
  - PG test: No interference by blood or meconium
  - LBC test: Interference by blood
  - TDX-FLMII: Interference by meconium

DIFFERENTIAL DIAGNOSIS
- Conditions that delay fetal lung maturity:
  - Poorly controlled type I maternal DM
- Conditions that accelerate fetal lung maturity:
  - Stressful conditions to the fetus
  - Maternal HTN
  - Intrauterine growth restriction
  - Maternal cigarette smoking
  - Premature rupture of membranes
  - Antenatal glucocorticoids administration

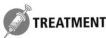

TREATMENT

GENERAL MEASURES
(See Corticosteroid Use for Fetal Lung Maturity.)
Antenatal corticosteroids should be administered to every pregnant patient:

- Between 24 weeks and 34 weeks gestation for preterm delivery
- Between 24 and 32 weeks in gestation with PROM

PREGNANCY-SPECIFIC ISSUES
Antenatal corticosteroids have shown to reduce:

- Neonatal death
- RDS
- Cerebro-ventricular hemorrhage
- Necrotizing enterocolitis
- Intensive care admissions
- Respiratory support need
- Systemic infections in the 1st 48 hours of life

Risks for Mother
Antenatal corticosteroids administration does not increase the risk of:

- Maternal death
- Chorioamnionitis
- Puerperal sepsis

Risks for Fetus
RDS:

- This condition is characterized by:
  – Acute respiratory difficulties
  – Subsequent apnea
  – Death if uncorrected
- Long-term sequelae include:
  – Chronic long disease requiring prolong ventilator
  – Extended oxygen therapy
  – Significant neurologic impairment

MEDICATION (DRUGS)
Antenatal corticosteroids:

- 12 mg of betamethasone IM repeated at 24 hours (preferred) OR
- 6 mg of dexamethasone IM repeated q12h for 4 doses total

FOLLOW-UP

- For practical and reliable evaluation of fetal lung maturity, the 1st test to be considered is LBC:
  – Results are usually available in 10–15 minutes.
  – Inexpensive
- In case of transitional results, the TDX-FLMII test or equivalent should be the next step:
  – Results are available in a few hours.
- If results are still at the transitional state, confirmation of fetal lung maturity can be achieved with L/S ratio test or phosphatidylglycerol levels:
  – Require several hours

DISPOSITION
Issues for Referral
Survival rates for preterm/very-low-birth weight infants and premature infants with pulmonary immaturity are higher in Level III centers; thus maternal transport may be indicated.

PROGNOSIS
Clinical outcome studies on neonates comparing 3 of the most commonly used tests of fetal lung maturity (LBC, TDX-FLMII, L/S ratio) have show similar results.

BIBLIOGRAPHY

ACOG Education Bulletin No. 230 Assessment of Fetal Lung Maturity. Washington DC: ACOG; Nov. 1996.

Gabbe SG. *Obstetrics. Normal and Problem Pregnancies*, 5th ed. New York: Churchill Livingstone; 2005.

Neerhof MG. Lamellar body counts: A consensus protocol. *Obstet Gynecol.* 2001;97:318–320.

Ventolini G. Update on assessment of fetal lung maturity. *J Obstet Gynecol.* 2005;25(6):535–538.

MISCELLANEOUS

CLINICAL PEARLS

- Lung maturity in multiple gestations occurs at a GA equivalent to that of singleton gestation.
- Lung maturity may be discordant among multiple fetuses.

- The smallest fetus is generally the most stressed, consequently the more mature therefore only assess for lung maturity the larger fetus.
- PG can be determined in AF collected from a vaginal pool in patients with PROM.
- Fetal lungs are almost always mature 1 week after the tests results were transitional.
- Poor man's test of turbidity: Place a transparent test tube with AF against a newspaper page; the test is positive when you are not able to read the letters through the tube.

ABBREVIATIONS

- ACOG—American College of Obstetricians and Gynecologists
- AF—Amniotic fluid
- FSI—Foam stability index
- GA—Gestational age
- HTN—Hypertension
- LBC—Lamellar body count
- L/S—Lecithin/Sphingomyelin ratio
- PG—Phosphatidyl glycerol
- RDS—Respiratory distress syndrome
- TDX-FLMII—Surfactant to albumin ratio

CODES

ICD9-CM
644.2 Early onset of delivery before 37 completed weeks

PATIENT TEACHING

ACOG Patient Education Pamphlet on Preterm Labor. Available at: http://www.acog.org

PREVENTION
Prevention of iatrogenic prematurity:

- At least 36 weeks of a positive pregnancy test
- US crown-rump length at 6–11 weeks supports ≥39 weeks
- US at 12–20 weeks of gestation supports ≥39 weeks
- Fetal heart tones documented for 20 weeks by fetoscope or for 30 weeks by Doppler

FETAL SURGERY AND PROCEDURES

Annette E. Bombrys, DO
Jeffery C. Livingston, MD

 BASICS

DESCRIPTION

- Placement of fetal shunt:
  - A shunt allows drainage of the malformation into the amniotic cavity.
- Fetoscopy:
  - Trocar is placed in the amniotic cavity under direct US guidance.
  - Fetal diagnosis or intervention is performed with direct visualization.
  - Fetoscopic laser ablation is used to treat twin-twin transfusion syndrome (see topic).
- Open fetal surgery:
  - Uterus is exposed and direct access to amniotic cavity is gained through uterine incision.
- EXIT procedure:
  - High-risk fetus is delivered by cesarean section; prior to delivery the fetal airway and/or venous access is obtained while utero placental gas exchange is preserved.
- Fetal cardiac procedures:
  - Percutaneous transthoracic pacemakers can be placed for fetal arrhythmias. (Note: Currently limited success with this technique.)
  - Open fetal surgery has been performed for structural fetal heart disease.
  - Balloon angioplasty for aortic stenosis

Indications

- Fetal shunting procedure:
  - Fetal indications:
    - Obstructive uropathy (posterior urethral valve, urethral atresia, prune belly syndrome, ureteropelvic junction obstruction, or renal dysplasia)
    - Cystic adenomatoid malformation of the lung
    - Aqueductal stenosis
    - Fetal pleural effusion
    - Ovarian cyst
    - Abdominal ascites
- Fetoscopic techniques:
  - Fetal indications:
    - Posterior urethral valve
    - Twin-twin transfusion syndrome
    - TRAP sequence; acephalic-acardiac twin syndrome
    - Myelomeningocele
    - Amniotic band syndrome
    - Diaphragmatic hernia
    - Sacrococcygeal teratoma

- EXIT procedure:
  - Fetal indications:
    - Reversal of tracheal occlusion
    - Fetal neck masses (cervical teratoma, congenital goiter, hemangioma, and neuroblastoma)
    - Lung masses (congenital cystic adenomatoid malformation, bronchopulmonary sequestration)
    - Mediastinal masses (teratoma, lymphangioma)
    - Immediate ECMO, referred to as EXIT to ECMO
- CDH
- Congenital heart disease:
  - CHAOS

Site (Office, Surgical Center, OR)

Operating room with obstetrical/neonatal capabilities

ASSOCIATED CONDITIONS

Fetal anomalies may be syndromic, with multiple associated anomalies.

 TREATMENT

PREGNANCY-SPECIFIC ISSUES

Risks for Mother

- Bleeding
- Infection
- Preterm labor and side effects of tocolytics
- EXIT procedure:
  - Same as risks associated with cesarean section (bleeding, infection, damage to bowel, bladder or major blood vessels) and prolonged surgical time (DVT)

Risks for Fetus

- Prematurity
- Preterm delivery
- Direct trauma from trocar insertion
- Intrauterine infection
- Death:
  - Not usually from fetoscopic procedure
  - Usually a result of worsening fetal condition from anomaly
- EXIT procedure:
  - Hypoxia
  - Death

SURGERY

- TTTS:
  - Amnioreduction: US-guided procedure in which a needle is inserted into polyhydramnios sac and AF removed until largest vertical pocket is normal (<5 cm). Some authors believe that an inadvertent microseptostomy is performed at the same time.
  - Microseptostomy: Fetoscopic procedure (in utero) by which a laser is used to make a small hole in the intertwin membrane in an effort to restore the AF to normal
  - Fetoscopic laser photocoagulation: In utero surgery that can be either selective (only direct vascular connections are photocoagulated) or nonselective (all vessels crossing the intertwin membrane are coagulated).
    - The nonselective technique may sacrifice vessels not responsible for TTTS, leading to an increased death rate of the donor twin (acute placental insufficiency)
  - Fetoscopic cord coagulation: US-guided procedure by which the umbilical cord is occluded, sacrificing 1 fetus (usually the fetus with dismal prognosis) to arrest the syndrome. This improves the outcome for the surviving fetus.
  - Sequential treatment:
    - Perform the least invasive procedure 1st and proceed with more invasive procedures once others have failed.
- Bladder outlet obstruction:
  - Serial bladder taps (3) to determine renal function:
    - Establishes a clear pattern of increasing or decreasing hypertonicity (hypotonic urine is associated with good function)
    - β2-Microglobulin allows identification of fetuses at risk for renal damage by unrelieved obstruction even if the AF is normal.
    - Prognostic criteria: Good prognosis if sodium <100 mEq/L, chloride <90 mEq/L, osmolarity <210 mEq/L, calcium <2 mmol/L, phosphorous <2 mmol/L, and β2-microglobulin <2 mg/L
  - Vesicoamniotic shunt:
    - Restores AF and avoids potential complications due to oligohydramnios (especially pulmonary hypoplasia)
    - Effects on renal function unclear
    - Increased incidence of gastroschisis
  - Fetoscopy: Laser posterior urethral valves

- EXIT procedure (steps):
  – Abdomen is entered via a low transverse skin incision or a midline fascial incision.
  – The uterus is examined for adequate myometrial relaxation (inhaled agents are adjusted to maintain adequate relaxation).
  – Sonographic mapping of placental edges
  – Hysterotomy with specially designed stapling device
  – Limited exposure of fetus (head, neck, and shoulders) while establishing an airway
  – After securing the airway, the fetus is then ventilated by hand.
  – Fetal umbilical artery and venous line are established.

FOLLOW-UP

DISPOSITION
Issues for Referral
- All cases should be referred to specialist in the field of MFM.
- Fetal intervention is performed at a limited number of specialized institutions.

PROGNOSIS
Dependent on GA at diagnosis and etiology of disease

COMPLICATIONS
- Fetal demise
- Preterm labor
- Preterm premature rupture of membranes
- Bleeding (maternal or fetal)
- Intrauterine infection

BIBLIOGRAPHY

Crombleholme TM, et al. Fetal intervention in obstructive uropathy: Prognostic indicators and efficacy of intervention. *Obstet Gynecol*. 1990; 162:1239–1244.

Harkness UF, et al. Twin-twin transfusion syndrome: Where do we go from here? [Review.] *Semin Perinatol*. 2005;29(5):296–304.

Johnson MP, et al. Fetal uropathy. *Curr Opin Obstet Gynecol*. 1999;11:185–194.

Lyerly AD, et al. Toward the ethical evaluation and use of maternal-fetal surgery. *Obstet Gynecol*. 2001;98(4):689–697.

Marwan A, et al. The EXIT procedure: Principles, pitfalls, and progress. *Semin Pediatric Surg*. 2006;15(2):107–115.

MISCELLANEOUS

SYNONYM(S)
- Fetal procedures
- Fetal surgery

CLINICAL PEARLS
Maternal-fetal surgery raises ethical issues related to maternal risks and benefits, informed consent, distinguishing lethal from nonlethal conditions, withholding unproven treatments, entrepreneurship, and prioritization. – Lyerly AD, et al. *Obstet Gynecol*. 2001.

ABBREVIATIONS
- AF—Amniotic fluid
- CDH—Congenital diaphragmatic hernia
- CHOAS—Congenital high airway obstruction syndrome
- DVT—Deep venous thrombosis
- ECMO—Extracorporeal membrane oxygenation
- EXIT—Ex utero intrapartum treatment
- GA—Gestational age
- MFM—Maternal-fetal medicine
- TRAP—Twin reverse arterial perfusion
- TTTS—Twin-twin transfusion syndrome

CODES

ICD9-CM
- 658.5x Congenital heart disease
- 648.6x Other cardiac disease (specify)
- 753.6 Bladder outlet obstruction
- 753.21 Congenital obstruction of ureteropelvic junction
- 753.29 Hydronephrosis
- 762.3 Placental transfusion syndromes
- 776.4 Polycythemia neonatorum due to donor twin transfusion

FORCEPS DELIVERY AND VACUUM EXTRACTION

Laetitia Poisson De Souzy, MD
Aaron B. Caughey, MD, PhD

BASICS

DESCRIPTION
- In an operative vaginal delivery, the deliverer uses forceps or vacuum to assist the delivery of the fetal head.
- Historically, the use of instruments to assist delivery of the newborn dates back to at least 1500 BC, when it was described in Sanskrit writings:
  - Credit for design of modern forceps in 1600 is given to Peter Chamberlen of England.
  - Vacuum extractors were 1st described in the early 1800s. In 1954, Malmström patented the metal-cup extractor, and vacuum extraction became more common.

Indications
- The following indications for operative delivery apply only when the cervix is fully dilated and the fetal head is engaged:
  - Prolonged 2nd stage:
    - Nulliparous women: Failure to progress for 3 hours with regional anesthesia or 2 hours without regional anesthesia.
    - Multiparous women: Failure to progress for 2 hours with regional anesthesia or 1 hour without regional anesthesia.
  - Immediate fetal distress (e.g., prolonged fetal heart rate decelerations) in the 2nd stage of labor, and high probability of successful expedient operative vaginal delivery.
  - Shortening the 2nd stage for maternal indications (e.g., maternal cardiac disease, maternal exhaustion)
- Both absolute and relative contraindications exist for operative vaginal delivery:
  - Absolute contraindications:
    - Position of the fetal head is unknown.
    - Fetal head is not engaged.
    - Fetal bone demineralization disorder (e.g., osteogenesis imperfecta)
    - Fetal collagen disorder (e.g., Ehlers-Danlos)
    - Fetal coagulopathy (e.g., alloimmune thrombocytopenia)
    - Gestational age <34 weeks (for vacuum deliveries)
  - Relative contraindications:
    - Fetal scalp sampling or multiple fetal scalp electrode placements
    - Suspected fetal macrosomia

EPIDEMIOLOGY
- Operative vaginal delivery rates are declining in the US.
  - 2004: 5.2% of all deliveries were performed via forceps or vacuum.
  - 2000: 7%
  - 1989: 9%
  - The majority of operative vaginal deliveries are now vacuum-assisted:
    - 2004: Vacuum deliveries accounted for 4.1% of all births.
    - 1989: 3.5% of all births
  - Forceps births continue to decline:
    - 2004: 1.1% of all births
    - 1989: 5.5% of all births

- In contrast, cesarean rates are increasing in the US:
  - 2005: Delivery by cesarean increased to an all-time high of 30.2% of all births, as rates of primary cesarean increased and vaginal birth after cesarean decreased.

TREATMENT

PROCEDURE
Informed Consent
- Before placing forceps or vacuum, the following conditions must be met:
  - Fetus is in vertex presentation (unless used to aid in delivery of aftercoming head in breech delivery).
  - Cervix is fully dilated.
  - Fetal membranes are ruptured.
  - Fetal head is engaged and exact position is known (i.e., direction of occiput and asynclitism).
  - Maternal pelvis is adequate.
  - Maternal anesthesia is adequate.
  - Maternal bladder is empty.
  - Deliverer is experienced OR
  - Is immediately available for cesarean if operative vaginal delivery is not successful.
- Consent should include a thorough discussion and documentation of the indications, risks, benefits, and alternatives of operative vaginal delivery. The deliverer should also document fetal and maternal assessments.
- Indications (as above)
- Maternal/Fetal assessments:
  - Maternal: Clinical pelvimetry demonstrates adequate pelvis.
  - Fetal: GA, estimated fetal weight, position, presentation, lie, engagement, asynclitism

Risks
- There are potential risks to both mother and fetus of operative vaginal delivery, although these risks may have more to do with abnormal labor (i.e., the indication for operative vaginal delivery) than the operative vaginal delivery itself.
- Maternal risks:
  - Lower genital tract lacerations, including risk of 3rd- and 4th-degree lacerations
  - Hematomas
  - Urinary retention
  - Postpartum perineal pain
  - Postpartum hemorrhage
  - Delayed complications: urinary or fecal incontinence
- Fetal risks:
  - Skin bruising, abrasions, lacerations
  - Ocular injury (e.g., retinal hemorrhage)
  - Cephalohematoma
  - Subgaleal hemorrhage
  - Intracranial hemorrhage
  - Facial nerve palsies
  - Shoulder dystocia
  - Brachial plexus injuries
  - Hyperbilirubinemia

- Risk profile of forceps vs. vacuum:
  - Forceps:
    - Higher risk of perineal 3rd- or 4th-degree lacerations
  - Vacuum:
    - Higher risk of shoulder dystocia
    - Higher risk of cephalohematoma
    - Higher risk of postpartum hemorrhage
- FDA public health advisory in 1998 regarding the risk of neonatal intracranial injury with vacuum extraction:
  - The evidence suggests that there is no significant difference between forceps, vacuum, or cesarean following labor in the risk of subdural or cerebral hemorrhage.
  - This suggests that abnormal labor is the biggest risk factor for serious neonatal intracranial injury.

Benefits
- Potential benefits to mother and fetus of operative vaginal delivery are mostly related to shortening of the 2nd stage and avoiding the need for cesarean.
- A prolonged 2nd stage is associated with increased risk of:
  - Cesarean, operative vaginal delivery, 3rd- and 4th-degree tears, and chorioamnionitis
- Cesarean delivery itself is associated with increased risk of:
  - Endomyometritis, wound complications, hemorrhage, postpartum maternal death, need for future cesarean, IUFD in future pregnancies, and placenta previa, and accrete
- Maternal benefits:
  - Quicker recovery
  - Lower risk of chorioamnionitis and endomyometritis
  - Decreased risk of hemorrhage
  - Mother-infant bonding
  - Shorter hospital stay
- Fetal benefits:
  - Mother-infant bonding

Alternatives
- The alternatives depend on the indication for operative vaginal delivery.
- Cesarean
- Spontaneous vaginal delivery (if indication is not emergent).
- The data does NOT support the use of sequential methods of operative vaginal delivery (e.g., going from forceps to vacuum) since this is associated with a higher risk of neonatal intracranial hemorrhage and maternal 3rd- and 4th-degree perineal lacerations.

Surgical
- Classification of forceps and vacuum deliveries is based on fetal station and angle of rotation used.
- Outlet:
  - Scalp is visible at introitus, without separating the labia.
  - Fetal skull is at pelvic floor.

– Sagittal suture is in AP diameter, ROA/LOA or posterior position.
– Fetal head is at or on perineum.
– Rotation is 45 degrees or less.
* Low:
– Leading point of fetal skull is at +2 station or beyond, but not on the pelvic floor.
– Rotation is 45° or less (from LOA/ROA to OA, or LOP/ROP to OP).
– Rotation is >45°.
* Mid:
– Leading point of fetal skull is above +2 station but head is engaged.
* High: Not included in classification, as no longer advisable to perform.

Choice of Instrument
* Use of forceps vs. vacuum depends on:
– Clinician's skill's and comfort level
– Maternal preference, based on informed consent discussion.
* Type of forceps depends on deliverer's experience, indication, and fetal anatomy (head molding and estimated fetal weight):
– Tucker-McLane: Used for unmolded fetal head. Rotation possible, if fetal head is flexed.
– Simpson: Used when fetal head is molded. Rotation possible, if fetal head is flexed.
– Luikart-Simpson: Similar to Simpson, but blade is semifenestrated.
– Eliotts: Similar to Simpson, with a lock to avoid head compression.
– Kielland: Mid-pelvic rotation possible. Can correct asynclitism.
– Piper: Aid in delivery of aftercoming head in breech delivery.
* Type of vacuum extractor used is mostly regional. In the US, the metal cup is nearly obsolete, and most providers use soft-cup vacuum extractors.
– Metal cups: Higher success rate, but higher rate of neonatal scalp injuries
– Soft cups (CMI Tender Touch, Mityvac, Silastic): Lower success rate, but lower rate of neonatal scalp injuries
– Kiwi: Vacuum tube inserts into side of vacuum disc, allowing appropriate placement on fetal head even with severe asynclitism.

Technique
* Forceps:
– Empty maternal bladder
– Choose appropriate forceps (as above). Biparietal diameter of fetal head should be equal to greatest distance between blades of forceps.

– Forceps placement: Place blades directly along the sides of the fetal head in the occipitomental diameter.
– Traction: Pull in line with pelvic axis; steady intermittent traction coordinated with maternal push.
– Stop if no progress occurs after 2 pulls along with uterine contractions or there is no progressive descent.
* Vacuum:
– Empty maternal bladder.
– Cup placement: Place center of cup over the sagittal suture and 3 cm in front of the posterior fontanelle towards the face. Make sure cup is free of maternal soft tissue.
– Traction: Pull in line with pelvic axis, steady intermittent traction coordinated with maternal push.
– Stop if ≥3 pop-offs occur, there is no progressive descent, or fetal scalp trauma occurs.

Postoperative Care
* Thorough examination of the mother and newborn.
* Maternal postoperative care:
– Examine maternal tissues (vaginal, cervical, perineal, and rectal) for injury.
– Ice and stool softeners for comfort
– Pelvic and rectal examination prior discharge
* Newborn postoperative care:
– Examine newborn for lacerations, hematomas, retinal hemorrhage, brachial plexus injuries, and fractures.
– Notify pediatricians of the mode of delivery, so they can monitor for possible delayed complications.

 ## FOLLOW-UP

Unless complications occur, maternal follow-up care is routine, with a postpartum examination within 4–6 weeks.

COMPLICATIONS
* Potential for early and delayed maternal and fetal complications.
* For routine operative vaginal deliveries, there is a low risk of delayed complications.
* Delayed maternal complications are mostly related to injury to pelvic support structures:
– Urinary incontinence
– Fecal incontinence
– Anal sphincter injury
– Pelvic organ prolapse

BIBLIOGRAPHY

ACOG Practice Bulletin. Operative Vaginal Delivery. Washington DC: ACOG; 2007 Compendium of Selected Publications 2007, 543–550.

Bofill JA, et al. A randomized prospective trial of the obstetric forces versus the M-cup vacuum extractor. *Am J Obstet Gynecol.* 1996;175:1325–1330.

Caughey AB, et al. Forceps compared with vacuum: Rates of neonatal and maternal morbidity. *Obstet Gynecol.* 2006;107(2 Pt 1);426–427.

Center for Devices and Radiological Health. FDA Public Health Advisory: Need for caution when using vacuum assisted delivery devices. 1998 May 21.

Cheng YW, et al. How long is too long: Does a prolonged 2nd stage in labor in nulliparous women affect maternal and neonatal outcomes? *Am J Obstet Gynecol.* 2004;191(3):933–938.

Demissie K, et al. Operative vaginal delivery & neonatal and infant adverse outcomes: Population based retrospective analysis. *Br Med J.* 2004; 329(7465):547.

Kuit JA, et al. A randomized comparison of vacuum extraction delivery with a rigid and pliable cup. *Obstet Gynecol.* 1993;82:280–284.

Martin JA, et al. Births: Final data for 2004. *Natl Vital Stat Rep.* 2006;55(1):1–101.

Silver R, et al. Maternal morbidity associated with repeat cesarean deliveries. *Obstet Gynecol.* 2006;107(6):1226–1232.

Smith GC, et al. Cesarean section and risk of unexplained stillbirth in subsequent pregnancies. *Lancet.* 2003;362(9398):1779–1784.

Towner D, et al. Effect of mode of delivery in nulliparous women on neonatal intracranial injury. *N Engl J Med.* 1999;341(23):1709–1714.

 ## MISCELLANEOUS

ABBREVIATIONS
* GA—Gestational age
* IUFD—Intrauterine fetal demise

CODES
ICD9-CM
72 Forceps, vacuum, and breech delivery:
* 72.0 Low/Outlet forceps operation
* 72.1 Low/Outlet forceps operation with episiotomy
* 72.2 Mid forceps operation
* 72.3 High forceps operation
* 72.4 Forceps rotation of the fetal head
* 72.7 Vacuum extraction

 ## PATIENT TEACHING

Patient discharge instructions:
* Activity:
– Pelvic rest for 6 weeks postpartum
– Keep area clean and dry.
– Use stool softeners (in case of 3rd- or 4th-degree laceration).

Section V

HYDATIDIFORM MOLE

Vernon T. Cannon, MD, PhD
Jean A. Hurteau, MD

BASICS

DESCRIPTION
- GTN (see topic) defines a neoplastic process that is derived from trophoblastic proliferation of the placenta during pregnancy. It includes a spectrum of disease comprising:
  - Hydatidiform moles (molar pregnancies)
  - Persistent moles
  - Invasive moles
  - Gestational choriocarcinomas
  - Placental-site trophoblastic tumors
- Over the past 25 years cytogenetic studies have clarified the existence of 2 distinct types of hydatidiform moles: Complete and partial moles with markedly different pathologic features and clinical course.
- Invasive moles are a form of GTN that is locally invasive into the myometrium of the uterus:
  - 5–10% of all GTN are invasive moles.
  - Diagnosis of invasive mole is made by pathologic evaluation of the uterus after hysterectomy performed due to continued vaginal bleeding or persistently elevated serum β-hCG levels.
- Choriocarcinoma is the malignant form of GTN:
  - 3–5% of all GTN
  - Progresses rapidly and metastasizes hematogenously to the brain, lungs, liver, kidneys, GI tract, and lower genital tract

Age-Related Factors
- Incidence higher in women <20 and >40
- Maternal age does not affect the risk of partial mole.
- Paternal age or race does not affect risk of hydatidiform mole.
- Malignant differentiation occurs in older women.

Staging
NIH Classification of Postmolar GTN
- Nonmetastatic GTN
- Metastatic GTN:
  - Good prognosis:
    - β-hCG <40,000
    - Symptoms <4 months
    - No brain or liver metastases
    - No prior chemotherapy
    - Pregnancy event is not a term pregnancy.
  - Poor prognosis:
    - β-hCG >40,000
    - Symptoms >4 months
    - Brain or liver metastasis
    - Prior chemotherapeutic failure
    - Antecedent term pregnancy

New FIGO Staging
The identification of a patient's stage is expressed by a Roman numeral for the FIGO stage and an Arabic numeral for the WHO risk score separated by a colon, for example, II:2.
- FIGO staging of GTN:
  - Stage I: Disease confined to the uterus
  - Stage II: GTN extends outside the uterus but is limited to the genital structures (adnexa, vagina, broad ligament).
  - Stage III: GTN extends to the lungs with or without genital tact involvement.
  - Stage IV: All other metastatic sites
- FIGO risk scoring:
  - Score 0: Age <40, molar antecedent pregnancy, interval months from index pregnancy <4, pretreatment β-hCG <1,000, lung metastasis
  - Score 1: Age $\geq$ 40, antecedent pregnancy an abortion, 4–<7 months from index pregnancy, pretreatment β-hCG 1,000–<10,000, largest tumor size 3–<5 cm, spleen and/or kidney metastasis, number of metastasis 1–4
  - Score 2: Term antecedent pregnancy, interval months from index pregnancy 7–<13, pretreatment β-hCG 10,000–<100,000, largest tumor size >5 cm, GI metastasis, number of metastasis 5–8, previous failed single-drug chemotherapy
  - Score 4: Interval months from index pregnancy $\geq$13, pretreatment serum β-hCG >100,000, liver and/or brain metastasis, number of metastasis 5–8, previous failed $\geq$2 chemotherapy drugs

EPIDEMIOLOGY
- Incidence of complete mole is 1 per 1,945.
- Incidence of partial mole is 1 per 695.
- Highest incidence in Asia, Africa, and Latin America
- Lowest incidence in North America, Europe, and Australia

RISK FACTORS
- Young maternal age
- Advanced maternal age
- Prior molar pregnancy
- Prior spontaneous abortion
- Diet deficient in vitamin A
- Asian ethnicity
- Histocompatibility between patient and partner may be associated with increased risk of metastatic GTN.

Genetics
- Most complete moles are 46, XX of paternal origin.
- Most partial moles are triploid: 69, XXY or 69, XXY or 69, XXX.

PATHOPHYSIOLOGY
- Complete mole:
  - Absent embryo/fetus
  - Round villous outline
  - Marked hydropic swelling, cisterns present, all villi involved
  - Variable to marked trophoblastic proliferation
  - Trophoblastic atypia often present
  - Staining for p57 negative or weakly positive
  - ~25% will develop post molar GTN.
- Partial mole:
  - Embryo/Fetus present
  - Scalloped villous outline
  - Hydropic swelling less pronounced and focal, cisterns less prominent, villous fibrosis
  - Focal and minimal trophoblastic proliferation
  - Trophoblastic atypia absent
  - Staining for p57 diffusely positive
  - 0.5–4% develop postmolar GTN

ASSOCIATED CONDITIONS
- Hyperthyroidism
- Preeclampsia <24 weeks
- Hyperemesis gravidarum
- Respiratory failure secondary to trophoblastic embolization
- Anemia secondary to vaginal bleeding
- 1 study has shown a possible correlation between infection with adeno-associated virus and GTN.
- Fertility drugs may increase risk of hydatidiform moles by an increase in multiple pregnancies.

DIAGNOSIS

SIGNS AND SYMPTOMS
History
- Vaginal bleeding is the most common symptom.
- Passage of vesicles
- Hyperemesis due to increased β-hCG
- Preeclampsia <24 weeks
- Pelvic pain from theca-lutein cysts

Review of Systems
Symptoms of hyperthyroidism

Physical Exam
- General exam: Tremulousness, diaphoresis, anxiety, and nervousness with hyperthyroidism
- Pulmonary exam: Wheezing and rhonchi from trophoblastic embolization
- Abdominal exam: Uterus size > dates, absent fetal heart tones

- Pelvic exam: Vaginal bleeding with or without protruding vesicles:
  - Cervix: Possibly dilated with bleeding and protruding vesicles
  - Uterus: Size > dates
  - Adnexa: Masses from theca-lutein cysts

TESTS
EKG may reveal cardiac arrhythmias such as supraventricular tachycardia associated with hyperthyroidism.

Lab
Serum quantitative β-hCG

ALERT
- Rare occurrence of false-positive hCG:
  - Confirmatory tests with urine, serial dilution, different assay
- CBC with differential
- Coagulation studies (PT and PTT)
- Thyroid function tests
- Type and crossmatch
- Some studies have suggested increases in serum inhibin A and B levels in patients with hydatidiform moles.

Imaging
- Pelvic US:
  - Classic "snowstorm" appearance
- CXR (PA and lateral)

DIFFERENTIAL DIAGNOSIS
- Spontaneous abortion
- Ectopic pregnancy
- Germ cell tumor

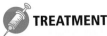 TREATMENT

GENERAL MEASURES
- Stabilize hemodynamically, if necessary.
- Transfuse, if severe anemia is present.
- Correct coagulopathy.
- Treat preeclampsia/HTN and hyperthyroidism, if necessary.

PREGNANCY-SPECIFIC ISSUES
- Preeclampsia <24 weeks
- Hyperemesis gravidarum
- In the case of twins (complete mole + fetus with normal placenta), increased risk of metastasis:
  - Termination of pregnancy is recommended.
  - If pregnancy is continued, risk of maternal hemorrhage, HTN, preeclampsia, and thyrotoxicosis has been documented, requiring termination.
  - Fetal karyotype is also recommended.

By Trimester
- Preeclampsia prior to 24 weeks gestation
- Hyperemesis gravidarum usually occurs in the 1st trimester.

Risks for Mother
- Hemorrhage
- Preeclampsia/HTN
- Thyrotoxicosis secondary to hyperthyroidism
- Trophoblastic embolization
- Postmolar GTN

Risks for Fetus
- Complete mole: No fetus/embryo
- Partial mole: Fetal parts are present but fetus is nonviable
- In the case of twinning, termination is recommended; however, careful maternal surveillance is warranted for continuation of pregnancy.

MEDICATION (DRUGS)
- Molar pregnancies:
  - Prostaglandin or oxytocin induction are not recommended for molar pregnancies.
  - Chemotherapy is usually reserved for persistent or metastatic post molar GTN.
- Postmolar GTN:
  - Methotrexate and actinomycin-D for low risk (WHO scores 0–6).
  - EMA-CO for high risk (WHO score $\geq$7)

SURGERY
- Suction D&C
- Hysterectomy considered in those who do not desire future fertility. Will decrease the risk of postmolar GTN from ~25% to 5% in complete molar pregnancies.

 FOLLOW-UP

DISPOSITION
Issues for Referral
- Increasing or persistent β-hCG levels after evacuation of molar pregnancy, spontaneous abortion, ectopic pregnancy, or subsequent to term pregnancy or noted placental abnormality on pathology
- Diagnosis of postmolar GTN:
  - β-hCG level plateau +/–10% of baseline recorded over a 3-week duration (days 1, 7, 14, 21)
  - hCG level rise >10% above baseline recorded over a 2-week duration (days 1, 7, 14)
  - Persistence of detectable hCG for >6 months after molar evacuation

COMPLICATIONS
Complications that can occur following uterine evacuation include:
- Uterine perforation
- ARDS with uteri >14–16-week size

- With clinical hyperthyroidism, thyroid storm can occur secondary to anesthesia and surgery. β-blockers should be administered preoperatively.
- Postmolar GTN

PATIENT MONITORING
- After uterine evacuation, a serum β-hCG should be obtained within 48 hours:
  - Repeat weekly until 3 normal values are obtained.
  - Then every 2 weeks for 3 months
  - Monthly for 6–12 months
- CXR should be performed both pre- and postevacuation.
- Pelvic exam to assess uterine size after evacuation.

BIBLIOGRAPHY

ACOG Committee Opinion No. 278. Avoiding Inappropriate Clinical Decisions Based on False-Positive Human Chorionic Gonadotropin Test. October 2002. Available at: www.acog.org/publications/committee opinions/co278.cfm.

Hurteau JA. Gestational trophoblastic disease: Management of hydatidiform mole. *Clin Obstet Gynecol.* 2003;46(3):557–569.

Ngan HYS. The practicability of FIGO 2000 staging for gestational trophoblastic neoplasia. *Intern J Gynecol Cancer.* 16:(2):882–883.

Soper JT. Gestational trophoblastic disease. *Obstet Gynecol.* 2006;108(1):176–187.

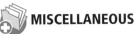 MISCELLANEOUS

ABBREVIATIONS
- ARDS—Adult respiratory distress syndrome
- FIGO—Federation of Gynecologic Oncologists
- GTN—Gestational trophoblastic neoplasia
- hCG—Human chorionic gonadotropin
- PT—Prothrombin time
- WHO—World Health Organization

CODES
ICD9-CM
630 Hydatidiform mole

 PATIENT TEACHING

- NCI Patient education Gestational Trophoblastic Tumors. Available at: www.cancer.gov/cancertopics/pdq/treatment/gestationaltrophoblastic/patient
- ACOG Patient Education Pamphlet Early Pregnancy Loss: Miscarriage and Molar Pregnancy. Available at: www.acog.org/publications/patient education/bp090.cfm

PREVENTION

ALERT
Effective contraception should be prescribed during the surveillance period following an evacuation to prevent intercurrent pregnancy that would preclude monitoring of hCG levels.

HYDRAMNIOS
Nancy Chescheir, MD

 BASICS

DESCRIPTION
- The presence of excessive AF

Age-Related Factors
- Not directly related to maternal age.
- More common in the late 2nd and 3rd trimesters

EPIDEMIOLOGY
In 1 study in which 40,000 US scans were reviewed, the incidence of hydramnios was 1%:
- The perinatal mortality rate in this study was 49 per 1,000 births if hydramnios was present, compared with 14 per 1,000 births in the control group.

RISK FACTORS
- Macrosomia
- Diabetes, gestational and pre-existing
- Twins
- Fetal anomalies

PATHOPHYSIOLOGY
- AF volume is regulated by the fetus.
- Excessive AF can result from of excess production of AF or diminished absorption of fluid.

ASSOCIATED CONDITIONS
- Maternal:
  - Respiratory compromise, ureteral obstruction, uterine rupture (prior uterine scar), preterm labor, PROM, dysfunctional labor, postpartum hemorrhage
- Fetal:
  - Malpresentation, fetal anomalies, prematurity

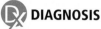 **DIAGNOSIS**

SIGNS AND SYMPTOMS
History
- General: Uterine contractions, shortness of breath, mother notices she "feels big"
- Acute polyhydramnios: Sudden increase in the size of the uterus, usually in the late 2nd trimester.

Physical Exam
- Size > dates by >3 cm in a normal-size woman
- Inability to easily outline the fetus on physical exam in the 3rd trimester
- Easily ballotable fetus in the late 3rd trimester

TESTS
Lab
Once diagnosis is made and if the following have not been completed recently:
- Screen for gestational diabetes; syphilis test
- Consider fetal karyotype of structural abnormalities or SGA fetus + polyhydramnios

Imaging
- Diagnostic role:
  - Diagnosis of polyhydramnios is made using semiquantitative measures or subjective evaluation.
  - MVP of fluid:
    ○ MVP ≥8 cm is diagnostic
  - AFI >20 cm is always above the 95th percentile.
  - Severe polyhydramnios: AFI >30 cm
- Causation identification:
  - Careful anatomic evaluation of the fetus is recommended for anatomic or functional abnormalities.

DIFFERENTIAL DIAGNOSIS
- Idiopathic (usually mild)
- Fetal abnormalities:
  - Proximal GI tract obstruction (to the level of the ileum)
  - Neurologic abnormalities:
    ○ Structural, such as anencephaly, hydrocephalus, holoprosencephaly
    ○ Functional, such as myotonic dystrophy, Peno-Shokeir syndrome
  - Twins
  - Macrosomia
  - Aneuploidy

Infection
- Syphilis
- Fetal infections causing hydrops, such as parvovirus

Hematologic
Fetal anemia:
- Parvovirus
- Isoimmunization

Metabolic/Endocrine
Maternal hyperglycemia

Immunologic
Immune hydrops

Tumor/Malignancy
Placental chorioangioma

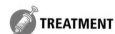 **TREATMENT**

PREGNANCY-SPECIFIC ISSUES
- For symptomatic relief remote from term, possible amnioreduction
- For idiopathic polyhydramnios <32 weeks' gestation: 3-day course of indomethacin
- Consider scheduling delivery at term for monitored amniotomy.

Risks for Mother

Discomfort, premature contractions, PROM with possible abruption; respiratory compromise; ureteral obstruction; dysfunctional labor; cesarean delivery for malpresentation, abruption

Risks for Fetus

Prematurity; underlying fetal anomaly; malpresentation

MEDICATION (DRUGS)

Consider timely steroids if prematurity is likely.

 ## FOLLOW-UP

DISPOSITION

Issues for Referral

Consider perinatal consultation if diagnosis is unclear or anomaly is detected.

PROGNOSIS

Related to age at delivery and underlying fetal status

PATIENT MONITORING

Mother

Monitor for premature cervical dilation, maternal symptoms.

Fetus

Fetal position, growth

BIBLIOGRAPHY

Martinez-Frias ML, et al. Maternal and fetal factors related to abnormal amniotic fluid. *J Perinatol.* 1999:19(7):514–520.

Ott WM. Reevaluation of the relationship between amniotic fluid volume and perinatal outcome. *Am J Obstet Gynecol.* 2005;192(6):1803–1809.

 ## MISCELLANEOUS

SYNONYM(S)

Polyhydramnios

CLINICAL PEARLS

- Once identified, look for the cause of the problem.
- Prepare for complications, including cord prolapse, at time of amniorrhexis if head is not engaged.

ABBREVIATIONS

- AF—Amniotic fluid
- AFI—Amniotic fluid index
- MVP—Maximal vertical pocket
- PROM—Premature rupture of membranes
- SGA—Small for gestational age

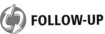

ICD9-CM

- 657.XX Polyhydramnios
- 761.3 Polyhydramnios affecting the fetus

PATIENT TEACHING

- Discuss etiologies, risk of anomalies, or other problems associated with severe but presumably idiopathic hydramnios
- Preterm labor identification information

PREVENTION

- Polyhydramnios is not preventable.
- Complications from polyhydramnios may not be preventable.

HYPEREMESIS GRAVIDARUM

Alice Stek, MD

 BASICS

DESCRIPTION
- Hyperemesis represents the extreme end of the continuum of nausea and vomiting of pregnancy.
- No single accepted definition for hyperemesis gravidarum, but generally includes:
  – Persistent vomiting without other etiology
  – Measure of acute starvation, such as large ketonuria
  – Weight loss, usually at least 5% of prepregnancy weight

EPIDEMIOLOGY
- Nausea and vomiting of pregnancy affects 70–85% of pregnant women
- Hyperemesis gravidarum in ~0.5–2% of pregnant women

RISK FACTORS
- Increased placental mass (e.g., molar gestation, multiple gestation)
- Family history
- History of hyperemesis in previous pregnancy
- Women with history of nausea and vomiting after estrogen exposure (such as OCPs)
- History of motion sickness or migraine
- Female fetus

Genetics
Women whose mothers or sisters had hyperemesis are more likely to experience hyperemesis themselves.

PATHOPHYSIOLOGY
- Etiology is poorly understood.
- Higher hCG and estrogen levels correlate with hyperemesis.

ASSOCIATED CONDITIONS
- hCG is a thyroid stimulator; up to 70% of women with hyperemesis have elevated free thyroxine and low TSH.
- Rarely, Wernicke encephalopathy due to vitamin B_1 deficiency, esophageal rupture, or pneumothorax
- Depression

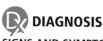 **DIAGNOSIS**

SIGNS AND SYMPTOMS
History
- Nausea and vomiting, typically starting before 9 weeks' gestation
- Clinical diagnosis of exclusion
- Typically no pain, fever, or headache

Physical Exam
- Clinically diagnosis of exclusion
- No fever, no tenderness, no neurologic findings, no goiter

TESTS
Labs
- Liver enzymes:
  – May be slightly elevated (<300 U/L)
- Serum bilirubin:
  – May be slightly elevated (<4 mg/dL)
- Amylase and lipase:
  – May be slightly elevated (<5 times ULN)
- Electrolytes, chemistry:
  – Hypochloremic metabolic alkalosis is possible
- UA:
  – Elevated specific gravity, ketonuria
- If hyperthyroidism suspected:
  – TSH, free thyroxine, free triiodothyronine

Imaging
Obstetric US for GA, evaluate for multiple gestation, molar gestation

DIFFERENTIAL DIAGNOSIS
If patient experiences nausea and vomiting for 1st time after 9 weeks' gestation, consider alternate diagnosis.

Infection
- Gastroenteritis
- Pyelonephritis
- Appendicitis
- Hepatitis

Metabolic/Endocrine
- Diabetic ketoacidosis
- Hyperthyroidism
- Addison's disease

Tumor/Malignancy
- CNS tumors
- Ovarian torsion

Drugs
Drug toxicity or substance abuse

Other/Miscellaneous
- GI conditions:
  – Peptic ulcer disease, gastroparesis, pancreatitis, obstruction, hepatitis, appendicitis
- GU tract:
  – Nephrolithiasis, pyelonephritis
- Neurologic:
  – Pseudotumor cerebri, migraines, CNS tumor
- Psychologic
- Acute fatty liver of pregnancy

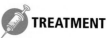 **TREATMENT**

GENERAL MEASURES
- Exclude other etiologies.
- Treat early manifestations to reduce need for hospitalization.

PREGNANCY-SPECIFIC ISSUES
Risks for Fetus
- The drugs listed below are generally considered safe, with the exception of corticosteroids, which may be associated with oral clefts.
- Little safety data on ondansetron in pregnancy
- Increased risk for prematurity and low birth weight if poor maternal weight gain

SPECIAL THERAPY
Complementary and Alternative Therapies
- Ginger 250 mg powder capsules 4/d or fresh: In randomized trials, powdered ginger was more effective for relieving the severity of nausea and vomiting of pregnancy than placebo and of comparable efficacy to vitamin B_6.
- High-protein, low-carbohydrate, low-fat meals
- Hypnosis has possible efficacy.
- Often recommended, but no proven efficacy: Rest; frequent small meals; bland, low-fat foods; acupressure to wrist

MEDICATION (DRUGS)
- Start with 1st listed, and if no response, continue to next treatment:
  – Vitamin B_6 10–25 mg t.i.d./q.i.d.
  – Vitamin B_6 + doxylamine 10–12.5 mg t.i.d./q.i.d.
  – Vitamin B_6 + doxylamine + promethazine 12.5–25 mg q4h PO or rectal
  – Add metoclopramide 5–10 mg q8h, IM or PO, or promethazine 12.5–25 mg q4h IM, PO, or rectal, or trimethobenzamide 200 mg q6–8h rectal
- If dehydrated:
  – IV fluids with correction of ketosis and vitamin deficiencies, thiamine
  – Dimenhydrinate 50 mg IV q4–6h, or metoclopramide 5–10 mg IV q8h, or promethazine 12.5–25 mg IV q4h
  – Add methylprednisolone 16 mg q8h for 3 days; taper to stop or to lowest effective dose over 2 weeks, or ondansetron 8 mg IV q12h
  – If unable take food PO and losing weight:
    ○ Peripheral parenteral nutrition with high-lipid formula for several days only
    ○ TPN for longer-term needs. Consider PICC line.

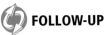 **FOLLOW-UP**

DISPOSITION

Issues for Referral
Hospitalization if IV hydration and therapy needed

PROGNOSIS
Prognosis for resolution of symptoms and normal pregnancy outcome is good. However, there is a risk for recurrence with subsequent pregnancy.

COMPLICATIONS
- Depression
- Wernicke encephalopathy
- Complications of hospitalization/intravenous treatments/TPN
- Transient hyperthyroidism

PATIENT MONITORING
- Hydration status
- Weight gain
- Electrolytes
- Evaluate for anemia
- Monitor for preterm labor

BIBLIOGRAPHY

ACOG Practice Bulletin No. 52: Nausea and Vomiting of Pregnancy. Washington, DC: ACOG; April 2004.

Borrelli F, et al. Effectiveness and safety of ginger in the treatment of pregnancy-induced nausea and vomiting. *Obstet Gynecol.* 2005;105:849–856.

Dodds L, et al. Outcomes of pregnancies complicated by hyperemesis gravidarum. *Obstet Gynecol.* 2006;107:285–292.

Safari HR, et al. The efficacy of methylprednisolone in the treatment of hyperemesis gravidarum: A randomized, double-blind, controlled study. *Am J Obstet Gynecol.* 1998;179:921–924.

Smith C, et al. A randomized controlled trial of ginger to treat nausea and vomiting in pregnancy. *Obstet Gynecol.* 2004;103:639–645.

Vutyavanich T, et al. Ginger for nausea and vomiting of pregnancy: Randomized, double-masked, placebo-controlled trial. *Obstet Gynecol.* 2001;97:577–582.

Vutyavanich T, et al. Pyridoxine for nausea and vomiting of pregnancy: A randomized, double-blind, placebo-controlled trial. *Am J Obstet Gynecol.* 1995;173:881–884.

 MISCELLANEOUS

CLINICAL PEARLS
- Nausea and vomiting of pregnancy is very common and may progress to hyperemesis.
- Early treatment is beneficial.
- Effective treatment, thought to be safe for the fetus, is available and prognosis is good.

ABBREVIATIONS
- GA—Gestational age
- hCG—Human chorionic gonadotropin
- OCPs—Oral contraceptive pills
- PICC line—Peripherally inserted central catheter
- TPN—Total parenteral nutrition
- TSH—Thyroid-stimulating hormone

CODES

ICD9-CM
- 643.0 Mild hyperemesis gravidarum
- 643.1 Hyperemesis gravidarum with metabolic disturbance
- 643 Excessive vomiting in pregnancy

 PATIENT TEACHING

- Reassurance about favorable pregnancy outcome
- Dietary advice
- Ginger
- Possible acupressure

PREVENTION
- Daily multivitamin: Women taking daily multivitamin at the time of conception had less severe hyperemesis.
- Small, high-protein meals
- Evaluate and treat nausea and vomiting of pregnancy early.

Section V

HYPERTENSIVE DISORDERS OF PREGNANCY

Annette E. Bombrys, DO
Baha Sibai, MD

 BASICS

DESCRIPTION
- HTN:
  - Elevated BP ≥140 mm Hg systolic and/or ≥90 mm Hg diastolic on at least 2 occasions at least 6 hours apart but within 1 week
- Proteinuria:
  - 0.1 g/L or more in at least 2 random urine specimens or ≥0.3 g in 24-hour specimen
- GHTN:
  - BP for 1st time in pregnancy or within 24 hours postpartum
  - BP ≥140 systolic or ≥90 diastolic before 20 weeks' gestation.
  - HTN present on 2 occasions 6 hours apart but within 1 week
  - BP must return to normal by 6 weeks postpartum
- Preeclampsia:
  - GHTN with proteinuria (≥300 mg in 24-hour urine collection or ≥30 mg/dL (≥1+ dipstick) in at least 2 random urine samples collected at least 6 hours apart
  - In the absence of proteinuria, preeclampsia should be considered when GHTN is associated with persistent cerebral symptoms, epigastric or RUQ pain with nausea and vomiting, or thrombocytopenia (platelets ≤100,000/mm³) and abnormal LFTs
  - Severe preeclampsia:
    ○ Protein excretion of ≥5 g in 24-hour urine collection, presence of multiorgan involvement such as PE, seizures, oliguria (≤500 mL/24 h), thrombocytopenia, abnormal LFTs, RUQ pain, or persistent CNS symptoms
    ○ BP ≥160 mm Hg systolic and/or ≥110 mm Hg diastolic
- Chronic HTN:
  - HTN prior to pregnancy, HTN prior to 20 weeks' gestation, or HTN persisting longer than 12 weeks postpartum
- Chronic HTN with superimposed preeclampsia:
  - Patients with chronic HTN without proteinuria at <20 weeks gestation, defined as new-onset proteinuria of ≥0.3 g in 24-hour specimen
  - Patients with chronic HTN and preexisting proteinuria before 20 weeks gestation, defined as severe BP in a previously well-controlled patient, and/or headache, blurred vision, epigastric pain, elevated liver enzymes, or thrombocytopenia

Age-Related Factors
Incidence increases with advancing maternal age

EPIDEMIOLOGY
- HTN is the most common medical disorder of pregnancy.
- Hypertensive disorders complicate 12–22% of pregnancies.

- Incidence:
  - CHTN: 0.6– 2.0% (women 18–29 years) to 4.6–22.3% (women 30–39 years). Incidence higher in African Americans
  - GHTN: 6–17% (nulliparous women) and 2–4% (multiparous women)
  - Preeclampsia: 6–8%, 14% in multifetal gestation, and 18% in those with a previous history of preeclampsia
  - Eclampsia: 1 in 2,000 pregnancies

RISK FACTORS
- Nulliparity
- Multifetal gestation
- Obesity
- Family history of preeclampsia, eclampsia
- Preeclampsia in previous pregnancy
- Abnormal uterine Doppler studies at 18 and 24 weeks
- Pregestational DM
- Presence of thrombophilia
- HTN
- Renal disease
- Infertility
- PCOS
- Recurrent miscarriages
- Thrombophilia
- Smoking (protective)

Genetics
Increased risk of developing preeclampsia or eclampsia if there is a positive family history.

PATHOPHYSIOLOGY
- Abnormal placentation or trophoblastic invasion of uterine blood vessels
- Immunologic intolerance between fetoplacental and maternal tissues
- Maladaptation to cardiovascular changes or inflammatory changes of pregnancy
- Dietary deficiency
- Genetic abnormalities

DIAGNOSIS

SIGNS AND SYMPTOMS
History
- Headache
- Scotoma
- Blurred vision
- Nausea
- Vomiting
- Abdominal pain
- RUQ pain
- Increased edema/swelling

Physical Exam
- Hyperreflexia
- RUQ pain or abdominal pain
- Generalized edema

TESTS
US:
- GA, estimated fetal weight, and AFI

Lab
- Renal:
  - Increased creatinine, urea, uric acid
  - Decreased creatinine clearance
  - Proteinuria
- Hematologic:
  - Increased fibrinogen, D-dimer, bilirubin, lactic dehydrogenase, hematocrit
  - Decreased antithrombin III activity, platelets
- Hepatic:
  - Increased liver enzymes

DIFFERENTIAL DIAGNOSIS
- Common conditions that can present similar to preeclampsia at <20 weeks' gestation:
  - Hydatidiform mole
  - Choriocarcinoma
- Common conditions confused with HELLP syndrome:
  - Acute fatty liver of pregnancy
  - Hepatitis
  - Exacerbation of system lupus erythematous
  - Cholestasis
  - Cerebral hemorrhage
  - Migraine
  - Pancreatitis

Hematologic
- HELLP syndrome (see topic)
- Altered hematocrit secondary to hemoconcentration (elevated hematocrit) or hemolysis (decreased hematocrit)
- Increased lactate dehydrogenase

Other/Miscellaneous
- Hepatic changes:
  - Elevation of ALT and/or AST
  - Hyperbilirubinemia
  - Subcapsular hematoma with hepatic rupture (associated with high mortality rate)
- Vascular changes:
  - Hemoconcentration with contraction of intravascular space
  - HTN
  - Intense vasospasm
  - Decreased oncotic pressure along with capillary leakage leading to increased edema
- Neurologic and cerebral manifestations:
  - Intracranial hemorrhage
  - Temporary blindness

- Renal changes:
  - Oliguria
  - Increase serum creatinine and BUN
  - Decreased glomerular filtration rate and renal blood flow
- Fetal changes:
  - IUGR
  - Oligohydramnios
  - Placental abruption
  - Nonreassuring fetal heart tracing

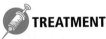

TREATMENT

GENERAL MEASURES
- Initial diagnosis requires inpatient admission for minimum of 24 hours.
- Labs (CBC with differential, renal panel, DIC panel, LFTs, LDH, urine dipstick for protein, 24 urine collection for protein)
- Fetal evaluation including GA assessment, US for estimated fetal weight and AFI, NST or BPP
- Preterm patient <34 weeks' gestation: Administer glucocorticoids for lung maturation.
- After initial admission, mild preeclampsia can be managed as an outpatient until term with weekly physician office visits, biweekly NST or weekly modified BPP (NST + AFI), weekly labs, and weekly 24-hour urine evaluation (at physician discretion).
- Magnesium sulfate is usually started at the time of initial evaluation following diagnosis of severe preeclampsia. If preterm, give corticosteroids and deliver. If patient is term, then deliver.

PREGNANCY-SPECIFIC ISSUES
Preeclampsia is a disease specific only to pregnancy.

By Trimester
- 1st-trimester preeclampsia is rare; consider molar pregnancy or choriocarcinoma prior to 20 weeks' gestation
- 2nd trimester: Preeclampsia is associated with increased maternal and perinatal morbidity and mortality. Consultation with specialist in MFM is recommended.
- 3rd-trimester preeclampsia is the most common GA at presentation, and is associated with good maternal and perinatal outcomes

Risks for Mother
- HELLP syndrome
- Eclampsia
- Pulmonary edema
- Pleural effusion
- Acute renal failure
- Abruptio placentae
- Subcapsular liver hematoma
- Intracerebral hemorrhage
- Death

Risks for Fetus
- IUGR
- Preterm delivery
- Hypoxia
- Fetal heart rate abnormalities
- Placental insufficiency

MEDICATION (DRUGS)
- Magnesium sulfate 4-g bolus with 2-g continuous infusion for the prevention of tonic-clonic seizures in severe preeclampsia. Magnesium is continued for 24 hours postpartum.
- Magnesium toxicity symptoms include loss of patellar reflex, feelings of warmth and flushing, somnolence, slurred speech, muscular paralysis, respiratory difficulty, and cardiac arrest:
  - Treat magnesium toxicity with calcium gluconate 10 mL of 10% solution.
- BP ≥160 mm Hg systolic and/or ≥105 mm Hg diastolic must be treated with antihypertensive agents to prevent maternal stroke:
  - Hydralazine 5–10 mg IV q20min
  - Labetalol 20–40 mg IV q10min or 1 mg/kg as needed
  - Nifedipine 10–20 mg PO q20–30min
  - Nicardipine 5–15 mg/h IV

ALERT
Diuretic therapy is avoided in preeclampsia because of the decreased intravascular volume. Diuretics are only used in cases where preeclampsia is complicated by pulmonary edema.

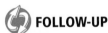

FOLLOW-UP

DISPOSITION
Issues for Referral
All the following should be referred to a specialist trained in MFM:
- Severe preeclampsia at any GA
- Preeclampsia with any complication

PROGNOSIS
- GHTN: Prognosis is similar to that seen in normotensive pregnancies.
- Preeclampsia: Prognosis depends on GA at onset and at delivery, severity of disease, presence of multiple gestations, and presence of pre-existing medical conditions.

BIBLIOGRAPHY

Barton JR, et al. Mild gestational hypertension remote from term: Progression and outcome. *Am J Obstet Gynecol.* 2001;184:979–983.

Coetzee EJ, et al. A randomized controlled trial of intravenous magnesium sulfate versus placebo in the management of women with severe preeclampsia. *Br J Obstet Gynaecol.* 1998;105:300–303.

Reports of the National High Blood Pressure Education Program. Working group report on high blood pressure in pregnancy. *Am J Obstet Gynecol.* 2000;183:S1–S22.

Sibai BM. Diagnosis and management of gestational hypertension and preeclampsia. *Am J Obstet Gynecol.* 2003;102:181–192.

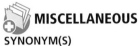

MISCELLANEOUS

SYNONYM(S)
Toxemia

ABBREVIATIONS
- AFI—Amniotic fluid index
- BPP—Biophysical profile
- GHTN—Gestational hypertension
- HELLP—Hemolysis, Elevated Liver function tests, Low Platelets
- HTN—Hypertension
- IUGR—Intrauterine growth restriction
- LFT—Liver function tests
- MFM—Maternal-fetal medicine
- NST—Nonstress test
- PCOS—Polycystic ovary syndrome
- PE—Pulmonary embolism
- RUQ—Right upper quadrant

CODES
ICD9-CM
- 642.0X—Benign essential HTN complicating pregnancy, childbirth, and the puerperium
- 642.3X—Transient HTN of pregnancy
- 642.4X—Mild or unspecified preeclampsia
- 642.5X—Severe preeclampsia
- 642.7X—Preeclampsia or eclampsia superimposed on pre-existing HTN

PATIENT TEACHING

PREVENTION
- No current prevention strategies
- Evidence based review has provided the following recommendations:
  - Insufficient evidence to recommend the use of fish-oil supplementation and other sources of fatty acids, diet and exercise, protein or salt restriction, or the use of antioxidant vitamins (C, E).
  - No evidence to recommend magnesium or zinc supplementation, heparin or low-molecular-weight heparin, or antihypertensive agents in women with CHTN.
  - Low-dose aspirin can be considered in high risk population.
  - Calcium supplementation is recommended in women at high risk for GHTN in communities with low dietary calcium intake.

INTRAUTERINE FETAL DEMISE

Bonnie J. Dattel, MD

 BASICS

DESCRIPTION
- Fetal death can occur at any GA.
- Etiologies differ by GA; causes include:
  - Chromosomal abnormalities
  - Fetal anemia secondary to alloimmunization or fetal-maternal hemorrhage
  - Cord accidents
  - Fetal infection
  - Antiphospholipid antibody syndrome
  - Maternal thrombophilias
  - Obstetric disorders:
    - Preeclampsia
    - Abruption
    - IUGR secondary to utero placental insufficiency

Age-Related Factors
Certain conditions associated with perinatal risk are more common in advanced maternal age:
- Chromosomal aneuploidies
- Preeclampsia/Chronic HTN
- DM

RISK FACTORS
Risk factors are related to both exogenous and endogenous conditions:
- Maternal age and increased risk for fetal aneuploidy and hypertensive diseases
- Inherited conditions such as thrombophilias
- DM and uteroplacental insufficiency
- Occupations with high risk for exposure to certain infections (e.g., preschool teachers and parvovirus)
- Multiple gestations with TTTS

Genetics
Fetal aneuploidy is the most common reason for 1st trimester loss and should be considered in cases of recurrent fetal loss (>3 consecutive spontaneous losses):
- 3–5% 1 of the parents has a balanced translocation
- Unbalanced karyotype in up to 40% of abortus specimens
- Recurrent aneuploidy especially if the 1st abortus was chromosomally abnormal.

PATHOPHYSIOLOGY
- The pathophysiology, outside of aneuploidy, for IUFD depends on underlying cause.
- Uteroplacental insufficiency leading to fetal hypoxemia and ultimately circulatory failure:
  - Chronic HTN
  - Preeclampsia/Eclampsia
  - DM
  - Abruptio placenta
  - Infections with overwhelming fetal sepsis and death, including fetal anemia
  - Autoimmune disease/thrombophilia with placental infarction/thromboses and relative uteroplacental insufficiency
  - Fetal-maternal hemorrhage with fetal anemia and circulatory failure leading to death
  - Trauma with acute placental circulation disruption
  - Cord "accidents" (true knots, occult prolapse) with interrupted fetal circulation and fetal hypoxemia leading to in utero death

ASSOCIATED CONDITIONS
Associated conditions that can increase the rate of in utero fetal death include:
- Multiple gestations
- Uterine anomalies
- Any maternal disease that can interfere with uteroplacental circulation

 DIAGNOSIS

SIGNS AND SYMPTOMS
History
The medical history associated with fetal loss depends on trimester of pregnancy:
- 1st-trimester complaints often involve bleeding and cramping as a sign of fetal loss.
- 2nd-trimester complaints can also include bleeding and cramping; however, fetal movement may also no longer be recognized by the mother.
- The most common complaint in the 3rd trimester is the loss of appreciated fetal activity:
  - IUFD can occur with no maternal symptoms and may be found incidentally.

Physical Exam
- The physical findings of IUFD all involve the absence of a fetal heart rate, regardless of GA. This absence should be confirmed by US.
- 3rd-trimester findings may also involve low AF levels and collapse of fetal structures when visualized on US.
- 1st and 2nd-trimester losses may involve significant uterine bleeding requiring surgical intervention.

TESTS
In very early pregnancy, loss prior to the ability to visualize a fetal heart rate by US, a falling β-hCG level may be the only indicator of fetal loss.

Labs
Recommended laboratory evaluation when a late 2nd- or 3rd-trimester IUFD is diagnosed:
- Indirect Coombs test
- Fetal karyotype
- Kleihauer Betke
- Serologic test for syphilis
- Toxicology screen
- Autopsy
- Antiphospholipid antibodies
- TORCH titers including parvovirus
- Thrombophilia workup
- Thyroid function tests
- Glucose tolerance testing (HbA1C)

Imaging
US with failure to visualize fetal heart rate and activity is the gold standard for diagnosis of IUFD.

DIFFERENTIAL DIAGNOSIS
The most important differential diagnosis when suspecting fetal death in the 1st trimester is to exclude ectopic pregnancy, which can be life-threatening to the mother.
- US evaluation of the adnexa
- Serial β-hCG levels to determine appropriate rise (or fall)

Infection
- Infectious etiologies must always be considered with IUFD. TORCH viral infection has been expanded to include parvovirus infection because of its association with fetal anemia.
- Infections cause fetal death by placental involvement causing a relative utero placental insufficiency and by direct fetal infection leading to organ system failure.

Hematologic
Fetal anemia either secondary to infection or direct fetal-maternal bleed should be considered in fetal death.
- Other causes of fetal anemia are alloimmunization and isoimmunization.
- These cause profound fetal anemia via direct attack on fetal blood cells and resulting bleeding (platelet consumption) or organ system failure (such as with Rh isoimmunization or other red cell antigens).

Metabolic/Endocrine
The most common metabolic disease to lead to IUFD is DM. This occurs due to placental failure generally in uncontrolled maternal diabetes.

Immunologic
New technologies have elucidated the relationship between maternal immunologic dysfunction and fetal loss. These conditions generally result in uteroplacental insufficiency that leads to fetal death:
- Antiphospholipid antibody syndrome
- Thrombophilias (Factor V Leiden, antithrombin III deficiency, prothrombin gene mutation, lupus anticoagulant):
  - Placental infarctions or thromboses interfering with fetal circulation

Tumor/Malignancy
Malignancies are an uncommon cause of fetal death. Rarely, maternal tumors such as melanoma can metastasize to the fetus and placenta.

Trauma
- Blunt force trauma as from a motor vehicle accident is a known cause of catastrophic fetal death. This usually results from an acute placental separation and loss of maternal fetal circulation.
- Maternal condition must be managed immediately.
- Often associated with DIC

Drugs
- Maternal drug use is also known to be associated with fetal death. The most common association is between cocaine use and IUFD. This occurs secondary to the blood flow changes that accompany cocaine ingestion and result in placental abruption.
- Chronic use of any substance, including nicotine, can result in placental infarcts which, if extensive enough, can result in fetal demise.

Other/Miscellaneous
Virtually any underlying abnormality can result in fetal loss, however, these would be rare entities.

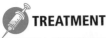

TREATMENT

GENERAL MEASURES
Treatment of IUFD begins with its identification. Further treatment measures are dependent on GA age of the discovery.

PREGNANCY-SPECIFIC ISSUES
Mothers experiencing a fetal death most desire to know the cause of the death. This is extremely important in counseling for future pregnancies. An autopsy and placental pathology are the 2 most useful pieces of information for the pregnant woman who has had an IUFD.

By Trimester
1st- and early 2nd-trimester fetal death can be treated either conservatively with uterine evacuation agents such as misoprostol or surgically with D&C. In the 3rd trimester, induction of labor with prostaglandins or oxytocin is the mainstay of treatment.

Risks for Mother
Risks for the mother involve the associated risks of the treatments involved. These include:
- Blood loss, surgical trauma, infection
- In cases of acute abruption, maternal DIC can be life-threatening and requires intensive maternal care.
- Rarely, cases of prolonged fetal death can be associated with maternal DIC and require prompt and aggressive intervention to save the mother.

Risks for Fetus
After a fetal death, the information gleaned toward determining the cause of the loss can be invaluable for prevention of the loss of future fetuses.

SPECIAL THERAPY
Complementary and Alternative Therapies
In addition to the use of agents for induction of labor or uterine evacuation, attention must be paid to the psychological well-being of the mother who has experienced the loss. Regardless of GA, IUFD is accompanied with profound psychological components. The mother should receive appropriate bereavement counseling and close follow-up to detect the development of associated depressive disorders.

MEDICATION (DRUGS)
The medications used for induction of labor are similar to those used for IUFD. Caution must be used to avoid uterine rupture.

SURGERY
In general, delivery of a dead fetus by cesarean section should be reserved for life-saving circumstances in the mother or the failure to accomplish safe vaginal delivery.

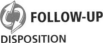

FOLLOW-UP

DISPOSITION
Issues for Referral
- Women who have experienced an IUFD should receive appropriate postpartum follow-up.
- An evaluation in the postpartum period should include not only the routine physical examination but a discussion of the events that occurred and information that has been obtained in the workup of the fetal death.
- Evaluation for depression should be part of every follow-up exam.
- Referral to parents' groups or individual counseling may be helpful.

PROGNOSIS
- Prognosis for recovering from a fetal loss is usually excellent. Most women recover from sporadic 1st-trimester losses relatively easily, as they can be assured that 90% of women with a single early pregnancy loss go on to have normal pregnancies in the future.
- For women with recurrent pregnancy loss or 3rd-trimester losses, the recovery time frame is longer (months–years). For many women there are trigger dates, such as the date of the loss or the due date of the pregnancy. Many of these women will benefit from outpatient counseling.

COMPLICATIONS
The main complications of IUFD are related to the underlying cause. In women with acute abruption, DIC, and circulatory collapse long-term sequelae may occur, involving renal failure as in shock/trauma cases. These are rare, however.

PATIENT MONITORING
- Patients should be monitored during labor as are parturients with a live fetus.
- Patients with acute abruption and DIC require intensive surveillance and blood product replacement.
- Postpartum, patients should be monitored and screened for depression.

Fetus
- No fetal monitoring is required in cases of IUFD.
- However, in subsequent pregnancies, antenatal fetal surveillance should be instituted near the time of a 3rd-trimester loss.
- Pregnancies complicated by prior utero placental insufficiency, regardless of etiology, should have serial US for fetal growth.
- Pregnancies complicated by thrombophilia should receive anticoagulant therapy.
- These pregnancies are best referred to MFM specialists due to their high-risk nature.

BIBLIOGRAPHY

Reece EA, et al., eds. *Medicine of the Fetus and Mother*. Philadelphia: Lippincott-Raven; 1999.

Creasey RK, et al. *Maternal-Fetal Medicine*, 4th ed. Philadelphia: W.B. Saunders; 1999.

MISCELLANEOUS

CLINICAL PEARLS
The occurrence of an IUFD is a life-altering experience for a pregnant woman. Considerations at this time include patient bereavement, appropriate delivery, and evaluation for discoverable causes of the demise that may impact future reproduction.

ABBREVIATIONS
- AF—Amniotic fluid
- DIC—Disseminated intravascular coagulation
- GA—Gestational age
- hCG—Human chorionic gonadotropin
- IUGR—Intrauterine growth restriction
- IUFD—Intrauterine fetal demise
- MFM—Maternal-fetal medicine
- TORCH—Toxoplasmosis, other, rubella, cytomegalic virus, and herpes
- TTTS—Twin-twin transfusion syndrome

CODES
ICD9-CM
646.4 Intrauterine death

PATIENT TEACHING

All pregnant women should be counseled regarding normal fetal activity, avoidance of high-risk behaviors (including smoking and substance use), avoiding infectious complications (parvo exposure, *Listeria* exposure), and symptoms to report to their care providers that could signal fetal danger.

PREVENTION
The prevention of IUFD rests on the provision of prenatal care to identify pregnancies at risk or in jeopardy. Careful evaluation of a prior fetal death can provide invaluable information to allow appropriate intervention and surveillance of future pregnancies to prevent loss.

Section V

INTRAUTERINE GROWTH RESTRICTION

Paula J. Adams Hillard, MD

 BASICS

DESCRIPTION

- FGR, also called IUGR, was previously termed intrauterine growth retardation.
- These terms describe a fetus that has not reached its growth potential.
- A common definition is a fetus weighing below the 10th percentile for GA.
- May be caused by fetal, placental, and maternal factors
- Terms that are not synonymous, but used to describe small babies include:
  - SGA
  - LBW
- It has been suggested that as many as 70% of babies weighing <10th percentile are constitutionally small because of female sex, maternal ethnicity, parity, or BMI:
  - These babies are not at the same high risk for perinatal mortality and morbidity as are growth-restricted fetuses.
- Patterns of FGR:
  - Symmetric FGR: 20–30% proportional decrease in all organs
  - Asymmetric FGR: Greater decrease in abdominal size, with sparing of head circumference, related to sparing of growth of the brain and heart as vital organs
- Fetal growth restriction (FGR)
- Previously termed intrauterine growth retardation

RISK FACTORS

- Fetal etiologies:
  - Chromosomal abnormalities
  - Congenital anomalies: 22% of anomalous fetuses were FGR in 1 series.
  - Multiple gestation
- Placental abnormalities:
  - Single umbilical artery
  - Bilobed placenta
  - Velamentous insertion of the cord
  - Placenta previa
  - Placental abruption
  - Thrombophilia-related placental pathology
- Maternal etiologies:
  - Poor nutrition:
    - Underweight
    - Poor weight gain
  - Maternal hypoxemia:
    - Cyanotic heart disease
    - Sickle cell anemia
    - Pulmonary disease
    - Living at high altitude

- Diminished uteroplacental perfusion:
  - Chronic HTN
  - Preeclampsia
- Thrombosis:
  - Antiphospholipid syndrome
  - Maternal thrombophilias
- Infection:
  - Toxoplasmosis, rubella, cytomegalovirus, varicella-zoster
  - Possibly bacterial infections listeria, TB, *Chlamydia*, mycoplasma
- Maternal substance abuse:
  - Alcohol, tobacco, other dugs
  - Smokers have 3.5-fold increased risk SGA infants
- Medications:
  - Warfarin, anticonvulsants, antineoplastic agents, folic acid antagonists
- Other maternal factors statistically associated:
  - Race, young adolescent or older gravidas, previous infant with FGR, ART pregnancy

Genetics

- Genetic factors are estimated to contribute 40% of the variation in birth weight, with ~60% environmental.
- Abnormal karyotype in 5–20% FGR, typically resulting in symmetric FGR, seen early in pregnancy.
- Chromosomal abnormalities include:
  - Trisomies:
    - Trisomy 21, 18, 13
  - Autosomal deletions:
    - Cri du chat syndrome
  - Other

PATHOPHYSIOLOGY

Multiple, from placental vasculature abnormalities, thrombosis

ASSOCIATED CONDITIONS

See "Risk Factors."

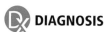 **DIAGNOSIS**

- Because FGR is associated with increased fetal morbidity and mortality, screening for FGR is a key component of prenatal care.
- Screening for risk factors
- Serial measurement of fundal height as a measure of fetal growth
- US exam if FGR suspected

SIGNS AND SYMPTOMS

History

- GA must be accurately established (See Establishing Estimated Date of Delivery)
- LMP
- Correlation with uterine size
- Discrepancies addressed by early US

Physical Exam

May be useful in screening in low risk pregnancies:

- Fundal height (FH):
  - Most useful if same examiner and in normal-weight individual
  - Further assess if FH in cm < GA by 3 cm

TESTS

Indicated to assess fetal well-being once FGR noted

Imaging

- Indicated to screen for FGR with high-risk conditions or if suspected based on physical exam
- Sonographic parameters include:
  - Abdominal circumference is the most sensitive single morphometric indicator.
  - EFW calculated on the basis of ≥2 body measurements
  - Body proportions:
    - HC/AC ratio
    - FL/AC ratio
    - Customized weight centile based on fetal gender, maternal parity, ethnicity, height, weight, age
  - AF volume:
    - Oligohydramnios is sequela of FGR (see chapter)
- Doppler US to assess fetal and maternal hemodynamics:
  - FGR associated with abnormal Doppler in both maternal and fetal vessels, including uterine and umbilical arteries
  - Cochrane review found the use of Doppler US associated with a trend toward fewer perinatal deaths, with fewer labor inductions.

DIFFERENTIAL DIAGNOSIS

See "Risk Factors."

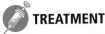 **TREATMENT**

GENERAL MEASURES

- Detection of FGR is useful to identify fetuses at risk for perinatal complications.
- History, including conditions associated with FGR plus physical exam with serial measurement of FH plus US evaluation as indicated can lead to diagnosis of FGR.
- After diagnosis of FGR, increased fetal surveillance:

  - Biophysical profile
  - Serial fetal weight/growth assessment
  - AF volume assessment
  - Doppler velocimetry
  - Antenatal steroids
- Timing of delivery determined by fetal status and GA, balancing the risks of prematurity with the risks of fetal death.
- Induction of labor with fetal monitoring, with cesarean delivery if fetal intolerance of labor vs. cesarean delivery

PREGNANCY-SPECIFIC ISSUES

By Trimester
Fetal karyotyping if early or severe FGR, if hydramnios, or structural anomalies.

Risks for Mother
Maternal risks of the conditions that can lead to FGR: HTN, preeclampsia, pulmonary disease, etc.

Risks for Fetus
- Fetal, neonatal, and perinatal mortality are increased, with greater mortality associated with greater growth restriction. Risks of preterm birth, whether spontaneous or induced.
- Potential deleterious effects on adult health:
  - HTN, hypercholesterolemia, impaired glucose tolerance, cardiovascular disease

 MEDICATION (DRUGS)

- Medical interventions have been suggested to improve fetal outcome, but none has proven consistently beneficial.
- Nutritional supplements, volume expansion, low-dose aspirin, heparin, bed rest, β-mimetics, calcium channel blockers

SURGERY

Cesarean delivery as indicated for fetal compromise

 FOLLOW-UP

DISPOSITION

Issues for Referral
Consultation with MFM specialist may be indicated.

PROGNOSIS

Risk of recurrent FGR in subsequent pregnancy.

PATIENT MONITORING

Fetal monitoring with US and antenatal surveillance, as well as intrapartum fetal monitoring are indicated.

BIBLIOGRAPHY

ACOG Practice Bulletin No. 12. Intrauterine Growth Restriction. Washington DC: ACOG; January 2000.

Divon MY, et al. Fetal growth restriction: Diagnosis. UpToDate Online 15.2. Available at www.utdol.com. Accessed 09/18/07.

Resnik R. Fetal growth restriction: Evaluation and management. UpToDate Online 15.2. Available at www.utdol.com. Accessed 09/18/07.

Vison MY, et al. Fetal growth restriction: Etiology. UpToDate Online 15.2. Available at www.utdol.com. Accessed 09/18/07.

 MISCELLANEOUS

ABBREVIATIONS

- AC—Abdominal circumference
- AF—Amniotic fluid
- ART—Assisted reproductive technologies
- EFW—Estimated fetal weight
- FGR—Fetal growth restriction
- FH—Fundal height
- FL—Femur length
- GA—Gestational age
- HC—Head circumference
- IUGR—Intrauterine growth restriction or intrauterine growth retardation (Outdated)
- LBW—Low birth weight
- LMP—Last menstrual period
- MFM—Maternal-fetal medicine
- SGA—Small for gestational age
- US—Ultrasound

CODES

ICD9-CM
764.9 Fetal growth retardation, unspecified

 PATIENT TEACHING

PREVENTION

No supplements of treatments have been shown to be effective in the prevention of FGR.

Section V

LOW BIRTHWEIGHT

Brooke Friedman, MD

 BASICS

DESCRIPTION
- By definition:
  - LBW: <2,500 g
  - VLBW: <1,500 g
  - ELBW: <1,000 g
- GA should be stated, as LBW infants may be born at term or preterm:
  - Clarify if AGA, SGA, or LGA

Age-Related Factors
Preterm delivery accounts for majority of LBW infants.

EPIDEMIOLOGY
- In 2004, 8.1% births were LBW; 1.5% were VLBW.
- Higher rates among African Americans than Caucasians

RISK FACTORS
- Tobacco
- Illicit drug use
- Inadequate maternal weight gain
- Hyperthyroidism
- Advanced maternal age
- Poverty/Stress
- IVF

Genetics
Birth defects (chromosomal or structural) associated with LBW and preterm delivery

PATHOPHYSIOLOGY
Majority of LBW infants result from:
- Preterm delivery
- IUGR

ASSOCIATED CONDITIONS
Preterm delivery and its associated conditions (See Prematurity.)

 DIAGNOSIS

Defined solely by weight at time of birth

 TREATMENT

GENERAL MEASURES
- Optimal mode of delivery for LBW infant is controversial:
  - Insufficient evidence to recommend routine cesarean delivery
- Efforts should be made to deliver infants with expected LBW at facility with appropriate level of neonatal nursery.

PREGNANCY-SPECIFIC ISSUES
Risks for Mother
VLBW or ELBW may prompt low vertical or fundal (classical) cesarean/hysterotomy incision with increased risk of uterine rupture and requirement for repeat cesarean in subsequent pregnancy.

Risks for Fetus
- Respiratory abnormalities:
  - Bronchopulmonary dysplasia, RDS
- Symptomatic PDA (30% LBW)
- Intraventricular hemorrhage (30% VLBW)
- Necrotizing enterocolitis (2–10% VLBW)
- Infection/Late-onset sepsis
- Hypothermia
- Hypoglycemia

MEDICATION (DRUGS)
Survival has improved, due to:
- Corticosteroids in women at risk of preterm delivery (See Corticosteroid Use for Fetal Lung Maturation.)
- Surfactant therapy
- Improved neonatal resuscitation
- Delivery at facilities with experienced personnel

 FOLLOW-UP

DISPOSITION
Issues for Referral
Referral may be indicated for delivery at hospital facility with appropriate level of neonatal nursery.

PROGNOSIS
- High mortality risk with weight 1,500–2,500 g, higher if <1,500 g, even in term infants
- VLBW and ELBW associated with long-term neurodevelopmental disability

COMPLICATIONS
Fetal origins hypothesis controversial:
- Some studies suggest LBW associated with diseases in later life (e.g., HTN)

PATIENT MONITORING
Fetus
Continuous fetal heart rate monitoring of suspected LBW fetus is recommended.

BIBLIOGRAPHY

Cifuentes J, et al. Mortality in low birth weight infants according to level of neonatal care at hospital of birth. *Pediatrics*. 2002;109:745.

Cunningham G, et al., eds. *Williams Obstetrics*, 22nd ed. New York: McGraw-Hill; 2005.

Hack M, et al. Outcomes in young adulthood for very-low-birth-weight infants. *N Engl J Med*. 2002;346:149.

Huxley RR, et al. The role of size at birth and postnatal catch-up growth in determining systolic blood pressure: A systematic review of the literature. *J Hypertension*. 2000;18:815.

Jackson RA, et al. Perinatal outcomes in singletons following in vitro fertilization: A meta-analysis. *Obstet Gynecol*. 2004;103:551.

Lemons JA, et al. Very low birth weight outcomes of the National Institute of Child Health and Human Development Neonatal Research Network, January 1995 through December 1996. NICHD Neonatal Research Network. *Pediatrics*. 2001;107:E1.

Martin JA, et al. Births: Final data for 2001. *Natl Vital Stat Rep*. 2002;51:1–102.

Williams RL, et al. Fetal growth and perinatal viability in California. *Obstet Gynecol*. 1982;59:624.

 MISCELLANEOUS

CLINICAL PEARLS

If expected birth weight <2,000 g, infants should be delivered at tertiary facility:

- In utero transfer to tertiary facility associated with improved outcomes

ABBREVIATIONS

- AGA—Appropriate for gestational age
- ELBW—Extremely low birth weight
- GA—Gestational age
- HTN—Hypertension
- IUGR—Intrauterine growth restriction
- IVF—in vitro fertilization
- LBW—Low birth weight
- LGA—Large for gestational age
- PDA—Patent ductus arteriosus
- RDS—Respiratory distress syndrome
- SGA—Small for gestational age
- VLBW—Very low birth weight

CODES

ICD9-CM

- V21.3 Low birth weight status (excludes history of perinatal problems V13.7)
- V21.30 Low birth weight status, unspecified
- V21.31 Low birth weight status, <500 g
- V21.32 Low birth weight status 500–999 g
- V21.33 Low birth weight status 1,000–1,499 g
- V21.34 Low birth weight status 1,500–1,999 g
- V21.35 Low birth weight status 2,000–2,500 g

PATIENT TEACHING

PREVENTION

- Appropriate prenatal and primary care
- Adequate nutrition
- Avoidance of smoking and illicit drugs

Section V

MACROSOMIA
Tania F. Esakoff, MD
Naomi E. Stotland, MD

BASICS

DESCRIPTION
- Fetal macrosomia is defined as excessive birth weight, usually 4,000 g or 4,500 g independent of GA
- LGA also describes excessive fetal growth, and is defined at >90th percentile for a given GA.

EPIDEMIOLOGY
- 10% of US liveborn infants weigh >4,000 g
- 1.5% of US liveborn infants weigh >4,500 g

RISK FACTORS
- Prior history of macrosomia
- Maternal prepregnancy weight
- Weight gain during pregnancy
- Pregestational and gestational diabetes
- Multiparity
- Male sex of fetus
- GA >40 weeks
- Ethnicity:
  − Latina women have a higher incidence of macrosomia compared to any other group
- Maternal birth weight
- Maternal height
- Maternal age <17 and advanced age
- Abnormal 1-hour GLT with normal 3-hour GTT

Genetics
Genetic, racial, and ethnic factors influence birth weight:
- Parental height and race interact with environmental factors during pregnancy.

PATHOPHYSIOLOGY
Depends on the underlying risk factor:
- In diabetic patients, likely etiology is hyperglycemia in the fetus resulting in hyperinsulinemia and increased fat and glycogen deposition.
- In obese women with normal glucose tolerance, relatively higher serum glucose levels may lead to larger birth weights via the same mechanism.
- In postdates pregnancy, longer gestation results in a larger size

ASSOCIATED CONDITIONS
- Pregestational diabetes
- Gestational diabetes
- Maternal obesity

Pediatric Considerations
Macrosomic infants born to obese mothers have increased body fat and decreased lean body mass:
- Increased risk of obesity in adolescence and adulthood
- Increased risk of type II diabetes and metabolic syndrome

DIAGNOSIS

Prenatal diagnosis is imprecise. Neonatal birth weight is the only accurate diagnostic sign.

SIGNS AND SYMPTOMS
History
Parous women can predict likely weight of the newborn better than physicians or imaging studies.

Physical Exam
- Fundal height
- Leopold maneuvers

TESTS
Lab
Higher rate of macrosomia among women with 1 abnormal value on 3-hour GTT (compared to women with all normal values)

Imaging
US can estimate fetal weight but has been unreliable:
- It can be +/− 500 g off at term.

DIFFERENTIAL DIAGNOSIS
Fundal height measurements > expected for GA may occur with multiple pregnancy. US exam will easily rule out this possibility.

TREATMENT

GENERAL MEASURES
- For mothers with diabetes, some evidence suggests that adding insulin to the diet regimen can decrease the incidence of macrosomia 3-fold.
- In women with excessive gestational weight gain but no diabetes, it is controversial whether caloric restriction or other dietary interventions can help.
- Labor and vaginal delivery are not contraindicated for women with estimated fetal weights up to 5,000 g in the absence of maternal diabetes.
- Suspected fetal macrosomia is not a contraindication to attempted vaginal birth after a previous cesarean delivery.

PREGNANCY-SPECIFIC ISSUES
Risks for Mother
Maternal complications include:
- Increased risk of cesarean delivery: Risk is twice as high when weight >4,500 g
- Postpartum hemorrhage: Almost twice as high at a birth weight of 4,000 g
- 3rd- and 4th-degree vaginal lacerations, especially if shoulder dystocia present
- Infection

Risks for Fetus
Fetal/Neonatal complications:
- Shoulder dystocia and, as a result, fracture of the clavicle (10-fold increase) and brachial plexus injury (Erb palsy)
- Low 5-minute Apgar
- Increased rate of NICU admission
- Risk of obesity in adolescence/adulthood
- Among infants weighing ≥5,000 g, significantly increased neonatal mortality

MEDICATION (DRUGS)

Suspected fetal macrosomia is not an indication for induction of labor:

- Induction does not improve maternal or fetal outcomes

SURGERY

- There are no sufficiently good studies from which to pick a weight cut-off at which cesarean delivery would be recommended to avoid complications of macrosomia.
- Level C recommendation from ACOG:
  - Consider prophylactic cesarean delivery with estimated fetal weight >5,000 g in nondiabetics.
  - Consider prophylactic cesarean delivery with estimated fetal weight >4,500 g in diabetics.
- Except in extreme emergencies, cesarean delivery should be done in the cases of midpelvic fetal arrest in the setting of macrosomia.

BIBLIOGRAPHY

ACOG Practice Bulletin, No. 22. Fetal Macrosomia. Washington DC: ACOG; November 2000.

Boulet SL, et al. Macrosomic births in the United Status: Determinants, outcomes, and proposed grades of risk. *Am J Obstet Gynecol*. 2003;188(5): 1372–1378.

Catalano PM. Management of obesity in pregnancy. *Obstet Gynecol*. 2007;109(2.1):419–433.

Kolderup LB, et al. Incidence of persistent birth injury in macrosomic infants: Association with mode of delivery. *Am J Obstet Gynecol*. 1997;177(1):37–41.

McLaughlin GB, et al. Women with one elevated 3-hour glucose tolerance test value: Are they at risk for adverse perinatal outcomes? *Am J Obstet Gynecol*. 2006:194(5);e16–e19.

Stotland NE, et al. Risk factors and obstetric complications associated with macrosomia. *Int J Gynaecol Obstet*. 2004;87(3):220–226. Erratum: *Int J Gynaecol Obstet*. 2005;90(1):88.

 MISCELLANEOUS

CLINICAL PEARLS

Optimization of prepregnancy body weight and avoidance of excessive pregnancy weight gain may reduce the risk of macrosomia.

ABBREVIATIONS

- ACOG—American College of Obstetricians and Gynecologists
- GA—Gestational age
- GLT—Glucose load test
- GTT—Glucose tolerance test
- LGA—Large for gestational age
- US—Ultrasound

 CODES

ICD9-CM
766.0 for LGA

 PATIENT TEACHING

ACOG Patient Education Pamphlets. Available at: www.acog.org:

- What to Expect after Your Due Date
- Diabetes and Pregnancy
- Good Health before Pregnancy

PREVENTION

- Screen high-risk populations for GDM and treat accordingly.
- Obese women should be screened for glucose intolerance (with 1-hour GLT) in the 1st trimester and again at 24–28 weeks' gestation.
- Preconception optimization of BMI
- Surveillance of gestational weight gain with nutritional counseling

MASTITIS AND GALACTOCELE

Ruth A. Lawrence, MD

BASICS

DESCRIPTION
- Mastitis:
  - Inflammation of the breast, whether or not a bacterial infection is present.
  - Tender, hot, swollen, wedge-shaped area of breast associated with:
    ○ Fever (≥38.5°C)
    ○ Chills
    ○ Flu-like aching
    ○ Systemic illness
- Galactocele:
  - A cyst in the breast that fills with milk during lactation.
  - A firm, nontender, smooth, round, moveable mass in the breast during lactation often associated with a plugged duct

EPIDEMIOLOGY
- Mastitis:
  - Common condition in lactating women.
  - Majority of cases occur in the 1st 6 weeks postpartum.
  - Prevalence of 20% in the 1st 6 months postpartum.
  - Mastitis can occur any time during lactation.
- Galactocele:
  - Common condition during lactation
  - Majority of cases occur in women with pre-existing breast cysts.
  - Can occur any time during lactation
  - Can recur

RISK FACTORS
- Mastitis:
  - Poor latch
  - Infrequent feeds
  - Missed feeds
  - Scheduled frequency or duration of feeds
  - Milk oversupply
  - Rapid weaning
  - Pressure on the breast (e.g., tight bra)
  - Damaged nipple
  - Blocked nipple duct
  - Maternal or infant illness
  - Maternal stress and fatigue
- Galactocele:
  - Cystic disease
  - Plugged ducts
  - Milk oversupply
  - Pressure on breasts from tight clothing

PATHOPHYSIOLOGY
- Mastitis:
  - Milk stasis is often the initiating factor, for whatever reason
  - There have been few research trials in this area.
  - Evidence for associations other than milk stasis is inconclusive, as is an association with sore nipples.
- Galactocele:
  - Cysts fill with milk
  - Plugged ducts

DIAGNOSIS

SIGNS AND SYMPTOMS
History
- Mastitis:
  - Red, painful breast
  - Usually unilateral
  - Subjective fever/chills
  - Most often within 6 weeks postpartum
  - If bilateral, it is an emergency.
- Galactocele:
  - Solitary nontender lump in the breast
  - Usually unilateral
  - No systemic symptoms

Physical Exam
- Mastitis:
  - Fever
  - Ill-appearing
  - Exquisitely tender, firm, red breast
  - +/− Nipple abnormality
- Galactocele:
  - Nontender breast lump
  - Well-appearing
  - Normal vital signs

TESTS
- Mastitis:
  - Primarily a clinical diagnosis
  - Laboratory investigations and other diagnostic procedures are NOT routinely needed.
- Galactocele:
  - Clinical diagnosis
  - US not indicated unless lump does not disappear in a week with massaging.

Labs
Mastitis:
- Breast milk culture and sensitivity testing should be undertaken only if:
  - No response to antibiotics within 48 hours
  - Mastitis recurs
  - Mastitis is hospital-acquired
  - Case is severe or unusual
  - Case is bilateral
- To obtain a culture:
  - 1st cleanse the nipple
  - Then collect a mid-stream, clean-catch sample of hand-expressed breast milk into a sterile cup.
  - Take care not to touch the inside of the container.

DIFFERENTIAL DIAGNOSIS
Mastitis and galactocele:
- Breast abscess
- Breast mass
- Inflammatory or ductal carcinoma

TREATMENT

GENERAL MEASURES
- Focuses primarily on frequent and effective milk removal
- Effective milk removal:
  - Breastfeed more frequently, starting on the affected side.
  - If pain interferes, start breastfeeding on the unaffected side and promptly switch to the affected side as soon as milk let down occurs.
  - Position the infant so that the chin or the nose points to the blockage.
  - During the feed, massage the breast from blocked area towards nipple.
  - After the feed, consider expressing by hand or pumping.
- Supportive measures:
  - Rest
  - Adequate fluids and nutrition
  - Practical help at home
  - Direct application of heat prior to feeding may help milk flow.
  - Direct application of cold packs after feeding may reduce pain and swelling.
- Galactocele:
  - Frequent and effective milk removal as above
  - Massage area toward nipple.
  - Manually express breast to remove plug.
  - If plugged ducts frequent, massage and express plugs.
  - Check clothing for tight straps.

MEDICATION (DRUGS)
Mastitis
- Analgesia:
  - Anti-inflammatory agents such as ibuprofen may help with the milk ejection reflex and be more effective than simple analgesics such as acetaminophen.
    ○ Ibuprofen is safe during breastfeeding
    ○ Doses up to 1.6 g/d are not detected in breast milk.
- Antibiotics:
  - A 10–14-day course is indicated if:
    ○ Symptoms are not improving after 12–24 hours of conservative measures OR
    ○ If a woman is acutely ill
  - The most common pathogen is penicillin-resistant *Staphylococcus aureus*:
    ○ Less common are streptococcus or *Escherichia coli*.
    ○ Bilateral infection is usually strep.
  - Consider the possibility of MRSA or ORSA community- or hospital-acquired organisms.

– Possible treatment regimens include:
  ○ Cephalexin 500 mg PO b.i.d. OR
  ○ Dicloxacillin 500 mg PO q.i.d. OR
  ○ Flucloxacillin 500 mg PO q.i.d. OR
  ○ Clindamycin 300 mg PO q.i.d. (for women with severe penicillin hypersensitivity)

Galactocele
• Usually not indicated
• If visible fatty plugs can be expressed; add lecithin to diet as oil or capsules (dose: 1 Tbs or 3 capsules/d)

SURGERY
Galactocele:
• If massage and removal of plugged ducts are unsuccessful, check by US.
• Can be drained by needle aspiration, but they will refill during lactation.
• Postweaning, can be surgically removed.

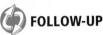 FOLLOW-UP

DISPOSITION
Mastitis:
• Initial clinical response to antibiotics is usually rapid, within 1–2 days but treatment must be continued for a minimum of 10 days.
• Consider hospital admission for IV antibiotic therapy if a woman is extremely ill or has inadequate support at home:
  – If hospitalized, rooming baby with the mother is mandatory so that breastfeeding can continue.

Issues for Referral
• Mastitis:
  – Consider a certified licensed lactation consultation for anyone with mastitis.
  – Consider surgical or infectious disease evaluation for the mother if she does not improve in 48 hours or has had >1 episode.
• Galactocele:
  – Breast surgeon if removal required postlactation
  – Aspiration or biopsy if US is suspicious.

COMPLICATIONS
Mastitis:
• Early cessation of breastfeeding (which may actually exacerbate mastitis)
• Breast abscess (diagnosed on physical exam and confirmed with breast US)
• Fungal infection (in which case treatment is needed for both mother and baby)
• Recurrent mastitis usually is due to inadequate treatment.

ALERT
• Mastitis more than twice in the same location warrants evaluation for an underlying mass.
• Galactocele:
  – May become inflamed and infected as a mastitis

BIBLIOGRAPHY

Academy of Breastfeeding Medicine Clinical Protocol No. 4. Mastitis, February 2, 2002. Available at: www.bfmed.org/protocol/mastitis.pdf. Accessed 02/01/07.

Hale T. *Medications and Mother's Milk: A Manual of Lactational Pharmacology,* 12th ed. Texas: Pharmasoft Medical Publishing; 2006.

Lawrence RA and Lawrence RM. *Breastfeeding: A Guide for the Medical Profession,* 6th ed. New York: Mosby-Elsevier; 2005.

MISCELLANEOUS

SYNONYMS
• Mastitis:
  – Breast infection
  – Nipple pain
  – Abscess, breast
• Galactocele:
  – Milk cyst
  – Lactocele
  – Galactocele
  – Plugged ducts

CLINICAL PEARLS
• The clinical diagnosis of mastitis is made when a lactating woman has a tender, hot, swollen, wedge-shaped area of breast associated with fever and chills.
• Women with mastitis should continue to breastfeed:
  – Stasis is often the initiating factor.
  – Most important management is frequent and effective milk removal.
• Often a 10–14 day course of cephalexin, dicloxacillin, flucloxacillin, or clindamycin is needed to treat penicillin-resistant *S. aureus.*

ABBREVIATIONS
• MRSA—Methicillin-resistant staphylococcus aureus
• ORSA—Oxacillin-resistant staphylococcus aureus

CODES

ICD9-CM
• 675.14 Mastitis (purulent)
• 675.24 Mastitis (nonpurulent)
• 676.8 Other disorders of lactation, galactocele
• 611.71 Mastodynia/breast pain

PATIENT TEACHING

• Breastfeeding Helpline. Available at: www.4woman.gov/Breastfeeding/index.cfm?page=ask
• Breastfeeding for Parents. La Leche League. Available at: http://www.lalecheleague.org/nb.html
• ACOG Patient Education Pamphlet. Available at: www.acog.org/publications/patient education/bp029.cfm
• New Mothers Guide to Breastfeeding: American Academy of Pediatrics, Joan Meek, ed., 2002.

PREVENTION
Mastitis
• Effective management of breast fullness and engorgement:
  – Improve latch
  – Do not restrict feeds
  – Teach mothers to hand-express milk:
    ○ Before the feed if the breasts are too full for the baby to attach
    ○ After the feed if the baby does not relieve breast fullness
• Prompt attention to any signs of milk stasis:
  – Teach mothers to check their breasts for lumps, pain, or redness
  – Any signs of milk stasis, mother needs to:
    ○ Increase the frequency of breastfeeding.
    ○ Apply heat to breast.
    ○ Massage any lumpy areas towards the nipple.
• Attention to other difficulties with breastfeeding by skilled professionals in a timely fashion
• Rest as much as possible.

Galactocele
• Effective management of breastfeeding, engorgement, and duct drainage:
  – Teach mothers manual expression of the breast.
  – Urge mother to manually express any plugged ducts.
  – Assistance from certified licensed lactation consultant

MULTIFETAL PREGNANCY

Charles Rittenberg, MD
Roger B. Newman, MD

 BASICS

DESCRIPTION
Twins, triplets, and higher-order multiples

Age-Related Factors
More common in older gravidas (peak, 35 years)

EPIDEMIOLOGY
- Spontaneous twins (~1/80 pregnancies):
  - Hellin-Zeleny hypothesis: If naturally occurring rate of twins in a population is 1/n; triplets estimated by $1/n^2$; quadruplets $1/n^3$.
  - Ethnic variation in rate largely dizygotic twins
  - Monozygotic twins fairly consistent at 4/1,000 live births
- Increasing rate in US since 1970s:
  - 2002, US:
    - 31.1 twins per 1,000 live births
    - 1.8/1,000 live births triplets or higher-order

RISK FACTORS
- Increasing maternal age responsible for ~1/3 of US increase in multiple births
- ART responsible for ~2/3 of US increase:
  - In vitro fertilization
  - Ovulation induction +/− intrauterine insemination
- African American race
- Personal or family history
- High parity
- Recent discontinuation of birth control pills

Genetics
Increased incidence by maternal lineage

PATHOPHYSIOLOGY
- Dizygotic (fraternal) twins:
  - Fertilization of 2 separate ova
  - Same or different sexes
  - Always diamniotic/dichorionic
  - Placentas may fuse
- Monozygotic (identical) twins:
  - Fertilized ovum divides into separate zygotes
  - Always same sex
  - Amnionicity/Chorionicity:
    - 18–36% diamniotic/dichorionic (<3 days)
    - 60–70% diamniotic/monochorionic (3–8 days)
    - 1% monoamniotic (8–12 days)
- Higher-order multiples:
  - 3 or more fetuses
  - May be combination of fraternal/identical

ASSOCIATED CONDITIONS
- Unique to multiples:
  - TTTS
  - Discordant growth
  - Vanishing twin
  - Retained dead fetus syndrome
  - Acardiac twin/TRAP sequence
  - Conjoined twins
- More common in multiples:
  - Spontaneous and indicated preterm birth
  - IUGR
  - Fetal anomalies
  - Preeclampsia/Gestational HTN
  - Gestational diabetes
  - Anemia

- Placental abruption
- 2-vessel cord/vasa previa
- Hyperemesis
- Cerebral palsy
- Malpresentation
- Cesarean delivery

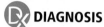 **DIAGNOSIS**

SIGNS AND SYMPTOMS
History
- Fertility treatments
- Personal or family history of twins
- Excessive weight gain
- Increased fetal activity
- Hyperemesis gravidarum

Physical Exam
- Size > dates
- Auscultation of >1 fetal heart rate

TESTS
Definitive diagnosis is made by US. Virtually all are diagnosed by routine sonography.

Labs
- Unexplained, severe anemia:
  - Iron deficiency most common (microcytic)
  - Folate/B_{12} deficiency (macrocytic)
  - Poor nutrition
  - Dilutional
- Elevated MSAFP
- Hypercoagulable state:
  - Increased vitamin K-dependent clotting factors
  - Increased venous stasis
  - Increased risk of trauma (cesarean)

Imaging
- Management requires serial US exams, usually every 4 weeks in the 2nd and 3rd trimesters.
- 1st trimester:
  - Determine fetal number
  - Diagnose vanishing twin syndrome
  - Determine placentation:
    - Amnionicity, chorionicity, zygosity
  - Establish GA
  - NT: Prenatal diagnosis
- Early 2nd trimester (14–20 weeks):
  - Diagnose congenital anomalies
  - Aneuploidy screening
  - Evaluate fetal growth and concordance
  - Confirm placentation
  - TVCL
- Late 2nd trimester (20–28 weeks):
  - Evaluate fetal growth and concordance
  - Measure AF volumes
  - Repeat TVCL (<25 mm: Increased risk preterm birth)
- 3rd trimester (>28 weeks):
  - Evaluate fetal growth and concordance
  - Measure AF volumes
  - Umbilical artery Doppler if IUGR (<10 percentile) or growth discordance (>20%)
  - Determine fetal lie
  - Biophysical profile assessment of fetal status

DIFFERENTIAL DIAGNOSIS
Other causes of size > dates (easily resolved with pelvic US): Ovarian tumor; uterine fibroids

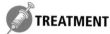 **TREATMENT**

GENERAL MEASURES
- Increased risk for numerous complications, thus more frequent surveillance is required.
- Multiples increase nutritional demands. Adequate nutrition and weight gain have beneficial impact on fetal growth, length of gestation, fetal well-being, and maternal health. Recommendations for twins:
  - Underweight (BMI <19.8):
    - Daily intake: 4,000 calories, 200 g protein, 400 g carbohydrates, 178 g fat
    - Weight gain: 25–35 lb by 20 weeks, 37–49 lb by 28 weeks, 50–62 lb by 38 weeks
  - Normal weight (BMI 19.8–26):
    - Daily intake: 3,500 calories, 175 g protein, 350 g carbohydrates, 156 g fat
    - Weight gain: 20–30 lb by 20 wks, 30–44 lb by 28 weeks, 40–55 lb by 38 weeks
  - Overweight (BMI 26.1–29):
    - Daily intake: 3,250 calories, 163 g protein, 325 g carbohydrates, 144 g fat
    - Weight gain: 20–25 lb by 20 weeks, 28–37 lb by 28 weeks, 38–47 lb by 38 weeks
  - Obese (BMI >29):
    - Daily intake: 3,000 calories, 150 g protein, 300 g carbohydrates, 133 g fat
    - Weight gain: 15–20 lb by 20 weeks, 21–30 lb by 28 weeks, 29–38 lb by 38 weeks
- Encourage heme-iron rich sources (red meat), nonheme iron sources (iron fortified bread, leafy green vegetables, nuts, blackstrap molasses)

PREGNANCY-SPECIFIC ISSUES
- Antepartum care requires attention to signs and symptoms of PTL. Most options for singletons at increased risk are similarly effective including: cervicovaginal fibronectin, TVCL, tocolysis, and antenatal corticosteroids.
- Weekly 17-α-hydroxy progesterone caproate (17P) has not improved outcomes in multiples.
- Bed rest is commonly recommended, but has not been proven to improve outcomes. Bed rest is reserved for patients with preterm labor, TVCL ≤25 mm, positive fetal fibronectin, preeclampsia, or abnormal fetal growth.

By Trimester
- 1st trimester:
  - 1st visit:
    - US to establish fetal number, EDD, chorionicity, amnionicity
    - Usual prenatal H&P and prenatal labs
  - Discuss expected weight gain targets by BMI. Discuss progress each visit.
  - 1st trimester screening:
    - NT alone vs. NT plus serum analytes (If not available, consider age 33 at EDD to be advanced maternal age unless known to be monochorionic twins
  - Discuss multifetal reduction in higher-order multiples or special circumstances with twins (history of singleton spontaneous preterm birth, psychosocial stressors).

– Educate on increased risks of multiples, especially the importance of nutrition and the signs and symptoms of PTL.
- 2nd trimester:
  - NTD +/− aneuploidy screening (quad screen)
  - Fetal anatomic evaluation at 18–20 weeks
  - Fetal echocardiography at 22–24 weeks
  - TVCL with anatomy scan. Repeat with subsequent US for growth (every 4 weeks) or more frequently if cervical shortening.
  - Begin visits once every 2 weeks to include digital cervical exam at 18–20 weeks.
  - No benefit to routine cerclage in twins
- 3rd trimester:
  - Begin weekly visits, including digital cervical exam if increased risk of preterm birth. Others, every 2 weeks, then weekly from 32–34 weeks
  - US for fetal growth every 4 weeks
  - TVCL with growth US until 28–30 wks; more frequently for cervical shortening
  - Symptoms or signs of PTL can be assessed by cervicovaginal FFN or TVCL. Negative FFN and TVCL >3 cm each have negative predictive value of >95% for delivery in the next 2 weeks.
  - Antenatal corticosteroids with PTL (24–34 wks) or PPROM (24–32 weeks)
  - Gestational diabetes screening, CBC at 24–28 wks; evaluate and treat anemia if present.
  - Address contraception alternatives including tubal sterilization early in the 3rd trimester.
  - Counsel patient regarding mode of delivery.
  - Assess for gestational HTN and preeclampsia at every visit: BP, urine protein, weight
  - Weekly fetal testing (NST +/− BPP) by 32 weeks for monochorionic twins and 34 weeks for dichorionic twins:
    ○ Monoamniotic twins require earlier and more frequent testing: Risk of cord entanglement
  - Delivery advised at 38 weeks if undelivered

Risks for Mother
- Cesarean delivery
- Operative vaginal delivery
- Uterine atony and postpartum hemorrhage
- 1st trimester increased β-hCG:
  - Nausea/Vomiting of pregnancy
  - Cross-reactivity with TSH may cause biochemical hyperthyroidism
  - Bilaterally enlarged ovaries
- 2nd and 3rd trimester increase in HPL and other anti-insulin hormones:
  - Worsen pregestational diabetes
  - Increase risk of gestational diabetes

Risks for Fetus
- Prematurity
- Growth restriction
- Fetal anomaly
- Cord prolapse
- Breech extraction (nuchal arm)
- Interlocking twins (rare)

SPECIAL THERAPY
Complementary and Alternative Therapies
Nausea and vomiting may respond to ginger, vitamin B_6, lemon heads/lemon sours, or sea wristbands.

MEDICATION (DRUGS)
- Prenatal vitamins
- Iron or folate if documented deficiency
- Ca 333 mg; Mg 133 mg; Zn 5 mg supplementation (1 t.i.d. in 1st trimester, 2 t.i.d. in 2nd trimester, 3 t.i.d. in 3rd trimester)

SURGERY
- Cervical cerclage:
  - Not effective with routine use
  - Recommended for classical history of cervical insufficiency
  - Option if TVCL <15 mm prior to 22 weeks
- Cesarean delivery:
  - Not generally recommended for vertex/vertex twins (40%)
  - Recommended if baby A is nonvertex (20%)
  - Option for vertex/nonvertex twins (40%) if operator or patient not comfortable with breech extraction of 2nd twin
  - Generally recommended for triplets
- External cephalic version of twin B is possible; but less reliable and greater risk than either elective cesarean or breech extraction.

 FOLLOW-UP

DISPOSITION
Postpartum care is important due to increased risk of cesarean, complicated contraceptive needs with history of infertility, breastfeeding, and increased risks of postpartum depression, exhaustion, or sense of being overwhelmed.

PROGNOSIS
Overall excellent but risk of serious complications.

COMPLICATIONS
Increased postpartum risk compared to singletons for:
- Postpartum preeclampsia
- Idiopathic cardiomyopathy
- DVT/PE
- Postpartum depression
- Exhaustion
- Rectus muscle diastasis and abdominal wall laxity (need for abdominoplasty)
- Weight retention

PATIENT MONITORING
Postpartum follow-up: 1–2 week telephone call, 2- and 6-week postpartum visit with assessment of:
- Mood alterations and emotional support
- Contraception
- Breastfeeding issues
- Appropriate pediatric follow up for infants

BIBLIOGRAPHY

Goldenberg RL, et al. The preterm prediction study: Risk factors in twin gestations. *National Institute of Child Health and Human Development Maternal-Fetal Medicine Units Network*, Am J Obstet Gynecol. 1996;175:1047–1053.

Luke B, et al. *When You're Expecting Twins, Triplets, or Quads, Revised Edition: Proven Guidelines for a Healthy Multiple Pregnancy*, New York: Harper Collins; 2004.

Luke B, et al. Body mass index-specific weight gains associated with optimal birth weights in twin pregnancies. *J Reprod Med.* 2003;48:217–224.

Newman R. Multiple Gestation. In: Scott JR, et al., eds. *Danforth's Obstetrics and Gynecology*, 9th ed. Philadelphia: Lippincott Williams & Wilkins; 2003.

Newman RB, et al. *Multifetal Pregnancy: A Handbook for Care of the Pregnant Patient*. Philadelphia: Lippincott Williams & Wilkins; 2000.

Rabinovici J, et al. Randomized management of the second nonvertex twin: Vaginal delivery or cesarean section. *Am J Obstet Gynecol.* 1987;156:52–56.

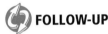 **MISCELLANEOUS**

ABBREVIATIONS
- AF—Amniotic fluid
- ART—Assisted reproductive technology
- BPP—Biophysical profile
- DVT—Deep venous thrombosis
- EDD—Estimated date of delivery
- FFN—Fetal fibronectin
- GA—Gestational age
- hCG—Human chorionic gonadotropin
- HPL—Human placental lactogen
- IUGR—Intrauterine growth restriction
- IVF—In vitro fertilization
- MSAFP—Maternal serum α-fetoprotein
- NST—Nonstress test
- NTD—Neural tube defect
- NT—Nuchal translucency
- PE—Pulmonary embolism
- PPROM—Preterm premature ruptured membranes
- PTL—Preterm labor
- TRAP—Twin-reversed arterial perfusion
- TSH—Thyroid-stimulating hormone
- TTTS—Twin-twin transfusion syndrome
- TVCL—Transvaginal cervical length

CODES
ICD9-CM
- 651.0 Twin pregnancy
- 651.01 Twin pregnancy delivered
- 651.03 Twin pregnancy antepartum
- 651.13 Triplet pregnancy antepartum
- 656.83 Fetal placental problem other antepartum (twin-twin transfusion syndrome)

 PATIENT TEACHING

- Luke B, et al. When You're Expecting Twins, Triplets, or Quads, Revised Edition: Proven Guidelines for a Healthy Multiple Pregnancy, 2004. Available at: www.DrBarbaraLuke.com
- National Organization of Mother of Twins Clubs, Inc. Available at: www.nomotc.org

PREVENTION
See ART topic on embryo transfer with IVF.

OLIGOHYDRAMNIOS

Nancy Chescheir, MD

 BASICS

DESCRIPTION
Oligohydramnios (oligo) refers to pathologically low volumes of AF.

Age-Related Factors
- Not uniquely related to maternal age
- Rare in 1st trimester

EPIDEMIOLOGY
The incidence of oligohydramnios ranges from 0.5–5% or more, depending on the patient population, high risk factors, and GA.

RISK FACTORS
- Vascular compromise
- PROM
- Medication use:
  – ACE inhibitors
  – NSAIDs

PATHOPHYSIOLOGY
- Abnormal production of AF:
  – Poor placental perfusion in response to decreased intravascular volume or BP, fetus preferentially perfuses vital organs, decreases GFR, reduces urine production (prerenal)
  – Abnormal fetal renal function: Any problem that prevents bilateral renal function or causes complete lower urinary tract obstruction (postrenal)
  – Renal toxicity (ACE inhibitors, NSAIDs) nephrosis; (renal)
- Loss of fluid:
  – PROM
- Prolonged early severe oligo can results in pulmonary hypoplasia, facial and limb abnormalities.
- Cord compression with severe oligo

ASSOCIATED CONDITIONS
- HTN
- Severe diabetes
- Lupus
- Smoking
- Unexplained MSAFP elevation
- IUGR
- Post-dates pregnancy
- Placental abnormality:
  – Chronic abruption
  – Infarction
  – Circumvallate
- Fetal abnormality:
  – Bilateral renal disease:
    ○ Agenesis, multicystic dysplastic kidneys
    ○ Lower urinary tract obstruction
    ○ Posterior urethral valves

 DIAGNOSIS

SIGNS AND SYMPTOMS
History
Typically not helpful
Physical Exam
Size < dates by ≥3 cm in normal-sized woman

TESTS
Imaging
US required to make diagnosis:
- Fetal crowding
- MVP <1 cm is strictest definition
- AFI <5 cm
- With subjective oligohydramnios, use color Doppler to confirm that "fluid pocket" isn't really loop of cord
- Search for anomalies.

- May require amnioinfusion to see well
- "Blue tap" with indigo carmine if PROM is suspected but unconfirmed.
- Doppler may be useful; color confirms renal artery presence; umbilical artery assessment if IUGR

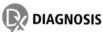 **TREATMENT**

GENERAL MEASURES
- Weigh risks of continuing pregnancy vs. neonatal morbidity and mortality risks and consider delivery.
- Efforts to improve perfusion:
  – Avoid smoking, ACE inhibitors, NSAIDs
  – Decrease maternal stress
  – Complete bed rest not likely helpful, but avoid aerobic exercise.
  – PROM therapy with latency antibiotics if appropriate
- Maternal fluid hydration not useful except for severe maternal dehydration

PREGNANCY-SPECIFIC ISSUES
Make as complete a diagnosis as possible.

By Trimester
- With absent fetal renal function or urine output, oligohydramnios occurs after ~16 weeks.
- With known risk factors, actively assess AF volume at intervals after intervention is considered.

Risks for Mother
Increased risk for cesarean delivery

Risks for Fetus
- Related primarily to etiology, duration
- Cord compression with IUFD, possible CNS injury possible

MEDICATION (DRUGS)
Steroids if anticipate preterm birth

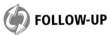 **FOLLOW-UP**

DISPOSITION
Issues for Referral
Perinatal consultation if known or suspected fetal anomaly, severe IUGR, severe maternal vascular disease

PROGNOSIS
Related to underlying cause, duration, and severity of oligohydramnios

PATIENT MONITORING
Fetus
- If potentially viable fetus, consider fetal monitoring:
  – Cord compressions: Variable decelerations
  – Placental insufficiency: Late decelerations, loss of variability
- Consider amnioinfusion in labor
- Prepare for pulmonary hypoplasia if severe oligohydramnios from 20 weeks or so.

 MISCELLANEOUS

CLINICAL PEARLS
- Oligohydramnios is a sign of another problem—find the problem.
- Send the placenta to pathology lab if etiology not known.
- High index of suspicion for IUGR, placental insufficiency

ABBREVIATIONS
- ACE—Angiotensin-converting enzyme
- AF—Amniotic fluid
- AFI—Amniotic fluid index
- GA—Gestational age
- GFR—Glomerular filtration rate
- IUGR—Intrauterine growth restriction
- MSAFP—Maternal serum α-fetoprotein
- MVP—Maximal vertical pocket
- PROM—Premature rupture of membranes

 CODES

ICD9-CM
- 658.0 Oligohydramnios
- 761.2 Oligohydramnios affecting fetus or newborn.

PATIENT TEACHING

- Stop smoking
- Perform fetal kick counts
- Details related to underlying diagnosis if known
- Limitations of US: Not a good predictor of pulmonary hypoplasia
- Cord accidents can be sudden, unpredictable, lethal

POSTPARTUM DEPRESSION

Nada L. Stotland, MD, MPH

BASICS

DESCRIPTION
- Depressive disorder occurring within 6–12 months of delivery
- Distinguish from:
  - "Baby blues":
    - Occurs within days of delivery
    - Heightened emotionalism
    - Self-limited
  - Postpartum psychosis:
    - Occurs within days of delivery
    - Delusions and/or hallucinations
    - Severe agitation, disorientation, confusion
    - Risk of infanticide and maternal suicide

ALERT
- Postpartum psychosis is a medical emergency. Patients should be hospitalized immediately.
- Bipolar disorder must be ruled out before medication is prescribed. Antidepressants can precipitate manic episodes.
- Suicidality must be ascertained.

Age-Related Factors
Reproductive-age women

Pediatric Considerations
Postpartum adolescents at increased risk

EPIDEMIOLOGY
- "Baby blues":
  - Up to 90% of new mothers
- Postpartum depression:
  - ~10% of new mothers
- Postpartum psychosis:
  - <0.1% of new mothers

RISK FACTORS
- Previous depression
- Family history of depression
- PMS
- History of or current abuse
- Lack of social supports
- Unwanted pregnancy
- Alcohol or substance abuse

Genetics
Clear evidence of family loading

PATHOPHYSIOLOGY
- Vulnerability to hormonal change
- Environmental stressors

ASSOCIATED CONDITIONS
- Anxiety disorders
- Alcohol and substance abuse
- Dysthymic disorder

DIAGNOSIS

SIGNS AND SYMPTOMS
History
5 of the following, most of the day, every day, for 2 weeks:
- Depressed or irritable mood
- Inability to enjoy (anhedonia)
- Changes in sleep:
  - Cannot sleep when baby sleeps
- Changes in appetite
- Guilt
- Hopelessness and helplessness
- Decreased concentration
- Decreased energy
- Thoughts of death
- Concerns about harm coming to baby

Physical Exam
Psychomotor agitation (especially for psychosis) or retardation

TESTS
Edinburgh Post-Partum Depression Scale

Lab
Consider a thyroid panel to rule out hypothyroidism.

Imaging
Differences between normal and depressed brain can be seen on brain imaging but this is not used diagnostically.

DIFFERENTIAL DIAGNOSIS
- Distinguish from bipolar disorder
- Manic-depression usually presents in depressed phase:
  - Ask all patients about episodes of:
    - Heightened mood, energy, overconfidence

Hematologic
Anemia

Metabolic/Endocrine
- Hypothyroidism
- Other endocrine disorders

Immunologic
Autoimmune disorders

Tumor/Malignancy
Depression is associated with lung cancer, but not especially postpartum.

Trauma
PTSD:
- Traumatic delivery

Drugs
Many drugs, prescribed and illicit, depress the CNS.

Other/Miscellaneous
Psychiatric disorders:
- Anxiety disorders
- Personality disorders
- Psychotic disorders

TREATMENT

GENERAL MEASURES
- For mild-moderate cases, medication and psychotherapy are equally effective.
  - CBT and interpersonal psychotherapies have most empirical support.
- For moderate-severe cases, medication is usually necessary:
  - Choice of antidepressant is determined by:
    - Previous positive response
    - Positive response in family members
    - Side effects (sedating or energizing)
    - Convenience (once-daily dosing) and cost
- See Depression topic for specific medications and doses:
  - Combined medication and psychotherapy produces best outcomes
- Reassurance of patient and family is essential.
- Breastfeeding mothers may prefer to use psychotherapy 1st to avoid exposure of infant:
  - Sertraline produces lowest levels in breast milk
- Any risks of treatment must be weighed against known risks of untreated depression:
  - Suffering and disability of mother
  - Developmental/Emotional effects on infant

PREGNANCY-SPECIFIC ISSUES
- Most cases begin during pregnancy.
- All pregnant patients should be screened.

Risks for Mother
Prepartum, poor adherence to nutritional, exercise advice

Risks for Fetus
Maternal depression during pregnancy:
- Growth retardation
- Premature delivery

SPECIAL THERAPY
Complementary and Alternative Therapies
- Light therapy if symptoms have been seasonal
- St. John's wort:
  - Unknown percentages of active ingredients in various preparations
  - Efficacy questionable
- ECT:
  - Safe and effective for severe cases
- Magnetic deep brain and vagus nerve stimulation:
  - Subspecialty expertise
  - Very severe cases
  - Controversial and expensive

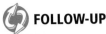 **FOLLOW-UP**

DISPOSITION

Issues for Referral

- Suicidality:
  - Risk factors:
    - Previous attempts
    - Family history of suicide
    - Lack of social supports
    - Alcohol/Substance abuse
  - Assessment:
    - Have you ever thought of harming yourself?
    - Are you thinking about that now?
    - Do you have a plan? Means?
  - Obtain emergency psychiatric consultation
- Worsening symptoms
- No improvement despite treatment
- Explain referral to patient on the basis of signs and symptoms:
  - Reassure her she is not "crazy" or lazy
- If patient is referred, maintain contact
- Refer to support group:
  - Depression After Delivery www.depressionafterdelivery.com
  - Postpartum Support International www.postpartum.net

PROGNOSIS

Prognosis is excellent:

- However, depression is a recurring condition

COMPLICATIONS

Suicide in up to 15% of cases of depression if untreated.

PATIENT MONITORING

- Patients should be treated until restored to premorbid condition, not only until improvement.
- Patients prescribed antidepressants:
  - Patient call in 2–3 days to report side effects
  - See patient at 1 week and weekly until response.
  - Treat for at least 9 months.

- Advise patient that abrupt cessation of an SSRI causes discontinuation syndrome:
  - Discontinuation should be under medical supervision: Gradual taper over 2 weeks.
- If less than full response after 6–8 weeks, increase dose to maximum, change medication, or augment with lithium or thyroid.
- Monitor patients for suicidal ideation/intent:
  - "Contracts" promising no self-harm are ineffective.

BIBLIOGRAPHY

Burt VK, et al., eds. *Concise Guide to Women's Mental Health*, 2nd ed., Washington DC: APPI; 2001.

Cox JL, et al. Detection of postnatal depression: Development of the 10-item Edinburgh Postnatal Depression Scale. *Br J Psych*. 1987:150:782–786.

Flynn HA. Epidemiology and phenomenology of postpartum mood disorders. *Psych Ann*. 2005;35: 544–551.

Miller L, ed. *Postpartum Mood Disorders*. Washington DC: APPI; 2001.

 MISCELLANEOUS

CLINICAL PEARLS

- All postpartum patients should be screened for depression.
- Most postpartum depression is a continuation of depression during and before pregnancy.

ABBREVIATIONS

- CBT—Cognitive behavioral therapy
- ECT—Electroconvulsive therapy
- PMS—Premenstrual syndrome
- PTSD—Post-traumatic stress disorder
- SSRI—Selective serotonin reuptake inhibitor

CODES

ICD9-CM

- 311 Depressive disorder NOS
- 296.2 Major depressive disorder, single episode
- 648.44 Mental postpartum condition or complication

 PATIENT TEACHING

- Address stigma of psychiatric diagnosis and treatment:
  - Depression is a real disease; treatment works
- Provide written materials for patient perusal:
  - Mental Health America. Available at www.mentalhealthamerica.net
  - American Psychiatric Association. Available at www.psych.org
  - National Institutes of Mental Health (several languages). Available at www.nimh.gov
  - Down Came the Rain: My Journey Through Postpartum Depression, Brooke Shields, 2005.
- Offer teaching to family at patient request:
  - Family members, especially children, tend to blame themselves for maternal depression
  - Advise family to bolster patient's confidence in mothering:
    - Help with housework and let mother care for baby
- Advise recovered patient to monitor herself for recurrent symptoms and to seek care at 1st sign

PREVENTION

- Discontinuation of antidepressants during pregnancy: 65% chance of relapse.
- Start previously effective antidepressant immediately after delivery.
- Help patients obtain needed psychosocial support.

POSTTERM PREGNANCY

Alice Stek, MD

BASICS

DESCRIPTION
- Postterm pregnancy is defined as a pregnancy that has extended to or beyond 42 weeks OR:
  - 294 days from LMP OR
  - EDD +14 days (see Establishing Estimated Date of Delivery)
- Postdates is not the same as postterm:
  - Postdates is a poorly defined term and should be avoided.
  - Postdates can mean any GA after the EDD

EPIDEMIOLOGY
- Determining the frequency of postterm gestation is difficult due to common inability to accurately determine GA.
- Reported frequency in US ~.7%

RISK FACTORS
- Error in dating is the most frequent cause.
- Cause of true postterm gestation is usually unknown.
- Primiparity
- Prior postterm pregnancy:
  - Risk of recurrence ~20%
- Fetus of male sex
- Genetic predisposition
- Regular heavy exercise may increase risk
- Rarely: Placental sulfatase deficiency, fetal anencephaly

Genetics
- Possible paternal component:
  - Reduced risk of recurrence with new partner
- Black mothers have lower risk for postterm delivery and recurrence

PATHOPHYSIOLOGY
- Pathophysiology is poorly understood; cause is usually unknown.
- Known risk factors and causes are listed above.

ASSOCIATED CONDITIONS
- Dysmaturity syndrome in 20% of postterm deliveries:
  - Similar to IUGR due to uteroplacental insufficiency, with neonatal complications
- Fetal macrosomia in 2.5–10%

DIAGNOSIS

SIGNS AND SYMPTOMS
History
- Accurate pregnancy dating is critical:
  - LMP, regular cycles, contraception?
  - Early US?
- Review GA of prior deliveries
- Review complications of prior deliveries
- Same partner as prior pregnancies?

Physical Exam
- Digital exam of cervix/Bishop score
- Estimate of fetal weight

TESTS
See section on patient monitoring for tests used to monitor fetal well-being and to determine timing of delivery.

Imaging
US for estimated fetal weight, AF volume, and fetal position

DIFFERENTIAL DIAGNOSIS
Inaccurate dates:
- EDD is most accurately determined early in pregnancy.
- LMP in women with regular, normal cycles
- 1st trimester US variation <7 days; up to 20 weeks <7 days; late 2nd trimester 14 days; and 3rd trimester 21 days
- If discrepancy between LMP and US estimate of GA exceeds the above, pregnancy should be redated based on US measurements.

TREATMENT

GENERAL MEASURES
- Conflicting evidence from literature regarding most appropriate management:
  - When to start fetal monitoring
  - Whether to manage expectantly or to induce labor
  - When to induce labor
  - Risk of complications
- Most studies show no differences between induced and monitored groups in neonatal outcome, maternal complications, or mode of delivery:
  - Delivery was effected by 43 weeks in these studies.

- Due to increased perinatal mortality, uteroplacental insufficiency, meconium aspiration, low umbilical artery pH, low 5-minute Apgar scores, and neonatal mortality with postterm pregnancies, the current trend is toward delivery at 41 weeks.

PREGNANCY-SPECIFIC ISSUES
Risks for Mother
- Maternal complications lowest at 38–39 weeks; highest postterm (cesarean delivery, operative vaginal delivery, hemorrhage)
- Fetuses born postterm are often larger; potentially increasing risk of labor dystocia, cesarean delivery, perineal injury:
  - Earlier induction of labor does not decrease risk of complications due to macrosomia.
- Maternal anxiety with expectant management

Risks for Fetus
- Perinatal/Neonatal complications, in general, lowest at 39 weeks and higher postterm:
  - Complications include: Death, low Apgar scores, low umbilical cord pH, meconium aspiration
- Perinatal mortality doubles after 42 weeks and increases 6-fold after 43 weeks
- Infant mortality increased in postterm deliveries

SPECIAL THERAPY
Complementary and Alternative Therapies
- Breast and nipple stimulation at term has not decreased incidence of postterm pregnancy.
- Conflicting data on efficacy and safety of stripping/sweeping membranes.

MEDICATION (DRUGS)
- Induction of labor with oxytocin and amniotomy if cervix is favorable
- If cervix unfavorable (Bishop score <6), prostaglandin cervical ripening indicated, followed by oxytocin and/or amniotomy:
  - Misoprostol (effective and inexpensive, but not licensed for labor induction, although much data exist on this use)
  - Dinoprostone

ALERT
Avoid prostaglandins in women with prior cesareans, due to increased risk of uterine rupture in some groups.

SURGERY

- Scheduled cesarean for >1 prior cesarean or other obstetric indication should be done prior to EDD.
- Although studies are not all in agreement, induction of labor at ≥41 weeks does not appear to increase the rate of cesarean delivery or operative vaginal delivery.

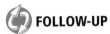 **FOLLOW-UP**

PROGNOSIS

With careful monitoring of fetal well-being, prognosis is good.

PATIENT MONITORING

Mother

Monitor closely for signs of preeclampsia or other maternal complications; at weekly or twice-weekly prenatal clinic visits.

Fetus

- Although no RCT has demonstrated an effect of fetal monitoring on perinatal mortality, close monitoring is standard of care.
- Most common monitoring is by twice-weekly NST + AFI, starting at 40 weeks.
- Other options: BPP, contraction stress test
- Deliver if:
  - Oligohydramnios (AFI <5 or deepest vertical pocket of AF <2 cm)
  - Worrisome fetal heart rate tracing
  - 42 or 43 weeks (current standard 41 weeks)
  - Some advise delivery as soon as cervix is favorable.

BIBLIOGRAPHY

ACOG Practice Bulletin No. 55. Management of postterm pregnancy. *Obstet Gynecol*. 2004;104: 639–646.

Heimstad R, et al. Outcomes of pregnancy beyond 37 weeks of gestation. *Obstet Gynecol*. 2006;108: 500–508.

Heimstad R, et al. Induction of labor or serial antenatal fetal monitoring in postterm pregnancy: A randomized controlled trial. *Obstet Gynecol*. 2007; 109:609–617.

 MISCELLANEOUS

CLINICAL PEARLS

- Increased risk of maternal and perinatal complications with postterm pregnancies
- Outcomes are good with careful surveillance (NST + AFI twice weekly).
- Delivery should be effected if oligohydramnios or fetal compromise.
- Expectant management with close monitoring is acceptable; however, antepartum testing starting between 40 and 41 weeks, and delivery at 41 weeks has become the most common management.
- Cervical ripening with prostaglandins is a valuable component of induction.
- Consider induction once cervix is favorable after 41 weeks.

ABBREVIATIONS

- AF—Amniotic fluid
- AFI—Amniotic fluid index
- BPP—Biophysical profile
- EDD—Estimated date of delivery; due date; 40 weeks from LMP
- GA—Gestational age
- IUGR—Intrauterine growth restriction
- LMP—Last menstrual period; generally 1st day of period
- NST—Nonstress test
- RCT—Randomized controlled trial

CODES

ICD9-CM

645.2 Prolonged pregnancy

 PATIENT TEACHING

- Importance of good fetal movement daily
- Need for close monitoring, antepartum testing
- Anticipation of induction of labor at 41–42 weeks
- ACOG Patient Education Pamphlets:
  - What to Expect after Your Due Date
  - Labor Induction

PREVENTION

Accurate determination of GA early in pregnancy will decrease number of pregnancies classified as postterm.

Section V

PREMATURE RUPTURED MEMBRANES

Mounira Habli, MD
Helen How, MD

BASICS

DESCRIPTION
- PROM is defined as rupture of amniotic membranes >1 hour before the onset of labor.
- Term PROM: After 37 weeks' gestation
- PPROM: Before 37 weeks:
  – PPPROM: >24 hours without delivery.
- Latency is the interval from time of rupture to onset of labor:
  – Latency is inversely proportional to GA.
  – Between 20–26 weeks, mean latency 12 days
  – Between 32–34 weeks, mean latency 4 days

Age-Related Factors
More common in mothers <18 years and >40 years old

EPIDEMIOLOGY
- PPROM occurs in 3–5 % of all pregnancies.
- Accounts for 25–40% of all preterm deliveries.
- Accounts for ~50% of adverse long-term outcomes and 60% of perinatal mortality
- Between 20–36 weeks, 60–70% of patients with PPROM deliver with in 48 hours.
- At 33–36 weeks, 80% deliver within 48 hours.
- 13.5% risk of recurrence:
  – 13.5 times greater when previous episode PPROM was <28 weeks' gestation

RISK FACTORS
- 50% have no risk factors.
- Prior PPPROM or preterm birth
- Bleeding in 1st trimester, GU tract infection, black race, low prepregnancy weight, age <18, pregnancy <6 month previously
- Smoking, frequent contractions, psychiatric disorders
- Uterine anomaly.
- Nulliparous women at greater risk of PPROM if working during pregnancy with medical complications and a short cervix ≤25 mm.
- Hemoglobin <11.1 g/dL (OR 4.33)
- Low socioeconomic status (OR 3.1)
- Bacterial vaginosis is NOT associated

Genetics
PPROM is a multifactorial condition with interplay of genetic and environmental factors.

PATHOPHYSIOLOGY
- Etiology is multifactorial. It is unknown in >50%.
- Many mechanisms are proposed: membrane collagen degradation, local inflammation, choriodecidual infection due to increased susceptibility to ascending infection, decreased membrane collagen content, localized membrane defects, membrane stretch (uterine overdistension), programmed cell death

ASSOCIATED CONDITIONS
- Amniocentesis
- Cervical cerclage, cervical insufficiency
- Chronic abruption placenta, abnormal placentation
- LEEP, cervical conization
- Uterine overdistension

DIAGNOSIS

SIGNS AND SYMPTOMS
History
- Identify risk factors
- Patients usually present with gush or leakage of fluids, continuous dripping, wet pants, increase in vaginal discharge, light vaginal bleeding, and labor pain.

Physical Exam
- Vital signs:
  – Temperature (>38.0° C): Check for a source of infection.
  – Blood pressure and pulse (if tachycardiac, rule out intrauterine infection)
- Abdominal exam: Assess for uterine tenderness, height of fundus measurement, fetal presentation.
- Vulvar exam: Check for lesions.
- Sterile speculum exam to confirm PPROM. Combination of ≥2 tests (Ferning, Nitrazine, or patient history) provide an accuracy of 93.1%.
  – Ferning testing: Microscopy of vaginal fluid:
    ○ Performed on the midvaginal or posterior fornix fluid.
    ○ False-positive results due to cervical mucus.
    ○ Allowed to dry for a minimum of 10 minutes.
    ○ Unaffected by meconium or change in PH
  – Nitrazine paper test (pH):
    ○ Blue color due to alkaline pH
    ○ False-positive results from: Blood, semen, alkaline urine, soap, antiseptic solutions.
- Pelvic exam:

ALERT
Avoid digital exam unless imminent delivery suspected:
- Visual assessment of cervix
- ≥2 digital exams resulted in shorter latency (3 vs. 5 days) but did not worsen maternal or neonatal outcome.

TESTS
Fetal monitoring:
- NST to assess fetal well being
- Uterine tocodynamometry for uterine contractions.

Labs
- CBC with differential, platelets; fibrinogen if bleeding
- UA, culture, sensitivities, toxicology screen
- Cervical culture for *Neisseria gonorrhea*, *Chlamydia trachomatis*
- Check for bacterial vaginosis and trichomonas by either vaginal swab or DNA probe.
- GBS cultures from lower 1/3 of vagina and perineum
- Biochemical testing has been used, but none is very useful clinically in *diagnosis* of PPROM:
  – FFN:
    ○ AF contains >50,000 ng/mL FFN
    ○ Extracellular glycoprotein that attaches the fetal membranes and uterine decidua

○ Normally absent between 22 and 37 weeks.
○ If no cervical exam or sexual intercourse in the last 24 hours, do the test between 24–34 weeks.
○ When history, Ferning test, and Nitrazine are equivocal then FFN has a role.
○ Sensitivity 94%, specificity 97%, PPV 97%, NPV 94%
  – AFP
  – Diamino-oxydase

Imaging
- US testing:
  – To assess for GA, fetal presentation, estimated fetal weight, AFI, rule out obvious fetal anomalies, placenta location
- Amniocentesis under US guidance:
  – Dye test (indigo carmine test) is the gold standard for diagnosis.
  – Indigo carmine dye is instilled via amniocentesis; if vaginal tampon turns blue, PROM is confirmed
  – If intrauterine infection suspected
  – If fetal lung maturity is clinically indicated
  – Send for WBC, Gram stain, culture, glucose
  – IL-6 is the best marker for intrauterine infection.

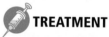 TREATMENT

GENERAL MEASURES
- Preventive treatment to prevent preterm delivery
- Transport mother to appropriate facility for fetal care.
- Corticosteroids to reduce risk of RDS, IVH
- Antibiotic for GBS prophylaxis and to increase latency period

PREGNANCY-SPECIFIC ISSUES
Upon arrival to triage:
- Confirm diagnosis
- Assess fetal status and presentation (NST, US)
- Bed rest, IV hydration, fluid bolus if dehydrated
- Take cultures before starting antibiotics

By Trimester
- After the diagnosis of PPROM is confirmed, deliver regardless of GA if evidence of clinical intrauterine infection, fetal death, nonreassuring fetal status, or advanced labor.
- Otherwise management is based on GA:
- If <24 weeks:
  – Counsel patient about risks of PPROM at <24 weeks (see below)
  – Consider termination
  – Monitor and bed rest with serial US if patient elects conservative management.
  – If persistent oligohydramnios (AFI <5 cm) again discuss options of termination of pregnancy or conservative management:
    ○ In conservative management, consider antibiotics for 7 days.
    ○ Discharge patient home with infection precautions and readmit at viability (24 weeks).

- Between 24–31 6/7 weeks:
  – If recurrent labor, consider amniocentesis to rule out infection.
  – Otherwise, modified bed rest
  – Corticosteroids (dexamethasone 6 mg IM q12h for total of 4 doses or betamethasone 12 mg IM q24h for 2 doses):
    ○ Tocolysis for 48 hours
  – Antibiotics per NIH protocol:
    ○ IV ampicillin (2-g dose q6h) and erythromycin (250–mg dose q6h) for 48 hours followed by oral amoxicillin (250–mg dose q8h) and erythromycin tablets (333–mg dose q8h) for 5 days
    ○ Composite morbidities (RDS, early sepsis, severe IVH, severe NEC) decreased by 53–44%
    ○ Decrease in amnionitis and prolongation of the latency period by >1 week
  – Serial evaluation for intrauterine infection, labor, abruption placenta
  – Serial evaluation for fetal well-being: NST at least twice a week, fetal growth evaluation q2–3 weeks
  – Delivery upon evidence of chorioamnionitis (clinically or by amniocentesis), nonreassuring fetal status, or at 32–34 weeks
  – Repeat tocolysis is not recommended beyond 28 weeks.
- Between 32–34 weeks:
  – Check for fetal lung maturity:
    ○ If lung maturity results from AF (transabdominally or transvaginally) are positive (lecithin/sphingomyelin >2.0 or lamellar body count ≥30 K), deliver
    ○ If lung maturity results are negative, consider conservative management until steroids and antibiotic are given.
  – Delivery at 34 weeks
- Intrapartum management:
  – Induction of labor
  – Mode of delivery is SVD, caesarian if obstetrically indicated.
  – Broad-spectrum antibiotics for intrauterine infection (ampicillin and gentamicin; add clindamycin if caesarian delivery)
  – Antibiotic for GBS prophylaxis

ALERT
Universal GBS prophylaxis is recommended (see topic on Preterm Labor).

Risks for Mother
Maternal sepsis, DIC from placenta abruption, postpartum hemorrhage requiring blood transfusion, hysterectomy.

Risks for Fetus
- Prematurity
- Infection:
  – Risk of neonatal sepsis is inversely related to GA.
  – Increased 10-fold with PPROM:
    ○ Chorioamnionitis in 0.55–71% of pregnancies with PPROM, depending on population
    ○ Risk of intrauterine infection ~36% at <26 weeks' gestation.
    ○ 31–33 weeks: 4-fold increased risk of intrauterine infection
  – Pulmonary hypoplasia if <24 weeks:
    ○ Depends on GA at time of PPROM; most critical period of lung development is before 22 weeks but may continue up to 25 weeks.
  – Restrictive deformations:
    ○ Including spadelike hands and flexion contractions of elbows, knees, and feet
  – Fetal akinesia
  – Amniotic bands

SPECIAL THERAPY
Complementary and Alternative Therapies
Amnioinfusion:
- No adequate controlled trial to support neonatal benefits
- Suggested benefits:
  – Decreased maternal and neonatal morbidity
  – Decreased fetal distress
- Risks:
  – Cord prolapse
  – Uterine overdistension, fetal bradycardia
  – Abruption, infection, PTL

MEDICATION (DRUGS)
See Preterm Labor.

 FOLLOW-UP

DISPOSITION
Issues for Referral
All patients should be referred and comanaged by a MFM specialist.

PROGNOSIS
Based on GA and associated medical conditions

COMPLICATIONS
- Short term: Feeding and growth difficulties, infection, apnea, neurodevelopmental difficulties, retinopathy, transient dystonia
- Long term: Cerebral palsy, sensory deficits, special needs, incomplete catch-up growth, school difficulties, behavioral problems, chronic lung disease

PATIENT MONITORING
Mother
- Vital signs for evidence of infection
- Contraction monitoring

Fetus
NST

BIBLIOGRAPHY

Gabbe SG, et al. Obstetrics: Normal and Abnormal Pregnancies. In: Iam J, ed. *Preterm birth*, 4th ed. Philadelphia: Churchill-Livingstone; 2002;755–827.
Iams JD, et al. Maternal-Fetal Medicine: Principles and Practice In: *Preterm Labor and Delivery*, 5th ed. 2004;623–663.

 MISCELLANEOUS

Outpatient management is not recommended.

ABBREVIATIONS
- AF—Amniotic fluid
- AFI—Amniotic fluid index
- AFP—α-Fetoprotein
- DIC—Disseminated intravascular coagulopathy
- FFN—Fetal fibronectin
- GA—Gestational age
- GBS—Group B streptococcus
- IL-6—Interleukin 6
- IVH—Intraventricular hemorrhage
- LEEP—Loop electrosurgical excision procedure
- MFM—Maternal-fetal medicine
- NEC—Necrotizing enterocolitis
- NIH—National Institutes of Health
- NPV—Negative predictive value
- NST—Nonstress test
- PPV—Positive predictive value
- PROM—Premature rupture of membranes
- PPROM—Preterm premature rupture of membranes
- PPPROM—Prolonged preterm premature rupture of membranes
- PTL—Preterm labor
- RDS—Respiratory distress syndrome
- SVD—Spontaneous vaginal delivery

CODES
ICD9-CM
- 644.03, 644.21 Preterm labor
- 658.1, 658.2 PPROM

 PATIENT TEACHING

- Provide written information about preterm-infant development.
- Support group web sites. Available at www.shareyourstory.org
- Help parents to develop confidence in caring for their preterm infants.

Section V

PREMATURITY

Yasser Y. El-Sayed, MD
Justin Collingham, MD

 BASICS

DESCRIPTION

- A premature or preterm delivery occurs prior to 37 completed gestational weeks.
- Preterm births as grouped by GA:
  – 32–36 weeks: Moderately preterm
  – <32 weeks: Very preterm
- Premature infants grouped by birth weight:
  – LBW: <2,500 g
  – VLBW: <1,500 g
  – ELBW: <1,000 g
- Spontaneous preterm birth accounts for 80% of preterm delivery:
  – 50% of preterm deliveries are a result of PTL.
  – 30% of preterm deliveries are a result of PPROM.
- Remaining 20% of preterm deliveries are iatrogenic; they occur as a result of intervention for maternal or fetal conditions.

Age-Related Factors
An increased risk of prematurity is observed with increasing maternal age partially secondary to:

- Increased use of ART and subsequent multiple gestations
- Increased risk of spontaneous multiple gestation
- Increased iatrogenic preterm delivery rate

EPIDEMIOLOGY

- US preterm delivery rate in 2004 rose to 12.5%, an 18% increase from the 10.6% preterm delivery rate in 1990.
- LBW birth rate in the US in 2004 rose to 8.1%, a 16% increase from the 7% LBW birth rate in 1990.
- Increase in preterm delivery rate and LBW birth rate due in part to increase in multiple gestations

RISK FACTORS

Risk factors for a premature delivery include:

- Risk factors for spontaneous preterm birth:
  – Low socioeconomic status
  – Multiple gestation
  – Polyhydramnios
  – Cervical insufficiency
  – Prior preterm delivery
  – Uterine anomaly
  – Maternal infection
- Risk factors for iatrogenic preterm delivery:
  – Placental abnormalities such as placenta previa or accreta
  – Preeclampsia and maternal conditions that increase the risk of preeclampsia
  – IUGR and maternal conditions that increase the risk of IUGR

PATHOPHYSIOLOGY

- Multiple pathways are suspected in preterm delivery.
- Premature activation of the fetal HPA axis leads to increased fetal CRH and increased fetal ACTH.
  – Increased ACTH leads to increased placental estrogens that may stimulate labor.
- Decidual hemorrhage and resultant thrombin can stimulate myometrial activity.
- Uterine distention secondary to multiple gestation or polyhydramnios can contribute to increased myometrial activity.
- Inflammatory cytokines (IL-1, -6, -8, and TNF) in the setting of chorioamnionitis induce prostaglandins in the amnion, decidua, and cervix.
- Some bacterial species produce proteases and collagenases that can degrade fetal membranes, leading to PPROM.

ASSOCIATED CONDITIONS

- PPROM
- Cervical insufficiency
- Chorioamnionitis

 DIAGNOSIS

SIGNS AND SYMPTOMS
Physical Exam

- PTL may be determined by the presence of contractions and cervical change by digital exam.
- PPROM may be determined by speculum exam with pooling present and positive Nitrazine and Fern testing.
- Signs of chorioamnionitis include maternal and fetal tachycardia, a tender uterine fundus, foul-smelling vaginal discharge.

TESTS
Labs

- Determining the presence or absence of FFN in cervicovaginal secretions may help assess the risk of preterm delivery in those patients with symptoms of PTL.
- Although PPV of test for preterm delivery within 7 days is only 13–32%, the NPV of >98% for delivery within 7–14 days may provide reassurance for those patients who test negative.

Imaging
US if GA in question

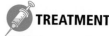 **TREATMENT**

GENERAL MEASURES

- Hydration
- Assess for infection
- Uterine activity monitoring

PREGNANCY-SPECIFIC ISSUES
Risks for Fetus

- Neonatal mortality rates in premature infants are inversely proportional to birth weights and GAs:
  – 85% mortality at <500 g in US in 2003.
  – 25% mortality at <1,500 g
  – 5.9% mortality at <2,500 g
- Neonatal morbidities related to prematurity are numerous and increase in incidence and severity as GA decreases. These morbidities include:
  – Hypothermia
  – PDA
  – Hypoglycemia
  – NEC
  – RDS
  – ROP
  – ICH

MEDICATION (DRUGS)

- Betamethasone 12 mg IM q24h for 2 doses OR dexamethasone 6 mg IM q12h for 4 doses in patients at risk for preterm delivery between 24 and 34 weeks
- Tocolytics as necessary for PTL (see Preterm Labor and Preterm Contractions)
- Antibiotic treatment to increase the length of latency in PPROM (see Premature Ruptured Membranes)
- GBS prophylaxis

SURGERY
The choice of uterine incision at the time of cesarean delivery may be influenced by GA and size of the fetus:

- A poorly developed lower uterine segment may preclude a low transverse incision of adequate size to effect delivery, and a low vertical or classical incision may be necessary for delivery.

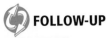 **FOLLOW-UP**

DISPOSITION
Issues for Referral
With PTL, transfer mother to facility with appropriate-level nursery facility

PROGNOSIS
See Risks for Fetus.

PATIENT MONITORING
Monitor for cervical change to diagnose PTL:

• No evidence exists to support the use of tocolytic therapy, home uterine activity monitoring, elective cerclage, or narcotics to prevent preterm delivery in women with contractions but no cervical change.

BIBLIOGRAPHY

Antenatal corticosteroids revisited: Repeat courses. NIH Consensus Statement, 2000;17(2):1–10.

Hamilton BE, et al. Births: Preliminary data for 2004. Natl Vital Stat Rep. 2005;54(8):1–18.

Mathews TJ, et al. Infant mortality statistics from the 2003 period linked birth/infant death data set. Natl Vital Stat Rep. 2005;54(16):1–30.

Meis PJ, et al. Prevention of recurrent preterm delivery by 17-alpha hydroxyprogesterone caproate. N Engl J Med. 2003;348:2379–2385.

Tekesin I, et al. Assessment of rapid fetal fibronectin in predicting preterm delivery. Obstet Gynecol. 2005; 105(2):280–284.

 MISCELLANEOUS

ABBREVIATIONS
• ACTH—Adrenocorticotropic hormone
• ART—Assisted reproductive technologies
• ELBW—Extremely low birth weight
• FFN—Fetal fibronectin
• GA—Gestational age
• GBS—Group B streptococcus
• HPA—Hypothalamic pituitary adrenal axis
• ICH—Intracranial hemorrhage
• IL—Interleukin
• IUGR—Intrauterine growth restriction
• LBW—Low birth weight
• NEC—Necrotizing enterocolitis
• PDA—Patent ductus arteriosus
• PTL—Preterm labor
• PPROM—Preterm premature rupture of membranes
• RDS—Respiratory distress syndrome
• ROP—Retinopathy of prematurity
• TNF—Tumor necrosis factor
• VLBW—Very low birth weight

CODES

ICD9-CM
• 765.0 Extreme prematurity (birthweight <1,000 g)
• 765.1 Other preterm infants (birthweight of 1,000–2,499 g)
• 765.2 Weeks of gestation:
  – 765.20 Unspecified weeks of gestation
  – 765.21 <24 completed weeks of gestation
  – 765.22 24 completed weeks of gestation
  – 765.23 25–26 completed weeks of gestation
  – 765.24 27–28 completed weeks of gestation
  – 765.25 29–30 completed weeks of gestation
  – 765.26 31–32 completed weeks of gestation
  – 765.27 33–34 completed weeks of gestation
  – 765.28 35–36 completed weeks of gestation

PATIENT TEACHING

• ACOG Patient Education pamphlet: Preterm Labor
• Review symptoms of PTL during prenatal visits: Painful and regular contractions, pelvic or back pain that waxes and wanes, vaginal bleeding, or increased vaginal discharge.

PREVENTION
In patients with a history of a prior preterm delivery, weekly injections of 17-hydroxyprogesterone caproate 250 mg IM starting at 16–20 weeks in a subsequent pregnancy and continuing to 36 weeks has been shown to decrease the incidence of preterm delivery and decrease neonatal morbidity.

Section V

PRETERM LABOR AND PRETERM CONTRACTIONS

Mounira Habli, MD
Helen How, MD

BASICS

DESCRIPTION
- PTL:
  - Labor resulting in birth before 37 weeks gestation (WHO)
  - Frequent contractions (>6–8/hr) in presence of cervical change (effacement, dilation)
- Spontaneous PTL (75%):
  - Early PTL before 32 weeks gestation
  - Later PTL after 32 weeks gestation
- Indicated PTL (25%) due to maternal or fetal conditions:
  - LBW: <2,500 g at delivery
  - VLBW: <1,500 g at delivery
  - ELBW: <1,000 g at delivery

Age-Related Factors
- 12.3% all ages
- 15.9% <18 years of age
- 16.3% >40 years of age

EPIDEMIOLOGY
- PTB in the US increased from 10.2% to 12.3% of live births in 2003.
- More common in unmarried women, low socioeconomic status, African American ancestry
- 70% of all neonatal mortality and morbidity
- 7–8% of all pregnancies
- Recurrence rate 25–50%
- US #1 cause of neonatal mortality (<28 days)
- US #2 cause of infant mortality (<1 year)
- US #1 cause of infant mortality for non-Hispanic black infants
- US #2 cause of neonatal death
- 57.4% premature birth rate among twins; 93.7% among higher-order multiples

RISK FACTORS
- Spontaneous PTL risk factors:
  - 50% have no risk factors.
  - Prior PTB, periodontal infection (OR, 4)
  - Bleeding in 1st trimester, GU tract infection, black race, low prepregnancy weight, age <18, interval pregnancy <6 month (OR, 2)
  - Smoking, frequent contractions, psychiatric disorders (OR, 1.5)
- Indicated PTL risk factors:
  - Uterine anomaly (OR, 7)
  - Hypertensive disorders (OR, 5)
  - Prior stillbirth (OR, 3.5)

Genetics
- PTB involves interplay of genetic and environment conditions.
- Clusters in families
- Does NOT show Mendelian inheritance
- Multifactorial condition

PATHOPHYSIOLOGY
- Inflammation:
  - Decidual: Chorioamnionic or systemic inflammation caused by GU tract or systemic infection (40%)
- Premature activation of the maternal–fetal HPA axis:
  - Fetal or maternal stress (30%)
- Decidual hemorrhage or abruption (20%)
- Pathologic uterine distension (10%)

ASSOCIATED CONDITIONS
- Abruption, PPROM
- Uterine over distension, multiple gestations, uterine anomalies, DES exposure
- Abdominal surgery during pregnancy
- Short cervix (<2.5 cm), substance abuse, LEEP, conization of cervix

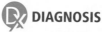

DIAGNOSIS

SIGNS AND SYMPTOMS
History
- Identify risk factors.
- Symptoms: Low back pain, pelvic pressure, persistent contractions(painful or painless), increased vaginal discharge, spotting, menstrual cramps, any respiratory or urinary tract infections symptoms, leakage of vaginal fluid

Physical Exam
- Vital signs: Temperature, BP, pulse
- Physical exam: Check for source of infection:
  - Abdominal exam: Assess for uterine tenderness, FH, presentation
  - Vulvar exam: Check for lesions
  - Cervical exam: Cervical dilation, effacement, position, consistency

TESTS
- Fetal monitoring:
  - NST to assess fetal well being
  - Uterine tocodynamometry for uterine contractions
- FFN:
  - Extracellular glycoprotein that attaches the fetal membranes and uterine decidua.
  - Normally absent between 22 and 37 weeks
  - If no cervical exam or sexual intercourse in the last 24 hours, do the test between 24–34 weeks.
- Cervical length ≤25 mm and FFN ≥50 ng/mL: PPV of preterm delivery <7 days is only 21%.

Lab
- CBC with differential, platelets, fibrinogen if bleeding
- UA, C&S, urine toxicology screen
- Cervical culture for *Neisseria gonorrhea* and *Chlamydia trachomatis*
- Check for bacterial vaginosis and trichomonas by either vaginal swab or DNA probe
- GBS cultures from lower 1/3 of vagina and perineum
- Biochemical markers experimental, not useful clinically: C-reactive protein, corticotropin releasing hormone, AFP, plasma granulocyte colony-stimulating factor

Imaging
- US:
  - To assess GA, presentation, estimated fetal weight, AFI, rule out obvious fetal anomalies, placenta location
- Cervical length assessment:
  - Likelihood of PTD inversely proportional to cervical length
  - Cervical length ≤ 2.5 cm
- Amniocentesis under US guidance:
  - If intrauterine infection suspected
  - If breakthrough tocolysis
  - If fetal lung maturity clinically indicated
  - WBC, Gram stain, culture, glucose

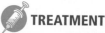

TREATMENT

GENERAL MEASURES
- Transport mother to appropriate facility for fetal care.
- Corticosteroids to reduce risk of RDS, IVH
- Antibiotic for GBS prophylaxis
- Upon arrival to triage:
  - Confirm diagnosis
  - Assess fetal status and presentation (NST, US)
  - Bed rest; IV hydration and fluid bolus if dehydrated
  - Take cultures before starting antibiotics.

PREGNANCY-SPECIFIC ISSUES
By Trimester
- Preterm labor <24 weeks: Expectant management; no evidence of benefits for steroids, tocolysis; antibiotics if evidence of infection
- Patients with PTL at 24–34 weeks:
  - Corticosteroids (dexamethasone 6 mg IM q12h for a total of 4 doses or betamethasone 12 mg IM q24h for 2 doses)
  - Antibiotic for GBS prophylaxis
  - Tocolysis if appropriate for 48 hours
  - Mode of delivery is SVD, caesarian if obstetrically indicated
  - Amniocentesis to rule out infection

Risks for Fetus

> **ALERT**
> **Recommendation of universal prenatal GBS prophylaxis:**
> - Screen ALL women for vaginal and rectal GBS colonization at 35–37 weeks' gestation.
> - Penicillin is 1st-line for intrapartum antibiotic prophylaxis; ampicillin is an acceptable alternative.
> - Penicillin G, 5 M units IV initially, then 2.5 M units IV q4h until delivery. Alternative regimen: Ampicillin; 2 g IV initially, then 1 g IV q4h until delivery

- During prenatal care, assess for penicillin allergy. Intrapartum for penicillin-allergic women:
  - Women not at high risk for anaphylaxis: Cefazolin, 2 g IV, then 1 g IV q8h until delivery
  - Women at high risk for anaphylaxis: Clindamycin and erythromycin susceptibility testing, if available, performed on isolates obtained during GBS prenatal carriage screening:
    - If clindamycin- and erythromycin-susceptible isolates, either clindamycin, 900 mg IV q8h until delivery; OR erythromycin, 500 mg IV q6h until delivery
    - If susceptibility testing not possible, susceptibility results not known, or isolates are resistant to erythromycin or clindamycin: Vancomycin, 1 g IV q12h until delivery.
  - If culture results not known, manage with risk-based approach per obstetric risk factors (ie, delivery at <37 weeks' gestation, duration of membrane rupture ≥18 hours, or temperature ≥100.4°.
- If negative vaginal and rectal GBS screening cultures within 5 weeks of delivery, intrapartum antimicrobial prophylaxis for GBS is not required, even if obstetric risk factors develop (i.e., delivery at

<37 weeks' gestation, duration of membrane rupture ≥18 hours, or temperature ≥100.4°F).
- If GBS bacteriuria in any concentration during current pregnancy or previous infant with GBS disease, give intrapartum antibiotic prophylaxis
- If no GBS UTI, antibiotics should not be used to treat asymptomatic GBS colonization.
- Routine intrapartum antibiotic prophylaxis not recommended for GBS-colonized women with planned cesarean deliveries who have not begun labor or had rupture of membrane.

MEDICATION (DRUGS)
- Magnesium sulfate:
  - Mechanism of action:
    - Direct effect on uterine smooth muscle by antagonizing calcium at cellular level and intracellular space
  - Pharmacokinetics:
    - Half-life ~600 minutes
    - Crosses placenta and readily distributes into AF and fetal compartments
    - Renal excretion
    - 6 g loading dose IV, then 2 g/hr as maintenance
  - Contraindications:
    - Absolute: Myasthenia gravis
    - Relative: Known myocardial compromise or cardiac conduction defect
    - Adjust dose for renal impairment.
  - Adverse effects:
    - Maternal flushing, nausea, vomiting, diplopia, blurred vision, and headache, ileus, hypocalcemia, pulmonary edema, subendocardial ischemia, cardiac arrest, maternal death
    - Fetal lethargy, respiratory depression, hypotonia
- Calcium channel antagonists (Nifedipine):
  - Mechanism of action:
    - Blockage of transmembrane flow of Ca2+ ions through voltage-gated L-type (slow inactivating) channels causing smooth muscle relaxation
    - Type 2 calcium channel antagonist; has minimal effects on cardiac conducting system
  - Pharmacokinetic:
    - Half-life 90 minutes, with 6 hour duration of action
    - Crosses placenta (cord blood/maternal ratio = 0.93)
    - Doses: 20 mg PO q30min for 1 hour, then 20 mg q2–8h
  - Contraindications:
    - Use with caution if left ventricular dysfunction, congestive heart failure, or other cardiac diseases.
  - Adverse effects:
    - Maternal nausea, flushing, headache, dizziness, palpitations, hypotension, and reflex tachycardia
    - Most favorable maternal side effect profile of current tocolytics
    - No fetal adverse side effects.
- β-Adrenergic agonists:
  - Mechanism of action:
    - Smooth muscle relaxation from disruption of actin-myosin interaction

- Pharmacokinetics:
  - Half-life 6–7 minutes
  - Readily crosses placenta
  - Tachyphylaxis common (receptors develop tolerance)
  - Doses: 250 μg SC q4–6h
  - Maintenance dose 2.5 or 5 mg PO q2–4h: Titrate to heart rate >100/min ≤120/min
- Contraindications:
  - Relative contraindication with cardiac disease, poorly controlled DM, or hyperthyroidism
- Adverse effects:
  - Maternal tachycardia, hypotension, palpitations, chest discomfort, shortness of breath, tremor, pulmonary edema, hypokalemia, hyperglycemia
  - Neonatal tachycardia, hyperinsulinemia, hyperglycemia
- NSAIDs (Indomethacin):
  - Mechanism of action:
    - Inhibit prostaglandin synthesis
    - Nonselective COX antagonist
  - Pharmacokinetics:
    - Half-life 2 hours
    - Doses: 50 mg PO/rectally then 25 mg PO/rectally q6h
    - Rectal route faster absorption but not available commercially
    - Crosses placenta
  - Contraindications:
    - Maternal: Platelet dysfunction or bleeding disorder, gastric ulcerative disease, hepatic or renal dysfunction, and asthma
    - Fetal: GA >32–34 weeks, oligohydramnios
  - Adverse effects:
    - Maternal: Nausea, vomiting, gastritis
    - Fetal: Constriction of ductus arteriosus, in utero pulmonary HTN, oligohydramnios
- Oxytocin receptor antagonist

 FOLLOW-UP

DISPOSITION
Issues for Referral
All patients should be referred and comanaged by MFM specialist

PROGNOSIS
Based on GA and associated medical conditions

COMPLICATIONS
- Short term: Feeding and growth difficulties, infection, apnea, neurodevelopmental difficulties, retinopathy, transient dystonia
- Long term: Cerebral palsy, sensory deficits, special needs, incomplete catch-up growth, school difficulties, behavioral problems, chronic lung disease

PATIENT MONITORING
Mother
- Vital signs for evidence of infection
- Contraction monitoring

Fetus
NST

BIBLIOGRAPHY
Gabbe SG, et al. Obstetrics: Normal and Abnormal Pregnancies. In: Iams J, ed. *Preterm Birth*, 4th ed. Philadelphia: Churchill Livingstone; 2002:755–827.

Hamilton BE, et al. Births: Preliminary data for 2004. *Natl Vital Stat Rep.* 2005;54(8):1–18.

Mathews TJ, et al. Infant mortality statistics from the 2003 period linked birth/infant death data set. *Natl Vital Stat Rep.* 2005;54(16):1–30.

Meis PJ, et al. Prevention of recurrent preterm delivery by 17-alpha hydroxyprogesterone caproate. *N Engl J Med.* 2003;348:2379–2385.

Tekesin I, et al. Assessment of rapid fetal fibronectin in predicting preterm delivery. *Obstet Gynecol.* 2005;105(2):280–284.

 MISCELLANEOUS

Outpatient management if local resident, cervix <4 cm dilation, singleton pregnancy, cephalic presentation, compliant patient

ABBREVIATIONS
- AF—Amniotic fluid
- AFI—Amniotic fluid index
- AFP—α-Fetoprotein
- COX—Cyclooxygenase
- DES—Diethylstilberol
- ELBW—Extremely low birth weight
- FFN—Fetal fibronectin
- FH—Fundal height
- GA—Gestational age
- GBS—Group B streptococcus
- HPA—Hypothalamus pituitary adrenal axis
- IVH—Intraventricular hemorrhage
- LBW—Low birth weight
- LEEP—Loop electrosurgical excision procedure
- MFM—Maternal-fetal medicine
- NST—Nonstress test
- OR—Odds ratio
- PPROM—Preterm premature rupture of membranes
- PPV—Positive predictive value
- PTB—Preterm birth
- PTL—Preterm labor
- RDS—Respiratory distress syndrome
- VLBW—Very low birth weight
- WHO—World Health Organization

CODES
ICD9-CM
- 644.03, 644.21 Preterm labor
- 658.1, 658.2 PPROM

 PATIENT TEACHING

- Provide written information about preterm-infant development.
- Support group Web sites. Available at www.shareyourstory.org

PREVENTION
- Identify high-risk patients
- 17-hydroxy-progesterone caproate 250 mg IM weekly starting at 16–21 weeks to 36 weeks

PYELONEPHRITIS DURING PREGNANCY

Bonnie J. Dattel, MD

 BASICS

DESCRIPTION
Women are more likely to develop infections of the urinary tract during pregnancy and postpartum due to physiologic changes unique to pregnancy:
- Mechanical compression-ureteral dilation
- Bladder compression
- Urinary stasis
- Muscle relaxation secondary to high progesterone levels (contributing to stasis and "reflux")

Pregnancy Considerations
- Pyelonephritis in pregnancy is a serious complication affecting up to 1–2% of pregnancies.
- More common in 2nd and 3rd trimesters

ALERT
Serious complications include life-threatening urosepsis and ARDS:
- Aggressive management with antibiotics
- Imaging studies for unresponsive infections
- High index of suspicion for ARDS:
  – Pulse oximetry
  – CXR
  – Arterial blood gases

Age-Related Factors
The prevalence of bacteriuria (>100,000 bacteria or more per milliliter of urine) increases at the rate of 1% per each decade of life from age 5 and older. mainly related to Increased sexual activity.

EPIDEMIOLOGY
Bacteriuria is reported in up to 10% of pregnant women and has associated predictive epidemiology:
- Lower socioeconomic status
- Poor prenatal care

RISK FACTORS
Pregnancy is the most important risk factor for development of pyelonephritis but other factors play a role as well:
- Sickle cell trait/disease
- Increasing parity
- Prior pyelonephritis
- History of frequent UTIs (>3 per year)

Genetics
In general, genetics plays little role in the development of pyelonephritis in pregnancy with rare exceptions:
- Congenital renal malformations
- Inherited immune abnormalities

PATHOPHYSIOLOGY
- All of the factors that predispose to UTIs are precursors to the development of pyelonephritis.
- Unrecognized asymptomatic bacteriuria progresses to symptomatic UTI including pyelonephritis in 40% of pregnant women.
- This progression is attributed to the unique physiologic factors of pregnancy:
  – Stasis
  – Compression
  – Ureteral dilation
  – Hormonal alterations

ASSOCIATED CONDITIONS
Women with sickle cell trait have ~2-fold increased risk for asymptomatic bacteriuria that, if left untreated, can develop into pyelonephritis.

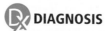 **DIAGNOSIS**

SIGNS AND SYMPTOMS
History
- By definition, asymptomatic bacteriuria is >100,000 bacteria/mL without symptoms.
- Acute cystitis includes symptoms of frequency, urgency and dysuria (burning on urination)
- Women with acute pyelonephritis present with fever, chills, and back pain.

Physical Exam
Although patients with asymptomatic bacteriuria and acute cystitis have few physical findings, pregnant women with pyelonephritis have significant physical findings:
- Fever
- CVA tenderness on the side of the involved kidney

TESTS
The diagnosis of pyelonephritis is based on a combination of history, physical exam, and specific laboratory criteria.
- Pyuria:
  – Bacteriuria
  – Elevated WBC count

Lab
Urine culture with sensitivity testing is the gold standard for diagnosis:
- >100,000 bacteria/mL of urine
- In symptomatic high-risk patients, lower colony counts with a single significant pathogen (50,000 col/mL) should be treated.
- The bacteria responsible for the development of simple UTIs are the same responsible for pyelonephritis.
- Organisms commonly found in pregnant women with pyelonephritis:
  – *Escherichia coli* 90%
  – *Proteus mirabilis*
  – *Klebsiella pneumoniae*
  – Enterococci
  – Less commonly *Pseudomonas aeruginosa*

Pregnancy Considerations
Imaging studies should be limited to special circumstances:
- Persistent fever despite adequate antimicrobial treatment
- Suspicion of renal calculi
- Suspicion of renal anomaly (associated with uterine anomalies):
  – Renal US can be helpful in identifying ureteral dilation out of proportion to expected pregnancy-related dilation.
  – IV pyelogram ("1 shot" to minimize fetal exposure) can identify the presence of anomalies, calculi or other masses, abscess, tumor.

DIFFERENTIAL DIAGNOSIS
The differential diagnosis for a pregnant woman with CVA tenderness, elevated WBC count, and fever should always include pyelonephritis, but other pregnancy-related causes must be considered:
- Intra-amniotic infection
- Intraperitoneal process (appendicitis, ovarian torsion)
- Pneumonia
- Any other infectious process

Hematologic
- A slight elevation in WBC count is common in pregnancy. Women with pyelonephritis have WBCs elevated beyond the expected pregnancy levels.
- Generally >10,000 WBC
- Left shift common

Metabolic/Endocrine
- In simple cases of pyelonephritis, other organ systems remain uninvolved.
- In untreated or advanced infection, multiple organ system involvement is common. Much of this is due to the dehydration, nausea, and vomiting that many patients experience with urosepsis. In these cases, abnormalities in laboratory studies can point to a more serious infection and thus should always be evaluated when pyelonephritis is suspected:
  – Elevation in serum creatinine:
    ○ Markedly abnormal serum creatinine suggests an obstruction as an underlying etiologic event for the pyelonephritis.
  – Abnormalities in liver enzymes

Immunologic
- Immunologic abnormalities are uncommon in normal pregnancy.
- There does not appear to be a difference in virulence or immune response to strains of bacteria responsible for pyelonephritis.
- Women who are immunocompromised (SLE, AIDS) may develop sepsis more rapidly than immunocompetent pregnant women.

Other/Miscellaneous
The presence of GBS bacteriuria at any time in pregnancy demonstrates heavy carriage of the organism.
- All of these patients should receive antibiotic prophylaxis in labor.
- Penicillin-allergic patients must have sensitivity testing because of organisms resistant to second-line antimicrobial agents.
- Patients scheduled for elective cesarean delivery do not require prophylaxis for the neonate if no labor or rupture of membranes occurs.
- A positive urine culture for GBS obviates the need for vaginal/perineal culture at 35 weeks.

TREATMENT

GENERAL MEASURES

- The 1st rule for the treatment of pyelonephritis in pregnancy is prevention. The known association between the presence of asymptomatic bacteruria and ascending renal infection mandates a high index of suspicion for the possible development of pyelonephritis.
- All pregnant women should have a urine culture performed on their 1st prenatal visit.
- The presence of urinary pathogens (>100,000 bacteria/mL) should be treated with appropriate antibiotics.
- The urine should be recultured to assure adequate eradication of bacteriuria.
- All women with a diagnosis of pyelonephritis should be hospitalized for IV antibiotics:
  - 10-day course of oral antibiotics instituted after IV antibiotics and afebrile for >24 hours
  - Oral antibiotic suppression is indicated for the remainder of pregnancy to prevent recurrence (nitrofurantoin 100 mg/d OR ampicillin 500 mg/d)

PREGNANCY-SPECIFIC ISSUES

By Trimester

- 1st trimester screening reveals up to 6% of women have asymptomatic bacteruria, presumably antedating the pregnancy.
- By 20 weeks (2nd trimester), the enlarging uterus contributes more to ureteral obstruction.
- 3rd trimester brings further mechanical obstruction and a physiologic "reflux" that can facilitate the development of pyelonephritis.

Risks for Mother

~10% of women with pyelonephritis in pregnancy develop urosepsis with pulmonary involvement (ARDS), which can be life-threatening.

Risks for Fetus

- Maternal infection and particularly sepsis is associated with an increased risk for preterm labor and delivery.
- In addition, bacteremia can be associated with the development of chorioamnionitis.

SPECIAL THERAPY

Complementary and Alternative Therapies

- No complementary or alternative therapies are effective for the treatment of pyelonephritis.
- Alternative or adjunct treatment may be helpful in prevention of UTIs and therefore, pyelonephritis:
  - Increased fluid intake
  - Good perineal hygiene (wipe front to back)
  - Emptying bladder after intercourse

MEDICATION (DRUGS)

- Medications used to treat pyelonephritis are directed at the specific causative organisms.
- Empiric therapy should be instituted as soon as the diagnosis is suspected, and broad-spectrum coverage for intestinal flora should be used.
- Common selections that are safe for use in pregnancy include: Ampicillin 1 g IV q6h, cephalosporin 1 g IV q6h, and aminoglycosides on a weight-based dosage schedule.

SURGERY

- Surgery is rarely needed in the treatment of uncomplicated pyelonephritis in pregnancy.
- The presence of urinary obstruction may require the placement of ureteral stents to alleviate infection.
- Presence of abscess in the renal parenchyma may require surgical/percutaneous drainage.

 ## FOLLOW-UP

DISPOSITION

Issues for Referral

- Pregnant women with recurrent or refractory pyelonephritis should be evaluated by a urologist to exclude underlying disorders that may require immediate surgical intervention.
- Postpartum follow-up can then also be arranged.

PROGNOSIS

The overwhelming majority of pregnant women treated for pyelonephritis have no sequelae.

COMPLICATIONS

Urosepsis is the most common complication of pyelonephritis in pregnancy and can be life-threatening.

PATIENT MONITORING

- All pregnant women with a diagnosis of or suspected pyelonephritis should be hospitalized for careful monitoring and IV antibiotics as noted above.
- This differs from the management of nonpregnant patients because of the underlying physiologic differences that predispose to urosepsis for pregnant women.

Mother

Mothers should be monitored for changes in vital signs that signify impending sepsis including pulse, temperature, and pulse oximetry.

Fetus

Depending on the GA, the fetus may require electronic fetal monitoring in cases of pyelonephritis accompanied by preterm labor.

BIBLIOGRAPHY

Creasy R, et al. *Maternal-Fetal Medicine*, 4th ed. Philadelphia: W.B. Saunders; 1999.

Harris RE. Urinary Tract Infections in Pregnancy. In: Sciarra ed. *Gynecology and Obstetrics*. 1998;1–9.

McNeely SG. Urinary Tract Infections in Pregnancy. In: Sciarra ed. *Gynecology and Obstetrics*. 1998;1–4.

 ## MISCELLANEOUS

CLINICAL PEARLS

The single most useful preventive strategy for pyelonephritis in pregnancy is identification and treatment of pregnant women with asymptomatic bacteriuria.

ABBREVIATIONS

- ARDS—Acute respiratory distress syndrome
- CVA—Costovertebral angle
- GBS—Group B streptococcus
- SLE—Systemic lupus erythematosus

CODES

ICD9-CM

646.6 Infections of genitourinary tract in pregnancy

 ## PATIENT TEACHING

Patients should be instructed in the signs and symptoms of cystitis so that prompt treatment can be instituted to prevent ascending infection. Other preventative strategies for women include:

- Voiding after intercourse
- Proper wiping techniques after voiding or bowel movements to prevent contamination
- Avoidance of dehydration

PREVENTION

Pyelonephritis is best prevented by identifying women at risk for its development:

- Urinary culture on 1st obstetric visit.
- Treatment of asymptomatic bacteruria
- Follow-up cultures to assure clearance of bacteruria
- Treatment of high-risk women with suppressive antibiotic therapy throughout pregnancy:
  - Sickle cell disease
  - Prior pyelonephritis during the pregnancy
  - Known renal anomalies predisposing to infection (duplication of the collecting system)
  - Women with frequent (>3) UTIs per year

RH SENSITIZATION AND PREVENTION

Joyce Fu Sung, MD
Paula J. Adams Hillard, MD

 BASICS

DESCRIPTION

- RhD is a RBC antigen.
- RhD sensitization or alloimmunization occurs when RhD negative women are exposed to RhD positive RBCs.
- Anti-D immune globulin (RhIG) is used to prevent RhD sensitization in subsequent pregnancies.
- RhD alloimmunization
- Hemolytic disease of the fetus and newborn

PREVENTION

- Administer Anti-D immune globulin (RhIG) to RhD-negative women.
- At delivery:
  - If given within 72 hours of delivery, reduces RhD sensitization rate by 90%
  - Can still have some benefit up to 13–28 days postpartum
  - If delivery occurs <3 weeks from antenatal RhIG administration, do not need to repeat.
  - Dose of 300 μg covers 30 mL of fetal RhD-positive blood (15 mL of RBC)
  - Check Rosette and KB test to determine if fetomaternal hemorrhage exceeds 30 mL, and therefore if extra doses of RhIG are needed.
- At 28–29 weeks:
  - When added to postpartum administration, reduces RhD-sensitization in the 3rd trimester from 2% to 0.1%
  - Check maternal type and screen before administration to detect Rh sensitization.
  - If not delivered in 12 weeks, consider repeat dose.
- At any procedures or events associated with fetomaternal hemorrhage:
  - Spontaneous abortion
  - Elective abortion
  - Ectopic pregnancy
  - Amniocentesis
  - Chorionic villous sampling
  - Fetal blood sampling
  - Threatened abortion (controversial)
  - Molar pregnancy
  - Blunt abdominal trauma
  - External cephalic version
  - 2nd or 3rd trimester hemorrhage
- Characteristics of RhIG:
  - Standard dose is 300 μg, covers 15 mL fetal RBC
  - 50 μg dose is effective in 1st trimester, covering 2.5 mL fetal RBC
  - Half-life, 24 days
  - Collected by apheresis of volunteer donors with high levels of anti-RhD antibodies
  - Formulations available in US:
    - RhoGAM and BayRho-D are given IM (contain small amounts IgA antibodies and other plasma proteins)
    - Rhophylac and WinRho-SDF can be given IV or IM (contain only IgG)

EPIDEMIOLOGY

- Incidence of RhD sensitization:
  - 14% without use of RhIG prophylaxis
  - 2% with routine postpartum RhIG prophylaxis
  - 0.1% with routine postpartum *and* antenatal RhIG prophylaxis
- Prior to RhIG, 10% of pregnancies affected by Rh hemolytic disease
- Decades after introduction of RhIG, 1/1,000 infants affected by Rh hemolytic disease
- RhD antigen incompatibility:
  - 10% of Caucasian and African American pregnancies
  - Rare in Asian pregnancies (RhD negative phenotype is rare)
- Among RhD positive infants with detectable maternal anti-D antibodies:
  - ~50% unaffected or mildly affected, need no treatment
  - ~20% severely affected in utero
  - ~10% require intrauterine transfusion prior to 34 weeks' gestation.

RISK FACTORS

Genetics

2 genes, RhD and RhCE, encode the 3 major rhesus RBC antigen groups (D, C/c, E/e). The Rh locus is on chromosome 1, inherited autosomally. Fetal RhD antigen status is positive if heterozygous or homozygous for RhD gene.

PATHOPHYSIOLOGY

- Fetomaternal hemorrhage results in maternal exposure to RhD antigen on fetal RBCs, stimulating production of anti-D antibodies in an RhD-negative mother:
  - At delivery: 90%
  - Antenatal (mostly 3rd trimester): 10%
- Subsequent pregnancy results in increased titers of anti-RhD IgG antibodies.
- Anti-RhD IgG antibodies cross the placenta and destroy RhD-positive fetal RBCs, causing fetal anemia.
- Fetal anemia can lead to hydrops fetalis and IUFD.
- Causes of fetomaternal hemorrhage:
  - Therapeutic abortion (4–5% risk sensitization)
  - Spontaneous abortion (1.5–2% risk sensitization)
  - Ectopic pregnancy
  - Threatened abortion (rare)
  - CVS (14% rate of fetomaternal hemorrhage, unknown risk sensitization)
  - Amniocentesis (7–15% rate of fetomaternal hemorrhage, unknown risk sensitization)
  - External cephalic version (2–6% fetomaternal hemorrhage, unknown risk sensitization)
  - Trauma

ASSOCIATED CONDITIONS

- IUFD
- Hydrops fetalis

 DIAGNOSIS

TESTS

- Routine antenatal testing for blood type and Rh antigen
- Amniocentesis indicated to check fetal RhD status or monitor fetal anemia (see "Patient Monitoring"):
  - PCR to determine fetal genotype:
    - 98.7% sensitive, 100% specific
    - Check maternal blood sample to rule out RhD pseudogene in African females (false positive)
    - At time of amniocentesis, also check paternal blood sample to rule out rearrangement of paternal RhD gene locus (false negative)
  - Indirectly assess fetal erythrocyte hemolysis by measuring AF bilirubin levels (as ΔOD_{450}); plotted against GA:
    - Liley curve (1961): 3 zones, 27–40 weeks' gestation: I (very low risk); II (mild-moderate hemolysis; low risk of severe fetal anemia); III (severe fetal anemia; high probability fetal death in 7–10 days)
    - Queenan curve (1993): 4 zones, 14–40 weeks' gestation: Rh negative (unaffected); indeterminate; Rh positive (affected); intrauterine death risk
- Cordocentesis (PUBS): See "Patient Monitoring" for indications:
  - Can be used to determine fetal hematocrit, fetal blood type, reticulocyte count, bilirubin level
  - 1–2% rate of fetal loss

Lab

- Maternal antibody titer:
  - Critical titer varies at each institution, usually 8–32
- Paternal blood type
- Free fetal DNA in maternal serum (not used in US)
- In nonsensitized pregnancies, Rosette and KB test are used to determine excessive fetomaternal hemorrhage, and thus dosage of RhIG to prevent sensitization.

Imaging

- US (see "Patient Monitoring" for indications)
- Peak velocity of fetal MCA:
  - >1.5 multiples of the median for GA is associated with moderate to severe anemia
- Fetal hydrops reflects end-stage hemolytic disease:
  - Fetal ascites, pleural effusions, scalp edema
  - Fetal hemoglobin ≤1/3 of normal

DIFFERENTIAL DIAGNOSIS

Infection

- CMV
- Toxoplasmosis
- Parvovirus B19
- Syphilis
- Herpes
- Rubella

Hematologic
- α-Thalassemia
- Fetomaternal hemorrhage
- G6PD deficiency
- In utero hemorrhage

Immunologic
Red cell alloimmunization from other RBC antigens

Other/Miscellaneous
- Cardiac malformations
- Cardiac arrhythmias
- Thoracic masses
- TTTS
- Chromosomal abnormalities

TREATMENT

GENERAL MEASURES
- Rh immune globulin is used to prevent RhD sensitization. However, in an Rh-sensitized pregnancy, monitor for fetal anemia (see Patient Monitoring) and treat with intrauterine transfusion when needed.
- Intravascular transfusion is more effective than intraperitoneal transfusion.
- Target hematocrit: 40–50%
- Average hematocrit drop 1%/day

PREGNANCY-SPECIFIC ISSUES

By Trimester
- 1st trimester: Blood type and antibody screen are checked as part of routine prenatal labs.
- 2nd trimester: Monitoring of sensitized pregnancies (see "Patient Monitoring")
- 3rd trimester:
  - Administration of RhoGAM to Rh negative mothers at 28 weeks
  - Monitoring of sensitized pregnancies (see "Patient Monitoring")

Risks for Fetus
Hemolytic disease of the fetus and newborn, resulting from RhD sensitization, is associated with:
- Anemia
- Fetal hydrops: Total body edema, hepatosplenomegaly, heart failure
- IUFD
- Hyperbilirubinemia postnatally

MEDICATION (DRUGS)
Rh immune globulin (RhIG) is used to prevent RhD sensitization.

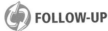

FOLLOW-UP

DISPOSITION
Issues for Referral
Patient with RhD-sensitized pregnancy should have consultation with or referral to a MFM specialist.

PROGNOSIS
Subsequent Rh-sensitized pregnancies are more severely affected.

COMPLICATIONS
Risks of amniocentesis and cordocentesis include pregnancy loss and premature labor.

PATIENT MONITORING
Mother
- In 1st RhD-sensitized pregnancy:
  - Check maternal titers monthly until 24 weeks' gestation, then every 2 weeks.
  - When critical maternal titer is found (varies at each institution), check fetal RhD status. If RhD-positive fetus, see "Fetus" below.
- If previously affected pregnancy:
  - Serial maternal titers not as helpful
  - Check fetal RhD status earlier, via amniocentesis at 15 weeks; if RhD positive, see "Fetus" below.

Fetus
- 1st RhD-sensitized pregnancy:
  - At 24 weeks' gestation, check serial MCA peak velocity (Doppler US) every 1–2 weeks:
    - Or, amniocentesis for ΔOD_{450}
  - If peak MCA velocity >1.5 MoM (or ΔOD_{450} in "affected" zone of Queenan curve or zone III of Liley curve): Cordocentesis to determine fetal hematocrit, and transfusion if <30%
- If previously affected pregnancy:
  - Serial MCA peak velocities (or amniocenteses for ΔOD_{450}) starting at 18 weeks' gestation, every 1–2 weeks.
  - If peak MCA velocity >1.5 MoM (or ΔOD_{450} in affected zone): Cordocentesis to determine fetal hematocrit, and transfusion if <30%
- NST/BPP starting at 32 weeks' gestation

BIBLIOGRAPHY

ACOG Practice Bulletin No. 4. Prevention of RhD Alloimmunization. Washington, DC: ACOG; May 1999.

Eder AF. Update on HDFN: New information on long-standing controversies. *Immunohematology*. 2006;22:188–195.

Jones ML, et al.*Br J Obstet Gynaecol*. 2004;111: 892–902.

Moise KJ Jr. Management of Rh Alloimmunization in Pregnancy. In: Queenan JT, ed. *High-Risk Pregnancy*. Washington, DC: ACOG; 2007;225–237.

Stockman JA 3rd. Overview of the state of the art of Rh disease: History, current clinical management, and recent progress. *J Pediat Hematol Oncol*. 2001;23:554–562.

MISCELLANEOUS

CLINICAL PEARLS
- Rh blood group system was discovered in the 1930s.
- In 1968, RhIG was introduced in the US for postpartum use.

ABBREVIATIONS
- AF—Amniotic fluid
- BPP—Biophysical profile
- CMV—Cytomegalovirus
- CVS—Chorionic villus sampling
- GA—Gestational age
- HDFN—Hemolytic disease of the fetus and newborn
- IUFD—Intrauterine fetal demise
- KB—Kleihauer-Betke
- MCA—Middle cerebral artery
- MFM—Maternal-fetal medicine
- MoM—Multiples of the median
- NST—Nonstress test
- OD—Optical density
- PCR—Polymerase chain reaction
- PUBS—Percutaneous umbilical blood sampling
- Rh—Rhesus
- RhIG—Anti-RhD immune globulin
- TTTS—Twin-twin transfusion syndrome

CODES

ICD9-CM
773.0 Hemolytic disease due to Rh isoimmunization

PATIENT TEACHING

- ACOG Patient Education Pamphlet (AP027): The Rh Factor: How It Can Affect Your Pregnancy
- Rh Sensitization During Pregnancy. Available at: www.healthbanks.com

SPONTANEOUS ABORTION

Lisa Keder, MD, MPH
Michelle M. Isley, MD

 BASICS

DESCRIPTION

- Spontaneous abortion is a pregnancy that ends before the fetus has reached a viable GA. This typically corresponds with a GA of <20 weeks based on the date of the 1st day of the LMP. An alternate definition is the delivery of a fetus that weighs <500 g.
- Threatened abortion: Bleeding in early pregnancy, when pregnancy loss does not always follow.
- Spotting or bleeding in early pregnancy:
  – Is common: 30–40% of pregnancies during the 1st 20 weeks
  – May be slight or heavy
  – May persist for days
  – May be painless or associated with minimal cramping
  – On exam, the uterus is appropriate size for GA and cervical os is closed. Cardiac activity is detected by Doppler or US if expected for GA.
  – ~85% of pregnancies will survive if cardiac activity is present.
- Inevitable abortion: Imminent expulsion of the conceptus:
  – Heralded by increased vaginal bleeding, increased cramping pain, or ruptured membranes in the 2nd trimester.
  – On exam, cervical os dilated and POC may be visible in cervix or lower uterine segment on US.
- Incomplete abortion: Expulsion of a portion of POC:
  – Amount of bleeding varies, but can be severe.
- Complete abortion: Passage of all POC:
  – The cervical os is closed.
  – Vaginal bleeding is minimal or decreasing.
  – Cramping is also decreasing or resolved.
- Missed abortion: In-utero death of embryo or fetus prior to 20 weeks without expulsion of any of the pregnancy tissue.
  – The uterus may be smaller than expected for GA.
  – Vaginal bleeding or spotting may be present.
  – Cervical os is closed.
  – Missed abortion remaining in uterus >5 weeks increases risk of consumptive coagulopathy.

Age-Related Factors
The overall risk for spontaneous abortion increases with increasing maternal age.
- 9.7% risk for abortion age 20–29
- 42.2% risk with maternal age >40

EPIDEMIOLOGY

- Spontaneous abortion is the most common complication of early pregnancy.
- Incidence:
  – ~15% (range 8–20) of clinically recognized pregnancies <20 weeks
  – True incidence of total human embryonic loss is much higher because of the loss of clinically unrecognized pregnancies.
  – 80% occur in 1st 12 weeks
  – Rate decreases with increasing GA

RISK FACTORS

- Advancing maternal age
- Previous spontaneous abortion
- Environmental factors:
  – Maternal smoking >10–14 cigarettes per day
  – Alcohol, cocaine, or caffeine use
  – Irradiation
- Increased parity
- Maternal infection
- Congenital uterine anomalies:
  – Unicornuate uterus, the least common uterine anomaly, is associated with the greatest incidence of spontaneous abortion: ~50%
  – Septate or bicornuate uterus: 25–30%
- DES exposure
- Immunologic factors:
  – Lupus anticoagulant
  – Anticardiolipin antibody
  – Activated protein C resistance (factor V Leiden)
  – Hyperhomocysteinemia
- Maternal endocrinopathies:
  – Uncontrolled DM
  – Thyroid dysfunction
  – Cushing syndrome
  – PCOS

Genetics
- Chromosomal abnormalities are present in ~50% of embryo or fetuses from spontaneous abortions:
  – Autosomal trisomy: 50–65%
  – Monosomy 45,X: 7–15%,
  – Triploidy (15%), tetraploidy (10%), structural abnormalities (5%)
- With ≥2 spontaneous abortions, a 3% rate of major chromosomal abnormality is possible in either parent; this is 5–6 times higher than in the general population.
  – Perform karyotypes in both members of couples with ≥2 spontaneous abortions:
    ○ If abnormal, genetic counseling is indicated.
    ○ May consider use of donor gametes if subsequent pregnancies are attempted.
  – Chromosomal abnormalities occur in the female parent about twice as often as in the male.

PATHOPHYSIOLOGY

- 1/3 of spontaneous abortions at ≤8 weeks gestation are anembryonic ("blighted ovum")
- Chromosomal abnormalities as above
- Exposure to teratogens:
  – Hyperglycemia due to poor glycemic control of DM
  – Drugs
  – Physical stresses, such as fever
- Trauma
- Uterine structural abnormalities can interfere with optimal implantation and growth:
  – Congenital uterine anomalies
  – Uterine submucosal leiomyoma
  – Intrauterine adhesions
- Hypercoagulable state due to inherited or acquired thrombophilia and abnormalities of the immune system can lead to immunologic rejection or placental damage.

- Cervical incompetence can be a cause of early 2nd-trimester pregnancy losses.
- Unexplained

ASSOCIATED CONDITIONS

- Septic abortion (see topic)
- Recurrent abortion defined ≥3 spontaneous abortions

 DIAGNOSIS

SIGNS AND SYMPTOMS

History
- Vaginal bleeding is the cardinal sign:
  – May be light, heavy, intermittent, or constant
- Other common symptoms are a history of amenorrhea and pelvic pain or cramping
- For missed abortion, the patient may report cessation of early pregnancy symptoms, such as nausea and breast tenderness.
- Fetal or embryonic demise may be an incidental finding at the time of US.

Physical Exam
- Vital signs with hypotension and/or tachycardia if severe bleeding, suggesting hypovolemia.
- Fever suggests septic abortion
- Abdominal exam for localization of pain
- Pelvic exam:
  – External genitalia as possible source of bleeding
  – Speculum exam: Remove clots and POC as needed to visualize vaginal walls and cervix
  – Internal digital exam after speculum exam to assess cervix, uterus, adnexa
  – Attempt to determine uterine size
  – Assess pain/discomfort and presence of masses
- Any tissue found on exam or brought by patient should be examined carefully and sent for pathology exam:
  – Visualization of chorionic villi can be facilitated by floating the tissue in water

TESTS

- Doppler for fetal heart tones if the pregnancy is ≥10 weeks of gestation:
  – Inability to detect fetal heart tones can be due to clinician error or error in dating

Labs
- Urine pregnancy test
- Hemoglobin/Hematocrit
- WBC count if fever present
- Blood type and screen:
  – Administer RhoGAM if Rh negative
- Send tissue for pathologic exam to confirm POC.
- If high suspicion for chromosomal abnormality, send POC for chromosomal analysis with patient consent.

Imaging
- US is the most useful test:
  - TVUS preferred for 1st trimester pregnancies
  - Assess if pregnancy is intra- or extrauterine
  - Establish estimated GA based on size of gestational sac, yolk sac, or fetus
  - Determine the presence or absence of fetal cardiac activity to establish viability
  - Diagnosis of a nonviable intrauterine pregnancy based on either:
    - Absence of fetal cardiac activity if embryo crown-rump length >5 mm
    - Absence of fetal pole if mean sac diameter is >25 mm measured transabdominally or >18 mm by the transvaginal technique

DIFFERENTIAL DIAGNOSIS
- Ectopic pregnancy
- Cervical ectropion

Infection
- Vaginitis
- Cervicitis

Tumor/Malignancy
- Molar pregnancy
- Vaginal warts
- Vaginal cancer
- Cervical polyps, warts, or fibroids
- Cervical neoplasms

Trauma
- Vaginal or cervical lacerations
- Foreign body

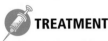

TREATMENT

GENERAL MEASURES
- No therapeutic intervention will prevent spontaneous abortion.
- IV fluids and/or blood products to maintain BP for patients with hypovolemia.
- Threatened abortion should be managed expectantly until symptoms resolve, a definitive diagnosis of nonviable pregnancy can be made, or there is progression to inevitable, incomplete, or complete abortion.
- Completed abortion can be managed as outpatient. Confirm that uterus is empty with US and that bleeding is lessening or stopped.
- Incomplete abortion usually requires surgical evacuation.
- Missed abortion can be managed expectantly, medically, or surgically, based on patient preference:
  - Expectant management for up to 4 weeks is acceptable if the woman is <13 weeks' gestation, stable, and without infection. If spontaneous expulsion does not occur, medical or surgical management can be administered.
  - Surgical management with D&C or D&E
  - Medical management with misoprostol:
    - Misoprostol is not approved by the FDA for treatment of early pregnancy failure.
    - Varying regimens: 1 regimen uses 800 μg once vaginally, with repeat dose if expulsion has not occurred by day 3.
    - Surgical evacuation may still be required.

- For septic abortion:
  - Stabilize the patient.
  - Obtain blood and cervical cultures.
  - Administer broad-spectrum antibiotics.
  - Surgically evacuate uterine contents.

MEDICATION (DRUGS)
- Consider doxycycline for prevention of infection: 100 mg PO q12h for 2 doses
- Consider oral ergonovine maleate (methedrine) 0.2 mg q6h for 1–2 days to decrease bleeding
- Consider iron sulfate 325 mg qd-tid for anemia
- Rh(D)-immune globulin if Rh (D) negative

SURGERY
- D&C for 1st-trimester incomplete or missed abortions:
  - Suction is preferred to sharp curettage.
- D&E for 2nd-trimester incomplete or missed abortions
- Prompt surgical evacuation is essential if suspected septic abortion or retained POC.

 ## FOLLOW-UP

DISPOSITION
Issues for Referral
- Manage as outpatient if hemodynamically stable and without signs/symptoms of infection
- Couples with recurrent abortion who desire future pregnancy should have evaluation including karyotype of both members of the couple.
- Referral for grief counseling is appropriate and should be offered.

PROGNOSIS
- Risk for future spontaneous abortion ~20% after 1 failed pregnancy, 28% after 2 failed pregnancies, and 43% after 3 or more failed pregnancies.

COMPLICATIONS
- Excessive vaginal bleeding can lead to hemodynamic instability and need for blood products for stabilization.
- Complications of surgical management include uterine perforation, intrauterine adhesions, cervical trauma, infection, and the risks of anesthesia.

PATIENT MONITORING
- Monitor for signs/symptoms of infection
- Monitor for heavy vaginal bleeding or signs of hemodynamic instability
- Monitor for signs/symptoms of depression

BIBLIOGRAPHY

Cunningham FG, et al. Abortion. In: Seils A, et al., eds. *Williams Obstetrics*, 21st ed. New York: McGraw-Hill; 2001:855–869.

Filly RA. Ultrasound Evaluation during the First Trimester. In: Callen PW, ed. *Ultrasonography in Obstetrics and Gynecology*, 3rd ed. Philadelphia: W.B. Saunders; 1994:63.

Knudsen UB, et al. Prognosis of a new pregnancy following previous spontaneous abortions. *Eur J Obstet Gynecol.* 1991;39.

Mishell DR. Spontaneous and Recurrent Abortion. In: Stenchever MA, et al., ed. *Comprehensive Gynecology*, 4th ed. Philadelphia: Mosby; 2001: 413–441.

Regan L, et al. Epidemiology and the medical causes of miscarriage. *Baillieres Best Pract Res Clin Obstet Gynecol.* 2000;14:839.

Zhang J, et al. A comparison of medical management with misoprostol and surgical management for early pregnancy failure. *N Engl J Med.* 2005;353:761.

 ## MISCELLANEOUS

SYNONYM(S)
Miscarriage

ABBREVIATIONS
- D&E—Dilation and evacuation
- DES—Diethylstilbestrol
- GA—Gestational age
- LMP—Last menstrual period
- PCOS—Polycystic ovary syndrome
- POC—Products of conception
- TVUS—Transvaginal ultrasound

CODES
ICD9-CM
- 629.9 Unspecified disorder of female genital organs
- 632 Missed abortion
- 634.91 Spontaneous abortion without mention of complication, incomplete
- 634.92 Spontaneous abortion without mention of complication, complete
- 640.03 Threatened abortion, antepartum condition or complication

PATIENT TEACHING

- For medical or expectant management of missed abortion, report to a medical facility if heavy bleeding or symptoms of hypotension.
- Report fever, chills, abdominal pain, or purulent discharge.
- Expect light-medium bleeding for up to 2 weeks:
  - Call if heavy bleeding develops.
  - Pelvic rest for 2 weeks
- Report signs or symptoms of depression:
  - Acknowledge patient's (and partner's) grief, and provide empathy and support.

PREVENTION
- No therapeutic interventions prevent 1st trimester pregnancy loss.
- If an early 2nd-trimester pregnancy loss is attributed to cervical incompetence, a cervical cerclage can be considered.
- Aspirin and/or heparin may decrease risk if lupus anticoagulant or anticardiolipin is present.

TORCH INFECTIONS
Brooke Friedman, MD

 BASICS

DESCRIPTION
- Perinatal infections account for 2–3% of all congenital anomalies.
- Infections acquired in utero contribute significantly to neonatal mortality and childhood morbidity.
- TORCH is an acronym for 5 perinatal infections with similar clinical presentations:
  - Toxoplasmosis
  - Other (syphilis):
    - Some have suggested that HIV, parvovirus B19, varicella, EBV, and hepatitis also be included under "Other"
  - Rubella
  - CMV
  - HSV

EPIDEMIOLOGY
- Toxoplasmosis:
  - 1/3 women have been exposed to parasite.
- Syphilis:
  - Neonatal rate: 1.1/100,000 (2002)
  - Associated with no prenatal care
- Rubella:
  - Neonatal rate: 0.1/100,000 (1999)
  - Little clinical importance in absence of pregnancy; devastating to fetus
- CMV:
  - Most common congenital infection (0.5–2% of all births)
- HSV:
  - 45 million Americans infected

RISK FACTORS
Syphilis, CMV, HSV associated with:
- History of high-risk sexual behavior, STDs, drug abuse

PATHOPHYSIOLOGY
- In utero fetal infection via placental transmission of parasite, virus, or bacteria or via virus exposure during birth process.
- Fetus is vulnerable; does not benefit from passive immunity from mother
- Toxoplasmosis:
  - Protozoan parasite *Toxoplasma gondii*
  - Increasing GA increases fetal infection but decreases severity:
    - 1st trimester: 10–15%
    - 2nd trimester: 25%
    - 3rd trimester: 60%
- Syphilis:
  - Spirochete *Treponema pallidum*
  - Untreated early syphilis: 40% cases lead to spontaneous abortion

- Rubella:
  - RNA togavirus
  - Rate of fetal infection:
    - <11 weeks: 90%
    - >16 weeks: 0%
  - Risk of fetal anomalies:
    - 1st trimester: 25%
    - 2nd trimester: 1%
- CMV:
  - DNA herpesvirus
  - 1st trimester infections associated with symptomatic neonates
  - 2nd trimester infections associated with initially asymptomatic infants
- HSV:
  - Risk of vertical transmission:
    - 30–60% if primary genital HSV lesion at delivery
    - 3% if recurrent genital lesion at delivery

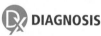 **DIAGNOSIS**

SIGNS AND SYMPTOMS
History
Maternal presentation:
- Toxoplasmosis:
  - Usually asymptomatic
- Syphilis:
  - 3 stages: Primary stage with painless chancre, then progresses to disseminated disease (See Sexually Transmitted Diseases (STDs): Syphilis.)
- Rubella:
  - Rash, lasting 3 days, occurs 2–3 weeks postexposure; "3-day measles"
- CMV:
  - Usually asymptomatic
- HSV:
  - Asymptomatic or painful ulcerative lesions (See Sexually Transmitted Diseases: Herpes Simplex Virus.)

Physical Exam
- Neonatal/Infant presentation
- Toxoplasmosis:
  - Triad:
    - Chorioretinitis
    - Hydrocephalus
    - Intracranial calcifications
- Syphilis:
  - Most asymptomatic at birth
  - If symptomatic, early findings include:
    - Cutaneous lesions, hepatosplenomegaly, jaundice
  - Late includes:
    - Frontal bossing, short maxilla, Hutchinson's triad (blunted upper incisors, interstitial keratitis, deafness), saddle nose
    - Osteitis on long bone radiography
- Rubella:
  - "Blueberry muffin" purpuric skin lesions
  - Hearing loss
  - Cataracts
  - Cardiac malformations (e.g., PDA)

- CMV:
  - Most asymptomatic at birth
  - If symptoms present:
    - Microcephaly, mental retardation, chorioretinitis, cerebral calcifications, petechial rash
- HSV:
  - Local skin, eye, mouth disease (45% cases)
  - CNS disease (30% cases)
  - Disseminated disease involving multiple organs (25% cases)

TESTS

> **ALERT**
> The TORCH acronym is widely recognized; in the past, routine screening with "TORCH titers" was common when IUGR was diagnosed. However, the value of this routine screening has been questioned, and it has been suggested that the Other category should include more pathogens. TORCH titers are not routinely recommended because of issues of reliability, cost effectiveness, and the availability of other diagnostic techniques.

- Diagnose infections via:
  - Maternal serologic response (TORCH titers):
    - May be inconclusive, not 100% sensitive
    - IgG antibodies: Persist long after pathogen exposure
    - IgM antibodies: Usually represents more recent exposure
    - IgM in newborn: Likely congenital infection (IgM cannot cross placenta)
  - Direct antigen testing:
    - Only performed in research labs; technically challenging for many TORCH organisms

Lab
Serology screening at 1st prenatal visit is recommended by ACOG for:
- Rubella
- Syphilis

Imaging
US findings associated with fetal infection:
- IUGR
- Echogenic bowel
- Intracranial or intrahepatic calcifications
- Hydrocephalus
- Microcephaly
- Isolated ascites
- Pericardial or pleural effusions
- Nonimmune hydrops
- Enlarged or reduced placental size
- Increased or decreased amniotic fluid volume

DIFFERENTIAL DIAGNOSIS
Infection
US findings as noted above frequently prompt evaluation for TORCH infections. Some authors have concluded that the yield of workup for TORCH infections among infants with IUGR is poor and does not justify the incurred costs.

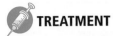 **TREATMENT**

GENERAL MEASURES

Treatment of maternal infection frequently does not substantially decrease fetal morbidity.

PREGNANCY-SPECIFIC ISSUES

By Trimester

- Infections in the 1st trimester generally cause more severe fetal consequences by impairing organogenesis.
- 2nd- and 3rd-trimester infections can lead to neurologic and growth compromise.

MEDICATION (DRUGS)

- Toxoplasmosis:
  – Spiramycin to treat acute infection in pregnancy for the prevention of congenital toxoplasmosis (limited evidence)
  – If prenatal fetal toxoplasmosis, pyrimethamine and sulfadiazine may be recommended
- Syphilis:
  – Penicillin G
- Rubella:
  – No treatment
- CMV:
  – No treatment
- HSV:
  – Acyclovir, Valacyclovir

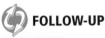 **FOLLOW-UP**

PROGNOSIS

- Toxoplasmosis:
  – Poor if overt disease at birth
- Other (syphilis):
  – Intrauterine death: 25%
  – Perinatal mortality: 25% (if untreated)
- Rubella:
  – Overall very poor
- CMV:
  – 30% severe infections die
  – 80% survivors with severe neurologic morbidity
- HSV:
  – 30% mortality for disseminated disease
  – 4% for CNS disease

COMPLICATIONS

- Toxoplasmosis:
  – 55–85% of infected fetuses have sequelae:
    ○ Microcephaly, chorioretinitis, hearing loss, mental retardation, seizures
- Syphilis:
  – Stillbirth, hydrops fetalis, prematurity, physical stigmata
- Rubella:
  – Deafness, neurologic sequelae (e.g., behavior disorders and mental retardation)
- CMV:
  – Mental retardation, hearing loss, visual impairment, seizures
- HSV:
  – 20% survivors with long-term neurologic sequelae

PATIENT MONITORING

Fetus

Once maternal infection diagnosed, close fetal surveillance indicated

BIBLIOGRAPHY

ACOG Committee Opinion No. 281. Rubella Vaccination. *Obstet Gynecol*. 2002;100(6):1417.

ACOG Practice Bulletin No. 20. Perinatal Viral and Parasitic Infections. Washington DC: ACOG; September 2000.

ACOG Practice Bulletin No. 82. Management of Herpes in Pregnancy. Washington DC: ACOG; June 2007.

ACOG Technical Bulletin No. 171. Rubella and Pregnancy. Washington DC: ACOG; August 1992.

Centers for Disease Control and Prevention. Sexually transmitted diseases treatment guidelines, 2006. *MMWR*. 2006;55(RR-11):1–100.

Crino JP. Ultrasound and fetal diagnosis of perinatal infection. *Clin Obstet Gynecol*. 1999;42:71–80.

Cunningham G, et al., eds. *Williams Obstetrics*, 22nd ed. New York: McGraw-Hill; 2005.

Hollier LM, et al. Cytomegalovirus, Epstein-Barr virus, and varicella zoster virus. *Clin Perinatol*. 2005;32(3):671–696.

Newton ER. Diagnosis of perinatal TORCH infections. *Clin Obstet Gynecol*. 1999;42:59–70.

 MISCELLANEOUS

CLINICAL PEARLS

- Most TORCH infections cause mild maternal disease, but serious perinatal morbidity.
- Suspect fetal infection if US findings include growth restriction, multiple organ system abnormalities.

ABBREVIATIONS

- ACOG—American College of Obstetricians and Gynecologists
- CMV—Cytomegalovirus
- EBV—Epstein-Barr virus
- GA—Gestational age
- HIV—Human immunodeficiency virus
- HSV—Herpes simplex virus
- IUGR—Intrauterine growth restriction
- MMR—Measles mumps rubella
- PDA—Patent ductus arteriosus
- STD—Sexually transmitted disease

CODES

ICD9-CM

- 054 Herpes simplex
- 0.90.2 Early congenital syphilis, unspecified
- 771.0 Congenital rubella
- 771.1 Congenital cytomegalovirus
- 771.2 Congenital toxoplasmosis

 PATIENT TEACHING

PREVENTION

- Toxoplasmosis:
  – Safe food preparation: Cook raw meat and wash produce
  – Avoid handling cat litter.
- Syphilis:
  – Serology screening at 1st prenatal visit
  – Safe sex practices
- Rubella:
  – Girls should be vaccinated against rubella before the childbearing years.
  – If immunization status unknown, rubella serology testing can be performed at preconception visit with immunization at least 3 months prior to conception.
  – Serology screening at 1st prenatal visit
  – Rubella susceptibility noted in pregnancy should prompt MMR vaccination postpartum.
- CMV:
  – Good hygiene (e.g., hand washing), especially for mothers of children in daycare
- HSV:
- Suppressive viral therapy at ≥36 weeks gestation for women with active recurrent genital herpes
- Cesarean delivery if active genital lesions or prodromal symptoms

Section V

TWIN-TWIN TRANSFUSION SYNDROME

William J. Polzin

 BASICS

DESCRIPTION
- TTTS is a disease of reproductive-age women that affects monochorionic twin pregnancies.
- Affects 10–20% of monochorionic twin pregnancies.
- It is most commonly identified when polyhydramnios is seen in 1 twin's sac and oligohydramnios is seen in the other twin's sac.
- It can have an indolent course that becomes evident in the 3rd trimester and requires no intervention except delivery close to term.
- It can also arise in the early 2nd trimester and progress so rapidly that hydrops and death of 1 or both twins occurs in a matter of weeks despite all treatment attempts.
- If present in the 2nd trimester and no treatment is rendered, the natural history is such that mortality rates for both twins approximate 90%.

Staging
- The Quintero staging system provides a useful shorthand for discussing the disease:
  - Stage I: Polyhydramnios/Oligohydramnios
  - Stage II: Urine not visible in the donor twin's bladder
  - Stage III: Abnormal Doppler velocimetry
  - Stage IV: Ascites or hydrops present in either twin
  - Stage V: Death of either or both twins
- Modified staging system that stratifies Stage III is more descriptive of disease severity:
  - Critical Doppler abnormalities (AEDF or REDF in UA, reverse flow in DV, pulsatile UV)
  - Mild to moderate cardiomyopathy*
  - Severe cardiomyopathy*

*AV valve incompetence, thick ventricular wall, decreased ventricular function

EPIDEMIOLOGY
- ~1 in 100 pregnancies are twin gestations.
- The prevalence of monochorionic twins is 1/400 pregnancies.
- 10–20% of monochorionic twins develop TTTS.
- 80% of monochorionic twins have arteriovenous connections visible on the placental surface:
  - These facts highlight the unknown etiology of TTTS

PATHOPHYSIOLOGY
- Unidirectional arteriovenous connections of placental circulations
- Inadequate bidirectional compensation:
  - Hypervolemic, hypertensive cardiomyopathy in the larger (recipient) twin
  - Hypovolemic, hypotensive circulatory pattern in the smaller (donor) twin

- Donor findings may be consistent with uteroplacental insufficiency:
  - Significant size differences can be seen
  - Abnormal umbilical artery and venous Doppler velocimetry
- Recipient findings may be consistent with plethoric, hypervolemic state in recipient:
  - Abnormal venous Doppler velocimetry in the ductus venosus
  - Cardiomyopathy
- Neurodevelopmental injury in ~22% of survivors:
  - About equal distribution of injury in recipients and donors
  - Better long-term outcome if born as surviving twins rather than a singleton survivor after a co-twin has died.

ASSOCIATED CONDITIONS
- PPROM due to hydramnios
- Preterm labor and delivery
- IUGR in donor
- Hemorrhagic or thrombotic brain lesions occurring antenatally
- Cardiomyopathy in recipient
- Hydrops fetalis in recipient
- Death of 1 twin with 15–50% morbidity or mortality in co-twin
- >90% mortality of both twins, if TTTS is untreated

 DIAGNOSIS

SIGNS AND SYMPTOMS
- Rapid change in FH
- Premature contractions
- Sudden onset of pelvic pressure
- Shortness of breath

History
Known monochorionic twin gestation

Physical Exam
- FH > dates
- Rapid interval growth in FH

TESTS
Labs
- For diagnosis of hydramnios:
  - TORCH titers in mother
  - Amniotic fluid culture and PCR evaluation
  - Thyroid function testing
  - Fetal karyotype

Imaging
- Weekly US evaluation of AF volume beginning at 16 weeks
- Monthly US evaluation of fetal size and changes in anatomy
- Monthly Doppler velocimetry evaluation of umbilical artery

DIFFERENTIAL DIAGNOSIS
TTTS is readily identified, if it is anticipated and suspected in monochorionic twin pregnancies. A number of other conditions should be considered and ruled out using readily available US and laboratory testing.

ALERT
Rule out premature labor. PROM and severe uteroplacental insufficiency can cause oligohydramnios. Previously identified congenital anomalies such as TE fistulas can cause hydramnios (see Hydramnios).

Infection
- TORCH titers in mother
- AF culture and PCR evaluation

Hematologic
Isoimmunization

Metabolic/Endocrine
- Thyroid conditions in mother
- Pregestational or gestational diabetes

Immunologic
SLE

Tumor/Malignancy
Placental or umbilical cord tumors

Trauma
Placental abruption

Drugs
Illicit drug use

Other/Miscellaneous
- Congenital fetal anatomic abnormalities
- Genetic syndromes
- Karyotype abnormalities

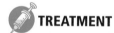 **TREATMENT**

PREGNANCY-SPECIFIC ISSUES
Bed rest is recommended:
- Helps with discomfort of hydramnios
- May be adjunct to treating PTL
- May promote better circulation to the placenta of the smaller twin

MEDICATION (DRUGS)
- Tocolytics for premature labor
- Indomethacin to reduce degree of hydramnios:
  - Special caution to identify cardiovascular side-effects and discontinue

SURGERY
- Amnioreduction:
  - May work effectively in up to 20% of cases
  - Survival of 1 or both twins approximates 60%; better than untreated
  - Little risk to mother
  - Chorioamnionic separation takes option of laser therapy off the table
  - Abruption or rupture of membranes may lead to pregnancy loss
- Microseptostomy:
  - Has been used primarily
  - Has been used adjunctively
  - Often an unintentional result of amniocentesis
- Laser photocoagulation of unidirectional arteriovenous anastomoses:
  - Bidirectional arterioarterial anastomoses may be protective
  - Performed through operating fetoscope
  - Selective treatment of 1-way anastomoses whether direct or via cotyledons
  - Survival of 1 or both twins approximates 90%
  - Reduced survival with advancing stage of disease
  - Treatment risk borne more heavily by mother
  - Fewer abnormal head US findings (6% vs. 18% in amnioreduction)
  - No difference in long-term neurologic morbidity compared to amnioreduction
- Bipolar or radiofrequency ablation of a previable, dying twin's cord can be protective of the surviving co-twin.

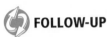 **FOLLOW-UP**

DISPOSITION
- Home bed rest is usually sufficient.
- Evaluate response to therapy at least once a week.
- Delivery usually occurs by 32 weeks' gestation.
- Route of delivery determined by usual obstetric indications

Issues for Referral
- Regional centers may offer more comprehensive evaluations and detect subtle cardiovascular changes that may upstage the disease and change recommendations for initiating or continuing treatment regimens.
- Important to refer to an experienced treatment center if not available at the primary care site:
  - Regional sites are available to evaluate, especially if laser is requested by the patient or required due to failure of amnioreduction.
- Detecting early cardiovascular changes requires an experienced fetal echocardiographer.

PROGNOSIS
- Prognosis is poor (<10% survival) if disease occurs at a previable GA and is untreated.
- Prognosis with early-stage disease and aggressive treatment can improve survival significantly.
- Overall survival of 1 or both twins approximates 90% when treated aggressively.

PATIENT MONITORING
Mother
Observe for PTL.

Fetus
The surviving neonates should be followed closely by physicians experienced in detecting subtle variations from normal development. Early and aggressive interventions can help mitigate the effects of injury from TTTS.

BIBLIOGRAPHY

Banek CS, et al. Long-term neurodevelopmental outcome after intrauterine laser treatment for severe twin-twin transfusion syndrome. *Am J Obstet Gynecol*. 2003;188:876–880.

Harkness UF, et al. Twin-twin transfusion syndrome: Where do we go from here? *Semin Perinatol*. 2005; 29:296–304.

Hecher K, et al. Endoscopic laser surgery versus serial amniocenteses in the treatment of severe twin-twin transfusion syndrome. *Am J Obstet Gynecol*. 1999;180:717–724.

Huber A, et al. Stage-related outcome in twin-twin transfusion syndrome treated by fetoscopic laser coagulation. *Obstet Gynecol*. 2006;108:333–337.

Quintero RA, et al. Staging of twin-twin transfusion syndrome. *J Perinatol*. 1999;19:550–555.

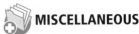 **MISCELLANEOUS**

SYNONYM(S)
Polyhydramnios/Oligohydramnios syndrome

ABBREVIATIONS
- AEDF—Absent end diastolic flow
- AF—Amniotic fluid
- AV—Atrial ventricular
- DV—Ductus venosus
- FH—Fundal height
- IUGR—Intrauterine growth restriction
- PCR—Polymerase chain reaction
- PPROM—Preterm premature rupture of membranes
- PTL—Preterm labor
- REDF—Reverse end diastolic flow
- SLE—Systemic lupus erythematosus
- TORCH—Toxoplasmosis, other, rubella, CMV, HSV
- TTTS—Twin-twin transfusion syndrome
- UA—Umbilical artery
- UV—Umbilical vein

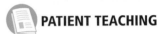 **CODES**

ICD9-CM
- 651.03 Twin pregnancy, antepartum
- 663.83 Other umbilical cord complications, antepartum

PATIENT TEACHING

Instruct patient to report the following:
- Rapid change in FH
- Premature contractions
- Sudden onset of pelvic pressure
- Shortness of breath

Section V

VAGINAL BIRTH AFTER CESAREAN DELIVERY

Jason N. Hashima, MD, MPH
Jeanne-Marie Guise, MD, MPH

BASICS

DESCRIPTION
A vaginal delivery in a woman who had a prior CD.

EPIDEMIOLOGY
The CD rate in the US was 5.5% in 1970. In response to rising CD rates, the NIH and WHO concluded that VBAC was a safe alternative to repeat CD. While VBAC rates peaked to 28.3% in 1996, they have steadily declined to 9.2% in 2004. Inversely, the CD rate in 2004 had risen as high as 29%.

- Contributing factors to recent trends:
  - Increase in the number of older and nulliparous women, who are at higher risk for CD
  - Breech vaginal deliveries contraindicated
  - Increased used of fetal monitoring
  - Patient preference
  - Medical-legal concerns
- TOLAC success rates are based on several large observation studies:
  - 60–80% success rate
  - Success rates may fall outside this commonly quoted range for selected patient populations.

RISK FACTORS
- History of cesarean delivery
- Pregnancy

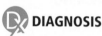

DIAGNOSIS

SIGNS AND SYMPTOMS
History
- Take a careful history regarding both obstetric and medical conditions.
- Obstetric history:
  - Number of prior VDs:
    - Birth weights
  - Number of prior CDs:
    - Type of uterine incision: Low transverse, vertical, classical, T-shaped
  - Prior CD indication:
    - Recurrent: Failure to progress, arrest of labor, cephalopelvic disproportion
    - Nonrecurrent: Breech, non-reassuring fetal heart tracing, bleeding, and all other conditions not listed as a recurrent indication
  - Interdelivery interval: Time between deliveries
- Maternal medical conditions that preclude vaginal delivery
- Future fertility: Determining a patient's desire for future fertility (i.e., desired sterilization) could affect the decision to attempt a TOLAC.

Physical Exam
Routine prenatal care exam

TESTS
Lab
Routine prenatal labs (See Prenatal Laboratory Testing, Routine.)

Imaging
- US:
  - Routine fetal exam
  - GA: Accurate estimation of GA is important in situations where repeat CD is being planned.
  - Placental location: Prior CD increases the risk of abnormal placentation, especially if the placenta is anterior:
    - Placenta previa
    - Placenta accreta/increta/percreta
- Pelvimetry:
  - X-Ray and MRI pelvimetry are ineffective in reliably predicting TOLAC success.

TREATMENT

GENERAL MEASURES
- A thorough review of the patient's past medical and obstetric history, as well as consideration of her current pregnancy issues is pertinent to patient counseling and patient selection for TOLAC.
- Advantages of a VBAC compared to ERCD:
  - Shorter hospital stay and quicker recovery
  - Decreased operative morbidity:
    - Less blood loss and fewer transfusions
    - Less infections
    - Fewer thromboembolic events
- Risks of a VBAC compared to ERCD:
  - Uterine rupture
  - Risk of hysterectomy is equal in both groups
  - Neonatal morbidity
- Candidates for a TOLAC:
  - 1 prior CD
  - Clinically adequate pelvis
  - No other uterine scars or previous rupture
  - Available resources for emergent CD
  - Other conditions associated with a slightly increased risk of failed TOLAC, but still considered to be relatively safe:
    - 2 prior CDs with a prior VD history
    - Unknown uterine scar type
    - Suspected macrosomia
    - Gestation >40 weeks
    - Twin gestation
- Contraindications for a TOLAC:
  - Previous classical or T-shaped uterine incision
  - Previous uterine rupture
  - Medical or obstetric complications that preclude VD
  - Inability to perform an emergent CD
  - 2 prior CDs without a prior VD history

PREGNANCY-SPECIFIC ISSUES
Risks for Mother
- Morbidity:
  - Uterine rupture
  - Uterine dehiscence
  - Hysterectomy
  - Bleeding, requiring transfusion
  - Infection
- Mortality is rare, but could be attributed to uterine rupture.

Risks for Fetus
- Morbidity:
  - Hypoxia
  - Encephalopathy
  - Other neurologic deficits
- Mortality is rare, but increases with TOLAC compared to ERCD (13–90/10,000 TOLAC vs. 1–50/10,000 ERCD).

MEDICATION (DRUGS)
- Prostaglandins are contraindicated for cervical ripening or induction of labor. Demonstrated increased risk of uterine rupture, especially if oxytocin is required for augmentation.
- Oxytocin use is considered reasonable in TOLAC induction and augmentation.
- Epidural is not contraindicated in TOLAC.

SURGERY
Cesarean delivery (See Cesarean delivery.):
- Elective
- Emergent

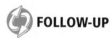

FOLLOW-UP

DISPOSITION
Issues for Referral
Referral might be indicated if patient strongly desires VBAC and local facility is unable to perform emergent CD.

PROGNOSIS
- As above; likelihood of successful TOLAC is 60–80%.
- Maternal and neonatal morbidity and mortality is associated with a failed TOLAC, not TOLAC in general.
- Factors associated with increased likelihood of VBAC:
  - Past obstetric factors associated with TOLAC success:
    - Prior VD/VBAC history
    - Fewer number of CD
    - Nonrecurrent CD indication
    - Interdelivery interval >18 months

– Current obstetric factors associated with TOLAC success:
  ○ Maternal age <35 years old
  ○ Maternal BMI <30
  ○ GA <40 weeks
  ○ Estimated fetal weight <4,000 g
  ○ Spontaneous labor
  ○ Favorable cervical exam
- Several predictive tools have been devised to identify those who will succeed at TOLAC. The AHRQ review identified 2 predictive tools for use at the time of labor admission that were rated as good to fair, however, no tool has been widely accepted for the everyday clinical setting to date. Factors within the tools include:
  – Flamm and Geiger Scoring Tool:
    ○ Maternal age
    ○ Prior VD
    ○ Prior CD indication
    ○ Cervical effacement at admission
    ○ Cervical dilation at admission
  – Troyer and Parisi Scoring Tool:
    ○ Previous dysfunctional labor
    ○ No prior VD
    ○ Nonreassuring fetal heart tracing at admission
    ○ Induction of labor

COMPLICATIONS
- In general, composite complication rates appear to be increased in those with a TOLAC compared to those with an ERCD.
- Complications appear to be associated with a failed TOLAC.

PATIENT MONITORING
- Patients should be counseled to report any potential signs or symptoms of uterine rupture, including abdominal or incisional pain, vaginal bleeding, maternal tachycardia, or decreased fetal movement.
- Continuous fetal monitoring is strongly recommended to monitor for signs of potential rupture.
- Fetal bradycardia is the most common sign of symptomatic uterine rupture.

BIBLIOGRAPHY

ACOG Practice Bulletin No. 54. Vaginal Birth After Previous Cesarean Delivery. Washington, DC: ACOG; July 2004.

ACOG Practice Bulletin No. 342. Induction of Labor for Vaginal Birth After Cesarean Delivery. Washington, DC: ACOG; August 2006.

Centers for Disease Control and Prevention statistics. Available at: www.cdc.gov.

Flamm BL, et al. Vaginal birth after cesarean delivery: An admission scoring system. *Obstet Gynecol*. 1997;90:907.

Guise JM, et al. Safety of vaginal birth after cesarean: A systematic review. *Obstet Gynecol*. 2004; 103(3):420.

Hashima JN, et al. Predicting vaginal birth after cesarean delivery: A review of prognostic factors and predictive tools. *Am J Obstet Gynecol*. 2004;190:547.

Troyer LR, et al. Obstetric parameters affecting success in a trial of labor: Designation of a scoring system. *Am J Obstet Gynecol*. 1992;167:1099.

 MISCELLANEOUS

See also: Term labor, Cesarean delivery, Labor augmentation, Labor, induced, Uterine rupture

CLINICAL PEARLS
- Carefully review patient obstetric and medical history.
- VBAC success rates are roughly between 60% and 80%, with some variation depending on specific patient characteristics
- Selection criteria for a TOLAC are established and should be followed for patient safety.
- Prostaglandins should be avoided in those wishing to attempt a TOLAC.
- The increased rate of complications associated with a TOLAC are mainly attributed to those who have a failed TOLAC.

- Uterine rupture can be a catastrophic TOLAC complication associated with maternal and neonatal morbidity and mortality. Fetal bradycardia can be the most reliable sign of uterine rupture.
- No individual perinatal factor has sufficient sensitivity and specificity to predict TOLAC outcome. When combined in certain predictive tools, more information is provided, but the applicability of current predictive tools is limited to the time of labor admission.

ABBREVIATIONS
- CD—Cesarian delivery
- ERCD—Elective repeat cesarean delivery
- GA—Gestational age
- TOLAC—Trial of labor after cesarean
- VBAC—Vaginal birth after cesarean
- VD—Vaginal delivery

CODES
ICD9-CM
- 650 Normal delivery
- 654.2 Previous cesarean delivery
- 763.4 Cesarean delivery

 PATIENT TEACHING

- Discussions should be held with the patient throughout her pregnancy regarding her options for delivery method (i.e., TOLAC or repeat CD).
- Counsel patients on likelihood of VBAC, risks associated with a TOLAC, and their options, including a repeat CD.
  – In some settings, the option of a VBAC may not be available to the patient, secondary to medical staff and hospital resources.
- Discuss warning signs for uterine rupture.

Section V

Section VI

Pregnancy with Underlying Medical Conditions

ANTIPHOSPHOLIPID ANTIBODY SYNDROME AND PREGNANCY

Lavenia B. Carpenter, MD

 BASICS

DESCRIPTION

- An autoimmune syndrome characterized by recurrent venous/arterial thromboembolic disease and/or pregnancy morbidity in the form of recurrent fetal loss or premature birth in association with persistently positive aPL.
- Types:
  - Primary: Patients without clinical evidence of another autoimmune disease
  - Secondary: Patients with evidence of another autoimmune disease such as SLE
- Spectrum of illness:
  - Asymptomatic aPL positivity:
    ○ Not APS
    ○ No treatment
  - Pregnancy morbidity only
  - Vascular events:
    ○ DVT, arterial thrombosis, PE, TIA, stroke, renal infarction, etc.
  - Nonthrombotic manifestations:
    ○ Raynaud phenomenon, livedo reticularis, cardiac valvular abnormalities, thrombocytopenia, transverse myelitis, multiple sclerosis–like disease
  - Catastrophic APS:
    ○ Severe disseminated vascular occlusions
    ○ Multiorgan ischemia and infarction

Geriatric Considerations
Look for other causes of thromboembolic events in this age group.

Pediatric Considerations
- Suspect in young patients with TIA/stroke
- 2/3 of children with idiopathic cerebral ischemia and acute infarction have evidence of elevated aPL antibodies.
- Factor V Leiden heterozygosity
- Retinal vaso-occlusion

Pregnancy Considerations
- Pregnancy loss at all stages
- Placental dysfunction in the 3rd trimester
- IUGR
- Preeclampsia

EPIDEMIOLOGY
- aPL antibodies are present, at some point, in almost every individual.
- Clinical criteria and persistently positive aPLs are required for diagnosis.
- 50% present with primary form.

Incidence
- 15% of recurrent pregnancy loss
- 35% with primary disease have cardiac valvular abnormalities
- 50% with SLE and APS have evidence of valvular abnormality

Prevalence
- 1–5% healthy young adults have aPLs
- 50%+ of patients with SLE with positive aPLs will develop this syndrome.

RISK FACTORS
- Family history of autoimmune disease
- Family history of aPL positivity
- Personal history of thrombosis
- Infection induction

Genetics
- Unknown
- HLA class II polymorphism and induction of aPL?
- β2-Glycoprotein I cofactor for aPL binding associated with clinical manifestation of disease gene located on chromosome 17

PATHOPHYSIOLOGY
- Any organ can be involved.
- Thrombosis is the primary etiology of all nonpregnancy manifestations:
  - Activation of endothelial cells, oxidant mediated injury of the vascular endothelium, interference with phospholipid binding proteins:
    ○ Intercellular adhesion molecule-1, vascular cell adhesion molecule-1, and P-selectin
    ○ Disruption of the annexin-V shield around cells and trophoblasts
    ○ Interference with protein C antithrombotic pathway
    ○ Complement activation
  - Interference with prostacyclin thromboxane balance:
    ○ Inhibition of AA release
    ○ AA essential for prostacyclin production
    ○ Prostacyclin potent vasodilator and inhibitor of thromboxane aggregation
  - Affects the adhesion molecules between trophoblastic elements of syncytiotrophoblast:
    ○ Damage unrelated to thrombosis

ASSOCIATED CONDITIONS
- SLE
- Raynaud phenomenon
- Malignant HTN
- Nephrotic syndrome
- Cardiac valvular abnormalities

 DIAGNOSIS

Sapporo criteria for diagnosis:
- Clinical criteria (at least 1 of following):
  - Vascular thrombosis:
    ○ $\geq$1 clinical episodes of arterial, venous, or small vessel thrombosis occurring within any tissue or organ
  - Complication of pregnancy:
    ○ $\geq$1 unexplained deaths of morphologically normal fetuses at or after the 10th week of pregnancy OR
    ○ $\geq$1 premature births of morphologically normal neonates at or before the 34th week of pregnancy OR
    ○ $\geq$3 unexplained spontaneous abortions before the 10th week of pregnancy
- AND at least 1 laboratory criterion:
  - Anticardiolipin IgG or IgM antibodies present in moderate or high levels in the blood on $\geq$2 occasions at least 6 weeks apart
  - Lupus anticoagulant detected in the blood on $\geq$2 occasions at least 6 weeks apart

SIGNS AND SYMPTOMS
- Arthralgias
- Thrombosis
- Livedo reticularis

History
- Family history of connective tissue disease
- Patient history of thromboembolic disease
- Pregnancy morbidity:
  - Prior pregnancy loss or preterm delivery
  - History of preeclampsia

Physical Exam
- Evidence of thromboembolic disease
- DVT most common initial manifestation of the disease

TESTS
- ELISA test for anticardiolipin antibodies:
  - IgG, IgM, IgA
  - IgG most predictive
- Clotting test for lupus anticoagulant
- β_2-Glycoprotein 1 may be in future screens

Lab
- Labs are poorly standardized and lead to widely ranging aPL levels.
- Thrombocytopenia
- Leukopenia

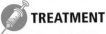 TREATMENT

GENERAL MEASURES
- Risk modification:
  - Smoking cessation
  - Control of HTN, diabetes, hyperlipidemia
  - Avoid OCP use
- Prophylaxis during high-risk periods (surgery, immobilization, pregnancy)

PREGNANCY-SPECIFIC ISSUES
Pregnancy with history of recurrent fetal loss:
- Aspirin 81 mg/d prior to conception or at confirmation of pregnancy
- UH 5,000–10,000 U SC b.i.d. vs. LMWH prophylaxis:
  - More studies exist on UH
  - Not enough data to determine benefit of 1 over the other
- Start at confirmation of fetal cardiac activity

By Trimester
- 1st trimester: Start heparin and aspirin when fetal cardiac activity detected (consider aspirin sooner, but not heparin because of risk for osteoporosis)
- 2nd trimester: Continue aspirin and heparin
- 3rd trimester: Continue heparin and aspirin; discontinue both just before delivery
- Postpartum: DVT prophylaxis, therapeutic anticoagulation in mothers with a history of prior thrombosis

Risks for Mother
- Thrombosis
- Preeclampsia

Risks for Fetus
- Preterm delivery
- Fetal growth restriction
- Death

MEDICATION (DRUGS)
Nonpregnant:
- Warfarin treatment of moderate intensity (to achieve an INR of 2.0–3.0) significantly reduces the rate of recurrent thrombosis:
  - Duration of treatment is lifelong.
- Corticosteroids and azathioprine for treatment of symptoms of lupus in patients with secondary form of the syndrome
- In patients who develop new thromboses despite moderate-intensity anticoagulant therapy and for patients with catastrophic APS:
  - Plasmapheresis
  - IV immunoglobulin

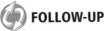 FOLLOW-UP

DISPOSITION
Issues for Referral
- Rheumatologic workup
- Anticoagulation monitoring and duration

PROGNOSIS
- Pulmonary HTN, neurologic involvement, myocardial ischemia, nephropathy, gangrene of extremities, and catastrophic APS are associated with a worse prognosis.
- Most patients experience recurrences months or years after the initial event.
- Mortality rate is ~50% in patients presenting with the catastrophic type, and death is due to multiorgan system failure.

COMPLICATIONS
- Discontinuation of warfarin results in increased risk of thromboembolic disease, particularly in the 1st 6 months after stopping treatment.
- Therapeutic anticoagulation is recommended in postpartum period for all women with history of thromboembolic disease.

PATIENT MONITORING
As warfarin therapy is lifelong, patients must have regular monitoring to maintain INR in the therapeutic range (between 2.0 and 3.0).

BIBLIOGRAPHY

Alarcon-Segovia D, et al. Prophylaxis of the antiphospholipid syndrome: A consensus report. *Lupus*. 2003;12(7):499–503.

Carp H. Antiphospholipid syndrome in pregnancy. *Curr Opin Obstet Gynecol*. 2004;16:129–135.

Francis J, et al. Impaired expression of endometrial differentiation markers and complement regulatory proteins in patients with recurrent pregnancy loss associated with antiphospholipid syndrome. *Molecul Human Reprod*. 2006;12(7):435–442.

Lim W, et al. Management of antiphospholipid antibody syndrome. *JAMA*. 2006;295:1050–1057.

Noble L, et al. Antiphospholipid antibodies associated with recurrent pregnancy loss: Prospective, multicenter, controlled pilot study comparing treatment with low molecular weight heparin versus unfractionated heparin. *Fertil Steril*. 2005;83(3):684–690.

Tincani A, et al. Treatment of pregnant patients with antiphospholipid syndrome. *Lupus*. 2003;12(7):524–529.

 MISCELLANEOUS

CLINICAL PEARLS
- Like any autoimmune disease, APS can have a wide range of presentations depending on the organ system primarily effected.
- In pregnancy, thrombosis may be secondary to dysfunctional trophoblast invasion for recurrent pregnancy loss.
- APS is still poorly understood and research is needed on the appropriate treatment; watch current literature.

ABBREVIATIONS
- AA—Arachidonic acid
- aPL—Antiphospholipid antibodies
- APS—Antiphospholipid antibody syndrome
- DVT—Deep venous thrombosis
- ELISA—Enzyme-linked immunosorbent assay
- IUGR—Intrauterine growth restriction
- LMWH—Low molecular weight heparin
- OCP—Oral contraceptive pill
- PE—Pulmonary embolism
- SLE—Systemic lupus erythematosus
- TIA—Transient ischemic attack
- UH—Unfractionated heparin

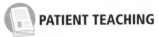 CODES

ICD9-CM
- 795.79 Other, unspecified, nonspecific, immunologic finding
- 286.9 Other, unspecified, coagulation defect

PATIENT TEACHING

PREVENTION
- Risk modification:
  - Smoking cessation
  - Control of HTN, diabetes, hyperlipidemia
  - Avoid OCP use
  - Prophylaxis during high-risk periods (surgery, immobilization, pregnancy)
- Pregnancy with history of recurrent fetal loss:
  - Aspirin 81 mg/d prior to conception or at confirmation of pregnancy
  - UH 5,000–10,000 U SC b.i.d. vs. LMWH prophylaxis:
    ○ More studies with UH
    ○ Not enough data to determine benefit of 1 over the other
    ○ Start at confirmation of fetal cardiac activity

Section VI

ASTHMA AND PREGNANCY

Mitchell Dombrowski, MD

 BASICS

DESCRIPTION
Asthma may be the most common potentially serious medical condition to complicate pregnancy. Current medical management for asthma emphasizes treatment of airway inflammation to decrease airway responsiveness and prevent asthma symptoms.

- Asthma severity classification:
  - Mild intermittent asthma: Symptoms < twice/week, nocturnal symptoms < twice/month, and PEFR or FEV1 >80% predicted
  - Mild persistent asthma: Symptoms > twice/week but not daily, nocturnal symptoms > twice/month and PEFR or FEV1 >80% predicted
  - Moderate persistent asthma: Daily symptoms, nocturnal symptoms > once/week and PEFR or FEV1 >60%–<80% predicted
  - Severe persistent asthma: Continuous symptoms/frequent exacerbations, frequent nocturnal symptoms and PEFR or FEV1 <60% predicted

EPIDEMIOLOGY
~4–8% of pregnancies are complicated by asthma.

RISK FACTORS
Positive history of asthma or bronchial hyper-responsiveness, respiratory infection, and environmental and seasonal factors

Genetics
Familial predisposition

PATHOPHYSIOLOGY
Asthma is characterized by chronic airway inflammation with increased airway responsiveness to a variety of stimuli, and airway obstruction that is partially or completely reversible.

ASSOCIATED CONDITIONS
Reflux esophagitis and allergies

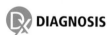 **DIAGNOSIS**

- Wheezing, cough, shortness of breath, chest tightness with temporal relationships (fluctuating intensity, worse at night), increased by triggers (e.g., allergens, exercise, infections)
- With a clinical picture consistent with asthma, a positive response to asthma therapy suffices to establish the diagnosis during pregnancy until more definitive testing can be completed postpartum, if indicated.
- Dyspnea of pregnancy can usually be differentiated from asthma by its lack of cough, wheezing, chest tightness, or airway obstruction.

SIGNS AND SYMPTOMS
History
- The patient should be asked to identify known triggers of her asthma.
- Identify uncontrolled rhinitis, sinusitis, or reflux that may be contributing to asthma intensity.

- Severity/Control should be assessed in terms of exacerbations and impairment.
- Identify a history of prior hospitalizations (especially with intensive care unit admission or intubation), emergency department, or other unscheduled asthma visits, or oral corticosteroid requirements.

Physical Exam
Wheezing on auscultation

TESTS
- Clinical evaluation includes pulmonary function tests or at least a measure of peak flow rate.
- Methacholine challenge is contraindicated during pregnancy.

Lab
Routine pregnancy tests

Imaging
- Consider US for fetal growth in patients with persistent asthma.
- CXR is only indicated in presence of suspicion of a pulmonary process other than asthma.

 TREATMENT

GENERAL MEASURES
- Allergy shots may be continued, but should not be initiated during pregnancy.
- Avoidance of triggers:
  - Avoid tobacco smoke.
  - Use allergen-impermeable mattress and pillow covers.
  - Remove carpeting.
  - Wash bedding in hot water weekly.
  - Reduce indoor humidity.
  - Leave the house when vacuumed.
  - Remove furry pets from home (or at least bedroom).
  - Control cockroaches by traps and eliminating exposed food or garbage.
  - Treat reflux esophagitis.

PREGNANCY-SPECIFIC ISSUES
- The effects of pregnancy on the course of asthma are variable: 23% improved and 30% become worse during pregnancy.
- Nonselective β-blockers, carboprost (15-methyl PGF2-α), ergonovine, and methylergonovine (Methergine) can trigger bronchospasm. Indomethacin can also induce bronchospasm in the aspirin-sensitive patient.
- PGE2 or PGE1 can be used but respiratory status should be monitored. Magnesium sulfate and calcium channel blockers should be well tolerated in pregnant asthmatic subjects.

By Trimester
- 2nd trimester may have least asthma symptoms.
- Intrapartum management:
  - Asthma medications should not be discontinued during labor and delivery.
  - Asthma is usually quiescent during labor; consideration should be given to assessing PEFRs upon admission and at 12-hour intervals.

- The patient should be kept hydrated and should receive adequate analgesia to decrease the risk of bronchospasm.
- An elective delivery should be postponed if the patient is having an exacerbation.

Risks for Mother
- Asthma exacerbations may cause morbidity and/or mortality.
- Increased risk for preeclampsia if daily symptoms
- Increased risk for cesarean delivery if moderate or severe asthma
- Increased risk of gestational diabetes if oral steroids

Risks for Fetus
- Morbidity and mortality if uncontrolled asthma or severe exacerbations
- Preterm delivery if severe or oral steroids
- SGA if daily symptoms
- Fetal distress

MEDICATION (DRUGS)
- Mild intermittent asthma:
  - No daily medications, albuterol as needed
- Mild persistent asthma:
  - Preferred: Low-dose inhaled corticosteroid
  - Alternative: Cromolyn, leukotriene receptor antagonist, or theophylline (serum level 5–12 μg/mL)
- Moderate persistent asthma:
  - Preferred: Low-dose inhaled corticosteroid and salmeterol, or medium-dose inhaled corticosteroid or (if needed) medium-dose inhaled corticosteroid and salmeterol
  - Alternative: Low-dose or (if needed) medium-dose inhaled corticosteroid and either leukotriene receptor antagonist or theophylline (serum level 5–12 μg/mL)
- Severe persistent asthma:
  - Preferred: High-dose inhaled corticosteroid and salmeterol and (if needed) oral corticosteroid
  - Alternative: High-dose inhaled corticosteroid and theophylline (serum level 5–12 μg/mL) and oral corticosteroid if needed
- Specific drugs and classes of drugs:
  - Budesonide preferred; other inhaled corticosteroids may be continued if good control by these agents prior to pregnancy
  - Salmeterol is preferred add-on controller therapy when asthma not well-controlled (symptoms > twice/week, nocturnal symptoms > twice/month, or PEFR or FEV1 <80% predicted). Alternative add-on therapies are theophylline, montelukast, or zafirlukast.
  - For patients not well-controlled on medium-dose inhaled corticosteroids and salmeterol, inhaled corticosteroids should be increased to high-dose.

    - For severe symptoms, a course of oral corticosteroids may be necessary to attain control, along with a step-up in therapy.
    - Regular oral corticosteroids may be required for some patients with severe asthma.

– If systemic corticosteroids have been used in the previous 4 weeks, IV corticosteroids (e.g., hydrocortisone 100 mg q8h) should be administered during labor and for the 24 hours after delivery to prevent adrenal crisis.
– Intranasal corticosteroids are the most effective for allergic rhinitis:
  ○ Loratadine (Claritin) or cetirizine (Zyrtec) are recommended 2nd-generation antihistamines.
  ○ Oral decongestants in 1st trimester have been associated with gastroschisis; thus, intranasal decongestants or intranasal corticosteroids should be considered 1st.
• Breast-feeding:
  – Prednisone, theophylline, antihistamines, inhaled corticosteroids, β_2 agonists, and cromolyn are not considered to be contraindications for breast-feeding.
  – Among sensitive individuals, theophylline may cause toxic effects in the neonate.

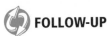 **FOLLOW-UP**

DISPOSITION
Issues for Referral
Consider consultation or referral to asthma specialist and/or perinatologist for patients with persistent asthma.

PROGNOSIS
• Patients with mild asthma had an exacerbation rate of 12.6% and hospitalization rate of 2.3%
• Moderate asthma: 25.7% and 6.8%
• Severe asthma: 51.9% and 26.9%

COMPLICATIONS
• Management of asthma exacerbations
• Initial assessment and treatment:
  – History, exam, PEFR or FEV1, pulse oximetry
  – Consider fetal monitoring and/or BPP if fetus is potentially viable.

ALERT
• If severe (FEV1 or PEFR <50% with severe symptoms at rest) then high-dose albuterol by nebulizer q20min or continuously for 1 hour and inhaled ipratropium bromide and systemic corticosteroid
• Albuterol by MDI or nebulizer, up to 3 doses in 1st hour
• Oral corticosteroid if no immediate response or if patient recently treated with systemic corticosteroid
• Oxygen to maintain saturation >95%
• Repeat assessment: Symptoms, physical exam, PEFR, oxygen saturation
• Continue albuterol q60min for 1–3 hours provided improvement occurs.
• Repeat assessment:
  – Symptoms, physical exam, PEFR, oxygen saturation, other tests as needed
  – Continue fetal assessment
• Good response:
  – FEV1 or PEFR ≥70%
  – Response sustained 60 minutes after last treatment
  – No distress, physical exam normal
  – Reassuring fetal status
  – Discharge home

• Incomplete response:
  – FEV1 or PEFR ≥50% but <70%
  – Mild or moderate symptoms
  – Continue fetal assessment until patient stabilized
  – Monitor FEV1 or PEFR, oxygen saturation, pulse
  – Continue inhaled albuterol and oxygen
  – Inhaled ipratropium bromide
  – Systemic (oral or intravenous) corticosteroid
  – Individualize decision for hospitalization
• Poor response:
  – FEV1 or PEFR <50%
  – $P_{CO_2} > 42$ mm Hg
  – Severe symptoms, drowsiness, confusion
  – Continue fetal assessment
  – Admit to ICU
• Impending or actual respiratory arrest:
  – Admit to ICU
  – Intubation with 100% oxygen
  – Nebulized albuterol plus inhaled ipratropium bromide
  – IV corticosteroid
• Discharge home:
  – Continue treatment with albuterol
  – Oral systemic corticosteroid if indicated
  – Initiate or continue inhaled corticosteroid until review at medical follow-up
  – Patient education: Review medicine use, review/initiate action plan, recommend close medical follow-up

PATIENT MONITORING
Mother
Determine FEV1 or PEFR for asthma symptoms or exacerbations.

Fetus
• Consider early US for dating. Consider NST (starting at 32 weeks) and serial US if suboptimally controlled or moderate to severe asthma, and after a severe exacerbation.
• Intensity of antenatal surveillance should be considered on the basis of the severity of the asthma as well as any other high-risk features of the pregnancy.
• Instruct all patients to be attentive to fetal activity.

BIBLIOGRAPHY

Bracken MB, et al. Asthma symptoms, severity, and drug therapy: A prospective study of effects on 2205 pregnancies. *Obstet Gynecol*. 2003;1024:739–752.
Dombrowski MP, et al. Asthma during pregnancy. *Obstet Gynecol*. 2004;103:5–12.
National Asthma Education and Prevention Program Expert panel report. Managing asthma during pregnancy: Recommendations for pharmacologic treatment - 2004 update. NHLBI, NIH #05-3279. Available at: www.nhlbi.nih.gov/health/prof/lung/asthma/astpreg.htm.

 MISCELLANEOUS

Goals of asthma therapy during pregnancy:
• Maintain adequate oxygenation of the fetus by prevention of maternal hypoxic episodes
• Minimal or no symptoms or exacerbations
• No limitations on activities
• Maintenance of (near) normal pulmonary function
• Minimal use of short-acting inhaled β_2-agonists

CLINICAL PEARLS
• It is safer for pregnant women with asthma to be treated with asthma medications than it is for them to have asthma symptoms and exacerbations.
• Clinical evaluation of asthma includes subjective assessments and pulmonary function tests.
• Identifying and controlling or avoiding such factors as allergens and irritants, particularly tobacco smoke, can lead to improved maternal well-being with less need for medication.
• Step-care therapy uses the principle of tailoring medical therapy according to asthma severity.
• Women on asthma medications may breast-feed.
• Asthma self-management education, including self-monitoring, correct use of inhalers, and an action plan, are part of optimal gestational asthma therapy.

ABBREVIATIONS
• BPP—Biophysical profile
• FEV1—Forced expiratory volume at 1 second
• PGE—Prostaglandin
• MDI—Metered dose inhaler
• NST—Nonstress test
• PEFR—Peak expiratory flow rate
• SGA—Small for gestational age

CODES
ICD9-CM
• 493.00 Extrinsic asthma, unspecified
• 493.10 Intrinsic asthma, unspecified
• 493.90 Asthma, unspecified

 PATIENT TEACHING

Patients should know the interrelationships between asthma and pregnancy, and understand the need for self-monitoring, correct use of inhalers, and following a plan for managing asthma long-term and for promptly handling signs of worsening asthma.

Section VI

BREAST CANCER AND PREGNANCY

Vicki L. Seltzer, MD

BASICS

DESCRIPTION
- Diagnosing and treating breast cancer during pregnancy presents many challenges.
- Prognosis is better than had previously been reported.

EPIDEMIOLOGY
- Worldwide, breast cancer occurs in from 1 in 3,000–1 in 10,000 pregnancies
- Breast cancer is among the most commonly diagnosed cancers in pregnancy, along with cervical cancer.
- Only 0.2–3.8% of breast cancers in women <50 are detected during pregnancy or postpartum.
- 10–20% of breast cancers in women ≤30 are discovered in pregnancy or the year after delivery.

RISK FACTORS
- Age:
  - Increasing risk with advancing age
  - 1st pregnancy after age 30 also increases risk
  - With demographic trend toward delay of 1st pregnancy, rates of breast cancer during pregnancy could be expected to increase.
- Family history:
  - Family history, particularly if breast cancer occurred in 1st-degree relatives, increases risk.
  - 1st-degree relatives with *premenopausal* breast cancer further increases risk.
- Early menarche
- 75% of women with breast cancer have no high risk factors; thus all breast complaints must be evaluated.

Genetics
- BRCA1 and BRCA2 mutation carriers have greatly increased risk of breast cancer overall, and may be more likely to develop breast cancer during pregnancy.
- Multiparity appears protective in BRCA1 carriers.
- Increasing parity may be associated with increasing risk in BRCA2 carriers.

PATHOPHYSIOLOGY
Pregnancy Considerations
- Physiologic breast changes during pregnancy (engorgement, hypertrophy), make physical exam and interpretation of findings more difficult.
- Majority of tumors are invasive ductal carcinomas, as in nonpregnant women.
- 40–80% present with poorly differentiated tumors, although a case-control study suggested no greater percentage than in nonpregnant women.
- Perhaps higher rate of inflammatory tumors than in nonpregnant women
- More commonly present with lymph node involvement, large tumors
- More likely to present at advanced stage
- May be less likely to be estrogen and/or progesterone receptor–positive tumors

DIAGNOSIS

SIGNS AND SYMPTOMS
History
- All breast complaints during pregnancy must be investigated. Do not assume that a breast complaint is physiologic or merely related to pregnancy.
- Common history for breast cancer in pregnancy is that patient palpates a mass:
  - Any mass in the breast during pregnancy must be addressed promptly.
- With inflammatory breast cancer, history may include edema, warmth, and breast complaints suggestive of infection.

Physical Exam
- Exam and interpretation of findings may be more difficult.
- Inspect and palpate breasts with patient sitting up and lying down.
- Evaluate for adenopathy.

TESTS
- See Imaging.
- After appropriate imaging has been performed, a biopsy should be done unless malignancy has been ruled out.
  - 10–15% of women with breast cancer will have normal mammograms. This percentage of false-negative mammograms is even higher in pregnant women.
  - If a lesion is clinically questionable, a normal mammogram is insufficient to rule out malignancy.
- Do not delay an indicated biopsy because the patient is pregnant. Delay in diagnosis can worsen the prognosis.
- Staging is indicated to rule out metastases.

Labs
- Tissue diagnosis of clinically suspicious mass is required for definitive diagnosis.
- Core, incisional, or excisional biopsy may be performed, preferably under local anesthesia.

Imaging
- Mammography:
  - Screening mammography is not performed during pregnancy.
  - Diagnostic mammography with fetal shielding is appropriate when needed, unless other modalities have been able to fully evaluate the problem, and a diagnosis is obtained.
  - Mammography is less sensitive during pregnancy.
- US:
  - Useful in distinguishing between a cyst and a solid lesion
  - May be helpful in identifying lesions suspicious for malignancy
  - False-negatives for malignancy not uncommon
  - When mammography is required, a normal US does not negate the need for the mammogram.
- MRI:
  - May be helpful in the assessment

DIFFERENTIAL DIAGNOSIS
- Galactocele (milk retention cyst), abscess, fibroadenoma, lactating adenoma, cystic changes, lobular hyperplasia, lipoma, hamartoma
- Rarely: Lymphoma, phyllodes tumor, sarcoma, neuroma, TB

TREATMENT

GENERAL MEASURES
- Breast cancer during pregnancy should be diagnosed and treated promptly, using many of the same general principles as in the nonpregnant woman.
- Abortion may not necessarily be required, but may be performed, with subsequent treatment as in the nonpregnant woman.
- Mastectomy with axial node dissection is traditionally considered the treatment choice when the patient elects to continue the pregnancy.
- If a small breast cancer is diagnosed very late in pregnancy, the woman may be able to decide to have a lumpectomy, with radiation initiated soon after delivery.
- Radiation generally is avoided in pregnancy because of risk of teratogenicity and induction of childhood malignancies and hematologic disorders.
- Decisions regarding systemic therapy and timing of initiation depend upon the disease characteristics and the stage of gestation. The patient will make this decision in conjunction with the medical oncologist, surgical oncologist, obstetrician-gynecologist, and others.
- Risks to the fetus from particular chemotherapeutic systemic agents must be a key consideration; most are pregnancy category D.

By Trimester
- 1st trimester: The period of exposure to chemotherapy is critical, with the greatest risk during period of organogenesis.
- 2nd and 3rd trimester:
  - Low incidence of malformations from chemotherapy
  - Several additional risks, some of which are agent-specific
  - Risk of IUGR, prematurity, LBW in ~1/2

Risks for Mother
The biggest risk to the mother is a delay in diagnosis or delay in treatment. This potentially will have an adverse impact on cure rates.

Risks for Fetus
- At present, radiation is not utilized due to risks of congenital anomalies and oncogenesis.
- Surgery and anesthesia exposure are not associated with high risk.

MEDICATION (DRUGS)
Systemic therapy is individualized based upon stage, disease characteristics, trimester, and risks of systemic therapy to the fetus vs. risk to the mother of delaying systemic therapy. Systemic therapy during pregnancy may be advised for patients with advanced disease. The choice of drugs would be those which minimize risk to the fetus during the particular gestational stage.

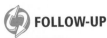 FOLLOW-UP

DISPOSITION

Issues for Referral
Postpartum, the woman will continue to receive care from her oncology team and her obstetrician-gynecologist.

PROGNOSIS
- Breast cancer diagnosed during pregnancy is associated with larger tumors and a greater likelihood of positive lymph nodes.
- Many older series showed a very poor prognosis for breast cancer diagnosed during pregnancy.
- When all disease characteristics are identical, and diagnosis and treatment are prompt, breast cancer during pregnancy has been shown in some recent series to have the same prognosis as breast cancer in the nonpregnant woman.

COMPLICATIONS
The worst complication is the failure to make the diagnosis, resulting in a more advanced stage and a worse prognosis.

PATIENT MONITORING

Fetus
- Confirmation of GA is critical for planning.
- Assessment of fetal pulmonary maturity may be required if preterm delivery is considered.

BIBLIOGRAPHY

Leslie KK, et al. Breast cancer and pregnancy. *Obstet Gynecol Clin North Am*. 2005;32(4):547–558.

Petrek J. et al. Breast cancer in pregnant and postpartum women. *J Obstet Gynaecol Canada*. 2003;25:944–950.

Seltzer V. Breast disease work-up for the generalist. *Obg Mgt*. 2006;18:58–76.

Seltzer VL, et al. The breast. In: Seltzer VL, et al., eds. *Women's Primary Health Care,* 2nd ed. New York: McGraw-Hill; 2000:793–823.

 MISCELLANEOUS

SYNONYM(S)
- Gestational breast cancer
- Pregnancy-associated breast cancer

CLINICAL PEARLS
- Any mass in the breast of a pregnant woman must receive the same prompt attention as a mass in a nonpregnant woman.
- Breast cancers diagnosed during pregnancy more often are diagnosed at an advanced stage.

- Recent information suggests that when disease stage and all clinical and pathologic characteristics are identical, the prognosis for breast cancer diagnosed during pregnancy may be as favorable as that in the nonpregnant woman.

ABBREVIATIONS
- GA—Gestational age
- IUGR—Intrauterine growth restriction
- LBW—Low birth weight

 CODES

ICD9-CM
648.9 Other conditions complicating pregnancy

 PATIENT TEACHING

As in the nonpregnant patient, when a patient identifies a mass in her breast or any other breast problems, this must promptly be brought to the attention of her physician.

Section VI

CONGENITAL HEART DISEASE AND PREGNANCY

Annette E. Bombrys, DO
Jeffery C. Livingston, MD

 BASICS

DESCRIPTION
Types of CHD:
- VSD
- ASD
- PDA
- Pulmonary stenosis
- COA
- Tetralogy of Fallot
- Transposition of the great vessels

Age-Related Factors
Because of advances in pediatric cardiology and cardiovascular surgery, as well as advances in the neonatal and pediatric care of infants with CHD, an increasing number of women with CHD are reaching reproductive age in relatively good health. Thus ob-gyns are more likely to see pregnant women with CHD than in years past.

EPIDEMIOLOGY
Among pregnant women with CHD, the incidence of specific types is:
- VSD: 13%
- ASD: 9%
- PDA: 2.7%
- Pulmonary stenosis: 8%
- Aortic stenosis: 20%
- COA: 8%
- Tetralogy of Fallot: 12%
- Transposition: 5.4%

RISK FACTORS
- Maternal DM, phenylketonuria, connective tissue disease, or exposure to drugs (lithium, alcohol, and anticonvulsants)
- Maternal infection with rubella, coxsackie virus, and CMV is associated with CHD.

Genetics
- Maternal CHD increases the risk of fetal CHD from 1% to 4–6%.
- 1 affected sibling increases risk 1–3%.
- >1 affected sibling increases risk 5–15%.

ASSOCIATED CONDITIONS
Eisenmenger syndrome: Pulmonary-to-systemic shunting associated with cyanosis and increased pulmonary pressures:
- Can develop from septal defects or PDA

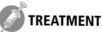 **DIAGNOSIS**

SIGNS AND SYMPTOMS
History
- Classic symptoms of heart disease include palpitations, shortness of breath with exertion, and chest pain.
- Worsening dyspnea, especially at rest, shortness of breath, irregular heart rate, or rapid heart rate

Physical Exam
- VSD: Harsh systolic murmur that radiates to the left sternal border but not to the carotids
- ASD: Split S2 that is fixed with respiration
- PDA: Continuous murmur at the upper left sternal border

TESTS
Imaging
- Color flow Doppler echocardiography
- CXR if CHF is suspected.
- Event monitoring and ECG if a cardiac arrhythmia is suspected.

DIFFERENTIAL DIAGNOSIS
- Any diastolic murmur and any systolic murmur greater than grade 3/6 or that radiates to the carotids should be considered pathologic.
- Systolic flow murmur is normal in pregnancy.

Drugs
Lithium is associated with Ebstein anomaly.

 TREATMENT

GENERAL MEASURES
- Screening for bacteriuria and vaccination against influenza and pneumococcus are appropriate for pregnant women with CHD.
- Treatment or prophylaxis of anemia with iron and folate is recommended.
  - Avoid excessive blood loss.

PREGNANCY-SPECIFIC ISSUES
- Most common associated conditions that require hemodynamic monitoring are severe preeclampsia, ARDS, pneumonia, previously undiagnosed heart disease, and fluid management after resuscitation from obstetric hemorrhage.
- Induction of labor at term with a favorable cervix is ideal.
- Cesarean delivery is recommended for obstetric indications only.
- Adequate anesthesia is a must.
- Avoid maternal pushing; use a low forceps or vacuum delivery.
- Aggressive diuresis postpartum is necessary.
- Increased risk of pulmonary edema
- Increased risk of PE from arrhythmias

Risks for Mother
- Significant maternal mortality is associated with Eisenmenger syndrome, pulmonary HTN with right ventricular dysfunction, and Marfan syndrome with aortic root dilatation. Pregnancy outcomes with other cardiac disease is favorable with aggressive treatment and lifestyle modification.
- Pulmonary edema
- CHF
- Arrhythmias
- HTN
- Maternal death

Risks for Fetus
- Increased risk of CHD
- PTL
- IUGR

MEDICATION (DRUGS)
- β-Blocker: Heart rate control
- Diuretics: CHF/Pulmonary edema
- ACE inhibitors if not breastfeeding

SURGERY
Surgical correction of cardiac anomaly is recommended prior to conception.

 FOLLOW-UP

DISPOSITION
Issues for Referral
All patients with CHD should be followed in conjunction with a specialist in the field of MFM and a cardiologist.

PROGNOSIS
- Poor prognosis:
  - Significant maternal mortality is associated with Eisenmenger syndrome, pulmonary HTN with right ventricular dysfunction, and Marfan syndrome with aortic root dilatation.
  - Pregnancy with cyanosis have a poorer outcome than pregnancies without.
- Good prognosis:
  - Pregnancy outcomes with other cardiac disease is favorable with aggressive treatment and lifestyle modification.

COMPLICATIONS
- Pulmonary edema
- CHF
- Arrhythmias
- HTN
- Maternal death
- Heart failure
- IUFD

PATIENT MONITORING
Mother
ECG in 3rd trimester

Fetus
Fetal ECG at 20–22 weeks' gestation

BIBLIOGRAPHY

Bonow R, et al. ACC/AGA guidelines for the management of patients with valvular heart disease. Executive summary: A report of the American College of Cardiology/American Heart Association Task Force on practice guidelines (committee on management of patients with valvular heart disease). *J Heart Valve Dis*. 1998;7:672.

Easterling R, et al. Heart Disease. In: *Obstetrics: Normal and Problem Pregnancies*. Philadelphia: Elsevier Health Sciences; 2001:1005–1030.

Reimond SC, et al. Valvular heart disease in pregnancy. *N Engl J Med*. 2003;349:52–59.

 MISCELLANEOUS

ABBREVIATIONS
- ACE—Angiotensin converting enzyme
- ARDS—Acute respiratory distress syndrome
- ASD—Atrial septal defect
- CHD—Congenital heart disease
- CHF—Congestive heart failure
- CMV—Cytomegalovirus
- COA—Coarctation of the aorta
- IUFD—Intrauterine fetal demise
- IUGR—Intrauterine fetal growth restriction
- MFM—Maternal-fetal medicine
- PE—Pulmonary embolism
- PDA—Patent ductus arteriosis
- PTL—Preterm labor
- VSD—Ventricular septal defect

CODES
ICD9-CM
648.5X Congenital heart disease (specify)

 PATIENT TEACHING

PREVENTION
- Pregnancy should be discouraged in patients with Eisenmenger syndrome, pulmonary HTN with right ventricular dysfunction, and Marfan syndrome with aortic root dilatation:
  - Counseling regarding effective forms of contraception or sterilization is necessary for women with these conditions.
- Preconception counseling and pregnancy planning is appropriate for ALL women with CHD.

Section VI

DIABETES AND PREGNANCY

Kimberly W. Hickey, MD
Menachem Miodovnik, MD

 BASICS

DESCRIPTION
- Type 1 DM:
  - Absolute insulin deficiency due to pancreatic β-cell destruction.
- Type 2 DM:
  - Insulin resistance and insulin deficiency
- GDM:
  - Insulin resistance and relative insulin deficiency associated with pregnancy
- A major cause of maternal and fetal morbidity and mortality

EPIDEMIOLOGY
Types 1, 2, and GDM, affect 14% of pregnancies:
- 10% of these have pregestational DM
- 90% with GDM:
  - 3% of these have undiagnosed Type 2 DM
  - Type 1 DM affects 1 in 300 women.

RISK FACTORS
- Risk factors:
  - History of GDM
  - Obesity
  - Age >25
  - 1st-degree relative with DM
  - Ethnic groups:
    - Hispanic, African, South or East Asian, Pacific Island, or Native American
  - History of macrosomia, shoulder dystocia, or unexplained stillbirth
- Risk factors are also suggested criteria for early screening for GDM.

Genetics
- Complex interaction of genes identified for Type 1 and Type 2 DM:
  - Up to 18 different regions on the human genome have been linked to Type 1 DM.
  - These regions (IDDM1–IDDM 18) are located on chromosomes 1,2, 5, 6, 10, 14, 15, and 18.
  - HLA Class II alleles have been identified in region IDDM 1 and are present in up to 40% of patients with Type 1 DM.
  - 40% of those with Type 2 DM have a parent with DM, suggesting a strong genetic basis.
- No single marker occurring only in those destined to develop DM has yet been identified.
- In utero environment (imprinting) may affect risk of DM as adult (Barker hypothesis).

PATHOPHYSIOLOGY
- Pregestational DM:
  - Type 1 DM:
    - Pancreatic β-cell destruction
    - Majority of cases thought to be autoimmune
  - Type 2 DM:
    - Failure of insulin to maintain glycemic homeostasis
    - Insulin resistance with progressive insulin secretory defect
    - Postprandial hyperglycemia that progresses to persistent hyperglycemic state
- GDM:
  - Increasing insulin resistance associated with advancing GA and placental hormones

ASSOCIATED CONDITIONS
- Maternal complications of DM:
  - Diabetic retinopathy
  - Diabetic nephropathy
  - Coronary artery disease
  - Chronic HTN
  - Diabetic neuropathy
  - Maternal hypoglycemia
  - Obesity
- Complications associated with DM and pregnancy:
  - Diabetic embryopathy:
    - Decreased rate of fertility
    - Increased rate of spontaneous abortion
    - Increased rate of major and minor congenital malformations
  - Abnormal fetal growth:
    - Macrosomia
    - Fetal growth restriction
  - Hypertrophic cardiomyopathy
  - Neonatal metabolic disturbances:
    - Hypocalcemia
    - Hypomagnesemia
    - Hypoglycemia
    - Polycythemia
    - Hyperbilirubinemia
  - Neonatal respiratory decompensation:
    - Increased rate of respiratory distress syndrome with poor glycemic control
    - Increased rate of transient tachypnea of the newborn
- Obstetric complications associated with DM:
  - Gestational HTN
  - Preeclampsia
  - Preterm delivery
  - Polyhydramnios
  - Infectious morbidity
  - Uteroplacental insufficiency
  - Stillbirth
  - Acute worsening of diabetic retinopathy

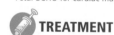 **DIAGNOSIS**

SIGNS AND SYMPTOMS
History
Pregestational DM:
- Polyuria
- Polydipsia
- Unexplained weight loss
- Ketoacidosis
- Polyhydramnios in absence of fetal anomalies

TESTS
- Diagnostic criteria for pregestational DM:
  - Symptoms of DM and random plasma glucose of ≥200 mg/dL
  - Fasting plasma glucose level of ≥126 mg/dL
  - 2-hour plasma glucose ≥200 mg/dL during an OGTT:
    - 75 g anhydrous glucose dissolved in water
- Screening and diagnostic criteria for GDM:
  - Screening at 24–28 weeks EGA (unless risk factors for early screening)
  - 1-hour 50-mg OGTT
  - If plasma glucose ≥130 mg/dL, do 3-hour OGTT

- Diagnosis with 3-hour 100-mg OGTT:
  - GDM diagnosed if 2 abnormal plasma glucose values:
    - Fasting ≥95 mg/dL
    - 1 hour ≥180 mg/dL
    - 2 hour ≥155 mg/dL
    - 3 hour ≥140 mg/dL
- Assessment of end-organ involvement for preventive care and health maintenance in 1st trimester if pregestational DM:
  - Exam by ophthalmologist for retinopathy
  - EKG if ≥35 years old, obese, hypertension, renal disease, hypercholesterolemia, or DM for >10 years
  - Stress test if EKG suggests CVD
  - 24-hour urine for protein and creatinine with serum creatinine to assess renal function and estimate GFR
  - Thyroid panel for autoimmune disease
  - Hemoglobin A1C to assess glycemic control prior to conception or at the 1st visit
- Glucose monitoring:
  - Use glucometer with memory to provide feedback on targets of glycemic control
  - Self-monitored plasma glucose concentrations on waking (fasting), before each meal, postprandial, and nighttime: 7 measurements a day.
  - Consider 3 a.m. plasma glucose if unexplained persistent fasting hyperglycemia
  - Targets: Fasting ≤60–90 mg/dL, pre-meal ≤80–95 mg/dL, 1-hour postprandial ≤140 mg/dL, or 2-hour postprandial ≤120 mg/dL
  - Hemoglobin A1C as close to normal (≤6%) as possible without hypoglycemia

Imaging
- US:
  - Serial sonograms for fetal growth
- Fetal ECHO for cardiac malformations

 TREATMENT

GENERAL MEASURES
- Interdisciplinary team for management
- Intensive glycemic control:
  - Dietary regulation:
    - Reduce carbohydrates to 40–50% of total calories OR focus on low glycemic index carbohydrates as 60% of total calories
    - Total calories based on prepregnancy BMI. BMI ≤20, 35–38 kcal/kg; BMI 20–25, 30 kcal/kg; BMI ≥26, 20–25 kcal/kg.
    - Calories as 3 meals and up to 4 snacks, adjusting for lifestyle and work schedule
- Control of chronic HTN
- Photocoagulation for proliferative retinopathy, prior to pregnancy
- Recommended exercise: 20 minutes a day, 3–4 times a week

PREGNANCY-SPECIFIC ISSUES

- Preconception measures:
  - Intensive glucose control, as majority of birth defects occur before pregnancy is recognized
- Renal disease:
  - Pregnancy is not a risk factor for development or progression of nephropathy.
  - Proteinuria may increase due to physiologic changes of pregnancy.
- Progression of retinopathy associated with rapid normalization of glucose levels, transient.

By Trimester

- Routine prenatal labs PLUS:
- Each trimester:
  - Hgb A1C to assess glycemic control
  - Evaluation of renal function
- 1st trimester:
  - US for accurate dating
  - Evaluation for CVD
  - Exam by ophthalmologist for retinopathy
- 2nd trimester:
  - Sonogram to screen for fetal anomalies
  - If pregestational DM, fetal ECHO 18–20 weeks EGA
  - Sonograms for fetal growth every 4 weeks
- 3rd trimester:
  - Sonograms for fetal growth every 4 weeks
  - Antepartum fetal testing with NST and AFI or BPP twice weekly starting at 32 weeks EGA or 28 weeks EGA if other obstetric complications
- Intrapartum:
  - Usual evening dose of insulin injection or insulin pump overnight until arrival
  - Hold the morning dose of insulin.
  - Assess initial glucose concentration; then q1h in labor
  - Goal of plasma glucose concentrations between 70 and 100 mg/dL throughout labor
  - Continuous insulin drips during labor:
    - Consult MFM or endocrinology for protocol
- Postpartum:
  - Pregestational doses of insulin or pump rates

Risks for Mother

- Diabetic ketoacidosis at much lower glucose levels (i.e., 250 mg/dL)
- Proliferative retinopathy associated with rapid normalization of glucose levels
- Increased frequency of hypoglycemic episodes, frequently asymptomatic
- Increased risk for preeclampsia and gestational HTN
- PTL
- Increased risk of infection including pyelonephritis, endometritis, and postpartum wound infections

Risks for Fetus

- Risks associated with poor glycemic control:
  - Fetal growth restriction or macrosomia with difficulty maintaining euglycemia in the immediate postpartum period
  - Major congenital anomalies:
    - Higher hemoglobin A1C associated with higher rates of congenital anomalies: NTDs, cardiac malformations
    - Caudal regression syndrome highly associated with poor glycemic control.
  - Macrosomia with increased risk of shoulder dystocia and fetal injury: Brachial nerve palsies, hypoxic neurologic insults, and death

---

- Hypertrophic cardiomyopathy, with thickened ventricular septum and walls
  - Neonatal hypocalcemia and/or hypomagnesemia
  - Neonatal hypoglycemia
- Neonatal polycythemia with risks related to hyperviscosity
- Hyperbilirubinemia
- Stillbirth

MEDICATION (DRUGS)

- Pregestational diabetes should be treated with an insulin regimen as first-line therapy:
  - Type I DM: 0.9 U/kg/d in 1st trimester; 1 U/kg/d in 2nd trimester; and 1.2 U/kg/d in 3rd trimester
  - Type II DM: 0.9 U/kg/d in 1st trimester; 1.2 U/kg/d in 2nd trimester; 1.6 U/kg/d in 3rd trimester
- If GDM doesn't respond to exercise and diet, begin with oral hypoglycemic agents (glyburide):
  - Glyburide (sulfonylurea): Starting dose 2.5 mg PO in a.m. If target concentrations not obtained, add 2.5 mg to a.m. dose. If after 3–7 days, targets not reached, then add a 5-mg PO evening dose with titration up to 10 mg PO b.i.d.
- If glycemic control not adequate with glyburide initiate insulin therapy:
  - Biphasic insulin requirements: Increasing dose up to 30 weeks then stabilizing. Estimate dose based on BMI. BMI ≤25, 0.8 U/kg/d; BMI ≥25, 1 U/kg/d.
- Insulin dosing:
  - 2/3 of total dose in morning, 1/3 in evening:
    - Morning dose 2:1 intermediate/rapid acting
    - Evening dose 1:1 intermediate/rapid acting
- Insulin pumps, carbohydrate counting with use of Lispro (fast-acting insulins), or use of Lantus (once or twice daily dosed insulin) should be undertaken with an MFM or endocrinologist consultation. These new insulins have not yet been approved for use in pregnancy.

 FOLLOW-UP

DISPOSITION

Issues for Referral

- Ophthalmology for retinopathy
- Endocrinology or MFM for comanagement for nontraditional insulin therapies, and to establish good life-long diabetes care
- Subspecialist, either perinatology (MFM) or pediatric cardiology, for fetal ECHO
- Perinatology regarding neonatal care

PROGNOSIS

- Pregestational DM: Excellent with strict glycemic control
- Gestational DM: Excellent although increased risk for developing DM and recurrent GDM

COMPLICATIONS

Progression of proliferative retinopathy

PATIENT MONITORING

Mother

- Hemoglobin A1C for long-term glycemic control
- Self-monitoring blood glucose concentrations to achieve good glycemic control

Fetus

Antepartum fetal testing beginning in the 3rd trimester

BIBLIOGRAPHY

ACOG Practice Bulletin No. 60. Pregestational Diabetes Mellitus. Washington DC: ACOG; 2005.

American Diabetes Association. Standards of Medical Care in Diabetes–2007. *Diabetes Care.* 2007;30:S4–S65.

Gabbe S, et al. Management of diabetes mellitus complicating pregnancy. *Obstet Gynecol.* 2003; 102:857-868.

Langer O, ed. *The Diabetes in Pregnancy Dilemma,* 1st ed. Lanham MD: University Press of America; 2006.

 MISCELLANEOUS

CLINICAL PEARLS

Preconceptional counseling and glycemic control are key to successful pregnancy outcome.

ABBREVIATIONS

- BPP—Biophysical profile
- DM—Diabetes mellitus
- CVD—Cardiovascular disease
- ECHO—Echocardiogram
- EGA—Estimated gestational age
- GA—Gestational age
- GDM—Gestational diabetes mellitus
- GFR—Glomerular filtration rate
- MFM—Maternal-fetal medicine
- NST—Nonstress test
- NTD—Neural tube defect
- OGTT—Oral glucose tolerance test
- PTL—Preterm labor
- AFI—Amniotic fluid index

CODES

ICD9-CM

- 250.1 DM with ketoacidosis
- 250.4 DM with renal manifestations
- 250.5 DM with retinopathy
- 250.6 DM with neuropathy
- 648.0 DM, complicating pregnancy, childbirth, puerperium
- 648.8 GDM
- 775.0 Maternal DM affecting the fetus or newborn

 PATIENT TEACHING

PREVENTION

- Effective contraception to prevent unintended pregnancies
- Preconception counseling
- Strict glycemic control prior to conception

EATING DISORDERS IN PREGNANCY

Barbara E. Wolfe, PhD, APRN
M. Colleen Simonelli, PhD(c), RN

BASICS

DESCRIPTION
- Diagnostic characteristics of AN:
  - Refusal to maintain normal body weight (<85% expected for age and height)
  - Excessive fear of weight gain or becoming fat
  - Distorted body image
  - Amenorrhea (for postmenarchal females)
  - Types:
    - Binge eating/purging: Regular binge eating and/or purging behavior (e.g., SIV, laxative use, diuretic use, enemas)
    - Restricting: No recurring binge eating and/or purging behavior. May use other compensatory behaviors (e.g., fasting, excessive exercising)
- Diagnostic characteristics of BN:
  - Repeated binge eating and compensatory behaviors that occur ≥2 twice a week for 3 months
  - Significant influence of weight and body shape on sense of self
  - ≥ Normal body weight for age and height
  - Types:
    - Purging: Regular use of SIV, laxatives, diuretics, or enemas to avoid weight gain
    - Nonpurging: No recurring binge eating or purging behavior. May use other compensatory behaviors (e.g., fasting, excessive exercising)
- Diagnostic characteristics of EDNOS:
  - Does not meet criteria for AN or BN but experiences disturbed eating-related behavior
  - Examples include:
    - Regular binge eating, but no compensatory behaviors while ≥ normal weight
    - Regular compensatory behaviors, but no binge eating while ≥ normal weight
    - Low body weight with regular menstrual cycles

EPIDEMIOLOGY
- Predominant age: Childbearing
- Prevalence:
  - AN and BN are thought to occur in ~1% of young women; EDNOS may occur at higher rates.
  - Prevalence estimates for ED are higher for women attending fertility clinics.
  - Onset of ED during pregnancy can occur, although patients may have active symptoms prior to pregnancy.

RISK FACTORS
- Eating disorders in pregnancy:
  - History of AN, BN, or EDNOS
- Pregnancy in eating disorders:
  - Knowledge deficit regarding risk for pregnancy in the presence of oligomenorrhea (BN)
  - Increased weight gain and normalized hormonal regulation associated with early recovery (AN)
  - Knowledge deficit regarding birth-control practices

Pregnancy Considerations
Recovery from ED prior to conception reduces perinatal morbidity and mortality.

Genetics
Not well studied for the occurrence of eating disorders in pregnancy

PATHOPHYSIOLOGY
- AN: Pregnancy is uncommon due to anovulation; rare occurrences have been reported and may be associated with weight gain and associated normalization of hormonal regulation.
- BN: Although oligomenorrhea and amenorrhea are common, menstrual cycle irregularities do not appear to have long-term influences on ability to conceive.

DIAGNOSIS

SIGNS AND SYMPTOMS
- Absence of expected weight gain associated with pregnancy
- Weight loss or body weight <85% expected for age and height
- Weight gain greater than expected with pregnancy
- Significant weight fluctuations
- Preoccupation with, and fear of, pregnancy-related weight gain
- Shame related to body weight or shape

History
- Body weight:
  - Low and high weight
  - Weight fluctuations
  - Satisfaction with body weight
  - Fear of weight gain, becoming fat
- Eating behavior:
  - Dietary intake and eating patterns
  - Presence of binge eating episodes
  - Presence of compensatory behaviors
- Menstrual cycle:
  - Menarche; delayed onset with low weight may be associated with history of AN
  - Frequency, duration, and amount of flow
  - History of amenorrhea and /or oligomenorrhea
- Sexual history:
  - Number of partners, contraception
- Past medical history:
  - Hospitalizations
  - Surgeries
- Past psychiatric history:
  - Treatments
  - Medications
- Alcohol and substance use

Review of Systems
- Special attention to systems affected by malnutrition or compensatory behaviors:
  - Cardiovascular
  - Endocrine and metabolism
  - GI (e.g., diarrhea, constipation)
  - Neurologic (e.g., syncope, vertigo)
  - Dermatologic
  - Musculoskeletal (bone fractures, osteopenia, osteoporosis)
  - Mental status (e.g., insight, mood, affect; thought process; preoccupations with body shape and weight; distorted body image)

Physical Exam
- General
- Appearance
- Orthostatic VS and BP
- Body mass index (BMI)
- Dermatologic:
  - Dry skin, brittle nails, hair loss, lanugo (malnutrition)
  - Russell sign: Dorsal metacarpal abrasions (SIV)
- ENT:
  - Enamel erosion and tooth sensitivity (SIV)
  - Parotid gland enlargement (SIV)
- Chest and abdomen:
  - AN: Decreased abdominal girth, protruding ribs and iliac crests

TESTS
- ECG may show prolonged QT interval; U waves, and change in S-T wave
- Echocardiogram (e.g., mitral valve prolapse)

Lab
- Blood chemistries:
  - CBC with differential
  - ESR
  - Electrolytes
  - Sodium bicarbonate:
    - Increase is associated with SIV-induced metabolic acidosis.
    - Decrease is associated with laxative-induced metabolic acidosis.
  - BUN
  - Creatinine
  - TSH test
  - AST/ALT, alkaline phosphatase
- UA
- ECG, in the presence of severe malnutrition and ED symptoms

Imaging
- Consider pelvimetry
- US:
  - Congenital anomaly scan
  - Serial US for fetal growth

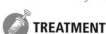

TREATMENT

GENERAL MEASURES
- Medical stability
- Stability of ED symptoms
- Adequate nutritional and fluid intake
- Adequate weight gain

PREGNANCY-SPECIFIC ISSUES
- High-risk pregnancy
- Increased incidence of obstetric complications associated with low and high BMI and poor weight gain in pregnancy:
  - BMI <19:
    - SAB, congenital anomalies, LBW
  - BMI >30:
    - Increased infant mortality

By Trimester
- 1st trimester:
  - Increased risk of SAB
  - Increased risk of congenital anomalies:
    - NTDs
    - Hyperemesis gravidarum
- 2nd trimester:
  - Preeclampsia
  - Gestational diabetes
  - IUGR
  - Prematurity
- 3rd trimester:
  - IUGR
  - Prematurity
  - SGA

Risks for Mother
- SAB
- Hyperemesis gravidarum
- Preeclampsia
- Cesarean birth
- Osteoporosis
- Relapse or exacerbation of ED symptoms
- Return to ED behaviors postpartum
- Postpartum depression

Risks for Fetus
- Congenital anomalies:
  - Cleft lip/palate
  - NTDs
- Premature birth
- IUGR
- SGA/LBW
- Breech presentation
- Decreased 5-minute APGAR score
- Increased perinatal mortality

MEDICATION (DRUGS)
- Folic acid, calcium, iron supplements
- Prenatal vitamins
- SSRI (BN; may be necessary, although not generally recommended during pregnancy, particularly 1st trimester):
  - Careful consideration of risk to child vs. maternal health

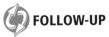 FOLLOW-UP

DISPOSITION
Issues for Referral
- Active ED symptoms:
  - Starvation/Restrictive dieting
  - Binge eating, purging
  - SIV, laxative, diuretic use
  - Excessive exercise pattern
  - Poor weight gain
- Psychiatric comorbidity:
  - Anxiety disorder
  - Alcohol, tobacco, substance abuse
  - Depression
- IUGR

PROGNOSIS
BMI >19, <30, and normal weight gain associated with pregnancy outcomes of general population

COMPLICATIONS
- Symptoms of active ED at diagnosis of pregnancy is associated with return or worsening of ED symptoms in postpartum period.
- Increased risk of postpartum depression (history of AN and/or BN)

PATIENT MONITORING
Mother
- Normal pregnancy weight gain:
  - Assess weight at every prenatal visit
  - AN: Maintain BMI >19
  - BN: Maintain BMI in normal range
- Symptoms of ED behaviors
- Fear of vaginal delivery:
  - Counsel regarding risks/benefits of vaginal vs. cesarean birth
- Symptoms of postpartum depression

Fetus
Serial US:
- Normal growth and development
- Presentation

BIBLIOGRAPHY

American Psychiatric Association. *Diagnostic and Statistical Manual of Mental Disorders*, 4th ed., text revision. Washington, DC: APA; 2000.

American Psychiatric Association Workgroup on Eating Disorders. *Practice Guideline for the Treatment of Patients with Eating Disorders*, 3rd ed. Washington, DC: APA; 2006.

Bulik CM, et al. Fertility and reproduction in women with anorexia nervosa: A controlled study. *J Clin Psychiatry*. 1999;60:130–135.

Carmichael SL, et al. Dieting behaviors and risk of neural tube defect. *Am J Endocrinol*. 2003;158: 1127–1131.

Crow SJ, et al. Long-term menstrual and reproductive function in patients with bulimia nervosa. *Am J Psychiatry*. 2002;159:1048–1050.

Franko DL, et al. Pregnancy complications and neonatal outcomes in women with eating disorders. *Am J Psychiatry*. 2001;158:1461–1466.

 MISCELLANEOUS

CLINICAL PEARLS
- Nondisclosure of ED is likely in OB/GYN and primary care settings.
- Thorough history and review of systems may uncover hidden ED.
- History of amenorrhea or oligomenorrhea may be masked by concurrent contraceptive use.
- In AN, appearance may be deceiving, as individuals attempt to disguise weight.

- Monitor for relapse and/or increase in ED symptoms in postpartum period.
- Active ED is often accompanied by comorbid psychiatric disorder including anxiety, mood, and /or substance use disorder, requiring referral.
- Treatment from mental health ED specialist should begin prior to delivery.
- Throughout prenatal care, include close collaboration with:
  - Nutritionist/Dietary counselor
  - Consulting or treating psychiatric clinician
  - Primary care provider
- Eating behavior must be assessed in all women seeking fertility assistance:
  - Those diagnosed with active AN should not be offered ovulation induction but counseled on weight restoration to restore fecundity.
- Mothers with an ED may have greater difficulties with infant feeding.

ABBREVIATIONS
- AN—Anorexia nervosa
- BN—Bulimia nervosa
- ED—Eating disorder
- EDNOS—Eating disorder not otherwise specified
- IUGR—Intrauterine growth restriction
- LBW—Low birth weight
- NTD—Neural tube defect
- SAB—Spontaneous abortion
- SGA—Small for gestational age
- SIV—Self-induced vomiting
- STD—Sexually transmitted disease

CODES
ICD9-CM
- 307.1 Anorexia nervosa
- 307.51 Bulimia nervosa
- 307.50 Eating disorder unspecified

PATIENT TEACHING

- If not currently engaged in therapy for ED, discuss referral and need for treatment.
- Provide information on amount and timing of weight gain and postpartum weight loss:
  - Prenatal weights done with women facing away from scale
- Counsel women that attempts at caloric restriction may directly affect fetus:
  - Minimum weight gain of 10.5 kg is recommended.
  - Maintenance of BMI >19 is associated with improved outcomes.
- Refer for patient-education on infant feeding
- ED Patient Education pamphlet. Available at http://www.4woman.gov/faq/

PREVENTION
- Primary: Not well-established
- Secondary: Reduce risk of unplanned pregnancy and STDs

GALLBLADDER DISEASE IN PREGNANCY

John D. Scott, MD
Michael S. Nussbaum, MD

BASICS

DESCRIPTION
- Wide differential of diseases related to gallbladder dysfunction and cholelithiasis during pregnancy.
- Asymptomatic cholelithiasis
- Biliary dyskinesia: Biliary colic in absence of gallstones
- Acute cholecystitis: Inflammation of the gallbladder
- Gallstone pancreatitis: Obstruction of the pancreatic duct by gallstones
- Choledocholithiasis: Obstruction of the common bile duct by gallstones, causing ductal dilatation
- Acute cholangitis: Ascending bactibilia caused by distal ductal obstruction, causing bacteremia

EPIDEMIOLOGY
Incidence
Occurs in 1 in 2,000–1 in 4,000 pregnancies

Prevalence
During obstetric US, 2–4% of women are found to harbor asymptomatic gallstones, but only 0.05–0.1% will become symptomatic during the course of their pregnancy.

RISK FACTORS
Independent risk factors for gallstone-related hospitalization during pregnancy and postpartum:

- Strong association:
  - Maternal race: Significantly higher in Native Americans but lower in Asian/Pacific Islanders
  - Age: Maternal age is inversely related to risk
  - Obesity: Risk is significantly increased in pregnant women who are overweight.
  - Pregnancy weight gain: Inversely related to risk
  - Estimated GA: Inversely related to risk
- Weak association:
  - DM
  - History of hormonal contraceptive use
  - Family history
  - Ileal dysfunction (Crohn's disease, bypass surgery)
  - Sedentary lifestyle

Genetics
- Cholesterol gallstones are 2–5 times more common in 1st-degree relatives of patients with known gallstones.
- Asymptomatic women <25 are more likely to have gallstones if they have a positive family history.

PATHOPHYSIOLOGY
- Bile facilitates the intestinal absorption of lipids and fat-soluble vitamins.
- Gallstones are caused by a disruption of the equilibrium between biliary solutes, cholesterol, and calcium salts.
- Cholesterol stones:
  - Most common stone
  - Caused by the supersaturation of bile with cholesterol
- Pigment stones:
  - Smaller, less common gallstone
  - Brown stones are associated with disorders of biliary motility and resultant bacterial infection.

Pregnancy Considerations
In pregnancy, altered physiology related to estrogen and progesterone exacerbates hypomotility and causes a more lithogenic bile.

DIAGNOSIS

SIGNS AND SYMPTOMS
History
- Family history
- Risk factor analysis
- Location, timing, and severity of pain:
  - Intermittent RUQ abdominal pain +/− radiation to right shoulder
  - Nausea
  - Intolerance with fatty foods
  - Gradual improvement

Physical Exam
- A benign physical exam is associated with biliary colic.
- Physical findings associated with complicated gallbladder pathology:
  - Murphy sign, inspiratory arrest with palpation of the gallbladder (acute cholecystitis)
  - Hypotension, tachycardia (ascending cholangitis)
  - Jaundice (biliary obstruction)
  - Fever (acute cholecystitis, cholangitis)
  - Mental status changes (cholangitis)

ALERT
Abdominal pain, fever, and jaundice is known as Charcot triad and is indicative of ASCENDING CHOLANGITIS, which requires emergent drainage of the biliary tract and is associated with a 10% mortality rate if undetected.

TESTS
Lab
LFTs:
- Elevation of alkaline phosphatase, total bilirubin, and direct bilirubin are suggestive of obstruction.

Pregnancy Considerations
Due to placental production, alkaline phosphatase is elevated in the 3rd trimester, often to twice the upper limit of normal.
- CBC:
  - Leukocytosis may indicate the presence of cholecystitis or cholangitis.
- Pancreatic enzymes:
  - An elevated amylase and lipase level suggests biliary pancreatitis.

Imaging
- US:
  - Safe, noninvasive, cost-effective
  - Most commonly used diagnostic modality, with high sensitivity
  - 98% sensitivity for uncomplicated gallstones
  - Can evaluate for ductal dilatation
  - Pericholecystic fluid, gallbladder wall thickening, and the US Murphy sign are hallmarks of acute cholecystitis.

- CT scan:
  - Little role in the evaluation of the gallbladder since most stones are radiolucent, but CT can be used to exclude other pathologies.
  - Fetal exposure to ionizing radiation
- Endoscopic US:
  - Invasive technique
  - Used in patients with biliary obstruction secondary to mass effects.
  - Rarely used in pregnant patients
- Cholecystokinin cholecystoscintigraphy (HIDA scan):
  - Nonvisualization of gallbladder is indicative of cholecystitis
  - Also used to in the post-cholecystectomy setting to rule out bile leaks
  - Diminished gallbladder ejection fraction may be indicative of biliary dyskinesia.

Pregnancy Considerations
- ERCP:
  - Used to detect and remove bile duct stones (choledocholithiasis) and drain the biliary system
  - Requires endoscopy and exposure to radiation
- Deemed safe in the 2nd and 3rd trimester. Minimize fetal exposure with shielding and monitor fetus during anesthesia.
- MRCP:
  - Used in the detection of choledocholithiasis
  - Gadolinium, which crosses the placenta, is used as a contrast agent. The ESUR has confirmed the safety of gadolinium usage in small doses in pregnancy.

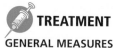 TREATMENT

GENERAL MEASURES
- Uncomplicated biliary pain:
  - Pain meds, IVF, NPO
- Septic patient with history of gallstones:
  - Evaluate for cholangitis, start immediate IV antibiotics
- Diet:
  - Uncomplicated cholelithiasis: Avoid fatty foods
  - Cholecystitis: NPO until pain resolved
- Nursing care
- Monitor vital signs
- Supportive care

PREGNANCY-SPECIFIC ISSUES
Fetal monitoring as appropriate

MEDICATION (DRUGS)

- UDCA, 5 mg/kg b.i.d.
  - Used to dissolve gallstones if <10 mm and normal gallbladder motility
  - UDCA has not been studied in pregnancy.
- Ketorolac 30–60 mg IV and ibuprofen 400 mg PO t.i.d. have been traditionally used to relieve pain, but these are contraindicated in pregnancy.
- Antibiotics:
  - Broad-spectrum antibiotics with enterococcal coverage are required if cholangitis or acute cholecystitis is suspected.
  - 1st line: Ampicillin and gentamicin, piperacillin-tazobactam
  - 2nd line: Imipenem

Pregnancy Considerations
Fluoroquinolones are contraindicated in pregnancy.

> **ALERT**
> Ascending cholangitis is a true emergency, and delay in initiation of antibiotic therapy can lead to fetal demise.

SURGERY

Laparoscopic cholecystectomy:

- Preferred treatment for symptomatic cholelithiasis and acute cholecystitis
- Safest when performed in the 2nd trimester
- Medical management for uncomplicated disease is recommended in the 1st and 3rd trimesters with a delayed cholecystectomy.
- Indications for surgery in pregnancy:
  - Acute cholecystitis
  - Recurrent biliary colic
  - Choledocholithiasis (in combination with ERCP)

Pregnancy Considerations
Surgical management of symptomatic cholelithiasis in pregnancy is safe, decreases hospital stay, and decreases labor induction and preterm delivery.

- ERCP:
  - Indications
    - Ascending cholangitis
    - Choledocholithiasis
    - Gallstone pancreatitis

> **ALERT**
> Untreated gallstone pancreatitis has a maternal mortality rate of 37%.

- Complications:
  - Pancreatitis
  - Bleeding
  - Perforation

> **ALERT**
> Post-ERCP pancreatitis is associated with a significant fetal demise rate (5–7%).

 FOLLOW-UP

DISPOSITION

- Most patients do not require inpatient admission for biliary colic.
- Patients can be discharged home with educational material regarding a healthy diet and risks of recurrent attacks.

Issues for Referral
- Surgical consultation for suspected cholecystitis and cholangitis
- Gastroenterological consultation for choledocholithiasis, pancreatitis, and cholangitis

PROGNOSIS
For uncomplicated cholelithiasis, laparoscopic cholecystectomy in the 2nd trimester is curative.

COMPLICATIONS
From nonoperative management:

- Patients with symptomatic cholelithiasis have a high rate of relapse.
- In patients who have an attack of biliary colic during pregnancy, 38% of women have recurrent attacks and 23% of women will eventually have complications related to their disease.

> **ALERT**
> Medical management of gallstone pancreatitis has a reported maternal mortality rate of 15% and a fetal demise rate as high as 60%.

From surgical management:

- Spontaneous abortion rate of 12% with open cholecystectomy in the 1st trimester, which drops to 5% and 0% in the 2nd and 3rd trimesters, respectively.
- The risk of PTL in the 2nd trimester is close to 0%, this rises to 40% in the 3rd trimester.
- Laparoscopic cholecystectomy in the 2nd trimester is the safest and preferred surgical technique.

BIBLIOGRAPHY

Halkic N, et al. Laparoscopic management of appendicitis and symptomatic cholelithiasis during pregnancy. *Langenbecks Arch Surg*. 2006;391: 467–471.

Juran BD, et al. Genetics of hepatobiliary disease. *Clin Gastroenterol Hepatol*. 2006;4:548–557.

Kahaleh M, et al. Safety and efficacy of ERCP in pregnancy. *Gastrointest Endoscopy*. 2004;60(2): 287–292.

Ko CW. Risk factors for gallstone-related hospitalization during pregnancy and the postpartum. *Am J Gastroenterol*. 2006;101: 2263–2268.

Lowe SA. Diagnostic radiography in pregnancy: Risks and reality. *Aust N Z J Obs Gyn*. 2004;44:191–196.

 MISCELLANEOUS

ABBREVIATIONS

- ERCP—Endoscopic retrograde cholangiopancreatography
- ESUR—European Society of Urogenital Radiology
- HIDA—Hepatobiliary hydroxyiminodiacetic acid scan
- MRCP—Magnetic resonance cholangiopancreatography
- PTL—Preterm labor
- RUQ—Right upper quadrant
- UDCA—Ursodeoxycholic acid

CODES

ICD9-CM
- 574.0 Nonobstructive cholelithiasis
- 574.1 Obstructive cholelithiasis
- 574.2 Biliary pain
- 574.3 Choledocholithiasis
- 575.0 Acute cholecystitis
- 576.1 Acute cholangitis

Section VI

HEADACHES DURING PREGNANCY: TENSION/MIGRAINE

Michael Marmura, MD
Stephen D. Silberstein, MD

 BASICS

DESCRIPTION
- Migraine and tension headaches are seen in all types of patients and are common in women of child-bearing age.
- Migraine is a moderate or severe headache usually worsened by movement, often unilateral, with a pulsating quality. It is often associated with nausea or vomiting and sensitivity to light, sounds, or odors.
- Tension headaches are usually mild or moderate in intensity with a pressing quality.
- Most primary headache disorders involve genetic and environmental factors.

EPIDEMIOLOGY
- Migraine and tension-type headaches are common.
- Migraine has a 1-year prevalence of 18% in women, 6% in men.
- Migraine usually presents in 1st 3 decades of life, but may present up to age 50.
- Prevalence is highest for ages 35–45.
- Migraine prevalence decreases with advanced age. Women with natural menopause may improve, whereas patients with surgical menopause often worsen.
- Tension headache has a yearly prevalence of 38% in the general population.

RISK FACTORS
Include family history, obesity, affective disorders

Genetics
- Both tension and migraine are increased in 1st-degree relatives of probands.
- There are some clearly autosomal dominant forms of migraine such as familial hemiplegic migraine.
- Chronic tension-type headache is also most common in 1st-degree relatives.

PATHOPHYSIOLOGY
- Migraine involves activation of the trigeminovascular system, which includes large intracranial vessels and dura mater.
- Trigeminal nerve activation ensues, and plasma proteins and neuropeptides are released.
- The trigeminal nucleus in the brainstem receives the afferents and may produce alteration of pain and sensory input, leading to nausea and sensory sensitivity.
- Aura results from neuronal suppression or dysfunction called cortical spreading depression.
- Tension headache physiology is poorly understood but may be similar to migraine.

ASSOCIATED CONDITIONS
- Affective disorders
- Epilepsy
- Stroke
- Functional bowel disorders
- Raynaud phenomenon

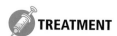 **DIAGNOSIS**

SIGNS AND SYMPTOMS

History
- Migraine may be diagnosed when the patient has 5 lifetime attacks of the following:
  - Headache lasting 4–72 hours
  - At least 2 of the following:
    - Unilateral location
    - Pulsating quality
    - Moderate or severe intensity
    - Aggravation by physical activity
  - During headache at least 1 the following:
    - Nausea and/or vomiting
    - Photophobia and phonophobia
  - No evidence of organic disease
  - Migraine with aura may be diagnosed if patients have at least 2 attacks with at least 3 of the following characteristics:
    - 1 or more fully reversible symptoms indicating brain dysfunction
    - At least 1 symptom develops gradually over 4 minutes or ≥2 symptoms occur in succession.
    - No aura symptom lasts >60 minutes.
    - Headache follows aura in <60 minutes. Headache may occur before or during aura.
  - Migraine auras may be prolonged in some cases.
  - Less common variants of migraine include basilar migraine with brainstem symptoms and hemiplegic migraine.
  - Chronic migraine refers to patients with ≥15 days of migraine per month, and is often associated with medication overuse.
  - Migraine patients may experience a prodrome before an attack that may present with depression, euphoria, irritability, yawning, food cravings, or neck stiffness.
  - Many patients have worsening migraine with menses. This is likely due to estrogen withdrawal. Menstrual migraine is defined as an attack occurring up to 1 day before and up to 4 days after menses.
  - "Status migrainosis" refers to a migraine headache that lasts >72 hours.
- Tension-type headache is diagnosed in patients with at least 10 lifetime attacks of the following:
  - Headache lasting from 30 minutes to 7 days
  - At least 2 of the following:
    - Mild or moderate intensity
    - Bilateral location
    - Pressing or tightening quality
    - Not aggravated by movement
  - Both of the following:
    - Nausea and vomiting absent
    - Photophobia and phonophobia cannot both be present
  - No evidence of organic disease

- Patients with attacks <15 days a month have episodic tension-type headache.
- Patients with episodic tension headache rarely present to a physician for evaluation.
- Patients with ≥15 headaches per month may be diagnosed with chronic tension-type headache.

Physical Exam
- General exam including vital signs is usually normal.
- Neurologic and musculoskeletal exams should be performed.

TESTS
Usually not required in most patients unless secondary causes are suspected

Labs
- No specific lab tests are available to confirm a diagnosis of migraine or tension headache.
- Routine labs to ensure no metabolic disturbance, anemia, etc.
- ESR/CRP if temporal arteritis is suspected
- Lumbar puncture for suspected meningitis or encephalitis
- Toxicology screen, as indicated

Imaging
- Indicated for suspected secondary causes
- CT for suspected hemorrhage, hydrocephalus or sinusitis
- MRI for suspected mass lesion or infection
- MRA or angiography for suspected aneurysm
- MRV for suspected venous thrombosis

ALERT
Patients with sudden-onset "thunderclap" headaches, systemic disease, focal deficits, or an abrupt change in headache pattern warrant further investigation for secondary causes of headache.

TREATMENT

GENERAL MEASURES
- Determine attack frequency, severity, and disability with attacks.
- Note any comorbidities (medical, neurologic and psychiatric) to determine treatment.
- Review previous treatments and outcomes.
- Identify and avoid triggers for headache for each individual patient:
  - Foods including alcohol
  - Weather changes
  - Sleep alterations
  - Head trauma
  - Menses
  - Stress
- Develop plan for treatment of acute attacks of variable severity.
- Consider prevention for frequent or disabling attacks.

PREGNANCY-SPECIFIC ISSUES

- Many women with migraine improve during pregnancy after the 1st trimester, but a minority may worsen or even 1st present with migraine during pregnancy.
- Medication use should be limited due to risk to the fetus, but may be used. This especially applies to patients with vomiting and dehydration, which may lead to fetal compromise. Risks of treatment should be discussed with the patient and given with their consent.
- Preventative medications should be used only in refractory cases or to treat a comorbid illness such as depression, HTN, or epilepsy.
- Acute symptomatic treatment:
  – Ice, massage, relaxation for moderate attacks
  – Acetaminophen
  – NSAIDs in 1st trimester
  – Metoclopramide
  – Prochlorperazine, promethazine (oral or suppositories)
  – Prednisone taper for refractory cases
- Preventative medications:
  – Magnesium
  – β-Blockers
  – Calcium channel blockers
  – Strongly consider biofeedback or relaxation therapy in patients with migraine, especially during pregnancy.

By Trimester
Migraine may worsen in the 1st trimester of pregnancy but significantly improve later in pregnancy.

Risks for Mother
Headache is a cause of significant disability for many patients. Migraine may also cause significant neurologic dysfunction in addition to head pain.

Risks for Fetus
Both medications taken and maternal distress from vomiting and dehydration may place the fetus at risk. However, women with migraine do not have increased rates of miscarriages, toxemia, or congenital abnormalities.

MEDICATION (DRUGS)

- Acute:
  – Triptans (treating early in attack): Pregnancy category C
  – Ergots and DHE should not be used in pregnancy: Pregnancy category X
  – Acetaminophen: Pregnancy category B
  – NSAIDS: Pregnancy category B
  – Aspirin and aspirin containing compounds: Pregnancy category D
  – Metoclopramide: Pregnancy category B
  – Neuroleptics (promethazine, prochlorperazine): Pregnancy category C
  – Barbiturates, benzodiazepines should be limited due to issues of withdrawal and overuse; also category D
  – Isometheptene and combination agents (i.e., Midrin): Pregnancy category C
  – Opioids with limits: Pregnancy category C
  – Occipital nerve blocks and trigger point injections
  – IV valproic acid: Pregnancy category D
  – IV magnesium, IV ketorolac: Pregnancy category C
  – Steroids for "status migranosis"

- Preventative:
  – β-Blockers: Pregnancy category C
  – Anticonvulsants (topiramate): Pregnancy category C, valproic acid: Pregnancy category D, gabapentin: Pregnancy category C
  – Calcium channel blockers: Pregnancy category C
  – Neuroleptics: Pregnancy category C
  – TCAs: Pregnancy category C
  – MAOIs: Pregnancy category C
  – SSRIs, SNRIs: Pregnancy category C with caution (paroxetine, D)
  – ACE inhibitors: Pregnancy category C/D/D for many
  – Angiotensin-receptor blockers: Pregnancy category C/D/D
  – Riboflavin, magnesium, butterbur
  – Botulinum toxin: Pregnancy category C
  – OCPs may induce, change or alleviate headache in different patients; obviously not relevant for pregnancy management.
  – Estrogen replacement therapy may exacerbate migraine or prevent natural improvement; pertains to menopausal women.

 FOLLOW-UP

DISPOSITION

Issues for Referral
Issues that require neurologic referral include:

- Medication overuse
- Significant disability
- Abnormal neurologic exam
- Poor response to acute attack medication
- Multiple preventative medications

PROGNOSIS
No cure for migraine exists, but patients may derive great improvement in symptoms and quality of life with treatment.

COMPLICATIONS
- Economic and quality-of-life impact is significant.
- Patients may experience significant neurologic dysfunction with or without radiologic evidence of infarction.

PATIENT MONITORING
- Monitor for effectiveness of acute-attack medications and/or preventatives and for medication side effects.
- This may include asking about GI symptoms, weight changes, monitoring of ECG, CBC, or LFTs on certain medications.

Mother
Per routine. Monitor the amount of acute medication used and effectiveness of the treatments.

Fetus
Per routine

BIBLIOGRAPHY

Ashkenazi A, et al. Hormone-related headache: Pathophysiology and treatment. *CNS Drugs*. 2006;20(2):125–141.

Headache Classification Subcommittee of the International Headache Society. *The international classification of headache disorders*, 2nd ed. Cephalalgia; 2004;24S1.

Silberstein SD, et al., eds. *Wolff's Headache and Other Head Pain*, 7th ed. New York: Oxford University Press; 2001.

 MISCELLANEOUS

CLINICAL PEARLS
- Most severe headaches are migraine.
- Severe headaches with neck pain are usually migraine not tension.
- "Sick" headaches or "sinus headaches" are usually migraine.
- Beware of red flags:
  – Sudden onset
  – Older age of 1st onset
  – Systemic illness such as immunosuppression
  – Alteration of consciousness
  – Focal neurologic deficits

ABBREVIATIONS
- ACE—Angiotensin-converting enzyme
- CRP—C-reactive protein
- ESR—Erythrocyte sedimentation rate
- MAOI—Monoamine oxidase inhibitor
- MRA/MRV—Magnetic resonance arteriography/venography
- OCP—Oral contraceptive pill
- SNRI—Selective norepinephrine reuptake inhibitor
- SSRI—Selective serotonin reuptake inhibitor
- TCA—Tricyclic antidepressant

CODES

ICD9-CM
307.81 Tension headache
346.0 Migraine with aura
346.1 Migraine without aura

PATIENT TEACHING

- Consider nonpharmacologic approaches such as biofeedback, relaxation, acupuncture, and physical therapy in selected patients, and particularly during pregnancy.
- Develop strategies for managing acute attacks, including options for moderate and severe attacks.
- Offer rescue therapy to prevent emergency room visits and increased disability.
- Encourage use of headache calendars for patients with frequent attacks.
- Preventative medications require an adequate trial of a few months to assess efficacy.

PREVENTION
- Avoidance of triggers when possible
- Regular sleep patterns
- Regular exercise
- Smoking cessation
- Avoiding overuse of acute attack medications
- Maintaining good general health
- Maintaining healthy weight

Section VI

HIV AND AIDS IN PREGNANCY

Jyothsna Bayya, MD
Howard Minkoff, MD

BASICS

DESCRIPTION
- HIV-1 and HIV-2 are retroviruses with RNA genomes; they are the etiologic agents of HIV infection and AIDS.
- AIDS, a syndrome 1st described in 1981, is the result of progressive immune debilitation.
- Unique importance to ob-gyns as HIV may affect women in their care and can be transmitted from pregnant women to their neonates.

EPIDEMIOLOGY
- >40 million people infected with HIV worldwide, of which 50% are women
- CDC estimates 40,000 new infections per year in US; ~70% among men, 30% among women
- ~2,000 new infections/d in children <15 years
- Due to effective retroviral therapy, increasing number of individuals with chronic HIV, despite decline in new infections in the 1990s
- ~15% of HIV-infected pregnant women in the US obtain no prenatal care.
- HIV is transmitted via:
  - Sexual contact:
    - Male to female transmission more efficient than female to male
    - Anal receptive sex more likely to transmit than vaginal sex
  - Exposure to infected blood:
    - Parenteral exposure via transfusions or sharing needles
    - Occupational exposure, risk of transmission is 0.3% after percutaneous exposure to HIV-infected blood; 0.09% after mucous-membrane exposure. With needlestick injury, risk of transmission is 1/300.
  - Breast milk transmission:
    - Overall risk in breast-fed children as high as 30–40%
  - Perinatally: In utero or during labor/delivery:
    - 20% of transmission occurs <36 weeks; 50% in days before delivery, 30% intrapartum
    - Risk of infected infant is ~20%; increased rate of transmission if low CD4 counts or > viral titers and previous diagnosis of AIDS
    - Vaginal delivery, especially with ROM >4 hours, increases risk of infant infection.
    - Untreated STDs, prematurity, and chorioamnionitis, increase the risk of mother-to-child transmission of HIV.
    - With optimal therapy, the rate of perinatal transmission is 1–2%.
- HIV is not believed to be transmitted by:
  - Bites
  - Sharing utensils, bathrooms, bathtubs
  - Exposure to urine, feces, vomitus (except if grossly contaminated with blood, and even then transmission is rare, if at all)
  - Casual contact in home, school, or day care

RISK FACTORS
- Sexual activity
- Injection drug use
- Recipients of blood products
- Children of HIV infected women
- Occupational exposure

PATHOPHYSIOLOGY
- The HIV outer envelope protein has a strong affinity for CD4 surface antigen on specific T lymphocytes, macrophages, and monocytes.
- The virus attaches to the CD4 molecule, as well as cytokine coreceptors.
- The virus then penetrates these cells, followed by transcription (using viral reverse transcriptase) of viral RNA into double-stranded DNA.
- This viral DNA is then integrated into the host cell genome and will remain there for the lifetime of the cell.
- Over time, the number of T cells drops insidiously.
- Active viral replication continues after the primary infection:
  - Even during the clinically latent period, $>10^6$ viral particles are produced daily.
  - Over time, the host immune system loses the ability to contain viral replication and replace lost CD4 cells.

ASSOCIATED CONDITIONS
- AIDS-defining illnesses include:
  - Invasive cervical cancer
  - Candidiasis
  - Recurrent pneumonia
  - PCP
  - Wasting syndrome
  - Kaposi sarcoma
- Syphilis may be more aggressive in HIV-infected patients.
- Tuberculosis is co-epidemic with HIV.
- Hepatitis C co-infected patients have more rapid progression to cirrhosis.
- Herpes recurrences may be more common and more widespread.
- When CD4 count drops below 200 mm³, patient is prone to opportunistic infections (e.g., toxoplasma, PCP, Kaposi sarcoma).

DIAGNOSIS

SIGNS AND SYMPTOMS
- Incubation period from exposure to HIV infection syndrome: Days to weeks
- Acute illness lasts <10 days, presenting as fever, night sweats, rash, headache, fatigue, nausea, vomiting, diarrhea, pharyngitis, myalgias, arthralgias, lymphadenopathy
- After symptoms subside, chronic viremia is established.
- In the absence of treatment, progression from asymptomatic viremia to AIDS is ~10 years.

TESTS
In US, 50–75% of pregnant women are tested when "opt-in" testing is used; 75–95% are tested when "opt-out" testing is used.

Lab
- Benefits of testing:
  - Selection of treatment
  - Prevention of mother-to-child transmission
  - Prevention of transmission of infection to others

- Types of tests:
  - Standard tests:
    - ELISA test is the standard testing protocol. Sensitivity and specificity >98%
    - Positive screening test confirmed with Western blot or IFA
  - Rapid tests recommended for patients who arrive in labor with unknown status.
- Screening: CDC and ACOG recommend universal but voluntary screening using the "opt-out" approach.
- Repeat HIV testing recommended in 3rd trimester if prevalence >1/1,000 person years. 2nd test may be required at delivery.

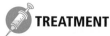
TREATMENT

GENERAL MEASURES
- Appropriate care requires coordination between an HIV specialist and an obstetrician.
- Decisions regarding the use of antiretroviral drugs during pregnancy should be made by the woman after discussions regarding known and unknown benefits and risks of therapy.
- HAART should be considered for all HIV-infected women with viral loads >100,000 or CD4 counts <350 mm³. It is recommended for all women before the CD4 count drops below 200 mm³.
- Resistance testing:
  - All antiretroviral-naïve pregnant women before initiating treatment or prophylaxis
  - Those on antenatal antiretroviral therapy with virologic failure with persistently detectable HIV RNA levels or who have suboptimal viral suppression after initiation of antiretroviral treatment.
- Types:
  - Phenotypic testing is a measure of activity of virus under set conditions.
  - Genotypic testing is a measure of structure.
- Empiric initiation of antiretroviral therapy before results of resistance testing are available may be warranted if diagnosis is made in late pregnancy, with adjustment as needed after the results are available.

PREGNANCY-SPECIFIC ISSUES
- 2 indications for medications:
  - Treatment of maternal HIV-1 infection
  - Chemoprophylaxis for PMTCT of HIV-1
- Treatment:
  - Highly active antiretroviral combination therapy to maximally suppress viral replication during pregnancy is the most effective strategy to prevent the development of resistance and to minimize the risk of perinatal transmission.
  - Counsel all pregnant women about adherence to reduce the potential for resistance.
  - Therapeutic goals are suppression of viral load to undetectable levels and restoration and preservation of immunologic function.
  - HAART:
    - The standard of treatment includes combination of antiretrovirals (NRTIs, NNRTIs, PIs, FIs).
    - Didanosine and stavudine: Causes mitochondrial toxicity, sometimes fatal

- Chemoprophylaxis:
  – PMTCT of HIV
- Prediction:
  – Maternal viral load is best predictor of neonatal infection.
  – Prolonged ROM increases risk.
- Medication:
  – Start HAART if patient meets criteria or viral load is >1,000 copies. Most would recommend for all HIV-infected pregnant women.
  – ZDV in labor if possible, along with established antiretroviral regimens, and oral ZDV for infant according to the PACTG 076 protocol
  – PACTG 076 3-part ZDU regimen:
    o Antepartum: Start at 14 weeks; continue through pregnancy, 100 mg PO 5 times daily
    o Intrapartum: In labor, loading dose 2 mg/kg over 1 hour, then 1 mg/kg maintenance
    o Neonate: Begin at 6–12 hours of age, ZDV syrup 2 mg/kg q6h for 6 weeks
    o If viral load is <1,000, maternal option of HAART or ACTG 076 (ZDV only)
    o ZDV as monotherapy reduces exposure to potentially toxic drugs, but may increase risk of resistance.
- For untreated women in labor: Intrapartum and neonatal components of ACTG 076:
  – ZDV/Lamivudine (3TC) recommended regimen:
    o 600 mg ZDV and 150 mg 3TC PO at onset of labor, then ZDV 300 mg PO q3h and 150 mg 3TC PO q12h
    o Infant: ZDV 4 mg/kg PO q12h and 3TC 2 mg/kg PO q12h for 7 days. Transmission is reduced by 42%.
  – Nevirapine single-dose 200 mg PO at the onset of labor and single 2-mg/kg PO dose to newborn at age 48–72 hours.
    o Inexpensive and easy to administer.
    o Risk of transmission reduced by ~50%.
    o Consider 3TC/ZDV "tail" for 3–7 days postpartum to reduce the likelihood that resistance will develop.
  – Both nevirapine and zidovudine: IV ZDV as 2-mg/kg bolus then 1 mg/kg/h infusion until delivery; single 200-mg PO dose NVP at the onset of labor. ZDV 2 mg/kg PO q6h for 6 weeks to newborn; single-dose 2 mg/kg PO at the age of 48–72 hours.
  – Cesarean delivery:
    o If viral load is >1,000 copies, reduces MTCT by 59%.
    o Combined with antiretroviral therapy, 87% reduction.
    o Schedule at 38 weeks without amniocentesis.
    o Use prophylactic antibiotics.

Risks for Mother
- ZDV causes anemia, bone marrow depression
- PIs cause hyperglycemia, worsening diabetes, DKA
- Nevirapine, if given when CD4 >250/mL in a woman who never received antiretroviral therapy, can cause rash-associated hepatotoxicity that can be life-threatening.
- Nucleoside analogs can induce mitochondrial dysfunction manifested as neuropathy, myopathy, cardiomyopathy, hepatic steatosis, lactic acidosis.
- Abacavir causes rash in genetically predisposed individuals. Can be harbinger of a lethal reaction.

Risks for Fetus
Antiretroviral therapy has been associated with:
- Preterm birth, mutagenesis, febrile seizures, mitochondrial dysfunction presenting with neurologic symptoms
- 1st trimester Efavirenz causes NTDs

 FOLLOW-UP

DISPOSITION
Issues for Referral
Comprehensive care and support services are important for women and their families, including:
- Primary, obstetric, pediatric, HIV specialty care
- Family planning services
- Mental health services
- Substance-abuse treatment
- Coordination of care through case management

COMPLICATIONS
- Immunodeficiency
- Opportunistic infections
- Neuropsychiatric symptoms
- HIV-associated malignancies
- Increased risk of cervical cancer in HIV-infected women; perform Pap smears every 6 months.

PATIENT MONITORING
Mother
Monitor in pregnancy as when not pregnant. CD4+ percentage is more stable than CD4+ count and may more accurately reflect immune status during pregnancy:
- HIV-1 RNA levels each month until undetectable, then every trimester
- US PHS 2003 perinatal guidelines: CD4 count each trimester or every 3–4 months, HIV RNA levels 4 weeks after change in treatment, then monthly until undetectable, then every 3 months and near term to plan mode of delivery
  – With therapy, viral load should drop by >1 log in the 1st month and become undetectable within 6 months.
- Postpartum: Monitor for depression, adherence to antiretroviral regimens

Fetus
- CBC and differential as a baseline evaluation before administration of ZDV
- Repeat hemoglobin is required at a minimum after the completion of the 6-week ZDV regimen.
- Intensive monitoring of hematologic and serum chemistry in 1st few weeks of life in infants whose mothers received combination antiretroviral treatment

BIBLIOGRAPHY

AIDS information. Available at: www.aidsinfo.nih.gov

Blanche S, et al. Placental mitochondrial dysfunction and perinatal exposure to antiretroviral nucleoside analogues. *Lancet.* 1999;354(9184):1084–1089.

Centers for Disease Control and Prevention Preconception Care Work Group. Recommendations to improve preconception health and health care, United States. *MMWR.* 2006;55(RR-6):1–30.

Guay LA, et al. Intrapartum and neonatal single-dose nevirapine compared with zidovudine for prevention of mother-to-child transmission of HIV-1 in Kampala, Uganda: HIVNET 012 randomised trial. *Lancet.* 1999;354(9181):795–802.

Hammer S, et al. Treatment for adult HIV infection: 2006 recommendations of the international AIDS society, USA panel. *JAMA.* 2006;296:827–843.

Landesman SH, et al. Obstetrical factors and the transmission of human immunodeficiency virus type 1 from mother to child. *N Engl J Med.* 1996; 334(25):1617–1623.

Merhi Z, et al. Rapid HIV screening for women in labor [Review]. *Expert Rev Mol Diagn.* 2005;5(5): 673–379.

Minkoff H. HIV infection in pregnancy. *Obstet Gynecol.* 2003;101:797–810.

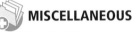 MISCELLANEOUS

ABBREVIATIONS
ELISA—Enzyme linked immunoabsorbent assay
FI—Fusion inhibitors
HAART—Highly active antiretroviral therapy
IFA—Immunofluorescence assay
NNRTI—Nonnucleoside reverse transcriptase inhibitors
NRTI—Nucleoside reverse transcriptase inhibitors
NTD—Neural tube defect
PCP—Pneumocystis carinii pneumonia
PI—Protease inhibitor
PMTCT—Prevention of maternal-to-child transmission
ZDV—Zidovudine

CODES
ICD9-CM
- 042 Human immunodeficiency virus (HIV) infection, symptomatic HIV infection, AIDS
- 795.71 Nonspecific serologic evidence of HIV, inconclusive HIV test
- v08 Asymptomatic HIV, HIV positive, NOS
- v1.79 Exposure to HIV
- v65.44 HIV counseling
- 079.53 HIV-2

PATIENT TEACHING

- The US Department of Health and Human Services: 1–877–696–6775, 1–202–619–0255
- AIDS Info Health Information Specialist: 1–800–448–0440 or www.aidsinfo.nih.gov
- National HIV Telephone Consultation Service (Warmline): 1–800–933–3413
- Pregnancy Registry that monitors HIV positive women during pregnancy and after delivery. Available at: www.fda.gov/womens/registries
- Antiretroviral Pregnancy Registry: 1–800–258–4263 or www.APRegistry.com

PREVENTION
- Avoid unscreened blood products.
- Avoid unprotected sexual intercourse.
- Use condoms.
- Avoid injection drug abuse.
- Needle exchange for active IV drug users

Prevention of Vertical Transmission
- Antiretroviral chemoprophylaxis
- Cesarean delivery

Section VI

OBESITY IN PREGNANCY

Sharon Phelan, MD

 BASICS

DESCRIPTION
- An excess of adipose tissue that contributes to complications in pregnancy
- Associated with caloric intake excessive to the energy expenditures needed by activity
- BMI defined as weight in kilograms (kg) divided by height in meters (m) squared:
  - Overweight: BMI 25–29.9 kg/m^2
  - Obesity: BMI 30 kg/m^2 or greater:
    - Type I: 30–34.9.
    - Type II: 35–39.9,
    - Type III/extreme obesity: >40

EPIDEMIOLOGY
- Rapidly increasing nationally
- Associated with maternal and perinatal complications
- "Dose-response" relationship between BMI change and increased risk of pregnancy complication (e.g., a doubling of relative risks with a 3-unit increase in BMI)
- Prevalence: 28% of women are overweight.
- 20% of reproductive-age women are obese.

RISK FACTORS
- Overweight or obese in childhood
- Increase intake of refined carbohydrates
- Decreased fresh fruits and vegetables
- Decreased physical activity both at work and daily activities
- Lower socioeconomic status
- Certain cultural influences (e.g., Hispanic patients often believe that if the mother does not eat foods she craves, the fetus will be damaged)
- Obese parents
- History of excessive weight gain in prior pregnancy, especially if weight not lost between pregnancies

Genetics
The human genome was developed in an environment of subsistence diet so there is no limit to the human body's ability to store calories as fat. This may be increased during pregnancy in the relative state of "starvation" induced by hPL.

PATHOPHYSIOLOGY
- Increased adipose tissue leads to increased insulin resistance, increased tissue insulin levels, and chronic hyperinsulinemia with resultant secondary HTN and hyperlipidemia.
- During pregnancy, craving for carbohydrates increases.

- Pregnancy is a pseudostarvation state, tending toward elevated glucose levels and increased risk of gestational diabetes.
- Excessive weight gain by mother tends to cause macrosomia in fetus, which is associated with overweight toddlers and children.

ASSOCIATED CONDITIONS
- HTN
- Type 2 diabetes
- Overall poor nutritional intake
- See Diet: Obesity.

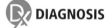 **DIAGNOSIS**

SIGNS AND SYMPTOMS
History
- Full medical history indicated with particular emphasis on:
  - Weight during key times in life: Adolescence, prepregnancy
  - Rate of weight gain, sudden weight gain concerning of medical problem (edema in pregnancy or preeclampsia)
  - Review of systems to check for any undiagnosed condition (although it is rare to have a major endocrine cause that has not been treated, since these pathologies are usually associated with infertility)
- Assess interest in changing behavior or initiating weight control activities:
  - Dietary patterns; food diary
  - Stressors that provoke/trigger eating

Physical Exam
Unlikely to have a significant endocrine source of obesity in presence of fertility and pregnancy

TESTS
Labs
Routine prenatal labs plus:
- 1-hour GTT screen for diabetes early as well as routine timing
- CBC for hematocrit since overnutrition often means poor nutrition

Imaging
- Consider early dating US since maternal obesity will make clinical sizing less accurate.
- May require serial US for fetal growth because of risk of macrosomia following excessive weight gain or decreased growth if hypertensive
- FH is distorted by maternal obesity and may not accurately reflect fetal growth.

 TREATMENT

- Prevention is the best management. Assess weight annually and alert patient if she is gaining excessive weight so she can modify habits prior to becoming overweight or obese.
  - This is key, because most interventions are not feasible during pregnancy and do not work well over the long term.
- Recommended pregnancy weight gain depends on prepregnant weight:
  - If starting pregnancy at <20 BMI: 30–40 lb gain
  - Normal BMI: 25–30 lb gain
  - BMI >30: 10–15 lb gain

GENERAL MEASURES
- Assess willingness to start on a major behavioral lifestyle modification. If not interested, let the patient know you are willing to help once she is ready.
- Pregnancy is not a time to attempt to lose weight but a time to gain only the ideal weight and to improve diet. Typically women who enter a pregnancy overweight gain > the recommended 15–20 lbs.
- Stress a healthy diet:
  - Recommend dietary change at once if overweight and sooner with excessive increasing weight gain
  - Behavioral aspects to diet:
    - This should be seen as a modification of life-long eating habits, not a short-term "punishment."
    - Encourage structured meals; no snacking and fast foods.
    - Eat slowly.
    - Decrease portion size, avoid all-you-can-eat restaurants and sugary drinks.
- Activity:
  - Exercise for 30–60 minutes daily for 5+ days/week. Start with activities that the patient can tolerate and sustain. Walking or swimming are the best overall activity initially when pregnant. Impact activities or those dependent on balance (bicycling) should be avoided in pregnancy.

PREGNANCY-SPECIFIC ISSUES
By Trimester
- 1st trimester:
  - Increased risk of spontaneous abortions
  - Twins
  - NTDs, other birth defects
- 3rd trimester and delivery:
  - Increased risk of trauma from macrosomic infant
  - Increased risk of operative delivery
  - Increased risk of caesarian delivery
  - Increased anesthesia risks
  - Increased risk of postpartum infections

Risks for Mother
- Gestational diabetes
- Hypertensive disorders such as preeclampsia
- Gall bladder disease
- Fatty liver disease
- Sleep apnea
- Thromboembolic disease

Risks for Fetus
- Birth defects
- Macrosomia
- Fetal or neonatal death
- Birth trauma from shoulder dystocia due to macrosomia
- Increase risk of metabolic syndrome or diabetes as adult
- Preterm delivery as a consequence of maternal disease such as diabetes and HTN

MEDICATION (DRUGS)
Not appropriate in pregnancy

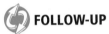

FOLLOW-UP

DISPOSITION
Issues for Referral
Involve nutritionist or nutritional counseling early in pregnancy for overweight women.

PROGNOSIS
- Long-term maintenance of weight loss is difficult. Patients tend to yo-yo, often gaining more weight than originally lost.
- If patient is not motivated to lose weight, attempts will not be successful.
- If patient does not lose excessive weight prior to next pregnancy, long-term prognosis poor.

COMPLICATIONS
Complications of obesity in pregnancy include:
- HTN and preeclampsia
- Gestational diabetes

- Gall bladder disease; may be worse with rapid weight loss
- Thromboembolism
- Sleep apnea
- Macrosomic infant with increase risk of birth trauma or operative delivery
- Stillbirth/IUFD
- Increase caesarian delivery rate
- Increase rate of DC/DA twins
- NTD in fetus

PATIENT MONITORING
Mother
- Weigh the patient at each prenatal visit. The weight will serve as a proxy for nutritional status during the pregnancy.
- Encourage breast-feeding, which assists in postpartum weight loss and tends to keep infant from getting obese.

Fetus
- Early dating US scan and then as needed to monitor growth
- Detailed anatomy scan to evaluate for birth defects
- Multiple marker screen should be encouraged.

BIBLIOGRAPHY

ACOG Committee Opinion No. 315. *Obesity in Pregnancy*. Washington DC: ACOG; September 2005.

Centers for Disease Control, Department of Health and Human Services. Overweight and Obesity. Available at: www.cdc.gov/nccdphp/dnpa/obesity/index.htm

Online BMI calculator. Available at: http://www.nhlbisupport.com/bmi

MISCELLANEOUS

CLINICAL PEARLS
- Understand cultural differences regarding dietary choices and cravings.
- Look at what the patient is drinking for a potential major source of empty calories.

ABBREVIATIONS
- BMI—Body mass index
- DC/DA—Dichorionic/Diamniotic
- FH—Fundal height
- GTT—Glucose tolerance test
- hPL—Human placental lactogen
- HTN—Hypertension
- IOM—Institute of Medicine
- IUFD—Intrauterine fetal demise
- NTD—Neural tube defect
- US—Ultrasound

CODES
ICD9-CM
649.1 Obesity complicating pregnancy

PATIENT TEACHING

- Educate the patient that only a couple hundred extra calories makes up the need for the developing fetus; in short, the baby doesn't need a piece of cake or an extra serving of fries.
- Have her realize that it is not just weight gain that is important but also the types of foods she is eating to gain the weight; nutrition is key.
- Target total weight gain to the IOM recommendations.
- This is not the time to diet but to eat healthy.
- Lose extra weight between pregnancies; breast-feeding helps.

PREVENTION
- Talk to patient about appropriate weight gain during pregnancy and monitor weight.
- Encourage weight loss prior to pregnancy or between pregnancies.

Section VI

RHEUMATOID ARTHRITIS AND PREGNANCY

Jonathan W. Weeks, MD

 BASICS

DESCRIPTION
- RA is a chronic, progressive autoimmune disease characterized by synovitis and joint destruction.
- Onset is typically in the 4th decade of life.
- Onset in childhood—JRA—now termed JIA by international experts
- Symmetric inflammatory arthritis
- Spreads from joint to joint:
  – Synovial inflammation results in cartilage and bone destruction.

EPIDEMIOLOGY
- RA is a relatively common condition:
  – Female > male; 4:1
  – Prevalence in the US is 1%
  – Worldwide prevalence is 0.5–1%
- Most patients develop symptoms in their 30s.

RISK FACTORS
- Family history of arthritis
- The following are thought to influence incidence, but are not causative:
  – Environmental factors
  – Nulliparity
  – Breastfeeding
  – Obesity
  – Tobacco
  – Coffee consumption

Genetics
Genetic risk factors include:
- HLA-DR4, HLA-DR1
- Twin studies have heritability of 60%.
- Siblings have 2–4-fold increased risk of developing RA.

PATHOPHYSIOLOGY
- Autoimmune process with complex interaction of cytokines, prostaglandins, and proteolytic enzymes
- Unknown antigen induces CD4+ T-cell immune response
- CD20+ B cells are activated:
  – Monocytes, macrophages, and fibroblasts are recruited, leading to production of TNFα and IL-1.
  – Matrix metalloproteinases and osteoclasts are activated, resulting in joint damage.

ASSOCIATED CONDITIONS
- Multiple coexisting conditions can impact prognosis:
  – Infection: Incidence doubled in RA
  – Osteoporosis: Incidence doubled in RA
  – CVD: Accounts for most of the mortality in RA
  – Malignancy risk increased 5-fold
  – Many patients experience depression.
- RA can have extra-articular manifestations:
  – Rheumatoid nodules
  – Pericarditis
  – Rheumatoid (restrictive) lung disease
  – Scleritis
  – Secondary Sjögren syndrome

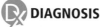 **DIAGNOSIS**

SIGNS AND SYMPTOMS
History
- Many syndromes, including self-limiting viral conditions, can mimic RA. Therefore, the presence of symptoms for at least 6 weeks is generally required.
- Joint pain and swelling, gradual, progressive
- Morning stiffness >1 hour
- Fatigue
- Inability to perform daily activities

Physical Exam
- Tenderness, warmth, and swelling of joints
- Hands are among the affected joints.
- Arthritis should be symmetric.
- Joint effusions
- Decreased ROM of affected joints
- Subcutaneous nodules (rheumatoid nodules)

TESTS
Labs
- RF:
  – Present in 60–85% of affected patients but low specificity
  – High titers predictive of severe disease, more joint destruction, and more extra-articular manifestations
- Anticyclic CCP:
  – Specificity 90–98%, sensitivity 50–70%
- May see elevated ESR, CRP
- May see anemia of chronic disease

Imaging
- At time of diagnosis, 30% of patients have radiographic findings. This increases to as high 60% by 2 years if good medical control has not been achieved.
- Radiographic findings:
  – Periarticular osteoporosis
  – Erosions and cysts
  – Loss of joint space
- MRI reveals joint changes earlier; up to 80% of patients may have changes at onset.

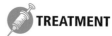 **TREATMENT**

GENERAL MEASURES
- Early treatment with appropriate medications improves pain, joint destruction, disability, and long-term prognosis:
  – Activity: Most patients with RA can participate in moderate-intensity aerobic exercise.
  – Physical therapy:
    ○ Flexibility, ROM, and aerobic exercise are all useful.
    ○ Joint protection and energy conservation is essential.
- Splinting of hands or wrists or use of lower-extremity orthotics can provide temporary pain relief.

PREGNANCY-SPECIFIC ISSUES

ALERT
- Few RA medications are safe in pregnancy. Ideally, patients will be in remission and well-controlled before conception.
- Antepartum course of RA: 75% remission rate during pregnancy.
- Postpartum course of RA: Symptoms commonly increase at 4–10 weeks postpartum.

Risks for Mother
- Some patients may suffer limited range of motion in the hip.
- The risk is particularly high in patients with JRA.
- Cesarean section may be necessary.

Risks for Fetus
Aside from the effects of drugs on the fetus, no excessive fetal wastage occurs among women with RA.

Breastfeeding
- Some case reports have suggested that breastfeeding may exacerbate symptoms.
- RA drugs compatible with breastfeeding:
  – Acetaminophen
  – NSAIDs
  – Sulfasalazine
  – Hydroxychloroquine

ALERT
- RA drugs incompatible with breastfeeding:
  – Gold
  – Methotrexate
  – Aspirin (usual RA dose is 3–4 g/d)
  – Azathioprine

MEDICATION (DRUGS)

Medical Management in Pregnancy

Ideally, patients should be in remission and off potential teratogens prior to conception. Most of these patients will do well in pregnancy with little need for medical therapy. When symptoms require maintenance meds in pregnancy, the following are recommended:

- Acetaminophen: Ensure that patient does not exceed recommended dosing.
- NSAIDs (e.g., Indocin, Ibuprofen, Naprosyn) can be used with caution in the 1st and 2nd trimesters:
  - If used regularly, US for AF assessment should be done every 2 weeks.
  - Oligohydramnios should prompt discontinuation.
- Corticosteroids:
  - Oral prednisone can be given daily (start with 5 mg/d PO). Maintenance doses above 10 mg/d increases the risk of PPROM.
  - Long-acting form can be injected into affected joints. This can sometimes bring months of symptomatic relief.
- Hydroxychloroquine

Medical Management in Nonpregnant Women

- In nonpregnant patients, relief and remission are best achieved with the use of DMARDs, many of which are teratogenic. Patients who conceive within 3 months of taking these drugs should be referred for genetic counseling and targeted US.
- Methotrexate is considered 1st-line unless contraindicated:
  - Should not be used in patients with underlying liver disease or history of heavy alcohol use
  - Concomitant use of folic acid (1–3 mg/d) significantly decreases side effects.
  - Adverse effects include myelosuppression and hepatic fibrosis and should monitor CBC, AST, ALT, albumin every 8 weeks.
- Leflunomide: Similar to methotrexate; long half life
- Sulfasalazine:
  - Safe to use in patients with liver disease
  - Adverse effects include myelosuppression; CBC monitored every 2 weeks for 1st 3 months, then every 3 months
- Hydroxychloroquine:
  - Very well tolerated; effective in mild RA or in combination therapy
  - Adverse effects include macular changes; patients should have funduscopic exam every year.
- TNFα antagonists are among the most effective treatments for RA, but they are costly and have several side effects to consider: Increased rate of infections, lymphoma, lupus-like autoimmune disease, MS-like demyelinating disease, and worsening of heart failure:
  - Etanercept: Soluble TNF-receptor fusion protein
  - Infliximab: Chimeric IgG anti-TNFα antibody
  - Adalimumab: Recombinant human IgG monoclonal antibody
- Rituximab: In combination with methotrexate, rituximab (Rituxan) is indicated for the treatment of RA in patients who have failed or cannot tolerate TNF immunomodulators:
  - Monoclonal antibody directed against B cells with the CD20 surface antigen
  - Selective reduction of CD20+ B cells, which play a role in promoting and maintaining the disease process of RA.
  - Cases of reactivated, fulminant hepatitis B have been reported with rituximab. Patients with a history of hepatitis B or C should be followed carefully. Antivirals are sometimes needed.

FOLLOW-UP

DISPOSITION

Issues for Referral

Arrange follow-up care with a rheumatologist:

- Antepartum if the patient's symptoms are not controlled with acetaminophen
- Postpartum in all cases, since symptoms commonly worsen postpartum
- Preconception to facilitate discontinuation of drugs that are teratogenic

PROGNOSIS

- Pregnancy does not influence the long-term prognosis of RA.
- In patients who desire birth control, OCPs are acceptable:
  - OCPs have good efficacy
  - Hormonal influence may assist in controlling disease.
- IUD should be avoided in women who require immunosuppressive therapy.

COMPLICATIONS

- Complications are generally not increased among pregnant women with RA.
- Patients with pulmonary disease may have a worsening of status in the 3rd trimester.
- Patients who require maintenance steroids may have poor healing and an increased risk of PPROM.

PATIENT MONITORING

Mother

- Recent DMARD use (within 3–6 months of conception) should have TB testing, LFTs, and an initial assessment of RF titers.
- Patients who require corticosteroids in pregnancy should have early glucose testing.

Fetus

Targeted US should be done for patients who conceive while on DMARDs or within 3 months of discontinuation.

BIBLIOGRAPHY

Chakravarty E, et al. The use of disease modifying antirheumatic drugs in women with rheumatoid arthritis of childbearing age: A survey of practice patterns and pregnancy outcomes. *J Rheumatol.* 2003;30(2):241–246.

Emery P. Treatment of rheumatoid arthritis. *Br Med J.* 2006;332:152–155.

Janssen N, et al. The effects of immunosuppressive and anti-inflammatory medications on fertility, pregnancy and lactation. *Arch Intern Med.* 2000;160(5):610–619.

Smolen J, et al. Consensus statement on the use of rituximab in patients with rheumatoid arthritis. *Ann Rheum Dis.* 2007;66(2):143–150.

Westwood O, et al. Rheumatoid factors: What's new? *Rheumatology.* 2006;45:379–385.

MISCELLANEOUS

Pierre-Auguste Renior, a 19th-century French painter and 1 of the world's most accomplished artists, suffered from RA. He was stricken in his 50s and, although the disease would render him wheelchair-bound and unable to grasp a brush without assistance, he continued to paint until he was beyond 70 years of age:

- "One must from time to time attempt things that are beyond one's capacity": Pierre-Auguste Renior.
  - Available at: http://arthritis.~.com/od/art/a/renoir.htm

CLINICAL PEARLS

- RA patients frequently have exacerbation of symptoms postpartum.
- Refer to a rheumatologist soon after delivery in anticipation of worsening symptoms.
- Consider OCPs, which may mimic the pregnant state.

ABBREVIATIONS

- AF—Amniotic fluid
- CCP—Cyclic citrullinated protein
- CVD—Cardiovascular disease
- DMARD—Disease-modifying antirheumatic drug
- JIA—Juvenile idiopathic arthritis
- JRA—Juvenile rheumatoid arthritis
- LFT—Liver function tests
- MS—Multiple sclerosis
- OCP—Oral contraceptive pill
- RA—Rheumatoid arthritis
- RF—Rheumatoid factor
- ROM—Range of motion

CODES

ICD9-CM

- 714.0 Rheumatoid arthritis
- 714.1 Felty syndrome (Rheumatoid arthritis with splenoadrenomegaly and leucopenia)
- 714.2 Rheumatoid arthritis with extra-articular involvement (e.g., carditis, pneumonitis)

PATIENT TEACHING

Better understanding of need for combination therapy and need to try various regimens:

- www.arthritis.org/conditions/diseasecenter/RA
- www.niams.nih.gov/hi/topics/arthritis/rahandout.htm

PREVENTION

Since many RA patients will be exposed to immunomodulators, they may be at increased risk for infections. Vaccination history should be carefully reviewed:

- Varicella
- Pneumococcal
- Hepatitis B
- Influenza
- Tuberculosis skin testing

Section VI

SEIZURE DISORDER AND PREGNANCY

Michael Privitera, MD
Jennifer Cavitt, MD

 BASICS

DESCRIPTION
- Epilepsy: 2 or more unprovoked seizures >24 hours apart
- Seizure: Sudden, abnormal, synchronous, rhythmic firing of neurons that may be associated with clinical manifestations corresponding to brain area involved
- Seizure types:
  - Generalized onset seizures begin involving the entire cortex diffusely at their onset:
    ○ "Primary" generalized tonic-clonic seizure
    ○ Tonic/Atonic "drop" seizures
    ○ Absence seizure
    ○ Myoclonic seizure
  - Partial seizures begin in 1 location and may or may not spread to involve other areas:
    ○ Simple partial seizure (consciousness intact)
    ○ Complex partial seizure (consciousness impaired)
    ○ "Secondarily" generalized tonic-clonic seizure

EPIDEMIOLOGY
- Epilepsy prevalence: 5–9 per 1,000
- 1.25–2 million people with epilepsy in US
- Epilepsy affects ~1% of population:
  - ~1 million US women of childbearing age
  - ~3–5 births/1,000 to women with epilepsy

RISK FACTORS
- Prior stroke
- Prior CNS infection
- TBI
- Congenital or developmental neurologic disorder
- Brain tumor
- Family history
- Degenerative disorder

Genetics
- Some syndromes with genetic component:
  - Primary generalized seizures/epilepsy have increased the risk of epilepsy in offspring.
  - With specific cause (e.g., TBI), risk in off-spring is unchanged from general population.
- Genetic factors may predispose to MCM, increasing further the risk with AEDs.

ASSOCIATED CONDITIONS
Women with epilepsy have increased risk for:
- Menstrual cycle disturbances
- PCOS
- Reduced fertility
- Fluctuations in seizure frequency related to menstrual cycle (catamenial epilepsy)
- Osteoporosis, fractures, osteomalacia:
  - Routine monitoring with DEXA is recommended.
  - Consider calcium and vitamin D supplementation for women taking AEDs.

 DIAGNOSIS

SIGNS AND SYMPTOMS
History
See Description.

Physical Exam
Usually normal unless affected by underlying condition

TESTS
EEG:
- Epileptiform discharges (spikes) characteristic, but absent in 1/3
  - Focal spikes support partial seizures.
  - Generalized spiking supports generalized onset seizure.

TREATMENT

GENERAL MEASURES
- The AED appropriate for seizure type that best controls seizures with the least adverse effects is drug of choice in childbearing years, and monotherapy is the goal if possible.
- Optimize therapy prior to conception.
- If seizure-free on AED >2 years, normal IQ, normal neurologic exam, and normal EEG, consider weaning off AED *prior* to conception:
  - Counseling on risk of seizure recurrence:
    ○ Greatest risk in 1st 6 months after discontinuation of AED
    ○ AED withdrawal should be completed at least 6 months prior to conception.
    ○ Do not wean off AED during pregnancy.

ALERT
- Enzyme-inducing AEDs increase the failure rate of hormonal contraceptives and unplanned pregnancies:
  - Phenobarbital, phenytoin, carbamazepine, oxcarbazepine, topiramate (>200 mg/d), primidone, felbamate, ethosuximide
- Breakthrough bleeding may signal drug interaction, and is more common with enzyme-inducing drugs.
- Higher estrogen OCPs and shorter interval for DMPA have been recommended.
- POP is not recommended.
- Barrier contraception should be used as backup.
- Mirena IUD is recommended.

ALERT
- Lamotrigine levels drop 25–70% in the presence of combined OCP:
  - Possible breakthrough seizures
  - Monitor levels and adjust dosage
- Treatment with some AEDs impairs folic acid absorption and/or increases its metabolism:
  - Folic acid deficiency linked to fetal malformations including NTDs in animals and humans
  - Folic acid supplementation 1–5 mg/d recommended in women of childbearing age.

PREGNANCY-SPECIFIC ISSUES
- Pregnancy is NOT contraindicated in women with epilepsy.
- >90% of women with epilepsy have good pregnancy outcomes.

Risks for Mother
- Obstetric complications are more frequent:
  - Spontaneous abortion: 3–5 times increased risk
  - Preterm labor, delivery: 3–5 times increased risk
  - Eclampsia
  - Pregnancy-induced HTN
  - Placental abruption
  - Anemia
  - Forceps-assisted or cesarean delivery
  - Hyperemesis gravidarum
  - Labor induction
- Seizures during pregnancy pose risks:
  - Both convulsive and nonconvulsive seizures may be detrimental to the fetus.
  - A minority with increased seizure frequency
  - Emphasize compliance.
  - Avoid known triggers (e.g., sleep deprivation).
- 2–4% have a convulsive seizure during labor or within 24 hours after delivery:
  - Delivery in hospital with facilities for maternal and neonatal resuscitation
- Majority with uncomplicated labor and delivery, but cesarean delivery and labor induction are performed twice as often.
  - Consider cesarean delivery in select patients:
    ○ When neurologic or cognitive impairment interferes with cooperation during labor
    ○ Poorly controlled seizures in 3rd trimester
    ○ Women with stress-induced seizures

Risks for Fetus
- Low Apgar scores
- Fetal hemorrhage
- Perinatal mortality (2 times increase)
- Stillbirth
- Increased incidence of MCM:
  - 4–8% in women with epilepsy (2 times increase):
    ○ Greater risk with multiple AEDs
    ○ Greater risk with higher doses
    ○ Greater risk with valproic acid: 10.7% with monotherapy, RR 7.3 (95% CI 4.4–12.2)
    ○ Risk with phenobarbital: 6.5% (RR 4.2, 95% CI 1.5–9.4)
  - Phenytoin, phenobarbital, primidone, and valproic acid have pregnancy risk category D rating; balance risk with benefits
  - Carbamazepine, ethosuximide, oxcarbazepine, felbamate, lamotrigine, gabapentin, topiramate, tiagabine, pregabalin, zonisamide, and levetiracetam have a pregnancy risk category C rating.
  - AED pregnancy registries collect prospective data on outcomes with specific AEDs.
- MCM: NTDs, congenital heart disease, orofacial clefts, intestinal atresia, urogenital defects
- Recommend testing with AFP levels at age 14–16 weeks' gestation
- Level II US at 16–20 weeks

- Amniocentesis if appropriate
- Minor malformations increased 2–3-fold:
  – 10–30% of AED-exposed fetuses
  – Minor malformations: Craniofacial dysmorphism, distal digit and nail hypoplasia, minor skeletal anomalies, umbilical and inguinal hernias
- Increased risk of developmental delay:
  – No data on relative risk of different AEDs
- Enzyme-inducing AEDs cause vitamin K deficiency in neonates:
  – Prenatal oral vitamin K supplementation 10–20 mg/d in the last month of pregnancy may help prevent early hemorrhagic disease.
  – ACOG/AAP recommend 1 mg vitamin K to the neonate (in addition to above).
- Majority of neonates born to women taking AEDs with no adverse effects (AEs) at birth:
  – Sedation, hypotonia, poor sucking, feeding difficulties, and rare respiratory depression have all been reported in 5–10%.
    ○ Such adverse effects typically resolve in 2–8 days.
  – Withdrawal symptoms have been reported in neonates exposed to barbiturates, phenytoin, and benzodiazepines.

MEDICATION (DRUGS)
- Changes in AEDs during pregnancy to reduce teratogenic risk are NOT recommended:
  – Risk of seizures
  – Most MCM occur in 1st month after conception, before prenatal care.
- AED levels may fluctuate during pregnancy.
- Baseline, preconception AED level recommended
- Frequent AED levels (monthly to every trimester) with dose adjustments, as clinically indicated
- Free drug levels are more reliable in monitoring levels of highly protein-bound AEDs.
- Lamotrigine clearance increases significantly (>65%) early and throughout pregnancy:
  – Close monitoring of LTG levels before, during, and after pregnancy with appropriate dose adjustment is recommended.

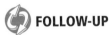 FOLLOW-UP

DISPOSITION
Issues for Referral
Collaborative care between neurology and obstetrics

PROGNOSIS
- >90% with good pregnancy outcomes
- Seizure control unchanged in >1/2
- 17–33% with increased seizure frequency
- Incidence of status epilepticus during pregnancy similar to the general epileptic population
- Increased risk for fetal/neonatal complications:
  – MCM, minor malformation, IUGR, developmental delay, hemorrhagic disease of newborn, isolated seizures, epilepsy

PATIENT MONITORING
Mother
- Continued monitoring of AED levels is required in the postpartum period.
- Some women may have required dosage increases during pregnancy.

- As physiologic changes of pregnancy reverse in the postpartum period, AED dosages usually may be reduced to prepregnancy doses within 1–2 months following delivery:
  – This may occur more quickly with some AEDs.
  – Toxicity may result from continuing higher AED dosages following pregnancy.

Fetus
AED therapy is not a contraindication to breast-feeding:
- All AEDs are detectable in breast milk, usually at a lower concentration than in maternal serum.
- Transfer through breast milk typically is much smaller than placental transfer.
- Drug elimination mechanisms are not fully developed in neonate, and accumulation of drug may occur, particularly with lamotrigine.
- Benefits of breast-feeding are felt to outweigh the small risk of adverse events caused by AEDs.
- Observe infant for signs and symptoms: Sedation, irritability, and failure to thrive

BIBLIOGRAPHY

Annegers JF. The epidemiology of epilepsy. In: Wyllie E, ed. *The Treatment of Epilepsy,* 3rd ed. Philadelphia: Lippincott Williams & Wilkins; 2001;131–138.

Crawford P. Best practice guidelines for the management of women with epilepsy. *Epilepsia.* 2005;46(9):117–124.

Foldvary N. Treatment of epilepsy during pregnancy. In: Wyllie E, ed. *The Treatment of Epilepsy,* 3rd ed. Philadelphia: Lippincott Williams & Wilkins; 2001; 775–786.

Holmes LE, et al. , for the AED Pregnancy Registry. The AED (antiepileptic drug) pregnancy registry: A 6-6-year experience. *Arch Neurol.* 2004;61: 673–678.

Morrow J, et al. Malformation risks of antiepileptic drugs in pregnancy: A prospective study from the UK Epilepsy and Pregnancy Register. *J Neurol Neurosurg Psychiatry.* 2006;77:193–198.

Practice parameter. Management issues for women with epilepsy (summary statement). Report of the Quality Standards Subcommittee of the American Academy of Neurology. *Neurology.* 1998;51: 944–948.

The EURAP Study Group. Seizure control and treatment in pregnancy: Observations from the EURAP Epilepsy Pregnancy Registry. *Neurology.* 2006;66:354–360.

Tran TA, et al. Lamotrigine clearance during pregnancy. *Neurology.* 2002;59:251–255.

Wyszynski DF, et al. , for the Antiepileptic Drug Pregnancy Registry. Increased rate of major malformations in offspring exposed to valproate during pregnancy. *Neurology.* 2005;64:961–965.

 MISCELLANEOUS

CLINICAL PEARLS
- Valproate, phenobarbital, and any AED combination confer highest risk of MCM; preconception counseling should address this.
- Limited data on risk of MCM for the 9 newer AEDs approved since 1993, but few trends show that they will pose a greater risk than older AEDs.
- AED levels often drop during all trimesters and should be monitored closely; adjust AED doses as needed.

- Enzyme-inducing AEDs increase the failure rate of hormonal contraceptives and the number of unplanned pregnancies.

ABBREVIATIONS
- AAP—American Academy of Pediatrics
- ACOG—American College of Obstetricians and Gynecologists
- AEDs—Antiepileptic drugs
- AFP—α-Fetoprotein
- CI—Confidence interval
- DEXA—Dual-energy x-ray assay
- DMPA—Depot medroxyprogesterone acetate
- IUGR—Intrauterine growth restriction
- MCM—Major congenital malformations
- NTD—Neural tube defect
- OCP—Oral contraceptive pill
- PCOS—Polycystic ovary syndrome
- POP—Progestin-only pill
- RR—Relative risk

CODES
ICD9-CM
649.4 Epilepsy complicating pregnancy, childbirth, or the puerperium

PATIENT TEACHING

Advise and counsel women regarding:
- Hormonal contraceptives may be less effective in women taking enzyme-inducing AEDs.
- $\geq$50 μg/d estrogen is recommended when OCP is prescribed, but contraceptive failure is still possible.
- Folic acid supplementation: At least 1 mg/d for all women of childbearing age with epilepsy
- Increased risk of MCM associated with AEDs during pregnancy.
- Risks posed to the fetus by seizures that may occur during pregnancy.
  – Emphasize the importance of compliance.
- AED therapy should be optimized 6 months prior to conception.
- Seizure frequency may change during pregnancy; advise on avoidance of known seizure triggers, such as sleep deprivation.
- Potential changes in AED levels that may occur during pregnancy and the need for close follow-up and drug monitoring
- Vitamin K supplementation during the last month of pregnancy when enzyme-inducing drugs are prescribed
- Risks and benefits of breast-feeding
- Infant care and seizure precautions:
  – Use a carrier or stroller when transporting infant, even in the house.
  – Use a pad on the floor for dressing and changing instead of a high changing table.
  – Never bathe infant without close supervision.
    ○ Patient education materials through the Epilepsy Foundation of America. Available at www.efa.org
    ○ Counsel about the existence of pregnancy registries, including the North American Antiepileptic Drug Pregnancy Registry. Available at www.massgeneral.org/aed or 1-888-233-2334.

SICKLE CELL DISEASE AND HEMOGLOBINOPATHIES IN PREGNANCY

Jill M. Zurawski, MD

 BASICS

DESCRIPTION
- SCA is the most common of a spectrum of major inherited hemoglobinopathies.
- In pregnancy, these diseases can have serious consequences for both mother and fetus, due to changes in the shape of abnormal hemoglobin chains:
  - Shortened lifespan of RBCs with hemolysis
  - Increased propensity to infection
  - Vaso-occlusive disease and end-organ damage, including placental involvement
  - Increased physiologic demands of uteroplacental flow

EPIDEMIOLOGY
- 1:12 African Americans are carriers of HgbS.
- 1:300 African American newborns have some form of the disease.

RISK FACTORS
Sickle hemoglobin is carried in people of African, African American, Mediterranean basin, Middle Eastern, or Indian descent.

Genetics
- Hemoglobin S results from a genetic mutation causing substitution of valine for glutamic acid from an A for T substitution on the β-globin gene.
- Autosomal recessive inheritance: If both parents are carriers, fetus has 25% chance of SCA.
  - Genetic counseling and discussion of prenatal diagnosis is recommended.
- Genotype frequencies: SCA-SS (60%), SCA-SC (25–30%), S-β-thalassemia, α-thalassemia and other lesser variants such as Hgbs C, D, and E.
- Phenotype is highly variable.

PATHOPHYSIOLOGY
- HgbS is poorly soluble when deoxygenated, resulting in distorted, sickle-shaped hemoglobin.
- This then leads to increased viscosity, red-cell hemolysis, anemia, further decreased oxygen tension, vasoocclusive crises with microvascular obstruction, and occasionally organ failure.
- Various morbidities and mortalities result depending on organ system and severity.
- Microinfarcts may occur in the placenta, impairing fetal oxygenation and growth.

ASSOCIATED CONDITIONS
- Increased incidence of miscarriage, IUGR, IUFD, preterm delivery, and perinatal mortality
- Increased incidence of pyelonephritis and UTI

- Cholecystitis, splenic infarcts, hepatitis, and hyposthenuria may confuse evaluation for preeclampsia.
- Pain crises with abdominal pain, cholecystitis, and appendicitis may present similarly to placental abruption.
- Acute chest syndrome (pleuritic chest pain, fever, cough, pulmonary infiltrates, hypoxia) is increased during pregnancy and can lead to more rapid decompensation due to decreased pulmonary expansion from growing uterus.
- Chronic disease can lead to stroke, severe cardiopulmonary compromise, and renal failure.
- Chronic hemolysis and/or transfusion may lead to iron overload.
- Alloimmunization may occur from transfusion; antibody screen is important both for fetus and to prevent transfusion reaction in future.

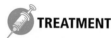 **DIAGNOSIS**

SIGNS AND SYMPTOMS
History
- Women of obstetric age may have had this diagnosis as children or even prenatally.
- Dyspnea should prompt close evaluation for acute chest syndrome or pneumonia.
- Pain crises may appear out of proportion to physical findings.
- Depression and narcotic addiction can be consequences of chronic disease and chronic pain.
- History of transfusion leaves pregnant women at risk of Rh or other isoimmunization from lesser-known antibodies; risks for hepatitis or transfusion-associated infections are increased.

Physical Exam
- Baseline funduscopic exam, cardiopulmonary exam and functions, and search for joint contractures or infections are imperative at initial prenatal visit and at any sign of infection.
- Scleral icterus, pallor, flow murmur are common due to acute and chronic hemolysis.
- Neurologic exam may indicate CNS infarction or hemorrhage.
- Lagging FH may indicate poor fetal growth.

TESTS
- Hemoglobin electrophoresis is definitive; test father to determine fetal risk.
- Various solubility screening tests are inadequate as they may miss less common hemoglobinopathies and cannot distinguish between SCA and SC trait.
- Preimplantation genetic diagnosis with IVF is available; prenatal diagnosis with CVS, amniocentesis, or cordocentesis is also available during pregnancy.

- CBC: Chronic mild to moderate anemia (iron and folate deficiencies should be considered).
- CXR and pulse oximetry should be checked for abnormal respiratory symptoms (acute chest syndrome, pneumonia).
- UA and frequent urine culture may (but does not always) decrease the increased incidence of pyelonephritis.
- US for dating and fetal growth
- Kick counts and fetal movement surveillance in 3rd trimester are imperative.
- No prospective studies on use of antenatal testing (NST, BPP, CST): Physicians should use discretion and clinical judgment.

Labs
- Hemoglobin electrophoresis at 1st visit; test father (see Genetics)
- Antibody screen
- CBC, iron, and folate studies as indicated
- UA and urine culture

Imaging
US should be used to follow fetal growth as patients are at increased risk of growth restriction (up to 45% incidence).

TREATMENT

GENERAL MEASURES
- Treatment is largely symptomatic. The main objective is to end pain crises, treat infection, and maintain a healthy uteroplacental environment.
- Oxygen may decrease intensity of sickling during a crisis.
- Rapid analgesia with narcotics may ease pulmonary demands, particularly with a large, gravid uterus.
- Transfusions may be considered on a case-by-case basis; they may shorten duration of severe crises (see below).

PREGNANCY-SPECIFIC ISSUES
- Some experts believe that prepregnancy course can predict maternal disease behavior during pregnancy.
- Serious pregnancy-specific issues such as ectopic implantation and abruption may be overlooked if women are presumed to be in pain crisis. Pain crisis should be an exclusionary diagnosis after all other diagnoses are systematically ruled out.
- Intense bone pain from marrow infarction is common and can be confusing, particularly with hip and back pain. Preterm labor and abruption may be difficult to distinguish in patient in pain.
- Exchange transfusion in pregnancy is controversial: No compelling evidence exists to transfuse prophylactically. However, transfusion should be considered for:
  - Symptomatic acute anemia
  - Acute chest syndrome with hypoxia
  - Surgery
  - Protracted, severe pain

- Pneumonia, particularly from *Streptococcus pneumoniae*, is more common due to autoinfection of the spleen.
- Baseline cardiac dysfunction and ventricular hypertrophy may be worsened by increased preload, decreased afterload, and increased cardiac output in pregnancy.

By Trimester
- 1st trimester: Educate patients of prenatal testing available; offer hemoglobin electrophoresis testing of father. Confirm dating by exam or US as fetal growth may lag with time.
- 2nd (and 3rd) trimester: Increased incidences of preterm labor, growth restriction, PROM
- 3rd trimester, particularly peripartum: Increased oxygen requirements, increased fetal intolerance to labor, chorioamnionitis, and endometritis. In labor, pay attention to oxygenation and hydration, as well as pain requirements. Be aware that patients may be tolerant of narcotics from past chronic pain crises; use regional anesthesia with caution secondary to volume state. Increased incidence of retained placenta.
- Influenza vaccination should be given annually regardless of trimester; vaccination against *Haemophilus influenza* B and *Pneumococcus* should be considered.

Risks for Mother
- Pain crises are more frequent (nearly 50% of women) for the woman with SCA due to increased physiologic demands.
- Nature of disease may lead to multiorgan system dysfunction or failure.
- Increased antepartum hospitalizations due to infection and preterm labor; increased postpartum endometritis may also prolong hospital stay.
- Maternal mortality is as high as 1–3%, due to infection, acute chest syndrome, CVA, MI, and acute anemia.

Risks for Fetus
- Inherited hemoglobinopathy
- Fetal growth restriction and preterm birth may lead to low birth weight.
- Perinatal death incidence may be as high as 6%.

MEDICATION (DRUGS)
- Folic acid requirements may be increased due to active hematopoiesis (1–4 mg).
- Acetaminophen may help mild pain.
- Severe pain or pain crisis often requires narcotic analgesia (may also be sedating to fetus). Chronic narcotic use may be necessary but watch for signs of withdrawal in neonate.
- Stool softeners are helpful in chronic narcotic use, as constipation is more common in pregnancy.

 FOLLOW-UP

DISPOSITION
Issues for Referral
- Psychiatric referral may be helpful for chronic pain and depression.
- Genetic counseling is appropriate, particularly prior to conception and in early pregnancy.
- Care should be coordinated with patient's primary physician and perinatal consultants.

PROGNOSIS
- Pregnancy state of disease may be predicted by prepregnancy state. However, both maternal and fetal outcomes vary widely.
- Maternal and fetal mortality is significantly increased.

COMPLICATIONS
- Multiple organ involvement and/or failure
- Premature delivery, LBW neonate
- Maternal death
- Fetal/Neonatal death

PATIENT MONITORING
Mother
Frequent prenatal visits with surveillance for pain, infection, and anemia

Fetus
- Serial US for fetal growth
- Antenatal testing has not been prospectively studied and should be individualized.

BIBLIOGRAPHY

Creasy R, et al. *Maternal-Fetal Medicine Principles and Practice*, 5th ed. Philadelphia: Saunders; 2004.

Cunningham FG, et al. *Williams Obstetrics*, 22nd ed. New York: McGraw Hill; 2005.

Mahomed K. Prophylactic versus selective blood transfusion for sickle cell anaemia during pregnancy. *Cochrane Rev Abstract*. 2006.

Serjeant GR, et al. Outcome of pregnancy in homozygous sickle cell disease. *Obstet Gynecol*. 2004;103(6):1278–1285.

World Health Organization. *Medical Eligibility Criteria for Contraceptive Use*, 3rd ed. Geneva, Switzerland: WHO, 2004;1–186. Available at www.who.org

 MISCELLANEOUS

- Life expectancy is decreased in women with SCD. Patients may wish to consider this in context of fertility and family planning.
- Bone marrow transplant can be curative for patients outside of pregnancy (replacement of marrow with normal hemoglobin-producing cells).

ABBREVIATIONS
- BPP—Biophysical profile
- COC—Combination oral contraceptive
- CST—Contraction stress test
- CVA—Cerebrovascular accident
- CVS—Chorionic villus sampling
- FH—Fundal height
- IUFD—Intrauterine fetal demise
- IUGR—Intrauterine growth restriction
- IVF—In vitro fertilization
- LBW—Low birth weight
- MI—Myocardial infarction
- NST—Nonstress test
- PROM—Premature rupture of membranes
- SCA—Sickle cell anemia
- SCD—Sickle cell disease

CODES
ICD9-CM
- 282.5 Sickle cell trait
- 282.6 Sickle cell anemia
- 282.41–41 Sickle thalassemia
- 282.69 Sickle cell with crisis

 PATIENT TEACHING

- Keeping mother well hydrated, oxygenated, and pain free will benefit developing fetus.
- Educate on signs and symptoms of preterm labor and kick counts are essential.

PREVENTION
- Avoid stress, cold, infection, and other known triggers of crisis.
- Unintended pregnancies should be avoided. Thus, contraception should be addressed prior to pregnancy, and during pregnancy, before delivery:
  - Progesterones are known to decrease the incidence of sickle cell pain crises (pills, injections, and implants are options).
  - Current evidence-based guidelines from the WHO suggest that:
    - COCs can be used safely in women with SCA
    - IUDs can be used safely in women with SCA, although the increased blood loss that may occur with copper IUDs may be problematic.
  - Sterilization may be considered.

Section VI

SPINAL CORD INJURY AND STROKE AND PREGNANCY

Julie Scott, MD
Kathryn L. Reed, MD

BASICS

DESCRIPTION

- SCI is an insult to the spinal cord resulting in any degree of sensory and/or motor deficit, autonomic dysfunction, and bladder/bowel dysfunction:
  - Acute and chronic
  - Temporary or permanent
  - Incomplete or complete:
    ○ Tetraplegia (replaces quadriplegia): Injury to the spinal cord in the cervical region affecting all 4 extremities
    ○ Paraplegia: Injury to spinal cord in the thoracic, lumbar, or sacral segments, including cauda equina and conus medullaris
- Stroke is the sudden onset of neurologic deficit resulting from infarction or hemorrhage within the brain:
  - Temporary or permanent

EPIDEMIOLOGY

- SCI:
  - 250,000–400,000 in US; 18% female
  - 11,000 new SCI/year-60% <30 years old
  - Highest per capita rate between ages 16 and 30
  - Men > women; 4:1
- Stroke:
  - No consensus on incidence in pregnancy; range 3–26/100,000 deliveries
  - Hemorrhagic/Ischemic about same frequency
  - Eclampsia occurs in 2% of pregnancies:
    ○ Associated with 24–47% of ischemic CVA and 14–44% of hemorrhagic CVA
- 1.8% recurrence rate in subsequent pregnancy if history of ischemic CVA
- Pregnancy-related stroke accounts for 5% of all maternal mortality (0.66/100,000 live births).

RISK FACTORS

- SCI:
  - MVA: 44%
  - Acts of violence: 24%
  - Falls: 22%
  - Sports (2/3 from diving): 8%
  - Other, including genetic, inflammatory, infectious, autoimmune, and vascular: 2%
- Stroke:
  - Age
  - Race: African American
  - Smoking
  - HTN
  - Diabetes
  - Preeclampsia/Eclampsia/HELLP
  - TTP
  - APA
  - Hyperlipidemia
  - Hyperhomocysteinemia
  - Atrial fibrillation
  - Cardiomyopathy
  - Family history
  - Illicit drug abuse

Genetics

- SCI:
  - Maternal congenital ONTD; polygenic
- Stroke:
  - Polygenic with a tendency to clustering of risk factors within families

PATHOPHYSIOLOGY

- SCI:
  - Depends on the mode of injury, with damage to the afferent and efferent pathways that travel from the peripheral nervous system to CNS
- Stroke:
  - Ischemic:
    ○ Carotid atherosclerotic disease
    ○ Cardiac: Arrhythmias, cardiomyopathy, valvular disease
    ○ HTN including chronic, preeclampsia/eclampsia
    ○ Cerebral artery or venous thrombus; thrombophilia associated
  - Hemorrhagic:
    ○ HELLP syndrome
  - Hypercoagulable:
    ○ Thrombophilias
  - Vascular malformations: AVMs, angiomas
  - Other: Vasculitis, traumatic, drug, tumors

ASSOCIATED CONDITIONS

- SCI:
  - Comorbid medical conditions
  - Depression
- Stroke related to APA syndrome:
  - Fetal loss >10 weeks
  - IUFD
  - Pregnancy morbidities including IUGR secondary to placental insufficiency, eclampsia, preeclampsia

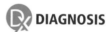

DIAGNOSIS

SIGNS AND SYMPTOMS

History
SCI

- Acute: Usually obtained by emergency medical staff to elucidate mode of injury
- Chronic: Important to assess any resolution of symptoms or return of function vs. loss of function
  - Coexisting medical issues as a result of chronic SCI:
    ○ Recurrent UTIs
    ○ Decubitus ulcers
    ○ Chronic constipation
    ○ Pulmonary deficiencies/infections
    ○ Musculoskeletal spasticity, decreased ROM
  - Risk of autonomic hyperreflexia with SCI above the T6 level

Stroke

- Stroke related to subarachnoid hemorrhage is usually the result of vascular malformation:
  - Cardinal features: Sudden severe headache, along with visual changes, cranial nerve abnormalities, focal deficits, or altered consciousness:
    ○ High mortality rate
- Other stroke signs and symptoms:
  - Hemiplegia, hemianesthesia, neglect, aphasia
  - Headache, nausea, vomiting, diplopia, facial paresis
  - Dysphagia, dysarthria
  - Impaired level of consciousness
  - Ataxia
  - Seizures
- History:
  - Prior episodes of symptoms
  - Any history of clots elsewhere in the body
  - Medication history if anticoagulated
  - Family history for genetic contribution

Physical Exam

- Complete physical exam
- Vital signs:
  - Hypotension, tachycardia or bradycardia, hypothermia
- Detailed neurologic exam:
  - Assessment of motor function of trunk and extremities
  - Assessment for sensory deficits:
    ○ Dermatomal distributions
- Assessment of centrally located lesions:
  - Vision changes
  - Speech quality, word usage
  - Cranial nerve exam
  - Funduscopic exam:
    ○ Papilledema, hemorrhages, A-V nicking

TESTS

- Acute SCI:
  - CBC with platelets
  - Coagulation studies
  - Illicit drug screening
- Stroke:
  - CBC with platelets
  - Coagulation studies
  - HELLP syndrome labs including LFTs, creatinine, LDH, haptoglobin, platelets followed serially
  - Thrombophilia evaluation: APA, LAC, ANA, factor V Leiden, prothrombin gene mutation, antithrombin III activity, protein S, protein C: Total and activity
  - Illicit drug screening

Imaging

- Acute SCI:
  - CT/MRI to evaluate level of injury
  - Deep peritoneal lavage to evaluate for coexistent internal injuries/hemorrhage
  - US evaluation of fetus:
    ○ EFM: Fetal status, maternal perfusion
- Stroke:
  - CT/MRI/MRA/MRV
  - Carotid artery duplex US
  - EKG and ECG
  - EEG for any associated seizure activity

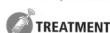

TREATMENT

GENERAL MEASURES

Acute SCI:

- Trauma protocol for stabilization

PREGNANCY-SPECIFIC ISSUES

Acute SCI:

- Maternal stabilization is primary goal.
- Spinal shock with hypoperfusion of the uterus
- Highest risk for thromboembolic events is from time of acute injury to 8 weeks later:
  - Thromboprophylactic measures
  - May last up to 3 weeks post injury

By Trimester

Acute SCI:

- Miscarriage dependent on coexistent injuries
- Abruption secondary to abdominal trauma

ALERT

- Prevent autonomic hyperreflexia:
  - Occurs in 85% if lesion at or above T6

- Monitor/assess "silent labor"; contractions may not be felt, based on level on SCI:
  - No evidence of higher risk of preterm labor

- Stroke:
  - Greatest risk in 3rd trimester and postpartum:
    ○ Higher rates of hemorrhage caused by AVM, other vascular abnormalities in 2nd trimester
  - Thrombophilia-related:
    ○ SAB, abruption, IUGR, preeclampsia
  - Hemorrhagic strokes:
    ○ Surgical repair needed near time of delivery—Cesarean delivery followed by craniotomy for complete repair
    ○ Surgical repair remote from delivery—no contraindication to vaginal delivery

Risks for Mother
- SCI:
  - Morbidity and mortality associated with acute injury and with chronic injury; autonomic hyperreflexia and comorbid conditions
  - No increased thrombotic risk except with acute injury within the 1st 8 weeks
- Stroke:
  - Depends on causative factors, neurologic extent, and arterial vs. venous vs. hemorrhagic pathology

Risks for Fetus
- Acute SCI:
  - Uterine hypoperfusion from spinal shock with fetal hypoperfusion and potential for loss
  - Maternal status/stabilization takes precedence; emergent delivery of viable fetus is considered only if stability is assured for mother.
- Chronic SCI:
  - >T10; "silent labor" with unattended delivery

MEDICATION (DRUGS)
Acute SCI
- Methylprednisolone within 8 hours to limit damage:
  - Bolus 30 mg/kg followed by infusion at 5.4 mg/kg/hr for 23 hours
- Cardiovascular/Hemodynamic support:
  - Dobutamine or dopamine

Chronic SCI
Autonomic hyperreflexia is life-threatening:
- Secondary to loss of hypothalamic control over sympathetic spinal reflexes in viable cord segment distal to the injury
- Symptoms: Facial flushing, HTN, diaphoresis, severe headache, cardiac arrhythmia, seizure, death
- Inciting events: Bladder distention, bladder catheterization, constipation, uterine contractions, cervical exam
  - Prevention is key
  - Manage HTN pharmacologically
  - Early epidural for labor
  - Bowel and bladder care

Stroke
Thrombotic:
- IV tPA 0.9 mg/kg within 3 hours of injury:
  - Controversial in pregnancy: Reported success; alternative is mechanical clot disruption
- Thrombophilias with clinical history of prior clots, poor pregnancy outcomes: Anticoagulate
- Valvular cardiac disease and hypokinetic cardiomyopathies: Anticoagulate

- Infectious etiologies: Antibiotic administration
Hemorrhagic:
- Neurosurgical clip ligation
- Analgesia for pain symptoms

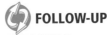 FOLLOW-UP
DISPOSITION
Issues for Referral
- Acute SCI:
  - Transfer to a tertiary-care center, preferably for complete care of mother and fetus
- Stroke:
  - Rapid-response team for stroke intervention to lessen morbidities and mortality

PROGNOSIS
- Acute SCI:
  - Depends on mode of injury and concurrent injuries
- Chronic SCI:
  - Pneumonia and pulmonary complications are leading cause of mortality, followed by septicemia and further trauma (suicide).
- Stroke:
  - Depends on timing of care, extent of injury, and continued loss of function

PATIENT MONITORING
Mother
- Chronic SCI:
  - Evidence of premature labor
  - Concurrent management of any comorbid medical illnesses:
    ○ Suppression therapy for recurrent UTIs
    ○ Aggressive bowel care to prevent constipation
    ○ Frequent position change/turning to prevent decubitus ulcers
- Stroke:
  - Monitoring of anticoagulation to achieve appropriate dosing:
    ○ Heparin/Lovenox dose increases to maintain same anticoagulation profile
  - BP, urinary protein for evidence preeclampsia:
    ○ Increased risk with diagnosis of thrombophilia

Fetus
- Acute SCI:
  - Continuous fetal monitoring if ongoing maternal instability and through period at highest risk of spinal shock
- Chronic SCI:
  - Usual antepartum fetal testing
- Stroke:
  - Thrombophilia related; assess for IUGR

BIBLIOGRAPHY

Jaigobin C, et al. Stroke and pregnancy. *Stroke.* 2000;31:2948–2951.

James AH, et al. Incidence and risk factors for stroke in pregnancy and the puerperium. *Obstet Gynecol.* 2005;106(3):509–516.

Johnson DM, et al. Thrombolytic therapy for acute stroke in late pregnancy with intra-arterial recombinant tissue plasminogen activator. *Stroke.* 2005;36:e53–e55.

Kang A. Traumatic spinal cord injury. *Clin Obstet Gynecol.* 2005;48(1):67–72.

Murugappan A, et al. Thrombolytic therapy of acute ischemic stroke during pregnancy. *Neurology.* 2006;66:768–770.

Pereira L. Obstetric management of the patient with spinal cord injury. *Obstet Gynecol Surv.* 2003;58(10):678–686.

Pope CS, et al. Pregnancy complicated by chronic spinal cord injury and history of autonomic hyperreflexia. *Obstet Gynecol.* 2001;97:802–803.

Shehata HA, et al. Neurological disorders in pregnancy. *Curr Opin Obstet Gynecol.* 2004;16:117–122.

 MISCELLANEOUS
CLINICAL PEARLS
Autonomic hyperreflexia is life-threatening:
- Early epidural prevents/reduces incidence
- Use of local/topical anesthesia for Foley catheter placement and cervical exams

ABBREVIATIONS
- ANA—Antinuclear antibody
- APA—Antiphospholipid antibody
- AVM—Arterial venous malformation
- CVA—Cerebrovascular accident
- EFM—Electronic fetal monitoring
- HELLP—Hemolytic anemia, elevated liver enzymes, low platelet count
- IUFD—Intrauterine fetal demise
- IUGR—Intrauterine growth restriction
- LAC—Lupus anticoagulant
- LDH—Lactate dehydrogenase
- LFT—Liver function tests
- MVA—Motor vehicle accident
- ONTD—Open neural tube defect
- ROM—Range of motion
- SAB—Spontaneous abortion
- SCI—Spinal cord injury
- tPA—Tissue plasminogen activator
- TTP—Thrombotic thrombocytopenic purpura
- UTI—Urinary tract infection

CODES
ICD9-CM
- 344.XX Paraplegia/Quadriplegia
- 434.01 Thrombotic CVA
- 434.11 Embolic CVA
- 434.91 Ischemic CVA
- 674.XX Embolism complicating pregnancy
- 806.XX Fracture of the vertebral column with spinal cord injury
- 852.XX Intracranial hemorrhage
- 952.XX Spinal cord injury without evidence of spinal bone injury

 PATIENT TEACHING

Chronic SCI:
- Prevention of autonomic hyperreflexia:
  - Bladder health
  - Bowel care
  - Uterine palpation/home uterine activity monitoring

PREVENTION
Stroke:
- Anticoagulation if hypercoagulable states are present; avoidance of estrogen-based contraceptives
- Management of coexistent maternal medical conditions: Antihypertensives, glycemic control, lifestyle modifications

Section VI

SYSTEMIC LUPUS ERYTHEMATOSUS AND PREGNANCY

Loralei Thornburg, MD
Ruth Anne Queenan, MD

 BASICS

DESCRIPTION
- SLE is an autoimmune disease characterized by fluctuating, chronic course.
- Varies in severity from mild to severe, and may be lethal.
- The most common connective tissue disease in pregnancy
- In general, women with SLE in pregnancy should be managed by an obstetrician with experience in high-risk pregnancies.

EPIDEMIOLOGY
- All age groups, 30–50 most common
- Normal fertility in most patients
- Female > male 10:1
- African American women have 2–5 times greater risk.
- Prevalence is ~1.22/1,000 for women ≥18 in the US
- Complicates 1 in 2,000 deliveries

RISK FACTORS
Almost all pregnancy complications are increased in patients with SLE.

Genetics
- Genetic predisposition to SLE supported by 10-fold greater risk in monozygotic twins.
- No increased risk of genetic or congenital anomalies from SLE

PATHOPHYSIOLOGY
Most cases are idiopathic.

ASSOCIATED CONDITIONS
Other autoimmune diseases occur in ~30% of SLE patients, including:
- Rheumatoid arthritis
- Hypothyroidism
- Diabetes
- Myasthenia gravis
- Autoimmune cirrhosis
- Celiac disease
- APA syndrome

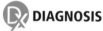 **DIAGNOSIS**

SIGNS AND SYMPTOMS
History
Patient history for complications of SLE should be carefully evaluated including:
- Length of time since diagnosis, and time in quiescence
- Previous biopsies and results
- Associated symptoms
- History of pregnancy loss
- History of venous or arterial thromboembolism
- History of renal transplantation
- Presence of nephritis or renal involvement
- Antibody status

Physical Exam
Initial evaluation of the pregnant patient should include baseline BP and UA, as well as routine prenatal assessment.

TESTS
US for dating should be performed in the 1st trimester:
- Performed in anticipation of growth restriction in the 2nd or 3rd trimester.

Lab
In addition to routine prenatal laboratory testing, patients should have baseline testing for:
- Renal function including:
  - GFR
  - 24-hour urine protein assessment or urine protein/creatinine ratio
  - Urinalysis
- CBC
- Anti-Ro/SSA
- Anti-La/SSB
- Lupus anticoagulant
- Anticardiolipin antibodies
- Anti–double stranded DNA (anti-dsDNA)
- Complement levels (CH50, C3, C4)
- TSH
- Early glucose tolerance testing may be indicated in women on steroid therapy.

Imaging
- US for pregnancy dating
- Serial US to assess fetal growth
- Women with anti-Ro or anti-La antibodies may benefit from serial fetal echocardiography to detect fetal heart block or fetal cardiomyopathy at an early stage.

 TREATMENT

GENERAL MEASURES
- In addition to routine prenatal care, women with SLE should be followed with:
  - Repeat assessment at least once in each trimester of:
    - GFR
    - Complement (C50, or C3 and C4) levels
    - Anti-DS DNA
    - Anticardiolipin antibodies
- Repeat assessments if there is evidence of activation of disease.
- ANA titers should NOT be followed as these do NOT correlate with disease activity.
- Monthly CBC

PREGNANCY-SPECIFIC ISSUES
- Chorea is a rare manifestation of lupus that may be estrogen induced, and is therefore more common in pregnancy.
- Pregnancy outcome:
  - Prognosis is best if the disease in good control for at least 6 months prior to conception.
  - Women without HTN, renal impairment, or APA syndrome have similar pregnancy outcomes to those without SLE (see chapter on APA syndrome).
- Flares of SLE disease during pregnancy:
  - 15–60% of patients experience flares.
  - Flares occur equally in all 3 trimesters.
  - Increased incidence of flairs postpartum
  - Can be difficult to distinguish from preeclampsia with HELLP syndrome

- Lupus nephritis:
  - Carries an increased pregnancy risk over other manifestations of SLE
  - Prognosis is best if:
    - Disease is in good control for at least 6 months prior to conception.
    - Serum creatinine is <1.5 mg/dL.
    - Proteinuria is <3 g/24 h.
    - No HTN
  - 25% of women experience renal deterioration during pregnancy; however most recover.
  - 8% of women have permanent renal deterioration during pregnancy.

By Trimester
- In addition to routine prenatal care and baseline laboratories, women with SLE should receive:
- 1st trimester:
  - Assessment of SLE status (see baseline labs and testing section)
- 2nd trimester:
  - Assessment of SLE serologies
  - Assessment of renal function
  - Assessment of fetal growth
  - Glucose tolerance screening
  - Serial fetal echocardiography for those with SSA/SSB seropositivity
- 3rd trimester:
  - Assessment of SLE serologies
  - Assessment of renal function
  - Assessment of fetal growth
  - Consider NTS and/or BPP testing based on above factors

Risks for Mother
- Pregnancy loss:
  - Risk of spontaneous loss <20 weeks is 4.7 times higher than general population.
  - Fetal death rates after 20 weeks are 4–15 times higher than general population.
- Preterm delivery:
  - 6.8 times rate of general population
  - Rates of PPROM may be as high as 40%.
- Preeclampsia:
  - Highest risk in those with lupus nephritis or APA syndrome
  - Can be very difficult to distinguish from a lupus flare
  - In general, complements will be low during a lupus flare and this may help to distinguish it from preeclampsia.
  - Renal histopathology may also be helpful, but biopsy carries increased risk in pregnancy.

Risks for Fetus
- IUGR:
  - Generally asymmetric
  - Not correlated with disease activity
- Heart block or cardiomyopathy:
  - Associated with maternal anti-Ro (SSA) and anti-La (SSB) antibodies
  - Treatment: Betamethasone or dexamethasone if develops
  - Prognosis is poor if hydrops is present.
  - Most infants will require postnatal pacemakers.
  - Affects ~2% of infants born to women with SLE:
    - However, after 1 infant with complete heart block, the recurrence risk is 15%.

MEDICATION (DRUGS)

- Medical therapy during pregnancy should be tailored to the individual patient and the disease manifestations. Consultation with a toxicologist may be helpful to assess the risks and benefits of therapy to both the mother and fetus.
- Immunosuppressants (mycophenolate, azathioprine, methotrexate, cyclophosphamide):
  – Not generally recommended
  – Assess individual risks and benefits.
  – IUGR, congenital anomalies, and immunosuppression have been reported
  – High rates of fetal loss
  – Azathioprine is the best choice if necessary.
- NSAIDs:
  – 1st trimester use may be associated with increased rates of fetal loss.
  – May be safe in late 1st and 2nd trimesters, in short courses
  – Should not be used near term due to risk of premature closure of the ductus arteriosus
- Glucocorticoids:
  – Relatively safe; lowest dose that controls symptoms should be used.
  – Can increase risk of cleft lip, maternal HTN, diabetes
  – Increased risk of PPROM, IUGR
  – Patients need stress doses in labor.
- Antimalarials:
  – Safety is uncertain.
  – Observational studies suggest safety.
  – Half-life is 1–2 months and therefore, to avoid fetal exposure, these must be stopped at least 6 months prior to pregnancy.
  – Not effective for SLE nephritis
- Antihypertensives:
  – Hydralazine, labetalol, and calcium-channel blockers are all considered safe in pregnancy.
  – Other agents may be used; individual risks should be assessed.

ALERT

- ACE inhibitors should not be used due to the risk of fetal renal failure and death.

- IVIG:
  – May be used to treat SLE associated thrombocytopenia
  – Generally considered safe in pregnancy
- Anticoagulation:
  – If indicated, heparin or LMWH are considered safe.
  – Aspirin is considered safe in pregnancy.
  – Warfarin should be avoided due to the risk of fetal anomalies.

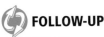 FOLLOW-UP

DISPOSITION

Issues for Referral

- In general, pregnant patients with SLE should be managed with the involvement of both a rheumatologist and an obstetrician/gynecologist with high-risk pregnancy experience.
- If the patient has other sequela of SLE, consultation and input from specialists in those organ systems involved should be sought.

PROGNOSIS

- Overall survival: 93% at 5 years after diagnosis, but worse for minority women.
- Pregnancy does not seem to alter the course or prognosis of SLE.

COMPLICATIONS

Pregnancy risks associated with SLE include an increased incidence of:

- Preterm labor
- Preterm birth
- Fetal loss
- Preeclampsia
- Fetal growth restriction
- DVT

Pediatric Considerations

Neonatal lupus syndrome:

- Rare disorder
- Affects 1–2% of infants born to women with SLE
- Caused by transplacental transfer of maternal antibodies
- Infants may present with malar rash, cardiomyopathy, heart block, cutaneous lupus lesions, hepatobiliary disease, and/or thrombocytopenia.
- Treatment is supportive care.
- Skin lesions generally resolve by 12 months.
- More frequent in infants born to mothers with anti-Ro/anti-La antibodies.

PATIENT MONITORING

See "Treatment."

Mother

In addition to routine prenatal care, women with SLE should receive:

- Assessment of SLE by serology each trimester
- Assessment of renal function each trimester
- Early glucose tolerance screening if on glucocorticoid therapy
- Careful assessment for associated pregnancy complications including preeclampsia and preterm labor

Fetus

- Dating US
- Assessment of fetal growth
- Serial fetal echocardiography for those with SSA/SSB seropositivity
- Weekly NST or BPP testing may be indicated.
- Continuous monitoring in labor if evidence of fetal compromise

BIBLIOGRAPHY

Creasy RK, et al., eds. *Maternal-Fetal Medicine*, 5th ed. Philadelphia: Elsevier; 2004.

Gabbe SG, et al. *Obstetrics, Normal and Problem Pregnancies*, 4th ed. Philadelphia: Churchill Livingstone; 2001.

Schur PH, et al. Pregnancy in women with systemic lupus erythematosus. In: Rose BD, ed. *UpToDate*. Waltham MA: UpToDate; 2006.

 MISCELLANEOUS

Breastfeeding is possible for most women:

- Some medications may enter the breast milk.
- Immunosuppressives should be avoided.
- NSAIDs, antimalarials, prednisone, warfarin and heparin appear to be safe.
- Anti-Ro and anti-La antibodies can be found in breast milk, but there is no evidence of neonatal lupus from breast-feeding.

CLINICAL PEARLS

- Anti-Ro/Anti-La antibodies may cause fetal heart block.
- Lupus nephritis carries a worse pregnancy prognosis.
- SLE should be well controlled for 6 months prior to attempting pregnancy.

ABBREVIATIONS

- ACE—Angiotensin-converting enzyme
- APA—Antiphospholipid antibody
- BPP—Biophysical profile
- GFR—Glomerular filtration rate
- HELLP—Hemolysis Elevated Liver Low Platelets
- IUGR—Intrauterine growth restriction
- IVIG—Intravenous immunoglobulin
- LMWH—Low molecular weight heparin
- NTS—Nonstress test
- PPROM—Preterm premature rupture of membranes
- SLE—Systemic lupus erythematosus
- TSH—Thyroid-stimulating hormone

CODES

ICD9-CM
710.0 Systemic lupus erythematosus

 PATIENT TEACHING

- National Institute of Arthritis and Musculoskeletal and Skin Diseases. Available at www.niams.nih.gov
- Lupus Foundation of America. Available at www.lupus.org

PREVENTION

- There is no way to prevent the onset of SLE.
- The 1/6th of patients with photosensitivity should avoid sun exposure.
- Good control for at least 6 months prior to pregnancy may prevent or delay the onset of complications during pregnancy.
- Pregnancy planning and contraception is essential to optimize pregnancy outcome:
  – Oral contraceptives do not increase risk of flare in women with stable disease:
    ○ Study excluded women with history of thrombosis, lupus anticoagulant, or anticardiolipin antibodies.

THROMBOCYTOPENIA/ITP AND PREGNANCY

Jonathan W. Weeks, MD

 BASICS

DESCRIPTION
- Thrombocytopenia is the 2nd most common hematologic condition in obstetrics.
- In pregnancy:
  - Normal platelet count: 150,000–400,000
  - Mild thrombocytopenia: <150,000
  - Moderate thrombocytopenia: <100,000
  - Severe thrombocytopenia: <50,000
  - Platelets <50,000 associated with increased risk of bleeding with surgery or trauma.
  - Platelets <20,000 associated with an increased risk of spontaneous bleeding.

EPIDEMIOLOGY
- By the 3rd trimester, 7–8% of pregnant mothers will have a platelet count of <150,000:
  - 75% have benign gestational thrombocytopenia.
  - 20% of cases are preeclampsia-related, HELLP syndrome (see "HELLP" topic).
  - 3% are immune disorders:
    - ITP (also termed ATP) with incidence ≤1/1,000 pregnancies
    - TTP
    - HUS
- Rarely, chronic thrombocytopenia due to folate acid deficiency or congenital conditions occurs.
- Thrombocytopenia may result from acute and chronic viral disorders (e.g., HIV, disseminated HSV) and malignancies (e.g., leukemia).

RISK FACTORS
Genetics
Rarely associated with congenital conditions:
- Fanconi anemia: Autosomal recessive condition characterized by short stature, skeletal anomalies, increased incidence of solid tumors and leukemias, bone marrow failure.
- Wiskott-Aldrich syndrome: Rare X-linked recessive disease characterized by eczema, thrombocytopenia, immune deficiency, and bloody diarrhea (due to thrombocytopenia).
- Congenital giant platelet disorders: May-Hegglin, Sebastian syndrome, Fechtner syndrome, Epstein syndrome, congenital macrothrombocytopenia

PATHOPHYSIOLOGY
- Thrombocytopenia can be a benign, self-limiting condition or secondary to autoimmune disease or serious medical conditions.
- The condition can occur due to:
  - Rapid consumption or destruction of platelets
  - Reduced production
- The likelihood of maternal morbidity and mortality is directly related to the platelet count, regardless of pathophysiology, and a favorable fetal outcome generally depends on a stable maternal condition.

- However, with ITP, maternal platelet-associated IgG can cross the placenta, with a direct effect on the fetus. In some cases, the fetal platelet count can be suppressed enough to result in risk for bleeding in the perinatal period.
  - ITP can be an acute or chronic disorder:
    - Acute ITP is self-limited, usually occurring in childhood, following a viral infection.
    - Chronic ITP occurs in the 2–3rd decades, with 3:1 female-to-male predilection.
  - Pathophysiologic events that affect mother and baby:
    - Autoimmune production of anti-platelet IgG
    - Leads to increased platelet destruction in the reticuloendothelial system, mostly in the spleen; other sites may be involved
    - Transplacental passage of maternal antiplatelet IgG can occur with fetal or neonatal thrombocytopenia. 12–15% of mothers with ITP deliver infants with platelet counts of <50,000.

ASSOCIATED CONDITIONS
- Diseases with rapid consumption:
  - Severe preeclampsia/HELLP syndrome
  - Immune thrombocytopenia:
    - ITP/ATP
    - SLE
  - DIC
  - Drug reaction
  - Massive thrombosis
  - Hemorrhage followed by transfusion
- Diseases with decreased production:
  - Congenital/Genetic disorders (see above)
  - Viral infections:
    - HIV
    - Hepatitis
    - CMV
- Bone marrow suppression by drugs, toxins, or cancers

 DIAGNOSIS

The diagnosis is straightforward; the challenge is in determining etiology, since the potential for maternal and fetal morbidity varies considerably depending on the source of the condition.

SIGNS AND SYMPTOMS
History
- Gestational thrombocytopenia:
  - No history of thrombocytopenia when not pregnant, and no underlying medical conditions are present as a cause.
  - Usually occurs in 3rd trimester
  - Resolves after pregnancy, confirming diagnosis

- ITP:
  - Thrombocytopenia often predates pregnancy.
  - Often, low platelet counts in early pregnancy
  - Counts may improve postpartum, but mild to moderate thrombocytopenia typically remains after delivery.
  - May have history of excessive menstrual bleeding, unusual postoperative bleeding, frequent epistaxis or easy bruising
  - Recent drug use may be causative.
- Preeclampsia/HELLP syndrome (see Hypertensive Disorders of Pregnancy and HELLP)
- TTP can be life-threatening; characterized by pentad of:
  - Fever
  - Microangiopathic hemolytic anemia
  - Renal impairment
  - Thrombocytopenia
  - Neurological signs or symptoms

Physical Exam
- Bleeding: Petechiae, purpura, oozing from venipunctures or incisions
- Hepatosplenomegaly (platelet sequestration)
- Jaundice and other signs of liver disease
- Evidence of thrombosis
- Arthritis, rash, signs of autoimmune disease

TESTS
- Platelets >115,000: Likely gestational thrombocytopenia. Repeat count every 2–4 weeks to ensure that the thrombocytopenia remains mild.
- Platelets <115,000 initially or with follow-up: Suggests ITP, TTP, or a significant medical disorder.

Lab
- Platelet-associated IgG is not specific enough to confirm gestational thrombocytopenia; reserve for patients with platelets counts <115,000:
  - Elevated platelet associate IgG in most patients with ITP
  - Normal in 10–30% of ITP, but elevated platelet-associated C3
- Diagnosis of ITP is largely 1 of exclusion:
  - This workup could be considered definitive:
    - Normal CBC except thrombocytopenia
    - Bone marrow with increased size and number of megakaryocytes
    - A blood smear with a large proportion of large platelets
    - Normal coagulation studies
    - No other obvious cause of thrombocytopenia
- Elevated PT, PTT, or bleeding time suggests DIC, liver disease, or platelet function disorder.

TREATMENT

GENERAL MEASURES
- If thrombocytopenia is due to medical or obstetric complications, treat primary disease.
- Gestational thrombocytopenia does not require treatment.
- If platelets <115,000, ITP is likely.
- Postoperative or postpartum bleeding risk is not increased until the platelet count is <50,000:
  - Treatment is indicated with platelets <50,000.

PREGNANCY-SPECIFIC ISSUES
- In ITP, antiplatelet autoantibodies cross the placenta with risk for fetal and neonatal thrombocytopenia and serious bleeding problems.
- A reliable, noninvasive method to identify fetuses at risk is not available:
  - Currently, no maternal treatment assuredly prevents neonatal thrombocytopenia.
  - Maternal labs and history do not accurately predict the fetal/neonatal platelet count:
    - Maternal antiplatelet antibody titers correlate poorly with neonatal platelet count.
    - Maternal splenectomy is not consistently protective of neonatal thrombocytopenia.
- Population-based studies and literature reviews reveal low probabilities of neonatal intracranial hemorrhage even with low platelets:
  - 12% risk of fetal platelet count <50,000
  - <1% risk of intracranial hemorrhage
  - Little evidence that risk of fetal intracranial hemorrhage is modified by delivery route.
  - Timing of occurrence of intracranial hemorrhage typically is not clear (before delivery, immediately after, or later):
    - Nadir of neonatal counts a few days after delivery; thus bleeding may occur then.
  - Case series have shown no improvement in the incidence of neonatal hemorrhagic complications with cesarean delivery.

Risks for Mother
- Gestational thrombocytopenia is not a threat.
- Moderate ITP with a platelet count of <100,000 precludes regional anesthesia.
- Severe ITP can increase the risk of excessive bleeding during and after delivery.

Risks for Fetus
- No risk with gestational thrombocytopenia.
- Potential risk for rapid destruction of fetal platelets due to maternal antiplatelet antibodies with ITP; in rare cases, the fetal platelets may be low enough to result in spontaneous bleeding.
- Generally delivery route (caesarian vs. vaginal) can be based on traditional obstetric indications:
  - Consider obtaining MFM consultation

MEDICATION (DRUGS)
- Prednisone is 1st line of treatment for ITP:
  - Initial dose is 1–2 mg/kg/d:
    - Transient remission in 75% of cases
    - Sustained response in only 14–33%
  - Once platelet counts are acceptable, decrease dose by 10–20%/wk to lowest dose necessary to maintain a count >50,000:
    - Response usually seen in 3–7 days
    - Maximum effect typically after 2–3 weeks

- If platelets remain <50,000 at 2–3 weeks, steroid treatment is unlikely to be successful.
- If prednisone is not effective, or when sustained remission is needed, use IVIG 0.4g/kg/d for 5 days. A significant rise in platelets can be seen in as little as 3 days. Can repeat monthly when a prolonged remission is needed.
- Splenectomy is commonly used in nonpregnant patients when steroids or medical treatment fail. In pregnancy, it is reserved as a last resort if platelet count <10–20,000 and steroids and IVIG have failed. Ideally, splenectomy should be done in the 2nd trimester:
  - Complete remission in 60–75%
  - Relapses can occur, most commonly within the 1st 2 years after splenectomy:
    - If relapse, look for accessory spleen with imaging

Emergency Treatment
In the rare ITP patient requiring emergency surgery or with life-threatening hemorrhage, the following acute interventions are recommended:
- IVIG 1 g/kg/d for 2 days
- Methylprednisolone 1 g/d for 3 days
- Platelet transfusions 5–6 units initially, followed by 5–6 units q4–6h until stable:
  - Rapid platelet destruction is expected, but less likely if the IVIG is administered 1st.

SURGERY
Recommendations as above if emergency surgery is required.

FOLLOW-UP

DISPOSITION
Issues for Referral
Gestational thrombocytopenia is a benign condition. However, in patients with platelet counts of <120,000 a referral to a MFM or hematology specialist is prudent.

PROGNOSIS
- With platelet counts >70,000, the prognosis is generally excellent.
- Patients with known ITP typically do well with careful follow-up and medical management.

COMPLICATIONS
Most complications of ITP are in the peripartum period:
- Platelet count too low for regional anesthesia
- Increased risk of incisional hematomas
- Increased blood loss
- Fetal thrombocytopenia possible with:
  - Petechiae
  - Internal hemorrhaging, including intracranial

PATIENT MONITORING
Mother
Frequent platelet counts for those with moderate or severe thrombocytopenia (every 2–4 weeks)

Fetus
Fetal scalp sampling is not recommended. Seek MFM consult for discussion of cordocentesis, especially in ITP patients whose babies experienced complications.

BIBLIOGRAPHY

ACOG Practice Bulletin No. 6. *Thrombocytopenia in Pregnancy.* Washington DC: ACOG; 1999.

Silver R, et al. Maternal thrombocytopenia in pregnancy: Time for a reassessment. *Am J Obstet Gynecol.* 1995;173(2):479–482.

Stasi R, et al. Management of immune thrombocytopenic purpura in adults. *Mayo Clin Proceed.* 2004;79(4):504–522.

MISCELLANEOUS

- The 1st case description for ITP has been attributed to Paul Gottlieb Werlhof, a 17th-century physician and poet.
- Werlhof described the disease in a 10-year-old girl and named it "Morbus haemorrhagicus maculosus" (purpura hemorrhagica):
  - www.whonamedit.com

SYNONYM(S)
Incidental thrombocytopenia

ABBREVIATIONS
- ATP—Autoimmune thrombocytopenia
- CMV—Cytomegalovirus
- DIC—Disseminated intravascular coagulation
- HELLP—Hemolytic anemia, elevated liver enzymes, low platelet count
- HSV—Herpes simplex virus
- HUS—Hemolytic-uremic syndrome
- ITP—Idiopathic thrombocytopenic purpura
- IVIG—Intravenous immune globulin
- MFM—Maternal-fetal medicine
- PT—Prothrombin time
- PTT—Partial thromboplastin time
- SLE—Systemic lupus erythematosus
- TTP—Thrombotic thrombocytopenic purpura

CODES
ICD9-CM
- 287.31 Immune thrombocytopenic purpura
- 287.5 Thrombocytopenia, unspecified
- 287.4 Thrombocytopenia, secondary:
  - Massive transfusion
  - Drugs
  - Dilutional
  - Platelet alloimmunization (immune)

PATIENT TEACHING

Patients with moderate or severe thrombocytopenia should:
- Avoid drugs that inhibit platelet function.
- Consider actions to reduce the risk of falls, especially when pregnant:
  - Avoid high heels.
  - Avoid carrying items in both hands when using stairs or walking on slippery surfaces.
  - Wear broad, rubberized shoes when walking in icy conditions.

BASICS

DESCRIPTION

- Hypo- and hyperthyroid disease have multiple etiologies and should be characterized and adequately treated in pregnancy.
- Overt hypothyroid disease:
  - Hashimoto thyroiditis is most common etiology in US:
    ○ Chronic autoimmune thyroiditis, often presenting as asymptomatic diffuse goiter
    ○ Often 1st detected after thyroid atrophy and hypothyroidism have occurred
  - Treated Graves disease with either radioactive iodine or thyroidectomy results in permanent hypothyroidism.
  - Lymphocytic thyroiditis:
    ○ Postpartum onset of goiter and/or hypothyroidism that may resolve spontaneously
  - Iodine deficiency is rare in US but is most common etiology worldwide.
- Subclinical hypothyroid disease:
  - Diagnosed in asymptomatic patient with normal T4 but elevated TSH. Unclear implication if diagnosed in pregnancy. Should not be routinely screened for during pregnancy.
- Overt hyperthyroid disease:
  - Graves disease most common etiology:
    ○ Autoimmune hyperthyroid disease caused by thyroid-stimulating antibodies

EPIDEMIOLOGY

- Overt hypothyroid disease:
  - Prevalence in pregnancy is 0.5%
- Hyperthyroid disease:
  - Prevalence in pregnancy is 0.1–0.4%:
    ○ Graves disease accounts for 85%.
    ○ Single toxic adenoma, multinodular toxic goiter, and thyroiditis account for remainder.

RISK FACTORS

- Overt hypothyroid disease:
  - Hashimoto thyroiditis:
    ○ Other autoimmune diseases
  - Iodine deficiency:
    ○ Country of origin particularly non US
- Hyperthyroid disease:
  - Graves disease:
    ○ Other autoimmune diseases
    ○ Family history of Graves disease

Genetics

Genetics of Graves disease is unclear, but strong association exists between family members.

PATHOPHYSIOLOGY

- Overt hypothyroid disease:
  - Hashimoto thyroiditis:
    ○ Thyroid autoantibodies cause hypothyroid function.
  - Iodine deficiency in diet causes hypothyroid disease and goiter.
  - Treated Graves disease with I131 or thyroidectomy usually causes permanent hypothyroid state.
- Graves disease:
  - TSIs, which are IgGs, cause stimulation of thyroid with increased free T4. They cross the placenta and can cause stimulation of fetal thyroid.

ASSOCIATED CONDITIONS

Hypothyroid disease and Graves disease:

- Other autoimmune diseases including type 1 diabetes

 DIAGNOSIS

SIGNS AND SYMPTOMS
History

- Hypothyroid disease:
  - Lethargy, cold sensitivity, constipation
- Graves disease:
  - Heat intolerance

Physical Exam

- Hypothyroid disease:
  - Weight gain, dry skin, hair loss, low heart rate, goiter:
    ○ Symptoms may be difficult to discern in pregnancy.
- Graves disease:
  - Tachycardia, tremor, weight loss, goiter, thyroid ophthalmopathy, pretibial myxedema

TESTS
Labs

- In pregnancy TT4 increases; to assess thyroid function in pregnancy multiply the TT4 by 1.5 or use free T4 or FTI.
- TSH in pregnancy does vary by trimester, but trimester-specific TSH is not routinely available so standard practice is to use laboratory nonpregnant norms.
- Hypothyroid disease:
  - TSH >4 mU/L and low FT4 or FTI
  - Thyroid autoantibodies not usually checked but can be used to confirm diagnosis of Hashimoto thyroiditis.
- Graves disease:
  - Suppressed TSH and elevated FT4 or FTI or T3
  - TSI: Pregnancy specific

Imaging

- If diffuse goiter is present, imaging is not usually needed.
- If thyroid nodule, then US followed by FNA.
- Radioisotope imaging is contraindicated in pregnancy.
- If thyroid cancer is diagnosed, refer to appropriate consultants for management.

 TREATMENT

GENERAL MEASURES

- Hypothyroid disease:
  - Goal is to treat with levothyroxine to maintain the TSH in the normal range.
- Graves disease:
  - Goal of medical treatment is to maintain the FT4 or FTI in the high normal range to minimize fetal exposure to antithyroid medications.
  - Propranolol may be needed on a short-term basis to control maternal tachycardia.
  - Thyroidectomy is acceptable in pregnancy if the patient has failed medical treatment and should be performed with multispecialty consultation including surgery, anesthesia, perinatology.

PREGNANCY-SPECIFIC ISSUES

- Hypothyroid disease:
  - Most women need an increase in levothyroxine treatment as early as 4–8 weeks' gestation:
    ○ May immediately increase dose by 30% once pregnancy is diagnosed, or obtain TSH as soon as possible and treat
- Graves disease:
  - TSI crosses the placenta and can cause fetal hyperthyroid disease independent of maternal treatment or thyroid function.
    ○ Controversial how useful levels of TSI are for managing Graves in pregnancy, although very elevated levels have higher association with fetal/neonatal Graves
    ○ Consider obtaining TSI on women with prior baby with Graves or treated Graves on thyroid replacement.
  - The maternal history of Graves disease should be clearly communicated to the pediatricians caring for the neonate.
- Women with any of the following should be screened for thyroid disease in pregnancy:
  - Personal or family history of thyroid disease
  - Goiter
  - Symptoms or clinical signs suggestive of thyroid disease
  - Type I diabetes
  - Other autoimmune disorders
  - Prior therapeutic head or neck irradiation

Risks for Mother
- Hypothyroid disease:
  - Untreated hypothyroid disease is associated with decreased fertility, preeclampsia, abruption, anemia.
- Graves disease:
  - Untreated Graves is associated with thyroid storm, preeclampsia, congestive heart failure.

ALERT
Thyroid storm occurs in 1% pregnant women with Graves, is an acute emergency, and usually requires ICU admission for management. Diagnosis is made by presence of tachycardia, sweating, fever, change in mental status, confusion, seizures, vomiting, diarrhea, or arrhythmia in a woman with hyperthyroidism. If untreated, it can progress to coma. If diagnosis is suspected, workup thyroid function tests and begin treatment. Drugs include PTU, SSKI, propranolol, dexamethasone, and phenobarbital. Consult with medicine and endocrine.

Risks for Fetus
- Hypothyroid disease:
  - Untreated severe disease is associated with neonatal and childhood cognitive deficits particularly in iodine-deficient hypothyroid disease.
  - Untreated disease is associated with preterm delivery, SGA.
- Graves disease:
  - Fetal/Neonatal Graves disease:
    - Occurs in ~1–5% of total and is more common with high (>130–150%) TSI or in mother with previously affected baby
    - May present in utero with fetal tachycardia, IUGR, hydrops, fetal goiter and, rarely, fetal death
    - Can confirm diagnosis with fetal percutaneous umbilical vein sampling
    - Can be treated in utero with maternal antithyroid medications and/or intrauterine medications
    - If diagnosis is considered, refer to MFM specialist.
  - Untreated Graves:
    - Associated with preterm delivery, SGA, fetal demise
  - Treated with antithyroid medications:
    - Fetal hypothyroid disease, goiter

MEDICATION (DRUGS)
- Hypothyroid disease:
  - Levothyroxine:
    - Begin with 100–150 μg/d PO
    - Check TSH in 4 weeks and adjust
    - Once therapeutic (TSH in normal range) repeat TSH every 8 weeks to every trimester
    - If patient is already on levothyroxine, increase dose by 30%, recheck in 4 weeks.
- Graves disease:
  - PTU:
    - 100 mg PO t.i.d.
    - Titrate to maintain FT4 in high normal range.
    - PTU crosses placenta and can cause hypothyroidism in fetus so use minimal effective dose.
  - Methimazole:
    - 15 mg PO b.i.d.
    - Also crosses placenta, so follow same principles as for PTU
- Although rare (<0.4%), agranulocytosis is the most serious side effect of both thioamides; presents with fever, sore throat, low WBC count; if diagnosed, stop medications immediately.
- Both PTU and methimazole are associated with low incidence of rash, nausea, anorexia.
- Methimazole may be associated with aplasia cutis and choanal/esophageal atresia so, if available, PTU is the preferred first-line medication.
- Both PTU and methimazole are safe in breast-feeding.

 FOLLOW-UP

DISPOSITION
Issues for Referral
- Thyroid storm
- Failed medical therapy of Grave disease

PROGNOSIS
For both hypothyroid and hyperthyroid disease, if women are made appropriately euthyroid, pregnancy outcomes are good.

PATIENT MONITORING
- Pregnant women with hypo- or hyperthyroid disease should have baseline thyroid function tests obtained at their 1st visit. Repeat as indicated depending on treatment.
  - In general ~4 weeks are necessary after any change in medication to determine effect of medication change on thyroid function.
- Obtain baseline 2nd trimester US for fetal growth and follow fetal growth, fetal heart rate carefully.
- Fetal Graves can present with fetal tachycardia, IUGR, or goiter.

BIBLIOGRAPHY

ACOG Practice Bulletin No. 37. *Thyroid disease in pregnancy.* Washington DC: ACOG; 2002.

Alexander EK, et al. Timing and magnitude of increases in levothyroxine requirements during pregnancy in women with hypothyroidism. *N Engl J Med.* 2004;351:241–249.

Belfort MA. Thyroid and other endocrine emergencies. In: Foley MR, et al., eds. *Obstetric Intensive Care Manual,* 2nd ed. New York: McGraw Hill; 2004;120–142.

Mestman JH. Hyperthyroidism in pregnancy. *Best Pract Res Clin Endocrinol Metab.* 2004;18:267–288.

 MISCELLANEOUS

ABBREVIATIONS
- FNA—Fine needle aspiration
- FTI—Free thyroxine index
- IUGR—Intrauterine growth restriction
- MFM—Maternal-fetal medicine
- PTU—Propylthiouracil
- SGA—Small for gestational age
- SSKI—Saturated solution of potassium iodide
- T4—Thyroxine
- TSH—Thyroid-stimulating hormone
- TSI—Thyroid-stimulating immunoglobulins
- TT4—Total thyroxine

CODES
ICD9-CM
- 242.9 Hyperthyroidism
- 244.9 Hypothyroidism
- 648.13 Thyroid disease

 PATIENT TEACHING

- ACOG Patient Education Pamphlet. Thyroid Disease. Available at http://www.acog.org
- Thyroid Disease and Pregnancy from the American Thyroid Association. Available at http://www.thyroid.org/patients/brochures/Thyroid_Dis_Pregnancy_broch.pdf

Section VI

HYPERTENSION IN PREGNANCY

Bryan E. Freeman, MD
Kathryn L. Reed, MD

See page 644.

Section VII
Obstetric and Gynecologic Procedures

ABDOMINAL INCISIONS

Deborah A. Simon, MD
Joseph P. Connor, MD

 BASICS

DESCRIPTION

Once it has been determined that a surgical procedure cannot be done successfully via laparoscopy, the surgeon must determine which type of skin incision to use for laparotomy. The choice of incision should be based on the planned and/or possible procedures with other considerations secondary.

- Transverse incisions:
  - Pfannenstiel:
    - Transverse elliptical incision just above the pubic symphysis through the rectus sheath with separation of the rectus muscles in the midline
  - Cherney:
    - Transverse incision similar to Pfannenstiel through the rectus sheath with removal of the rectus muscles from their insertion into the pubic symphysis
  - Maylard:
    - Transverse muscle-cutting incision through all layers of the anterior abdominal wall
  - Küstner:
    - Transverse elliptical incision with a midline fascial incision and separation of the rectus muscles in the midline
- Vertical incisions:
  - Midline:
    - Vertical incision through all layers of the anterior abdominal wall in the midline
  - Paramedian:
    - Vertical Incision through all layers of the anterior abdominal wall lateral to the midline
- Oblique incisions:
  - Gridiron incision of McBurney:
    - Oblique incision made over McBurney's point through the external oblique muscles, which are separated along muscle fibers

Indications

- Pfannenstiel:
  - Commonly used for cesarean deliveries and benign gynecologic surgery requiring exposure to the central pelvis
- Cherney:
  - Offers exposure of the pelvic sidewall and space of Retzius for urinary incontinence procedures
- Maylard:
  - Provides exposure to the lateral pelvic sidewalls for radical pelvic surgery
- Küstner:
  - Similar to indications for Pfannenstiel but less commonly used as it offers no distinct advantage
- Midline:
  - Commonly used when rapid abdominal entry is needed (emergency cesarean) or when upper abdominal as well as pelvic exposure is necessary, as when gynecologic malignancy is known or suspected
- Paramedian:
  - Same indications as for midline incision. May be preferred in patients at high risk for evisceration or for extraperitoneal procedures.
- Gridiron incision of McBurney:
  - Useful for extraperitoneal drainage of pelvic abscesses

Site (Office, Surgical Center, OR)

Inpatient or outpatient operating room or surgical center

Concurrent Procedures

Incision/Wound closure:

- When considering methods and materials for wound closure, consider closure techniques that will provide adequate tensile strength and tissue approximation for the duration of wound healing.

- Considerations when choosing suture material include tensile strength, knot security, tissue reaction, and suture absorbability.
- Randomized studies comparing continuous vs. interrupted suture closure techniques have found no differences in wound infection, dehiscence, and hernias. Continuous closures can be performed more quickly, making this the preferred method for closure in most patients.

Age-Related Factors

Surgeons often attempt to use more cosmetic incisions in younger patients. It is imperative to use the best incision for the procedure, regardless of the age of the patient.

EPIDEMIOLOGY

The most common incision for ob-gyn procedures is the Pfannenstiel incision.

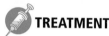 **TREATMENT**

PROCEDURE

Informed Consent

When obtaining consent for the planned surgical procedure, discuss the type of incision anticipated for the case as well as the potential incision-related complications or factors that might necessitate a different type of incision.

Patient Education

Postoperative wound care and signs/symptoms of wound infection or dehiscence should be reviewed prior to discharge.

Risks, Benefits

- Transverse incisions have the best cosmetic results, are stronger than vertical incisions, and are generally less painful. However, they are more time-consuming to perform, generally result in more blood loss, and provide less abdominal exposure than vertical incisions.
  - Pfannenstiel:
    - Most secure incision
    - Limited exposure
  - Cherney:
    - Excellent exposure
    - Higher risk for nerve injury
  - Maylard:
    - Excellent exposure to the pelvic sidewall
    - Patients with peripheral vascular disease may have ischemia due to ligation of the inferior epigastric arteries.
- Vertical incisions allow rapid entry with excellent exposure, can be easily extended, and result in less blood loss than transverse incisions. They are less cosmetic in appearance and have an increased risk of wound dehiscence and hernia.

Alternatives

Laparoscopy should be considered for all surgical cases and used when appropriate.

 FOLLOW-UP

Patients should be seen for postoperative exams as directed, based on the type of procedure. An exam of the incision is done at these visits. Patients should be cautioned to follow-up sooner if they are having erythema, serous or purulent drainage from the incision site, or other signs of infection, such as increased pain or fever.

COMPLICATIONS

Some of the conditions associated with wound complications include prior radiation to the abdomen or pelvis, immunosuppression, steroid use, obesity, DM, underlying vascular disease, neoplasm, infection, anemia, or general physical debilitation.

- Dehiscence (see Wound Dehiscence and Disruption)
- Infection (see Wound Infection)
- Hernia

BIBLIOGRAPHY

Colombo M, et al. A randomized comparison of continuous versus interrupted mass closure of midline incisions in patients with gynecologic cancer. *Obstet Gynecol*. 1997;89(5 Pt1):684–689.

Funt MI. Abdominal incisions and closures. *Clin Obstet Gynecol*. 1981;24:1175–1185.

Masterson BJ. Selection of incisions for gynecologic procedures. *Surg Clin North Am*. 1991;71: 1041–1052.

Richards PC, et al. Abdominal wound closure. A randomized prospective study of 571 patients comparing continuous vs. interrupted suture techniques. *Ann Surg*. 1983;197(2):2388–2343.

Rock JA, et al., eds. *Te Lind's Operative Gynecology*, 9th ed. Philadelphia: Lippincott Williams & Wilkins; 2003.

 MISCELLANEOUS

CLINICAL PEARLS

- Laparoscopy should be considered 1st and should be utilized if deemed adequate to successfully perform the procedure.
- Re-entry incisions should be made through the previous incision and not parallel to it, as devascularization of the wound may occur.
- The choice of incision should be procedure driven, with other considerations secondary.
- Langer skin lines reflect lines of skin tension and collagen fibers in the dermis. Surgical incisions along Langer lines heal with less scarring.

ABORTION, MEDICAL

Tessa Madden, MD, MPH
Paul D. Blumenthal, MD, MPH

 BASICS

DESCRIPTION
- Medical abortion, also sometimes called medication abortion, is the induced termination of an early intrauterine pregnancy without primary surgical intervention.
- Although medications can be used to induce abortion in both the 1st and 2nd trimesters, the most common setting is at <63 days estimated GA (calculated from the 1st day of the last menstrual period).
- 1 of the most commonly used regimens in the US and Europe (and the focus of this chapter):
  - The evidence-based regimen of 200 mg mifepristone (RU-486) followed by 800 μg misoprostol intravaginally 6–72 hours later. This is 96% effective up to 63 days.
- Other possible regimens include:
  - The FDA-approved regimen of 600 mg mifepristone followed by 400 μg misoprostol PO 48 hours later. This is 95% effective up to 49 days.
  - The evidence-based regimen of 200 mg mifepristone followed by 800 μg misoprostol buccally 6–48 hours later. This is 95% effective up to 56 days.
  - Methotrexate 50 mg PO or 50 mg/m^2 IM followed by misoprostol 800 μg intravaginally 3–7 days later. This is 94% effective up to 49 days.
  - Misoprostol alone 800 μg intravaginally q24h (may repeat up to 3 doses). This is 87% effective up to 56 days.
- The FDA-approved (2000) mifepristone in combination with misoprostol for medical abortion:
  - Mifepristone is an antiprogestin or SPRM that binds to the progesterone receptor with greater affinity than natural progesterone without activating it.
  - Due to the inhibition of progesterone, mifepristone causes the trophoblast to separate from the decidua and the endometrial lining to shed.
  - Additionally, mifepristone causes the cervix to soften and the uterus to become more sensitive to prostaglandins.
  - Studies have shown that the 200-mg dose of mifepristone is equally effective to the 600-mg dose approved by the FDA.
- Misoprostol is an inexpensive synthetic prostaglandin (E1 analog) that is stable at room temperature:
  - The peak serum levels of misoprostol differ depending on the route of administration:
    - Vaginal and buccal routes have lower peak serum levels than oral and sublingual routes, but greater bioavailability (the area under the curve).
    - Oral and sublingual dosing has higher peak serum levels, however these seem to be associated with an increase in the rate of GI side effects.

- Importantly, all these routes have been found to be acceptable to women, with oral, sublingual, and buccal being slightly more acceptable than vaginal.
  - The addition of misoprostol to mifepristone increases efficacy rates from 64–85% to ~95%.
  - Shortening the duration of time between administration of mifepristone and misoprostol is also associated with a decrease in side effects.

Indications
Undesired pregnancy at <63 days (depending on regimen) where patient desires pregnancy termination, has access to emergency care, and the provider can perform or refer for surgical procedure if necessary.

Site (Office, Surgical Center, OR)
Medical abortion can be provided in multiple locations including:
- Provider office
- Hospital-based clinic
- Free-standing clinic

Concurrent Procedures
- US to determine GA
- Check hematocrit; severe anemia is a contraindication to medical abortion.
- Type and screen to determine patient's blood type.

ALERT
Must administer RHOGAM prior to medical abortion if patient is Rh negative.

Age-Related Factors
Pediatric Considerations
Although multiple factors influence an individual's preference for medical vs. surgical abortion, medical abortion has been shown to be acceptable and safe among adolescents.

EPIDEMIOLOGY
In the US, >600,0000 women have used mifepristone for early pregnancy termination since it was approved in 2000. In 2003, the most recent year for which abortion surveillance data is available from the CDC, >800,000 abortions were performed in the US.
- 8% were medical abortions.
- 60% of these were performed at ≤56 days, this suggests more women are eligible for medical abortion than are currently utilizing it.

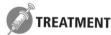 **TREATMENT**

PROCEDURE
- Women <63 days EGA who have decided to undergo pregnancy termination are evaluated by a trained clinician, including US if indicated.
- Blood count and typing are performed.
- Consents are signed, including manufacturers' consent.
- Mifepristone 200 mg is administered by the provider in the office.
- Patients are given 800 μg misoprostol to take intravaginally 6–72 hours later, at a time they choose (alternatively an 800-μg dose of misoprostol can be provided buccally or a 400-μg dose PO)
- Patients are given an appointment to follow-up in 5–14 days and are counseled regarding bleeding precautions.

Informed Consent
- Be sure patient understands she is taking medication to terminate the pregnancy.
- If using evidence-based regimens, explain this is a non–FDA approved use of the medications mifepristone and misoprostol.
- Risks and benefits of medical abortion and the alternative of surgical abortion must be discussed.

Conditions Requiring Caution
- No support person available
- Hct <28
- >1 hour from nearest ER
- No access to phone or emergency services
- Refuses surgical procedure if medical abortion is not successful

Patient Education
Counsel patients about what to expect during the medical abortion process:
- Bleeding like a heavy period or a miscarriage
- Heaviest bleeding in the 1st 2–6 hours after taking misoprostol
- *Bleeding precautions:* If soaking through >2 pads an hour for 2 hours or more, the patient must call her provider or go to the nearest ER.
- Average duration of bleeding after medical abortion is 9 days; however, bleeding may last as long as 45 days.

Risks, Benefits
- Risks:
  - Bleeding, including possible need for blood transfusion (<0.5%)
  - Infection, including postabortal endometritis (<1%) and possible risk of *Clostridium sordellii* TSS and death (<0.001%)
  - Surgical intervention (vacuum aspiration) in ~5% of cases

- Benefits:
  - Avoids surgical procedure
  - Increased flexibility of timing
  - Increased privacy of abortion process
- Contraindications to medical abortion with mifepristone and misoprostol:
  - Suspected ectopic pregnancy
  - Concurrent, long-term, systemic steroid use
  - Chronic adrenal failure
  - Severe anemia, use of anticoagulants, or bleeding disorder
  - Gestational trophoblastic disease
  - Pregnancy with IUD in place or obstruction or cervical canal
  - Allergy to mifepristone or misoprostol

Alternatives
- Surgical termination of pregnancy
- Continuation of pregnancy

Surgical
Patients must be willing to consent to a surgical procedure (vacuum aspiration) in the case of a failed medical abortion.

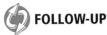 FOLLOW-UP

- Follow-up in 5–14 days to ensure that patient has expelled the pregnancy.
- If patient does not provide a history suggestive of having expelled the pregnancy (i.e., moderate to heavy vaginal bleeding), repeat US is warranted.

PROGNOSIS
- Successful completion of abortion occurs in 95–97% of patients.
- Overall risk of major complication is very low, <1.0%.

COMPLICATIONS
- Lower genital tract infection with abdominal pain, persistent bleeding, and offensive discharge
- Postabortal endometritis, possibly requiring admission and IV antibiotics. No evidence suggests administration of prophylactic antibiotics decreases postabortal infection rate.
- Heavy bleeding, possibly requiring blood transfusion

BIBLIOGRAPHY

Creinen MD, et al. A randomized comparison of misoprostol 6 to 8 hours versus 24 hours after mifepristone for abortion. *Obstet Gynecol*. 2005;103:851–859.

Fiala C, et al. The effect of non-steroidal anti-inflammatory drugs on medical abortion with mifepristone and misoprostol at 13 to 22 weeks gestation. *Human Reprod*. 2005;20:3072–3077.

Jain JK, et al. A prospective randomized, double-blinded, placebo-controlled trial comparing mifepristone and vaginal misoprostol to vaginal misoprostol alone for elective termination of early pregnancy. *Human Reprod*. 2002;17:1477–1482.

Kahn JG, et al. The efficacy of medical abortion: A meta-analysis. *Contraception*. 2000;61:29–40.

Middleton T, et al. Randomized trial of mifepristone and buccal or vaginal misoprostol for abortion through 56 days of last menstrual period. *Contraception*. 2005;72:328–332.

Peyron R, et al. Early termination of pregnancy with mifepristone (RU 486) and the orally active prostaglandin misoprostol. *N Engl J Med*. 1993;328:1509–1513.

Schaff EA, et al. Low-dose mifepristone followed by vaginal misoprostol at 48 hours for abortion up to 63 days. *Contraception*. 2000;61:41–46.

Strauss LT, et al. Abortion surveillance-United States, 2003. *MMWR*. 2006;55:1–32.

 MISCELLANEOUS

- Treatment of pain:
  - 75% of women will require narcotic analgesia, usually on the day of misoprostol administration.
  - Factors associated with narcotic use include higher GA, younger patient age, and nulliparity.
  - Use NSAIDs (either ibuprofen 800 mg q8h or naproxen 500 mg q12h) and narcotic (such as hydrocodone/APAP). There has been concern that the antiprostaglandin properties of NSAIDs may interfere with the mechanism of action of misoprostol; however, this has not been seen in clinical studies.
  - +/− Antiemetic
- Other uses of mifepristone currently being investigated include:
  - Contraception and EC
  - Treatment of leiomyomata
  - Treatment of endometriosis
  - Treatment of meningioma
  - Cushing syndrome
  - Breast cancer
  - Cervical ripening/labor induction

ALERT
C. sordellii TSS is an extremely rare, but life-threatening infection (<1 in 100,000 women undergoing medical abortion):

- Appears to be associated with pregnancy and childbirth; previous case reports after vaginal delivery and cesarean section
- Unclear association with medical abortion, risk factors for infection are not known.
- Typical clinical presentation includes:
  - Absence of fever
  - Abdominal pain
  - Hypotension
  - Tachycardia
  - Marked leukocytosis
  - Hemoconcentration

SYNONYM(S)
Medication abortion

CLINICAL PEARLS
Counseling patients about what to expect during the medical abortion process will greatly increase patient confidence and decrease the number of unnecessary phone calls or trips to the ER. Counseling points should include:

- Expect heavy bleeding "like a miscarriage" or "like a heavy period." Reinforce bleeding precautions.
- The heaviest bleeding is usually 2–6 hours after misoprostol administration, however may commence as soon as 20 minutes
- Expect cramping during the heaviest bleeding. Encourage NSAIDs and ensure that patient has prescription for narcotic pain medications if needed.
- Bleeding on average lasts 9 days after a medical abortion, but may last >1 month.
- Reinforce that the patient may have a surgical procedure at any point if she is not happy with the medical abortion process.

ABBREVIATIONS
- EC—Emergency contraceptives
- EGA—Estimated gestational age
- GA—Gestational age
- Hct—Hemocrit
- SPRM—Synthetic progesterone-receptor modulator
- TSS—Toxic shock syndrome

 CODES

ICD9-CM
635 Legally induced abortion

PATIENT TEACHING

Activity restrictions:
- Pelvic rest (nothing in the vagina including intercourse and tampons) for 2 weeks.
- No heavy exercise for 1 week.

Section VII

ABORTION, SURGICAL

Eve Espey, MD, MPH

BASICS

DESCRIPTION

Surgical abortion, the induced termination of pregnancy, encompasses several procedures. MVA, electric suction D&C, and D&E account for almost all surgical abortions in the US.

- MVA employs an inexpensive hand-held plastic syringe, available both as a disposable and a reusable product:
  - MVA may be used for termination of pregnancy up to ~10 weeks.
  - MVA has made abortion safer in developing countries where electricity or the ability to sterilize equipment is unavailable.
- Electric suction D&C employs a suction machine to achieve evacuation of pregnancy up to 13 weeks.
- D&E defines the pregnancy termination procedure after 13 weeks:
  - The D&E procedure is technically the same as a D&C up to 16 weeks' gestation.
  - The more advanced the GA, the larger the suction cannula.
  - At ~16 weeks and over, the fetus must be disarticulated with crushing clamps or forceps.
  - GA limits to D&E depend on the degree of cervical dilation, the experience of the operator, and state laws governing GA and abortion.
  - An alternative to D&E for later-term abortions is medical induction of labor, usually performed in a hospital setting with the use of vaginal misoprostol.
- Preparation of the cervix with osmotic dilators prior to surgical abortion after ~11 weeks' gestation makes the procedure safer.
- Later-term procedures may require a total of 1–3 days for cervical preparation prior to the procedure.
- Prophylactic antibiotics have been shown to reduce the likelihood of periabortal infection and are routinely used:
  - Doxycycline 100 mg PO b.i.d. is the standard antibiotic.
- Paracervical block with lidocaine is commonly used for pain control. Vasopressin or epinephrine may be added to the block for control of bleeding.
- Several analgesia regimens, both oral and parenteral, may be used.
- Determination that surgical abortion was successful may be confirmed in the following way(s):
  - Fetal tissue is floated in water with back lighting and inspected or sent to pathology for exam.
  - Intra- and/or postprocedure US is performed verifying an empty uterus.

PREVENTION

The most effective prevention for abortion is access to affordable and effective contraceptives. Public health strategies to reduce abortion include:

- Comprehensive sex education
- Universal health care access
- Promotion of reliable long-term methods such as intrauterine contraception and implants

ALERT

RhoGAM must be administered prior to surgical abortion or before discharge from the facility if the patient is Rh negative.

EPIDEMIOLOGY

- 1 of the most common procedures in the US. In 2003, over 800,000 abortions were performed.
- Over 33% of US women will have had an abortion by age 45.
- Abortion has low mortality except where it is illegal.
- 13% of maternal mortality worldwide is due to illegal, unsafe abortion.

RISK FACTORS

- In the US, abortions are more common in young, disadvantaged, unmarried women of color.
- Globally, 39% of women live in countries where abortion is illegal and unsafe.

Pediatric Considerations

- Laws governing parental notification and consent for abortion vary by state.
- It is important to be aware of the state's laws for those who refer for and provide abortion.

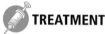

TREATMENT

PROCEDURE

- Women undergo counseling for the options of pregnancy termination, adoption, and continuing the pregnancy as a parent (see Unplanned Pregnancy and Options Counseling).
- Women who choose pregnancy termination are evaluated for GA, usually with US.
- Women are counseled about medical vs. surgical abortion. For those choosing surgical abortion:
  - Blood count and type are determined.
  - Patients are counseled about contraceptives.
  - Informed consent is signed.
  - Prophylactic antibiotics for up to 7 days.
- For MVA and D&C up to 11 weeks:
  - The cervix is cleansed with Betadine.
  - A paracervical block is administered.
  - Oral NSAIDs may be administered.

- IV or inhalation sedation may be offered. Several regimens are available:
  - A combination of fentanyl and versed
  - Nitrous oxide
  - The cervix is serially dilated to accommodate an appropriate-sized suction cannula.
  - Aspiration is accomplished with the MVA syringe or electric suction.
- For D&C from 11–16 weeks:
  - Osmotic dilators, either *Laminaria japonica* or synthetic dilators may be placed intracervically from 12–24 hours before the procedure.
  - Alternatively, vaginal misoprostol may be used 30 minutes prior to the procedure.
  - After removal of osmotic dilators, the procedure is carried out as above.
  - IV access is customary after ~15 weeks GA because of an increased risk of bleeding.
  - After ~11 weeks GA, intra-operative US guidance may improve the safety of the procedure.
- For D&E between 16 and 20+ weeks:
  - Osmotic dilators are used, often in serial fashion, requiring 2–3 days of preparation.
  - The cervix is cleansed, a paracervical block with oxytocin is administered, and sedation is offered.
  - Given the higher risk of bleeding in later gestations, other oxytocic medications may be given routinely or in case of excess bleeding
    - Methergine .2 mg IV, IM, or PO
    - Misoprostol 400–1,000 μg per rectum
  - The fetus is disarticulated and removed with specially designed crushing forceps.
  - Suction or forceps may be used to remove the placenta.

Nursing Care

- If sedation is administered, standard monitoring guidelines should be adhered to, including appropriate BP, pulse, and oxygen saturation monitoring.
- A nurse or medical assistant is often designated to monitor the patient's level of consciousness, check vital signs as needed, and give the patient verbal support during the procedure.

Conditions Requiring Caution

- Women with medical complications such as hypercoagulability, severe cardiac disease, or those on medications like Coumadin
- Consultation and planned location of procedure in the operating room rather than clinic setting should be considered for women with certain medical conditions.

- Rarely, a surgical procedure termed "hysterotomy" is necessary to accomplish an abortion. Hysterotomy involves a laparotomy incision with a uterine incision (like a cesarean section) to remove the fetus. This surgery is only performed only in exceptional circumstances such as:
  - A woman with an advanced gestation, a lower uterine segment fibroid, and intractable bleeding
  - A woman with an advanced gestation and a D&E complicated by perforation of the uterus

 FOLLOW-UP

Patients are given an appointment to follow-up in 5–14 days and are given contact numbers for possible complications. The follow-up visit focuses on contraception.

COMPLICATIONS

- Abortion is 1 of the safest surgical procedures for women.
- The overall risk of major complications with abortion is <1%.
- The risk of death with abortion is ~0.6/100,000 abortions.
- Risks include:
  - Heavy bleeding, including possible need for blood transfusion (<0.5%)
  - Risk of retained tissue and need to repeat the procedure
  - Infection, including postabortal endometritis (<1%)
  - Uterine perforation and possible injury to intra-abdominal structures

PROGNOSIS

- Long-term consequences of abortion are unusual.
- Specious epidemiologic associations have been made between abortion and certain conditions. In general, the evidence does not support a statistically greater risk for populations having an abortion and the subsequent development of:
  - Breast cancer
  - Depression
  - Infertility
  - Preterm labor

BIBLIOGRAPHY

Cates W, et al. The public health impact of legal abortion: 30 years later. *Perspect Sex Reprod Health*. 2003;35(1):25–28.

Finer LB, et al. Abortion incidence and services in the United States in 2000. *Perspect Sex Reprod Health*. 2003;35:6–15.

Henshaw SK, et al. The accessibility of abortion services in the United States, 2001. *Perspect Sex Reprod Health*. 2003;35(1):16–24.

Stubblefield PG, et al. Methods for induced abortion. *Obstet Gynecol*. 2004;104(1):174–185.

Women's State Health Facts. Mandatory waiting periods, Parental consent/notification. Available at: www.statehealthfacts.kff.org/. Accessed 08/31/07.

 MISCELLANEOUS

LEGAL ISSUES

- The Supreme Court decision, *Row v. Wade*, established a woman's right to a 1st-trimester abortion in the US in 1973. Several Supreme Court cases since then have allowed states to place certain restrictions on abortion:
  - 31 states require mandatory counseling:
    - Some direct the state health department to develop materials.
    - Some mandate specific information to be given.
  - >20 states require a delay, usually 24 hours but up to 48 hours, between counseling and the procedure.
  - >30 states require minors to notify 1 or both parents or to obtain parental consent for the abortion.
- The federal ban on "partial birth abortion" was upheld by the Supreme Court in 2007:
  - "Partial birth abortion" is a term that refers to an uncommon procedure. The procedure described as a "partial birth abortion" is the "intact D&X" procedure. In this procedure, used rarely, the cervix is dilated, a fetus is delivered as a breech with the fetal head remaining within the uterus. The fetal calvarium is punctured and evacuated, allowing delivery of the entire fetus.
  - Although "partial birth abortion" points to the intact D&X procedure, abortion providers fear they may be criminally liable for performing a standard D&E procedure. As the Supreme Court decision is recent, time will tell whether the "partial birth abortion" ban has an impact on availability and safety of abortion in the US.

Access to Abortion

- Abortion is rarely integrated into the spectrum of women's health care services in the US. 90% of abortions occur in free-standing dedicated clinics.
- The number of abortion providers has decreased over the last 20 years.
- 86% of US counties lack an abortion provider.
- No federal funds may be used for abortion except in the case of rape, incest, or as a life-saving procedure for the woman.
- 16 states allow state Medicaid funds to be used for "medically necessary" abortions, including those in which the woman's psychological health would be negatively impacted by continuing the pregnancy.

SYNONYM(S)

- Aspiration abortion
- Suction abortion
- Suction curettage
- Vacuum abortion

CLINICAL PEARLS

- Counseling about expected postprocedure bleeding will allay anxiety. Bleeding may be like a period but will taper over the following week.
- Postprocedure cramping is common and typically responds to NSAIDs or a heating pad.
- Patients vary in their need for narcotics but may be given a prescription prior to discharge if necessary.
- Initiate contraception as soon as possible:
  - IUDs may be inserted immediately postprocedure.
- Hormonal contraception may be initiated on the day of the abortion.

ABBREVIATIONS

- D&C—Dilation and curettage
- GA—Gestational age
- MVA—Manual vacuum aspiration

CODES

ICD9-CM
635.00 Legally induced abortion

PATIENT TEACHING

Activity restrictions:

- Pelvic rest (nothing in the vagina including intercourse and tampons) for 1–2 weeks.
- No heavy exercise for a few days to a week.
- Initiate contraception as instructed.

AMNIOCENTESIS

Nicole W. Karjane, MD
John W. Seeds, MD

 BASICS

DESCRIPTION

- Amniocentesis is an invasive procedure whereby a narrow-gauge needle is passed through the maternal abdominal wall into the gravid uterus and gestational sac to aspirate amniotic fluid.
- Generally performed for diagnostic purposes:
  - Most commonly to obtain desquamated fetal cells to grow in tissue culture for chromosomal analysis:
    - Typically performed between 15 and 20 weeks under US guidance
  - Also to obtain AF to verify fetal lung maturity before labor induction or cesarean delivery prior to 39 weeks
  - May be used to help diagnose intra-amniotic infection
  - May be used for monitoring fetal isoimmunization using optical density of fluid at 450-nm wavelength, which may correlate with fetal anemia.
    - Is often replaced by noninvasive MCA Doppler evaluation
- May be performed for therapeutic indications:
  - Amnio-reduction in cases of TTTS or other severe polyhydramnios

Indications

- Genetic amniocentesis is indicated in cases where the risk of fetal aneuploidy is estimated to be > the risk of fetal loss associated with the procedure (~1 in 200). These include the following:
  - Maternal age ≥35 at time of delivery (advanced maternal age)
  - Dizygotic twin pregnancy with maternal age ≥31 at time of delivery
  - Previous pregnancy with fetal trisomy
  - Patient or partner is carrier of a chromosome translocation or inversion
  - Patient or partner has aneuploidy
  - Abnormal 1st or 2nd trimester maternal serum screening test results
  - Fetal anatomic abnormality detected on US
- Indications for nongenetic amniocentesis include:
  - Elective induction or cesarean delivery prior to 39 weeks to confirm lung maturity
  - Concern for intra-amniotic infection when diagnosis is unclear
  - Fetal isoimmunization with rising maternal titer or abnormal middle cerebral artery study
  - TTTS with polyhydramnios.

Site (Office, Surgical Center, L&D)

- 2nd-trimester amniocentesis is generally performed in an office setting with US guidance.
- Amniocentesis performed after fetal viability (generally after 24 weeks) should be performed in a venue that has the ability to perform an emergent delivery, including neonatal resuscitation, if required.

Concurrent Procedures

Testing AF for assessment of fetal lung maturity

Age-Related Factors

- Pregnant women who will be ≥35 at the time of delivery are more likely to undergo diagnostic amniocentesis.
- Risk of fetal aneuploidy increases with maternal age.

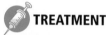 **TREATMENT**

PROCEDURE

Informed Consent

Prior to amniocentesis, a thorough discussion of risks and benefits should be documented, and the patient should sign an appropriate consent form that documents the risk of pregnancy loss.

Patient Education

All patients who are at increased risk of fetal aneuploidy should be counseled about the purpose of amniocentesis as well as the risks, benefits, alternatives, and limitations of the procedure.

Risks, Benefits

- Risks:
  - Vaginal spotting, AF leakage, pregnancy loss, infection, failure to obtain an adequate sample, and fetal injury
  - Fluid leakage after genetic amniocentesis often stops and the pregnancy continues.
- Benefits:
  - Ability to diagnose or exclude a fetal chromosomal abnormality in the mid trimester; and ability to confirm fetal lung maturity in later pregnancy

Alternatives

- Include noninvasive testing, alternative invasive testing, or no testing at all
- Noninvasive testing modalities include:
  - 1st trimester screening using maternal serum markers (PAPP-A and β-hCG) in combination with a fetal nuchal translucency.

- 2nd trimester maternal serum screening using hCG, AFP, uE3, and inhibin A.
- No noninvasive screening test confirms or excludes aneuploidy but may alter probability.
- Alternative invasive testing involves CVS between 9 and 12 weeks.
- Some women, both at low and high risk of a fetal chromosomal abnormality, may not wish to pursue fetal screening; however, all pregnant women should be counseled about the options and offered screening tests.

 FOLLOW-UP

- RhoGAM (300 μg dose) should be given to unsensitized Rh-negative mothers to prevent Rh sensitization following amniocentesis unless the father of the pregnancy is confirmed Rh-negative.
- Fetal heart rate should be documented after the procedure:
  - Electronic fetal and uterine monitoring should be considered if the procedure is performed after fetal viability.
- Women should be instructed that they may experience cramping, spotting, or leakage of fluid:
  - Any persistent leakage of fluid, bleeding, severe cramping, or fevers should be reported.

PROGNOSIS

- Loss rate attributable to the procedure has been shown to be ~1 in 180–200.
- Prognosis for the pregnancy largely depends on the indication for the procedure and the results of testing.
- Termination of pregnancy may be considered in situations where significant abnormalities are diagnosed.

COMPLICATIONS

Generally rare, but may include:
- Bleeding from puncture site
- Leakage of fluid
- Intra-amniotic infection
- Failure to obtain an adequate sample
- Injury to the fetus or umbilical cord
- Fetal loss

BIBLIOGRAPHY

ACOG Educational Bulletin No. 230. *Management of Fetal Lung Maturity.* Washington DC: ACOG; 1996;267–273.

ACOG Practice Bulletin No. 27. *Prenatal Diagnosis of Fetal Chromosomal Abnormalities.* Washington DC: ACOG; 2001;867–877.

Alfirevic Z, et al. Amniocentesis and chorionic villus sampling for prenatal diagnosis. *Cochrane Database Syst Rev.* 2003;3:CD003252.

Gabbe SG, et al., eds. *Obstetrics: Normal and Problem Pregnancies,* 5th ed. Philadelphia: Churchill, Livingstone, Elsevier; 2007.

Ghidini G. Amniocentesis: Technique and complications. UpToDate; 2006.

Seeds J. Diagnostic mid trimester amniocentesis: How safe? *Am J Obstet Gynecol.* 2004;191:608–616.

 MISCELLANEOUS

- Amniocentesis is not appropriate for diagnosing birth defects caused by environmental teratogens.
- Amniocentesis may increase risk of vertical transmission of HIV, hepatitis C, CMV, or toxoplasmosis.

ABBREVIATIONS

- AF—Amniotic fluid
- AFP—α-Fetoprotein
- CMV—Cytomegalovirus
- CVS—Chorionic villus sampling
- hCG—Human chorionic gonadotropin
- MCA—Middle cerebral artery
- PAPP-A—Pregnancy-associated plasma protein
- TTTS—Twin-twin transfusion syndrome
- uE3—Unconjugated estriol

 CODES

ICD9-CM

- V28.0 Screening for chromosomal anomalies by amniocentesis
- 655.83 Suspected or know fetal abnormality not elsewhere classified
- V23.81 Elderly primigravida
- V23.82 Elderly multigravida
- 758.4 Balanced autosomal translocation in normal individual
- 762.3 Placental transfusion syndromes

PATIENT TEACHING

- ACOG Patient Education Pamphlet: Diagnosing Birth Defects
- ACOG Patient Education Pamphlet: Birth Defects
- ACOG Patient Education Pamphlet: Later Childbearing
- ACOG Patient Education Pamphlet: The Rh Factor: How It Can Affect Your Pregnancy
- ACOG Patient Education Pamphlet: Genetic Disorders

Section VII

ASSISTED REPRODUCTIVE TECHNOLOGIES

Michael D. Scheiber, MD, MPH

BASICS

DESCRIPTION
- ART includes the wide array of techniques used to help couples conceive with advanced techniques beyond superovulation and insemination.
- Common to these techniques is the fact that the gametes and/or embryos are manipulated prior to fertilization and implantation.
- IVF-ET comprise the vast majority of ART procedures performed in the US:
  - Sometimes used in combination with other techniques:
    - ICSI
    - AH
- ART also includes:
  - GIFT
  - ZIFT
  - TET
  - FET
  - Oocyte donation
  - Gestational carriers
  - PGD

Indications
- Although ART has helped thousands of couples worldwide to conceive, ART is usually reserved for cases in which simpler or less expensive fertility therapy has failed.
- In some cases, such as severe tubal disease, severe male factor, or protracted infertility, ART may represent a 1st-line therapy choice.
- According to ASRM, ART accounts for <3% of infertility services and only 0.07% of US health care costs.

Site (Office, Surgical Center, OR)
- Most large ART centers perform IVF-ET in an outpatient office or ambulatory surgery center setting.
- Most physicians perform this procedure under moderate sedation with or without a paracervical block.
- Some physicians use general anesthesia for IVF.
- GIFT, ZIFT, and TET require a fully equipped laparoscopy suite with special equipment available for gamete handling.

Age-Related Factors
- The age of the woman providing the oocytes is the most predictive factor in ART outcome.
- Live birth rates per embryo transfer in the US fall from 43% in women <35 years of age to 15% in women 41–42 years old.
- The same rate was >50% for women undergoing oocyte donation.

EPIDEMIOLOGY
- Since its 1st use in the US in 1981, through the end of 2003, >300,000 babies have been born in the US through the use of ART.
- ~1% of all US births are now conceived through the use of ART, representing ~49,000 babies each year.
- >400 clinics in the US perform ART procedures (all data available at: www.cdc.gov).

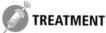

TREATMENT

PROCEDURE

Informed Consent
- Patients undergoing ART procedures should be informed of small risk of:
  - Infection
  - Adjacent organ damage with repair
  - Bleeding with transfusion
  - Anesthetic complications
  - Ovarian hyperstimulation syndrome
  - Multiple pregnancy
- The vast majority of babies born through ART are healthy and normal.
- There may be subtle increased health risks to the offspring of ART pregnancies that are difficult to separate from the primary effects of:
  - Infertility
  - Multiple pregnancy with preterm birth
  - Advanced maternal age

SURGICAL
- IVF-ET: Typically involves controlled ovarian stimulation combined with US and serum monitoring:
  - When oocyte maturity is reached, egg retrieval is performed via US-guided transvaginal needle aspiration in the outpatient setting:
    - Egg retrieval usually takes 20–25 minutes and typically requires no incisions, sutures, or scars.
  - Mature eggs that have been retrieved are then fertilized in the petri dish ("in vitro") either by placing sperm and eggs together or by directly injecting a single sperm inside of an egg (ICSI).
  - If fertilization is successful, embryos are then incubated for 2–6 days in the laboratory.
  - Some (usually 1–4 embryos depending on patient's age) or all of the embryos are transferred back to the uterus transcervically with a small flexible catheter, often under US guidance.
  - Embryos in excess of those desired for transfer can be frozen for later FET.
  - Luteal progesterone support is usually provided until a pregnancy test is obtained 12–14 days after embryo transfer.

- Trend is toward transferring fewer embryos so that high-order multiple pregnancy rates are dropping rapidly.
- Success rates are improving significantly.
- With GIFT, fertilization occurs in the fallopian tube:
  - Controlled ovarian stimulation is undertaken with US and hormonal monitoring.
  - When oocyte maturity is reached, laparoscopy is performed:
    - Oocytes are aspirated under direct visualization.
    - Both sperm and eggs are loaded into a catheter and placed via the laparoscope into 1 or both fallopian tubes.
  - Oocytes that are not transferred can be fertilized in vitro and resultant embryos cryopreserved for later FET.
  - Before refinement of laboratory IVF culture techniques, GIFT offered a moderate advantage in pregnancy rates over IVF-ET.
  - This gap has narrowed, and there is a trend away from GIFT:
    - GIFT is typically more expensive and significantly more invasive than IVF-ET.
  - Currently, <1% of ART cycles in the US are now GIFT procedures.
  - Other disadvantages of GIFT include unknown fertilization rates and its unsuitability for patients with tubal disease or significant male factor infertility.
- ZIFT and TET are similar procedures in which eggs are retrieved and mixed with sperm as for IVF:
  - Resultant zygotes or cleaved embryos are placed laparoscopically in fallopian tube.
  - Little advantage to ZIFT or TET over IVF-ET:
    - Combined risks and costs of both transvaginal egg retrieval and laparoscopy
    - Thus ZIFT and TET are more expensive and dangerous than either IVF-ET or GIFT alone.
    - Few of these procedures currently performed.
- FET is the transfer of previously cryopreserved embryos back to the uterus:
  - Embryos can be successfully frozen at the pronuclear, cleaved, or blastocyst stage.
  - Pregnancy rates somewhat inferior to fresh IVF-ET, but:
    - FET is totally noninvasive
    - Much less expensive than fresh IVF-ET
  - The endometrium is usually artificially prepared for implantation with exogenous estrogen and progesterone therapy:
    - FET can also be performed in a low-dose stimulated cycle or a natural cycle.

- During an *oocyte donation* cycle, medication (usually a GnRH-agonist) is given to both egg donor and recipient to synchronize their menstrual cycles. The donor then receives standard ovarian stimulation with egg retrieval. IVF is performed with the intended father's sperm, and resulting embryos are transferred to the recipient's uterus. The recipient's endometrium is supported with the sequential administration of exogenous estrogen and progesterone:
  - Indications for oocyte donation include:
    - Decreased ovarian reserve or hypergonadotropic anovulation
    - A history of poor ovarian response to stimulation
    - Repeated IVF failures
    - Inheritable genetic diseases
    - Some cases of recurrent pregnancy loss
    - Advanced female age (>42–43 years old)
  - Pregnancy rates from oocyte donation exceed 50–60% in most large centers:
    - Superior pregnancy rates compared to autologous IVF for women >40
    - A much reduced miscarriage rate
    - A much lower incidence of aneuploidy
- The technical aspects of *gestational (uterine) surrogacy* are identical to oocyte donation with the intended biologic parents serving as the gamete donors and the gestational carrier as the recipient:
  - Uterine surrogacy is indicated for women with:
    - Medical contraindications to pregnancy
    - An absent or abnormal uterus
    - Damaged endometrium (e.g., severe synechiae)
    - Some cases of recurrent pregnancy loss
    - Repeated IVF failures with high quality embryos
  - The legal aspects of surrogacy vary from state to state and even within counties.
  - Adequate legal preparation must be undertaken prior to surrogacy to protect the rights of the intended parents and the surrogate.

- With ICSI, a single sperm is injected directly into the cytoplasm of a mature oocyte using a micromanipulator under a high-powered microscope:
  - ICSI has revolutionized the treatment of severe male factor infertility.
  - Even sperm too few, too immotile, or too morphologically abnormal to fertilize an egg even in vitro can be used to achieve fertilization with reliably good results and excellent subsequent pregnancy rates.
  - Even sperm aspirated directly from the testicles can be used in cases of obstructive azoospermia.
  - ICSI should be reserved for cases in which it is absolutely necessary, due to the potential long-term unknown effects.
- AH refers to artificial thinning or partial removal of the zona pellucida surrounding the embryo in an effort to improve embryo implantation rates:
  - Accomplished mechanically with a micropipette, chemically with acid solution, or with a laser under the microscope.
  - A small risk of injuring underlying blastomeres
  - A very small risk of conjoined twinning
  - Unclear which patients will absolutely benefit, and criteria vary from center to center
- PGD can be indicated for those couples with inheritable diseases, those at risk for aneuploidy, or those with recurrent aneuploidic miscarriages (see chapter).

BIBLIOGRAPHY

ACOG Committee Opinion No. 324. Perinatal Risks Associated with Assisted Reproductive Technology. *Obstet Gynecol*. 2005;106:1143–1146.

Centers for Diseae Control. ART Report: National Summary. Available at: http://apps.nccd.cdc.gov/ART2003/nation03.asp

Fluker MR, et al. A prospective randomized comparison of zygote intrafallopian transfer and in vitro fertilization-embryo transfer for nontubal factor infertility. *Fertil Steril*. 1993;60:515–519.

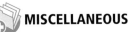

MISCELLANEOUS
ABBREVIATIONS

- AH—Assisted hatching
- ART—Assisted reproductive technology
- ASRM—American Society of Reproductive Medicine
- FET—Frozen embryo transfer
- GIFT—Gamete intrafallopian transfer
- ICSI—Intracytoplasmic sperm injection
- IVF-ET—In vitro fertilization-embryo transfer
- PGD—Preimplantation genetic diagnosis
- TET—Tubal embryo transfer
- ZIFT—Zygote intrafallopian transfer
- GnRH—Gonadotropin-releasing hormone

CODES
ICD9-CM

- 606.9 Male infertility, unspecified
- 628.2 Infertility, tubal
- 628.9 Infertility unspecified
- 628.8 Infertility other

PATIENT TEACHING

- ASRM Patient Fact Sheet on ART. Available at: http://www.asrm.org/Patients/patientbooklets/ART.pdf
- The SART website at http://www.sart.org offers specific outcomes data from infertility clinics around the country.

CERVICAL CERCLAGE

Mona Prasad, DO, MPH
Jay Iams, MD

 BASICS

DESCRIPTION

- Cervical cerclage is a surgical procedure in which suture or synthetic tape is used to reinforce the cervix.
- 3 common cerclage techniques:
  - McDonald:
    - Transvaginal approach
    - Purse-string, circumferential suture
  - Shirodkar:
    - Transvaginal approach
    - Dissect the vaginal epithelium anteriorly and posteriorly to the level of the internal os
    - Allows potentially higher placement of circumferential suture
  - Transabdominal:
    - Laparotomy approach
    - Suture is placed at the level of the uterine isthmus and internal cervical os.
    - Requires subsequent cesarean delivery and may remain in situ until cessation of childbearing

Indications
- Prophylactic:
  - Placed at 12–16 weeks gestation
  - Obstetric history of recurrent midtrimester loss
- Urgent:
  - Less obvious obstetric history
  - Cervical sonography identifies cervix <20 mm between 16 and 24 weeks
- Emergent/Rescue:
  - Cerclage placed when advanced cervical dilation and effacement are identified on digital or speculum exam.
- Transabdominal:
  - When vaginal approach is unlikely to succeed:
    - Minimal cervix noted vaginally
  - When transvaginal approach has failed repeatedly

Site (Office, Surgical Center, OR)
- Operating room
- Possible ambulatory, same day surgery
- Regional anesthesia preferred

Concurrent Procedures
- Regional anesthesia
- +/− Intraoperative transvaginal US:
  - Evaluate postprocedure cervical length
  - Evaluate bladder integrity

EPIDEMIOLOGY
The use of cerclage is estimated at 1/182–1/222 pregnancies.

 TREATMENT

PROCEDURE
Cervical cerclage is commonly placed after 1st trimester, after the time of greatest risk of SAB and prior to the time of viability.

Informed Consent
Informed consent is required for this procedure.

Patient Education
The efficacy of cerclage in prolonging pregnancy is unproven.

Risks, Benefits
- Risks:
  - Infection (chorioamnionitis/sepsis)
  - Bleeding
  - PROM
  - Preterm labor/preterm delivery
  - Postoperative suture displacement with cervical injury
  - Failure
- Benefits:
  - Correction of a structural weakness of the cervix
  - Possible prolongation of pregnancy

Alternatives
- Bed rest
- Pelvic rest
- Pessaries

Medical
17-hydroxyprogesterone supplementation:
- Used in patients with history of spontaneous preterm delivery
- 250 mg IM weekly, weeks 16–36
- Can be use as adjunct to cerclage or alternative therapy in conjunction with bed rest

Surgical
No surgical alternatives to cerclage are available.

 FOLLOW-UP

- Postoperation analgesia:
  - Mild narcotic, brief use of NSAIDs or acetaminophen for postoperative analgesia
- Follow cervix with US for cervical length every 2 weeks after cerclage placement:
  - Consider replacement of cerclage if membranes prolapse before 22 weeks
- Administer corticosteroids to facilitate lung maturity if cervical length <25 mm after 24 weeks' gestation
- Schedule cerclage removal 35–36 weeks if patient is candidate for vaginal delivery

PROGNOSIS
- Type of cerclage may affect outcome.
- Patients undergoing emergent cerclage have worse outcomes than those with prophylactic or urgent cerclage.
- Urgent and prophylactic cerclage have equal success rates in recent studies.
- Emergent cerclage with cervical dilation ≥3 cm have decreased perinatal survival.
- Emergent cerclage placed with visible membranes have increased rates of perinatal loss.

COMPLICATIONS

- Perioperative complications:
  - Iatrogenic rupture of membranes
  - Contractions
- Late complications:
  - Chorioamnionitis
  - PROM
  - Preterm labor/preterm delivery
  - Suture migration

BIBLIOGRAPHY

ACOG Practice Bulletin No. 48. Cervical Insufficiency. *Obstet Gynecol*. 2003;102:1091–1099.

Barss VA, et al. Cervical cerclage: Technique. Available at: www.uptodate.com. Accessed 11/01/06.

Creasy RK, et al., eds. *Maternal-Fetal Medicine Principles and Practice,* 5th ed. Philadelphia: Saunders; 2004.

 MISCELLANEOUS

ABBREVIATIONS

- PROM—Premature rupture of membranes
- SAB—Spontaneous abortion

CODES

ICD9-CM/CPT

- 593.20 CPT code transvaginal cerclage
- 593.25 CPT code transabdominal cerclage
- 598.71 CPT code cerclage removal
- 654.5

 PATIENT TEACHING

- 1st week after cerclage placement:
  - Rest most of the day.
  - Lie down on left side for 1 hour twice a day.
  - Find assistance for routine household activities.
- For the remainder of pregnancy:
  - Limit strenuous activity, difficult household chores
  - Pelvic rest
  - Prenatal visits every 1–3 weeks
- Notify physician if you have:
  - Menstrual-like cramps
  - Low backache
  - Contractions
  - Pelvic pressure
  - Change in vaginal discharge
  - Vaginal spotting, bleeding or tan discharge
  - Leaking fluid

Section VII

CERVICAL CONIZATION, LEEP, AND CRYOTHERAPY

Jack Basil, MD

BASICS

DESCRIPTION
- LEEP, LLETZ, CKC, and CO_2 laser cone are terms to describe techniques of surgical removal of the entire TZ and a portion of the endocervical canal.
- Conization can be both diagnostic and therapeutic.

Cryotherapy and CO_2 laser of the TZ are ablative procedures used to treat cervical dysplasia in cases where a biopsy specimen is not obtained.

Indications
- LEEP/LLETZ:
  - Treatment of CIN 2 or CIN 3 with negative ECC
- Conization (classic indications):
  - Microinvasive cervical cancer (<3 mm)
  - Abnormal (positive) ECC
  - Discrepancy of 2 grades between Pap and cervical biopsy with Pap worse than cervical biopsy (Cx Bx)
  - Inadequate colposcopy
  - Adenocarcinoma in situ
  - Expert colposcopist suspects invasion

Site (Office, Surgical Center, OR)
- LEEP cone, LLETZ, and CO_2 laser cone:
  - Office
  - Outpatient surgery center
  - Operating room
- CKC:
  - Outpatient surgery center
  - Operating room

Concurrent Procedures
- Colposcopy usually is performed with conization.
- Post-cone ECC is optional.

Age-Related Factors
- Begin Pap screening ~3 years after onset of intercourse, but no later than 21 years of age
- Consider a shallower depth cone in a younger patient.
- Consider more conservative management of CIN 2 in appropriately compliant adolescents.

EPIDEMIOLOGY
- Estimated 500,000 new cases of cervical dysplasia in the US
- Average age of cervical dysplasia 25–35 years

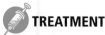

TREATMENT

PROCEDURE

Informed Consent
Standard informed consent should be obtained prior to performing a conization.

Patient Education
- Understand workup and management of abnormal Paps
- Understand cervical dysplasia
- Understand different conization techniques

Risks, Benefits
- Risks:
  - Bleeding
  - Infection
  - Potential subsequent preterm labor/delivery
- Benefits:
  - Prevention of cervical cancer
  - Treatment of cervical dysplasia

Alternatives
- Rates for clearance of squamous dysplasia of all grades are the same for laser therapy, LEEP, and cryotherapy:
  - Excisional procedures offer the advantage of a specimen for histologic exam.
- Ablative procedures should not be performed in patients with dysplasia on ECC.
- If 1 of the classic indications for a conization is present, a conization should be performed.

Medical
Research underway evaluating chemoprevention of cervical dysplasia with COX-2 inhibitors

Surgical
- LEEP cone:
  - Anesthetize the cervix:
    - Typically with intracervical local anesthetic block
  - Select settings (60:60 Blend 1)
  - Larger loop used to remove TZ and entire lesion
  - Smaller loop to remove portion of endocervix
  - Ball cautery to cone bed
  - Apply Monsel and/or Gelfoam
- CKC:
  - Anesthetize patient and cervix
  - Stay sutures in cervical-vaginal fold at 3 and 9 o'clock for traction and hemostasis
  - Use scalpel to excise cone biopsy (TZ and portion of endocervix)
  - Cauterize cone bed
  - Suture bed for hemostasis
  - Apply Monsel and/or Gelfoam
- Laser cone:
  - Anesthetize patient
  - Use CO_2 laser to excise cone (TZ and portion of endocervix)
  - Laser/Cauterize cone bed
  - Suture for hemostasis (optional)
  - Apply Monsel and/or Gelfoam

FOLLOW-UP

If no invasive cancer is present on cone specimen, it is customary to perform follow-up Pap in 3–6 months.

PROGNOSIS
- Overall, quite favorable if no invasive cancer is found
- Risk of recurrent or persistent dysplasia is ~10–25%.
- Risk of recurrence or persistence is independent of type of conization performed.

COMPLICATIONS
- Bleeding
- Infection
- Damage to surrounding tissue

BIBLIOGRAPHY

ACOG Practice Bulletin No. 66. *Management of Abnormal Cervical Cytology and Histology.* Washington DC: ACOG; September 2005.

Smith RA, et al. American Cancer Society Guidelines for early detection of cancer. *CA Cancer J Clin.* 2006;56:11–25.

 MISCELLANEOUS

SYNONYM(S)
- LEEP cone:
  - Technical variations:
    - 2 pass LEEP
    - LEEP with a top hat
- LLETZ
- Cold Knife Conization (CKC)
- Laser conization

CLINICAL PEARLS
- Apply Lugol solution to delineate extent of lesion on exocervix.
- Dilute vasopressin solution may decrease bleeding with a CKC.
- Gelfoam or Monsel solution applied after a conization may decrease bleeding.

ABBREVIATIONS
- CKC—Cold knife conization
- CIN—Cervical intraepithelial neoplasia
- COX—Cyclooxygenase
- Cx Bx—Cervical biopsy
- ECC—Endocervical curettage
- LEEP—Loop electrosurgical excision procedure
- LLETZ—Large loop excision of the transformation zone
- TZ—Transformation zone

CODES

ICD9-CM
- 233.1 Cervical dysplasia (severe)
- 622.1 Cervical dysplasia (mild/moderate)
- 795 Abnormal Pap smear

 PATIENT TEACHING

- It is paramount to stress the importance of cervical cancer screening guidelines.
- ACOG Patient Education Pamphlet: Loop Electrosurgical Excision Procedure. Available at: http://www.acog.org/publications/patient_education/bp110.cfm

CESAREAN DELIVERY

Paula J. Adams Hillard, MD

 BASICS

DESCRIPTION
- Delivery of fetus via abdominal and uterine incisions
- Uterine incision does not correspond to skin incision, and may be:
  - Low transverse: Most common
  - Low vertical: Occasional use with densely adherent bladder, lower uterine fibroid, fetal anomalies, fetal malpresentation
  - Classical: Extending to fundus
  - T-shaped: Resulting from dystocia after an initial low transverse excision required extension
- CD or CS can also be classified as:
  - Primary (1st)
  - Repeat after a previous CD
  - "Labored" CD after planned vaginal delivery
  - Elective:
    ○ CD on maternal request defined as a CD for a singleton pregnancy on maternal request at term in the absence of any medical or obstetric indications
    ○ Elective CD includes a planned CD for a range of maternal and fetal indications
  - Emergency

Indications
- Most common indications for CD:
  - Failure to progress in labor: 30%
  - Previous hysterotomy (CD, myomectomy, etc.): 30%
  - Fetal malpresentation: 11%
  - Nonreassuring fetal status: 10%
- Additional indications:
  - Abnormal placenta: Placenta previa, placenta accreta
  - Multiple gestation
  - Maternal infection (HSV, HIV)
  - LBW infant
  - Fetal anomaly
- Situations in which women with previous CD are not a candidate for a trial of labor:
  - Previous classical or T-shaped uterine incision or extensive transfundal uterine surgery
  - Previous uterine rupture
  - Medical or obstetric complication precluding vaginal delivery
  - Inability to perform emergency CD because of unavailable surgeon, anesthesia, sufficient staff, or facility
  - ≥2 cesarean births, unless previous vaginal delivery

- Term singleton breech delivery: ACOG notes that the decision regarding mode of delivery should depend on the experience of the health care provider, but that CD will be the preferred mode for most physicians because of the diminishing expertise in vaginal breech delivery.
- Scheduled CD may be indicated for HIV infected women (see topic).

Site (Office, Surgical Center, OR)
- Labor and delivery operating suite
- Operating room

Concurrent Procedures
- Sterilization
- Rarely, myomectomy
- As emergency, for intractable hemorrhage, cesarean hysterectomy

Age-Related Factors
Higher rates of CD on maternal request in older primiparous women

EPIDEMIOLOGY
- In 2004, 1.2 million or 29.1% of U.S. live births were by CD:
  - Rapid increases in CD in 1970s and early 1980s, with declines in late 1980s–1996, with subsequent increase
  - Factors to which rising rates are attributed include:
    ○ Changing physician and patient expectations
    ○ Changes in clinical practice (e.g., fewer vaginal breech births, fewer forceps deliveries)
    ○ Medicolegal concerns
    ○ Financial issues
    ○ Increasing maternal age
    ○ Increasing rates of multiple gestation
    ○ Maternal obesity
  - Declining rates of VBAC since 1996
  - Primary CD increasing in all ethnic and age groups
- International and domestic estimates of CD on maternal request range from 4–18% of all CDs, although these estimates are not believed to be based on solid data.
  - From US birth certificate data, "no indicated risk" in 5.5%
  - Higher rates in older primiparous women: 25.7% in women >40

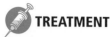 **TREATMENT**

PROCEDURE
Informed Consent
As with any surgical procedure, patients should be informed of indications, risk, and benefits. Ideally, these issues are considered prior to the onset of labor or requirement for emergency CD.

Patient Education
Patient-specific factors play a role in decisions about CD and impact risk as well.
- Age
- Childbearing plans
- Obesity
- Accuracy of GA assessment and estimated date of delivery (See Establishing Estimated Date of Delivery.)
- Personal factors:
  - Need for control
  - History of interpersonal violence, traumatic delivery, infant death, symptoms of PTSD
  - Depression, feelings of guilt
  - Fear of labor

Risks, Benefits
- Unplanned CD may be indicated for either maternal or fetal medical conditions, in which case the obstetrician makes the decision that the benefits of CD outweigh the potential risks. The maternal risk/benefit assessment includes factors different from the fetal/neonatal risk/benefit assessment.
- Risks: Typical risks associated with abdominal surgery:
  - Hemorrhage and need for transfusion
  - Infection
  - Injury to bowel, bladder, urinary tract
  - Elective CD entails the risk of iatrogenic prematurity.
  - Hemorrhage with planned CD < planned VD with unplanned CD
  - CD has a longer length of hospital stay than VD.
  - Infection rate > in all CD than VD
  - Placenta previa in subsequent pregnancies increases with the number of prior CDs, advancing age, and parity:
    ○ CD nearly double the risk of placenta previa
- Benefits:
  - SUI less likely after elective CD than with VD, but multifactorial
  - Lower risk of surgical complications with elective CD than with unplanned CD after attempted VD
  - Elective repeat CD associated with lower risks of uterine rupture than VBAC
  - Elective CD associated with lower risk of neonatal intracranial hemorrhage, neonatal asphyxia, and encephalopathy than operative vaginal delivery and CD in labor
  - CD associated with lower risk of brachial plexus injury

Alternatives

The modes of delivery are either VD or CD, although CD may occur as unplanned CD after attempted VD, elective CD at maternal request, or indicated elective CD. VD may be assisted with forceps or vacuum delivery.

Surgical

After the decision to perform a CD is made, the surgical procedure includes:

- Decisions about type of anesthesia (general, epidural, or spinal):
  - Cochrane review shows no evidence that regional anesthetic is superior to general regarding maternal or neonatal outcomes.
- Baseline CBC, type, and antibody screen
- Prophylactic antibiotics:
  - Cochrane review concluded a decreased risk of endometritis and wound infection after elective and nonelective CD with antibiotics.
  - Timing: Preoperative vs. after cord clamps; Cochrane concludes no RCT to guide choice
- Placement of urinary catheter, prep, and drape
- Left lateral uterine displacement with wedge:
  - Cochrane shows insufficient evidence to support
- Decisions about type of skin incision:
  - Most commonly Pfannenstiel transverse incision
  - Vertical incision is faster with less bleeding for emergency CD
- Skin, subcutaneous tissue, fascial incision, muscle separation, peritoneal entry
- Assess uterine rotation
- Develop bladder flap and retract inferiorly
- Uterine incision: Typically transverse, sufficiently large to allow atraumatic delivery, avoid laceration of uterine vessels
- Extend uterine incision laterally: Sharp or blunt dissection
- Delivery of fetus, flexing head, delivering through uterine incision:
  - Occasionally may require forceps or vacuum device
  - If head deeply is impacted in pelvis, assistant pushes head up through vagina
- Spontaneous delivery of placenta: Cochrane review shows an increased blood loss with manual removal.
- Decision to exteriorize uterus vs. repair in situ: Cochrane review draws no definitive conclusions.
- Single or 2-layer uterine closure: Cochrane review suggests no advantages or disadvantages except shorter operating time for single-layer closure.
- Peritoneal closures not required: Cochrane review shows nonclosure has less postoperative fever and reduced stay; long-term data not available.
- Closure of subcutaneous fat may reduce wound complications (Cochrane review).
- Skin closure: Cochrane review shows subcuticular closure may provide more cosmetic result; staples are faster.

 FOLLOW-UP

After CD, a follow-up visit is frequently schedule at 3–6 weeks postpartum.

PROGNOSIS

Prognosis for the health of mother and baby is excellent in developed countries with good prenatal care, healthcare facilities, and surgical options available as needed.

COMPLICATIONS

- Surgical complications as with any surgical procedure
- Additional maternal and fetal risks; see above.

BIBLIOGRAPHY

ACOG Practice Bulletin No. 54. Vaginal Birth after Previous Cesarean Delivery. Washington DC: ACOG; July 2004.

Afolabi DD, et al. Regional versus general anaesthesia for caesarean section. *Cochrane Database Syst Rev.* 2007. CD004350

Alderdice AE, et al. Techniques and materials for skin closure in caesarean section. *Cochrane Database Syst Rev.* 2007. CD003577

Anderson ER, et al. Techniques and materials for closure of the abdominal wall in caesarean section. *Cochrane Database Syst Rev.* 2007. CD004663

Bamigboye JS, et al. Closure versus non-closure of the peritoneum at caesarean section. *Cochrane Database Syst Rev.* 2007. CD000163

Capeless E, et al. Cesarean delivery. Available at: www.uptodate.com. Accessed 09/22/07.

Dodd LLAN, et al. Planned elective repeat caesarean section versus planned vaginal birth for women with a previous caesarean birth. *Cochrane Database Syst Rev.* 2007. CD004906

Enkin PL, et al. Single versus two-layer suturing for closing the uterine incision at Caesarean section. *Cochrane Database Syst Rev.* 2007. CD000192

Hopkins WH, et al. Antibiotic prophylaxis regimens and drugs for cesarean section. *Cochrane Database Syst Rev.* 2007. CD001136

Jacobs-Jokhan DD, et al. Extra-abdominal versus intra-abdominal repair of the uterine incision at caesarean section. *Cochrane Database Syst Rev.* 2004. CD000085

NIH. State-of-the Science Conference Statement: Cesarean delivery on maternal request. Washington DC: NIH; March 2006;27–29.

Wilkinson GG, et al. Manual removal of placenta at caesarean section. *Cochrane Database Syst Rev.* 2006. CD000130

Wilkinson JS, et al. Lateral tilt for caesarean section. *Cochrane Database Syst Rev.* 2007. CD000120

 MISCELLANEOUS

The evidence regarding risks and benefits of elective CD at maternal request are not of strong quality.

SYNONYM(S)

- Cesarean birth
- Cesarean delivery
- Cesarean section

CLINICAL PEARLS

- Increasing rates of CD are due to many factors other than medical, including cultural and societal expectations, perceptions of risks, delayed childbearing, trends in family size, health care provider types, professional experiences and training, philosophy regarding birth, medical-legal issues.
- Many ethical issues surround birth and how it is viewed—as a natural process or 1 that requires medical management.
- An ethical relationship exists between a woman and her clinician that requires the provision of information, a discussion of relative risks and benefits, a realistic assessment of potential complications and outcomes, as well as effective communication, an understanding of cultural and personal context, and individualized and shared decision-making.

ABBREVIATIONS

- CD—Cesarean delivery
- CS—Cesarean section
- GA—Gestational age
- HSV—Herpes simplex virus
- LBW—Low birth weight
- PTSD—Posttraumatic stress disorder
- RCT—Randomized controlled trials
- SUI—Stress urinary incontinence
- VBAC—Vaginal birth after cesarean
- VD—Vaginal delivery

CODES

ICD9-CM
763.4 Cesarean delivery

 PATIENT TEACHING

- ACOG Patient Education Pamphlets:
  - Cesarean Birth
  - Vaginal Birth after Cesarean Delivery

Section VII

CHORIONIC VILLUS SAMPLING

Tania F. Esakoff, MD
Aaron B. Caughey, MD, PhD

BASICS

DESCRIPTION
Aspiration of placental tissue to obtain fetal cells for genetic analysis. Approach is determined by placental location:

- Transabdominal approach
- Transcervical approach

Indications
CVS is indicated for any pregnant woman who desires a fetal karyotype in the 1st trimester of pregnancy. Since the decision to undergo prenatal diagnosis depends on a woman's preferences toward having a baby with aneuploidy or experiencing a procedure-related miscarriage as well as the risks of these 2 outcomes, the decision will vary from patient to patient. However, there are several groups of women who are at higher risk of aneuploidy.

- TCVS should be offered to the following types of pregnant women:
  - Women who will be ≥35 at delivery
  - Women with prior pregnancies with aneuploidy
  - The fetus is found to have a major structural defect on US.
  - If either parent has a chromosome translocation or inversion
  - Women who are deemed to be high risk on 1st trimester nuchal translucency, serum screening, or the combination of the 2
- Some women should not have CVS because of increased risk from the procedure or difficulty of the procedure.
  - Absolute contraindications:
    - Active cervical infections such as *Chlamydia* or herpes
  - Relative contraindications:
    - Vaginal infections
    - Vaginal bleeding or spotting
    - Extreme anteversion or retroversion of uterus
    - Patient body habitus precluding easy access to uterus

Site (Office, Surgical Center, OR)
- Usually performed in an office setting by a physician with special training in the procedure.
- Of note, it is generally thought that the learning curve for CVS is long, thus it is difficult for providers to become trained in the usual clinical setting. For example, providers will often train to do CVS procedures in the setting of elective pregnancy terminations. Because of this difficulty in training, not enough providers are trained to perform the procedure.

Concurrent Procedures
The procedure is performed under US guidance.

Age-Related Factors
CVS is usually performed at 10–12 weeks' gestation.

EPIDEMIOLOGY
- The risk of all aneuploidies increases with maternal age. For example, at age 33, the risk is 1:208; at age 35, the risk is 1:132; at age 45, the risk is 1:12.
- For women with a prior pregnancy complicated by autosomal trisomy, the risk of the same or a different autosomal trisomy is 1% until the age-related risk reaches 1%. At this point, her risk is equal to the age-related risk.
- Women with increasing numbers of SABs have an increased risk of karyotypic anomaly identified at the time of prenatal diagnosis:
  - A woman with an a priori risk for Down syndrome of 1:300, would have a risk of 1:204 if a history of 3 prior SABs was present.
  - In women with 1 prior SAB the risk of any aneuploidy is 1.67%, whereas this risk goes up to 2.18% in women with 3 prior SABs.
- For many years, maternal age of ≥35 was considered the cut-off age at which to offer chromosomal testing. This recommendation was based on:
  - The assumption that we had a limited number of sites and providers that could perform the procedures and laboratories to provide results.
  - Economic analysis showing that, at this age, screening for chromosomal anomalies was cost beneficial
  - Down syndrome data suggesting increased risk for this syndrome at age 35
  - Risk/Benefit analysis suggesting that the risk for the diseases should be greater than that of the procedure
- Recent studies have challenged these assumptions by demonstrating that:
  - It may be excessively stringent to propose that to be an acceptable health intervention like prenatal diagnosis has to save money.
  - Many women do not assign equal weights to miscarriage and Down syndrome.
  - Preferences vary widely between women.
- Current ACOG statement is that it is reasonable to offer invasive prenatal diagnosis to all women.

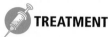

TREATMENT

PROCEDURE

Informed Consent
Patients should undergo a complete counseling session prior to the procedure.

Patient Education
- Occasionally, ambiguous results may occur in cases when mosaicism is present. When this occurs, follow-up testing may be necessary.
- Confined placental mosaicism: Although placenta and fetus have a common ancestry, they do not always reflect the same genotype.
- Mosaicism can occur through 2 mechanisms:
  - A meiotic error leads to a trisomic conceptus that would normally abort spontaneously. However, if during subsequent mitotic divisions some of the aneuploid cells lose the extra chromosome, a mosaic may result.
  - Mitotic postzygotic errors result in a mosaic morula or blastocyst with the distribution and percentage of aneuploid cells depending on timing of nondisjunction.
- Successful cytogenetic analysis results in 99.7% of cases.
- 1.1% of patients require follow-up testing (76% mosaicism, 21% laboratory failure, and 3% maternal contamination).

Risks, Benefits
- Risks:
  - Total pregnancy loss rates are 0.6–0.8% in excess of those associated with amniocentesis (generally thought to be 0.5%), although some institutions have shown no difference between CVS and amniocentesis in terms of loss rate.
  - An association between CVS and limb reduction and oromandibular defects exists when CVS is performed before 9 weeks.
- Benefits:
  - Cytogenetic diagnostic is accuracy >99%.
  - Results are available earlier in pregnancy than those from amniocentesis.

Alternatives
- Amniocentesis
- Other options that do not offer the same level of cytogenetic accuracy:
  - Nuchal translucency and 1st-trimester screening markers
  - 2nd-trimester maternal serum screening
  - US
  - No testing

Medical

Patient must have determination of ABO and Rh status determined prior to the procedure. All Rh-negative women whose partners are Rh-positive or who are unaware of their blood type should get RhoGAM, and anti-Rh IgG that protects the woman from becoming alloimmunized.

Surgical

- Transabdominal approach:
  - Patient is placed in supine position.
  - US is performed to locate the site, making sure to avoid bowel.
  - The skin is infiltrated with 5 mL of 1% lidocaine at the site and cleansed with iodine.
  - Under continuous US guidance, a 19-gauge spinal needle is introduced into the placenta.
  - The stylet is removed, a syringe is attached with cytogenetic transport medium.
  - 10–15 rapid aspirations are made.
  - Once complete, the catheter and syringe are removed under negative pressure.
- Transcervical approach:
  - Patient is placed in lithotomy position.
  - Speculum is placed.
  - Vagina is cleansed with iodine.
  - Under continuous US guidance, a plastic catheter with an inner, metal obturator is introduced transcervically into placenta.
  - Once placed, the obturator is removed, a syringe is attached filled with cytogenetic transport medium.
  - 10–15 rapid aspirations are made.
  - Once complete, the catheter and syringe are removed under negative pressure.
- Transabdominal vs. transcervical approach:
  - Generally, the decision between which approach is taken to perform the procedure is based upon placental location:
    - With anterior, lateral, or fundal placenta, the transabdominal approach is generally taken.
    - For a posterior placenta, this approach would require entering the amniotic sac and is generally thought to have a higher risk. For those posterior placentae that are low enough in the uterine cavity, a transcervical approach can be taken.
    - Even fewer providers are trained in the transcervical approach; thus, if the transabdominal approach is not feasible, these providers would have the patient delay diagnosis for several weeks until an amniocentesis is feasible.
- It appears that the pregnancy loss rate is higher after transcervical CVS.

FOLLOW-UP

- Document fetal heart tones before and after the procedure.
- How best to follow-up regarding the prenatal diagnosis is not clear. While giving telephone results is not optimal, it prevents having every patient return for a follow-up visit and is how the prenatal diagnosis information is usually conveyed. As the vast majority of women will have normal findings, this works well for them.
- For women with an abnormal finding on CVS, a follow-up visit with a prenatal geneticist is scheduled to review the diagnosis and possible need for further testing, and to outline a decision between continuing or terminating the pregnancy.

PROGNOSIS

Almost 99% have a successful procedure without complication.

COMPLICATIONS

- Pregnancy loss
- Infection
- Bleeding

BIBLIOGRAPHY

ACOG Practice Bulletin No. 27. Chorionic Villus Sampling. Washington DC: ACOG; May 2001.

Bianco K, et al. History of miscarriage and increased incidence of fetal aneuploidy in subsequent pregnancy. *Obstet Gynecol*. 2006;107(5):1098–1102.

Canadian Collaborative CVS-Amniocentesis Clinica Trial Group. Multicentre randomized clinical trial of chorion villus sampling and amniocentesis. *First Report Lancet*. 1989;1:1–6.

Caughey AB, et al. Chorionic villus sampling compared with amniocentesis and the difference in the rate of pregnancy loss. *Obstet Gynecol*. 2006;108(3.1):612–616.

Kuppermann M, et al. Who should be offered prenatal diagnosis? The 35-year-old question. *Am J Public Health*. 1999;89(2):160–163.

Ledbetter DH, et al. Cytogenetic results of chorionic villus sampling: High success rate and diagnostic accuracy in the United States collaborative study. *Am J Obstet Gynecol*. 1990;162:495–501.

Shulman LP, et al. Amniocentesis and chorionic villus sampling. *Fetal Med West J Med*. 1993;159:260–268.

Smidt-Jensen S, et al. Randomised comparison of amniocentesis and transabdominal and transcervical chorionic villus sampling. *Lancet*. 1992;340(8830):1237–1244.

Wapner RJ. Invasive prenatal diagnostic techniques. *Semin Perinatol*. 2005;29(6):401–404.

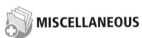

MISCELLANEOUS

SYNONYM(S)

- Biopsy, chorionic villi
- CVS

CLINICAL PEARLS

- Offer the procedure 1–2 weeks prior to the recommended GA, so that women can discuss the option with their partners and take time to make the best decision.
- Procedure should be performed by a highly trained and experienced physician.
- Patients must undergo counseling, preferably with a geneticist, prior to procedure.

ABBREVIATIONS

- CVS—Chorionic villus sampling
- GA—Gestational age
- SAB—Spontaneous abortion

CODES

ICD9-CM/CPT
75.33 Chorionic villus sampling

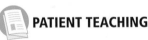

PATIENT TEACHING

- CVS is a way to obtain a fetal karyotype by biopsying or collecting cells from the placenta.
- CVS should be offered to all women who desire determination of fetal karyotype during the 1st trimester. It is performed between 10 and 12 weeks gestation.
- The procedure can only be performed by trained practitioners.
- There is a slightly increased risk of miscarriage over amniocentesis, although some sites have reported similar loss rates.
- Diagnostic accuracy is >99%.
- Patients usually undergo genetic counseling at the same time.

Section VII

COLPOSCOPY

Alan G. Waxman, MD, MPH
Meggan M. Zsemlye, MD

 BASICS

DESCRIPTION

- Exam of cervix and vagina under magnification
- Exam is considered "satisfactory" or "adequate" if entire TZ visualized:
  - Requires seeing the full extent of lesion and entire squamo-columnar junction
- Lesions are highlighted with 3–5% acetic acid wash.
- Lesion characteristics: Defined by color density, margins, topography, vascular pattern:
  - Color density: More opaque, dense white corresponds with higher-grade lesions.
  - Margins: Straight lesion margins correspond with higher-grade dysplasia; geographic or indistinct margins correlate with lower-grade lesions
  - Topography: Nodularity or ulceration should raise suspicion for cancer; peeling edges or "pasted on" appearance of lesion correlate with high-grade lesions.
  - Vascular pattern:
    ○ Mosaic and punctuation may exist in all grades of dysplasia; intercapillary distance and vessel diameter increase with higher-grade lesions.
    ○ Atypical vessels raise suspicion for microinvasive or invasive cancer.
- Lugol's iodine solution identifies non–glycogen containing tissues:
  - Dysplastic epithelium
  - Columnar epithelium
  - Atrophic tissues

Indications

- Abnormal Pap test:
  - ASC-US with positive high risk HPV test or LSIL:
    ○ Exceptions may include adolescents and postmenopausal women (see "Age-Related Factors")
  - ASC-H
  - HSIL
  - AGC
  - Suspicious for cancer
- Abnormal appearance of cervix, vagina, or vulva

Pregnancy Considerations

- Colposcopy may be delayed until postpartum if Pap shows LSIL or HPV-positive ASC-US.
- Because of physiologic changes, colposcopy in pregnancy should be performed by experienced provider.

Site (Office, Surgical Center, OR)
Usually performed in office

Concurrent Procedures

- Cervical biopsy of suspected lesions:
  - Biopsy the most severe-appearing lesion.
  - Diagnosis is improved with multiple biopsies.
  - Ferric subsulfate (Monsel's paste) or silver nitrate is applied for hemostasis.
- Endocervical assessment:
  - Endocervical speculum may aid in visualization of endocervical portion of lesion.
  - Endocervical curette and/or cytobrush is used to sample endocervix:
    ○ Valuable in unsatisfactory colposcopy or when lesion not seen
- Vaginoscopy (colposcopy of the vagina):
  - Indications
    ○ Abnormal cytology: Cervix absent
    ○ Abnormal cytology: No lesion seen on cervix
    ○ Lesion palpated or seen grossly on vagina
  - Both 3–5% acetic acid and Lugol's iodine are indicated for best visualization of lesions:
    ○ Lesions appear faint aceto-white or Lugol's-negative. Punctuation may be present; mosaic is rare.
  - Cervical biopsy forceps may be used for Lugol's-negative or aceto-white lesions:
    ○ Anesthesia important in lower 2/3 of vagina.
- Vulvoscopy (magnified exam of vulva):
  - Indications:
    ○ Visible lesion
    ○ Unexplained pain or itching
    ○ Follow-up of known or treated lesions
  - 5% acetic acid requires 3–5 minutes to take effect on cornified squamous epithelium.
  - Local anesthesia is required for biopsy.
- Endometrial biopsy:
  - Indicated for cytology showing AGC in women ≥35; if abnormal bleeding is present; or if otherwise at risk for hyperplasia.
  - Indicated for Pap in the presence of atypical endometrial cells

Pregnancy Considerations

- Biopsy indicated if HSIL or cancer is suspected:
  - Biopsy is safe in pregnancy.
  - Biopsy only worst area.
  - Monsel's paste provides effective hemostasis.
- Endocervical curettage is contraindicated in pregnancy.

Age-Related Factors

- Adolescents (up to age 21):
  - HPV positive ASC-US and LSIL on Pap test may be followed with cytology rather than immediate colposcopy:
    ○ Repeat Pap annually for 2 years. Colposcopy if HSIL or worse at 1 year, or if ASC-US or worse at 2 years

  - Follow-up with cytology and colposcopy at 6-month intervals for up to 24 months if colposcopy satisfactory as an alternative to treatment for adolescents and young women with CIN 2,3
  - Follow-up with cytology and colposcopy is preferred management of adolescents with HSIL cytology and colposcopy <CIN 2. Colposcopy must be satisfactory and ECC negative.
- Postmenopausal women:
  - LSIL may be followed with colposcopy, reflex HPV DNA testing with colposcopy if positive for high risk types, or cytology at 6 to 12 months with colposcopy if either is ≥ASC-US.

EPIDEMIOLOGY

- >50 million Pap tests per year in US
- >6 million abnormals require follow-up:
  - ~300,000 HSIL
  - ~1,250,000 LSIL
  - ~1,875,000 HPV-positive ASC-US
  - 2–3 million ASC-US
- 11,150 cervical cancers estimated in 2007, per ACS:
  - 3,670 deaths from cervical cancer in 2007

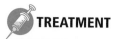 **TREATMENT**

PROCEDURE

Informed Consent

- Required before colposcopy
- Rules for minors vary on a state-by-state basis.

Patient Education
Discussion of HPV:

- Very common infection: 75–80% of sexually active adults have been exposed.
  - Long latent period; HPV infection is not evidence for partner infidelity.
  - Relationship of dysplasia to smoking; stress importance of smoking cessation.
  - Reassure patient that dysplasia is not cancer.
- Condoms offer partial protection from HPV transmission.
- Cannot be reinfected with same HPV type
- Male partner does not need evaluation unless gross lesions; penile cancer very rare
- Perinatal transmission is uncommon.

Risks, Benefits

- Risks:
  - Discomfort
  - Bleeding: Usually minimal or well controlled with Monsel paste
  - Heavy bleeding: Uncommon; rarely requires Surgicel or suture
  - Failure to diagnose existing dysplasia: 17–19% in ALTS study
- Benefits:
  - Increases specificity of diagnosis over cytology alone
  - Lesion identification allows effective treatment

Pregnancy Considerations

- Because of physiologic changes in pregnancy, accuracy of diagnosis is not as good as in nonpregnant women.
- Colposcopy is safe in pregnancy.
- Biopsy does not increase risk of pregnancy loss.
- Bleeding may be brisk with biopsy; apply Monsel paste immediately on taking biopsy:
  – Monsel paste is safe and effective in pregnancy.
- Most colposcopists limit number of biopsies in pregnancy.

Alternatives

HPV DNA testing or repeat Pap may be used in select situations:

- See "Age-related Factors."

Medical

None

Surgical

- 4-quadrant biopsy is less sensitive.
- Conization has higher cost and morbidity.
- "See and treat" LEEP without biopsy may be used with HSIL Pap plus HSIL colposcopic impression.

Pregnancy Considerations

- Treatment is not indicated in pregnancy unless invasive cancer is present.
- LEEP, CKC may be indicated for microinvasive squamous cancer:
  – Consult with gynecologic oncologist and perinatologist.

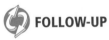 **FOLLOW-UP**

- If biopsy proves CIN 1:
  – Treatment is discouraged
  – Follow with Pap every 6 months (total of 2 exams) with colposcopy if ≥ ASC-US or follow with HPV in 12 months and colposcopy if high-risk positive.
- If biopsy proves CIN 2 or 3:
  – Treat with excision or ablation as appropriate.
  – Ablation requires satisfactory exam, lesion <3 quadrants, completely visualized, and no prior treatment.
- If ASC-US, LSIL, ASC-H on Pap and no CIN 2 or 3 on biopsy:
  – Follow with Pap every 6 months (total of 2 exams) or HPV in 12 months
- If HSIL on Pap and no CIN 2 or 3 on biopsy:
  – Diagnostic excision
  – If adolescent, may follow with Pap and colposcopy in 6 and 12 months
  – If pregnant, reassess postpartum
- If microinvasive or invasive cancer, consult gynecologic oncologist

---

- If AGC on Pap or atypical endocervical cells and no CIN 2 or 3, and no adenocarcinoma in situ on biopsy or endocervical sampling:
  – If HPV-negative, repeat Pap with HPV in 12 months
  – If HPV-positive, repeat Pap with HPV in 6 months
  – If HPV is not done, repeat Pap every 6 months (total of 4 exams)
- If adenocarcinoma in situ on Pap and no CIN 2,3, or adenocarcinoma in situ on biopsy:
  – Diagnostic excision procedure
- If adenocarcinoma in situ on biopsy or ECC, refer to gynecologic oncologist

PROGNOSIS

Cure rates after treatment of CIN:

- ~95% at 6 months
- ~85–90% at 24 months

COMPLICATIONS

- Bleeding:
  – Usually controlled with Monsel paste or silver nitrate
  – Suture rarely required
- Discomfort:
  – Usually well-controlled with NSAIDs
  – Frequently no treatment needed
- Vaso-vagal reaction rare
- Infection exceedingly rare
- Failure to diagnose:
  – Usually small lesions, subsequently found after follow-up cytology or HPV

BIBLIOGRAPHY

ASCUS-LSIL Triage Study (ALTS) Group. Results of a randomized trial on the management of cytology interpretations of atypical squamous cells of undetermined significance. *Am J Obstet Gynecol.* 2003;188:1383–1392.

Gage JC, et al. Number of cervical biopsies and sensitivity of colposcopy. *Obstet Gynecol.* 2006;108:264–272.

Guido R, et. al. Postcolposcopy management strategies for women referred with low-grade squamous intraepithelial lesions or human papillomavirus DNA-positive atypical squamous cells of undetermined significance: A two-year prospective study. *Am J Obstet Gynecol.* 2003;188:1401–1405.

Mosciski AB, et al. Regression of low-grade squamous intra-epithelial lesions in young women. *Lancet.* 2004;364:1678–834.

Wright TC, et al. 2006. Consensus guidelines for the management of women with abnormal cervical cancer screening tests. *Am J Obstet Gynecol.* 2007;197:346–355.

Wright TC, et al. 2006. Consensus guidelines for the management of women with abnormal cervical intraepithelial neoplasia or adenocarcinoma in situ. *Am J Obstet Gynecol.* 2007;197:340–346.

 MISCELLANEOUS

- Lesion mimics:
  – Metaplasia, inflammation:
    ○ May be mistaken for LSIL
  – Atrophy:
    ○ High-grade lesion may be mistaken for lower grade
  – Pregnancy:
    ○ Lower-grade lesion may have prominent mosaic or punctation patterns.
    ○ Higher-grade lesions may be less densely aceto-white than expected.

CLINICAL PEARLS

- Degree of aceto-white change is most predictive of severity of lesion.
- Green filter highlights vessels.
- Atypical vessels may be more easily seen before application of dilute acetic acid; examine 1st with saline wash.
- Sharp biopsy instruments are essential.

ABBREVIATIONS

- AGC—Atypical glandular cells
- ASC-H—Atypical squamous cells cannot exclude high-grade squamous intraepithelial lesion
- ASC-US—Atypical squamous cells of undetermined significance
- CIN—Cervical intraepithelial neoplasia
- CKC—Cold knife conization
- ECC—Endocervical curettage
- HPV—Human papillomavirus
- HSIL—High-grade squamous intraepithelial lesion
- LEEP—Loop electrosurgical excision procedure
- LSIL—Low-grade squamous intraepithelial lesion
- TZ—Transformation zone

CODES

ICD9-CM

- 233.1 CIN 3
- 622.10 Dysplasia of the cervix
- 622.11 CIN 1
- 622.12 CIN 2

 PATIENT TEACHING

- Reassure if cancer is not suspected.
- Anticipate some spotting; brown to blackish discharge if Monsel used; notify provider for heavy bleeding.
- Pelvic rest for several days, until discharge is absent
- Notify provider for fever or pelvic pain.
- Follow-up for results and discussion of management is important.

Section VII

ENDOMETRIAL ABLATION

Howard T. Sharp, MD

 BASICS

DESCRIPTION

- EA is aimed at ablating or destroying the endometrial lining of the uterus. It can be performed with a resectoscope (operative hysteroscope), or with 1 of 5 different nonhysteroscopic devices (global ablation devices, GEA).
- Resectoscopic endometrial ablation: Requires use of an operative hysteroscope to apply energy to the endometrium manually by way of rollerball, loop electrode resection, or laser. It also requires the use of a fluid distending medium compatible with the energy employed:
  - Rollerball: A rollerball electrode attachment is used with a resectoscope to apply radiofrequency current to coagulate the endometrium.
  - Endometrial resection: A loop electrode using radiofrequency current is used to resect the endometrial lining in chips.
  - Laser: A Nd:YAG laser fiber can be placed through the operating channel of a hysteroscope to apply laser energy to the endometrium.
- Global ablation devices: Devices designed to ablate the uterine endometrium without the use of a resectoscope. Several different energy sources have been developed using computer-controlled feedback.
  - Thermal balloon: A silicone balloon is inflated with fluid in the uterine cavity. Heated fluid is circulated within the balloon for an 8-minute cycle.
  - Cryoablation: A cryoprobe is inserted into the endometrial cavity and an iceball is created for 2 freeze cycles of 4 and 6 minutes.
  - Circulating heated fluid: A diagnostic hysteroscope with a plastic sheath allows circulation of heated fluid over a 10-minute period under low pressure to ablate the endometrium.
  - Bipolar radiofrequency: An electrode array is placed to the uterine fundus and expanded to conform to the endometrial cavity. Radiofrequency current is applied for ~90 seconds to achieve EA.
  - Microwave: An applicator wand is inserted to the uterine fundus and microwave energy is applied to the endometrium as the wand is moved from side to side throughout the endometrial cavity over 3–5 minutes.

Indications

- EA can be offered to women with idiopathic menorrhagia who have failed medical therapy or are intolerant or otherwise unable to be treated medically.
- Prerequisites to EA:
  - Perform endometrial sampling to rule out endometrial malignancy or hyperplasia.
  - Perform endometrial imaging (ideally sonohysterography or office hysteroscopy) to rule out a structural lesion of the endometrium such as a submucosal fibroid.
- Contraindications to EA:
  - Pregnancy
  - Desire to become pregnant in the future
  - Endometrial carcinoma
  - Premalignant change of the endometrium
  - Active PID
  - Prior classical cesarean delivery or transmural myomectomy
  - Uterine anomaly (septate uterus, bicornuate uterus)
  - IUD in place
  - Active genital tract infection

Site (Office, Surgical Center, OR)

- Resectoscopic endometrial ablation is performed in the operating room as an outpatient procedure with general or regional anesthesia.
- GEA can be performed in the operating room under general or regional anesthesia, but may also be performed in the office under conscious sedation.

Concurrent Procedures

- Hysteroscopy and D&C are frequently performed concurrently. This allows the surgeon to confirm a normal endometrium and endometrial cavity.
- Sterilization may also be performed at the time of EA.

Age-Related Factors
EA is performed in women of reproductive age.

Geriatric Considerations
In general, EA is not for use in geriatric patients.

Pediatric Considerations
In general, EA is not for use in pediatric patients.

Pregnancy Considerations
EA is contraindicated during pregnancy.

EPIDEMIOLOGY
~600,000 hysterectomies are performed annually (NCHS, 2002 data). This reflects a hysterectomy rate of 5.5 per 1,000 in the US. The impact of EA on the hysterectomy rate is currently unknown.

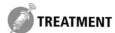 **TREATMENT**

PROCEDURE

Informed Consent
The patient should understand the potential risks and benefits associated with EA. She should also understand alternatives to EA.

Patient Education
- The patient should be informed that this may not eliminate bleeding but should reduce her bleeding to a satisfactory level.
- The patient should have an understanding of the basic anatomy of the uterus and cervix.

Risks, Benefits
- Risks:
  - Acute uterine or cervical bleeding
  - Infection of the uterus, cervix, fallopian tubes, or urinary tract
  - Uterine perforation
  - Injury to bowel or urinary tract.
  - Fluid overload syndrome (resectoscopic surgery only)
  - Possible need for additional surgery to correct bleeding in the case of failure:
    ○ Repeat procedure
    ○ Hysterectomy
  - Vaginal burns (heated circulating fluid)
- Benefits:
  - Absent or diminished uterine bleeding
  - Less invasive than hysterectomy

Alternatives
- No treatment
- Medical therapy (hormonal and nonhormonal medications) (see chapters on AUB)
- Levonorgestrel-containing IUD
- Hysterectomy

Medical
See Alternatives.

Surgical
See above.

FOLLOW-UP

Most patients will follow-up in the office within weeks to assess potential early complications. Progress and late-occurring complications are assessed in 2 or 3 months.

PROGNOSIS
- Rates of amenorrhea after EA: 13–50%
- Overall satisfaction rate: 80–90%
- Rates of hysterectomy after EU: 1–34%

COMPLICATIONS
The most commonly occurring late complications associated with EA include endometritis, hematometra, and UTI.

BIBLIOGRAPHY

Endometrial ablation: Where have we been? Where are we going? *Clin Obstet Gynecol*. 2006:49: 736–766.

Lethaby A, et al. Endometrial destruction techniques for heavy menstrual bleeding. *Cochrane Database Syst Rev*. 2005;4:CD001501.

Sharp HT. Assessment of new technology in the treatment of idiopathic menorrhagia and uterine fibroids. *Obstet Gynecol*. 2006;108:990–1003.

 MISCELLANEOUS

- A contraceptive plan should be agreed upon.
- A post-ablation tubal ligation syndrome has been reported. It consists of painful hematosalpinges resulting from active endometrial tissue near the corneal region and endometrial scarring preventing menstrual egress. This may be treated with bilateral salpingectomy or hysterectomy.

SYNONYM(S)
- Global endometrial ablation
- Rollerball ablation
- Transcervical endometrial resection-ablation

CLINICAL PEARLS
- When using GEA devices, strict adherence to the manufacturer's protocol is strongly recommended.
- In the case of resectoscopic EA, intraoperative distending fluid deficit must be monitored carefully as hyponatremia with fluid overload syndrome can occur. If the fluid deficit is 750–1,500 mL (depending on the patient's baseline), the procedure should be stopped and a stat serum sodium should be obtained.
- Hyponatremia at or below 125 mEq/L is considered severe and potentially life-threatening. Consultation with medical specialists with experience with hyponatremia in women should be sought.

- 5% mannitol is an iso-osmolar, nonelectrolyte solution used as a distending medium, which may be less likely to result in hypo-osmolality compared to hypo-osmolar solutions.

ABBREVIATIONS
- EA—Endometrial ablation
- GEA—Global endometrial ablation
- NCHS—National Center of Health Statistics
- Nd:YAG—Neodymium: Yttrium aluminum garnet laser
- PID—Pelvic inflammatory disease
- UTI—Urinary tract infection

CODES

ICD9-CM/CPT
68.23 Endometrial ablation

 PATIENT TEACHING

The patient should call her physician for heavy bleeding, fever >100.5°F, or increased pain after procedure.

ENDOMETRIAL SAMPLING/DILATION AND CURETTAGE

Howard T. Sharp, MD

BASICS

DESCRIPTION

Dilation of the cervix and curettage of the endometrium (referred to as D&C) is performed to obtain endometrial tissue in cases of abnormal uterine bleeding, postmenopausal bleeding, and abnormal cervical cytology such as abnormal or atypical glandular cells. Endometrial sampling with small-diameter cannulas may also be performed in the office without the need for dilation of the cervix.

- Endometrial sampling in the office can be accomplished by several devices including:
  – Plastic cannula with internal piston
  – Plastic cannula with syringe
  – Stainless steel cannula with a self-contained pump with handle
  – Stainless steel cannula with electric suction

Indications

- Endometrial sampling in the office is indicated for diagnosis in the following cases:
  – Abnormal uterine bleeding
  – Postmenopausal bleeding
  – Abnormal cervical cytology such as abnormal or atypical glandular cells
- D&C is indicated if endometrial sampling in the office is not possible due to:
  – Cervical stenosis
  – Patient intolerance
  – Inability to adequately access the cervix
- Although D&C can be effective as therapy for acute bleeding, its effect does not provide benefit in subsequent menstrual cycles.

Site (Office, Surgical Center, OR)

- Endometrial sampling can usually be performed in the office without cervical dilation using a 3-mm (outer diameter) cannula. Gentle dilation may be required and can also usually be performed in the office. This may be assisted by a paracervical block (see Miscellaneous).
- D&C is performed in the operating room under general or regional anesthesia. Conscious sedation may also be used.

Concurrent Procedures

Hysteroscopy is usually performed concurrently with D&C. This enables the surgeon to visualize endometrial pathology if present, whereas D&C alone is a blind procedure.

Age-Related Factors

Postmenopausal women have a higher incidence of cervical stenosis, which can increase the risk of uterine perforation during dilation.

Pediatric Considerations

D&C is rarely indicated in adolescents with acute menorrhagia. Hormonal management should be considered 1st, as likelihood of endometrial pathology is small.

Geriatric Considerations

Geriatric patients are at a higher risk of uterine perforation.

Pregnancy Considerations

Endometrial sampling and D&C are contraindicated in pregnancy. In premenopausal women, hCG should be considered prior to EMB/D&C.

EPIDEMIOLOGY

D&C is performed in 40.8/100,000 population, according to the 1995 survey of the NCHS. It is most commonly performed in the 15–44-year age group.

TREATMENT

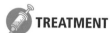

PROCEDURE

Informed Consent

The patient should understand the potential risks and benefits associated with endometrial sampling/D&C. She should also understand alternatives.

Patient Education

The patient should have an understanding of the basic anatomy of the uterus and cervix.

Risks, Benefits

- Risks:
  – Acute uterine or cervical bleeding
  – Infection of the uterus, fallopian tubes, or urinary tract
  – Uterine perforation
  – Injury to the intestinal tract
- Benefits:
  – The ability to rule out endometrial malignancy
  – Gaining a histologic diagnosis to assist in therapy
  – Therapeutic effect on acute bleeding (D&C only)

Alternatives

- No treatment
- US of the endometrium*
- Sonohysterography*
- Hysterosalpingogram*
- Hysteroscopy*

* May assist in diagnosing endometrial lesions but cannot provide a histologic diagnosis

Medical

Medical management of abnormal uterine bleeding may be hormonal or nonhormonal (see Bleeding, Abnormal Uterine).

Surgical

- Prior to performing endometrial sampling/D&C, a bimanual exam of the uterus should be performed prior to the procedure to determine the axis of the uterus. This is done to reduce the risk of uterine perforation.
- Endometrial sampling (in the office):
  – This performed with a vaginal speculum in place. Topical lidocaine or a submucosal lidocaine injection can be given at the cervix. A tenaculum is placed on the cervix. A cannula is then inserted carefully to the uterine fundus. Depending on the type of cannula, an internal piston is pulled, a syringe is aspirated, or electric suction is applied as the cannula is rotated along the length of the endometrial cavity.
- D&C:
  – This is performed under appropriate anesthesia. A weighted speculum is placed vaginally and a right-angle retractor is used to allow visualization of the cervix. A tenaculum is placed on the anterior cervix. A uterine sound is placed to the uterine fundus and the length of the uterine cavity is noted. The cervix is then gradually dilated until a curette can be inserted to the uterine fundus. This can usually be accomplished with dilation to 6–9 mm in diameter.
  – The most common types of dilators are either Pratt or Hegar dilators. Pratt dilators range from 13–43 Fr. The French unit is 0.33 mm in diameter. Pratt dilators have a more gradual taper at the ends. They require less dilating force compared to Hegar dilators. Hegar dilators come in sizes ranging from 1–26 mm and have a blunter dilating end.
  – Curettage is performed by applying pressure to the curette handle as the curette is withdrawn from the uterine fundus to the cervix. An attempt is made to scrape the entire endometrial cavity in a systematic fashion until a "uterine cry" (palpable resistance) is noted.
  – The cervix should be observed after the tenaculum is removed to assess bleeding, which may require treatment with silver nitrate or a suture.

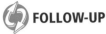 **FOLLOW-UP**

Most patients will follow-up in the office within weeks to assess potential early complications and to review endometrial histology.

PROGNOSIS

Prognosis after endometrial sampling/D&C is directly related to histologic findings (see chapters on endometrial hyperplasia/endometrial cancer).

COMPLICATIONS

The most commonly occurring late complications associated with endometrial sampling/D&C include endometritis, salpingitis, and UTI.

BIBLIOGRAPHY

Crane JM, et al. Use of misoprostol before hysteroscopy: a systematic review. *J Obstet Gynaecol Can.* 2006:28:373–379.

DeSimone CP, et al. Rate of pathology from atypical glandular cell Pap tests classified by the Bethesda 2001 Nomenclature. *Obstet Gynecol.* 2006;108:1285–1291.

Li HW, et al. Effect of lidocaine gel application for pain relief during suction termination of first trimester pregnancy: A randomized controlled trial. *Hum Reprod.* 2006:21:1461–1466.

 MISCELLANEOUS

A paracervical block can be administered by injecting 5 mL of 1% lidocaine or 0.25% bupivacaine at the ectocervix at both 5 and 7 o'clock. Prior to injection, aspiration of the syringe should be performed to avoid intravascular injection.

SYNONYM(S)

Endometrial biopsy

CLINICAL PEARLS

- The sharply anteverted uterus is at risk for a posterior perforation.
- The sharply retroverted uterus is a risk for an anterior perforation.
- In the reproductive-aged woman, pretreatment with misoprostol can aid in significant cervical preparation/"softening" and dilation.
- In patients with cervical stenosis, US guidance can be useful to assess the endocervical canal.
- Adolescents who present with acute menorrhagia may have a coagulopathy; D&C is rarely indicated in this age group.

ABBREVIATIONS

AUB—Abnormal uterine bleeding
D&C—Dilation and curettage
EMB—Endometrial biopsy
hCG—Human chorionic gonadotropin
NCHS—National Center of Health Statistics

CODES

ICD9-CM

- 581.00 Endometrial biopsy
- 581.20 Dilation & curettage

 PATIENT TEACHING

Postprocedure, the patient should call her physician for heavy bleeding, fever >100.5°F, or increased pain.

EPISIOTOMY

Jerry L. Lowder, MD, MSc
Anne M. Weber, MD, MS

 BASICS

DESCRIPTION
- Surgical enlargement of the vaginal introitus by an incision of the perineum using either scissors or scalpel.
- Purpose is to increase the diameter of the soft-tissue pelvic outlet to facilitate delivery.
- 3 types of episiotomy described:
  - Midline (or median) episiotomy:
    - A vertical incision through the posterior vaginal introitus. When the vagina and perineal body are cut, this is commonly referred to as a 2nd-degree episiotomy. If a part or all of the anal sphincter is cut or torn, this is 3rd-degree; if anorectal epithelium and anal sphincter are involved, 4th-degree. 3rd- and 4th-degree episiotomies are also called severe perineal lacerations.
    - Most frequent type of episiotomy performed in the US.
    - Associated with high risk of anal sphincter laceration
  - Mediolateral episiotomy:
    - An incision in the posterior vaginal introitus directed at least 45 degrees from the midline (to avoid the rectum and anal sphincter).
    - Decreased risk of anal sphincter laceration compared to midline episiotomy
    - Anecdotally associated with increased blood loss and perineal pain
  - J incision episiotomy:
    - An incision in the posterior vaginal introitus initially extending into the perineum and then curving away from the midline avoiding the anal sphincter and anorectum
    - Thought to combine advantages of both midline and mediolateral incisions while avoiding disadvantages

Indications
- Indications for episiotomy are not established.
- Episiotomy use is based on training, experience, and clinician judgment at each delivery.
- Situations in which episiotomy is commonly used:
  - Nonreassuring fetal heart rate pattern with delivery imminent
  - OVD
  - Shoulder dystocia
- Routine use of episiotomy is not clinically indicated.

Site (Office, Surgical Center, OR)
Usually performed in a labor and delivery room or operating room

Concurrent Procedures
OVD:
- Vacuum extraction
- Forceps (outlet, low)

Age-Related Factors
An increasing trend of episiotomy with increasing age has been demonstrated in some studies.

EPIDEMIOLOGY
The most commonly performed procedure in obstetrics in the US:
- Episiotomies performed more frequently than other common procedures in women: In 1979, 32.7 episiotomies per 1,000 women, compared to 18.7 per 1,000 women in 1997
- Episiotomy use is decreasing over time: Over 2 million episiotomies performed in the US in 1981, decreased to 1 million in 1997
- More recent data revealed episiotomy was performed in 61% of vaginal deliveries in 1981, compared to 39% in 2000.
- Performed in an average of 30–35% of vaginal births in the US (with wide variation by region, type of hospital, and other factors)

 TREATMENT

PROCEDURE
Informed Consent
- Timing of episiotomy during delivery often makes consent process difficult.
- Consider adding episiotomy to vaginal delivery consent form and include:
  - Increased risk of anal sphincter laceration with midline episiotomy
  - Risk of infection and breakdown/dehiscence
  - Potential increased postpartum pain
  - Risk of dyspareunia

Patient Education
- Patient education about vaginal delivery and episiotomy should occur during prenatal care.
- Patients should be informed of risks and potential benefits (see below) of episiotomy during prenatal care.

Risks, Benefits
- Risks:
  - Increased risk of anal sphincter laceration by extension of midline episiotomy
  - Increased blood loss
  - Episiotomy repair infection and breakdown/dehiscence
  - Increased postpartum pain
  - Dyspareunia
- Benefits:
  - Few data support benefits
  - Decreased anterior perineal trauma
  - Anecdotally easier surgical repair

Alternatives
- Restricted episiotomy use:
  - Expedite delivery for maternal and/or fetal indications
  - When likelihood of spontaneous laceration appears high
- No episiotomy use:
  - Allow lacerations to occur

Medical
Prophylactic antibiotics after episiotomy are not usually administered unless rectal involvement:
- IV antibiotics during repair
- PO antibiotics for 7 days post repair

Surgical
- Adequate analgesia/anesthesia mandatory:
  - Epidural anesthesia OR
  - Spinal anesthesia OR
  - Pudendal block AND/OR
  - Local injection
- Episiotomy performed with scissors or scalpel
- Typically performed when soft tissue of perineum is NOT under tension; avoid performing episiotomy during uterine contraction or as fetal head is crowning:
  - Incision type: Midline, mediolateral, or J incision
- Surgical repair of episiotomy typically performed after delivery of placenta and uterine tone/hemostasis obtained:
  - Adequate analgesia/anesthesia is mandatory
  - 2–3-layer running closure of incision and extension depending on surrounding tissue involvement
  - Less-reactive polyglycolic acid or monofilament suture preferable over chromic catgut (high tissue reactivity)

- Narcotic and/or NSAIDs and topical anesthetic sprays used for postprocedural and postpartum pain
- Daily Sitz baths and perineal care after voids and bowel movements recommended to decrease pain and improve perineal hygiene, possibly reducing risk of infection

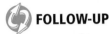

FOLLOW-UP

Timing of clinical follow-up depends on size and extension of episiotomy:

- Consider clinical follow-up in 1–2 weeks if episiotomy involved anal sphincter and/or rectum
- Evaluate for pain, signs of infection/dehiscence, and hematoma

PROGNOSIS

Follow patient clinically for signs and symptoms of:

- Hematoma
- Infection
- Wound breakdown
- Chronic pain/dyspareunia
- Anal incontinence

COMPLICATIONS

- Bleeding
- Hematoma formation
- Infection:
  – Abscess formation
  – Episiotomy repair breakdown/dehiscence
  – Necrotizing fasciitis

- Rectovaginal fistula formation:
  – Rare; consider primary bowel disease (Crohn's, ulcerative colitis)
- Perineal pain
- Dyspareunia
- Increased risk of anal incontinence:
  – Fecal incontinence
  – Flatal incontinence

BIBLIOGRAPHY

ACOG Practice Bulletin No. 71. Episiotomy. *Obstet Gynecol.* 2006;107(4):956–962.

Carroli G, et al. Episiotomy for vaginal birth. *Cochrane Database Syst Rev.* 2004. CD000081

Coats PM, et al. A comparison between midline and mediolateral episiotomies. *Br J Obstet Gynaecol.* 1980;87:408–412.

Cunningham FG, et al. *Williams Obstetrics,* 21st ed. New York: McGraw-Hill; 2001.

Curtin SC, et al. Preliminary data for 1999. National vital statistics reports. Vol. 48, No. 14. Hyattsville MD: National Center for Health Statistics; 2000.

DeFrances CJ, et al. 2003 National Hospital Discharge Survey. CDC Vital and Health Statistics-Advance Data. No. 359, July 8, 2005.

Hartmann K, et al. Outcomes of routine episiotomy: A systematic review. *JAMA.* 2005;293:2141–2148.

Robinson JN, et al. Predictors of Episiotomy use at first spontaneous vaginal delivery. *Obstet Gynecol.* 2000;96:214–218.

Signorello LB, et al. Midline episiotomy and anal incontinence: Retrospective cohort study. *Br Med J.* 2000;320;86–90.

Weber AM, et al. Episiotomy use in the United States, 1979–1997. *Obstet Gynecol.* 2002;100:1177–1182.

 MISCELLANEOUS

SYNONYM(S)

Episioproctotomy involves full thickness of perineal body including anal sphincter and anorectal mucosa.

CLINICAL PEARLS

- Indications for episiotomy are primarily clinical judgment and not well-supported by data.
- Routine use of episiotomy should be avoided.
- Restrict use of episiotomy for maternal or fetal indications.
- Episiotomy does not appear to protect against future pelvic organ prolapse/relaxation, or urinary incontinence.
- Risk of anal sphincter laceration, with subsequent anal incontinence, is increased with midline episiotomy.

ABBREVIATIONS

OVD—Operative vaginal delivery

CODES

ICD9-CM

- 72.1 Episiotomy with outlet forceps
- 72.71 Episiotomy with vacuum extraction
- 73.6 Episioproctotomy/Episiotomy with subsequent episiorrhaphy

 PATIENT TEACHING

- Discuss role of episiotomy in your clinical practice with your patient during prenatal care:
  – Not routinely used vs.
  – Restricted use vs.
  – Routine use
- Inform patient of potential indications, risks, and benefits of procedure.
- If episiotomy is performed, instruct patient on wound care and warning signs of infection and hematoma.

Section VII

FALLOPIAN TUBE SURGERY

Christopher P. Montville, MD, MS
Michael A. Thomas, MD

BASICS

DESCRIPTION
Encompasses procedures performed for infertility associated with tubal disease; ectopic pregnancy; reversal of tubal sterilization; and tubal abscess.

Tubal Anatomy
- 4 specific tubal regions: Proximal to distal
  - Interstitial: Origin in uterus at cornua
  - Isthmic: Origin uterine serosa; narrow lumen
  - Ampulla: Convoluted, larger lumen
  - Fimbria: Ciliated projections
- Contained within broad ligament:
  - Evagination of müllerian ducts and ovaries from pelvic sidewall:
    - Enclosed in peritoneal folds
    - Mesosalpinx: Peritoneum attaching tube to round ligament superiorly and ovary inferiorly
  - Tube is most cephalic structure (between broad ligament and ovary)
- Blood/Lymphatic/Neural supply:
  - Arterial:
    - Branches from ovarian artery (origin at anterior aorta)
    - Retroperitoneal, through infundibulo-pelvic ligament to ovary and tube
    - Fimbrial branch of ovarian artery
  - Venous:
    - Right tube: Venous plexus to IVC
    - Left tube: Plexus to left renal vein
  - Lymphatics:
    - Follow venous drainage to paraaortic nodes
  - Neural:
    - Sympathetic: Renal plexus (T10)
    - Parasympathetic: From vagus

Indications
- Majority of procedures are for tubal-factor infertility (occlusion, peritubal adhesions). Mechanisms of tubal damage include ascending infection/PID, adhesions related to endometriosis, prior pelvic surgery, and IBD.
- Specific factors include:
  - Salpingitis/Pelvic abscess:
    - STIs
    - Salpingitis isthmica nodosa
  - Prior tubal sterilization
  - Ectopic pregnancy or history of ectopic
  - Unknown cause
- If infertility is the primary diagnosis, consider risks and benefits of surgery vs. IVF

Site (Office, Surgical Center, OR)
- Majority of operative procedures in OR center.
- Diagnostic procedures may be office-based (hysteroscopy), or in radiology suite (HSG), depending on resources

Concurrent Procedures
- Hysteroscopy most common (diagnostic/operative) at time of laparoscopy.
- Ostial cannulation
- Chromopertubation
- Salpingoscopy, falloposcopy

Age-Related Factors
- Fecundability (probability of pregnancy during 1 menstrual cycle) decreases as maternal age increases.
  - Surgery is not advised for older women (>35) with tubal disease.
  - Accurate diagnosis is paramount for appropriate therapy.
  - Endometriosis more severe with time.
- Surgery applicable if:
  - Age <35
  - Tubal factor only
  - Ethical concerns regarding ART/IVF
- IVF advised if:
  - Significant tubal damage
  - Multifactorial infertility diagnosis:
    - Ovulatory
    - Male factor
  - General health comorbidities

EPIDEMIOLOGY
- Extent of tubal damage depends on etiology of disease (infectious vs. inflammatory, etc.).
  - Outcomes are primarily pregnancy rate and ectopic rate after surgery.
  - Fecundability of general population ~20%.
  - Actual fecundability vs. overall pregnancy rate of surgical therapy must be considered.
- Infectious etiology:
  - *Chlamydia trachomatis; Neisseria gonorrhoeae; Mycoplasma hominis* most common
  - PID: 10 cases per 10,000 age 15–39
    - 20% reduced fertility after single episode
    - Infertility approaches 60% if >2 episodes
- Ectopic pregnancy:
  - 19.7 cases per 1,000 pregnancies (1992)
    - 6–fold increase in PID
    - Prior tubal surgery: 2–18%
    - Reversal of tubal sterilization: ~4%
- Endometriosis:
  - Diagnosed in 20–40% of infertile women

Outcomes
- Pregnancy rates after surgery range from 10–60%, depending on extent of tubal damage:
  - Fecundability rates: 1–8%
- Ectopic rates after surgery: 1–24%:
  - Depend on extent of tubal damage and specific procedure

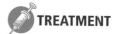

TREATMENT

Accurate diagnosis needed for proper intervention. For active infection (abscess) or ectopic pregnancy, indications of medical vs. surgical management should be carefully considered.

PROCEDURE
Informed Consent
Indications, risks, benefits, and alternatives should be discussed. Patients should be made aware of success rates of surgery compared to IVF; risks of ectopic pregnancy; risk that further surgery will be required.

Patient Education
Comparison of IVF success rates vs. surgical rates is often difficult.
- IVF success related to per-cycle pregnancy rate.
- Success of surgery depends on healing time after surgery and initiation of attempts at conception.

Risks, Benefits
- Decision to pursue surgery is patient-dependent and includes consideration of maternal age and future fertility/family considerations. In general, IVF success rates per cycle closely mimic fertile fecundability rates (~20%).
- Benefits:
  - Moderate success rates in patients with mild tubal disease; beneficial for patients desiring conservative therapy
- Risks:
  - Increased incidence of ectopic pregnancy
  - Iatrogenic adhesion formation
  - Surgical complications (general anesthetic)
  - Postoperative infection
  - Costs

Alternatives
- IVF:
  - Benefits:
    - Higher success rates, minimally invasive techniques, broader range of application
  - Risks:
    - Multiple gestation, ovarian hyperstimulation syndrome, cost of multiple cycles
- Medical therapy for endometriosis used primarily before surgical intervention

Medical
Appropriate medical therapy used in selected cases of PID, ectopic pregnancy, endometriosis

Surgical

- Tubal cannulation:
  - Hysteroscopic cannulation of proximal tubal occlusion. Performed at time of concurrent laparoscopy or interventional radiology
- Diagnostic laparoscopy:
  - Diagnosis and treatment. Required if proximal tubal occlusion for further evaluation of tubal patency using chromopertubation.
  - Survey of pelvic anatomy, adhesions, endometriosis with photodocumentation
- Lysis of tubo-ovarian adhesions with restoration of normal anatomy:
  - Pregnancy rate: 51–62%
  - Ectopic rate: 5–8%
- Fimbrioplasty:
  - Partial distal occlusion, prefimbrial phimosis, peritubal adhesions
  - Usually performed with salpingostomy:
    - Pregnancy rate: 40–48%
    - Ectopic rate: 5–6%
- Salpingostomy treatment of hydrosalpinx:
  - Creation of new tubal opening in completely occluded distal segment:
    - Laparotomy/Laparoscopy results are comparable.
    - Tube is distended with chromopertubation.
    - Incise central tube and extend toward ovary.
    - Serial incisions make new stoma.
    - Exposed flaps are sutured or desiccated with electrocautery.
  - Pregnancy rate: 20–37%
  - Ectopic rate: 5–18%
- Tubal reanastomosis:
  - Performed primarily for reconstruction after tubal sterilization
  - Critical end-points include tube length ≥4 cm, adequate vascular supply, chromopertubation demonstrates patency following procedure, tension-free mesosalpinx
  - Commonly performed with mini-laparotomy and microsurgical technique
  - Performed with laparoscopy in some centers
  - Appropriate patient selection
  - Contraindications: Advanced maternal age, prior use of electrocautery, extensive tubal damage, total tube length <4 cm
  - Surgical technique:
    - Proximal tube is distended with chromopertubation fluid.
    - Tube is excised from mesosalpinx to provide mobility.
    - Pediatric feeding tube is used to cannulate lumen.
    - Care must be taken not to damage/suture mucosa.
    - Vasopressin decreases bleeding.
  - Specific procedures:
    - Isthmic-isthmic: Lumen comparable in size; most common
    - Isthmic-ampullary: Ampullary opening often must be enlarged.
    - Ampullary-ampullary
    - Ampullary-infundibular: Often performed when distal ampullary segment was completely excised in prior procedure
    - Intramural-isthmic: Common after sterilization with little isthmic portion present

- Results:
  - Pregnancy rates: 40–80%
  - Ectopic rates: 2–12.5%
- Ectopic pregnancy (conservative procedure):
  - If future fertility desired:
    - Pregnancy rates: 60–80% after ectopic
    - Mean risk of repeat ectopic: 20%
    - If nulliparous, risk of 2nd ectopic: 33%
  - Appropriate patient selection: Failed medical therapy, pain, hemodynamic instability, prior history of ectopic pregnancy
  - Linear salpingotomy via laparotomy:
    - Incise distended serosa; expel contents of lumen. Irrigate.
    - Obtain hemostasis and reapproximate serosa and muscularis with interrupted suture.
    - Limit damage to mucosa.
  - Linear salpingotomy via laparoscopy:
    - Irrigate pelvis and identify site.
    - Incise at point of maximal distension with scissors/cautery (antimesenteric incision). Hydro-dissection is useful.
    - Express products.
    - If isthmus is involved, perform salpingectomy or segmental resection.
    - Tube may be left open to heal by secondary intention.
    - Follow β-hCG postoperatively.
- Ectopic pregnancy with salpingectomy:
  - Perform if ruptured ectopic and hemodynamically unstable, recurrent ectopic, marked tubal damage, completed childbearing
  - Salpingectomy via laparotomy:
    - Clamp and incise mesosalpinx close to tubal border.
    - Transect tube close to cornua. May over-sew round ligament at site of resection.
  - Salpingectomy via laparoscopy:
    - Isolate tubo-ovarian ligament. Coagulate tube with electrocautery, then transect proximal tube.
- Pelvic abscess:
  - Typically performed after failure of medical therapy
  - Consider extent of involvement of adnexal structures and course of infection.
  - Salpingectomy usually required if abscess within tube
  - Irrigation and lysis of adhesions if tube is not directly involved

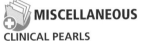 FOLLOW-UP

Usual postoperative care; pelvic rest for 4 weeks

PROGNOSIS

Success/Pregnancy rates vary depending on extent of tubal damage, length of tube at conclusion of surgery, use of bipolar cautery for sterilization (further decreased pregnancy rates).

- In general, success rates are higher with IVF.
- Patient selection is important.

COMPLICATIONS

- Similar to other pelvic surgeries.
- Surgery for tubal disease increases likelihood of iatrogenic pelvic adhesions and Increased risk of ectopic pregnancy (relative risk of ectopic may be as high as 4.5).

BIBLIOGRAPHY

American Society for Reproductive Medicine. The role of tubal reconstructive surgery in the era of assisted reproductive technologies. *Fertil Steril*. 2006; 86(Suppl 4):S31–S34.

Penzias AS, et al. Is there ever a role for tubal surgery? *Am J Obstet Gynecol*. 1996;174:1218–1221.

Rock JA, et al., eds. *Te Linde's Operative Gynecology*, 9th ed. Philadelphia: Lippincott Williams & Wilkins Publishers; 2003.

Stenchever MA, et al., eds. *Comprehensive Gynecology*, 4th ed. St. Louis: Mosby; 2002.

Taylor RC, et al. Role of laparoscopic salpingostomy in the treatment of hydrosalpinx. *Fertil Steril*. 2001;75(3):594–600.

MISCELLANEOUS

CLINICAL PEARLS

- Role of tubal surgery declining due to success rates and lower surgical morbidity of IVF.
  - Proper patient selection, multiple gestation with IVF, and desire for future childbearing are important considerations.
- Fallopian tube is the most cephalic structure, and is in the middle of adnexal structures with respect to the uterus.
- Presence of PID increases risk of ectopic pregnancy 6-fold:
  - Fertility decreases 20% after 1st episode of PID; approaches 60% with >2 episodes.
- Proximal occlusion on HSG requires evaluation with hysteroscopy/laparoscopy.
- Contraindications to reanastomosis include advanced maternal age, prior use of bipolar cautery, length <4 cm.
- Conservative surgery for ectopic is most prudent (salpingotomy) if patient is medically stable.

ABBREVIATIONS

ART—Assisted reproductive technologies
hCG—Human chorionic gonadotropin
HSG—Hysterosalpingogram
IBD—Inflammatory bowel disease
IVC—Inferior vena cava
IVF—In vitro fertilization
PID—Pelvic inflammatory disease
STI—Sexually transmitted infections

CODES

ICD9-CM

- 614.6 Infertility associated with adhesions
- 614.9 PID
- 628.2 Infertility tubal origin
- 633.10 Ectopic pregnancy
- V26.0 Tuboplasty after sterilization

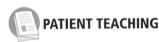 PATIENT TEACHING

Risks and benefits of IVF vs. surgery should be discussed.

HYSTERECTOMY, ABDOMINAL: TOTAL AND SUPRACERVICAL

Jerry L. Lowder, MD, MSc
Anne M. Weber, MD, MS

 BASICS

DESCRIPTION
- TAH is the surgical removal of the body of the uterus (uterine corpus) and uterine cervix.
- TAH is performed through an abdominal incision, usually a transverse (Pfannenstiel) or midline incision.
- SAH is the surgical removal of the body of the uterus (uterine corpus) and preservation of the uterine cervix. This procedure is also known as subtotal hysterectomy:
  - SCH is performed through an abdominal incision, usually a transverse (Pfannenstiel) or midline incision.

Indications
- General indications for hysterectomy:
  - Benign Indications:
    - Abnormal bleeding
    - Leiomyoma (fibroid)
    - Adenomyosis
    - Endometriosis
    - Recurrent CIN 2/3
    - Atypical endometrial hyperplasia
    - Pelvic organ prolapse
    - Pelvic inflammatory disease
    - Chronic pelvic pain
    - Pregnancy-related conditions
    - Miscellaneous
  - Malignant indications for hysterectomy:
    - Endometrial cancer
    - Ovarian cancer
    - Fallopian tube cancer
    - Gestational trophoblastic disease
- Indications for TAH:
  - Recurrent CIN 2/3
  - Atypical endometrial hyperplasia
  - Cervical leiomyomas (fibroids)
  - Patient's desire for removal of cervix
- Indications for supracervical abdominal hysterectomy:
  - Patient's desire to retain cervix (and understanding of ongoing need for cervical cancer screening)
  - Surgical conditions (e.g., limited visualization, altered anatomy, or excessive blood loss) that favor cervical preservation over removal

Site (Office, Surgical Center, OR)
Performed in an OR under general endotracheal or regional anesthesia

Concurrent Procedures
- Unilateral or bilateral salpingo-oophorectomy:
  - Ovarian pathology
  - Prophylactic oophorectomy
- Lysis of intraabdominal adhesions
- Removal of endometriosis

- Cystoscopy
- Prolapse procedure(s)
- Urinary incontinence procedure(s)
- Gynecologic cancer–related procedures:
  - Tumor debulking
  - Lymph node biopsy

Age-Related Factors
- Indications for hysterectomy vary throughout a woman's lifetime (see Indications).
- The median age of women undergoing total abdominal hysterectomy for benign conditions is 43 (interquartile range 37–51).
- The median age of women undergoing supracervical abdominal hysterectomy is 45 (interquartile range 38–61).

Pediatric Considerations
Not applicable unless a malignancy is involved.

Geriatric Considerations
Medical comorbidities and physiologic changes that occur with aging must be taken into consideration when planning for surgery.

Pregnancy Considerations
An abdominal hysterectomy may be performed after delivery in response to refractory uterine hemorrhage due to atony. The type of procedure chosen will depend on the indication and the surgeon's judgment, although supracervical (subtotal) hysterectomy may be technically easier if the cervix was fully dilated.

EPIDEMIOLOGY
- Most common major procedure performed by gynecologists
- 2nd most common major surgical procedure performed in the US
- Most common non–pregnancy-related procedure performed in women
- ~600,000 women undergo hysterectomy each year in the US.
- In 1997, the rate of hysterectomy was 5.6 procedures per 1,000 women.
- In 2003, the rate of hysterectomy had decreased to 3.4 procedures per 1,000 women.
- In 1993, TAHs accounted for 57% of all hysterectomies, whereas supracervical hysterectomies accounted for 7% of all hysterectomies performed.
- In 2003, TAHs accounted for 50% of all hysterectomies, whereas supracervical hysterectomies accounted for 20% of all hysterectomies performed.

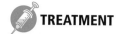 **TREATMENT**

PROCEDURE
Informed Consent
Hysterectomy is rarely a surgical emergency. The physician and patient should thoroughly discuss the risks, benefits, and alternative treatments:
- The patient should be clearly informed of the consequences of hysterectomy, including no chance of pregnancy.

Patient Education
Perioperative teaching:
- Patients should be thoroughly informed of the potential risks, benefits, and alternatives of hysterectomy.
- Patients should be aware:
  - That hysterectomy is major abdominal surgery
  - That hysterectomy may not definitively treat certain conditions such as chronic pelvic pain
  - Of the postoperative restrictions regarding diet (if any), physical activity including lifting, and operating motor vehicles or heavy machinery

Risks, Benefits
- Intraoperative risks:
  - Hemorrhage with possible transfusion
  - Injury to adjacent structures (i.e., ureter(s), bladder, bowel, pelvic nerves and vasculature
  - Peripheral nerve injury
  - Risks related to anesthesia
  - Death (1:1,000)
- Postoperative risks:
  - Hemorrhage with possible transfusion
  - Infection (e.g., urinary tract, wound, vaginal cuff, pneumonia)
  - Wound dehiscence with or without evisceration
  - DVT/PE
  - Fistula formation (vesicovaginal, ureterovaginal, or rectovaginal)
- Benefits:
  - Resolution of preoperative symptoms
  - Prevention of disease in removed organs

Alternatives
- Alternative treatments instead of hysterectomy depend on the indication.
- Abnormal bleeding:
  - Hormonal therapy (OCPs, levonorgestrel IUD, DMPA, GnRH agonist)
  - Endometrial ablation
- Leiomyomata (fibroids):
  - Hormonal therapy (OCPs, levonorgestrel IUD, DMPA, GnRH agonist)
  - Myomectomy
  - Uterine artery embolization

- Endometriosis:
  - Hormonal therapy (OCPs, levonorgestrel IUD, DMPA, GnRH agonist)
- Pelvic organ prolapse:
  - Pessary

Medical
- Treatment of existing infections before surgery:
  - Bacterial vaginosis
  - UTI
- Perioperative antibiotics should be administered 1 hour before the procedure (unless otherwise noted):
  - Cefazolin 1- or 2-g single dose, IV
  - Cefoxitin 2-g single dose, IV
  - Metronidazole 1-g single dose, IV
  - Tinidazole 2-g single dose, PO (4–12 hours before surgery)

Surgical
- General principles for AH:
  - Abdominal hysterectomy is usually performed under GETA; however, it can be performed under regional anesthesia (spinal or epidural).
  - Patient is positioned either in supine or low lithotomy.
  - Betadine or chlorhexidine scrub of abdomen, perineum, and vagina
  - Foley catheter for continuous bladder drainage
  - Abdominal cavity entered either through a transverse (Pfannenstiel) or midline incision
  - Abdomen and pelvis explored manually and visually for pathology
  - Self-retaining retractor placed and bowel packed into upper abdomen with moistened laparotomy sponges
  - The round ligaments and utero-ovarian ligaments are grasped with clamps for uterine manipulation.
  - The round ligament is ligated and divided bilaterally; the anterior leaf of the broad ligament is incised to the midline, allowing dissection of the bladder off the lower uterus and cervix.
  - When the ovaries are conserved, a window in the posterior leaf of the broad ligament is created so the utero-ovarian ligament can be ligated and transected.
  - The uterine arteries are skeletonized (dissected out) bilaterally, hysterectomy clamps are placed on the cardinal ligaments bilaterally.
  - Subsequent cardinal ligament pedicles will ligate the uterine artery, severing the main blood supply to the uterus.
  - At completion of the hysterectomy, cystoscopy may be performed to evaluate bladder integrity and ureteral patency.
  - The rectus fascia is closed with delayed absorbable suture, and the skin is closed with absorbable suture or skin clips.
- TAH:
  - Cardinal ligament pedicles are created to the level of the external cervical os, at which time curved hysterectomy clamps are placed across the upper vagina.
  - The cervix and uterus are amputated, and the vaginal cuff is closed with sutures.
- SAH:
  - At the level of the uterocervical junction, the uterine corpus is amputated, leaving the cervical stump to be oversewn (or electrocoagulated) for hemostasis.

 FOLLOW-UP

- The patient is usually asked to follow-up in 4–6 weeks after surgery.
- If a perioperative complication occurred or medical comorbidities are present, the patient may need to follow-up sooner.
- Until follow-up, the patient is asked to abstain from:
  - Heavy lifting
  - Operating motor vehicle or heavy equipment while requiring narcotics for pain control
  - Sexual intercourse
  - Douching or tampon use

PROGNOSIS
- The outcome of hysterectomy depends on the indication.
- Abnormal bleeding:
  - TAH will completely resolve all uterine bleeding.
  - SAH may result in cyclic spotting or bleeding from residual endometrial tissue in the cervical stump.
- Leiomyoma are smooth muscle tumors that can develop from any structure containing smooth muscle:
  - TAH will resolve leiomyoma of uterine origin.
  - After SAH, leiomyoma can develop from the cervical stump.
- Pain:
  - If pelvic pain is uterine in origin, hysterectomy should resolve symptoms.
  - Pelvic pain may also be of muscular (levator ani/obturator internus), bladder, or bowel origin and will not be addressed by hysterectomy.
- Uterine/Cervical cancer resolution depends on the stage of cancer.

COMPLICATIONS
- Intraoperative complications:
  - Hemorrhage with possible transfusion
  - Injury to adjacent structures (i.e., bladder, ureter, small or large bowels, nerves, or vasculature)
- Postoperative complications:
  - Fever
  - Infection (e.g., urinary tract, wound, vaginal cuff, pneumonia)
  - Abdominal wound infection/dehiscence
  - Vaginal cuff dehiscence
  - DVT/PE
  - Intra-abdominal adhesion formation
  - Fistula formation (vesicovaginal, ureterovaginal, or rectovaginal)

BIBLIOGRAPHY

ACOG Practice Bulletin No. 16. Antibiotic Prophylaxis for Gynecologic Procedures. *Obstet Gynecol.* 2001;97(1):1–9.

ACOG Practice Bulletin No. 65. Management of Endometrial Cancer. *Obstet Gynecol.* 2005;106(2): 413–425.

ACOG Practice Bulletin No. 66. Management of Abnormal Cervical Cytology and Histology. *Obstet Gynecol.* 2005;106(3):645–664.

ACOG Practice Bulletin No. 74. Antibiotic Prophylaxis for Gynecologic Procedures. *Obstet Gynecol.* 2006;108(1):225–234.

Farquhar CM, et al. Hysterectomy rates in the United States 1990–1997. *Obstet Gynecol.* 2002;99: 229–234.

Gilmour DT, et al. Rates of urinary tract injury from gynecologic surgery and the role of intra-operative cystoscopy. *Obstet Gynecol.* 2006;107:1366–1372.

Rock JA, et al., eds. *Te Linde's Operative Gynecology,* 9th ed. Philadelphia: Lippincott Williams & Wilkins; 2003.

 MISCELLANEOUS

SYNONYM(S)
Fibroid is used interchangeably with myoma or leiomyoma.

CLINICAL PEARLS
- If intraoperative visualization or access is diminished due to fibroids, a myomectomy can be performed to reduce uterine size. If bleeding from the myometrial bed occurs, the space can be closed by oversewing or placing a clamp to prevent blood loss until the uterus is removed.
- After the uterine arteries have been clamped, the upper uterus can be amputated and removed from the surgical field to improve access for the completion of the hysterectomy.

ABBREVIATIONS
- AH—Abdominal hysterectomy
- DMPA—Depot medroxyprogesterone acetate
- DVT—Deep venous thrombosis
- GETA—General endotracheal anesthesia
- OCP—Oral contraceptive pill
- PE—Pulmonary embolism
- SAH—Subtotal abdominal hysterectomy
- SCH—Supracervical hysterectomy
- TAH—Total abdominal hysterectomy
- UTI—Urinary tract infection

CODES
ICD9-CM
- 68.3 Supracervical or subtotal abdominal hysterectomy
- 68.4 Total abdominal hysterectomy

 PATIENT TEACHING

Postoperative instructions:
- Patients should be instructed to report warning signs of infection (e.g., fever, pain with urination), heavy vaginal bleeding, wound complications, and excessive pain.
- Patients should be instructed on general wound care.
- After supracervical (subtotal) hysterectomy, patients should continue to receive screening for cervical cancer at intervals appropriate to their level of risk.
- After TAH for benign indication(s), patients should be informed that they no longer require screening for cervical cancer.
- Women should be reminded to have regular pelvic exams as part of their overall health care.

HYSTERECTOMY, LAPAROSCOPIC AND LAPAROSCOPICALLY ASSISTED

Mary T. Jacobson, MD

 BASICS

DESCRIPTION

- The use of a laparoscope and accessory ports and instruments to perform all or parts of a hysterectomy
- Patient is under general anesthesia.
- Abdominal cavity accessed through 2–12 mm incision using Veress needle, direct trocar, open Hasson, or microlaparoscope
- Laparoscope functions as a telescope with light source and camera head attachments.
- Intraumbilical, infraumbilical, left upper quadrant most common entry sites
- Distension usually with CO_2 gas
- Image projected onto a video monitor
- 2–12 mm ancillary ports for instruments that act as extension of surgeon's hands
- Advantages over abdominal hysterectomy:
  - Magnification of operative field for optimal visualization
  - Shorter hospital stay
  - Quicker recovery
  - Less pain medication
  - Less adhesion formation
  - Less blood loss
- Advantages over vaginal hysterectomy:
  - Visualization of pelvis for diagnosis and treatment of pelvic pathology
  - Facilitation of vaginal hysterectomy
- Disadvantages:
  - More expensive and time-consuming
  - Higher complication rates vs. TVH

Indications

Diagnosis and/or treatment of concurrent pathology (i.e., adhesions, endometriosis, fibroids, uterine prolapse, urinary incontinence)

Site (Office, Surgical Center, OR)

- Outpatient surgical center
- Operating room
- Operating room equipped with sufficient video monitors
- Staff trained in laparoscopic surgery

Concurrent Procedures

Laparoscopic treatment of:
- Endometriosis
- Lysis of adhesions
- BSO
- Burch urethrocolpopexy

Age-Related Factors

Controversial as to whether to perform BSO at the time of hysterectomy for benign disease:
- BSO should be considered in women with a family history of ovarian cancer or >65 years of age.
- Surgical menopause has immediate risks of menopausal symptoms, sexual dysfunction, bone loss, and possibly CVD in women <65 years of age.

EPIDEMIOLOGY

Hysterectomy is the 2nd most common procedure performed in reproductive-age women in the US:
- 600,000 procedures performed in the US annually
- LAVH has increased from 13–28% of hysterectomies between 1994–1999.

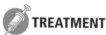 TREATMENT

PROCEDURE

Informed Consent

- Always include exam under anesthesia.
- Specify and mark side/site of concurrent ovarian procedures (e.g., right ovarian cystectomy).
- Include all procedures that may be performed:
  - Diagnostic laparoscopy and possible operative laparoscopy with treatment of endometriosis, lysis of adhesions, appendectomy, cystoscopy, sigmoidoscopy

Patient Education

- Explain procedure in detail using ACOG brochures, as well as cartoons, photographs.
- Suggest legitimate Web sites (e.g., www.AAGL.org, www.my-emmi.com)
- Review goals of surgery.
- Review patient goals and expectations.
- Make it clear to patient that she is recovering from surgery and is not sick!
- Familiarize patient with the surgical environment including the preoperative area, surgical suite, and postanesthesia care unit.
- Discuss postoperative recovery.

Risks, Benefits

- Risks:
  - Infection, bleeding, fistula similar to TVH. Trocar injury to blood vessel and bowel, herniation through trocar site, and urinary tract injuries higher in LH vs. TVH.
- Benefits:
  - Diagnosis and treatment, resolution or improvement of symptoms

Alternatives

Medical

- For menorrhagia as indication:
  - COCs, transdermal patch, vaginal ring, progestogens, DMPA
  - Mirena IUS
- For pain as indication:
  - Management of endometriosis with:
    - NSAIDs
    - COCs, transdermal patch, vaginal ring, aromatase inhibitor plus COC, DMPA, danazol, GnRHa
  - Pain management team
  - Pelvic floor physical therapy

Surgical

- For fibroids:
  - Uterine fibroid embolization
  - MR-guided US treatment
  - Hysteroscopic, laparoscopic, laparoscopic-assisted, abdominal myomectomy
- For bleeding:
  - Endometrial ablation
  - TVH
  - TAH
  - Laparoscopic or abdominal supracervical hysterectomy (SCH)

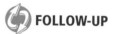 FOLLOW-UP

- 2-week postoperative appointment or sooner if patient experiences problems
- No lifting for 6 weeks
- Disability up to 6 weeks
- No driving until reflexes are not impaired and patient is off narcotics (generally 5–7 days).

PROGNOSIS

- 96% patient satisfaction; symptoms had completely or mostly resolved.
- Postdischarge complication necessitating readmission was important influence on patient dissatisfaction.
- Many women report improved sexual function after surgery but a sizeable minority report worsened sexual function:
  - Preoperative discussion about postoperative sexual function may decrease this.

COMPLICATIONS

- Higher with operative vs. diagnostic laparoscopy
- Entry-related injury most common:
  - Vascular
  - Bowel
  - Subcutaneous emphysema
  - Incisional hernia
- Nerve compression injury due to stirrups and positioning and length of procedure
- Other complications as with any hysterectomy, regardless of approach:
  - Wound infection (vaginal cuff abscess or cellulitis)
  - UTI
  - Atelectasis or pneumonia
  - DVT/PE
  - Fistula (vesicovaginal most common)

BIBLIOGRAPHY

Bateman BG. Complications with operative laparoscopy. *Fert Steril*. 1996;66(6):1045–1046.

Bradford A, et al. Sexual outcomes and satisfaction with hysterectomy: Influence of patient education. *J Sex Med*. 2007;4(1):106–114.

Centers for Disease Control. Hysterectomy surveillance-1994–1999. *MMWR*. 2002;51(SS05): 1–8.

Jansen FW, et al. Complications of laparoscopy: An inquiry about closed versus open-entry technique. *Am J Obstet Gynecol*. 2004;190(3):634–638.

Kjerulff KH, et al. Patient satisfaction with results of hysterectomy. *Am J Obstet Gynecol*. 2000;183(6): 1440–1447.

Nezhat CR, et al. *Operative Gynecologic Laparoscopy: Principles and Techniques*, 2nd ed. San Francisco: McGraw Hill; 2002.

Parker WH, et al. Ovarian conservation at the time of hysterectomy for benign disease. *Obstet Gynecol*. 2005;106(2):219–226.

Wetter PA. *Prevention and Management of Laparoendoscopic Surgical Complications*, 2nd ed. Miami: Society of Laparoendoscopic Surgeons, Inc.; 2005.

MISCELLANEOUS

CLINICAL PEARLS

- Use systematic routine for entry.
- Be familiar with equipment (i.e., energy sources, CO_2 settings, instrumentation).
- Know your technical limits.
- Foster open communication among surgical assistants, anesthesiologist, circulating nurse, and scrub technician.
- Have a very low threshold for immediately seeing any patient with a postoperative problem.

ABBREVIATIONS

- AAGL—American Association of Gynecologic Laparoscopists
- BSO—Bilateral salpingo-oophorectomy
- COCs—Combination oral contraceptives
- CVD—Cardiovascular disease
- DMPA—Depot medroxyprogesterone acetate
- DVT—Deep venous thrombosis
- GnRHa—Gonadotropin-releasing hormone agonist
- IUS—Intrauterine system
- LAVH—Laparoscopically assisted vaginal hysterectomy
- LH—Laparoscopic hysterectomy
- PE—Pulmonary embolism
- SCH—Supracervical hysterectomy
- TAH—Total abdominal hysterectomy
- TVH—Total vaginal hysterectomy
- UTI—Urinary tract infection

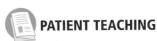

CODES

ICD9-CM/CPT

- LH-58550
- LAVH-58550
- SCH-58541 Laparoscopic

PATIENT TEACHING

Many women are confused about the term: *Total* hysterectomy, thinking this means removal of ovaries:

- Be sure to clarify that removal of ovaries is a separate issue from removal of entire uterus.

Section VII

HYSTERECTOMY, RADICAL

M. Heather Einstein, MD
Joseph P. Connor, MD

 BASICS

DESCRIPTION
- Radical hysterectomy is the en bloc excision of the uterus, cervix, upper 1/3–1/2 of the vagina, as well as the parametria (cardinal and uterosacral ligaments).
  - Radical hysterectomy requires complete dissection of the ureteric tunnel bilaterally and ligation of the uterine artery at its point of origin from the internal iliac artery.
- Modified radical hysterectomy is similar, except the parametria is only partially excised, medial to the ureter, and ureterolysis caudal to the uterine artery is not necessary. The uterine artery is ligated at the point where it crosses over the ureter.
- The distinction between "modified radical" and "radical" hysterectomy is determined on the extent of parametrectomy and vaginectomy, however these definitions vary from institution to institution.

Indications
- Early stage cervical cancer:
  - Stage IB1, select IB2, and minimal IIA
- Stage II endometrial cancer (cervical involvement)

Site (Office, Surgical Center, OR)
OR

Concurrent Procedures
- Common:
  - Pelvic lymphadenectomy, para-aortic lymph node sampling, staging
  - Suprapubic catheter placement
  - Ovarian transposition (premenopausal women)
  - Bilateral salpingo-oophorectomy (postmenopausal women)
- Investigational:
  - Sentinel lymph node sampling

> **ALERT**
>
> The procedure is often aborted in favor of chemoradiation therapy if:
> - Positive lymph nodes are identified.
> - Extrauterine disease is present.
> - The disease extends into the parametria toward the side-wall (and is therefore unresectable).

Age-Related Factors
Geriatric Considerations
- In older patients with multiple comorbidities, the risk of surgery may outweigh the benefit, making chemoradiation preferable.
- Healthy geriatric patients whose surgical risk is low should undergo radical hysterectomy to avoid the potential bowel, bladder, and sexual function complications of chemoradiation therapy.

Pregnancy Considerations
- Early cervical cancer diagnosed during pregnancy can be monitored until term and treated with radical hysterectomy at the time of a planned cesarean delivery.
- Patients desiring fertility may be candidates for radical trachelectomy (see "Alternatives"). Subsequent pregnancies would require cesarean delivery.

EPIDEMIOLOGY
(See Cervical and Endometrial cancers).

 TREATMENT

PROCEDURE
Informed Consent
- General surgical concerns:
  - Bleeding/Transfusion (higher risk than in simple hysterectomy due to vascularity of the parametria)
  - Injury to other organs
  - DVT/PE
- Urinary dysfunction
- Lymphedema or lymphocele

Patient Education
- Differing surgical approaches, expectation of recovery time, possible complications
- Possibility of aborting procedure based on intraoperative findings in favor of chemoradiation therapy
- Likelihood of short-term bladder dysfunction and use/care of suprapubic catheter or self-catheterization

Risks, Benefits
- Risks:
  - Risks of surgery (see "Informed Consent") and anesthesia
  - 1% risk of lasting urinary dysfunction
  - Urinary tract fistula (ureterovaginal, vesicovaginal)
- Benefits:
  - Less long-term bowel, bladder, or sexual dysfunction than chemoradiation therapy
  - In early stage cervical cancer, survival is equal after either radical hysterectomy or chemoradiation therapy.

Alternatives
- Chemoradiation therapy:
  - Recommended for patients with early-stage cervical cancer who do not have access to a gynecologic oncologist
  - Recommended for patients with comorbidities that limit surgical options
  - Recommended for patients with advanced cervical cancer

- Cone biopsy or simple hysterectomy:
  - Appropriate for patients with CIS or Stage 1A1 disease
- Radical trachelectomy:
  - Removal of the cervix, upper vagina, and part of the parametria while leaving the uterine corpus in situ
  - Indications: Patients with cervical cancer (<2 cm lesion) who desire fertility:
    - Only possible if frozen section margins of trachelectomy specimen are negative
  - Approach: Abdominal, vaginal, or laparoscopic-assisted vaginal

Medical
Chemoradiation therapy:
- Combination of external beam and internal brachytherapy with concomitant IV radiosensitizing chemotherapy, most often cis-platinum
- If administering chemoradiation, uterus and cervix should be left in situ to decrease risk of injury to bowel and bladder.

Surgical
- 3 possible procedures:
  - RAH:
    - Classical method
    - Vertical, Maylard, or Cherney incision
  - LRH
  - LARVH (Schauta procedure):
    - Lymphadenectomy done laparoscopically, as well as preparation for radical vaginal hysterectomy
- Approach is based on surgeon preference, patient body habitus, size of uterus, extent of disease.
- Recovery time is 6 weeks with the abdominal approach, 2–3 weeks with laparoscopic or vaginal approaches.
- Recovery of bladder function can be weeks to months in some cases, regardless of the radical procedure done.

 FOLLOW-UP

- 2-week postoperative check, then follow-up for cervical cancer as appropriate.
- Voiding trials: Goal of PVR depends on preoperative PVR:
  - If patient fails in-hospital voiding trial, send home with catheter (suprapubic or Foley).
  - Return to office for voiding trial the week following discharge from hospital.

PROGNOSIS

- Radical hysterectomy is usually well-tolerated by most patients.
- There is no evidence to suggest that surgical approach affects survival, although there may be increased complication rates with laparoscopy, especially early in the surgeon's learning curve.
- Patients who require adjuvant chemoradiation after surgery have a higher complication rate than those who had surgery or chemoradiation alone.
- (See Cervical Cancer.)
- Prognosis (see topic)

COMPLICATIONS

- Prolonged or lasting urinary dysfunction due to sympathetic denervation of the bladder:
  - Diagnosed by persistently elevated PVR or the inability to urinate
  - Treat with timed voiding; if not possible, timed catheterization
- Urinary tract fistula (ureterovaginal, vesicovaginal):
  - Diagnose with cystoscopy and retrograde dye study
  - Repair fistula and place ureteral stents as needed.
- Lymphocele or lymphocyst:
  - Can be asymptomatic or cause pain with or without a degree of infection
  - Diagnose with CT or US
  - Observation if asymptomatic without evidence of infection
  - If symptomatic and/or infected, treat with CT-guided drainage or surgical excision with or without antibiotics.
- DVT/PE:
  - Prophylaxis with sequential compression devices and heparin or LMWH
  - DVT:
    - Edema, erythema, and pain, usually in the lower extremity
    - Diagnosis by US or Doppler, CT, MRI
    - Treatment with long-term anticoagulation
  - PE:
    - Shortness of breath, tachycardia, chest pain sudden death
    - Diagnosed by CT angiogram or V/Q scan
    - Treatment with long-term anticoagulation and/or vena cava filter placement

BIBLIOGRAPHY

Hoffman MS. Extent of radical hysterectomy: Evolving emphasis. *Gynecol Oncol*. 2004;94(1):1–9.

Hoskins W, et al. *Principles and Practice of Gynecologic Oncology*, 3rd ed. Philadelphia: Lippincott Williams & Wilkins; 2000.

Ostergard D, et al. *Atlas of Gynecologic Surgery*. Philadelphia: W.B. Saunders; 2000.

Plante M, et al. Vaginal radical trachelectomy: An oncologically safe fertility-preserving surgery. An updated series of 72 cases and review of the literature. *Gynecol Oncol*. 2004;94(3):614–623.

Steed H, et al. A comparison of laparoscopic-assisted radical vaginal hysterectomy and radical abdominal hysterectomy in the treatment of cervical cancer. *Gynecol Oncol*. 2004;93(3):588–593.

 MISCELLANEOUS

- Controversy exists as to which stage of cervical cancer is best treated by radical hysterectomy:
  - It is clear that survival outcomes are equivalent between chemoradiation and radical hysterectomy in patients with Stage IBI or less.
  - In Stage IB2, the argument for surgery is the lower rate of bowel and bladder complications compared to chemoradiation.
- The argument against surgical therapy is that the rate of positive lymph nodes (and therefore need for adjuvant chemoradiation) in patients with a >4 cm lesion is high, leading to the use of combined modalities, with more morbidity.

SYNONYM(S)

- Type III hysterectomy: Radical abdominal hysterectomy; Wertheim hysterectomy
- Type II Hysterectomy: Modified radical abdominal hysterectomy
- Schauta procedure: Radical vaginal hysterectomy

ABBREVIATIONS

- DVT—Deep venous thrombosis
- LARVH—Laparoscopic-assisted radical vaginal hysterectomy
- LMWH—Low-molecular-weight heparin
- LRH—Laparoscopic radical hysterectomy
- PE—Pulmonary embolism
- PVR—Postvoid residual
- RAH—Radical abdominal hysterectomy

 CODES

ICD9-CM
58548 Radical hysterectomy

 PATIENT TEACHING

- Self-catheterization or care of suprapubic catheter, recording of PVRs
- No heavy lifting (>25 lb), nothing per vagina for 6 weeks
- Call provider for wound erythema, temperature >100.4°F, severe pain, vaginal bleeding > menses, or voiding difficulties with or without dysuria.

HYSTERECTOMY, VAGINAL

Paula J. Adams Hillard, MD
Joseph P. Connor, MD
M. Heather Einstein, MD

 BASICS

DESCRIPTION

- Removal of the uterus via the vagina with no abdominal incision
- Routes of hysterectomy for benign disease include:
  - Abdominal hysterectomy; TAH if cervix is removed with fundus
  - VH, also termed TVH
  - Laparoscopic hysterectomy:
    - LAVH, where vaginal hysterectomy is assisted by laparoscopic procedures that do not include uterine artery ligation
    - LH, where laparoscopic procedures do include uterine artery ligation
    - TLH, with no vaginal component and the vaginal vault is sutured laparoscopically
- A Cochrane review noted significantly improved outcomes for TVH, and stated that VH should be performed in preference to AH where possible.
  - Where VH is not possible, LH may avoid the need for AH.

Indications

- Indicated generally for benign uterine disease (1997 data); VH indications, including:
  - Uterine prolapse: 44.9%
  - Uterine leiomyomata: 17.1%
  - Menstrual disorders: 13.6%
  - Endometriosis: 7.2%
  - Cervical premalignant disease if indicated
- VH has been described for endometrial cancer for women with extreme obesity.
- Many gynecologists believe, in the absence of supporting data, that the following are contraindications for VH:
  - Nulliparity
  - Previous pelvic surgery (including cesarean section)
  - Need for oophorectomy
  - Pathology outside the uterus
- Surgeons choose AH on the basis of their experience, comfort, and preference:
  - Younger residents get less surgical experience with vaginal surgery than AH.
- No consensus on uterine size or weight that precludes VH:
  - ACOG has stated that VH is indicated for patients with a mobile uterus of <12 weeks' gestational size.
  - Laterally extending leiomyoma, especially with uterus high in the pelvis, may not allow vaginal approach to uterine arteries.
  - Uterine position and mobility may impact decision more so than size alone.
  - Vaginal capacity may impact decision.
  - VH is potentially feasible for larger uteri, and may be preferable to AH in experienced surgeon's hands:
    - Estimates suggest overall VH rate could be increased by ~12% if VH were performed up to 10 wks, by 24% up to 14 weeks, and by 30% if enlarged to 18 weeks.

Site (Office, Surgical Center, OR)

Inpatient surgical center:

- Same-day surgery, with discharge after a period of observation has been described.
- 23-hour admission is potentially feasible in the absence of complication.

Concurrent Procedures

- Oophorectomy: Unilateral or bilateral
- LAVH for lysis of adhesions, oophorectomy, etc. (see topic)

Age-Related Factors

The median age for VH in US in 1997 was 45.

Geriatric Considerations

Symptomatic uterine prolapse with a small mobile uterus is a frequent indication for VH.

EPIDEMIOLOGY

- In the US, rates of hysterectomy did not change from 1990–1997.
- International hysterectomy rates highest in US and lowest in Norway and Sweden.
- Rates of hysterectomy in 1997 in US were 5.6/1,000 women:
  - No change in rates of VH
  - Increase in LH with decline in AH
- Ratio of AH–VH range from 1:1–6:1 in North America.
- Ratio ~3:1 in Canada
- 23% of hysterectomies in US in 1997 were VH.

 TREATMENT

PROCEDURE

Informed Consent

Discuss type of procedure, indications, alternatives, expectations of outcome, risks, benefits, other planned procedures (e.g., oophorectomy) and document these discussions.

Patient Education

In addition to issues of informed consent, provide information about planned hospitalization duration, recovery period, and restrictions on postoperative activity.

Risks, Benefits

- Risks of VH:
  - Risks of surgery in general, and abdominal/pelvic surgery in particular:
    - Hemorrhage, possibly necessitating transfusion
    - Infection; minimized by the use of prophylactic antibiotics
    - Injury to bowel, bladder, pelvic organs
    - Venous thromboembolic disease: PE/DVT
    - Fistula
    - Necessity of reoperation
    - Adhesions
    - Small bowel obstruction
    - Failure to achieve the desired relief of symptoms
  - Risks of VH specifically include:
    - Bladder injury; may be increased in women with previous cesarean delivery
    - Injury to bowel/rectum

- Inability to complete procedure vaginally, necessitating conversion to AH
    - Fallopian tube prolapse
- Benefits of VH over AH noted in Cochrane review include:
  - Shorter duration of hospital stay
  - Speedier return to normal activities
  - Fewer infections or febrile episodes
  - Other benefits:
    - Typically shorter operative time for VH vs. AH
  - Cochrane review found no benefits of LH over VH
    - Increased operating time for LH

Alternatives

See specific conditions by indication
Medical
See specific conditions by indication
Surgical

- The surgical hysterectomy options include:
  - AH, TAVH, TLH, LH
- As with any surgical procedures, appropriate selection of the indications and type of procedure are important. The patient should participate in the decisions about whether, when, and what type of surgical procedure will be performed, based on accurate information.
- Prophylactic antibiotics:
  - In the early 1980s, perioperative prophylactic antibiotics for VH were shown to reduce postoperative infection:
    - Reduced febrile morbidity
    - Reduced pelvic/wound infection
    - Reduced duration of stay
    - Reduced total antibiotic use
- Prevent DVT (see ACOG guidelines by risk category).
- Appropriately position for dorsal lithotomy, with prep and draping.
- Perform bimanual exam after emptying bladder to confirm office exam, assess uterine mobility and descensus, and confirm decision to proceed with vaginal approach.
- Bladder catheter is inserted by physician preference.
- Appropriate retractors: Weighted, right-angle, Deaver
- Vasoconstrictors are injected into cervix by surgeon preference.
- Traction on cervix exerted using tenaculum.
- Circumferential incision made around cervix with mobilization of vaginal epithelium off cervix, bluntly or sharply.
- Expose posterior vaginal fornix and enter cul-de-sac sharply, identify peritoneum and tag with suture.
- If posterior peritoneal entry is difficult, ligate uterosacral and cardinal ligaments until posterior cul-de-sac can be entered, or alternatively enter anterior peritoneum.
- Clamp divide and ligate uterosacral ligaments.
- Mobilize and advance bladder, allowing visualization of vesicovaginal peritoneal reflection; identified by "silk sign" of peritoneal surface slipping over peritoneal surface.

- Enter anterior peritoneum and place retractor beneath bladder.
- Identify, clamp, cut, and suture ligate cardinal ligaments in a series of bites bilaterally, keep traction on cervix.
- Identify uterine vessels; clamp:
  - If possible, incorporate both anterior and posterior peritoneum
  - Some surgeons prefer to doubly clamp uterine vessels
  - May need to place 2nd clamp to control all uterine vessels
- Options for facilitating VH in presence of enlarged uterus after securing uterine vessels:
  - Bisection
  - Wedge morcellation
  - Coring
- Deliver uterine fundus posteriorly.
- Clamp and divide utero-ovarian ligament in pedicle including fallopian tube:
  - May doubly clamp with suture tie, followed by suture ligation of the distal pedicle
- Nonvascular pedicles may be held for later exam in assuring hemostasis.
- Salpingo-oophorectomy may then be performed by clamping infundibulopelvic ligament followed by tie and suture ligature of pedicle, assuring the ureter is well away from clamp/tie.
- Inspect pedicles for bleeding after placing lap sponge into abdomen:
  - Ligate bleeders
- May close peritoneum using purse-string suture circumferentially and incorporating pedicles and ligating uterosacral ligaments:
  - Many surgeons recommend culdoplasty to decrease risk of enterocele.
- Surgeon removes lap sponge and ties purse-string suture around her finger to assure no prolapse of intraabdominal organs.
- Close vaginal mucosa; may use continuous suture or interrupted through full thickness.
- Vaginal packing and bladder catheter are not routinely required.

FOLLOW-UP

- Hospital discharge on postoperative day 1 or 2, although some do same-day discharge
- Postoperative visit in 4–6 weeks

PROGNOSIS
- Outcome is assessed by:
  - Relief of symptoms
  - Patient satisfaction, dependent on:
    - Relief of symptoms
    - Sexual function
  - Preoperative psychiatric symptoms:
    - Depression or anxiety may be improved, although these factors have been associated with a higher risk of negative outcome.
    - Feelings about loss of fertility
- Overall high rates of satisfaction: 70–90%

COMPLICATIONS
- UK study reported severe intraoperative complications in 3.1% and postoperative complications in 1.2%.
- The most common complications included:
  - Ureteral, bowel, and bladder injuries
  - Hemorrhage
  - Infection
- Rate of unintended major surgical procedure: 3–5%
- Mortality overall 20/10,000 cases, but varies by age

BIBLIOGRAPHY

ACOG Practice Bulletin No. 84. Prevention of Deep Vein Thrombosis and Pulmonary Embolism. *Obstet Gynecol.* 2007;110(2 Pt 1):429–440.

Brill AI. Hysterectomy in the 21st century: Different approaches, different challenges. *Clin Obstet Gynecol.* 2006;49(4):722–735.

Farquhar CM, et al. Hysterectomy rates in the United States 1990–1997. *Obstet Gynecol.* 2002;99(2):229–234.

Johnson N, et al. Surgical approach to hysterectomy for benign gynaecological disease. *Cochrane Database Syst Rev.* 2006;(2):CD003677.

McCracken G, et al. Vaginal hysterectomy: Dispelling the myths. *J Obstet Gynaecol Can.* 2007;29(5): 424–428.

MISCELLANEOUS

SYNONYM(S)
Total vaginal hysterectomy (TVH)

CLINICAL PEARLS
It has been stated that, "Vaginal surgery, and vaginal hysterectomy in particular is the hallmark of a good gynecologic surgeon."

ABBREVIATIONS
- AH—Abdominal hysterectomy
- DVT—Deep venous thrombosis
- LAVH—Laparoscopically assisted vaginal hysterectomy
- LH—Laparoscopic hysterectomy
- PE—Pulmonary embolism
- TAH—Total abdominal hysterectomy
- TLH—Total laparoscopic hysterectomy
- TVH—Total vaginal hysterectomy
- VH—Vaginal hysterectomy

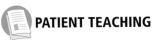 CODES

ICD9-CM
68.59 Vaginal hysterectomy

PATIENT TEACHING

ACOG Patient Education Pamphlet: Hysterectomy

HYSTEROSCOPY, DIAGNOSTIC AND OPERATIVE

Scott P. Serden, MD
Philip G. Brooks, MD

 BASICS

DESCRIPTION

- Endoscopic procedure to assist in the diagnosis and treatment of intrauterine pathology
- Developed as a visual adjunct to traditional D&C for greater diagnostic accuracy and treatment effectiveness
- Distension of uterine cavity with fluid or gas facilitates visualization
- Alternative minimally invasive management of women with AUB who would have undergone hysterectomy in the past

Indications
- Premenopausal AUB
- Postmenopausal bleeding
- Suspected intrauterine polyps, myomas, septae, or adhesions
- Recurrent pregnancy loss
- Lost IUD
- Assess uterine cavity size/shape during infertility evaluation

Site (Office, Surgical Center, OR)
May be performed in office, surgical center, or OR:
- Local, regional, or general anesthesia
- In some cases, no anesthesia is required

Concurrent Procedures
- Removal of endometrial polyps
- Resection of submucous myomas
- Endometrial ablation
- Diagnostic laparoscopy
- Insertion of intratubal sterilization devices

Age-Related Factors
Reproductive-age and postmenopausal

 TREATMENT

PROCEDURE

Informed Consent
The risks, benefits, alternatives, complications, and options should be discussed with the patient and documented in the medical record. Patient identity and procedure planned should be confirmed using OR or office "time out" confirmation.

Patient Education
- Complications occur in <1% of cases.
- Inform of risks and benefits

Risks, Benefits
- Risks and complications are either procedure-related (dependent on technical skills of hysteroscopist or dependent on instrumentation) or media-related.
- Procedure-related:
  - Uterine perforation: ~1%
  - Hemorrhage: <1%
- Media-related:
  - Gas embolism: 0.17%
  - Fluid overload: 0.14%
  - Electrolyte disorders

Alternatives
- D&C
- Other diagnostic and therapeutic procedures:
  - Laparoscopic sterilization
  - Myomectomy, laparoscopic, or laparotomy
  - Hysterosalpingography
  - Sonohysterography

Medical
- Hormonal management of abnormal bleeding prior to diagnostic procedures
- Management of uterine leiomyoma using GnRH analogs

Surgical
- Diagnostic hysteroscopy:
  - Rigid rod-lens or flexible optics:
  - 12°, 15°, and 30° angles of viewing assist in visualizing abnormalities in cornua or midline.
  - Distension media instilled via:
    - Syringe, gravity, or hysteroscopic fluid management systems (requires continuous-flow sheath)
  - Media:
    - Saline, CO_2, sorbitol/mannitolglycine/Hyskon
- Operative hysteroscopy:
  - Continuous flow with inflow rates > outflow to distend uterus and facilitate visualization
  - Need for accurate fluid monitoring due to large volumes of media
  - Energy source (mono- or bipolar) to treat abnormality and obtain hemostasis
  - Equipment:
    - 23–28 Fr, continuous flow hysteroscope
    - 5 mm rod-lens; 12°, 15°, and 30° optics
    - Monopolar energy through 90° loops, rollerballs, barrels, or vaporizing electrodes
    - Fluid-monitoring/pump systems allow for adjustable flow rates to maximize distention and monitor fluid deficit simultaneously to ovoid fluid overload and hyponatremia

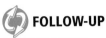

FOLLOW-UP

COMPLICATIONS

- Uterine perforation with sound, dilators, scope, or loop:
  - Perforation with energy source requires laparoscopy to rule out bowel injury.
- Fluid overload:
  - With no-electrolytic solutions, possible hyponatremia
  - Fluid monitoring systems standard of care
- Bleeding:
  - Pitressin in cervix to cause vasospasm
  - Intrauterine Foley balloon: 30 mL if excessive bleeding; leave for 2–4 hours
  - Infection is rare.
  - Failure to complete procedure

BIBLIOGRAPHY

Bradley LD. Complications in hysteroscopy: Prevention, treatment and legal risk [Review]. *Curr Opin Obstet Gynecol.* 2002;14(4):409–415.

DeCherney AH, et al. Endometrial ablation for intractable uterine bleeding: Hysteroscopic resection. *Obstet Gynecol.* 1987;70(4):668–670.

Loffer FD. Hysteroscopy with selective endometrial sampling compared with D&C for abnormal uterine bleeding: The value of a negative hysteroscopic view. *Obstet Gynecol.* 1989;73(1):16–20.

MISCELLANEOUS

- Endometrial polyps:
  - Use 90° resecting loops
  - Specimen removed with loop or polyp forceps after base/stalk severed
  - Some coagulation artifact on pathology
- Uterine myomas:
  - Use 90° resecting loops
  - As myoma is resected, myoma extruded into cavity if >50% intracavitary
  - Slow resection ensures greater coagulation and fluid loss

- Endometrial ablation:
  - For resection/coagulation, loop placed at fundus and full thickness of endometrium resected under direct visualization
  - Wattage setting: 80–120 W pure cutting and 60–70 W coagulation
  - Slow resection reduces bleeding and intravascular fluid loss
  - Resected bed coagulated with rollerbar at 100 W pure cutting or blend at less wattage

ABBREVIATIONS

AUB—Abnormal uterine bleeding

CODES

ICD9-CM/CPT

- 621.9 Endometrial polyp
- 218.9 Leiomyoma, uterus
- 626.2 Menorrhagia
- 626.8 Dysfunctional uterine bleeding
- 58555 Diagnostic hysteroscopy
- 58563 Operative hysteroscopy, endomaterial ablation
- 58561 Operative hysteroscopy, resection myoma
- 58558 Operative hysteroscopy, resection polyp

PATIENT TEACHING

ACOG Patient Education Pamphlet. Available at: http://www.acog.org

Section VII

INCONTINENCE SURGERIES

Soo Y. Kwon, MD

 BASICS

DESCRIPTION

- The definition of SUI was revised in 2001 by the International Continence Society.
- SUI is defined as the complaint of involuntary leakage with effort or exertion or on sneezing or coughing.
- When stress urinary incontinence is confirmed on UD, it is defined as UDSUI.
- UD is recommended to confirm the diagnosis of SUI prior to surgical treatment of SUI.
- Many surgical treatments are available including minimally invasive TVT.
- Less invasive procedures offer lower morbidity while maintaining treatment efficacy.
- SUI is often related to POP and anal incontinence.

Indications
- When conservative treatments have failed
- If the patient declines conservative treatments and desires definitive treatment instead
- When other causes of incontinence have been thoroughly evaluated and managed:
  - Overactive bladder

Site (Office, Surgical Center, OR)
- Office procedures:
  - Transurethral bulking agent
- Outpatient surgical center:
  - Transurethral bulking agent
  - TVT
- Inpatient surgery:
  - Burch retropubic urethropexy
  - Traditional sling procedure

Concurrent Procedures
- Surgical correction of POP
- Surgical correction of anal incontinence

Age-Related Factors
- Prevalence and severity increases with age.
- With increase in age, urge incontinence becomes more prevalent.
- SUI is more common in younger patient population (ages 30–49).

EPIDEMIOLOGY
SUI:
- 10–43% of community dwelling female population
- Up to 50% of nursing home population

 TREATMENT

PROCEDURE
Informed Consent
Options:
- Discuss success rates by procedure

Patient Education
Discuss:
- Benefits
- Success rates:
  - Short term
  - Long term
- Risks:
  - Surgical risks of injury
  - Recurrence
- Alternatives
- Decision making

Risks, Benefits
Specific to procedure

Alternatives
Medical and surgical
Medical
Prior to proceeding with surgery, conservative treatment options should be offered:
- Pelvic floor muscle training
- Bladder training
- Pessaries
- Duloxetine (currently under investigation)

Surgical
- Burch retropubic urethropexy:
  - Most widely performed retropubic procedure
  - Considered as "gold standard"
  - Indication:
    - UDSUI with urethral hypermobility
  - Route:
    - Laparotomy
    - Laparoscopic: Less invasive and equally efficacious
  - Success rate:
    - 80–90%
  - Complications:
    - Bladder, ureteral and bowel injury
    - De Novo urge UI
    - Voiding dysfunction of 0–22%

- TVT:
  - >500,000 procedures performed worldwide by 2003
  - Mechanism of action:
    - Probably by kinking of midurethra
  - Indication:
    - UDSUI with urethral hypermobility
    - ISD
  - Cure rate:
    - 85% at 5 years
    - Comparable to Burch urethropexy
  - Complications:
    - Bladder injury, 6%
    - Bowel injury, 1%
    - Vascular injury, <1%
    - De novo urge UI, 5%
    - Voiding dysfunction of 2–4%
    - Mesh erosion, <2%
    - UTI, 7%
- Traditional suburethral sling:
  - Not as commonly performed after emerging of TVT
  - More dissection and surgical time required compared to TVT
  - Various sling materials:
    - Autologous fascia
    - Cadaveric fascia
    - Others
  - Indication:
    - UDSUI with urethral hypermobility
    - ISD
  - Success rate
    - 88% in 5 yr with autologous fascia
  - Complications:
    - De novo urge UI, 7%
    - Voiding dysfunction, 2%
- Trans/Periurethral bulking agents
  - Indications:
    - UDSUI
  - Excellent treatment option for those with significant comorbidities and have surgical contraindications
  - Often need multiple injections
  - Skin testing should be performed at least 30 days prior to injection of collagen
  - Performed via cystoscope
  - Bulking agents:
    - Collagen; most widely utilized
    - Carbon coated zirconium oxide beads, calcium hydroxylapatite, ethylene vinyl alcohol

– Cure rate:
  o Short term, up to 94%
  o Long term, 45%
– Minimal risk of complications
• Needle suspension:
  – Poor long-term success, 18% at 4 years
  – Not widely performed

 FOLLOW-UP

• Those patients who are discharged with a transurethral catheter should return to the office for voiding trial within 1 wk of discharge.
• If the patient has post void residual volume >100 cc:
  – Either an indwelling catheter should be replaced
  – Or patient should be taught to start clean self catheterization.

Pregnancy Considerations
Complications related to pregnancy unknown after anti-incontinence surgery:

• Elective cesarean delivery has been advocated

BIBLIOGRAPHY

Balmforth, et al. Trends toward less invasive treatment of female stress urinary incontinence. *Urology*. 2003;62:52–60.
Dildy GA, et al. Cardiac arrest during pregnancy. *Obstet Gynecol Clin North Am*. 1995;22:303–314.
American College of Obstetricians and Gynecologists. Practice Bulletin: Urinary Incontinence in Women. 2006;991–1003.
Cost P, et al. Advancing the treatment of stress urinary incontinence. *Br J Urology*. 2006;97:911–915.
Luber KM, et al. Transactions of the 67th annual meeting of the Pacific Coast Obstetrical and Gynecological Society. *Am J Obstet Gynecol*. 2001;184:1496–1503.
Walters M, et al. *Urogynecology and Reconstructive Pelvic Surgery*. Philadelphia: Elsvier; 2007:172–233.

 MISCELLANEOUS

When to refer?
• Failed conservative treatment
• Prior pelvic surgery
• Consider physician's own surgical experience and practice type
• Community standards:
  – Availability of urogynecologist or urologist

ABBREVIATIONS
• SUI—Stress urinary incontinence
• UD—Urodynamics
• UDSUI—Urodynamic stress incontinence
• TVT—Tensionfree vaginal tape
• POP—Pelvic organ prolapse
• ISD—Intrinsic sphincter deficiency

 CODES

ICD9-CM
• 596.5 Overactive bladder
• 625.6 Stress urinary incontinence
• 788.2 Urinary retention, unspecified
• 788.21 Incomplete bladder emptying
• 788.34 Incontinence without awareness
• 788.31 Urge incontinence
• 788.380 Verflow incontinence
• 788.33 Mixed incontinence
• 788.41 Urinary frequency
• 788.63 Urinary urgency

PATIENT TEACHING

• Treatment should be offered if patient's quality of life is affected.
• Educating the patient is critical in achieving patient satisfaction.
• Pelvic floor exercises:
  – www.patients.uptodate.com/topic.asp?file= wom_issu/3002
• Urinary incontinence:
  – www.patients.uptodate.com/topic.asp?file= gen`hlth/6576

Section VII

INTRAUTERINE CONTRACEPTIVE (IUC) INSERTION

DeShawn L. Taylor, MD, MSc
Raquel D. Arias, MD

BASICS

DESCRIPTION

- ParaGard T 380A intrauterine copper contraceptive and Mirena levonorgestrel-releasing intrauterine system (LNG-IUS) are the 2 IUCs available in the US.
  - Both frames contain barium sulfate for detection by x-ray.
  - Monofilament polyethylene removal threads are attached at base of vertical stems.
- ParaGard T 380A Copper IUC:
  - T-shaped IUC with polyethylene frame
  - Copper wound around stem and transverse arms to create total surface area of 380 mm^2

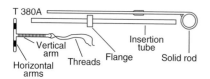

- Mirena LNG-IUS
  - T-shaped polyethylene IUS with reservoir that contains 52 mg of LNG
  - Sustained-release of LNG directly into the uterine cavity at an initial rate of 20 μg/d

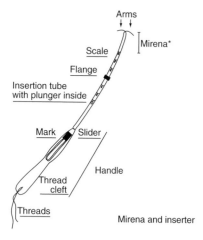

Mirena and inserter

Indications

Women desiring highly effective, long acting, reversible IUC

Site (Office, Surgical Center, OR)

Office

EPIDEMIOLOGY

- IUC prevalence: 1% in US
- IUC prevalence: 3–26 times higher in other developed countries:
  - Canada (3%), United Kingdom (6%), France (20%), Finland (26%)

TREATMENT

PROCEDURE

Informed Consent

- Discuss benefits, risks, and alternatives prior to IUC insertion.
- Signed consent forms are recommended.

Patient Education

- Protection against pregnancy begins immediately after insertion.
- Changes in menstrual patterns may occur and are expected.
- Use condoms to protect against STIs.
- Transient increased risk of pelvic infection in the 1st few weeks after insertion.
- IUC can be spontaneously expelled.

Risks, Benefits

- Risks:
  - Changes in menstrual bleeding patterns
  - Cramping and pain at time of IUC insertion
  - Expulsion of 2–10% in 1st year, then declines over time
  - Perforation 1/1,000 insertions:
    - Occurs at the time of insertion
  - Pelvic infection risk greatest in 1st 20 days after insertion due to contamination of endometrial cavity at time of insertion
- Benefits:
  - Highly effective
  - Long acting
  - Protective against ectopic pregnancy
  - Rapid return to fertility after discontinuation
  - Noncontraceptive benefits (see topic)

Alternatives

Medical

Reversible long-acting contraceptives:

- Injectable (Depo Provera)
- Implant (Implanon)

Surgical

Irreversible (sterilization):

- Tubal occlusion via laparoscopy, laparotomy, or hysteroscopy

FOLLOW-UP

Follow-up in 2–3 months after insertion to evaluate for pelvic infection and expulsion:

- Patient should return sooner if she experiences any problems.

COMPLICATIONS

- Excessive bleeding:
  - Bleeding due to copper IUC can be treated with NSAIDs.
  - Provide iron supplementation if hemoglobin declines.
  - Persistent abnormal bleeding requires clinical evaluation.
- Expulsion:
  - Suspect if following symptoms present: Unusual vaginal discharge, cramping or pain, intermenstrual or postcoital spotting, dyspareunia (male or female), absence or lengthening of IUC strings, and visualization of IUC at cervical os or in vagina

- Uterine perforation:
  - Copper induces adhesion formation in the peritoneal cavity that may involve adnexal, omentum, and bowel.
  - Prompt, preferably laparoscopic, removal recommended.
- PID:
  - No need to remove IUC during treatment.
- Pregnancy:
  - IUC should be removed at time pregnancy is diagnosed if strings visible regardless of patient's plan for the pregnancy.
  - 40–50% risk of spontaneous abortion if IUC left in place
  - 30% risk of spontaneous abortion after IUC removed

BIBLIOGRAPHY

Hatcher RA, et al. Contraceptive Technology, 18th ed. New York: Ardent Media; 2004.

Jensen JT. Contraceptive and therapeutic effects of the levonorgestrel intrauterine system: An overview. Obstet Gynecol Surv. 2005;60(9):604–612.

Kaunitz AM. Beyond the pill: New data and options in hormonal and intrauterine contraception. Am J Obstet Gynecol. 2005;192:998–1004.

Speroff L, et al. A Clinical Guide for Contraception, 3rd ed. Philadelphia: Lippincott Williams & Wilkins; 2001.

United Nations Population Division. World Contraceptive Use 2005. Available at: www.un.org/esa/population/publications/contraceptive2005/2005_World_Contraceptive_files/WallChart WCU2005.pdf.

MISCELLANEOUS

- IUC insertion technique, general preparation:
  - Perform bimanual exam to exclude active infection and determine position of uterus.
  - Insert speculum, view and cleanse cervix and vagina with antiseptic solution.
    - Local anesthetic may be appropriate but is not required for IUC insertion.
    - May inject only at site of tenaculum placement or may place a paracervical block
    - If using plain lidocaine, upper limit is 2 mg/lb, not to exceed 300 mg.
    - Anesthetize the cervix at the 12 o'clock position for tenaculum placement (1–2 mL).
    - Use tenaculum to move cervix laterally, revealing lateral vaginal fornix.
    - Inject 4–5 mL of anesthetic into cervical mucosa at the 5 and 7 o'clock positions ~2 cm lateral to cervical os.
  - Apply traction to tenaculum to straighten axis of uterus before sounding and measuring uterine depth:
    - Insertion tube may be used to sound the uterus.
    - Uterus should sound to depth of 6–9 cm.
    - Insertion into smaller uteri may increase incidence of expulsion, bleeding, pain, and perforation.

- ParaGard insertion (figures reproduced with permission from ParaGard package insert):
  - Step 1:
    - Do not remove ParaGard from inserter tube prior to placement in uterus.
    - Do not bend arms of ParaGard earlier than 5 minutes before introduction into uterus.
    - If sterile gloves are not being used, device can be loaded by folding arms inside of partially opened package.
    - Pull solid rod partially from package so it does not interfere with assembly.
    - Bend arms of ParaGard and maneuver insertion tube to pick up arms.
    - Introduce solid rod into insertion tube alongside threads until it touches bottom of ParaGard.
  - Step 2:
    - Adjust movable flange to indicate depth to which ParaGard should be inserted.
    - Horizontal arms of ParaGard and long axis of flange should lie in same horizontal plane.
    - Introduce loaded insertion tube through cervical canal and upward until ParaGard lies in contact with fundus.
    - Movable flange should be at cervix.
  - Step 3:
    - Holding solid rod stationary, withdraw insertion tube no more than $\frac{1}{2}$-inch to release arms of ParaGard.

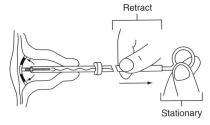

Retract

Stationary

- Step 4:
  - After arms are released, move insertion tube gently upward until resistance at fundus is felt.

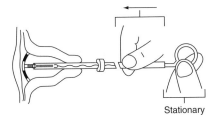

Stationary

- Step 5:
  - Hold insertion tube stationary and withdraw solid rod.

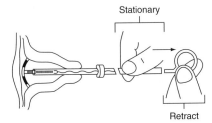

Stationary

Retract

- Step 6:
  - Withdraw insertion tube from cervix and trim strings 4 cm from external os.
  - Note length of strings in patient record.

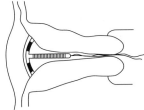

- Mirena insertion (figures reproduced with permission from Mirena package insert):
  - Pick up inserter containing Mirena and carefully release threads from slider.
  - Make sure that slider is positioned at top of handle nearest IUS.
  - Align arms of system horizontally using sterile surface or sterile gloved fingers.
  - Pull on both strings to draw Mirena into insertion tube.

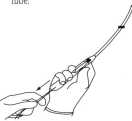

- Fix threads tightly in cleft at end of handle and set flange to depth measured by sound.

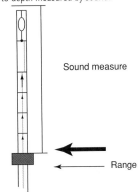

Sound measure

Range

- Hold slider firmly at top of handle and gently introduce inserter into cervical canal; advance into uterus until flange is 1.5–2 cm from external cervical os.

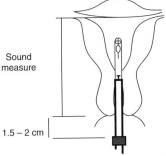

Sound measure

1.5 – 2 cm

- Hold inserter steady and release arms of Mirena by pulling slider back until top of slider reaches raised horizontal line on handle.

- Push inserter gently into uterine cavity until flange touches cervix.

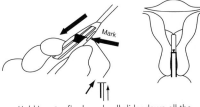

Mark

- Hold inserter firmly and pull slider down all the way to release Mirena.
- Remove inserter from uterus and cut strings 4 cm from external os.
- Note length of strings in patient record.

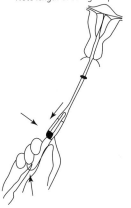

SYNONYM(S)
- Intrauterine device (IUD)
- Intrauterine contraceptive device (IUCD)
- IUS—Intrauterine system (Mirena)

CLINICAL PEARLS
- Take 2 IUCs in room with you for each insertion in case device is contaminated or dropped.
- DO NOT force sound if there is significant resistance.
- Allow patient to feel trimmed IUC strings so she knows what to check for at home.
- NSAIDs 1 hour prior to IUC insertion may reduce cramping/pain during and after insertion.

ABBREVIATIONS
- IUC—Intrauterine contraceptive
- LNG—IUS Levonorgestrel-releasing intrauterine system
- PID—Pelvic inflammatory disease
- STI—Sexual transmissible infection

CODES
ICD9-CM
- 69.7 Insertion of intrauterine contraceptive device
- 97.71 Removal of intrauterine contraceptive device

 PATIENT TEACHING

- Dispel myths about IUC.
- ACOG Patient Education Pamphlet: The Intrauterine Device. Available at: http://acog.org/publications/patient_education/bp014.cfm

Section VII

IN VITRO FERTILIZATION (IVF)

Jared C. Robins, MD

 BASICS

DESCRIPTION

- IVF is a process where a woman's eggs are retrieved from the ovaries and fertilized in the laboratory. The developing embryos can then be replaced in the uterus or cryopreserved.

Indications

IVF was initially developed for the treatment of tubal infertility. Over time, indications expanded to all aspects of infertility. The development of ICSI makes IVF/ICSI the most successful treatment for male-factor infertility.

Site (Office, Surgical Center, OR)

- Ovarian hyperstimulation is monitored in the office with serial US and hormone levels.
- Oocyte retrieval and transfer is typically performed in an outpatient surgical center.
- Fertilization of the oocytes is performed in a laboratory specially designed and equipped for IVF.

Concurrent Procedures

- See topic on ART
- ICSI:
  - Indicated for:
    - Male factor infertility
    - Prior fertilization failure
  - Single sperm is injected into the egg
  - May be associated with rare risk of birth defects
- Assisted hatching:
  - Process of thinning the zona pellucida prior to embryo transfer
  - Zona pellucida hardens with age.
  - Embryo hatching must occur prior to implantation.
  - Assisted hatching may improve pregnancy rates in:
    - Subjects >35
    - Subjects with prior failed IVF
    - Frozen embryo transfer
- Embryo cryopreservation:
  - May be used to preserve embryos for future transfers
  - Embryos can be frozen at the 2 pro-nuclear stage, cleaved stage, or blastocyst stage of development.
- Aspiration of hydrosalpinx:
  - Can be performed during oocyte aspiration
  - May be associated with improved pregnancy rates

Age-Related Factors

The success of IVF is inversely proportional to patient age. These rates are closely monitored by the CDC and SART. The statistics below were compiled from US fertility centers in 2003 and published by CDC/SART in 2005.

- Women age <35:
  - 43% of cycles result in pregnancy
  - 37% of cycles result in a live birth
  - 38% of live births have multiple infants:
    - 33% twins

- Women age 35–37:
  - 36% of cycles result in pregnancy
  - 30% of cycles result in a live birth
  - 32% of live births have multiple infants:
    - 28% twins
- Women age 38–40:
  - 27% of cycles result in pregnancy
  - 20% of cycles result in a live birth
  - 26% of live births have multiple infants:
    - 23% twins
- Women age 41–42:
  - 19% of cycles result in pregnancy
  - 11% of cycles result in a live birth
  - 17% of live births have multiple infants:
    - 15% twins
- IVF with donor eggs:
  - Indicated for:
    - Older patients
    - Patients with poor ovarian stimulation
    - History of recurrent abortion
  - The pregnancy rate is directly related to the age of the donor

EPIDEMIOLOGY

- >80,000 IVF cycles performed each year in the US:
  - 70% in women ≤37
  - 56% performed with ICSI
- Diagnoses:
  - Male factor: 17%
  - Tubal factor: 12%
  - Diminished ovarian reserve: 10%
  - Unexplained infertility: 10%
  - Ovulatory dysfunction: 6%
  - Other: 15%
- Multiple factors identified: 30% of cases:
  - Female factors only: 13%
  - Both female and male factors: 17%

 TREATMENT

PROCEDURE

- Treatment requires close monitoring by a specialist trained in ovarian hyperstimulation and oocyte retrieval. It also requires an embryology laboratory and staff trained in oocyte identification, oocyte and embryo manipulation, and tissue culture.
- Ovarian hyperstimulation:
  - Daily injections of gonadotropin containing FSH with or without LH
  - Follicular development is monitored with US and estradiol levels.
  - Ovulation is inhibited with a GnRH analogue or antagonist.
  - hCG is administered to initiate oocyte meiosis ~35 hours prior to retrieval.
- Oocyte retrieval:
  - Outpatient procedure, performed with conscious sedation or general anesthesia.
  - Follicles are aspirated transvaginally under US guidance with a needle fitted to the US probe.
  - Follicular fluid is given to the embryologist to identify the oocyte.

- Fertilization:
  - Egg and sperm are incubated together for ~16 hours (~150,000 sperm / oocyte).
  - Presence of 2 pro-nuclei indicates fertilization.
  - ICSI may be performed ~4 hours after retrieval.
- Embryo transfer:
  - Embryos are placed 1–1.5 cm from the uterine fundus with a plastic catheter.
  - May be performed with transabdominal US guidance
  - Typically performed 3–5 days after retrieval/fertilization

Informed Consent

Patients should be informed about the risks, benefits, and alternatives to IVF treatment. Separate consent should be obtained for the ovarian hyperstimulation, operative procedures including ovarian retrieval and embryo transfer, cryopreservation, and indicated concurrent therapies.

Patient Education

Intensive patient education is required to inform the patient of all the medications and procedures involved with their IVF cycle. This includes teaching the patients to prepare and inject the gonadotropin, GnRH agonist or antagonist, and/or hCG.

Risks, Benefits

- OHSS:
  - Affects 20% of IVF cycles
  - Severe in 3–5% of IVF cycles
  - Characterized by the development of ascites:
    - Leads to abdominal distention and pain
    - May restrict diaphragm causing respiratory distress
    - Oliguria may lead to electrolyte imbalance
  - Hemoconcentration may result in thrombosis
  - Treatment is supportive; paracentesis may improve respiratory status.
  - Condition worsens in pregnancy
- Vascular injury:
  - Anatomic position of the ovary is medial to the iliac vessels.
  - Arterial and venous puncture potential during retrieval
  - Treatment is typically observation:
    - May require transfusion
    - May require interventional radiology or vascular surgery
- Multiple pregnancy:
  - Involves 35% of all live births
  - Twin pregnancy most common
  - Associated with:
    - Pregnancy loss
    - Prematurity
    - Increased obstetric complications
    - Poor neonatal outcome
- Birth defects:
  - Increased risk of birth defects is controversial
  - Small increased risk noted in literature may be related to:
    - IVF procedures
    - Underlying infertility diagnosis
    - Small study populations studied

Alternatives

Alternative treatments for infertility depend on the patient's specific etiology. However, no alternative treatment will result in equivalent fecundity.

Medical

- Ovulation induction:
  - Subject must have normal reproductive anatomy with patent tubes.
  - May be effective for subjects with unexplained infertility or anovulation
  - Clomiphene citrate:
    - Selective estrogen receptor modulator
    - Induces pituitary FSH production by hypothalamic negative feedback
    - May have a negative effect on endometrial development
- Gonadotropin therapy:
  - FSH prepared by urinary purification or recombinant
  - May contain LH (urinary purified products)
  - Require daily injections and close monitoring
- hCG:
  - May be urinary purified or recombinant
  - Structurally similar to LH
  - Induces ovulation ~36 hours postinjection
- Insulin sensitizer

Surgical

- Establish tubal patency (see chapter on fallopian tube surgery)
- May be efficacious for proximal or distal tubal occlusion
- Not efficacious with multisite occlusion
- Procedures:
  - Tubal reanastomosis:
    - Connect distal and proximal fallopian tube remnants after tubal ligation
    - Pregnancy rate: 40–80%
  - Tubal cannulation:
    - Hysteroscopic procedure to repair proximal tubal occlusion
    - Pregnancy rate: 60%
  - Salpingostomy:
    - Create new tubal opening for distal tubal occlusion
  - Fimbrioplasty:
    - Reconstruct distal tube
    - Often performed with salpingostomy
  - Lysis of adhesions
- Laparoscopic ovarian diathermy:
  - Establish ovulation in PCOS
  - Laser drilling of the ovary
  - Ovulatory function restored: 80%

FOLLOW-UP

Patients are placed on progesterone for luteal support for the 1st 2–8 weeks after oocyte retrieval. This can be administered IM or vaginally. A pregnancy test is performed ~14 days after the transfer. US is performed at ~6.5 weeks estimated GA.

PROGNOSIS

Live birth rates are age-dependant as described. There is a slightly higher risk of low birth weight and pregnancy complications in pregnancies conceived by IVF. However, there are no recommendations regarding a greater degree of surveillance in these patients. There may be a greater probability of birth defects. The etiologies for these phenomena are unclear.

COMPLICATIONS

See "Risks, Benefits."

BIBLIOGRAPHY

Allen C, et al. Assisted reproductive technology and defects of genomic imprinting. *Br J Obstet Gynaecol.* 2005;112(12):158–194.

Barbieri RL. Female Infertility. In: *Yen and Jaffe's Reproductive Endocrinology: Pathophysiology and Clinical Management,* 5th ed. Philadelphia: Elsevier-Saunders; 2004.

Buckett WM, et al. Congenital abnormalities in children born after assisted reproductive techniques: How much is associated with the presence of infertility and how much with its treatment? *Fertil Steril.* 2005;84(5):1318–1319.

Klemetii R, et al. Complication of IVF and ovulation induction. *Human Reprod.* 2005;20(12): 3293–3300.

Wright VC, et al. Assisted reproductive technology surveillance-United States, 2003. *MMWR.* 2006; 55(SS04):1–22.

MISCELLANEOUS

SYNONYM(S)

- Assisted Reproductive Technology
- In vitro fertilization
- Test tube baby

CLINICAL PEARLS

- Pregnancy rates after IVF are improving:
  - Improved embryo handling
  - Better cycle management
- Numerous stimulation protocols have been developed to safely maximize the number of oocytes obtained from a given IVF cycle:
  - Poor responder
  - Hyper-responder
  - Use of agonist vs. antagonist

- IVF should be considered for infertility patients who have failed less invasive therapies.
- Multiple IVF cycles may be necessary to achieve success.
- Limiting the number of embryos transferred will reduce the number of higher-order multiple pregnancies.

ABBREVIATIONS

- ART—Assisted reproductive technology
- CDC—Centers for Disease Control
- FSH—Follicle-stimulating hormone
- GnRH—Gonadotropin-releasing hormone
- hCG—Human chorionic gonadotropin
- ICSI—Intracytoplasmic sperm injection
- IVF—In vitro fertilization
- LH—Luteinizing hormone
- OHSS—Ovarian hyperstimulation syndrome
- PCOS—Polycystic ovarian syndrome
- SART—Society for Assisted Reproductive Technology

CODES

ICD9-CM

- 256.39 Premature ovarian failure
- 256.4 Polycystic ovaries
- 628.X Infertility:
  - 628.0 Anovulatory
  - 628. 2 Tubal
  - 628.9 Unexplained
- V23.5 Pregnancy with history of infertility

PATIENT TEACHING

American Society for Reproductive Medicine Patient booklet: Assisted Reproductive Technologies. Available at: http://www.asrm.org/Patients/patientbooklets/ART.pdf

LABOR AUGMENTATION

John P. Horton, MD
Wendy F. Hansen, MD
James E. Ferguson, II, MD

 BASICS

DESCRIPTION
- *Induction* refers to any intervention used to initiate labor in a nonlaboring patient.
- *Augmentation* refers to any intervention used to intensify existing labor.
- *Cervical ripening* refers to any intervention used to prepare the cervix for induction of labor.

Indications
- Rare absolute indications for induction
- Consider GA, as well as maternal and fetal conditions.
- Indications may include:
  - Preeclampsia/Eclampsia
  - Postdates (>41–42 weeks)
  - PROM
  - Chorioamnionitis
  - IUGR
  - Nonreassuring fetal testing
  - Abruptio placentae
  - Fetal demise
- Induction is not indicated for maternal desire or lifestyle.
- Contraindications:
  - Placenta previa
  - Vasa previa
  - Pelvic obstruction

Site (Office, Surgical Center, OR)
With few exceptions, inductions should take place as an inpatient procedure with proper monitoring.

Concurrent Procedures
- Fetal monitoring:
  - External Doppler
  - Internal FSE
- Uterine monitoring:
  - External tocometer
  - IUPC
- Anesthesia:
  - Local
  - Intravenous
  - Epidural/Spinal

EPIDEMIOLOGY
- Induction of labor occurred in 20.6% of cases in the US in 2000.
- Rates vary according to patient population and hospital setting.

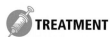 **TREATMENT**

PROCEDURE
Informed Consent
Patients must understand all indications, risks, benefits, and alternative procedures prior to initiating induction of labor.

Patient Education
Clinicians should provide information regarding:
- Mode/Method of induction
- Expected hospital course/stay
- Postpartum care

Risks, Benefits
- Risks:
  - Failed induction with need for surgical intervention
  - Bleeding
  - Infection
  - Anesthesia
  - Uterine rupture
  - Uterine hyperstimulation
  - Fetal intolerance to labor
- Benefits:
  - Shortened interval to delivery versus awaiting spontaneous labor

Alternatives
- Await spontaneous labor in the face of prescribed indications
- Consider close fetal surveillance

Medical
- Oxytocic agents:
  - Pitocin (synthetic oxytocin) IV
  - 0.5–40 mu/min, titrated to increasing dose at 15–30 minute intervals
- PGE1 agents:
  - Contraindicated in patients with previous cesarean section
  - Cytotec (misoprostol): Tablet (oral, buccal, vaginal)
  - 25 μg q3–4h, at term
  - >50 μg dosing associated with uterine hyperstimulation

- PGE2 agents:
  - Contraindicated in patients with previous cesarean section
  - Prepidil (dinoprostone): Cervical gel
  - 0.5 mg intracervical application q12h
  - Cervidil (dinoprostone): Vaginal insert
  - 10-mg insert placed vaginally q12h

Surgical
- Osmotic dilator (laminaria)
- Foley bulb
- Amniotomy (AROM)
- Membrane sweeping
- EASI

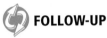 ## FOLLOW-UP

- Intrapartum:
  - Frequent monitoring of maternal and fetal status and well-being
- Postpartum:
  - Surveillance for abnormal bleeding or infection

PROGNOSIS
- Assessment of cervical status is the most important prognostic factor.
- The Bishop score is the most common cervical assessment tool in the US:
  - Bishop score (0–13):
    - Cervical dilation (0–3)
    - Cervical effacement (0–3)
    - Cervical consistency (0–2)
    - Cervical position (0–2)
    - Fetal station (0–3)
  - Bishop score ≥8:
    - High likelihood for vaginal delivery
  - Bishop score ≤5
    - ~50% risk of failed induction
- Multiparity, fetal weight <3,500 g, and a normal maternal BMI are associated with improved success rates.

COMPLICATIONS
- Uterine hyperstimulation
- Uterine rupture
- Nonreassuring fetal status
- Bleeding
- Chorioamnionitis
- Need for surgical intervention
- Hyponatremia/Water intoxication with prolonged oxytocin in high doses

BIBLIOGRAPHY

ACOG Practice Bulletin No. 10. Washington DC: ACOG; 1999.

Bishop EH. Pelvic scoring for elective induction. *Obstet Gynecol*. 1964;24:266.

Crane JM. Factors predicting labor induction success: A critical analysis. *Clin Obstet Gynecol*. 2006;49:573.

Martin JA. Births: Final data for 2002. National Center for Health Statistics. *Natl Vital Stat Rep*. 2003; 52(10):1–114.

 ## MISCELLANEOUS

CLINICAL PEARLS
- Assess fetal presentation:
  - Nonvertex lie may be considered a relative contraindication.
- Combining medical induction agents should be avoided secondary to increased risk for hyperstimulation.
- A low Bishop score may indicate need for cervical ripening prior to initiating induction.
- A low Bishop score also suggests a decreased overall success rate.

ABBREVIATIONS
- EASI—Extra-amniotic saline infusion
- GA—Gestational age
- FSE—Fetal scalp electrode
- IUGR—Intrauterine growth restriction
- IUPC—Intrauterine pressure catheter
- PGE—Prostaglandin E
- PROM—Premature rupture of membranes

 ## PATIENT TEACHING

- Teaching should center on explanations/description of induction method.
- Patients must understand all indications, risks, benefits, and alternative procedures prior to initiating induction of labor:
  - Expected hospital course/stay
  - Postpartum care, including any perineal care

Section VII

LABOR INDUCTION

Amanda L. Horton, MD
M. Kathryn Menard, MD, MPH

 BASICS

DESCRIPTION
Iatrogenic stimulation of uterine contractions prior to the onset of spontaneous labor to achieve a vaginal delivery

Indications
- Induction may occur for maternal or fetal indications when the risk of continuing the pregnancy is associated with a greater risk than delivery:
  - Maternal medical conditions:
    ○ DM
    ○ Chronic HTN
  - Fetal compromise:
    ○ Fetal growth restriction
    ○ Alloimmunization
  - Postterm pregnancy
  - Preeclampsia, eclampsia
  - Chorioamnionitis
- Labor may also be electively induced for various reasons:
  - Risk of rapid labor and delivery
  - Long distance from the hospital
  - Psychosocial reasons
- Should an elective induction take place, the best candidates are women with a favorable cervix and a well-dated pregnancy of at least 39 weeks documented by clinical criteria or with probable fetal lung maturity by amniocentesis.

ALERT
Contraindications to labor induction include:
- Transverse fetal lie
- Prior classical uterine incision
- Active genital herpes lesions
- Placenta previa
- Vasa previa

Site (Office, Surgical Center, OR)
Induction of labor should take place in a labor and delivery suite.

Concurrent Procedures
The fetal heart rate and uterine activity should be continuously monitored during labor induction.

Age-Related Factors
Maternal age has little impact on labor induction.

EPIDEMIOLOGY
- One of the most common obstetric procedures
- >20% of all deliveries are labor inductions.
- Induction rates are positively associated with:
  - Nulliparous women
  - White women
  - Higher formal education
  - Early prenatal care

 TREATMENT

PROCEDURE
A variety of methods and techniques exist for labor induction, including mechanical and pharmacologic methods.

Informed Consent
The patient should be counseled regarding the indication for induction, methods and techniques used for induction, and possible need for repeat induction or cesarean delivery.

Risks, Benefits
Nulliparous patients with an unfavorable cervix undergoing an elective induction have higher rates of operative and cesarean deliveries.

Alternatives
A preinduction assessment should confirm no contraindications to labor or vaginal delivery and to assess the likelihood of a successful induction:
- Cervical assessment
- Clinical pelvimetry
- Estimation of fetal weight
- Fetal presentation
- Confirmation of term gestation and probability of fetal lung maturity:
  - Fetal heart tones documented for 20 weeks by fetoscope or for 30 weeks by Doppler
  - 36 weeks have passed since a positive blood or urine hCG test
  - US measurement of a crown-rump length at 6–12 weeks or biometric marker between 13–20 weeks confirms GA of at least 39 weeks.
- Bishop score is a system that creates and assigns points and based on the following:
  - Cervical dilation
  - Effacement
  - Station
  - Position
  - Consistency
- A Bishop score of ≥ 5 indicates the likelihood of a vaginal delivery whether labor is induced or spontaneous.
- If the cervical score is unfavorable (≤ 5), patients may undergo techniques to ripen the cervix, to make it more favorable for induction.

Mechanical Methods
- Membrane sweeping:
  - Clinician's finger is placed beyond the internal cervical os and is rotated circumferentially along the lower uterine segment to detach the fetal membranes
  - Can be performed during an office visit
  - Associated with greater frequency of spontaneous labor and fewer inductions of postterm pregnancies

- Osmotic dilators:
  - Composed of hydrophilic materials
  - Absorb water and gradually stretch and dilate the cervix as they enlarge
  - 2 most common materials are sterile seaweed and synthetic hydrophilic materials
  - Placed in cervix through the internal cervical os
- Balloon catheter:
  - Transcervical Foley catheter
  - 14–26 gauge catheter
  - Placed through the internal cervical os
  - Inflated with 25–50 mL saline
  - Placed on traction by taping it to the inner aspect of the patient's thigh or placing a weight on the catheter

Medical
- Oxytocin:
  - Synthetic octapeptide hormone administered IV
  - Diluted 10 U in 1,000 mL of an isotonic solution for a concentration of 10 mU/mL
  - Uterine response begins 3–5 minutes after infusion.
  - Steady state is achieved in plasma by 40 minutes.
  - Uterine response depends on GA, with the highest sensitivity at term.
  - Low- and high-dose regimens
  - A maximum dose has not been established, although most labor units do not exceed 40 mU/min.
- Prostaglandins:
  - Effective for labor induction
  - Result in dissolution of collagen bundles and an increase in the submucosal water content of the cervix
  - Can be administered intracervically, intravaginally, and orally
  - Optimal type and dose for induction has not been determined.
  - Dinoprostone (PGE2) can be administered as:
    ○ Intracervical gel (0.5 mg in 2.5 mL) q6–12h, maximum of 3 doses
    ○ Vaginal insert (10 mg released 0.3 mg/hr) removed after onset of labor or after 12 hours
  - Misoprostol (PGE1) can be administered vaginally (25–50 μg) q3–6h.

ALERT
PGEs may increase the effect of oxytocin:
- 6–12 hours should pass after prostaglandin administration before initiating oxytocin.

ALERT
PGEs should not be used for cervical ripening or labor induction in women with prior uterine incisions due to the risk of uterine rupture.

Other Labor Induction Methods
- Nipple stimulation
- Amniotomy:
  - Artificial rupture of membranes
  - Can only be performed in women with a partially dilated cervix

ALERT
To reduce the risk of umbilical cord prolapse with amniotomy, the clinician should ensure fetal vertex is the presenting part and is well applied to the cervix.

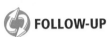 FOLLOW-UP

PROGNOSIS
- A multiparous woman with a favorable cervix, induction presents a high success rate for vaginal delivery.
- A nulliparous woman with an unfavorable cervix has a higher risk for prolonged labor and operative or cesarean delivery.
- Bishop score to assess cervical ripeness; higher score correlates with higher chance of successful induction

FACTOR	0	1	2
Dilation (cm)	0	1–2	3–4
Effacement (%)	0–30	40–50	60–70
Station	−3	−2	−1 or 0
Consistency	Firm	Medium	Soft
Position	Posterior	Mid	Anterior

- Bishop score ≥9 associated with successful induction; ≤5 increased risk of cesarean delivery

COMPLICATIONS
- All labor induction methods are associated with risk and complications that include:
  - Hyperstimulation:
    - Can occur with both oxytocin and prostaglandin use
    - ≥5 contractions in 10-minute period with evidence of fetal intolerance
  - Rates of hyperstimulation:
    - Intracervical PGE2 gel: 1%
    - Vaginal insert PGE2: 5%
    - Misoprostol PGE1: Rate varies based on dose and frequency of administration; ranges from 3–8%
    - Oxytocin: Rate varies
- Hyponatremia:
  - Oxytocin has a similar structure to vasopressin (antidiuretic hormone) and cross-reacts with the renal vasopressin receptor.
  - Should high doses of oxytocin be administered in large quantities of hypotonic solutions for prolonged periods of time (>24 hours), excessive water retention can occur and result in severe, symptomatic hyponatremia.
  - An electrolyte panel may be ordered if prolonged oxytocin is administered.
- Hypotension:
  - Can result from rapid IV injection of oxytocin
- Failed induction:
  - There are currently no standards for what marks a failed induction.
  - It is important to allow adequate time for cervical ripening and development of an active labor pattern before determining that an induction has failed.

BIBLIOGRAPHY

ACOG Practice Bulletin No. 10. Induction of Labor. Washington DC: ACOG; November 1999.

ACOG Committee Opinion No. 228. Induction of Labor with Misoprostol. Washington DC: ACOG; November 1999.

Boulvain M, et al. Mechanical methods for induction of labor. *Cochrane Database Syst Rev.* 2001; CD001233.

 ## MISCELLANEOUS

ABBREVIATIONS
- GA—Gestational age
- hCG—Human chorionic gonadotropin
- PGE—Prostaglandin

 ## PATIENT TEACHING

- ACOG Patient Education Pamphlet: Labor Induction. Available at: http://www.acog.org/publications/patient_education/bp154.cfm
- ACOG Patient Education Pamphlet: What to Expect after Your Due Date. Available at: http://www.acog.org/publications/patient_education/bp069.cfm

Section VII

LAPAROSCOPY, DIAGNOSTIC AND OPERATIVE

Mary T. Jacobson, MD

BASICS

DESCRIPTION
- Abdominal cavity is accessed through 2–10 mm incision using Veress needle, direct trocar, open Hasson, or microlaparoscope.
- Intraumbilical, infraumbilical, LUQ most common entry sites
- Distension usually with CO_2 gas
- Laparoscope is like a telescope, with light source and camera head attachments.
- Image projected onto a video monitor
- 2–12-mm ancillary ports for instruments act as extension of surgeon's hands.

Indications
Indications include various gynecologic diseases that were routinely treated with exploratory laparotomy in the past:
- Infertility
- Fibroids
- Ovarian cysts
- Endometriosis
- Hysterectomy
- Tubal reversal
- Malignancy
- Pelvic pain
- Pelvic floor disorders
- Urinary incontinence
- Lymph node dissection
- Surgical staging for malignancy

Site (Office, Surgical Center, OR)
- Outpatient surgical center for procedures that require no or a short (<1 day) hospitalization
- OR located within a hospital to accommodate larger and more complicated set-ups (e.g., robotic and transplant surgery, intraoperative radiation)
- Office for procedures that can be performed under conscious sedation, such as pain mapping and bilateral tubal ligation (rare).

Concurrent Procedures
- Gynecologic operative procedures performed via the laparoscope include:
  - Laparoscopic sterilization procedures
  - Ovarian cystectomy
  - Oophorectomy
  - Salpingectomy
  - Removal of ectopic pregnancy with salpingostomy
  - BSO
  - Oophoropexy
  - Myomectomy
  - Hysterectomy (includes supracervical and radical) with or without BSO
  - Appendectomy
  - Sacrocolpopexy
  - Burch urethropexy

  - Lysis of adhesions (enterolysis, ureterolysis, ovariolysis)
  - Treatment of endometriosis
  - Pelvic and abdominal lymph node dissection
  - Cerclage
  - Tubal reanastomosis
- Hysteroscopy
- Chromopertubation
- Pelvic exam under anesthesia
- Pelvic organ prolapse reconstructive procedures

Age-Related Factors
Pediatric Considerations
- Surgeons slow to adopt minimally invasive surgery because patients are smaller, operations are through smaller incisions, and conditions that require surgery are rare.
- RCTs comparing laparoscopy vs. laparotomy are difficult to perform because of parent, patient, and selection bias.
- Appears safe, with all the benefits of laparoscopy
- Improvement in techniques and development of smaller and shorter instruments allows laparoscopic procedures in small patients and the pediatric age group.

Pregnancy Considerations
- Favorable outcome data vs. laparotomy, with above advantages
- Nonemergent cases usually performed in early 2nd trimester
- Modify laparoscopic entry and trocar sites due to gravid uterus.
- Operate with patient in leftward tilt and with insufflation pressures of ≤ 12 mm Hg of CO_2 to maximize cardiac output and hepatic flow and minimize fetal acidosis.

Geriatric Considerations
- Consider comorbid conditions, such as cardiopulmonary compromise and acidosis.
- Overall decline in normal physiologic function
- Decreased recuperative reserve following surgical stress
- Safe, with benefits of laparoscopy as above

EPIDEMIOLOGY
- LAVH increased from 13% of all hysterectomies performed in the US in 1994 to 28% in 1999.
- Majority of surgical ectopic pregnancies are treated laparoscopically; from 41% in 1995 to 86% at 1 institution.
- Between 1994–1996, 89% of outpatient interval tubal sterilizations were performed laparoscopically.

TREATMENT
PROCEDURE
Informed Consent
- Always include exam under anesthesia on the consent form.
- Specify side (e.g., right ovarian cystectomy).
- Include all procedures that may be performed (e.g., diagnostic laparoscopy and possible operative laparoscopy with treatment of endometriosis, lysis of adhesions, appendectomy).
- Parental consent statutes for minors and emancipated minor vary by state.

Patient Education
- Explain procedure in detail using ACOG brochures, cartoons, photographs, videos, and authoritative web sites (e.g., www.AAGL.org).
- Review goals of surgery.
- Review patient expectations:
  - Familiarize patient with the surgical environment including preoperative area, surgical suite, and postanesthesia care unit.

Risks, Benefits
- Risks:
  - Infection
  - Bleeding
  - Bowel, bladder, ureter, nerve, vascular injury
  - Failure to improve symptoms
- Benefits:
  - Diagnosis and treatment
  - Resolution or improvement of symptoms
  - Optimization for fertility, incontinence, cancer treatment, sexual function

Alternatives

ALERT
Advantages over laparotomy:
- Magnification of operative field for optimal visualization
- Shorter hospital stay
- Quicker recovery
- Less pain medication
- Less adhesion formation
- Less blood loss

Surgical
- Can be divided into 3 parts: Entry, procedure, and exit
- Patient in dorsal lithotomy position and flat
- Foley catheter is placed in bladder.
- Stomach is decompressed.
- Entry site (e.g., intraumbilical) is selected.
- Entry technique is chosen (e.g., Veress).
- Incision site is preinjected with local anesthetic.

- Infraumbilical skin is elevated with a skin hook and intraumbilical incision made with scalpel (5–12 mm depending upon trocar diameter).
- Anterior abdominal wall is elevated with towel clips or surgeons' hands to optimize the distance between the anterior abdominal wall and the great vessels and bowel.
- Abdominal cavity is entered at a 90° angle:
  - Some authors recommend insertion angle of 45°.
  - Intraabdominal entry is confirmed using a laparoscope (i.e., 0° and 30° lenses differ by their angle of visualization; a 10-mm a 5-mm operative laparoscope allows the surgeon to use a laser and also allows passage of an instrument directly through the laparoscope).
- Abdominal cavity is insufflated with CO_2 gas to a pressure of 15 mm Hg.
- Evaluate area below entry site for trauma.
- Evaluate upper abdomen.
- Patient is placed in steep Trendelenburg to optimize visualization of pelvis.
- Ancillary incision sites (5–12 mm) are preinjected with local anesthetic.
- Lower quadrant trocars are placed lateral to the inferior epigastric vessels (at least 5 cm lateral from the midline to minimize risk of vascular injury) and at the level of the anterior superior iliac spine or above the uterine fundus, depending upon the procedure).
- Suprapubic trocar is placed 4 cm above the pubic symphysis to minimize risk of bladder injury.
- Instruments such as a suction irrigator, an energy source (e.g., bipolar, monopolar), traumatic and atraumatic graspers, scissors, morcellator, needle drivers are used interchangeably amongst these ports.
- A systematic evaluation of the pelvis is performed; landmarks such as the course of the ureters are evaluated and normal anatomy is restored to perform a successful procedure.
- Evaluate the surgical sites under 5 mm Hg intraumbilical pressure to assess for bleeding that may be tamponaded under higher pressures.
- Fascial incisions >5–10 mm are closed to minimize risk of hernia.
- Patient's abdomen is decompressed of CO_2 gas.
- Remaining trocars are removed under laparoscopic visualization.
- Laparoscope is removed while guarding against herniation of bowel or omentum.

FOLLOW-UP

- Both pre- and postoperatively, patient should be advised that she:
  - May experience transient (24–48 hours) nausea, vomiting, shoulder pain (i.e., due to CO_2 gas irritation of the phrenic nerve)
  - Should feel better each day and should call with symptoms (i.e., increasing abdominal pain, nausea/vomiting, fever, chest pain, shortness of breath, lower extremity pain)
  - Should not drive until at least 24 hours after surgery, and she is off of narcotics and reflexes are not inhibited from pain

- Should be physically active but defer exercise that increases intraabdominal pressure for 4–6 weeks
  - May remove wound dressings post-operative day 1
  - May take a shower after dressing removal
- Any new prescriptions and pain management plans should be reviewed with the patient preoperatively.
- Should follow-up in 2 weeks or sooner, if necessary
- Postoperative visit includes brief interim history, physical, suture removal (if necessary), discussion of procedure, operative findings, pathology report, and plan.

COMPLICATIONS

- Higher with operative vs. diagnostic laparoscopy
- Entry-related most common
- Types of injuries include:
  - Vascular (aorta, inferior vena cava, common iliac vessels, inferior epigastric vessels)
  - Bowel (small bowel, colon, duodenum, stomach)
  - Urinary tract (bladder, ureter)
  - Subcutaneous and omental emphysema
  - Infection, bleeding, ileus, bowel obstruction, adhesions, abdominal-pelvic pain

ALERT
Entry-related complications represent the majority of laparoscopic surgical complications.

BIBLIOGRAPHY

Bateman BG. Complications with operative laparoscopy. *Fert Steril*. 1996;66(6):1045–1046.

Hysterectomy Surveillance–U.S. 1994–1999. *MMWR*. 2002;51(SS05):1–8.

Jansen FW, et al. Complications of laparoscopy: An inquiry about closed versus open-entry technique. *Am J Obstet Gynecol*. 2004;190(3):634–638.

MacKay AD, et al. Tubal sterilization in the United States—1994–1996. *Fam Plan Perspect*. 2001;33(4):161–165.

Nezhat CR, et al., eds. *Operative Gynecologic Laparoscopy: Principles and Techniques*, 2nd ed. San Francisco: McGraw Hill; 2002.

Takacs P, et al. Laparotomy to laparoscopy: Changing trends in the surgical management of ectopic pregnancy in a tertiary care center. *JMIG*. 2006;13(3):175–177.

Wetter PA. *Prevention and Management of Laparoendoscopic Surgical Complications*, 2nd ed. Miami: Society of Laparoendoscopic Surgeons, Inc.; 2005.

MISCELLANEOUS
CLINICAL PEARLS

ALERT
- Use systematic routine for entry, ancillary port placements, and exit.
- Understand CO_2 opening insufflation pressure parameters, appropriate intraabdominal insufflation pressures, and CO_2 flow rate
- Accurately document intraabdominal fluid type, intake and output amounts, and deficit.
- Be familiar with equipment and new technology and mechanisms by which they work prior to the planned surgery:

  - Energy sources (monopolar, bipolar, radiofrequency, US, lasers)
  - Morcellator
  - Bags
  - Adhesive barriers
  - Hemostatic barriers
  - Meshes
  - Entry and closure devices
- Know your limits.
- Consider patient safety 1st.

ABBREVIATIONS
- BSO—Bilateral salpingo-oophorectomy
- LUQ—Left upper quadrant
- RCT—Random controlled trial
- LAVH—Laparoscopically-assisted vaginal hysterectomy

PATIENT TEACHING

ACOG Patient Education Pamphlets:

- Laparoscopy
- Sterilization by Laparoscopy
- Laparoscopically Assisted Vaginal Hysterectomy
- Endometriosis
- Dysmenorrhea
- Pain During Intercourse
- Treating Infertility
- Ovarian Cysts
- Uterine Fibroids
- Incontinence
- Pelvic Organ Prolapse
- Fibroids
- Pelvic Pain
- Abnormal Uterine Bleeding

LAPAROTOMY FOR BENIGN DISEASE

Thomas A. deHoop, MD

BASICS

DESCRIPTION

- Laparotomy is a surgical procedure to gain entry into the abdominal cavity for the diagnosis and/or treatment of surgical disease in the abdomen or pelvis. There are various ways to perform a laparotomy, and each is chosen depending on the urgency, indications, and associated perioperative conditions.
- Vertical skin incision:
  - Midline (median):
    - Skin incision is typically infraumbilical, but can be from xiphoid to symphysis.
    - Incise the fascia in the midline.
    - Incise peritoneum between the retracted rectus muscles.
    - Less blood loss and risk of hematoma
    - Rapid entry
  - Paramedian:
    - Skin and fascia are incised 1 cm lateral to midline.
    - Flap of fascia overlying the midline is dissected from the muscle to visualize linea alba.
    - Rectus muscles are retracted laterally to enter the peritoneal cavity between the rectus muscles, as in a median incision.
    - Possible increased infection rates and intraoperative bleeding
    - May reduce incisional hernias and rectus muscle nerve injury
    - Avoid midline skin incision in patients with previous paramedian, as blood supply between incision sites may be compromised.
- Transverse skin incision:
  - Pfannenstiel incision commonly used in gynecologic procedures:
    - Curvilinear skin incision (following Langer lines of skin tension) is made ~2 cm above symphysis
    - Rectus fascia is incised transversely and sharply dissected from rectus muscles superiorly and inferiorly.
    - Rectus muscles are retracted laterally in the midline, and the peritoneum is incised vertically.
    - Excellent cosmesis
    - Decreased risk of dehiscence compared with vertical incision
    - Increased blood loss and risk of subfascial hematoma
    - Limited exposure, especially to upper abdomen
    - Generally not used with malignant disease
  - Cherney:
    - Skin and fascia incision are similar to Pfannenstiel, but closer to symphysis.
    - Tendinous insertions of the rectus muscle to the symphysis are dissected and transected near the symphysis.
    - During closure, the rectus muscle tendons are reattached to the symphysis and lower edge of the rectus fascia.

- Better exposure than a Pfannenstiel, especially to the space of Retzius
- Pfannenstiel can be converted to a Cherney for better exposure.
  - Maylard:
    - Skin incision is 3–6 cm above the symphysis.
    - Fascia is incised, but not dissected from the rectus muscles; this prevents retraction of the muscles after transection.
    - Lateral edges of the rectus muscles are identified, and the muscles are gently dissected free posteriorly.
    - Isolation and ligation of the inferior epigastric vessels is made below the lateral edge of the muscles.
    - Muscle is transected with cautery.
    - Reapproximation of the fascia will bring the ends of the muscle in close proximity and create a tendinous insertion.
    - Avoid in patients with poor lower extremity circulation, as the inferior epigastrics may be important in the collateral flow.
    - Never convert a Pfannenstiel incision to a Maylard as the muscles will retract since they are detached from the rectus fascia.
    - Avoid a Maylard in a patient with a previous Pfannenstiel, as previous separation of the rectus sheath may allow retraction of the muscle.
    - Good exposure to pelvis
    - Low risk of subfascial hematoma

Indications

Access to the abdominopelvic cavity for the diagnosis or treatment of disease. Likely to be performed in concert with additional procedures.

Site (Office, Surgical Center, OR)

- Hospital-based operating room:
  - Postoperative care is required for at least 1–2 days, although "mini" laparotomy (small suprapubic incision) may be performed as same-day procedure
- Outpatient surgical center:
  - May be appropriate for "mini" laparotomy

Concurrent Procedures

- Cesarean delivery
- Exploration of abdominopelvic cavity
- Hysterectomy
- Salpingo-oophorectomy
- Salpingectomy
- Lysis of adhesions
- Myomectomy
- Tubal microsurgery
- Ovarian cystectomy

Age-Related Factors

With increasing age, many comorbid conditions must be considered when choosing the type of incision and closure:

- Obesity:
  - Avoid placing the incision in the moist, anaerobic subpannicular skin fold.
  - Retract the panniculus caudad to avoid incision into the subpannicular fold.
  - Midline paraumbilical incision may be necessary.
  - Consider subcutaneous sutures to close dead space if subcutaneous fat layer >2–3 cm.
- Risk of dehiscence:
  - Chronic lung disease, obesity, corticosteroid use, poor nutrition, diabetes, intraabdominal infections, age, previous abdominal surgery, and vertical incision
  - Mass closure of the anterior abdominal wall reduces incidence:
    - Suture passes through the fat, fascia, muscle, and peritoneum
    - Sutures tied loosely
    - Enter at least 1 cm from fascial edges
  - Consider retention sutures to reduce traction on incision.
  - Consider pelvic drain if surgical bed moist.

Pregnancy Considerations

- 1st trimester:
  - Spontaneous miscarriage rate is high and may be erroneously attributed to the procedure for incidental disease; avoid if possible.
  - Period of organogenesis and potential teratogenicity of medications
- 2nd trimester:
  - Ideal time to operate to avoid pitfalls of 1st and 3rd trimester
- 3rd trimester:
  - Greater risk of premature labor, PROM, and preterm delivery
  - Fetus more sensitive to hemodynamic shifts
  - Uterine size compromises exposure
  - For exploration, consider vertical incision

TREATMENT

PROCEDURE

Informed Consent
Required prior to laparotomy; the specifics depend on the indications and concurrent procedure(s) to be performed.

Patient Education
The specifics depend on the indications and concurrent procedure(s) to be performed.

Risks, Benefits
The specifics depend on the indications and concurrent procedure(s) to be performed.

Alternatives
- Varies depending on the indication
- Many procedures that have traditionally been performed with laparotomy are now performed with operative laparoscopy.
- Vaginal hysterectomy, if possible with less morbidity and shorter recovery than abdominal hysterectomy

Medical
- Hormonal management including progestin IUD to reduce menorrhagia may reduce need for hysterectomy.
- NSAIDs to reduce pain and inflammation
- GnRH agonist to induce menopause

Surgical
Conservative surgical approach with the excision of less unaffected organs:
- Laparoscopic or vaginal approach

 FOLLOW-UP

- Postoperative hospitalization for several days for pain control and hydration
- Discharge when pain is controlled with oral analgesics, voiding properly, and return of bowel function.
- Postoperative visit to the office in 1–2 weeks for wound evaluation

COMPLICATIONS
- Intraoperatively:
  - Injury to bowel requiring repair or colostomy
  - Injury to vessels
  - Injury to bladder requiring prolonged drainage
  - Excessive blood loss requiring transfusion
  - Cardiac or respiratory arrest secondary to complications from anesthesia
- Short-term:
  - Infection (wound, lung, bladder)
  - Wound dehiscence
  - Blood clot (DVT or PE)
  - Bowel dysfunction
- Long-term:
  - Pain as a result of scarring and/or adhesions
  - Failure to cure or diagnose
  - Need for additional surgery
  - Inability to complete planned procedure secondary to complications or unforeseen circumstances

BIBLIOGRAPHY

Gallup DG. Primary mass closure of midline incisions with a continuous polyglyconate monofilament absorbable suture. *Obstet Gynecol.* 1990;76:872–875.

Nichols DH, et al., eds. *Gynecologic, Obstetric, and Related Surgery,* 2nd ed. St. Louis: Mosby; 2000.

Rock JA, et al., eds. *Te Linde's Operative Gynecology,* 8th ed. Philadelphia: Lippincott, Williams & Wilkins; 1997.

 MISCELLANEOUS

SYNONYM(S)
Celiotomy

ABBREVIATIONS
- ACOG—American College of Obstetricians and Gynecologists
- DVT—Deep venous thrombosis
- GnRH—Gonadotropin-releasing hormone
- PE—Pulmonary embolism
- PROM—Premature rupture of membranes

CODES

ICD9-CM
ICD9 codes are based on the diagnosis and indications for surgery.

 PATIENT TEACHING

- Patient teaching specific to indications for procedure, alternatives, and specifics of postoperative recovery
- Written patient education brochures (ACOG or other) or videos specific to procedure
- Expectations regarding:
  - Time off work
  - Pain management
  - Scenarios that would dictate different intraoperative procedure
  - Risks, benefits, alternatives (surgical and nonsurgical)

Section VII

LAPAROTOMY FOR OVARIAN MALIGNANCY

Nita Karnik Lee, MD, MPH
Jonathan S. Berek, MD

 BASICS

DESCRIPTION

- Laparotomy via an adequate abdominal incision is indicated for known or suspected ovarian malignancy.
- A staging laparotomy should include:
  - Peritoneal washings for cytology
  - Total abdominal hysterectomy
  - Bilateral salpingo-oophorectomy
  - Infracolic omentectomy
  - Peritoneal biopsies
  - Retroperitoneal exploration including lymphadenectomy if no other evidence of extraovarian disease
  - Diaphragmatic sampling by biopsy or scraping for cytology

Indications

- Indications for laparotomy include large, complex adnexal or pelvic masses with clinical suspicion for malignancy on the basis of tumor size, tumor markers, patient age, or known malignancy.
- Laparotomy is generally performed to establish the diagnosis and stage the malignancy.
- The goal in patients with advanced disease is to achieve maximum cytoreductive surgery with little or no macroscopic residual disease
  - Optimal cytoreduction is defined as no residual lesions >1 cm.
  - Survival is directly related to the maximal size of residual tumor after initial laparotomy.
- Laparotomy (secondary debulking) can be considered for patients with recurrent disease in individualized cases.

Site (Office, Surgical Center, OR)

Exploratory laparotomy is performed in an OR with appropriate anesthesia support, monitoring, availability of blood products, and postoperative care resources, including intensive care units.

Concurrent Procedures

- Staging procedures generally performed at the time of laparotomy for ovarian malignancy include:
  - Omentectomy
  - Appendectomy
  - Peritoneal biopsies
  - Lymphadenectomy
- Other procedures depending on specific history and extent of disease include:
  - Hysterectomy
  - Bilateral salpingo-oophorectomy
  - Bowel resection
  - Pelvic tumor resection and debulking
  - Splenectomy
  - Placement of intraperitoneal port for appropriately selected patients

Age-Related Factors

- Age and patient comorbidities should be used to counsel patients regarding their individual perioperative risk factors.
- Advanced age alone is not a contraindication for appropriate exploration, staging, and attempts at maximal cytoreductive surgery.

EPIDEMIOLOGY

- In the US, the annual incidence of new cases of ovarian cancers is estimated to be 22,000. >16,000 women will die of their disease yearly.
- The lifetime risk of developing ovarian cancer is ~1.4%.
- 90% of all ovarian cancers are epithelial and primarily affect postmenopausal women.
- 10% are malignant germ cell or stromal tumors and are more common in younger reproductive-age women.

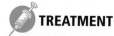 **TREATMENT**

PROCEDURE

Informed Consent

- Patients should sign consent for total abdominal hysterectomy, bilateral salpingo-oophorectomy, omentectomy, lymphadenectomy, appendectomy, tumor resection, and biopsies.
- The goal in patients with advanced disease is maximal cytoreductive surgery (tumor debulking).
- Any additional procedures based on preoperative imaging/survey of disease sites should be included on the surgical consent.

Risks, Benefits

- Risks:
  - General risks of laparotomy and staging for ovarian malignancy includes risks of infection, bleeding, need for blood transfusion, and damage to nearby organs including bower, bladder, blood vessels, or ureters.
- Benefits:
  - Accurate staging information which will direct appropriate adjuvant therapy and improved survival associated with maximal cytoreductive surgery.

Alternatives
Medical

- For patients with stage IV disease and/or those who are not surgical candidates, histological diagnosis of malignancy can be made via paracentesis, thoracentesis, or biopsy.
- Neoadjuvant chemotherapy followed by interval debulking surgery

Surgical

- Young women with early-stage disease who desire to maintain fertility options may opt to undergo unilateral salpingo-oophorectomy and staging with preservation of the uterus and opposite ovary:
  - This has been best studied in young women with germ cell tumors of the ovary, in which fertility preservation is standard.
- The role of laparoscopic staging in early ovarian cancers is being explored but is not current standard of care.

FOLLOW-UP

- Primary surgery is followed by adjuvant chemotherapy in patients with early-stage, high-risk disease and in all patients with advanced disease.
- Chemotherapy regimens vary with histology:
  - Epithelial ovarian cancer is treated with a taxane (paclitaxel) and a platinum-based drug (cisplatin or carboplatin).
  - Patients with advanced optimally cytoreduced epithelial ovarian cancer can consider intraperitoneal chemotherapy regimens.
  - Germ cell tumors of ovary requiring chemotherapy are traditionally treated with BEP (see Ovarian Tumors, Germ Cell).
- After initial surgery and chemotherapy, patients with ovarian malignancies should be followed closely with clinical exam, tumor markers, and imaging if indicated.

COMPLICATIONS

Retrospective data suggest that initial laparotomy:

- Major surgical morbidity: ~5%
- Surgical mortality: 1%
- Immediate perioperative complications include infection, bleeding, damage to nearby organs, and acute thromboembolic events.

BIBLIOGRAPHY

Berek JS, et al. Ovarian and Fallopian Tube Cancer. In: *Berek & Novak's Gynecology,* 14th ed. Philadelphia: Lippincott Williams & Wilkins; 2007;1457–1547.

Berek JS. Epithelial Ovarian Cancer. In: Berek JS, et al., eds. *Practical Gynecologic Oncology,* 4th ed. Philadelphia: Lippincott, Williams & Wilkins; 2005;443–509.

Bristow RE, et al. Survival effect of maximal cytoreductive surgery for advanced ovarian carcinoma during the platinum era: A meta-analysis. *J Clin Oncol.* 2002;20:1248–1259.

Chan JK, et al. Patterns and progress in ovarian cancer over 14 years. *Obstet Gynecol.* 2006;108:521–528.

Jemal A, et al. Cancer Statistics, 2007. *CA Cancer J Clin.* 2007;57(1):43–66.

MISCELLANEOUS

ABBREVIATIONS

BEP—Bleomycin, etoposide, and cisplatin

Section VII

LYSIS OF ADHESIONS

Tia M. Melton, MD

 BASICS

DESCRIPTION

- Adhesions are bands of fibrous tissue that form between or within tissues/structures of the body.
- They may be varied in appearance:
  - Thin and avascular
  - Thick, vascular or multilayered
  - Dense and inflexible
- Intraabdominal adhesions are common after surgery, and may span between:
  - Loops of bowel
  - Bowel and any other pelvic organs
  - Uterus, fallopian tubes, ovaries, bladder
  - Abdominal wall and pelvic/abdominal organs
  - Pelvic peritoneal surfaces
- Causes of adhesions include:
  - Previous surgery
  - Disease:
    - Endometriosis
    - IBD
  - Infections:
    - PID
  - Radiation therapy

Indications

- LOA in the asymptomatic or CPP patient remains controversial.
- LOA for patients with intestinal obstruction has clear benefits.
- Lysis of intrauterine synechiae/adhesions is recommended to treat infertility and improve pregnancy outcomes (see Asherman's Syndrome).
- Lysis of labial adhesions in the asymptomatic patient is not strongly recommended (see Labial Adhesions).

Pregnancy Considerations

In early pregnancy, an adnexal mass is an ectopic pregnancy until proven otherwise.

Site (Office, Surgical Center, OR)

- Lysis of abdominal/pelvic adhesions should generally take place in a surgical center or OR capable of managing the potential complications of the procedure.
- A few studies have advocated for 2nd and 3rd look LOA via mini/micro laparoscopy in the office or at a surgical center.

Concurrent Procedures

LOA may be performed at the time of laparotomy or laparoscopy and management of any other intraabdominal pathology.

EPIDEMIOLOGY

In most patients, intraabdominal adhesions do not cause a problem. Caution should be exercised in attributing pelvic pain to the presence of adhesions.

Incidence

- Studies suggest:
  - Up to 70% incidence of adhesions after multiple gynecologic surgeries
  - 50% incidence of adhesions in patient with a history of appendectomy
  - 20% incidence of adhesions in nonsurgical autopsied patients

PREVENTION

- There are no ways to completely eliminate or prevent abdominal/pelvic adhesions.
- Decrease the risk of adhesions by:
  - Using gentle surgical technique
  - Operating with powder free gloves
  - Minimizing bleeding
  - Using frequent irrigation
  - Achieving hemostatic without ischemia
  - Limiting the use of reactive foreign bodies (i.e., excessive suture, lint, talc, etc.)
- Adhesion-preventing agents include:
  - Intraperitoneal instillates
  - Adhesion barrier films

 TREATMENT

PROCEDURE

Informed Consent

The patient needs to be informed that LOA via laparoscopic or laparotomy may not "cure" her problem. Some studies have shown a 70% recurrence rate of adhesion formation. As with any surgical procedure, the risks, benefits, and alternatives must be discussed with the patient.

Patient Education

- The patient must be given information about her specific disease process.
- The success of LOA for infertility treatment depends on which other factors (endocrine or anatomical distortion) may be contributing to the patient's infertility.
- LOA for endometriosis is only 1 part of the overall treatment plan.

Risks, Benefits

- Risks:
  - Bowel perforation/damage to other internal organs:
    - Requiring prolonged hospital stays
    - Requiring an interval colostomy
  - Prolonged operating times
  - Bleeding
  - Infection
  - Fistula formation
  - Need for reoperation/additional surgeries and/or procedures
  - Incisional hernias
  - Continued CPP/endometriosis/infertility, etc.
  - Postoperative ileus

- Benefits:
  - Relief of bowel obstructions
  - Possible improved fertility
  - Possible relief of pain
    - Treatment of CPP with LOA has only been shown to be successful in observational studies.
    - Some studies have shown laparoscopy without LOA to be equally as effective as laparoscopy with LOA.

Alternatives
Medical

There are no medical alternatives for the treatment of adhesions; patients may elect to treat the underlying causes of their adhesions:

- Analgesics for CPP
- GnRH agonist for endometriosis
- Local anesthesia injections at trigger points identified during pain mapping surgery
- Physical therapy
- Acupuncture

Surgical

- If or when surgery is performed, it should be performed by a skilled, highly experienced operator.
- Adhesions are preferably taken down sharply, but blunt dissection is often necessary.
- Some studies suggest that laparoscopic LOA is preferable to laparotomy.
- Placement of an adhesion barrier (like INTERCEED) has been shown in some studies to decrease reformation of new adhesions.
- Clinical trials have shown no decrease in CPP with LOA except in those patients with severe/dense adhesive disease.

FOLLOW-UP

The usual postoperative surgical follow-up is recommended, although some studies advocate 2nd-look laparoscopic surgery to remove any new filmy adhesions.

PROGNOSIS

Adhesions tend to be a recurrent problem:

- As many as 11–21% of patients with LOA for bowel obstruction have a recurrence.
- Up to a 70% recurrence of new adhesion formation is possible.
- Surgery is both the cause and treatment of adhesive disease.

COMPLICATIONS

See Risks, Benefits; many complications are possible, including any related medical complications from anesthesia.

BIBLIOGRAPHY

Addis HM. Laparoscopic Lysis of Adhesions. In: Kavis MS, et al., eds. *Prevention and Management of Laparoendoscopic Surgical Complications*, 1st ed. Miami: Society of Laparoendoscopic Surgeons; 1999.

DeCherney AH. Preventing adhesions in gynecologic surgery. Available at: www.uptodate.com. Accessed 01/01/07.

Hammond A, et al. Adhesions in patients with chronic pelvic pain: A role for adhesiolysis. *Fertil Steril*. 2004;82:1483–1491.

Parker JD, et al. Adhesion formation after laparoscopic excision of endometriosis and lysis of adhesions. *Fertil Steril*. 2005;84:1457–1461.

Swank DJ, et al. Laparoscopic adhesiolysis inpatients with chronic abdominal pain: A blinded randomized controlled multi-centre trial. *Lancet*. 2003;361:1247–1251.

MISCELLANEOUS

CLINICAL PEARLS

- A thorough knowledge of the pelvic anatomy is a must.
- Place tension on the adhesion, not the underlying structure when performing adhesiolysis.
- Always clearly identify the surrounding pelvic organs before cutting adhesions (bowel, ureter).
- Be willing to stop the procedure, reassess and ask for help.
- Be able to use a retroperitoneal approach.
- Prepare the bowel.
- Provide adequate DVT prophylaxis.
- A complete preoperative assessment helps anticipate the level of difficulty of the procedure and what other specialist might need to be involved.
- Use caution when utilizing cautery or laser.

ABBREVIATIONS

- CPP—Chronic pelvic pain
- DVT—Deep venous thrombosis
- GnRH—Gonadotropin-releasing hormone
- IBD—Inflammatory bowel disease
- LOA—Lysis of adhesions
- PID—Pelvic inflammatory disease

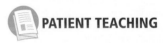

ICD9-CM

- 586.60 Lysis of adhesions, laparoscopically
- 587.40 Lysis of adhesions, open

PATIENT TEACHING

ACOG Patient Education Pamphlet: Pelvic Pain

MYOMECTOMY

Paula J. Adams Hillard, MD

 BASICS

DESCRIPTION

- Myomectomy is a surgical procedure to remove uterine leiomyomata (fibroids), leaving the uterus intact.
- The procedure can be performed via laparotomy, laparoscopy, or hysteroscopy.

Indications

- Symptomatic uterine leiomyomata in a woman who desires to preserve her uterus
- Traditionally, the procedure was felt to be indicated only in women who wanted to preserve child-bearing capability.
- Currently, there are women who desire uterine preservation for reasons other than planned future pregnancies.

Site (Office, Surgical Center, OR)

Typically performed in an operating suite

Concurrent Procedures

Additional procedures may be performed, depending on the indications and route:

- Laparoscopic lysis of adhesions
- Concurrent laparoscopy and hysteroscopy

Age-Related Factors

See note above regarding planned childbearing.

EPIDEMIOLOGY

- In 1999, 598,000 hysterectomies were performed in the U.S. for fibroids, compared to 30,000 myomectomies that year.
- Uterine fibroids were the indication for surgery in 33% of hysterectomies in 1999.

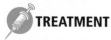 **TREATMENT**

Consideration should be given to treating preoperative anemia:

- Oral iron therapy
- GnRH agonist or other options for menstrual suppression
- Possible use of recombinant erythropoietin

PROCEDURE

- Surgical techniques for reducing blood loss with abdominal myomectomy:
  - A Cochrane review found limited evidence from a few RCTs that the following measures reduce intraoperative blood loss:
    ○ Misoprostol
    ○ Vasopressin
    ○ Bupivacaine plus epinephrine
    ○ Tourniquets
    ○ Chemical dissection

- Cochrane review found no support for oxytocin or morcellation
  - Incisions are placed transversely, parallel to arcuate vessels.
  - Dissection through myometrium and pseudocapsule can identify less vascular surgical plane.
  - Vascular casting studies indicate no vascular pedicle, but surrounding vascular layer.
  - Limiting the number of incisions has been suggested, but hemostasis within tunneled myometrial defects may be difficult.
  - Layered closure is placed promptly after removal of each myoma.
  - Cell savers should be considered to minimize need for blood transfusion or autologous blood donation.
- Laparoscopic myomectomy:
  - May be limited by the size, number, and location of myoma
  - Technically more difficult, involving laparoscopic suturing
- Prospective randomized studies comparing abdominal and laparoscopic myomectomies report:

  - Similar blood loss
  - Similar surgical times
  - Similar complication rates
  - Less postoperative pain, shorter stay and recover time with laparoscopic approach in selected patients
  - Possible lower rates of fever for laparoscopy
- Laparoscopic procedure:
  - Port placement is dictated by size and position of leiomyomas to be removed:
    ○ LUQ port if uterine size > umbilicus
  - Pitressin, as with abdominal approach
  - Transverse incision:
    ○ Dissection is in avascular plane after grasping myoma.
  - Alternatively, cryomyolysis or myolysis using bipolar, nd:YAG laser:
    ○ Myolysis may be accompanied by dense adhesions, impacting fertility
  - Bleeding is cauterized with bipolar cautery.
  - Several-layer closure is placed as needed.
  - Morcellation of myoma is performed under direct visualization.
  - Irrigation and suctioning
- Decreasing adhesions:
  - Unclear if fewer adhesions with laparoscopic approach
  - Adhesion barriers may be used:
    ○ Cochrane review found evidence for decreased adhesions with Interceed at laparoscopy or laparotomy; data are not sufficient to support improved fertility.

○ Gore-Tex may prevent adhesions, but must be affixed to uterus and later removed.
○ Limited evidence for Seprafilm
- Hysteroscopic myomectomy (See Hysteroscopy.)

Informed Consent

Patient should be informed of risks, benefits, alternatives, including risks of recurrence of fibroids, adhesions that may impact fertility, risk of conversion of laparoscopy to laparotomy, or laparotomy to hysterectomy.

Patient Education

Patient should be informed of size and location of uterine fibroids, as well as alternative procedures including observation or medical therapy.

Risks, Benefits

- While previous reports suggested greater risks of hysterectomy than myomectomy, recent reports do not support these concerns.
- Compared to hysterectomy, risks with myomectomy:
  - Case-control studies suggest less risk of intraoperative injury with myomectomy.
  - Longer operating times with myomectomy
  - Less blood loss with myomectomy
- Patients should be cautioned about the following surgical risks of myomectomy, which appear to be similar to the risks associated with hysterectomy:
  - Hemorrhage
  - Febrile morbidity
  - Unintended surgical procedure
  - Life-threatening events
  - Rehospitalization
- Additional risks of surgical procedures:
  - Bladder, ureteral injury
  - Bowel injury
  - Ileus
  - Pelvic abscess
  - Reoperation
  - Transfusion
- Patients should be counseled about the following future risks:
  - Persistent myomas
  - New myoma growth
  - Risk of adhesions that would impact fertility
  - Need for cesarean delivery in subsequent pregnancy
  - Risk of uterine rupture in subsequent pregnancy
- Risk of conversion of laparoscopic procedure to abdominal procedure
- Risk of subsequent surgical procedure

Alternatives

Many alternatives to myomectomy exist, both medical and surgical. Women should be informed of all options, their specific risks and benefits, as well as their applicability for their own specific situation.

Medical

Options for medical management depend on specific symptoms, but include:

- Observation
- NSAIDs
- GnRHa
- GnRH with add-back therapy
- Levonorgestrel-releasing IUS
- Oral progestins
- Combination OCPs, cyclic or continuous

Surgical

- Alternative routes for myomectomy:
  – Abdominal, laparoscopic, hysteroscopic
- Endometrial ablation
- Cesarean section and concurrent myomectomy
- Uterine artery embolization
- Newly approved technology of MR-guided focused US
- Hysterectomy (see topics):
  – Abdominal
  – Vaginal
  – Laparoscopically assisted

 FOLLOW-UP

- Clinical follow-up to assess recurrence of symptoms and quality of life may be the most important issue.
- US evaluation can detect new myomas, but may detect clinically insignificant myomas.

PROGNOSIS

- Relief of symptoms in up to 75%; depends on specific symptom, indications, comparison group
- Risk of persistent myomas in ~30% at 6 months
- Risk of new myomas may vary with:
  – Number originally removed
  – Use of preoperative GnRHa may make myomas more difficult to see and remove at surgery

  – Overall ~20–60% with new myomas
  – GnRHa may decrease risk of regrowth
- Risk of subsequent surgical procedure:
  – If single fibroid removed, subsequent surgery: 11%
  – Multiple myomas, subsequent surgery: 26%
  – Rates of hysterectomy after myomectomy: 4–17%
- Health-related quality of life was assessed in women with noncancerous pelvic problems (of whom 60% had fibroids):
  – Of those who had myomectomy, 51% were very satisfied with treatment, while 35% were bothered by adverse effects, and improvements in overall satisfaction were not significant.

COMPLICATIONS

See Risks.

BIBLIOGRAPHY

Banu NS, et al. Alternative medical and surgical options to hysterectomy. Bailliere's best practice and research. *Clin Obstet Gynaecol.* 2005;19(3): 431–449.

Kongnyuy EJ, et al. Interventions to reduce haemorrhage during myomectomy for fibroids. *Cochrane Database Syst Rev.* 2007;(1):CD005355.

Kuppermann M, et al., Effect of noncancerous pelvic problems on health-related quality of life and sexual functioning. *Obstet Gynecol.* 2007;110(3):633–642.

Parker WH. Laparoscopic myomectomy and abdominal myomectomy. *Clin Obstet Gynecol.* 2006;49(4): 789–797.

Parker WH. Uterine myomas: Management. *Fertil Steril.* 2007;88(2):255–271.

 MISCELLANEOUS

SYNONYM(S)

- Fibroids
- "Fireballs"
- Myomas
- Uterine leiomyoma
- Uterine leiomyomas
- Uterine leiomyomata

CLINICAL PEARLS

- Multiple alternatives exist for management of uterine myomas.
- In the absence of anemia or other medical sequelae, asymptomatic fibroids do not require treatment.
- Patients should be informed of medical and surgical options for management, which should be tailored toward specific symptoms.
- Perimenopausal women treated with GnRHa may remain amenorrheic.
- Surgeons should base recommendations on patient's needs, but be aware of own skills and limitations regarding techniques of surgery.

ABBREVIATIONS

- ACOG—American College of Obstetricians and Gynecologists
- ASRM—American Society for Reproductive Medicine
- GnRHa—Gonadotropin releasing hormone agonist
- IUS—Intrauterine system
- nd:YAG—Neodymium, yttrium, aluminum, garnet laser
- NSAIDs—Nonsteroidal anti-inflammatory drugs
- OCP—Oral contraceptive pill
- RCT—Randomized controlled trial

CODES

ICD9-CM

654.1 Tumors of body of uterus

 PATIENT TEACHING

- ACOG patient education pamphlets:
  – Fibroids
  – Dysmenorrhea
  – Pelvic Pain
  – Abnormal Uterine Bleeding
  – Hysteroscopy
  – Laparoscopically Assisted Vaginal Hysterectomy
  – Hysterectomy
- ASRM Patient Information Booklet: Fibroids

Section VII

OOPHORECTOMY AND SALPINGO-OOPHORECTOMY

Paula J. Adams Hillard, MD

BASICS

DESCRIPTION
- Oophorectomy, removal of the ovary, is often accompanied by salpingo-oophorectomy, which also involves removal of the adjacent fallopian tube.
- Elective oophorectomy or salpingo-oophorectomy may be performed at the time of hysterectomy in the absence of any ovarian disease; typically both ovaries and fallopian tubes removed—a BSO.
- Although oophorectomy may be indicated by disease, consideration should be given to the performance of an ovarian cystectomy with specific benign ovarian disease.

Indications
Indications depend on the presentation, acuity, timing in menstrual cycle, patient's age, likely pathology, findings on US, pelvic exam, and lab findings. Possible indications for oophorectomy include:
- Benign ovarian neoplasms in older woman
- Prophylactic oophorectomy at the time of hysterectomy (see Risks, Benefits)
- Prophylactic oophorectomy for women with inherited BRCA1/2 mutation associated with increased risk of breast and ovarian cancer
- TOA without adequate response to antibiotics
- Definitive surgery for endometriosis
- With GI malignancy, to present ovarian metastases
- Gonadial dysgenesis in phenotypic females with Y chromosome after puberty, to prevent risk of ovarian malignancy
- Other metastatic cancers: Breast, lung, melanoma
- Ovarian malignancies (See Ovarian Tumors.)

Site (Office, Surgical Center, OR)
Surgical center or OR

Concurrent Procedures
- Salpingectomy
- Appendectomy
- Lysis of adhesions
- Tubal sterilization

EPIDEMIOLOGY
- 90% of the 600,000 hysterectomies performed annually in US are for benign disease.
- From 1965 to 1999, the percentage of hysterectomies accompanied by oophorectomy increased from 25% to 55%.
  - 38% of women 18–44 have concurrent oophorectomy
  - 78% of women 45–60

TREATMENT

PROCEDURE
- If the preoperative assessment suggests benign disease, laparoscopy is a reasonable surgical approach, although the surgeon's judgment is based on patient's age, presentation, weight, and medical conditions.
- Intraoperative findings suggestive of malignancy mandate laparotomy with appropriate staging procedures (see Laparotomy for Malignancy).
- Laparoscopic procedure:
  - Inspect pelvis for signs of malignancy.
  - Isolate infundibulopelvic ligament and visualize ureter.
  - Control ovarian ligament and infundibular pelvic ligament using:
    - Pre-tied suture loops
    - Bipolar cautery
    - Stapling device
    - Harmonic scalpel
  - Place ovary in specimen bag.
  - Remove ovary through:
    - Laparoscopic port
    - Colpotomy incision
    - Minilaparotomy incision
- Laparotomy:
  - Divide round ligament and dissect retroperitoneal space to identify ureter.
  - Divide ovarian ligament.
  - Isolate infundibulopelvic ligament.
  - Doubly clamp, divide, and doubly ligate infundibular pelvic ligament.
  - If salpingectomy is also performed and tube is removed with the ovary, the ovarian ligament and fallopian tube are clamped together just lateral to the uterus.

Informed Consent
As with any surgical procedure, the indications, risks, benefits, and alternatives are discussed with the patient and documented.

Patient Education
The individual woman's risk for ovarian malignancy should be discussed. For women of average risk of ovarian cancer, the risks of prophylactic oophorectomy at the time of hysterectomy should be weighed against the potential risks.

Risks, Benefits
In a study of long-term mortality after elective oophorectomy in women of average risk for ovarian malignancy, using modeling, preservation of ovaries rather than oophorectomy was associated with higher survival rates.
- For women 50–54 years old with ovarian preservation at the time of hysterectomy, the probability of surviving to age 80 was 62% vs. 54% with oophorectomy:
  - Improved survival related to fewer women dying of cardiovascular disease and/or hip fracture
- After age 64, there was no survival advantage
- Risks: Oophorectomy has been linked to higher rates of:
  - Cardiovascular disease
  - Osteoporosis
  - Hip fracture
  - Dementia
  - Short-term memory impairment
  - Decline in sexual function
  - Decreased psychological well-being
  - Adverse skin and body composition changes
  - Adverse ocular changes
  - More severe hot flashes
  - Urogenital atrophy
- Benefits: Potential benefits of elective oophorectomy:
  - Prevention of ovarian cancer
  - Decrease in risk of breast cancer
  - Reduced risk of pelvic pain
  - Reduced risk of subsequent pelvic surgery

Alternatives

- Observation and expectant management of functional ovarian cysts
- Detorsion of adnexal torsion without oophorectomy (See Adnexal Torsion.)
- Ovarian cystectomy (See topic.)
- Preservation of ovary at time of hysterectomy, depending on age and risk/benefit analysis

Medical

- Observation is appropriate for even symptomatic ovarian cysts if the likely diagnosis is a functional cysts, as these cysts will resolve over time.
- Because OCPs prevent ovulation, the development of follicular and corpus luteal cysts is minimized.

Surgical

- If oophorectomy is indicated, decision must be made among laparoscopy vs. laparotomy vs. mini-laparotomy.
- Advantages of laparoscopic oophorectomy:
  – Decreased recovery time
  – Shorter hospital stay
  – Less expense
  – Less risk of pelvic adhesions, and thus potentially fertility preservation
  – Less febrile morbidity
  – Less postoperative pain
  – Fewer postop complications
- Disadvantages of laparoscopy:
  – Possible spill of tumor cells if malignant

 ## FOLLOW-UP

Depending on surgical approach, postoperative visit scheduled:

- Typically 2 weeks postoperatively if laparoscopy
- 3–6 weeks postoperatively if laparotomy

PROGNOSIS

Depends on indications

COMPLICATIONS

Complication rates are similar to other pelvic surgeries.

BIBLIOGRAPHY

Parker WH, et al. Ovarian conservation at the time of hysterectomy for benign disease. *Obstet Gynecol*. 2005;106(2):219–226.

Shoupe D, et al. Elective oophorectomy for benign gynecological disorders. *Menopause*. 2007;14(3 Pt 2):580–585.

Valea FA, et al. Oophorectomy, ovarian cystectomy, oophoropexy. Available at: www.uptodate.com. Accessed 09/22/07.

 ## MISCELLANEOUS

CLINICAL PEARLS

Oophorectomy, unless for malignant disease, should be avoided if at all possible. Situations in which alternatives to oophorectomy should be strongly considered include:

- Ovarian torsion
- Benign cystic teratoma
- Ruptured ovarian cyst

ABBREVIATIONS

- BSO—Bilateral salpingo-oophorectomy
- OCP—Oral contraceptive pill
- TOA—Tubo-ovarian abscess

 ### CODES

ICD9-CM/CPT

- 58150 TAH-BSO
- 58700 Salpingectomy
- 58940 Oophorectomy

PATIENT TEACHING

Up-to-date patient education materials are not currently available, given the very recent publication of analyses assessing the risks vs. benefits of elective oophorectomy.

Section VII

OVARIAN CYSTECTOMY

Paula J. Adams Hillard, MD

 BASICS

DESCRIPTION

Ovarian cystectomy is performed as an ovarian-conserving procedure when a benign cyst is removed from the ovary. Enucleation of a benign solid tumor can also be performed to preserve ovarian tissue. Oophorectomy may be performed if it is the surgeon's judgment that insufficient ovarian tissue would remain or that the ovary cannot be preserved.

Indications

Benign ovarian cyst requiring surgery, with anticipated sufficient normal ovarian tissue remaining, and patient desires attempted ovarian conservation

Site (Office, Surgical Center, OR)

OR, operating suite

Concurrent Procedures

- Typically performed as stand-alone procedure, although if other procedures indicated, could be combined (e.g., urogynecologic)
- If endometriosis, could be combined with laser or cautery ablation of endometriotic implants

Age-Related Factors

- Benign neoplastic cysts can occur in any age group.
- Ovarian tumors in the premenarchal and postmenopausal age group are more likely to be benign.

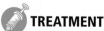 **TREATMENT**

- Avoid the removal of functional cysts, which resolve spontaneously without surgery (see Ovarian Cysts, Functional).
- With a persistent mass, surgery is indicated; the decision to perform cystectomy vs. oophorectomy can be challenging:
  - Cystectomy maximizes future ovarian follicle and functional capacity, and is generally preferable in young women.
    - Even a very thin capsule of ovarian cortex will typically contain stroma and follicles; remodeling of ovarian tissue typically occurs.
  - The normalcy of the contralateral ovary should be assessed at the time of surgery, but the possibility of a subsequent event compromising the other ovary should also be considered, such as:
    - Adnexal torsion
    - Benign or borderline tumor requiring oophorectomy
  - Oophorectomy should be performed if malignancy is likely.

- The preoperative assessment of likelihood of malignancy is based on patient's age, US characteristics of the ovarian mass, tumor markers if indicated as in postmenopausal women, the presence of ascites, or other characteristics suggesting malignancy (capsule excrescences, matted bowel, adenopathy, dense adhesions).
- Most ovarian cystectomies can be performed laparoscopically, particularly those in which the preoperative diagnosis is:
  - Probable dermoid
  - Endometrioma
  - Simple cysts that have not resolved with expectant management
- See chapter on laparoscopy regarding relative merits of laparoscopy vs. laparotomy, with shorter recovery time and hospital stay.
- Some clinical situations may be better managed via laparotomy, including mini-laparotomy. Situations in which many or most gynecologists would perform a laparotomy include:
  - Ovarian malignancy or strong suspicion of malignancy, in an effort to minimize the risks of spill of cancer cells
  - Large benign cystic teratomas (dermoids), to minimize the risks of cyst rupture and subsequent granulomatous/chemical peritonitis

PROCEDURE

Informed Consent

The patient should be informed of:

- Planned technique—laparoscopy vs. laparotomy—and the possibility of conversion of laparoscopy to an open procedure
- Usual risks associated with any surgery:
  - Infection
  - Bleeding, possibly requiring transfusion
  - Intraoperative injury to bowel, bladder, other pelvic organs
- The planned procedure—ovarian cystectomy—with information about what eventualities would lead to oophorectomy:
  - Findings suggesting malignancy
  - Inability to performed cystectomy with complete removal of pathology
  - Excessive bleeding or other intraoperative technical challenges

Patient Education

Patient should be informed of possible need for oophorectomy rather than cystectomy, but that if the other ovary is intact and normal, hormonal function should be unchanged:

- Regular menses
- Regular ovulation
- Fertility: Women with a single ovary do not generally have reduced fertility potential to conceive, either naturally or with IVF.
- Earlier menopause: 1 study found women with early menopause more likely to have had "incessant ovulation":
  - Earlier menarche, fewer pregnancies, less COC use, more likely to have had unilateral oophorectomy

Risks, Benefits

The benefits of preservation of ovarian tissue with ovarian cystectomy vs. the risks of incomplete removal of pathology and possible recurrence should be discussed.

Alternatives

- Oophorectomy is alternative to cystectomy
- Cyst aspiration is not recommended, as:
  - Recurrence rates are high (11–65%)
  - Malignant cyst fluid may be spilled
  - Cytology on cyst fluid is not reliable for diagnosis of malignancy (sensitivity 25–82%)
- Fenestration: Creating larger full-thickness window in a portion of the cyst wall may be less likely to result in reaccumulation, but cystectomy is generally preferable.

Medical

Observation for spontaneous resolution is indicated for ovarian masses with US characteristics suggesting functional cysts (see Ovarian Cysts, Functional).

Surgical

- Laparoscopic cystectomy:
  - Visualize pelvis and abdomen and assess whether laparoscopic cystectomy appears to be feasible and whether there appears to be any signs suggesting malignancy:
    - Biopsy suspicious sites and send for frozen section.
  - Determine port sites, typically infraumbilical, suprapubic, and contralateral to ovarian cyst or bilateral lower quadrant.
  - Obtain pelvic washings.

- Lyse adhesions if necessary.
- Stabilize utero-ovarian ligament.
- Incision is placed using unipolar cautery or harmonic scalpel through capsule and dissection of cyst wall:
  ○ Some surgeons perform aspiration or cystotomy, but intact cyst may be easier to dissect, depending on cyst type.
  ○ If spill of cyst occurs, irrigate copiously.
- Grasp wall of cyst and dissect from ovarian stroma using sharp or blunt dissection with:
  ○ Endoscopic scissors
  ○ Electrocautery, uni- or bipolar
  ○ Blunt probe
  ○ Laser
- Place cyst into specimen bag and remove through port (can aspirate in the bag) or through minilaparotomy or colpotomy incision.
- Assess for hemostasis.
- Cauterize as required for hemostasis, but minimize tissue damage.
• Laparotomy with cystectomy:
- As with laparoscopy, assess likelihood of malignancy, obtain pelvic washings, lyse adhesions.
- Longitudinal incision is placed in ovarian cortex in avascular area away from tube.
- Develop plane using blunt or sharp dissection to allow cyst to be shelled out, preferably intact.
- May need to cauterize base of cyst to obtain hemostasis.
- If spill of cyst occurs, irrigate copiously.
- If necessary, reapproximate ovarian tissue, keeping sutures within the deep tissue; avoid surface sutures that may increase the risks of adhesions.
- Gentle tissue handling is indicated.
- Some evidence of benefit of hyaluronic acid agents to decrease adhesions (Cochrane database).

 FOLLOW-UP

PROGNOSIS

The prognosis for ovarian function after cystectomy is good.

COMPLICATIONS

- Complications after ovarian cystectomy are similar to those typically seen with laparoscopy or laparotomy.
- With laparoscopy, ureteral injury can occur.
- Spill of malignant cyst fluid has been suggested as worsening the prognosis of early-stage ovarian cancer.
- Risk of chemical peritonitis due to spill of contents of ovarian benign cystic teratoma (dermoid)
- Adhesion formation may increase risks of:
  - Infertility
  - Ectopic pregnancy
  - Small bowel obstruction
  - Chronic pelvic pain

BIBLIOGRAPHY

ACOG Practice Bulletin No. 83. Management of Adnexal Masses. Washington DC: ACOG; July 2007.

Cramer DW, et al. Does "incessant" ovulation increase risk for early menopause? *Am J Obstet Gynecol*. 1995;172(2 Pt 1):568–573.

Lass A. The fertility potential of women with a single ovary. *Human Reprod Update*. 1999;5(5):546–550.

Valea FA, et al. Oophorectomy, ovarian cystectomy, and oophoropexy. Available at: www.uptodate.com. Accessed 09/28/07.

 MISCELLANEOUS

CLINICAL PEARLS

- Observation for 5–10 weeks is warranted if US appearance suggests functional cyst.
- Aggressive management of ovarian cysts with oophorectomy is generally to be avoided unless malignancy is present.
- Ovarian cystectomy is generally preferable to oophorectomy if surgery is indicated.
- Laparoscopy provides faster recovery for patient, but is not always feasible or appropriate.

ABBREVIATIONS

- COC—Combined oral contraceptive
- IVF—In vitro fertilization

 CODES

ICD9-CM/CPT

- 620.2 Other unspecified ovarian cyst
- 220 Benign neoplasm of ovary
- 620.0 Follicular cyst of ovary
- 620.1 Corpus luteum cyst of hematoma
- 58925 Ovarian cystectomy
- 58662 Laparoscopy, surgical, removal of cysts of ovaries

PATIENT TEACHING

ACOG Patient Education Pamphlet: Ovarian Cysts

OVULATION INDUCTION

Michael D. Scheiber, MD, MPH

 BASICS

DESCRIPTION

Normal folliculogenesis and subsequent ovulation is necessary for conception to occur. Disorders of ovulation are the most common cause of female infertility. Inducing normal ovulation in women with disordered ovulation will restore normal fertility potential in the absence of other etiologies of infertility. The use of medications to achieve ovulation in anovulatory or oligo-ovulatory women is known as OI.

- The goal of ovulation induction is the development of a single mature follicle with subsequent release of a single mature oocyte.
- OI should be differentiated from superovulation (or controlled ovarian stimulation) undertaken for the treatment of infertility related to factors other than anovulation, in which the goal of treatment is to induce the maturation of multiple follicles.

Indications

- Women with anovulation or oligo-ovulation who wish to conceive
- Most women with regular menses occurring 27–32 days apart accompanied by moliminal symptoms are ovulatory.
- Ovulation can easily be confirmed by a luteal-phase progesterone level of >3 ng/mL, although conception may be more likely in cycles with luteal-phase progesterone levels >10 ng/mL.
- In the absence of ovulation, OI is indicated, starting in the early follicular phase of the cycle.
- Anovulatory women with amenorrhea may require a progesterone withdrawal bleed prior to initiating therapy.
- Disorders of thyroid, prolactin, and weight should be addressed before starting OI.
- Evaluation of FSH levels can be helpful in choosing the appropriate choice of ovulation induction agents.

Pregnancy Considerations

It may be difficult for some women with irregular cycles to determine if they are pregnant. Therefore, either a urine or serum pregnancy test should be performed prior to starting any medications for OI if there is any doubt as to a patient's pregnancy status.

EPIDEMIOLOGY

- Ovulatory dysfunction accounts for almost 1/2 of female infertility.
- Based on FSH levels, 3 categories:
  - Hypogonadotropic:
    - Primarily due to hypothalamic disorders related to weight or body composition, excessive exercise, or severe emotional stress
    - Often poor response to oral agents like clomiphene; may require gonadotropin therapy
  - Normogonadotropic or eugonadotropic:
    - The most common type of anovulation
    - Often associated with hyperandrogenism and hyperinsulinemia suggesting PCOS
    - 4–8% of adult females have PCOS
  - Hypergonadotropic:
    - Anovulation often due to POF, which does not respond well to any stimulation protocol
    - Karyotype should be performed on women <35 with POF. These women may benefit from oocyte donation.

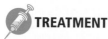 **TREATMENT**

PROCEDURE

- Several oral OI agents are available. All of the currently available gonadotropins are injectable via the self-administered SC route.
- Clomiphene citrate: Useful in eugonadotropic and rare cases of hypogonadotropic anovulation:
  - Nonsteroidal mixed estrogen agonist-antagonist with long half-life. Blocks hypothalamic estrogen receptors, causing an increase in endogenous FSH secretion
  - Starting dose: 50 mg/d for 5 days starting days 3, 4, or 5 of the full menstrual flow
  - Documentation of ovulation with serum progesterone levels or US monitoring
  - Coitus timed by US or urine LH monitoring or empirically every other day for 8 days starting on the 4th day after the last dose.
  - If ovulation occurs at a given clomiphene dose, the same dose is repeated with the menses.
  - No benefit to increasing dosage beyond the ovulatory dose for OI
  - If ovulation does not occur at a given dose, incremental increases of 50 mg/d are given to a maximum of 200 mg/d.

- In hyperandrogenic women (DHEAS >2 μg/mL) not responding to clomiphene, the addition of dexamethasone 0.5 mg/d may improve the response.
- Women who do not ovulate on high doses of clomiphene or who have not conceived after 3–4 ovulatory cycles should be referred to a reproductive endocrinologist.
- Twin rates: 7–8%
- High-order multiple pregnancies: <1%
- Common side effects: Hot flushes, mood changes, and a decrease in endometrial thickness or cervical fluid
- Metformin: An oral biguanide insulin-sensitizing agent useful for OI in patients with PCOS and insulin resistance (hyperinsulinemia):
  - Should not be initiated in patients with abnormal renal or hepatic function
  - Start at 500 mg/d and increase over 2–3 weeks (as GI tolerance allows) to 500 mg t.i.d.–q.i.d. Extended-release form may be better tolerated with 1,500–2,000 mg/d with the evening meal.
  - Periodic progesterone levels may be monitored to see if ovulation is occurring.
  - In the absence of ovulation after 12 weeks of therapy, can add clomiphene citrate therapy, as above.
  - Metformin may also be used to improve the response to gonadotropin therapy in clomiphene-resistant PCOS.
  - Category B drug in pregnancy
  - No increased risk of multiple pregnancy with metformin alone.
- Aromatase inhibitors: Not FDA approved but potentially useful in eugonadotropic anovulation and rare cases of hypogonadotropic anovulation:
  - Reduce estrogen levels in the hypothalamus thereby increasing release of endogenous gonadotropins
  - Fewer side effects than with clomiphene
  - May provide a superior uterine environment when compared to clomiphene
  - Similar pregnancy rates but lower twin rates than clomiphene
  - Letrozole 2.5–7.5 mg/d on cycle days 3–7
  - Monitoring and coitus same as clomiphene

- Gonadotropins: Useful in hypogonadotropic and eugonadotropic anovulation and rarely in hypergonadotropic anovulation:
  - All available products injected SC:
    ○ Purified human menopausal gonadotropins (containing both FSH and LH)
    ○ Recombinant human FSH and LH products
  - Stimulate the ovaries directly
  - Associated with >80% ovulation rates
  - Per cycle pregnancy rates: 15–30%
  - Following a baseline US evaluation, injections are started in the early follicular phase and usually administered daily.
  - Transvaginal US and serum estradiol levels are monitored serially until lead follicles reach maturity. Ovulation is then triggered by administration of an hCG shot that physiologically mimics the LH surge.
  - Multiple pregnancy rates are high (20–30%), including significant risk of higher-order multiples.
  - Rare risk of severe OHSS not present with the oral agents:
    ○ Severe OHSS may result in ARDS, renal failure, or even death.
  - Costs to the patient: Often $500–1,000/cycle.
  - Because of the risks and expense, gonadotropin therapy should only be managed by physicians with specialty training in their use.
- Dopaminergic agonists: Useful only in those patients with anovulation associated with hyperprolactinemia:
  - Evaluate etiology of hyperprolactinemia prior to initiating therapy.
  - Bromocriptine or cabergoline:
    ○ Restore normal prolactin levels.
    ○ Usually result in normal ovulation and fecundity
- GnRH agonists: Useful in patients with hypogonadotropic anovulation and some cases of eugonadotropic anovulation:
  - IV or SC infusion pump
  - Pulsatile administration restores ovulation in patients with hypothalamic amenorrhea and a normal pituitary.
  - Lower risk of OHSS or multiple pregnancy than gonadotropin therapy
  - Should only be attempted by those with specialty training in this area

Risks, Benefits
- Increased risk of multiple pregnancy from some OI medications
- Risk of OHSS
- 3–4 ovulatory cycles is an average time frame to conceive, depending on patient's age

Alternatives
Surgical
For patients with PCOS who do not conceive with medical OI, surgical therapy (either wedge resection or laparoscopic ovarian drilling) may be considered with expectation of reasonable success. Postoperative adhesions and surgical risks may complicate this treatment choice.

FOLLOW-UP

- Perform serum or urine pregnancy test ~14 days after presumed ovulation or with a missed menses.
- Some physicians elect to do a pelvic exam or baseline US before starting another round of clomiphene or letrozole.
- Pelvic exam or baseline US should always be done before initiating a subsequent cycle of gonadotropins.

PROGNOSIS
40–45% of couples using clomiphene citrate will become pregnant within 6 cycles.

COMPLICATIONS
See specific medications.

BIBLIOGRAPHY

Atay V, et al. Comparison of letrozole and clomiphene citrate in women with polycystic ovaries undergoing ovarian stimulation. *J Int Med Res*. 2006;34:73–76. *Cochrane Database Syst Rev*. 2005;20:CD001122.

Hull MG, et al. The value of a single serum progesterone measurement in the midluteal phase as a criterion of a potentially fertile cycle derived from treated and untreated conception cycles. *Fertil Steril*. 1982;37:355–360.

Palomba S, et al. Prospective parallel randomized, double-blind, double-dummy controlled clinical trial comparing clomiphene citrate and metformin as the 1st-line treatment for ovulation induction in nonobese anovulatory women with polycystic ovary syndrome. *J Clin Endocrinol Metab*. 2005;90:4068–4074.

MISCELLANEOUS

CLINICAL PEARLS
- There is no reason to increase the dose of an oral OI agent once ovulation has been achieved.
- The goal of OI for the anovulatory patient is monofollicular development, not superovulation.
- Anovulatory patients who have failed to conceive after 3–4 ovulatory treatment cycles should be referred to a reproductive endocrinologist.

ABBREVIATIONS
- ARDS—Acute respiratory distress syndrome
- ASRM—American Society for Reproductive Medicine
- DHEAS—Dehydroepiandrosterone
- FSH—Follicle-stimulating hormone
- GnRH—Gonadotropin releasing hormone
- hCG—Human chorionic gonadotropin
- LH—Luteinizing hormone
- OHSS—Ovarian hyperstimulation syndrome
- OI—Ovulation induction
- PCOS—Polycystic ovary syndrome
- POF—Premature ovarian failure
- SART—Society for Assisted Reproductive Technology

CODES
ICD9-CM
- 253.1 Hyperprolactinemia
- 256.1 OHSS
- 256.3 Premature ovarian failure
- 256.4 PCOS
- 611.6 Galactorrhea
- 626.0 Amenorrhea
- 626.8 Dysfunctional uterine bleeding
- 628.0 Anovulation
- 628.1 Pituitary-hypothalamic infertility

PATIENT TEACHING

- The ASRM web site at http://www.asrm.org has a patient information booklet on Medications for Inducing Ovulation and other topics related to infertility.

Section VII

PELVIC IMAGING: COMPUTED TOMOGRAPHY (CT)

Verghese George, MD
Shirley M. McCarthy, MD, PhD

 BASICS

DESCRIPTION

- CT is a medical imaging method in which a rotating gantry comprising an X-ray tube and detector array is used to generate a large series of 2–D cross-sectional images.
- CT produces a volume of data that can be manipulated to demonstrate various structures based on their ability to block the X-ray beam (attenuation).
- Although traditionally CT images are generated in the axial or transverse plane, modern scanners allow this volume of data to be reformatted in various planes or even as volumetric (3–D) representations.
- Helical CT scanners have evolved into newer versions incorporating multiple rows of detectors (multidetector CT or MDCT) and >1 X-ray tube (dual source CT).
- Sometimes, IV contrast agents, usually nonionic iodinated media, are administered for better visualization of vascular lesions such as tumors.
- In the imaging of the female pelvis, CT has largely been replaced by MRI owing to concerns regarding radiating dose and its inherently poor contrast resolution as compared to MRI.

ALERT

- Preliminary results of a recent study indicate that radiation exposure from medical devices in the US has increased by nearly 650% as compared to 1980 levels, most of this exposure resulting from the use of CT.
- The study, which has been described as the 1st large-scale review of US population radiation exposure since 1989, found that the number of CT scans done in the US has grown from 18.3 million in 1993 to 62 million in 2006.
- The study also suggested that the doses of medical radiation can be significantly reduced without reducing diagnostic accuracy.
- Most referring physicians are not educated enough on the magnitude of risk associated with increased medical radiation.

Pediatric Considerations

- The best available risk estimates indicate that pediatric CT results in significantly increased lifetime radiation risk over adult CT, both because of the increased dose per milliampere-sec, and the increased lifetime risk per unit dose.
- In the US, ~600,000 CT scans are performed annually in children <15 years:
  - Roughly 500 of these patients might ultimately die from cancer attributable to the CT radiation.
  - Careful consideration must be made of risk versus benefit issues when ordering a pediatric CT.
  - Additionally, lower milliampere-sec settings can be used for children without significant loss of information and should be employed whenever possible.

Geriatric Considerations

- Nonionic iodinated contrast agents used in CT are potentially nephrotoxic.
- The risk of renal damage is increased in patients with pre-existing renal insufficiency, diabetes, or reduced intravascular volume:
  - These risk factors are more common in the geriatric population.
- Departmental protocols should be applied when deciding on the use of contrast-enhanced CT scans on these patients.

Gynecologic Indications

- Acute pelvic pain:
  - Although US is the primary imaging modality in the evaluation of gynecologic causes of pelvic pain, the role of CT in these cases continues to expand.
  - CT is a superior option in the evaluation of pelvic pain of unexplained etiology, since nongynecologic causes of pain like diverticulitis, appendicitis, or bowel obstruction can also be evaluated.

- PID: CT is the technique of choice.
- CT is also useful in the diagnosis of:
  - Ovarian torsion, hemorrhagic ovarian cysts and ovarian hyperstimulation as causes of pelvic pain.
- Pelvic masses:
  - MRI has replaced CT to a large extent in the evaluation of pelvic masses.
  - Indeterminate pelvic lesions seen on CT or US are best evaluated by MRI for characterization and possible local staging.
- However, CT is superior for the assessment of distant metastases since it offers the most efficient scanning of the abdomen and pelvis, and also the chest, if necessary.
- Postoperative complications: CT is the ideal imaging modality for the assessment of postoperative complications like:
  - Fluid collections, hematomas, abscesses, and peritonitis:
    - Aspiration and drainage of such collections can be performed under CT guidance.

Obstetric Indications

- Acute abdomen in pregnancy:
  - Although being increasingly replaced by MRI, CT continues to be used for the evaluation of the acute abdomen and in the setting of trauma in pregnancy.
- CT is preferred in the critically unwell patient since MRI is more time-consuming and requires patient cooperation.
- Complications of HELLP syndrome are also best assessed on CT.
- CT pelvimetry is associated with less radiation exposure than conventional X-ray pelvimetry and is a reliable tool in the assessment of cephalopelvic disproportion.
- Postpartum complications:
  - CT is the modality of choice for the evaluation of peri- and postpartum complications such as:
    - Uterine perforation, hemorrhage, ovarian vein thrombosis and pelvic abscess formation

Pregnancy Considerations

- During pregnancy, the diagnostic utility of CT is limited by concern for radiation exposure to the fetus:
  - Although the risk of teratogenesis even in a 1st trimester scan is low, the risk of carcinogenesis is about doubled after fetal exposure to a pelvic CT.
  - Surgical conditions, such as appendicitis and cholecystitis, should be diagnosed sonographically, if possible.
- MRI is increasingly employed in the setting of life-threatening conditions like trauma and acute abdomen; however, CT may be indicated to assess for potentially fatal complications.
- Iodinated CT contrast is excreted through breast milk, and lactating postpartum mothers are usually advised to express and discard breast milk for 24 hours after a contrast enhanced CT.

Safety Issues

- Contrast allergy:
  - Although the nonionic, hypo-osmolar contrast agents used in CT today are much safer than their ionic predecessors, susceptible patients can get allergic reactions ranging from mild cutaneous reactions like itching and hives to full-blown anaphylaxis.
  - Anaphylaxis carts and CPR-trained staff should always be available to deal with contrast-induced allergic reactions.
  - Patients with known allergy to iodinated contrast should undergo premedication with steroids and antihistamines.
- Nephrotoxicity:
  - Risk of contrast media nephrotoxicity can be reduced in susceptible patients by:
    - Adequate hydration
    - Premedication with n-acetylcysteine and bicarbonate
    - Lower doses of iodinated contrast
    - Use of a more hypo-osmolar agent (e.g., iodixanol)
  - Departmental protocols should be applied in these situations.

Informed Consent

Whenever possible, informed consent should be obtained from a pregnant patient undergoing a CT scan. The justification of the study, and the risks and benefits associated with it must be clearly elucidated.

BIBLIOGRAPHY

Bennett GL, et al. Gynecologic causes of acute pelvic pain: Spectrum of CT findings. *RadioGraphics*. 2002;22:785–801.

Brenner D, et al. Estimated risks of radiation-induced fatal cancer from pediatric CT. *AJR Am J Roentgenol*. 2001;176:289–296.

Damilakis J, et al. Estimation of fetal radiation dose from computed tomography scanning in late pregnancy: Depth-dose data from routine examinations. *Invest Radiol*. 2000;35:527–533.

Mettler F. Proceedings of the 2007 National Council of Radiation Protection and Measurements meeting in Arlington, VA.

 MISCELLANEOUS

ABBREVIATIONS

- HELLP—Hemolysis, elevated liver enzyme levels, low platelet count
- PID—Pelvic inflammatory disease

Section VII

PELVIC IMAGING: MAGNETIC RESONANCE IMAGING (MRI)

Verghese George, MD
Shirley M. McCarthy, MD, PhD

 BASICS

DESCRIPTION

- MRI involves placing the patient in a powerful magnetic field and then directing RF pulses towards the area to be imaged. An electrical signal is thereby generated, which is processed by a computer to produce the MRI image.
- MRI relies on the difference in the density and bonding of hydrogen atoms in different tissues to produce images with exquisite detail and unparalleled contrast resolution.
- Sometimes, IV contrast agents, usually gadolinium chelates, are administered for better visualization of vascular lesions like tumors.
- Unlike CT, MRI does not involve ionizing radiation and hence has no known adverse effects.
- MRI has revolutionized imaging of the female pelvis and has multiple indications in current clinical practice.

ALERT

Emerging literature suggests that, very rarely, gadolinium chelates (used as MRI contrast agents) may be linked to the development of NSF in patients with advanced renal failure.

- NSF is a rare, multisystem fibrosing disorder that is disfiguring and potentially debilitating and fatal.
- FDA recommendations and departmental protocols should be applied while deciding on the use of contrast enhanced MRIs in patients with renal dysfunction.

Pediatric Considerations

As with the geriatric population, these patients are also less likely to be cooperative and can be difficult to image. "Feed and wrap," sedation, or even general anesthesia may be required to produce diagnostic images.

Geriatric Considerations

MRI scans require the patient to be cooperative and lie still for relatively long periods of time. Breath-hold sequences may also be required. These may be difficult for the geriatric patient, resulting in suboptimal imaging. Claustrophobia and the attendant risks of sedation may also be an issue.

Gynecologic Indications

- Uterine anomalies:
  - The superior contrast resolution offered by MRI makes it the procedure of choice in the classification of Müllerian developmental anomalies.
  - Septate and bicornuate uteri can be distinguished by evaluating the fundal contour, thus obviating the need for invasive laparoscopy or HSG for their diagnosis.
- Fibroid evaluation:
  - MRI is superior for the therapeutic evaluation of leiomyomas because their number, size, vascularity, location, and degeneration are well demonstrated.
  - Also the optimal technique to follow response to fibroid embolization
  - MRI-guided HIFU is also emerging as an alternative nonsurgical option for management of leiomyomas.
- Adenomyosis:
  - MRI is the only imaging modality that can reliably diagnose adenomyosis with a high degree of accuracy.
  - Focal and diffuse disease, as well as cystic adenomyosis and adenomyomas, can be readily identified.
  - Adhesions and implants related to concomitant endometriosis may also be visualized.
- Pelvic masses:
  - MRI is very useful in localizing masses equivocal on US to a uterine or ovarian location.
  - Signal behavior can be used to characterize most benign, solid ovarian masses such as dermoids, endometriomas, and fibromas.
  - However, a clearly cystic ovarian mass on US that is indeterminate for malignancy cannot be definitively characterized as benign or malignant by MRI:
    ○ MRI relies on the same morphologic criteria as US to label a cystic mass as malignant (e.g., thick septations, nodularity, etc.).
    ○ Gadolinium enhanced MRI can however, be used to differentiate tumor from blood clot within a cyst.

- Staging:
  - MRI is superior to CT for local staging of pelvic malignancies:
    ○ In ovarian malignancies, MRI is used in the evaluation of local tumor extent and tumor implants involving the diaphragm and liver surface.
    ○ For the local staging of cervical cancer, MRI is superior to CT in the assessment of tumor size, presence and depth of stromal invasion, and in assessing parametrial invasion.
    ○ In endometrial cancer, MRI can be used to evaluate depth of myometrial invasion.
  - Assessment for distant metastases is best performed by CT since it offers the most efficient scanning of the abdomen and pelvis, and the chest if necessary.
- Pelvic congestion:
  - While pelvic congestion is a diagnosis by exclusion clinically, MRI can be used to check for retrograde flow within the gonadal veins.
  - Dynamic post contrast sequences are performed to look for gonadal vein filling in the arterial phase, indicating reflux of contrast into the vein.
  - In a patient with unexplained pelvic pain, this finding is consistent with pelvic congestion.
- Pelvic floor imaging: Dynamic cine sequences are performed with the patient performing various maneuvers to evaluate for pelvic floor laxity. Pelvic floor dysfunction and degrees of organ descent can be assessed, thus aiding surgical planning.
- Urethral imaging:
  - High-resolution MRI is used to visualize the urethra for the evaluation of conditions like urethral diverticula, periurethral cysts, and malignancy.
  - MRI is also useful for the assessment of fistulae between the rectum and urogenital system.

Obstetric Indications

- Fetal anatomy:
  - While US continues to be the primary tool to evaluate fetal anatomy, MRI is being increasingly used in cases where US is equivocal.
  - This has been enabled by the recent development of ultra-fast sequences, thus eliminating the need to sedate the fetus.
  - The commonest use of fetal MRI is to better assess CNS and skeletal abnormalities.

- Placental evaluation:
  - MRI complements US in the diagnosis of placental abnormalities, especially placenta percreta.
  - A concomitant low-lying placenta can also be visualized.
- Acute abdomen in pregnancy:
  - While CT is the most effective way of evaluating the surgical abdomen in a nonpregnant patient, the radiation involved should deter its use in pregnancy.
  - MRI is rapidly emerging as a useful tool in such cases, especially in appendicitis, fibroid infarction, and trauma.
- MRI pelvimetry:
  - Assessment of cephalopelvic disproportion can be reliably made with MRI, thus eliminating the risks of radiation associated with X-ray or CT pelvimetry.

Pregnancy Considerations

- Although no feto-maternal adverse effects have been documented, MRI in pregnancy is usually reserved to answer questions not resolved by US.
- Whenever possible, it should be delayed until the 2nd or the 3rd trimester owing to the theoretical safety concerns regarding tissue overheating by RF pulses.
- IV contrast should not be administered, as gadolinium chelates cross the placenta and its long-term effects are not known.
- Gadolinium is excreted through breast milk; its effects on the breast-fed infant are unknown:
  - Lactating postpartum mothers are usually advised to express and discard breast milk for 24 hours after a contrast-enhanced MRI.

Safety Issues

- The high magnetic field used in an MRI necessitates stringent safety precautions.
- Implants:
  - Most medical and biostimulation implants are considered contraindications to an MRI:
    - Pacemakers, implanted defibrillators, cochlear implants, vagus nerve and thalamic stimulators malfunction in the magnetic field
- Ferromagnetic foreign bodies:
  - Shrapnel, aneurysm clips, and intraorbital metallic fragments are potential risks due to hazards posed by movement of these bodies in the magnetic field and thermal injury by RF-induced heating.
  - Metallic foreign bodies in or contiguous to the imaging field can also produce susceptibility artifacts leading to suboptimal images.
- Projectiles:
  - The high magnetic field of the scanner pulls ferromagnetic objects in its vicinity toward the center of the field. Objects such as oxygen cylinders can become dangerous projectiles.
  - Multiple levels of safety precautions exist in an MRI suite to avoid accidental introduction of ferromagnetic objects into the magnetic field.
  - All patient support and monitoring equipment used during a scan should be MRI compatible.
- Peripheral nerve stimulation:
  - Rapid switching on and off of magnetic gradients can occasionally cause peripheral nerve stimulation.

- Acoustic effects:
  - Gradient field switching causes loud noises, and appropriate ear protection should be used.
- Cryogens:
  - Emergency shutdown of a superconducting magnet ("quenching") may result in the introduction of helium into the scanner room, thus presenting an asphyxiation risk.
- Magnetic media:
  - The magnetic field can erase information contained on magnetic media such as floppy discs and even credit card stripes; these should not be introduced into the scan room.
- Contrast allergy:
  - Extremely rare
  - Susceptible patients should be premedicated with steroids and antihistamines.

BIBLIOGRAPHY

Kuo PH, et al. Gadolinium-based MR contrast agents and nephrogenic systemic fibrosis. *Radiology*. 2007;242(3):647–649.

McCarthy S. MR imaging of the uterus. *Radiology*. 1989;171:321.

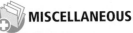 **MISCELLANEOUS**

ABBREVIATIONS

- HIFU—High-intensity focused US
- HSG—Hysterosalpingogram
- NSF—Nephrogenic systemic fibrosis
- RF—Radiofrequency
- US—Ultrasound

Section VII

Steven R. Lindheim, MD

 BASICS

DESCRIPTION

- SIS is the instillation of saline, and potentially other echogenic US contrast agents including air bubbles, into the uterine cavity during US to evaluate the uterine cavity and fallopian tubes.
- SIS has greater diagnostic accuracy compared to other diagnostic studies including HSG, EMB, and abdominal US and TVUS.

Indications

- SIS is used for diagnostic evaluation of the uterine cavity including:
  - AUB in both peri- and postmenopausal women:
    ○ AUB is a harbinger of endometrial cancer occurring in 0.1–0.2% of postmenopausal women per year.
    ○ Screening for AUB including D&C, endometrial sampling via suction devices and/or TVUS can miss a significant number of lesions, particularly isolated submucosal defects:
      ■ SIS has been shown to enhance the diagnostic accuracy.
      ■ Compared to TVUS, SIS has been shown to detect more pathology.
      ■ Compared to aspiration EMB, SIS has been shown to have similar specificity, but greater sensitivity in identifying lesions causing PMB.
      ■ Resolves discordance between TVUS and EMB
- Evaluation of endometrium that is thickened, irregular, difficult to measure, or poorly defined on conventional TVUS:
  - Postmenopausal breast cancer patients receiving tamoxifen:
    ○ Because tamoxifen induces subepithelial stromal hypertrophy, TVUS shows a poor correlation between endometrial thickness and abnormal pathology.
    ○ SIS has better sensitivity, specificity, and predictive value compared to endometrial sampling in symptomatic women on tamoxifen; thus surgery may be avoided.
  - Preoperative assessment of uterine leiomyomata:
    ○ SIS helps identify size, location, depth of myometrial involvement of submucosal fibroids, allowing better surgical planning for complete resection.
    ○ SIS is more accurate than TVUS and hysteroscopy.
  - Intraoperative SIS can help assure complete removal of deep intramural myoma(s).
- Infertility and recurrent miscarriage:
  - Studies suggest that SIS may be twice as accurate as HSG and TVUS in diagnosing abnormalities of uterus or fallopian tubes that occur in up to 40% of infertile women and up to 20% of those with recurrent miscarriage.
  - SIS is used by some as 1st-line screening for the evaluation of the uterus before embryo transfer in patients undergoing IVF, ovum donation, and IVF-surrogacy.

- With a history of recurrent abortion, SIS can demonstrate müllerian anomalies, as well as other uterine-cavity defects.
- Other:
  - As an alternative to HSG for assessing tubal anatomy and patency especially when added with Doppler US
  - Finding "lost" IUD (i.e., string cannot be visualized) and assessing if embedded
  - Documenting and removing fragments of laminaria, diagnosing postabortal remnants including placenta accreta, and visualization of previous cesarean delivery scars
- SIS is used for therapeutic indications including:
  - PLUG, for the treatment of selected cases of mild intrauterine adhesions
    ○ PLUG may reduce the need for operative hysteroscopy, although this indication requires further investigation.
  - Operative SIS:
    ○ Directed biopsies for small submucosal pathology using small graspers inserted through an access catheter or an aspiration catheter have been described.
    ○ The instrument's small size and limited rotation restrict this application, but may represent a cost-effective alternative to hysteroscopy and is deserving of further study.

Site (Office, Surgical Center, OR)
Office-based procedure

Concurrent Procedures
Pelvic US

 TREATMENT

PROCEDURE

- SIS is a simple procedure that provides detailed visualization of the endometrial lining and possible intracavitary defects including:
  - Polyps, submucosal leiomyoma(s), and endometrial carcinoma
- SIS timing:
  - Within 10 days of onset of menses or withdrawal bleeding
  - Avoid SIS during heavy bleeding (avoids false-positives).
  - If performed during bleeding and small lesions (<10 mm) are seen, repeat when bleeding-free.
- SIS instrument placement:
  - Comprehensive baseline US of entire pelvis is performed and TVUS probe removed.
  - Speculum is inserted and cervix cleansed with antiseptic solution.
  - Balloon catheter is introduced into uterine cavity just passing the internal os.
  - Placement in the cervix, particularly in nulliparous women, may minimize discomfort during the SIS and allows superior visualization of the entire endometrial cavity.

- Catheter should be primed with saline to minimize infusion of air bubbles that can cause image artifact and pain.
- When advancing catheter, avoid touching fundus of the uterus with the catheter tip as this can cause pain and/or vasovagal response.
- Many catheter systems are available, including rigid systems or flexible catheters without an attached balloon.
  ○ Balloon system is recommended to prevent distension media from escaping.
  ○ If cervix is patulous or incompetent, or uterus is enlarged, balloon is recommended.
- After careful removal of speculum to avoid dislodging of the catheter, US probe is placed in the proper position.
- If cervical stenosis is present, options include guidewires through the catheter or the use of a tenaculum to place traction on the cervix.
- SIS fluid instillation:
  - Solutions for instillation include saline, Ringer's lactate, and glycine 1.5%.
  - Warm the solution and connect to the catheter system.
  - Initial infusion rate should not exceed 5 mL/min and can be adjusted based on the patient's response and comfort level.
  - In RCTs, the use of intrauterine analgesics has not been demonstrated to reduce pelvic pain/discomfort.
- SIS procedure:
  - The uterus is scanned in the longitudinal plane, fanning from 1 cornu to the other, and in the transverse plane, from the top of fundus to cervix.
  - Inadequate distension may result in poor visualization; overzealous distension may obscure pathology or extent of disease.
  - Most cases should not require >10–20 mL of fluid.
  - All images should be recorded as still images or on videotape for permanent records.
  - The SIS should last on average 3–10 minutes.
  - After completion, and prior to removal of the catheter, the balloon should be deflated and fluid aspirated to minimize uterine cramping.
  - The patient should rest for 5–10 minutes to avoid postprocedure syncope.
- SIS pitfalls:
  - Common problems encountered during SIS include:
    ○ Air trapped in cavity: Can be prevented by flushing the catheter system prior to SIS
    ○ Mechanical shearing of endometrium: Due to overzealous placement of the catheter, as it can shear the endometrium and cause false-positive results
    ○ Mechanical interference with visualization: To avoid this, deflate the balloon at the conclusion of SIS to adequately assess the lower uterine segment and cervical canal so as not to miss any pathology. Use fluid instead of air to inflate the balloon.

Informed Consent

- Physician must inform patient about SIS, explaining benefits and potential complications including bleeding, infection, and perforation.
- Possible alternatives should be addressed and all questions answered.
- Consent form must be signed before procedure.

Patient Education

- The risk of infection is reported to be <1%.
- Prophylactic antibiotics with history of PID
- NSAID 30 minutes prior to SIS reduces discomfort.

Alternatives

- Hysteroscopy: Gold standard but may require OR with local or general anesthesia:
  - Risks include inadvertent uterine perforation, bowel or bladder injury, and costs.
- HSG: Remains standard, nonoperative diagnostic procedure to evaluate the female pelvis:
  - Long-standing historical acceptance
  - Problems associated with procedure include:
    ○ Cannot differentiate myomas from polyps or müllerian anomalies
    ○ Unlike TVUS, adnexa cannot be simultaneously visualized nor can myometrial images be assessed
    ○ Requires dedicated fluoroscopy
    ○ Risks include exposure to ionizing radiation, the potential for allergic reaction from iodinated contrast agents, higher costs, and patient discomfort.
- EMB:
  - Endometrial suction sampling devices may be inadequate for disease confined to a localized area or polyp.
  - Long-standing acceptance, but studies demonstrate that ≤15% of the endometrial cavity is actually assessed.

- TVUS: Valuable diagnostic tool for evaluation of uterine and pelvic pathology, particularly in patients with abnormal uterine bleeding:
  - Benefits include safe, noninvasive procedure, readily available in the office setting.
  - Findings on TVUS have been used to determine which patients should undergo further investigation.
  - TVUS has limited usefulness in evaluating the exact location of endometrial-cavity pathology.

 FOLLOW-UP

COMPLICATIONS

Concerns regarding flushing of malignant endometrial cells into the peritoneal cavity during procedures such as hysteroscopy, HSG, and SIS:

- Malignant cells can be extravasated from the fallopian tube during SIS in those diagnosed with endometrial carcinoma.
- In our experience, however, the mean volume at which spill occurs during SIS is 20.5 mL, and most SIS only require up to 5 mL for an adequate study; none of the disseminated cancer cells appear to be functionally viable.
- Thus, SIS has a low probability of cancer cell dissemination particularly if low volumes are used.

BIBLIOGRAPHY

Lindheim SR, et al. Sonohysterography: A valuable in tool in evaluating the female pelvis. *Obstet Gynecol Survey*. 2003;58(11):770–784.

Lindheim SR, et al. In: Hurd W, ed. *Ultrasonography and Sonohysterography*. New York: Elsevier; 2007;441–459.

 MISCELLANEOUS

SYNONYM(S)

- Hysterosonography
- Saline infused sonography
- Transvaginal sonography with fluid contrast augmentation

CLINICAL PEARLS

- SIS has definite value in the investigation of gynecologic disorders and has consistently been demonstrated to be equally or more accurate than HSG and TVUS.
- A number of definitive applications exist, including AUB, infertility, and pre- and intraoperative assessment.
- Other potential applications include directed biopsies (operative SIS), assessing the depth of endometrial carcinoma, and evaluation of tubal anatomy.
- SIS is a simple and inexpensive procedure that adds tremendously to our diagnostic acumen and should be considered as part of the routine assessment of the reproductive tract.

ABBREVIATIONS

- AUB—Abnormal uterine bleeding
- EMB—Endometrial biopsy
- HSG—Hysterosalpingogram
- IVF—In vitro fertilization
- PLUG—Pressure lavage under US guidance
- PMB—Postmenopausal bleeding
- RCT—Randomized controlled trial
- SIS—Saline infusion sonohysterography
- TVUS—Transvaginal US

 PATIENT TEACHING

ACOG Patient Education Pamphlets:

- US Exams
- Abnormal Uterine Bleeding
- Menopausal Bleeding

PELVIC IMAGING: ULTRASOUND (GYNECOLOGIC)

Leann E. Linam, MD
Sara M. O'Hara, MD

 BASICS

DESCRIPTION

- Sonography is the initial imaging modality of choice in the evaluation of gynecologic disease. TVUS and TAUS approaches are described here.
- Doppler sonography can be used to evaluate vascular structures and distinguish normal from abnormal blood flow.

Gynecologic Indications

Indications include, but are not limited to the following:

- Pelvic pain
- Dysmenorrhea
- Menorrhagia
- Metrorrhagia
- Menometrorrhagia
- Follow-up of previously detected abnormality (e.g., hemorrhagic cyst)
- Evaluation and/or monitoring of infertility
- Delayed menses or precocious puberty
- Postmenopausal bleeding
- Abnormal pelvic exam
- Further characterization of a pelvic abnormality noted on another imaging study (CT or MRI)
- Evaluation of congenital anomalies
- Excessive bleeding, pain, or fever after pelvic surgery or delivery
- Localization of intrauterine contraceptive device
- Screening for malignancy in patients with an increased risk

Pediatric/Adolescent Considerations

- TVUS is not appropriate for prepubertal or premenarchal girls
- Young adolescents may not be good candidates for TVUS; TAUS can be substituted
- Most adolescents who have been voluntarily sexually active can tolerate TVUS
- Many adolescents who are not sexually experienced can tolerate TVUS if the exam is done by a gentle (female) technologist who explains the procedure and takes time to coach the patient through the exam
- Adolescents with vaginal agenesis, imperforate hymen, or a vaginal septum may be able to tolerate a transperineal/translabial or transrectal US exam:
  - Transducer, covered by a sheath containing gel, is place directly onto the introitus or within rectum
  - Imaging in transverse and longitudinal planes

Comparison with Other Imaging Techniques

- Advantages:
  - Inexpensive
  - Noninvasive
  - Widely available
  - No radiation involved
  - Easily differentiates between cystic and solid structures
  - Doppler sonography can be used to evaluate vascular structures and distinguish normal from abnormal blood flow.
- Limitations:
  - Tissue differentiation is suboptimal; i.e., it cannot reliably identify cartilage, hair, etc. in a teratoma.
  - Cannot reliably distinguish benign from malignant masses
  - Not reliable in evaluating invasive or disseminated disease
  - Dependent on skill of sonographer
  - Bowel gas limits sonographic window

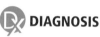 **DIAGNOSIS**

TESTS

Consent

- The exam should be explained to the patient, and verbal consent should be obtained.
- If the examiner is a male, a female staff member should be in the room throughout the entire exam as a chaperone.

Transabdominal Sonogram

- Distension of the urinary bladder:
  - Provides an acoustic window to view pelvic organs
  - Displaces small bowel and contained gas from the field of view
  - Serves as an internal reference for cystic structures
  - Bladder is considered fully distended when it covers the fundus of the uterus
  - If overdistended, may distort anatomy. In adults, have the patient partially empty the bladder and resume the study. This may not be possible in children or elderly patients.
  - 2 methods for filling urinary bladder:
    - Allow patient to drink and wait for bladder filling, checking periodically
    - Place bladder catheter and fill the bladder in a retrograde fashion; catheterization is recommended for emergency studies, as the bladder is filled quickly, the exam is expedited, and NPO status is maintained if surgery is indicated.

- Technique:
  - Use highest frequency transducer possible for depth of penetration required:
    - Generally 7.5 MHz for neonate
    - 5.0–MHz for child or thin teenager
    - 3.5–MHz for teenager or adult
  - Imaging of the uterus and ovaries should be performed in transverse and longitudinal planes.
  - Measure uterus and ovaries in 3 dimensions, calculating ovarian volume.
  - Measure endometrial stripe thickness on the longitudinal view of uterus.
  - Evaluate for free fluid or other pelvic abnormalities.
- Advantages:
  - Wider field of view allows for overview of entire pelvis and lower abdomen, if necessary.
- Limitations:
  - Patients unable to fill bladder, incontinent patients
  - Obese patients
  - Distance from adnexa limits optimal characterization of masses

Transvaginal Sonogram

- Urinary bladder is preferably empty:
  - Brings the pelvic organs into the focal zone of the transducer
  - May improve patient comfort
- Technique:
  - After preparing the transducer with US gel, it should be covered with a condom or other protective barrier:
    - Gel is applied to the outside of the barrier.
  - The transducer is inserted into the vagina by the patient or sonographer.
  - The exam should be performed with the patient supine with hips slightly elevated.
  - Imaging of the uterus and ovaries should be performed in transverse and longitudinal planes.
  - Measure uterus and ovaries in 3 dimensions, calculate ovarian volume.
  - Measure endometrial stripe thickness on the longitudinal view of uterus.
  - Evaluate for free fluid and pelvic abnormalities.
  - Evaluate cervix, vagina, and urethra as probe is being removed.
- Advantages:
  - Better spatial resolution
  - Allows exam of patients unable to fill bladder
  - Obese patients
- Limitations:
  - Field of view is limited
- Contraindications:
  - Virginal patients (see "Pediatric/Adolescent Considerations," above)
  - Patients who do not willingly consent
  - Immediately post vaginal delivery or vaginal surgery
- Sonohysterography (See Pelvic Imaging: Sonohysterography)

TREATMENT

- Imaging evaluation:
  - Uterus:
    - ○ Uterine size, shape, and orientation
    - ○ Document any abnormalities of the uterus
  - Endometrium:
    - ○ Evaluate thickness
    - ○ Document mass or fluid in cavity
  - Myometrium:
    - ○ Evaluate for contour, echogenicity, and masses
  - Cervix:
    - ○ Evaluate for contour, echogenicity, masses, endoluminal content, open/closed
- Adnexa:
  - Ovaries:
    - ○ Measurements with volume calculations
    - ○ Masses: Measure any mass in at least 2 dimensions
    - ○ Document if >12 follicles/ovary measuring 2–9 mm (criteria for PCOS)
    - ○ Document if follicles are primarily peripheral ("string of pearls" sign) as in PCOS
  - Fallopian tubes:
    - ○ Normal fallopian tubes are not typically identified.
- Cul-de-sac:
  - A small amount of fluid in the cul-de-sac is physiologic; larger volumes deserve comment on volume.
- Adjacent structures:
  - Bladder
  - Pelvic floor
  - Iliac vessels
  - Lymph nodes
  - Rectosigmoid colon

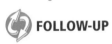 FOLLOW-UP

Normal Sonographic Anatomy

- Uterus (uterine anatomy changes with age and parity):
  - Neonatal uterus (0–1 year):
    - ○ Neonatal uterus and cervix are under the influence of maternal hormones; appear prominent.
    - ○ Cervix is the most prominent part of the uterus.
    - ○ Cervical length is generally twice the length of the fundus.
    - ○ Mean length of the neonatal uterus is 3.5 cm
  - Prepubertal uterus (1 year-menarche):
    - ○ Prepubertal uterus has a tubular configuration.
    - ○ AP diameter of the fundus is equal to the AP diameter of the cervix.
    - ○ Gradual growth between 3–8 years of age.
    - ○ Average uterine length is 4.3 cm in the 10–13-year-old premenarchal patient.
    - ○ With estrogen stimulation at puberty, the ratio of uterine fundus:cervix changes from 1:1 in a prepubertal girl to 2:1 or more post-puberty.
  - Postmenarchal/Premenopausal uterus:
    - ○ Pear configuration (fundus larger than cervix)
    - ○ 5–8 cm in length
- Endometrium:
  - Cyclical changes in premenopausal patients:
    - ○ 2–4 mm after menses; uniform echogenicity
    - ○ 10–14 mm at ovulation, appearing layered
    - ○ 10–14 mm after ovulation with more uniform echogenic appearance
  - Postmenopausal uterus:
    - ○ After menopause, the uterus atrophies
    - ○ Length from 3.5–6.5 cm in patients >65
    - ○ Endometrium should be thin (<5 mm if not on hormone therapy), homogeneous, and echogenic
- Ovaries:
  - Neonatal ovary (0–24 months):
    - ○ Mean ovarian volume in 1st year of life is ~1 mL.
    - ○ Ovarian volume decreases slightly in the 2nd year of life, to a mean volume of 0.67 mL.
    - ○ Ovaries of neonates contain numerous underdeveloped follicles, which can be seen sonographically.
    - ○ Larger follicles and even simple unilocular cysts can be seen.
  - Prepubertal ovary (2 years to menarche):
    - ○ In girls 2–6 years, average volume is 1 mL.
    - ○ Prepubertal girls 6–10, ovarian volume gradually increases, ranging from 1.2–2.3 mL.
    - ○ As girls approach menarche, volumes increase to close to 4 mL.
    - ○ Larger follicles and even simple unilocular cysts can be seen, but require observation and follow-up.
  - Postmenarchal/Premenopausal ovary.
- Ovarian volume averages 8 mL:
  - Standard deviation is large (5–6 mL).
  - PCOS present in 5–7% of adult population with currently defined criteria (2D US): Larger ovarian volume uni- or bilaterally.
  - Volume >20 cm³ suggested criterion
  - Peripheral follicles >12 of 2–9 mm
  - Further use of 3D US may provide future clinical, biochemical, and US correlation with different criteria.

ALERT

Early literature suggested that follicles and small cysts were abnormal in the prepubertal girl outside the neonatal period and in menopausal women. It has since been found that simple small cystic ovarian follicles can be seen in prepubertal girls as well as beyond menopause. Caution is advised in interpretation; observation with repeat exam may be warranted to rule out malignancy.

- Postmenopausal ovaries:
  - Ovarian atrophy can make ovaries difficult to see.

BIBLIOGRAPHY

American College of Radiology Practice Guidelines & Technical Standards: Guideline for the Performance of Pelvic Ultrasound in Females. At www.acr.org/s_acr/bin.asp?CID=539&DID=12223&DOC=FILE.PDF.

Cohen HL, et al. Ovarian cysts are common in premenarchal girls: A sonographic study of 101 children 2–12 years old. *Am J Roentgenol.* 1992;159:89–91.

Cohen HL, et al. Normal ovaries in neonates and infants: A sonographic study of 77 patients 1 day to 24 months old. *Am J Roentgenol.* 1993;160:583–586.

Garel L, et al. Ultrasound of the pediatric female pelvis: A clinical perspective. *Radiographics.* 2001;21:1393–1407.

Jeong YY, et al. Imaging evaluation of ovarian masses. *Radiographics.* 200;20:1445–1470.

Nalaboff KM, et al. Imaging the endometrium: Disease and normal variants. *Radiographics.* 2001;21:1409–1424.

Rataani RS, et al. Pediatric gynecologic ultrasound. *Ultrasound Q.* 2004;20(3):127–139.

Salem S, et al. Gynecologic Ultrasound. In: Rumack CM, et al., eds. *Diagnostic Ultrasound,* 3rd ed. St. Louis: Mosby; 2005;527–587.

William PL, et al. Ultrasound of abnormal uterine bleeding. *Radiographics.* 2003;23:703–718.

MISCELLANEOUS

CLINICAL PEARLS

If there is a question regarding the still images obtained by a technologist, the clinician should personally perform the scan to clarify.

ABBREVIATIONS

- TVUS—Transvaginal ultrasound
- TAUS—Transabdominal ultrasound
- PCOS—Polycystic ovary syndrome

CODES

ICD9-CM/CPT

- 765.75 Doppler
- 768.56 Pelvic ultrasound
- 768.17 Transvaginal ultrasound

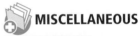 PATIENT TEACHING

- The findings should be documented in report form and conveyed to the ordering physician.
- Any abnormality that requires time-sensitive intervention should be personally conveyed to the ordering physician (via telephone or direct communication).
- It is at the discretion of the imaging physician whether to discuss imaging findings with the patient at the time of the study.

Section VII

PELVIC IMAGING: ULTRASOUND (OBSTETRICAL)

Pauline Chang, MD

 BASICS

DESCRIPTION

- US produces real-time imaging from sound waves reflected back from the imaged structure.
- 1st trimester US exam: For screening and diagnostic
- 2nd and 3rd trimester US exams: Standard, limited, or specialized:
  - Standard: Exam of fetal presentation, amniotic fluid volume, cardiac activity, placental position, fetal biometry, anatomy survey
  - Limited: Exam to answer a specific question (e.g., amniotic fluid volume, fetal presentation of laboring patient)
  - Specialized: Detailed anatomic exam when an anomaly is suspected from standard US, past history, or biochemical abnormalities:
    - Level 2 US, targeted US
    - Other specialized exams: Doppler, fetal echocardiography, BPP
- Accuracy of gestational age assessment by US:
  - 1st trimester: +/- 7 days
  - 2nd trimester: +/- 14 days
  - 3rd trimester: +/- 21 days
- Obstetric indications:
  - 1st-trimester US:
    - Evaluation of intrauterine pregnancy: GA, cardiac activity, and multiple gestation
    - Suspected ectopic pregnancy or molar pregnancy
    - Vaginal bleeding, pelvic pain, or pelvic masses
    - 1st-trimester screening: Nuchal translucency as adjunct to biochemical screening
    - Adjunct to CVS
  - 2nd- and 3rd-trimester US:
    - Evaluation of intrauterine pregnancy: GA (uncertain dates, late prenatal care), fetal growth, fetal presentation, fetal anatomy, and multiple gestation
    - Vaginal bleeding, pelvic pain, incompetent cervix, or uterine abnormality
    - Abruptio placentae, placental previa, or abnormal amniotic fluid volume
    - Suspected ectopic pregnancy, fetal death, or molar pregnancy
    - History of previous congenital anomaly, follow-up of identified fetal anomaly, or abnormal biochemical abnormalities
    - Size discrepancy on clinical exam
    - Adjunct to amniocentesis, external version, cervical cerclage placement, fetal reduction, or intrauterine fetal transfusion

- Site (office, surgical center, OR):
  - 1st-trimester US: Emergency room, obstetric office, radiology site
  - Limited/Standard US: Emergency room, radiology site, obstetric office, specialized obstetric centers (tertiary center), labor and delivery units
  - Specialized: Specialized obstetric centers
- Concurrent procedures:
  - US is used as adjunct to CVS, fetal reduction, amniocentesis, external version, cervical cerclage placement, or intrauterine fetal transfusion
  - Biophysical profile; with each component rated 0 or 2:
    - Fetal breathing
    - Fetal movement
    - Fetal tone
    - Amniotic fluid volume
    - Fetal heart rate acceleration with NST

Age-Related Factors
US used in screening and diagnostic tests for aneuploidy in patients with advanced maternal age (>35 years at time of delivery)

- 1st-trimester screening:
  - 11–13 + 6 weeks gestation age (CRL between 45–84 mm)
  - US nuchal translucency combined with biochemical screening (PAPP-A, β-hCG)
    - Nuchal edema associated with chromosomal abnormalities
    - Detection rate for trisomy 21:
      - 64–70% if only using nuchal translucency
      - 82–87% if using 1st trimester screening
      - 94–96% if integrating 1st trimester screening with 2nd-trimester quad screen (MSAFP, hCG, unconjugated estriol, inhibin A)
    - Not diagnostic of chromosomal abnormalities
    - This screening modality is available for all patients regardless of age
- 2nd-trimester US:
  - US markers associated with chromosomal abnormalities:
    - Echogenic bowel
    - Intracardiac echogenic focus
    - Dilated renal pelvis
    - Choroids plexus cysts
    - Abnormalities in extremities
    - Low sensitivity and specificity if used in low risk population, but 50–75% detection rates in high-risk populations

- CVS and amniocentesis:
  - US used for direct visualization of tissue/site during sample collection
  - Improves safety of these diagnostic techniques

EPIDEMIOLOGY
In the US, ~65–67% of pregnant women have at least 1 US exam.

 TREATMENT

- Basic fetal anatomy:
  - Head and neck: Cerebellum, choroid plexus, cisterna magna, lateral cerebral ventricles, midline falx, cavum septum pellucidi
  - Chest: 4-chamber heart, outflow tracts
  - Abdomen: Stomach, kidney, bladder, umbilical cord insertion, umbilical cord number
  - Spine: Rule out neural tube defects
  - Extremities: Presence of arms and legs
- Multiple pregnancies: Chorionicity, amnionicity, growth concordance, amniotic fluid volume, fetal sex

PREGNANCY-SPECIFIC ISSUES
- 16–20 weeks gestational age is optimal timing for a single US exam if no 1st trimester indications are present:
  - Anatomy can be assessed and, if abnormal, pregnancy termination can be performed within the allowable limits
- Specialized exam is indicated for patients with advanced maternal age or abnormal 1st- or 2nd-trimester biochemical marker screen.
- US should only be preformed with valid medical indication, with lowest exposure setting.
- 3-D US can provide additional information on fetal anatomy; improving visualization of structures such as face, ear, and extremities.

By Trimester
- 1st trimester:
  - Performed transvaginally or transabdominally
  - Evaluate for uterus, adnexa, and cul-de-sac for masses, anomalies, and fluid
  - Evaluate gestational sac (location and size), evidence of yolk sac, embryo, and fetal number
  - Evaluate for CRL for GA and cardiac activity:
    - Cardiac activity should be present in an embryo >5 mm.

- 2nd/3rd trimester:
  – Evaluate for fetal number, fetal presentation, cardiac activity, amniotic fluid volume, placental location, number of vessels in umbilical cord, and fetal anatomy
  – Estimate GA and fetal weight: Biparietal diameter, head circumference, femur length, and abdominal circumference
  – Evaluate uterus and adnexa, if possible.

Risks for Mother
If US markers associated with chromosomal abnormalities present, may increase diagnostic testing (CVS, amniocentesis) and patient anxiety.

Risks for Fetus
Fetal US considered safe when properly used. Under laboratory conditions, US can produce mechanical vibrations and increase tissue temperature, but no confirmed damaging biologic effects.

PROCEDURE
Informed Consent
- Detection of fetal anomalies varies based on the specific anatomic defect, the skill of sonographer, and time spent on exam. Maternal body habitus, fetal GA, and fetal position also can affect the quality of images.
- Routine US exam used as a screening tool does not detect all major or minor congenital abnormalities.

Patient Education
- Before an US exam is performed, patient should be counseled about the limitations of US.
- Chromosomal abnormalities are not always present even with positive ultrasonographic markers.
- Nonmedical use of obstetric US is discouraged because these exams can be misinterpreted by patients and providers.

Risks, Benefits
- Risks: See Risks for Mother, Risks for Fetus, above
- Benefits: Early diagnosis of congenital anomalies; improves safety of obstetric procedures and management

Imaging
- No imaging
- If anomalies suspected, diagnostic procedures (CVS, amniocentesis), fetal MRI, and fetal echocardiography can be used to assist with diagnosis.

 FOLLOW-UP

- Recurrent follow-up US exams are indicated in certain maternal–fetal conditions, such of evaluation of fetal growth in cases of intrauterine growth restrictions.
- Specialized exam indicated if standard US exam is concerning for congenital anomalies.

PROGNOSIS
- Chromosomal abnormalities are not always present even with positive US markers.
- Routine US exam for fetal anatomy is only a screening tool; does not detect all major or minor congenital abnormalities.

BIBLIOGRAPHY

Nonmedical use of obstetric ultrasonography. ACOG Committee Opinion No. 297. American College of Obstetricians and Gynecologists. *Obstet Gynecol.* 2004;104:423–424.

Normal Fetal Anatomy Survey. In: Nyberg DA, et al., eds. *Diagnostic Imaging of Fetal Anomalies.* Philadelphia: Lippincott Williams & Wilkins; 2003;1–29.

Nuchal Translucency and Chromosomal Defects. In: Nicolaides KH, et al., eds. *The 11–14– Week Scan.* New York: Parthenon Publishing Group; 1999;13–30.

Screening for fetal chromosomal abnormalities. ACOG Practice Bulletin No. 77. American College of Obstetricians and Gynecologists. *Obstet Gynecol.* 2007;109:217–227.

Ultrasonography and Doppler. In: Cunningham FG, et al., eds. *Williams Obstetrics,* 22 ed. New York: McGraw-Hill; 2005;389–400.

Ultrasonography in pregnancy. ACOG Practice Bulletin No. 58. American College of Obstetricians and Gynecologists. *Obstet Gynecol.* 2004;104: 1449–1458.

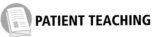 **MISCELLANEOUS**

SYNONYM(S)
Level 2 ultrasound: Specialized ultrasound

CLINICAL PEARLS
- 16–20 weeks GA is optimal timing for a single US exam if no 1st trimester indications are present.
- Specialized exam is indicated for patients with advanced maternal age, abnormal 1st- or 2nd-trimester biochemical marker screen, or history of previous chromosomal abnormalities.

ABBREVIATIONS
- β-hCG—β-Subunit of human chorionic gonadotropin
- BPP—Biophysical profile
- CRL—Crown-rump length
- CVS—Chorionic villus sampling
- GA—Gestational age
- MSAFP—Maternal serum α-fetoprotein
- NST—Non-stress test
- PAPP-A—Pregnancy associated plasma protein-A

CODES
ICD9-CM/CPT
- Based on indication or diagnosis for US
- CPT codes: 76801–76817 for obstetric ultrasounds

 PATIENT TEACHING

- Routine US exam for fetal anatomy does not detect all major or minor congenital abnormalities.
- Commercial, nonmedical use of obstetric US is discouraged.
- ACOG Patient Education Pamphlet: US Exam; Diagnosing Birth Defects

Section VII

PREIMPLANTATION GENETIC DIAGNOSIS

Stephan P. Krotz, MD
Sandra A. Carson, MD

 BASICS

DESCRIPTION
- PGD is the earliest form of prenatal diagnosis:
  - Performed during IVF; requires DNA from biopsied polar bodies, blastomeres or blastocysts
  - DNA analyzed with FISH, PCR, DNA sequencing or DNA linkage analysis
  - Detects genetic aberrations from single base pairs to chromosomal abnormalities

Used to minimize or eliminate risk of genetic problems in transferred embryos.

Disorders Detectable by PGD
- Theoretically any single-gene disorder whose molecular basis is known is testable, as are all aneuploidies and other translocations.
- Disorders commonly tested listed by mode of genetic transmission:
  - Autosomal dominant disorders:
    - Myotonic dystrophy
    - Huntington disease
    - Charcot-Marie-Tooth
    - Others, including: Adenomatous polyposis coli, Marfan syndrome, Li-Fraumeni syndrome (p53)
  - Autosomal recessive disorders:
    - Cystic fibrosis
    - Thalassemia
    - Spinal muscular atrophy
    - Others, including: Fanconi anemia, Tay-Sachs disease, β-thalassemia, sickle cell disease, Gaucher disease, phenylketonuria, epidermolysis bullosa, Rh(D), PLA-1 isoimmunization
  - X-linked disorders:
    - Fragile-X
    - Duchenne/Becker muscular dystrophy, hemophilia
    - Others, including: Lesch-Nyan syndrome, retinitis pigmentosa, ornithine transcarbamoylase deficiency, severe combined immunodeficiency, ocular albinism 1
  - Chromosomal disorders:
    - Aneuploidy of chromosomes 13,16,18,21,22, X, Y and others
    - Unbalanced translocations

Indications
- Recurrent miscarriage/poor IVF outcomes:
  - ≥ 2 unexplained miscarriages
  - Multiple failed IVF cycles
- Unexplained infertility:
  - Chromosomal abnormalities or rearrangements in either partner may cause infertility.
- Advanced maternal age:
  - Women of advanced age have a higher risk of producing genetically aneuploid oocytes.
  - Genetically abnormal oocytes lead to higher implantation failure and miscarriage rates, and higher risk of children born with birth defects or genetic syndromes (e.g., Down syndrome)
- Male factor infertility:
  - 4–7% of sperm in men with normal semen analysis parameters are aneuploid.
  - 10–23% of sperm in men with azoospermia (no sperm) or oligospermia (low sperm count) on semen analysis are aneuploid.
  - Men with azoospermia or oligospermia are at high risk of having chromosomal abnormalities.
- Family history:
  - Used to identify parents who are carriers or affected by segregating genetic disorders and thus prevent transfer of affected embryos
  - Transfer of female embryos to avoid X-linked recessive disorders
- HLA-typing:
  - Used to produce unaffected, HLA-type–compatible sibling for purposes of bone marrow or hematopoietic transplantation in older sibling affected by disorder
  - Termination unacceptable
  - Preimplantation diagnosis allows couples to avoid the ethical, moral, or religious dilemma created when an invasive diagnostic procedure detects abnormalities in pregnancy.

Concurrent Procedures
IVF

Age-Related Factors
See Indications.

EPIDEMIOLOGY
- Can be performed on any woman planning to undergo in vitro fertilization
- Can be used to assess genetic contribution from both partners

 TREATMENT

PROCEDURE
Informed Consent
All risks and benefits of IVF and the effects of preimplantation genetics on an IVF cycle should be discussed with the patient prior to the 1st cycle.
- Patients should meet with a genetic counselor or medical geneticist to discuss proposed testing and potential outcomes before each cycle.
- Patients may also benefit from psychologic counseling, given the stress associated with genetic testing in addition to IVF.

Patient Education
- Patient education should occur through counseling with the physician, genetic counselor, and office staff.
- Literature with general information and information specific to each patient's circumstance can be provided.

Risk, Benefits
- Benefits:
  - Earliest available form of genetic diagnosis
  - Maximize chances of healthy pregnancy in couples with risk factors
  - May avoid need for clinical termination of genetically affected offspring
- Risks:
  - Possible reduction in implantation potential, blastocyst formation and quality
  - Loss of biopsied embryos
  - Genetic mosaicism in embryo may lead to incorrect diagnosis, resulting in implantation of abnormal embryos or destruction of normal embryos.
  - Parents may acquire knowledge of own disease carrier status (e.g., Huntington).

Alternatives
- Amniocentesis
- 2nd-trimester maternal serum screening
- CVS
- 1st-trimester serum screening and US for nuchal translucency or nasal bone width
- Sequential serum screening in 1st and 2nd trimester
- 2nd-trimester anatomy US alone or in combination with above methods
- Pregnancy termination if diagnostic results unfavorable and desired by parents

Biopsy Methods

- Polar body biopsy:
  - Removal of polar body 1 and/or 2 from oocyte
  - Can identify single-gene mutations or chromosomal errors of meiosis I or II
  - Limited to identification of maternal genetic abnormalities
  - Unable to determine sex
  - Recombination may require analysis of polar body 1 and polar body 2.
  - Technically challenging
- Blastomere biopsy:
  - Performed at day 3 on 4–9-cell stage embryos
  - Zona pellucida mechanically or chemically dissociated followed by pipette aspiration of 1 or 2 cells
  - Most common form of PGD
- Blastocyst (trophectoderm) biopsy:
  - Excision of 10–30 cells from an embryonic pole of day 5–6 blastocyst, allowing more cells for analysis
  - In vitro culture of blastocysts difficult
  - Increased rate of monozygotic twinning in nonbiopsied embryos

Laboratory Methods

- FISH:
  - Multicolor probes bind chromosome-specific regions or centromeres
  - Probes used on interphase nuclei to determine number of chromosomes
  - ~95% sensitivity
  - Not useful for single-gene defects or detecting mutations in DNA sequence
- PCR:
  - Applicable for single-gene defects
  - Amplification of embryonic DNA sequence of interest
  - Multiple protocols including nested PCR, fluorescent PCR, and DNA sequencing
  - Linkage analysis concurrent to mutation analysis to minimize errors due to allele drop-out
  - Requires parental DNA for comparison

FOLLOW-UP

PROGNOSIS

- Pregnancy outcomes:
  - Outcomes for pregnancies after PGD similar to those for ART
  - Pregnancy loss rate for ART in the US is ~18–20% vs. 12% for non-ART cycles
- Surveillance for anomalies:
  - Complete obstetric information and outcomes of PGD patients should be kept and compared to general patient population to verify safety.
  - Obstetric information to be kept includes:
    ○ Sociodemographic history
    ○ Ethnic information
    ○ Occupational history
    ○ Exposure to drugs and other teratogens
    ○ Obstetric, medical, and family history
    ○ Pregnancy complications
    ○ Timing of fetal loss

COMPLICATIONS

- Procedural risk:
  - Possible reduction in implantation potential, blastocyst formation, and quality
  - Loss of biopsied embryos
  - Risk of incorrect diagnosis and sequelae of action taken based on results
- Risk of anomalies:
  - No increased risk of anomalies after PGD compared to conventional ART

BIBLIOGRAPHY

Simpson JL, et al. Preimplantation Genetic Diagnosis. In: Simpson JL, et al., eds. *Genetics in Obstetrics and Gynecology*, 3rd ed. Philadelphia: Saunders; 2003; 413–431.

Verlinsky Y, et al. *Practical Preimplantation Genetic Diagnosis*. Singapore: Springer-Verlag; 2005.

MISCELLANEOUS

ETHICAL CONCERNS

Currently, concern and ongoing debate exists about preimplantation genetic testing for the purposes of sex selection or for screening for nonmedical characteristics.

SYNONYM(S)

- Preimplantation genetics
- Other related terms: PGD; preimplanation genetics; prenatal diagnosis; in vitro fertilization (IVF); chromosome; genetic disease; FISH; PCR; polar body biopsy; blastocyst biopsy; blastomere biopsy; first trimester screening; chorionic villus sampling (CVS); amniocentesis; Triple Screen; Quadruple Screen; first trimester ultrasound; second trimester ultrasound

ABBREVIATIONS

- ART—Assisted reproductive technologies
- CVS—Chorionic villus sampling
- FISH—Fluorescence in situ hybridization
- HLA—Human leukocyte antigen
- IVF—In vitro fertilization
- PCR—Polymerase chain reaction
- PGD—Preimplantation genetic diagnosis

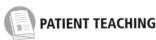 CODES

ICD9-CM/CPT

89290 Biopsy, oocyte polar body or embryo blastomere, microtechnique (for preimplantation genetic diagnosis); less than or equal to 5 embryos

89291 Biopsy, oocyte polar body or embryo blastomere, microtechnique (for preimplantation genetic diagnosis); greater than 5 embryos

PATIENT TEACHING

Information regarding risks, benefits, and limitations of PGD should be discussed with the patient.

STERILIZATION, FEMALE

Amy E. Pollack, MD
Lisa J. Thomas, MD

 BASICS

DESCRIPTION

- Female sterilization is one of the safest, most effective, and most cost-effective contraceptive methods, providing permanent contraception in 1 simple surgical procedure.
- Female sterilization involves cutting or mechanically blocking the fallopian tubes to prevent the sperm and egg from uniting.
- For the past 20 years, the most common method of female sterilization in the US has been interval tubal sterilization using laparoscopy or postpartum tubal sterilization using a subumbilical mini-laparotomy approach.
- In 2002, the US FDA approved the Essure micro insert device for interval tubal sterilization:
  - This device is placed transcervically through a hysteroscope, and may be placed in the office under local anesthesia as an interval procedure.
  - This represents a significant change in the sterilization delivery system.
- Timing:
  - Can be performed at the time of cesarean delivery, postpartum, after spontaneous or therapeutic abortion, or as an interval procedure (unrelated in time to pregnancy). The timing of the procedure influences both the surgical approach and the method of tubal occlusion.
- Options for approach:
  - Transabdominal:
    - Mini-laparotomy: Most commonly used for postpartum procedures prior to involution of the uterus
    - Laparoscopy: Most commonly used for interval sterilization and is usually performed as an outpatient procedure
  - Transcervical (see "Essure" above): Involves gaining access to the fallopian tube via the cervix:
    - Special training is needed, and this can only be done as an interval procedure.
    - Because effectiveness depends on the formation of tubal scar tissue, an alternate method of reliable contraception must be used for 3 months following placement, until a HSG demonstrates that the device is correctly placed and the tubes are occluded. Essure is the only FDA-approved transcervical method, although several other transcervical devices are under development.

- Choice of occlusion method:
  - Tubal occlusion at the time of cesarean delivery, mini-laparotomy, or laparotomy is usually performed by ligation and resection of a portion of both of the fallopian tubes:
    - The Pomeroy and Parkland methods are most commonly used.
    - The Uchida and Irving methods require special training and are rarely used.
  - Laparoscopic procedures use special instruments to apply clips, bands, or electrocoagulation for complete occlusion:
    - Unipolar electrocoagulation is not as commonly used because of an association with thermal bowel injury.
    - Use of a current meter during bipolar coagulation more accurately indicates complete coagulation and is associated with improved efficacy rates.
    - The silastic band (Falope Ring) is 1 of the most commonly used tubal sterilization devices worldwide. It is possible to lacerate the tube and/or surrounding vessels, and application may be more difficult in tubal abnormalities such as adhesions or edema.
    - The Filshie Clip is easier to use than other occlusion devices, destroys a minimal amount of the fallopian tube, and has a high efficacy rate. Studies do not support the routine application of multiple clips per tube.
- Anesthesia and pain management:
  - Short-acting general anesthesia or regional anesthesia is most frequently used for female transabdominal sterilization procedures in the US, although the procedure can be performed using local anesthetic with sedation.
  - The transcervical device (Essure) may be provided under local anesthesia with oral premedication or minimal IV sedation.
  - Advantages of local anesthesia include lower complication rates, lower cost, quicker recovery, better postoperative course with fewer or milder side effects.

Indications

- Female sterilization is ideal for those women who are certain they wish no further children and need a reliable contraceptive method.
- No medical condition absolutely restricts a woman's eligibility for sterilization.
- All surgical procedures carry some risk specific to the nature of the surgery and anesthetic used:
  - Higher probability of the pregnancy being ectopic if the method fails
  - Lack of protection against STIs, including HIV

Site (Office, Surgical Center, OR)
Typically performed in surgical center OR

Age-Related Factors

- Most women who choose sterilization do not regret their decision; however, women who undergo sterilization before the age of 30 are at greater risk for regret.
  - Thorough and effective counseling is crucial in reducing regret.
- The presence of strong risk factors (such as age) should not be used to uniformly restrict sterilization:
  - These risk factors should be indicators for more extensive counseling before undergoing sterilization.

EPIDEMIOLOGY

- Sterilization is the most commonly used contraceptive method in the US, with 15 million US women relying on either female or male sterilization.
- ~700,000 tubal sterilizations are done in the US annually.
- In 2002, female sterilization accounted for 27% of method use in all women age 15–44 who were using a contraceptive method.

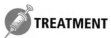 **TREATMENT**

PROCEDURE

Informed Consent

- The permanence of sterilization is a significant consideration with respect to counseling and informed consent.
- Information must be provided to the client that is in a language that can be understood, and a consent form should be signed or marked.
- Arbitrary decisions by healthcare professionals to restrict access violates the legal rights of women.
- Knowledge of state and local guidelines is important in informed consent.
- Consent information should include the following:
  - Alternative highly effective, long-acting, and temporary methods of contraception are available to women, and male sterilization should also be considered as an option when appropriate.
  - Laparoscopic and postpartum tubal sterilization require surgery (details to be explained before obtaining consent).
  - If the procedure is successful, the woman will not be able to have any more children. Women should be screened for risk factors for regret to enhance counseling.
  - Although tubal sterilization is permanent, there is a small risk of failure.
    - If failure occurs, early medical attention is necessary to establish that the pregnancy is intrauterine.
  - Tubal sterilization does not provide protection against HIV or other STIs.

Patient Education

- Tubal sterilization should be considered a permanent end to fertility. Although tubal reversal or ART may enable a previously surgically sterilized woman to become pregnant, these interventions are expensive, require technically demanding procedures, and carry some associated risks. Results cannot be guaranteed.
- Transcervical sterilization with the Essure device is not surgically reversible, and the safety of pregnancy using ART has not been established.
- Although tubal sterilization is highly effective, it is not 100% successful. Sterilization failure occurs even years after.
- If poststerilization failure occurs, an estimated 30% of failures will be ectopic. Ectopic pregnancy can be a life-threatening event if not evaluated and treated.

Risks, Benefits

- Risks:
  - Deaths from transabdominal (laparoscopic or postpartum) sterilization are rare (1–4 per 100,000), and most are associated with anesthetic complications.
  - Complications are estimated to be 0.9–1.6 per 100 procedures and vary by type of surgery and anesthesia.
  - Risk factors include previous abdominal or pelvic surgery, obesity, and diabetes.
  - Risk of regret is highest in women undergoing sterilization before age 30, following postpartum sterilization, and following interval sterilization within 1 year of delivery.
- Benefits:
  - Permanent contraception; requires only 1 procedure
  - Sterilization is 1 of the safest and most cost-effective contraceptive methods.
  - The risk of ovarian cancer is reduced following surgical tubal sterilization.

Alternatives
Medical

- Reversible or temporary contraceptive methods: Pills, IUDs, injectables, implants, patches, rings, diaphragms, and sponges
- Natural family planning
- Male-dependent methods: Condoms or withdrawal

Surgical
Male sterilization: Vasectomy (See Contraception: Sterilization, Male)

FOLLOW-UP

- Patients undergoing laparoscopic or postpartum sterilization return to their provider 1 week following surgery to assess wound healing. Patients treated with transcervical sterilization may not be required to return until 3 months postprocedure for an HSG to verify occlusion.
- Following surgical sterilization:
  - Rest for 24 hours
  - Avoid intercourse for 1 week
  - Avoid strenuous lifting for 1 week

PROGNOSIS
Women can resume most normal activities after 2–3 days, although strenuous physical exercise should be avoided for ~1 week.

COMPLICATIONS

- Intraoperative complications: Damage to bowel, bladder, or major vessels may require laparotomy and/or blood transfusion.
- Postoperative complications: Wound infection or prolonged pelvic pain
- Reported complications of transcervical sterilization using the FDA-approved Essure device include:
  - Hysteroscopy-associated hypervolemia in <1%
  - Perforation in 1.1%. Perforation may require laparoscopy or laparotomy for removal.

BIBLIOGRAPHY

Kjaer S, et al. Tubal sterilization and risk of ovarian, endometrial and cervical cancer. A Danish population-based follow-up study of more than 65,000 sterilized women. *Int J Epidemiol.* 2004;33:596–602.

Peterson HB, et al. The risk of pregnancy after tubal sterilization: Findings from the U.S. Collaborative Review of Sterilization. *Am J Obstet Gynecol.* 1996;174:1161–1168.

Pollack AE, et al. Female and male sterilization. In: *Contraceptive Technology,* 19th ed. New York: Ardent Media; 2007:363–403.

MISCELLANEOUS

SYNONYM(S)

- Laparoscopic tubal
- Tied tubes
- Tubal ligation:
  - Bilateral tubal ligation (BTL)
- Tubal sterilization

CLINICAL PEARLS

- No medical condition absolutely restricts eligibility for sterilization, although some conditions indicate special precautions:
  - Women with contraindications to laparoscopy may be candidates for mini-laparotomy under local or regional anesthesia or transcervical sterilization under local anesthesia.

- Although the risk of ectopic pregnancy when tubal sterilization fails is estimated to be 30%, the overall risk of ectopic pregnancy is lower than in the noncontracepted population because the failure rate of sterilization is low.
- The long-term health effects of tubal sterilization on menstrual pattern disturbance (post-tubal ligation syndrome) appear to be negligible.
- Women who undergo tubal sterilization are 4–5 times more likely to have a hysterectomy than partners of vasectomized men, although there is no known biologic causal mechanism.

ABBREVIATIONS

- ART—Assisted reproductive technologies
- BTL—Bilateral tubal ligation
- HSG—Hysterosalpingogram
- STI—Sexually transmitted infections

CODES
ICD9-CM

- 66.2 Bilateral endoscopic destruction or occlusion of fallopian tubes by culdoscopy, endoscopy, hysteroscopy, laparoscopy peritoneoscopy, endoscopic destruction of solitary fallopian tube
- 66.6 Other salpingectomy (includes salpingectomy by: cauterization, coagulation, electrocoagulation, excision; excludes: fistulectomy)
- 66.32 Other bilateral ligation and division of fallopian tubes: Pomeroy operation
- 66.39 Other bilateral destruction or occlusion of fallopian tubes: Female sterilization operation NOS

PATIENT TEACHING

After tubal sterilization, women should receive clear instructions about:

- Postoperative care
- Actions to take if complications occur
- Sites where they can access emergency care
- That failure can occur even many years after tubal sterilization and that, because of the risk of ectopic pregnancy, care should be sought immediately
- That tubal sterilization does not protect against STIs, including HIV
- The time and place for the follow-up visit

SUBDERMAL CONTRACEPTIVE IMPLANT INSERTION

Melissa Kottke, MD
Carrie Cwiak, MD, MPH

 BASICS

DESCRIPTION

Implanon is the only subdermal contraceptive implant available in the US:

- 4 cm x 2 mm flexible rod
- Contains 68 mg of 3–keto desogestrel, which is metabolized to etonogestrel, in a ethylene vinyl acetate core
- Provides 3 years of contraception

Indications

- Use in reproductive-age women seeking highly effective, long-term contraception.
- Safe in lactating women.
- Good for those who cannot use estrogen.
- Contraindications include active thrombosis, pregnancy, hepatic tumors, active liver disease, undiagnosed abnormal vaginal bleeding, suspected current or personal history of breast cancer, and hypersensitivity to any component of Implanon.
- Efficacy may be reduced in patients taking hepatic metabolism–inducing medicines.

Site (Office, Surgical Center, OR)

Insertion and removal can occur in the office.

Concurrent Procedures

Insertion of contraceptive implant can occur during the same visit as removal of previous implant or IUD.

Age-Related Factors
Pediatric Considerations

- This method has only been studied in women >18 years. However, safety and efficacy after menarche are expected to be the same as in adult women.
- May be used in women >35 who smoke; however, all women who smoke should be encouraged to stop.

EPIDEMIOLOGY

The cumulative Pearl index was 0.38 pregnancies per 100 women-years of use.

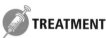 **TREATMENT**

PROCEDURE
Informed Consent

- Perform history and physical exam to ensure candidacy.
- Review risks, benefits, and side effects of the implant.
- Review other appropriate contraceptive methods.
- Review insertion and removal procedure in detail.
- Have patient sign a written consent for the placement of a contraceptive implant.

Patient Education

- No protection from STIs
- Must be inserted and removed by trained clinician
- May be removed in the office at the request of the patient

Risks, Benefits

- Risks:
  - Possible pain, infection, bruising, or scar formation at insertion site
  - Complications with insertion and/or removal
  - Irregular and unpredictable bleeding changes
  - Ovarian cysts, which often resolve spontaneously
  - Ectopic pregnancy:
    - Although less likely to become pregnant, if pregnancy occurs with an implant in situ, it is more likely to be ectopic.
  - Rare adverse reactions include weight increase, headache, acne, emotional lability, breast pain, and depression.
- Benefits:
  - Long-term effective contraception
  - Rapidly reversible
  - Safe with breastfeeding
  - Safe for those who cannot use estrogen
  - Safe for many women with medical conditions in whom pregnancy may be dangerous

Pregnancy Considerations

Current pregnancy is a contraindication to insertion of a contraceptive implant. If a woman who has an Implanon in situ is pregnant and plans to continue the pregnancy, the implant should be removed.

Alternatives

A patient may choose any contraceptive method suitable to her.

Medical

Anesthetize insertion site along planned insertion tunnel:

- Anesthetic spray OR
- 2 cc 1% lidocaine

ALERT

Clinicians must attend and complete an Organon-sponsored training program in order to prescribe, insert, or remove Implanon.

- Timing of insertion:
  - Between days 1–5 of menstrual cycle
  - When switching from combined hormonal contraception within 7 days of last dose
  - When switching from progestin-only method within last day of pill, on day of removal of implant or IUS, or when next injection due
  - Within 5 days of 1st-trimester miscarriage or abortion
  - 21–28 days following delivery (after 28 days if exclusively breastfeeding) or 2nd-trimester abortion

- Tools needed:
  - Exam table
  - Sterile gloves, drape, antiseptic, marker
  - Local anesthetic, needle, syringe
  - Sterile gauze, adhesive bandage, pressure bandage
- Patient positioning:
  - Lying on back with nondominant arm flexed at elbow so that her wrist is parallel to her ear and hand is near her head
  - Insertion site is 6–8 cm above elbow crease on the inner upper arm in the groove between the biceps and triceps.
  - Mark insertion site and a guiding mark 6–8 cm more proximal with a marker.
- Preparation:
  - Cleanse insertion site with antiseptic.
  - Anesthetize the insertion site and track with local anesthetic as above.
  - Remove implant applicator from packaging.
  - Keeping cap on, visually confirm rod is in applicator:
    - If rod is not visible, gently tap needle shield to bring the rod to the needle tip
    - Following visual confirmation, lower the rod back into the applicator by gently tapping it while holding the applicator upright.
  - Remove cap. HOLD UPRIGHT, as implant can fall out of needle.
- Implant placement:
  - Apply countertraction to the skin.
  - Insert needle tip, bevel up, at a slight (<20°) angle.
  - Lower the applicator to a horizontal position.
  - Lift skin up with needle tip. Keeping the needle in the subdermal tissue, tent up the skin and insert the full length of the needle.
  - Keep needle parallel to the surface of the skin during insertion.
  - Break the seal of the applicator by pressing the obturator support.
  - Rotate the obturator 90° in either direction.
  - Hold the obturator in place.
  - Fully retract the needle, leaving the implant behind.
- After implant placement:
  - Confirm implant placement:
    - Check needle tip for absence of rod. The grooved tip of the obturator should be visible.
    - Palpate the rod in the patient's arm.
    - Palpation of the implant in the patient's arm must be confirmed prior to relying on the implant for contraception.
  - Place adhesive bandage over insertion site to stay in place 3–5 days.
  - Have patient palpate implant in her arm.
  - Apply pressure bandage to decrease bruising (keep in place 24 hours).

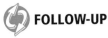 **FOLLOW-UP**

- If placed according to recommended timing, no back-up contraception is needed.
- If placed at other times when pregnancy can be ruled out, back-up contraception or abstinence is necessary for 7 days.
- Routine follow-up is appropriate.

PROGNOSIS
Irregular, unpredictable, sporadic, and erratic bleeding or spotting may occur; women should be advised about this prior to insertion.

COMPLICATIONS
- Local skin reactions:
  - Infection is very rare and can be treated with oral antibiotics:
    ○ Very rarely will the implant need to be removed secondary to infection not responding to antibiotics.
  - Hematomas are rare but can occur:
    ○ May be reduced by pressure bandage and ice
  - Pain post-insertion is often mild and can be managed with oral analgesics.

- Inability to palpate implant in patient's arm:
  - Ensure rod is not still in applicator.
  - Patient should use nonhormonal back-up method until implant is localized:
    ○ Locate rod using 10 MHz US (most in-office US is NOT 10 MHz) or MRI.
    ○ Implant is not radio-opaque and will not be seen with X-ray or CT.

BIBLIOGRAPHY

Implanon (Etonogestrel Implant) package insert labeling.

 MISCELLANEOUS

SYNONYM(S)
- Implanon
- Subdermal contraceptive implant

CLINICAL PEARLS
- Placement is the opposite movement of an injection:
  - Do not push the obturator.
  - Hold the obturator in place and pull back on the cannula.
  - The implant will be left behind in the patient's arm.

- Do not place too deeply:
  - Ideal placement is just beneath the skin.
  - Too deep a placement can make removal difficult or impossible.

ABBREVIATIONS
STI—Sexually transmitted infection

CODES
ICD9-CM/CPT
- V25.5 Insertion of implantable subdermal contraceptive
- 11975 Insertion of implantable contraceptive capsules vs
- 11981 Insertion, nonbiodegradable drug delivery implant
- 11976 Removal of implantable contraceptive capsules
- 11977 Removal and reinsertion of implantable contraceptive capsules

 PATIENT TEACHING

- Complete User Card and give to patient.
- Remind patient to have implant removed after 3 years.
- May be removed at any time pregnancy is desired prior to 3 years, with immediate return to baseline fertility.

VULVAR ABCESS: INCISION AND DRAINAGE

S. Paige Hertweck, MD

 BASICS

DESCRIPTION

In the I&D procedure, an incision is made in the vulvar epithelium over an area of fluctuance over deep vulvar tissue infection; this results in release of purulent material and resolution of pain and infection.

Indications

- Significantly tender unilateral labial mass with visible erythema, induration, warmth, and pain
- Typically, abscess begins to "point" or "come to a head" and may drain spontaneously.
- Incision and drainage may be required if:
  - Rapidly (over 24 hours) expanding cellulitis surrounding painful labial fluctuant swelling
  - Patients with a tender labial swelling and signs of systemic illness with fever and/or signs of sepsis (i.e., hypotension)

Site (Office, Surgical Center, OR)

- Office or emergency department setting:
  - For smaller abscesses without significant or expansive areas of associated cellulitis
- Surgical center or OR:
  - For larger labial abscesses, cases with expanding margins and concerns for MRSA
  - Pediatric cases requiring general anesthesia
  - Significant pain or anxiety precluding procedure in office or emergency department

Pediatric Considerations

Manage in the operating room for best pain and anxiety control.

PATHOPHYSIOLOGY

- Most vulvar infections are related to aerobic and anaerobic organisms commonly seen in the vaginal and cervical flora.
- Organisms gain access to soft tissue through a break in the epithelium, which may or may not be apparent.
- Tissue breakdown releases toxins, triggering an inflammatory reaction with an increase in WBC infiltrate and blood flow.
- Community-acquired MRSA is an increasingly seen pathogen in labial abscesses, especially in children.
- Bartholin gland abscesses typically have both anaerobic and aerobic organism on culture but also have association with *Gonorrhea* and *Chlamydia*.

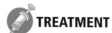 **TREATMENT**

PROCEDURE

Informed Consent

Counsel patient regarding postoperative:

- Pain
- Spread of infection
- Bleeding
- Failure to achieve resolution and need for repeat I & D
- Anesthetic complications including death
- Scarring

Risks, Benefits

Counsel about probably benefits:

- Likely improvement of pain
- More rapid resolution of infection

Alternatives

Allow for spontaneous drainage:

- Initiate antibiotic coverage
  - Antibiotic coverage for both aerobic and anaerobic organisms, as well as MRSA
- Apply local treatment: Sitz baths/heat
- Initiate NSAIDs

Medical

Antibiotics:

- Oral antibiotics are not routinely given to treat skin abscesses that are draining or have been drained unless there is an associated cellulitis, systemic symptoms such as fever, or the patient is immunocompromised.
- With rapidly expanding cellulitis over 24 hours, antibiotics to cover MRSA is indicated (Clindamycin 300 mg PO q.i.d.)

Surgical

- After adequate local or general anesthesia:
  - Prep the labial area.
  - Use 18 mL needle to aspirate purulent material to send for aerobic and anaerobic culture and sensitivity.
  - Use No. 11 or 15 scalpel to make incision:
    - Length of incision depends on extent of abscess
    - Bartholin abscess incision often 4 mm if Word catheter is to be left in place
  - Probe the abscess cavity first with a hemostat to break up loculations and check for presence of foreign body.
  - If incision length allows, probe with finger to check extent of cavity.
  - Irrigate wound completely.

- Pack with gauze, leaving 1–2 cm outside the cavity for wicking and easy removal of packing.
- Alternatively, place Word catheter.
- Cover with absorbant dressing if geometry of anatomy allows.
- Alternative surgical approach:
  - Give a single dose of intraoperative clindamycin.
  - Follow with incision, curettage, and primary suture under general anesthesia.
  - After exposing the abscess cavity and curetting lining, pass interrupted polypropylene sutures beneath but not through the cavity and close the defect.
  - Remove sutures on 6th day.

 ## FOLLOW-UP

In 24 hours, reevaluate wound:
- If drainage continues, unpack and repack wound.
- If drainage stopped, remove the packing.

PROGNOSIS

Good:
- Most abscesses resolve with I&D alone, with no antibiotics.
- Pain is relieved with the decompression of the abscess cavity.

COMPLICATIONS

Uncommon but include:
- Local extension
- Necrotizing fasciitis
- Damage to adjacent structures
- Scarring
- Pain

BIBLIOGRAPHY

Larsen T, et al. Treatment of abscesses in the vulva. *Acta Obstet Gynecol Scand*. 1986;65:459–461.

 ## MISCELLANEOUS

If patient has need for SBE prophylaxis:
- Decisions about antibiotic therapy must address both the need for endocarditis prophylaxis and for therapy of the abscess.

ABBREVIATIONS

- I&D—Incision and drainage
- MRSA—Methicillin-resistant *Staphylococcus aureus*
- NSAIDs—Nonsteroidal anti-inflammatory drugs
- OR—Operating room
- SBE—Subacute bacterial endocarditis

CODES

ICD9-CM
- 616.4 Vulvar abscess

 ## PATIENT TEACHING

- Patient must:
  - Soak wound b.i.d. to t.i.d.
  - Watch for resolution or worsening of condition.
  - Expect healing over next 7–10 days.
- Instruct patient to call if:
  - Fever or chills
  - Recollection of pus in the area
  - Increased pain or redness
  - Red streaks

Section VII

VULVAR BIOPSY

Martina Chiodi, MD
Paula J. Adams Hillard, MD

 BASICS

DESCRIPTION
Vulvar biopsy establishes a pathologic diagnosis of uncertain or symptomatic vulvar skin lesions (see Vulvar Signs and Symptoms: Vulvar Masses and Rashes).

Indications
- Skin lesions of uncertain diagnosis or significance:
  - Suspected malignancy
  - Pigmented lesion
- Persistent symptoms:
  - Irritation
  - Itching

Age-Related Factors
- Pediatric:
  - Malignancy less likely
  - Office biopsy less feasible except in adolescents
- Geriatric:
  - Malignancy more likely

EPIDEMIOLOGY
- Skin disorder
- Infectious
- Cancerous

 TREATMENT

PROCEDURE

Informed Consent
- Explain procedure, risk, benefits, and alternatives.
- Patient may ask questions or decline.
- Document discussion and obtain patient signature.

Patient Education
- Discuss need for diagnosis and specific management tailored to diagnosis.
- Anesthetics (local):
  - Inquire about allergies.

Risks, Benefits
- Benefits:
  - Establishes accurate diagnosis for effective management
  - Biopsy may be excision, and thus is both diagnostic and therapeutic.
- Risks:
  - Infection or bleeding (low risk)

Alternatives
- Empiric therapy without establishing diagnosis
- Biopsy if empiric therapy not effective

Surgical
- Determine if biopsy is intended to be excisional (possible for small lesions) or incisional/sampling.
- Determine location to biopsy:
  - Colposcopy of the vulva may be helpful in visualizing abnormal areas requiring biopsy; 5% acetic acid may highlight abnormal epithelium
  - Representative sites:
    ○ Avoid biopsy of clitoris, urethra, labia minora if possible
  - Consider biopsy of nodularity, granulation tissue, ulceration
- May use topical EMLA cream:
  - Apply to area for 1 hour prior to biopsy
  - With occlusive dressing for 1 hour, analgesia to 3 mm
- Prep skin using iodine.
- Localize lesion, pinch it between 2 fingers, and inject with 1–2 mL 1% lidocaine (+/− epinephrine).
- Use Keyes punch 2–6 mm for full-thickness core biopsy of the epithelium.
- Rotate clockwise/counterclockwise.
- Grasp the biopsy with forceps and, if it is still attached, at the base, cut it with scissors.
- Hemostasis can be obtained with:
  - Pressure
  - Silver nitrate
  - Monsel's solution
  - Cautery
  - Very seldom is a stitch (4–0 absorbable; e.g., polygalactic acid) required.

- If no Keyes punch is available, biopsy can be performed with scalpel/scissors.
- Provide information to pathologist about site, symptoms, suspected diagnosis, patient data (age, previous therapy).
- 2% lidocaine jelly may be applied p.r.n. for 2–3 days to provide analgesia.

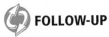

FOLLOW-UP

Follow-up office visit should be scheduled to discuss results of biopsy and planned therapy based on biopsy results.

COMPLICATIONS

- Rarely, infection of the biopsy site
- Uncommon reactions to local anesthetic

BIBLIOGRAPHY

Apgar BS, et al. Differentiating normal and abnormal findings of the vulva. *Am Fam Physician*. 1996;53(4): 1171–1180.

Foster DC. Vulvar disease. *Obstet Gynecol*. 2002; 100:145.

Illustration of vulvar biopsy technique. Available at: www.brooksidepress.org. Accessed 11/17/07.

 MISCELLANEOUS

CLINICAL PEARLS

- If biopsy site is likely to be exposed to urine, application of 2% lidocaine jelly 5 minutes prior to urination can be helpful in controlling pain.
- Pigmented vulvar lesions should be excised, as the site is difficult for patient and physician to adequately monitor.
- Vulvar lesions may be excised at the time of vaginal delivery if an epidural anesthetic is planned.

ABBREVIATIONS

EMLA—Eutectic mixture of local anesthetics lidocaine and prilocaine

 CODES

ICD9-CM/CPT
56605–Vulvar biopsy

PATIENT TEACHING

- ACOG Patient Education Pamphlet: Disorders of the Vulva
- If lesion is likely to be exposed to urine, application of 2% lidocaine jelly 5 minutes prior to urination can be helpful in controlling pain.

Section VII

Section VIII

Obstetric and Gynecologic Emergencies

ABDOMINAL TRAUMA IN PREGNANCY

Shirley L. Wang, MD

 BASICS

DESCRIPTION

- Trauma is the most common cause of nonobstetric death in pregnant women in the US.
- Because there are 2 patients involved, the mother and fetus, evaluation of the pregnant trauma patient present unique challenges:
  – Main principle guiding therapy: Resuscitating the mother will resuscitate the fetus.
- Physiologic changes in pregnancy can affect the interpretation of vital signs and thus the management of the gravid patient.
- Often requires a multidisciplinary approach involving an emergency physician, trauma surgeon, obstetrician, and neonatologist

DIFFERENTIAL DIAGNOSIS

Types of trauma:

- Blunt abdominal trauma:
  – Influence of GA:
    ○ >18–20 weeks, compression of IVC and aorta in supine position lead to increased likelihood for hypotension and decreased uterine perfusion.
    ○ <13 weeks, uterus is protected by bony pelvis; therefore direct injury is less likely and usually does not result in pregnancy loss.
- Pelvic fractures:
  – May result in significant retroperitoneal bleeding
  – Intraperitoneal bleeding leading to hypovolemic shock
  – Bladder and urethral disruption
- Penetrating trauma:
  – Gunshot wound or stab wound
  – Fetal loss usually due to:
    ○ Direct injury
    ○ Injury to umbilical cord
    ○ Injury to placenta

EPIDEMIOLOGY

- Trauma affects 6–7% of pregnancies in the US.
- 0.3% of pregnant women require hospital admission because of trauma.
- MVA, DV, and falls are the most common causes of blunt trauma in pregnancy:
  – MVA accounts for 2/3 of all trauma during pregnancy.
  – DV, up to 25% prevalence in pregnancy:
    ○ Physicians only detect 4–10% of cases.
    ○ 60% of victims report ≥2 episodes during pregnancy.
- Penetrating trauma accounts for as many as 36% of maternal deaths.
- Overall maternal mortality in gunshot wounds to the pregnant abdomen is low (3.9 %), but fetal mortality is high, ranging 40–70%.

 TREATMENT

MEDICAL MANAGEMENT

- Trauma assessment for all injuries
- Assess maternal stability
- Assess GA
- Assess fetus with FHTs

Primary Survey

- ABCs: Airway/Cervical spine control, breathing and circulation
- Treat the mother immediately for cardiovascular or respiratory compromise:
  – Displace the uterus to the left:
    ○ If >20–week size, place a wedge under the woman's right side, positioning the woman on her left side.
    ○ Avoids compression of the IVC and maximizes cardiac preload and uteroplacental blood flow.
  – Cricoid pressure to prevent aspiration until the airway has been protected with a cuffed endotracheal tube.
- Aggressive fluid resuscitation:
  – 2 large-bore IV lines (14–16 gauge)
  – Replacement is preferable to vasopressors for BP support (vasopressor can compromise uterine blood flow).
- Supplemental oxygen by nasal cannula, oxygen mask, or endotracheal intubation as needed

Secondary Survey

- Extent of trauma via physical exam and history
- Any treatment required to save the mother's life or treat her critical status should be undertaken, regardless of her pregnancy.
- Any diagnostic imaging deemed necessary:
  – 1st trimester:
    ○ US: No radiation, preferred method
    ○ DPL: Supraumbilical, open technique to avoid injury to the gravid uterus, but invasive
    ○ CT scan
  – 2nd trimester:
    ○ US or CT scan
    ○ DPL difficult to perform because of uterine size, but very useful
  – 3rd trimester:
    ○ US and CT scan
- Call obstetric consult to evaluate fetal age, viability, and need for fetal monitoring or delivery:
  – Attempt continuous fetal monitoring if the fetus is ≥24 weeks' GA.

Drugs

Regarding fluid resuscitation: Try to avoid vasopressors, as they compromise uterine blood flow:

- Should not be withheld if needed in resuscitation.

Other
Fetal Monitoring

- Continuous electronic fetal monitoring after trauma is the current standard of care with a viable fetus.
- May be predictive of placental abruption.
- Initiated as soon as possible after maternal stabilization.
- ≥8 uterine contractions/hr for >4 hours is associated with placental abruption.
- Optimal length of monitoring is unclear.
- Recommended minimum time of 4 hours
- Monitoring should be prolonged if:
  – Uterine contractions
  – NRFHT
  – Vaginal bleeding
  – Significant uterine tenderness of irritability
  – Serious maternal injury
  – ROM
- Upon discharge, patient must be given precautions. Return if you have:
  – Vaginal bleeding
  – Leakage of fluid
  – Decreased fetal movement
  – Severe abdominal pain

Fetal-Maternal Hemorrhage

- Administer 300 μg of IgD to all D-negative trauma victims.
- Kleihauer-Betke assay is useful in identifying unsensitized D-negative patients who require >30 mL transfusion.
  – Administer 300 mg of IgD for every 30 mL of whole blood transfused:
    ○ Give within 72 hours following hemorrhage

SURGICAL MANAGEMENT
Informed Consent

- Consent obtained urgently, as with any trauma
- Patient should be informed of necessity for management of her trauma, as fetal salvage depends on her survival and management.
- Patient informed of potential risks to fetus

Risks, Benefits

- Risks to fetus with surgical management must be discussed, but primary concern is maternal management.
- Consider urgent cesarean delivery pregnancies ≥24 weeks of gestation if:
  - Imminent maternal death
  - CPR has not been effective within 5 minutes
  - Stable mother with a NRFHT
- Perimortem cesarean delivery:
  - For optimum infant survival, delivery should be initiated within 4 minutes of maternal cardiac arrest.
- GA <24 weeks, emergency cesarean delivery is usually not performed because the fetus is too small to survive and the delivery is unlikely to have much effect on maternal hemodynamics.

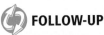 **FOLLOW-UP**

COMPLICATIONS

- Fetal loss depends on severity of trauma.
- Placental abruption or other placental injury:
  - Accounts for 50% of fetal loss
  - Mechanism of injury: Shearing force of placenta from myometrium, displacement of AF, and distension of other parts of the uterus
  - 67–75% rate of fetal mortality in abruptions after trauma
  - If significant placental abruption occurs, a viable fetus should be delivered immediately.
- Direct fetal injury:
  - <1% of all pregnancies complicated by trauma
- Uterine rupture:
  - 0.6% of all trauma injuries during pregnancy
  - Results from direct abdominal impact with substantial force
  - Results in serosal hemorrhage
  - Avulsion of uterine vasculature with hemorrhage
  - Disruption of myometrial wall with extrusion of fetus, placenta, or umbilical cord into abdomen
  - 75% involve uterine fundus
- Maternal shock or death: In severe MVA, maternal loss of life was the most frequent cause of death to the fetus.
- NRFHT:
  - Bradycardia or repetitive late decelerations unresponsive to intrauterine resuscitation also require immediate delivery, if the mother is stable.

BIBLIOGRAPHY

ACOG Educational Bulletin No. 251. Obstetric Aspects of Trauma Management. *Int J Gynecol Obstet*. 1999;64:87–94.

Baerga-Varela Y, et al. Trauma in pregnancy. *Mayo Clin Proc*. 2000;75:1243–1248.

Connolly AM, et al. Trauma and pregnancy. *Am J Perinatol*. 1997;14:331–336.

Drost TF, et al. Major trauma in pregnant women: Maternal/fetal outcome. *J Trauma*. 1990;30:574–578.

Hedin LW, et al. Domestic violence during pregnancy. The prevalence of physical injuries, substance use, abortions and miscarriages. *Acta Obstet Gynecol Scand*. 2000;79:625–630.

Jacob S, et al. Maternal mortality in Utah. *Obstet Gynecol*. 1998;91:187–191.

Katz VL, et al. Perimortem cesarean delivery. *Obstet Gynecol*. 1986;68(4):571–576.

Rogers FB, et al. A multi-institutional study of factors associated with fetal death in injured pregnant patients. *Arch Surg*. 1999;134:1274–1277.

Shah KH, et al. Trauma in pregnancy: Maternal and fetal outcomes. *J Trauma*. 1998;45:83–86.

 MISCELLANEOUS

CLINICAL PEARLS

Resuscitating the mother will resuscitate the fetus.

ABBREVIATIONS

- AF—Amniotic fluid
- DPL—Diagnostic peritoneal lavage
- DV—Domestic violence
- FHT—Fetal heart tones
- GA—Gestational age
- IVC—Inferior vena cava
- MVA—Motor vehicle accident
- NRFHT—Nonreassuring fetal heart tones
- ROM—Rupture of membranes

 CODES

ICD9-CM

- 761.9 Unspecified maternal complication of pregnancy affecting fetus or newborn
- 867 Injury to pelvic organs
- 868 Injury to other intraabdominal organs

PATIENT TEACHING

PREVENTION

- MVA and DV are common preventable causes of trauma in pregnancy:
  - Proper seat belt use is the most significant modifiable factor in decreasing maternal and fetal injury and mortality after MVA.
  - Seat belt–restrained women who are in MVA have the same fetal mortality rate as women who are not in MVA.
  - Unrestrained women who are in crashes are 2.8 times more likely to lose their fetuses.
  - Prenatal care must include 3-point seat belt instruction:
    - Lap belt should be placed under the gravid abdomen, snugly over the thighs, with the shoulder harness off to the side of the uterus, between the breasts and over the midline of the clavicle.
    - Seat belts placed directly over the uterus can cause fetal injury.
    - Airbags should not be disabled during pregnancy.
- Screen all patients for DV:
  - Be familiar with the community resources for helping patients who experience domestic abuse.
  - Screening of younger patients is particularly important, because they have higher rates of MVA and DV.
  - Resource materials in waiting rooms and restrooms allow patients to gather information without confrontation.

Section VIII

ABNORMAL FETAL HEART RATE TRACING IN LABOR

Ernest M. Graham, MD
Joel D. Larma, MD

 BASICS

DESCRIPTION

- EFM may be done either externally through the maternal abdominal wall with Doppler or internally by attaching a bipolar spiral electrode directly to the fetal scalp.
- External: Ultrasonic waves undergo a shift in frequency as they are reflected from moving fetal heart valves and pulsatile blood ejected during systole.
- Internal: The R wave of the electrical fetal cardiac signal is amplified, and the time in milliseconds between fetal R waves is used to calculate the FHR.
- With internal EFM continuous R to R wave FHR computation is known as beat-to-beat variability.
- External monitoring may not give a valid indication of beat-to-beat variability because the Doppler signal is broad and slurred, so that an artificial short-term variability is portrayed.
- Normal FHR is 110–160 bpm:
  - Bradycardia: Baseline FHR <110 bpm
  - Tachycardia: Baseline FHR >160 bpm
- Acceleration: A visually apparent abrupt increase (onset of acceleration to peak in <30 seconds) in FHR above the baseline
- Late deceleration: A smooth, gradual, symmetrical decrease in FHR beginning at or after the peak of the contraction and returning to baseline only after the contraction has ended. Indicates uteroplacental insufficiency.
- Early deceleration: A gradual decrease and return to baseline associated with a contraction. Indicates fetal head compression, which is a normal part of labor.
- Variable deceleration: Abrupt decrease in FHR whose onset varies in relation to the onset of successive contractions:
  - The most common deceleration patterns seen during labor
  - Related to cord compression
  - ACOG has defined significant variable decelerations as those decreasing to <70 bpm and lasting >60 seconds.

- Sinusoidal pattern: Smooth, sinewave-like pattern of regular frequency and amplitude. Is associated with fetal anemia.
- The National Institute of Child Health and Human Development research planning workshop agreed on FHR patterns that are normal and confer an extremely high predictability of a normally oxygenated fetus:
  - Normal baseline rate
  - Moderate variability
  - Presence of accelerations
  - Absence of decelerations
- The research workshop agreed on several patterns that are predictive of current or impending fetal asphyxia so severe that the fetus is at risk for neurologic and other fetal damage or death:
  - Recurrent late or variable decelerations
  - Substantial bradycardia with absent FHR variability
- The research workshop stated that many fetuses have FHR tracings that are intermediate between these 2 extremes, and their presumed condition and clinical management are controversial.

DIFFERENTIAL DIAGNOSIS

If fetal bradycardia is suspected by external monitoring, check the maternal pulse to make sure that you are not confusing a normal maternal pulse with fetal bradycardia.

EPIDEMIOLOGY

- EFM is the most common obstetric procedure in the US, occurring in 85% of all births.
- Since the introduction of EFM in the late 1960s, the incidence of cesarean delivery has increased from 5% to 29% in 2004 with around 10% of these cesareans being done for nonreassuring fetal status.
- Intrapartum management based on EFM is no better in reducing the risk of cerebral palsy or perinatal death than that based on intermittent heart rate auscultation.

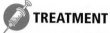 **TREATMENT**

MEDICAL MANAGEMENT

- A nonreassuring FHR during labor has a very high false-positive rate, so other tests can be done to identify the fetus that is truly developing hypoxia-ischemia.
- Fetal scalp pH:
  - pH >7.25 is normal: Continue to observe labor.
  - pH 7.2–7.5: Repeat pH within 30 minutes.
  - pH <7.2: Immediate delivery is indicated.
  - This procedure is now used uncommonly because fetal scalp stimulation can provide the same information noninvasively.
- Scalp stimulation:
  - When the fetal scalp is stimulated manually through the dilated cervix during labor, the elicitation of an acceleration provides reassurance that the fetus is not acidotic.
  - Even when no acceleration can be elicited, only 30% have a scalp pH <7.2.

Resuscitation

- In the presence of a nonreassuring intrapartum FHR tracing, in utero resuscitation is preferred to immediate delivery when possible.
- Repositioning the mother to either side or onto her hands and knees may relieve cord compression and improve oxygen delivery to the fetus.
- Administering oxygen to mother by face mask may improve oxygen delivery to the fetus.

Drugs

- If an abnormal FHR tracing develops during labor with frequent repetitive contractions due to an induction with Pitocin or cervical ripening with dinoprostone or misoprostol, these drugs can be immediately stopped or removed.
  - When the contractions decrease, oxygen delivery to the fetus will improve, and the FHR tracing may become reassuring.
- If the nonreassuring FHR tracing is associated with spontaneous frequent repetitive contractions, a tocolytic such as subcutaneous terbutaline may be given to break the contractions.

Other

If the nonreassuring FHR tracing persists despite scalp stimulation, maternal repositioning, and oxygen administration, and the cervix is completely dilated with the fetal head engaged, an operative delivery with either vacuum or forceps should be considered.

SURGICAL MANAGEMENT

Informed Consent

If the nonreassuring FHR tracing persists despite the above steps and delivery cannot be accomplished vaginally, then immediate cesarean delivery is indicated. The patient should be consented either on admission in labor for possible cesarean should it become necessary or during labor at the time the indication arises.

Surgical

- If immediate cesarean delivery is indicated, anesthesia can be administered using general endotracheal anesthesia, redosing the epidural, or by placing a quick spinal.
- An emergent cesarean delivery can be performed using either a vertical or Pfannenstiel incision and either a low transverse or classical uterine incision, depending on the clinical situation.

ALERT

- The term "fetal distress" should be replaced with "nonreassuring fetal status" followed by a further description of findings such as repetitive variable decelerations, fetal tachycardia or bradycardia, late decelerations, or low BPP.
- The term "birth asphyxia" should only be used in the presence of damaging acidemia, hypoxia, and metabolic acidosis.

 FOLLOW-UP

In the presence of an abnormal intrapartum FHR tracing, a team of clinicians (Pediatrics/nursing) should be present at the delivery to attend to the neonate.

PROGNOSIS

- A reassuring FHR tracing is very reliable in predicting a fetus with normal oxygenation.
- A nonreassuring FHR tracing has a very high false-positive rate in identifying the compromised fetus.
- Most fetuses delivered emergently because of a nonreassuring FHR tracing have a normal outcome.

BIBLIOGRAPHY

ACOG Committee Opinion No. 326. Inappropriate use of the terms fetal distress and birth asphyxia. Washington DC: ACOG; Dec 2005.

ACOG Technical Bulletin No. 207. Fetal Heart Rate Patterns: Monitoring, Interpretation, and Management. Washington DC: ACOG; 1995.

Alfirevic Z, et al. Continuous cardiotocography (CTG) as a form of electronic fetal monitoring (EFM) for fetal assessment during labour. *Cochrane Database Syst Rev.* 2006. CD006066

American College of Obstetricians and Gynecologists, American Academy of Pediatrics. Neonatal Encephalopathy and Cerebral Palsy: Defining the pathogenesis and pathophysiology. 2003.

Elimian A, et al. Intrapartum assessment of fetal well-being: A comparison of scalp stimulation with scalp pH sampling. *Obstet Gynecol.* 1997;89:373–376.

National Institute of Child Health and Human Development Research Planning Workshop. Electronic fetal heart rate monitoring: Research guidelines for interpretation. *Am J Obstet Gynecol.* 1997;177:1385–1390.

 MISCELLANEOUS

A task force from ACOG and the AAP has produced criteria to define an acute intrapartum event sufficient to cause cerebral palsy:

- Essential criteria:
  - Umbilical arterial pH <7.0 or base deficit ≥12 mM
  - Early-onset moderate-severe neonatal encephalopathy in infants born at ≥34 weeks
  - Cerebral palsy of the spastic quadriplegic or dyskinetic type
  - Exclusion of other identifiable etiologies such as trauma, coagulation disorders, infectious conditions, or genetic disorders
- Criteria that collectively suggest intrapartum timing but are nonspecific to asphyxial insults:
  - Sentinel (signal) hypoxic event occurring immediately before or during labor
  - A sudden and sustained fetal bradycardia or the absence of FHR variability in the presence of persistent late or variable decelerations, usually after a hypoxic sentinel event when the pattern was previously normal.
  - Apgar scores of 0–3 beyond 5 minutes
  - Onset of multisystem involvement within 72 hours of birth
  - Early imaging study showing evidence of acute nonfocal cerebral abnormality

ABBREVIATIONS

- AAP—American Academy of Pediatricians
- ACOG—American College of Obstetricians and Gynecologists
- BPP—Biophysical profile
- EFM—Electronic fetal monitoring
- FHR—Fetal heart rate

CODES

ICD9-CM

- 656.8 Abnormal fetal acid-base balance
- 659.7 Abnormality in fetal heart rate or rhythm

Section VIII

ACUTE PELVIC PAIN

Geri D. Hewitt, MD

 BASICS

DESCRIPTION

- Acute pelvic pain is a relatively common complaint of reproductive-aged women, but can occur in premenarchal and postmenopausal patients as well.
- Acute pelvic pain is the sudden onset of pain in the lower abdominal and pelvic region and is typically due to ischemia or injury to a viscous organ with autonomic reflex responses.
- In addition to pain, patients may experience nausea/vomiting, fever/chills, restlessness, sweating, or back pain depending on the etiology and/or intensity of the pain.
- Most commonly, acute pelvic pain has a gynecologic, urologic, or gastroenterologic cause.

DIFFERENTIAL DIAGNOSIS

- Gynecologic:
  - Ectopic pregnancy
  - Ruptured ovarian cyst
  - Adnexal torsion
  - Degenerating uterine fibroid
  - PID
  - Mid-cycle ovulatory pain—Mittelschmerz
- Urologic:
  - Cystitis/Pyelonephritis
  - Urolithiasis
- GI:
  - IBD
  - Ischemic bowel disease
  - Irritable bowel syndrome
  - Appendicitis
  - Diverticulitis/Diverticulosis
  - Constipation

Pregnancy Considerations

ALERT

All reproductive-aged women with acute pelvic pain should have a pregnancy test to rule out ectopic pregnancy, a life-threatening condition.

EPIDEMIOLOGY

~10% of all women are using no method of contraception, and thus at high risk for unintended pregnancy:

- Acts of unprotected sexual intercourse can lead to ectopic pregnancy and PID.

PATHOPHYSIOLOGY

- Acute pelvic pain results from damage, ischemia, inflammation, or infection to any internal organs.
- An ectopic pregnancy may cause swelling in the fallopian tube from the pregnancy mass or bleeding, resulting in activation of the autonomic nervous system and pain.
- Visceral perforation from a ruptured ectopic pregnancy or ruptured appendix similarly results in pain.
- Infection such as PID also results in pain.

 DIAGNOSIS

TESTS

Lab

- Most commonly indicated labs include:
  - Pregnancy test (to rule out ectopic pregnancy)
  - CBC with differential (looking for signs of infection or acute blood loss)
  - UA (looking for signs of infection or hematuria)
  - Cervical or urine testing for STIs is indicated if the patient is sexually active and PID is a concern.
- UA looking for evidence of infection, blood, or stones is important if the patient has any urinary complaints.

Imaging

- If a gynecologic cause is suspected or the pelvic exam is abnormal, a pelvic US may be useful to access for free fluid in the pelvis, and uterine or adnexal abnormalities:
  - Using Doppler flow of the adnexa can be helpful if adnexal torsion is suspected.
- Abdominal-pelvic CT scan may be indicated to evaluate for appendicitis or other gastroenterologic abnormalities and kidney stones.

 TREATMENT

MEDICAL MANAGEMENT

- Pain medication may be indicated while the diagnostic evaluation is being completed; it's important not to overmedicate the patient with narcotics, which would interfere potentially with the evaluation.
- If PID is diagnosed, antibiotics for either outpatient or inpatient treatment should be started as indicated by the current CDC guidelines:
  - Patients being treated for outpatient PID should have follow up ~48 hours later to make sure their symptoms have improved.
- Antibiotics are also indicated in patients with cystitis/pyelonephritis or diverticulitis.
- Ectopic pregnancy may be treated with IM methotrexate (50 mg/m^2) in select patients.
- Other:
  - IV fluids may be required if the patient is dehydrated, hemodynamically unstable, or has physical findings suggestive of an "acute (surgical) abdomen"—rebound tenderness indicative of peritoneal irritation. Normal saline is adequate.

SURGICAL MANAGEMENT

Informed Consent

- The suspected diagnoses and surgical options should be outlined to the patient, describing the most likely findings and procedures, as well as best- and worst-case scenarios.
- For example, a suspected ruptured ovarian cysts maybe managed with the following options, depending on the findings at the time of surgery:
  - Observation for a ruptured corpus luteum cyst with no further bleeding
  - Detorsion, if the finding is torsion
  - Ovarian cystectomy for a benign cystic teratoma
  - Oophorectomy for a large benign cyst or a germ cell tumor
  - Total abdominal hysterectomy and bilateral oophorectomy if the findings are disseminated ovarian cancer

Medical Alternatives

- If the working diagnosis, based on clinical history of pain in the luteal phase of the cycle, findings on US, and a negative hCG, is pain from a corpus luteum cyst, the preferred option is observation with close follow-up.
- Pain from a corpus luteum cyst resolves within several days to a week, and a repeat US demonstrates resolution of this functional cyst.

Surgical Alternatives

- Diagnostic laparoscopy may be indicated for both diagnostic and therapeutic reasons.
- Patients with ectopic pregnancy may undergo laparoscopic salpingectomy or salpingostomy.
- Patients with an acute abdomen but an uncertain diagnosis (PID vs. appendicitis, for example) often benefit from a diagnostic laparoscopy to confirm the diagnosis with certainty.
- Acutely symptomatic adnexal masses, suspected adnexal torsion, and hemoperitoneum are also relatively common indications for laparoscopy.
- Ovarian cystectomy, hemostasis, oophorectomy, and untwisting adnexa can all be accomplished laparoscopically.
- Laparoscopy may be indicated in patients with ectopic pregnancy, hemoperitoneum, ruptured ovarian cysts, or acutely painful ovarian cysts, appendicitis, or uncertain diagnosis.
- Oophorectomy, cystectomy, salpingostomy, salpingectomy, untwisting adnexal torsion with adnexal-pexy, and appendectomy can all be done laparoscopically.
- A patient who is hemodynamically unstable with a hemoperitoneum may benefit from an urgently performed exploratory laparotomy.

FOLLOW-UP

- All surgical specimens are sent for a pathologic evaluation and the final pathologic diagnosis should be reviewed at the time of follow-up.
- Hematosalpinx or chorionic villi in the fallopian tube confirms the presence of an ectopic pregnancy.
- The exact nature of the ovarian tumor (hemorrhagic corpus luteum, dermoid cyst, etc.) can be confirmed on pathologic exam.
- Appendicitis can be confirmed with a pathologic exam.
- The vast majority of adnexal lesions in young women are benign.
- Patients diagnosed with a gynecologic cause of their acute pelvic pain would benefit from follow-up with a gynecologist.
- Patients with recurrent kidney stones may need to see an urologist.
- A gastroenterologic cause of the acute pain may necessitate referral to a GI specialist.

PROGNOSIS
- Patients most commonly need admission to the hospital:
  - If they require surgery
  - Are unable to tolerate PO pain medications or antibiotics
  - Have an uncertain diagnosis, or meet the criteria for inpatient treatment of PID (see CDC guidelines)
- Discharge from the hospital is feasible after the correct diagnosis is made, treatment initiated, and the patient's symptoms have improved.

COMPLICATIONS
- Ectopic pregnancy can result in rupture, hemorrhage, and death.
- Infectious causes of acute pelvic pain can result in overwhelming sepsis.
- Adnexal torsion can be associated with tissue necrosis and loss of function.

- Surgical complications of laparoscopy include anesthetic complications, bleeding, infection, wound infection, DVT/PE, and damage to other organs, particularly thermal injury to the bowel or damage to bladder or ureters.
- Surgical patients need a 2-week postoperative evaluation as an outpatient.
- Patients receiving methotrexate for ectopic pregnancy need follow-up lab work in 3–4 days.
- Patients with the diagnosis of ruptured ovarian cyst should have outpatient follow up in 7–10 days to confirm improvement of their symptoms.
- All patients should be instructed to return if their symptoms do not improve or if they worsen.

BIBLIOGRAPHY

Brosens I, et al. Bowel injury in gynecologic laparoscopy. *J Am Assoc Gynecol Laprosc.* 2003: 10(1):9–13.

Center For Disease Control. Pelvic inflammatory disease. Sexually Transmitted Disease Treatment Guidelines–2006. Available at: www.cdc.gov/std/treatment/2006/pid.htm. Accessed 06/04/07.

Lipscomb GH, et al. Nonsurgical treatment of ectopic pregnancy *N Engl J Med.* 2000;343(18):1325–1329.

Wang PH, et al. Major complications of operative and diagnostic laparoscopy for gynecologic disease. *J Am Assoc Gynecol Laparosc.* 2001;8(1):68–73.

 MISCELLANEOUS

ABBREVIATIONS
- PID—Pelvic inflammatory disease
- IBD—Inflammatory bowel disease
- STI—Sexually transmitted infection
- hCG—Human chorionic gonadotropin
- DVT—Deep venous thrombosis
- PE—Pulmonary embolism

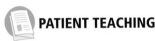

ICD9-CM
- 218.9 Degenerating uterine fibroid
- 220 Dermoid cyst
- 541 Appendicitis
- 557.0 Ischemic bowel
- 558.9 IBD
- 562.11 Diverticulosis
- 564.00 Constipation
- 564.1 IBS
- 568.81 Hemoperitoneum
- 590.80 Pyelonephritis
- 592.9 Urolithiasis
- 595.9 Cystitis
- 614.9 PID
- 620.2 Ruptured ovarian cyst
- 620.5 Adnexal torsion
- 625.2 Mid-cycle ovulatory pain
- 625.9 Pelvic pain
- 633.1 Ectopic pregnancy

PATIENT TEACHING

ACOG Patient Education Pamphlet: Pelvic Pain. Available at: www.acog.org

ADNEXAL TORSION

Michelle Moniz, BA
Tassawan Rungruxsirivorn, MD
Diane F. Merritt, MD

 BASICS

DESCRIPTION

Adnexal torsion refers to excessive rotation of the ovary, fallopian tube, or both, which produces a mechanical impediment to vascular flow. This well-known yet difficult to recognize entity is a true gynecologic emergency, because it can compromise adnexal blood supply.

- Torsion disrupts lymphatic and venous flow, resulting in adnexal edema and enlargement, which can progress to ischemia and necrosis.
- The catastrophic outcome of late or missed diagnosis is loss of ovarian and/or tubal function and compromise of future fertility.
- The exact duration of compromised flow that produces irreversible damage is unknown.
- Torsion is often associated with an underlying ovarian or paraovarian lesion, but can also occur in the setting of a normal tube and ovary.
- Etiology: Various theories advanced include:
  - Anatomic theory: Predisposing anatomic abnormalities: Long mesosalpinx, long accessory ostia, paraovarian cysts, increased weight of fallopian tube with hydrosalpinx or hematosalpinx, ovarian cysts and benign tumors, functional cysts, or polycystic ovaries. Malignant tumors and inflammatory lesions less prone to torse, as adhesions are likely to limit motility.
  - Hemodynamic theory: Unequal pressures in the arteries and veins of the ovarian mesentery may predispose to torsion.
  - Sellheim theory: Accounts for torsion with dancing, gymnastics, intercourse, abdominal trauma, coughing, and defecation; proposes that body movements are transmitted to internal organs
  - Physiologic theory: Suggests that follicular growth, ovulation, a corpus luteum, increased midcycle tubal motion, or any disturbance of the regular peristaltic movements of fallopian tube or surrounding intestines may precipitate torsion.
  - Pregnancy: May predispose due to increased vascularity, tubal pregnancy, corpus luteum of pregnancy, or displacement of adnexa by growing uterus, fetal movements, labor, or diminution in pelvic contents following labor
  - Mechanical factors: Possible initiating events may include bladder distension and evacuation, descent of feces into the rectum, intestinal peristalsis, vomiting, enemas, or even gynecologic exams
  - Gynecologic Surgery: Tubal ligations and hysterectomies may be destabilizing to remaining tube and ovary
  - OHSS: Cystic stimulated ovaries with ovulation induction and ART may be prone to torse

DIAGNOSIS

SIGNS AND SYMPTOMS

- Preoperative diagnosis of adnexal torsion is often challenging, so it is important to maintain a high index of suspicion.
- Sudden-onset, severe, unilateral lower abdominal pain at the ileac fossa (90%), sharp and stabbing in nature that intermittently worsens over hours. May

wax and wane with torsion-detorsion. May radiate to groin, flank, or thigh. 25% present with bilateral lower quadrant pain.
- Nausea and vomiting in 70–80% (often accompanies pain in torsion, while it is a late sign in appendicitis)
- Unilaterally enlarged adnexal mass (nearly 100% on US, palpable in 20–30%)
- Anorexia, constipation, tenesmus, or dysuria
- Fever (20%; late finding, often concurrent with ovarian necrosis)

History

Last menstrual period, history of ovarian mass, and onset of pain during exercise, recent episodes of milder abdominal pain. Generally, nonspecific and highly variable.

Physical Exam

- Unilateral, tender enlarged adnexa +/−
- Uterus may be pulled toward the torsion or displaced away from the enlarged adnexa.
- Peritoneal signs/symptoms are late signs

TESTS

Diagnostic tests: Pregnancy test (required in all woman of reproductive age with pelvic pain), UA, rapid hemoglobin

Labs

- No specific laboratory findings; WBC may be elevated, but ischemia doesn't correspond
- May present with variable and often nonimpressive findings; the paucity of objective findings can support the diagnosis.

Imaging

- US: Transabdominal or transvaginal sonography is indicated; findings consistent with torsion include: A unilateral, enlarged adnexa, stromal edema, free peritoneal fluid, ovarian mass, hemorrhage within the ovary with peripheral follicles. A twisted vascular pedicle is highly predictive. Transvaginal sonography is most helpful, but may be technically impossible when dealing with a young child or adolescent.
- Color Doppler sonography: Abnormal flow in a twisted vascular pedicle is highly predictive of torsion, but normal flow does not rule out torsion. Absent flow in the adnexa is not diagnostic of torsion, as it is consistent with other diagnoses, such as hemorrhage of corpus luteum or ovarian follicle.
- MRI: Imaging of choice for pregnant patients with RLQ pain when US and color Doppler sonography are nondiagnostic.
- CT: Can demonstrate enlarged ovary; primarily used to rule out other causes of abdominal pain (appendicitis).

DIFFERENTIAL DIAGNOSIS

- Acute appendicitis
- PID
- Ectopic pregnancy
- Gastroenteritis
- Pelvic endometriosis, endometrioma of ovary
- Ovarian mass (hemorrhagic corpus luteum, cyst, benign or malignant tumor)
- Acute degeneration of a uterine fibroid tumor
- Ovarian vein thrombophlebitis
- UTI, renal colic
- Meckel diverticulum

- Acute bursitis of the hip
- Small or large bowel obstruction
- Mesenteric ischemia
- Diverticular disease

Geriatric Considerations

With older age, presentation is often nonclassical.

Pediatric Considerations

- >50% of children and adolescents with torsion have normal ovaries and fallopian tubes.
- Preoperative diagnosis is particularly difficult, so a high index of suspicion is required.
- Ovarian lesions in newborns and infants are found on abdominal exam rather than as pelvic masses, due to the small size of the pelvis.
- Rectal exam may detect a mass at the brim of the pelvis or lower abdomen.
- Pain may refer to the T10 level, due to the ovary's embryonic origins.
- In premenarcheal girls, the diagnostic sign of *abdominal* pain must include not only appendicitis and gastroenteritis, but also adnexal torsion.

ALERT

Ovarian torsion is a *clinical diagnosis*, and workup must be thorough. Normal Doppler imaging must not be used to exclude diagnosis. Doppler sonography can miss the diagnosis of torsion in up to 60% of cases. With high clinical suspicion of torsion based on H&P, workup must proceed to diagnostic laparoscopy, as delay in diagnosis may lead to loss of the ovary and tube.

EPIDEMIOLOGY

Predominant age: Adnexal torsion is most common in the reproductive age group (12–45), but nearly 20% of cases occur in premenarcheal or postmenopausal women.

Incidence

Torsion makes up 3% of acute gynecologic complaints and is the 5th most common condition necessitating emergency gynecologic surgery. It may represent up to 3% of acute abdominal pain in children.

RISK FACTORS

- Pregnancy
- History of pelvic surgery, especially tubal ligation or hysterectomy
- Known ovarian cyst or neoplasm
- Paraovarian cyst
- Ovulation induction with ART
- Elongated mesovaria or fallopian tube (more common in children)
- Risk factors for isolated tubal torsion include hematosalpinx, hydrosalpinx, pregnancy, and paraovarian cysts

Pregnancy Considerations

The literature suggests that 12–25% of women with adnexal torsion are pregnant, and torsion may complicate 1:1,800 pregnancies; most often occurring in the 1st and early 2nd trimesters, but possible at any GA. Often secondary to ovarian enlargement with corpus luteum cyst and tissue laxity. Detorsion has not demonstrated adverse fetal effects. Laparoscopy has been successfully used up to 20 weeks.

TREATMENT

Treatment of suspected torsion is strictly surgical; medical management does not play a role.

SURGICAL MANAGEMENT

ALERT
Diagnostic laparoscopy is indicated for suspected torsion as soon as possible for the best chance of confirming the diagnosis, detorsing the adnexa, and preserving ovarian function and future fertility.

Risks, Benefits
- Surgical risks include bleeding, infection, and damage to surrounding structures.
- The magnitude of potential benefit, including preservation of ovarian function and reproductive capacity, far outweighs the potential risks of the detorsion operation.

Surgical
- Immediate laparoscopy is indicated to confirm the diagnosis and detorse the adnexa.
- Surgical findings may include torsion without strangulation, massive edema of the ovary, or gangrenous changes in the affected tube and/or ovary.
- Treatment aims to salvage the ovary and tube.
- Whenever possible, the adnexa should be manipulated with atraumatic instruments.
- Once the ovary is detorsed, the adnexa may show signs of reperfusion (color change from deep blue-black or purple-pink mottling) in minutes.

ALERT
- The often necrotic macroscopic appearance of the twisted adnexa is not a reliable indicator of viability.

- Postoperative assessment of viability has consistently demonstrated that grossly black, edematous ovaries can recover function in 88–100% after detorsion.
- Detorsion is often the only procedure that ought to be performed initially, and adnexectomy should be avoided.
- Rare indications for oophorectomy include visible ligament detachment or ovarian tissue decomposition.
- Extirpation is also acceptable in postmenopausal women.
- Cystectomy should be avoided because excess handling of the friable adnexa may further damage the ovary.
- A large percentage of ovarian masses are functional cysts that do not require removal:
  - Interval cystectomy has a higher rate of success without ovarian dysfunction.
- PE is an extremely uncommon complication of adnexal torsion (incidence, 0.2%), and may be the result of prolonged preoperative immobilization rather than the operative treatment:
  - Immobilization and preoperative delay represent significant risk factors for adnexal necrosis, as well as for PE.
  - Thus, timely laparoscopy with detorsion should be the procedure of choice.

- Oophoropexy is a controversial topic:
  - It can be recommended with repeat torsion (which can be seen with PCOS), but there is no consensus as to whether the normal contralateral adnexa should be pexied at the time of laparoscopy and detorsion.
  - Some recommend elective contralateral oophoropexy in all children with torsion:
    ○ Long-term follow-up of prophylactic oophoropexy is not currently available.
    ○ Theoretical risks include compromising the blood supply to the adnexa and creation of adhesions that might compromise future function and fertility.
  - To fix, place 2 ovarian sutures, 1 at the infundibulopelvic ligament pole, and the other at the ovarian ligament pole. Attach the ovary to adjacent lateral pelvic sidewall, or posterior wall of the uterus.

FOLLOW-UP

- Patients with torsion in the presence of a functional ovarian cyst may benefit from COCs to avoid recurrence of functional cyst.
- Postoperative sonography at 6 weeks can verify resolution of functional cyst, identify persistent cyst or tumor, and, in reproductive-age women, document presence of follicular function.

PROGNOSIS
Multiple studies have documented functional ovarian recovery by Doppler, flow, follicular development, 2nd-look laparoscopy, and pregnancy rates. >90% of patients can expect normal follicular development following detorsion.

COMPLICATIONS
- Surgical complications are rare and include infection, peritonitis, sepsis, adhesions, and chronic pain. Fever is the most common.
- Recurrent torsion is well documented, as is autoamputation in untreated cases, antenatal torsion, and bilateral torsion, either simultaneous or subsequent.
- If diagnosis is delayed, fertility is compromised by loss of ovary or fallopian tube.

BIBLIOGRAPHY

Abes M, et al. Oophoropexy in children with ovarian torsion. *Eur J Pediatr Surg.* 2004;14:168–171.

Breech LL, et al. Adnexal torsion in pediatric and adolescent girls. *Curr Opin Obstet Gynecol.* 2005; 17:483–489.

Canning DA. Ovarian torsion: To pex or not to pex? Case report and review of the literature. *J Urol.* 2005;173:1364.

Hibbard LT. Adnexal torsion. *Am J Gynecol.* 1985; 152:456–461.

Houry D, et al. Ovarian torsion: A fifteen-year review. *Ann Emerg Med.* 2001;38:156–159.

Levy T, et al. Laparoscopic unwinding of hyperstimulated ischaemic ovaries during the 2nd trimester of pregnancy. *Hum Reprod.* 1995;10: 1478–1480.

McGovern PG, et al. Adnexal torsion and pulmonary embolism: Case report and review of the literature. *Obstet Gynecol Surv.* 1999;54:601–608.

Merritt DF. Torsion of the uterine adnexa: A review. *Adolesc Pediatr Gynecol.* 1991;4:3–13.

Oelsner G, et al. Adnexal torsion. *Clin Obstet Gynecol.* 2006;49;3:459–463.

Pena JE, et al. Usefulness of Doppler sonography in the diagnosis of ovarian torsion. *Fertil Steril.* 2000;73:1047–1050.

Rackow B, et al. Successful pregnancy complicated by early and late adnexal torsion after in vitro fertilization. *Fertil Steril.* 2007;87(3):697. e9–e12.

Rody A, et al. The conservative management of adnexal torsion: A case-report and review of the literature. *Eur J Obstet Gynecol Reprod Biol.* 2002;101:83–86.

MISCELLANEOUS

SYNONYM(S)
Ovarian torsion

CLINICAL PEARLS
- Torsion often presents elusively, with nonspecific signs of acute abdomen; early detection and appropriate emergent surgical treatment is critical to preserve ovarian function and fertility.
- Suspect adnexal torsion with lower abdominal pain, nausea/vomiting, and an adnexal mass.
- With suspected torsion, expeditious intervention ensures the best chance for ovarian and reproductive reclamation.
- If torsion is suspected, laparoscopy is the diagnostic and therapeutic method of choice.

ABBREVIATIONS
- ART—Assisted reproductive technologies
- COC—Combination oral contraceptive
- GA—Gestational age
- OHSS—Ovarian hyperstimulation syndrome
- PCOS—Polycystic ovary syndrome
- PE—Pulmonary embolism
- PID—Pelvic inflammatory disease
- RLQ—Right lower quadrant
- UTI—Urinary tract infection

CODES

ICD9-CM
620.5 Torsion of ovary, ovarian pedicle, or fallopian tube

PATIENT TEACHING

- Explain that torsion is the twisting of the ovary and tube leading to loss of blood flow.
- Adnexal torsion is an emergency because it can result in death of the ovary or tube, and result in loss of hormonal and reproductive function.
- >90% of patients treated with detorsion can expect full recovery of ovarian function and reproductive ability postoperatively.
- Even if 1 ovary or tube is lost to torsion, the unaffected ovary and tube function normally.
- Recommend routine gynecologic visits to monitor ovarian function and diagnose adnexal pathology.
- Consider COCs to minimize risk of functional cysts.
- If known ovarian mass (hemorrhagic corpus luteum, hyperstimulated ovary, ovarian teratoma) is present, have patient limit activities that might lead to torsion of the enlarged adnexa.

AMNIOTIC FLUID EMBOLISM

Gary D. V. Hankins, MD
Angela D. Earhart, MD

 BASICS

DESCRIPTION
Uncommon obstetric disorder and a leading cause of maternal mortality:

- Complex presentation (findings with incidence 80–100%):
  - Hypoxia/Respiratory failure
  - Hypotension/Cardiogenic shock
  - Altered mental status
  - Coagulopathy:
    - These findings with incidence 80–100%
- Sudden fetal compromise:
  - Deterioration of fetal heart rate
- Syndrome most commonly occurs after maternal intravascular exposure to fetal tissue during normal labor, or during or shortly after vaginal or cesarean section delivery:
  - 70% cases occurred in labor per national registry data.
  - 30% occurred after delivery:
    - After vaginal delivery: 11%
    - After cesarean section: 19%
- Time from delivery to clinical presentation: 15–45 minutes
- Rarely occurs 48 hours postpartum, following 1st- or 2nd-trimester abortions, or amniocentesis
- Time from collapse to death: 1–7 hours
- No evidence of tumultuous labor
- No causative link between hypertonic contractions, oxytocin use, or hyperstimulation
- 13% developed syndrome after AROM, IUPC placement
- Rapid patient deterioration and death often results.

DIFFERENTIAL DIAGNOSIS
- Remains a clinical diagnosis of exclusion.
- Other obstetric complications:
  - Placental abruption, eclampsia, hemorrhage
- Nonobstetric complications:
  - Pulmonary (thrombo) embolism (PE), air embolism, septic shock, myocardial infarction, anaphylaxis, aspiration, transfusion reaction, cardiomyopathy
- Anesthetic complications:
  - Total spinal anesthesia, systemic local anesthetic toxicity

EPIDEMIOLOGY
- Mortality: 60–80%:
  - As high as 50% in 1st hour after presentation
- 10% of all maternal deaths in US
- 21% perinatal mortality
- Worldwide, incidence between 1 in 8,000 and 1 in 80,000 live births:
  - In US, 1 in 20,000 to 1 in 30,000 deliveries

RISK FACTORS
- Not easily identified
- Male fetus
- Prior history of drug allergies (41%)

PATHOPHYSIOLOGY
- Unclear etiology; uncommon event
- Animal models:
  - AF into venous circulation resulted in transient pulmonary HTN, acute cor pulmonale:
    - Secondary to occlusion and vasospasm of maternal pulmonary vasculature
  - Followed by left ventricular dysfunction, systemic hypotension, and shock
- Hemodynamic data from humans: Biphasic pattern:
  - Breech in barrier between maternal circulation and AF:
    - AF enters maternal circulation through endocervical veins, placental insertion site, or site of uterine trauma
  - Early phase: Transient pulmonary HTN, right heart dysfunction as result of occlusion and release of vasoactive substances:
    - Low cardiac output, leading to V/Q mismatch, hypoxemia, hypotension
    - Duration <30 minutes
  - 2nd phase:
    - Left ventricular failure
    - Return of normal right-heart function
    - Cardiogenic pulmonary edema
    - Cardiogenic shock
    - Severe hemodynamic instability
- Disruption of normal clotting cascade (40%):
  - Unclear etiology:
    - Substances in AF
    - Or later from systemic inflammatory response
- Inflammatory response:
  - Exposure to atypical substances in AF:
    - Leukotrienes, arachidonic acid metabolites
  - Host immune responses:
    - Endogenously released mediators
    - Fetal antigens insulting maternal circulation
    - Elevated serum tryptase levels
    - Increased pulmonary mast cell activity in some patients

Pathological Findings
Historically, identification of AF debris (squamous and trophoblastic cells, mucin, lanugo) in samples from distal port of pulmonary artery catheter or at autopsy:

- However, several recent studies suggest similar findings in normal pregnant women and nonpregnant women.
- Therefore, histologic findings are not pathognomonic.

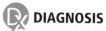 **DIAGNOSIS**

SIGNS AND SYMPTOMS
- Acute, dramatic, profound shock and severe respiratory compromise during labor or immediately postpartum
- Hypoxemia:
  - Early findings are present in 93%.
  - Results from severe V/Q mismatching or severe left ventricular dysfunction
  - Accounts for ~50% deaths in 1st hour
  - Up to 70% who survive later develop noncardiogenic PE with improvement in left ventricular dysfunction.
  - Anoxic encephalopathy causes neurologic deficiencies and brain death.
- Cardiovascular collapse:
  - ~86% die from cardiogenic shock or its complications.
  - Results from left ventricular failure
  - Cardiac dysrhythmias may occur: Pulseless electrical activity, bradycardia, ventricular fibrillation, asystole
  - Diminished cardiac output
  - Left ventricular stroke work index severely reduced
  - Elevated left heart filling pressures
  - Small increases in pulmonary vascular resistance
- DIC:
  - As many as 80%
  - 1/2 develop DIC within 4 hours
  - Profound hemorrhage, hemorrhagic shock
  - Early and late occurrences seen
- Altered mental status:
  - Encephalopathy
  - Impaired oxygen delivery to brain
  - Seizure activity in up to 50%
- Other symptoms:
  - Agitation
  - Fetal distress: Late decelerations, bradycardia
  - Constitutional: Fever, chills, nausea, vomiting, headache

TESTS
Labs
- No specific lab tests confirms diagnosis
- PT/PTT:
  - Increased
- Fibrinogen:
  - Decreased
- Fibrin split products:
  - Decreased

- Recommended lab tests:
  - CBC/Platelets
  - Electrolytes, BUN, creatinine, glucose, calcium, magnesium
  - Arterial blood gases:
    ○ Oxygen, acid base status
  - Creatine phosphokinase isoenzymes
  - Troponin levels
- ECG:
  - Signs of ischemia and infarction
  - Tachycardia
  - ST and T-wave abnormalities
  - Right ventricular strain
  - Arrhythmias with severe cardiovascular collapse

Imaging
- Not diagnostic
- CXR:
  - Pulmonary edema
  - Interstitial and alveolar infiltrates, bilaterally
- Transesophageal echocardiogram:
  - Acute left heart failure
  - Diminished left ventricular contractility

TREATMENT
MEDICAL MANAGEMENT
- Monitoring:
  - Continuous pulse oximetry
  - Continuous cardiac telemetry
  - Continuous electronic fetal monitoring if undelivered
  - Arterial BP monitoring:
    ○ Systolic BP >90 mm Hg
  - Pulmonary artery catheterization:
    ○ Pulmonary capillary wedge pressure
    ○ Cardiac output
- Prevention of fetal hypoxia:
  - Maternal PO_2 in range of 65 mm Hg acceptable for adequate fetal oxygenation
  - If inadequate oxygenation or unconscious, prompt endotracheal intubation:
    ○ Most require mechanical ventilation
- Noncardiogenic pulmonary edema:
  - Aggressive fluid management
  - Application of PEEP in intubated patients
  - Avoid barotrauma

Resuscitation
- Nonspecific, supportive care.
- 3 goals: Oxygenate, maintain cardiac output and BP, combat coagulopathy. Never delay giving medications.
- Maternal:
  - Immediate delivery of 100% oxygen
  - Face mask, bag-valve mask, or endotracheal intubation
  - Aggressively treat hypotension initially with IV fluids.
  - Vasopressors for refractory hypotension
  - ACLS medications per protocol for arrhythmias
  - Displace uterus to left during resuscitation
  - Treat left heart failure with fluids, inotropic drugs
  - Treat DIC, coagulopathy with FFP, cryoprecipitate, fibrinogen, factor replacement
  - RBC transfusion for hemorrhage
  - Platelets for thrombocytopenia
  - Admission to ICU after stabilization

- Fetal:
  - ~65% cases are undelivered patient
  - Immediate delivery within 4 minutes with asystole or malignant arrhythmia
  - Prevent further hypoxic damage to fetus.
  - Facilitate maternal resuscitation.

Drugs
- Cardiogenic shock requires use of inotropic and vasoactive agents.
- Maintenance of cardiac output and BP:
  - Norepinephrine 2–12 μg/min IV infusion:
    ○ Start 0.5–1 μg/min IV. Refractory shock may require up to 30 μg/min
  - Dopamine 1–50 μg/kg/min IV:
    ○ Increase by 1–4 μg/kg/min q10–30min. Titrate response.
- Severe left ventricular dysfunction:
  - Dobutamine 2–20 μg/kg/min IV:
    ○ Start 0.5–1 μg/kg/min. Maximum of 40 μg/kg/min:
    ○ Increases low cardiac output
    ○ Decreases high filling pressures
    ○ Use vasopressor (norepinephrine) to prevent resulting hypotension

IV-Fluids
- Use pulmonary artery catheter to guide volume resuscitation
- Use both crystalloid and colloid:
  - Isotonic solutions
- Urine output >25 mL/hr
- Transfusion for significant coagulopathy and hemorrhage:
  - Monitor for uterine atony
- High-dose corticosteroids

FOLLOW-UP
PROGNOSIS
- Improvement in mortality with early recognition, prompt resuscitation
- High morbidity:
  - Neurologic impairment, encephalopathy
  - Only 15% remain neurologically intact
- Neonatal survival is 79%:
  - Only 50% were neurologically intact
- No data showing recurrence with subsequent pregnancies
- Unpreventable and unpredictable

COMPLICATIONS
- Cardiac failure:
  - Left ventricular impairment
  - Cardiogenic PE
  - Myocardial ischemia and infarction
  - Decreased systemic vascular resistance
- Respiratory failure:
  - Noncardiogenic PE
  - Refractory bronchospasm
- Neurologic compromise:
  - Seizures
  - Altered mentation
- Acute renal failure:
  - Oliguric or nonoliguric
  - Acute tubular necrosis
- Hematologic compromise:
  - DIC
  - Hemorrhage
  - Thromboses

BIBLIOGRAPHY
Clark SL, et al. Amniotic fluid embolism: Analysis of the national registry. *Am J Obstet Gynecol.* 1995;172:1158–1169.

Dildly GA, et al. Anaphylactoid syndrome of pregnancy (amniotic fluid embolism). In: Dildy GA, ed. *Critical Care Obstetrics*, 4th ed. Boston: Blackwell Science; 2004;463–471.

Malinow AM. Embolic Disorders. In: Chestnut DH, ed. *Obstetric Anesthesia, Principles and Practice*, 2nd ed. St. Louis: Mosby; 1999.

Moore J, et al. Amniotic fluid embolism. *Crit Care Med.* 2005;33:S279–S285.

Tuffnell DJ. Amniotic fluid embolism. *Curr Opin Obstet Gynecol.* 2003;15:119–122.

MISCELLANEOUS
Newer strategies:
- Anecdotal reports, small case reports:
  - Intra-aortic balloon counterpulsation
  - Extracorporeal membrane oxygenation
  - Cardiopulmonary bypass
  - Plasma exchange transfusions
  - Uterine artery embolization
  - Continuous hemofiltration
  - Cell-salvage combined with blood filtration
  - Serum protease inhibitors
  - Inhaled nitric oxide
  - Inhaled prostacyclin

SYNONYM(S)
Anaphylactoid syndrome of pregnancy

ABBREVIATIONS
- ACLS—Advanced cardiac life support
- AF—Amniotic fluid
- AFE—Amniotic fluid embolism)
- AROM—Amniotomy
- DIC—Disseminated intravascular coagulation
- IUPC—Intrauterine pressure catheter
- PE—Pulmonary embolism
- PEEP—Positive expiratory end pressure
- PT—Prothrombin time
- PTT—Partial thromboplastin time

CODES
ICD9-CM
- 673.11 Delivered
- 673.13 Antepartum

PATIENT TEACHING
PREVENTION
- No prophylactic measures
- Constant vigilance of parturient
- Monitor patient for restlessness, agitation, complaints of dyspnea

APPENDICITIS IN PREGNANCY

Yair Blumenfeld, MD

 BASICS

DESCRIPTION
- By definition, inflammation of the appendix
- Suspected appendicitis in pregnancy poses both diagnostic and treatment challenges to the treating physician.

EPIDEMIOLOGY
- Incidence in pregnancy is 0.1–0.2%.
- The most common etiology of abdominal surgery in pregnancy
- High false-positive rates (15–40%)
- Often causes preterm labor and delivery (15–30%)
- Fewer cases during pregnancy:
  – Possible protective effect
- Slightly higher rates in the 2nd trimester
- More likely to rupture in pregnancy due to delay in diagnosis and treatment

ASSOCIATED CONDITIONS
- May precipitate preterm labor and delivery
- Ruptured appendix may lead to maternal morbidity and neonatal demise

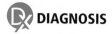 **DIAGNOSIS**

- Diagnosis is difficult to make in pregnancy.
- Classic signs and symptoms of appendicitis are not sensitive or specific in pregnancy.
- Vast differential diagnosis
- High false-positive rates
- Delayed diagnosis may increase maternal and neonatal morbidity

SIGNS AND SYMPTOMS
History
- Abdominal pain:
  – Location may change due to migration of appendix toward upper abdomen with progressing GA.
  – Pain may be in the RLQ or higher in the 2nd and 3rd trimesters.
  – Sharp in nature and unremitting
- GI symptoms:
  – Nausea/Vomiting
  – Decreased appetite
  – Altered bowel function

Physical Exam
- Fever
- Abdominal tenderness
- Rebound/Guarding
- Preterm labor may be present (uterine contractions, cervical change)
- Absence of other obstetric, urinary, GI findings

TESTS
Lab
- Limited utility except to rule out alternative diagnoses
- Leukocytosis:
  – Values as high as 20,000 cells/mm^3 may also be found in normal pregnancies.
- UA may occasionally show WBCs, due to peritoneal inflammation and proximity of appendix to ureter; pyuria is seen in up to 1/3 of those with acute appendicitis.

Imaging
- US:
  – Previously thought to be the gold standard in pregnancy
  – Sensitivity and specificity originally reported as high as 90% (newer studies report sensitivity and specificity of 80–90%)
  – Uterine size and appendix location make correct diagnosis difficult.
- CT scan:
  – The gold standard in nonpregnant patients
  – Should be considered in equivocal cases
  – Usual ionizing radiation exposure 300 mrad to 1.5 rads (well below the amount known to cause congenital abnormalities)
- MRI:
  – May be utilized in centers where experienced radiologists are available
  – Limited case series describe sensitivity and specificity as high as 95–100%.

DIFFERENTIAL DIAGNOSIS
- Urinary tract abnormalities:
  – Renal stones
  – UTI
  – Pyelonephritis
- GI abnormalities:
  – Gastroenteritis
  – Cholecystitis
  – Choledocholithiasis
- Pelvic structure pathologies:
  – Uterine fibroids
  – Ruptured ovarian cysts
  – Adnexal torsion
- Obstetric-related abnormalities:
  – Chorioamnionitis
  – Round ligament pain
  – Preterm labor
  – Placental abruption
  – Uterine rupture
  – Ectopic pregnancy

 TREATMENT

- Accurate diagnosis is paramount, but false-positive rates are unavoidable.
- True appendicitis in pregnancy is a surgical emergency.
- A multidisciplinary approach is optimal, including surgery, maternal-fetal medicine, neonatology, and anesthesiology.

MEDICAL MANAGEMENT
- Patient resuscitation and optimization for surgery
- Medical treatment of preterm labor if present

Resuscitation
- IV fluid hydration
- Correct electrolyte abnormalities

Drugs
- Antibiotics:
  – No specific regimen is recommended in pregnancy.
  – Different regimens are available based on intact vs. ruptured appendix.
- Narcotics for pain
- Tocolytics for preterm labor

Other
Continuous fetal and uterine contraction monitoring beyond mid-trimester

SURGICAL MANAGEMENT
Informed Consent
- False-positive rates: 15–40%
- Risk of preterm labor: 15–30%
- Increased miscarriage rates in 1st trimester
- No increase in congenital abnormalities, stillbirth following surgery
- Cesarean delivery rarely indicated at the time of surgery

Surgical
- Decision to perform laparotomy vs. laparoscopy is often influenced by surgeon comfort, experience, and GA.
- Important to consider uterine size, appendix location
- No difference in intraoperative complications, preterm delivery rates between laparotomy and laparoscopy
- Possible decreased length of stay with laparoscopy
- Limit uterine manipulation with either approach

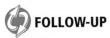 FOLLOW-UP

PROGNOSIS
- Overall good maternal prognosis if appendix excised prior to rupture or abscess formation
- 15–30% risk of postoperative preterm labor regardless of true or negative pathology

COMPLICATIONS
- Appendicitis-related complications:
  – Appendiceal rupture
  – Appendiceal abscess
- Surgical complications:
  – Bleeding
  – Postoperative infection
  – Requirement for reoperation
  – Incisional hernia
  – Trauma to intestine, bladder
- Obstetric complications:
  – Preterm labor
  – Preterm delivery
  – Neonatal morbidity as a result of prematurity

BIBLIOGRAPHY

Al-Quedah S, et al. Appendectomy in pregnancy: The experience of a university hospital. *J Obstet Gynaecol*. 1999;19(4):362–364.

Andersson RE, et al. Incidence of appendicitis during pregnancy. *Int J Epidemiol*. 2001;30:1281–1285.

Blumenfeld Y, et al. Laparotomy versus laparoscopy for antenatal appendectomy. *Am J Obstet Gynecol*. 2005;193:S81.

Castro MA. The use of helical computed tomography in pregnancy for the diagnosis of acute appendicitis. *Am J Obstet Gynecol*. 2001;184:954–957.

Mazze RI, et al. Appendectomy during pregnancy: A Swedish registry of 778 cases. *Obstet Gynecol*. 1991;77(6):835–840.

Mazze RI, et al. Reproductive outcome after anesthesia and operation during pregnancy: A registry study of 5405 cases. *Am J Obstet Gynecol*. 1989;161(5): 1178–1185.

Pedrosa I, et al. MR imaging evaluation of acute appendicitis in pregnancy. *Radiology*. 2006;238(3): 891–899.

Reedy MB, et al. Laparoscopy during pregnancy: A study of 5 fetal outcome parameters with use of the Swedish Health Registry. *Am J Obstet Gynecol*. 1997;177(3):673–679.

Rollins MD, et al. Laparoscopy for appendicitis and cholelithiasis during pregnancy. *Surg Endosc*. 2004;18:237–241.

Ueberrueck T, et al. Ninety-four appendectomies for suspected acute appendicitis during pregnancy. *World J Surg*. 2004;28:508–511.

MISCELLANEOUS

CLINICAL PEARLS
- Appendicitis in pregnancy is a difficult diagnosis to make.
- Vast differential diagnosis and limited utility of laboratory values result in high false-positive rates.
- Encourage liberal use of CT or MRI imaging in equivocal cases in order to reduce inappropriate surgery.
- Decision to proceed with laparotomy or laparoscopy is largely based on surgeon comfort, experience.
- Postoperative preterm labor rates are as high as 15–30% regardless of appendix pathology.

ABBREVIATIONS
- GA—Gestational age
- RLQ—Right lower quadrant
- UTI—Urinary tract infection

Section VIII

BOWEL INJURY, INTRAOPERATIVE

Rebeccah L. Brown, MD

 BASICS

DESCRIPTION

- Potential exists for intraoperative bowel injury during any obstetric or gynecologic procedure. The risk increases substantially in the presence of infection/inflammation and with reoperative surgery due to formation of adhesions.
- Contributing factors:
  - Infection/Inflammation
  - Radiation therapy
  - Reoperative surgery/adhesions
- Mechanisms of injury:
  - Injury upon entry into the peritoneal cavity:
    ○ Veress needle injury
    ○ Trocar injury
    ○ Inadequate insufflation during laparoscopy
    ○ Adhesions of bowel to abdominal wall or old scar
  - Electrocautery injury
  - Difficult dissection due to extensive adhesions
- Types of injuries:
  - Serosal tears
  - Intestinal lacerations
  - Mesenteric tears/lacerations

EPIDEMIOLOGY
Incidence
- 1.3/1,000 cases
- Small bowel (58%)
- Colon (32%)
- ~1/2 caused by electrocautery
- Majority of injuries (55–70%) are not identified at the time of surgery.

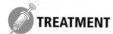 **TREATMENT**

MEDICAL MANAGEMENT
- Not indicated
- Ideally, injury should be recognized at time of surgery and treated appropriately.

SURGICAL MANAGEMENT
Informed Consent
Informed consent for any obstetric or gynecologic procedure should include the risk of injury to the intestines or other adjacent organs. For laparoscopy, informed consent should include the risk of injury due to introduction of the Veress needle or trocars into the peritoneal cavity.

Surgical
- Consider early intraoperative consultation with general surgeon once intestinal injury or significant potential for intestinal injury is identified.
- Serosal tears:
  - Repair with interrupted Lembert sutures if possible
  - If extensive serosal tear, consider resection of involved piece of intestine
- Intestinal lacerations:
  - Small (<1/2 of intestinal circumference):
    ○ Repair primarily with 2–layer closure in a transverse direction
  - Large (>1/2 of intestinal circumference):
    ○ Consider resection of involved piece of intestine with primary anastomosis
  - If extensive contamination with enteric contents, especially colonic, consider diverting ileostomy or colostomy
- Mesenteric lacerations:
  - Control bleeding
  - Assess intestinal viability
  - Consider bowel resection if significant vascular compromise due to mesenteric injury

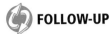 **FOLLOW-UP**

PROGNOSIS

- If injury is identified intraoperatively and appropriately treated, prognosis should be good.
- Delayed recognition of intestinal injury portends a worse prognosis and increases risk for litigation.

COMPLICATIONS

- Peritonitis due to unrecognized perforation or leak
- Bowel obstruction due to stricture or adhesions
- Short gut syndrome due to extensive bowel resection
- Enterocutaneous fistulae
- Prolonged ileus

BIBLIOGRAPHY

Bishoff JT, et al. Laparoscopic bowel injury: Incidence and clinical presentation. *J Urol*. 1999;161(3): 887–890.

El-Bann M, et al. Management of laparoscopic-related bowel injuries. *Surg Endosc*. 2000;14(9):779–782.

Mendez LE. Iatrogenic injuries in gynecologic cancer surgery. *Surg Clin North Am*. 2001;81(4):897–923.

Tarik A, et al. Complications of gyneacological laparoscopy: A retrospective analysis of 3572 cases from a single institution. *J Obstet Gynaecol*. 2004;24(7):813–816.

Wang PH, et al. Major complications of operative and diagnostic laparoscopy for gynecologic disease. *J Am Assoc Gynecol Laparosc*. 2001;8(1):68–73.

 MISCELLANEOUS

CLINICAL PEARLS

- Key to good outcome is intraoperative recognition of injury with appropriate treatment.
- Consider early intraoperative consultation with general surgeon once intestinal injury or potential for injury is identified.
- Consider preoperative mechanical bowel prep if adhesions are anticipated or risk of bowel injury considered higher than typical, although limited evidence from RCTs suggest that if bowel anastomosis is required, mechanical bowel prep may increase the risk of anastomosis leakage.

ABBREVIATIONS

RCT—Randomized controlled trial

CODES

ICD9-CM
998.2 Accidental puncture or laceration during a procedure

Section VIII

CESAREAN DELIVERY, EMERGENCY

Kimberly W. Hickey, MD
Menachem Miodovnik, MD

 BASICS

DESCRIPTION
- Immediate need for intervention and delivery for maternal and/or fetal well being
- Alternative definition: All acute nonscheduled CD

DIFFERENTIAL DIAGNOSIS
- Maternal Indications:
  - Abruptio placenta: Shearing of the placenta from the uterus
  - Placenta previa: The placenta covers part or all of the internal os, with or without hemorrhage in labor
  - Placenta accreta, increta, percreta: Abnormal invasion of the placenta into the uterine wall in labor
  - Vasa previa: Fetal vessels traverse and cover the internal os, with or without hemorrhage in labor.
  - Uterine rupture
  - Trauma with abruptio placenta or uterine rupture
- Fetal indications:
  - Abnormal FHT
  - Transverse lie with advanced cervical dilation
  - Breech presentation with advanced cervical dilation
  - Prolapsed umbilical cord
  - Uterine rupture
  - Shoulder dystocia unrelieved by traditional maneuvers (Zavanelli maneuver involves reversing the mechanisms of labor by rotating the fetal head to the occiput anterior position, flexing the fetal head, and replacing the fetal head within the vagina)
  - Fetal anemia
  - Fetal bleeding due to vasa previa (as indicated by a positive Apt test)

EPIDEMIOLOGY
- Prevalence of clinical scenarios requiring immediate intervention
- 18% of maternal mortality is associated with maternal hemorrhage:
  - Abruptio placenta occurs in ~1:100 pregnancies. Abruptio placenta with fetal death occurs in 1:1,600 pregnancies.
  - Recurrence of abruptio placenta: 15–20%
- Uterine rupture:
  - 0.7% of women with 1 low transverse segment scar in spontaneous labor vs. 0.9% if 2 prior CDs
  - 0.9% with low transverse scar with Pitocin augmentation
- Cord prolapse:
  - Risk of prolapse is 5% with complete breech presentation or 15% in footling breech presentation.
- Placenta previa occurs in 0.3–0.5% of all pregnancies. Incidence is 4.5% with 1 prior CD; 45% with 4 prior CDs.
- Cumulative risk for placenta accreta/increta/percreta with placenta previa present: 3% after 1 CD, 11% after 2, 40% after 3, 61% after 4, 67% after ≥5 CD
- Vasa previa occurs in 1:1,000–5,200 pregnancies.

 TREATMENT

MEDICAL MANAGEMENT
In these emergent situations, management is aimed at optimizing maternal and fetal status while moving expeditiously to the OR for operative delivery.

Resuscitation
Practices to optimize maternal and fetal status:
- Left lateral displacement of uterus to increase venous return
- Oxygen at 6–8 L/min through a tight-fitting mask. If indicated, assisted ventilation by anesthesia to maintain maternal hemoglobin saturation at ≥90%
- Obtain IV access. If bleeding, consider insertion of 2 large-bore IV catheters.
- Call for help: Nursing, attending, anesthesia, pediatrics
- Stop labor augmentation or induction agents
- If bleeding, administer Ringer's lactate solution for volume expansion.
- If blood products readily available, draw, type, and cross-match for 2–4 units of packed RBCs.

Drugs
- In patients with uterine hypertonus, consider muscle relaxants as follows:
  - Administer terbutaline, 0.25 mg SC or IV. This agent may cause uterine atony and therefore increase bleeding after delivery.
- In cases of severe hemorrhage consider uterotonics after delivery:
  - Oxytocin (Pitocin), 10–40 U in a 1 L bag of Ringer's lactate solution or 10 U IM if no IV access
  - Methylergonovine (Methergine), 0.2 mg IM q2–4h; use with caution in patients with HTN.
  - 15–methyl PGF2α (Hemabate), 0.25 mg IM or intrauterine q15–90min up to 8 doses; use with caution in patients with asthma.
  - Misoprostol (Cytotec), 800–1,000 μg per rectum
  - Dinoprostone (Prostin E2), 20 mg per rectum q2h; avoid if patient is hypotensive
- Consider antibiotic administration at cord clamping for prevention of maternal infection:
  - Consider antibiotic prophylaxis for 24 hours if the surgery is not performed under aseptic conditions.

Other
- Order initial laboratory evaluation on arrival to labor and delivery as follows:
  - CBC, PT/PTT, fibrinogen, fibrin split products, Kleihauer-Betke, UA, and vaginal pool for Apt test
- Order packed RBCs, FFP, and/or cryoprecipitate for massive hemorrhage.
- Consider medications the patient may have ingested that require reversal, such as narcotics or anticoagulants.
- In case of uncontrollable DIC, trauma, or the need to reverse LMWH, consider administering recombinant Factor VIIa. In most institutions, the blood bank will provide this agent.

SURGICAL MANAGEMENT
Informed Consent
- If consent not obtained on admission, verbal counseling and informed consent should be obtained as the patient is taken to the OR.
- Unresponsive patients may be treated in emergent situations with family's consent or without consent if family members are not available.

Patient Education
- General prenatal education:
  - Discuss any relevant obstetric complications and care-specific options.
  - Patients should be advised to contact their care provider for the following complaints:
    ○ Decreased or absent fetal movement
    ○ Vaginal bleeding
    ○ Rupture of membranes
    ○ Abdominal/Epigastric pain
    ○ Severe headaches
    ○ Intractable nausea and emesis
    ○ Any other concerns
  - Educate the patient on common practices that they should expect upon admission to labor and delivery:
    ○ Continuous fetal heart rate monitoring, external or internal
    ○ Uterine monitoring, tocometer or IUPC
    ○ Agents used for induction and/or augmentation of labor
  - Discuss method of delivery:
    ○ Vaginal
    ○ CD
    ○ Operative vaginal delivery (vacuum extraction vs. forceps)
    ○ Emergent CD
- Specific instructions for known pregnancy complications:
  - Vaginal bleeding with placenta previa or vasa previa:
    ○ Avoid digital exam in cases of bleeding or premature rupture of membranes. Obtain US to evaluate for abnormal placentation, fetal presentation, and AF volume.
  - In cases of persistent breech presentation, discuss the recommendations for CD and the complications of vaginal breech delivery if patient declines surgical management:
    ○ If premature labor and breech presentation, and patient declines surgical management, then discuss the risk of head entrapment.
    ○ Discuss the risk of cord prolapse with subsequent management.

Risks, Benefits

- Risks:
  - Infection
  - Injury to maternal tissues and internal organs
  - Injury to fetus at delivery
  - Need for application of vacuum or forceps to expedite delivery in cesarean section.
  - 10% of patients undergoing emergent CD require transfusion due to severe maternal hemorrhage.
  - Risks of transfusion reactions and acquired infections from blood products
  - Risk of hysterectomy for intractable uterine hemorrhage
  - Risk from administration of anesthesia
- Benefits:
  - Decrease in short- and long-term fetal morbidity
  - In cases of severe maternal hemorrhage, maternal morbidity and mortality are decreased.

Alternatives

In the case of intractable hemorrhage, no alternatives exist to emergent CD. These situations all require immediate intervention and delivery. Delay may compromise maternal and fetal well-being.

Surgical

- Consider the type of abdominal or uterine incision that will allow good exposure, expedite delivery, and minimize maternal complications. Vertical skin incision is the best choice in severe maternal hemorrhage.
- Abdominal incisions:
  - Midline (vertical)
  - Paramedian
  - Pfannenstiel
  - Maylard
  - Supraumbilical
- Uterine incisions:
  - Low segment transverse:
    - May attempt vaginal birth in subsequent pregnancies
    - May be extended superiorly to increase area for delivery ("T" incision). In subsequent pregnancies, a trial of labor is contraindicated.
  - Low segment vertical:
    - Useful for minimizing damage to extremely preterm infants
    - In subsequent pregnancies, a trial of labor is contraindicated.
  - Classical:
    - Useful for minimizing damage to extremely preterm infants
    - Useful in transverse lie, back-down presentation
    - Useful to deliver the fetus in cases of abnormal placentation, avoiding excessive maternal bleeding
    - In subsequent pregnancies, a trial of labor is contraindicated.
  - Fundal:
    - Useful in avoiding the site of abnormal placentation
    - In subsequent pregnancies, a trial of labor is contraindicated.

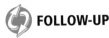 **FOLLOW-UP**

Discharge instructions:

- Discuss breast-feeding and access to lactation consultants.
- Discuss care for operative site.
- Follow-up appointments:
  - Postoperative incision evaluation in 7–14 days
  - Postpartum/Postoperative visit in 4–6 weeks
- Indications for earlier follow-up:
  - Bleeding
  - Signs and symptoms of operative site, uterine, or breast infection
- Contraceptive counseling should be offered prior to discharge. If not discussed prior to discharge, then this should be discussed at the postpartum visits as above.

PROGNOSIS

Prognosis depends on intrapartum and intraoperative complications:

- Majority of patients have no short- or long-term complications

COMPLICATIONS

- Infection:
  - Wound infection
  - Wound dehiscence
  - Wound seroma
  - Wound hematoma
  - Uterine infection, endometritis
  - Pneumonia
  - UTI
  - Pyelonephritis
  - Mastitis
- Thromboembolic events:
  - DVT/PE
  - Septic pelvic thrombophlebitis
- Hemorrhage/Bleeding:
  - Fatigue
  - Orthostatic hypotension with syncope
  - Iron deficiency
  - Need for transfusion
  - Need for hysterectomy
  - Maternal mortality
- Injury to internal organs:
  - Bladder injury requiring prolonged catheterization
  - Ureteral injury
  - Bowel injury with or without colostomy
  - Bowel resection due to extensive injury
  - Excision of fallopian tube and/or ovary for the control of severe hemorrhage
- Risk of anesthesia:
  - Aspiration of gastric contents
  - High spinal with need for endotracheal intubation
  - Inability to ventilate with maternal hypoxia and brain injury
  - Maternal mortality due to hypoxia or cardiovascular collapse

BIBLIOGRAPHY

ACOG Practice Bulletin No. 54. Vaginal Birth after Previous Cesarean Delivery. Washington DC: ACOG; 2004.

ACOG Practice Bulletin No. 76. Postpartum Hemorrhage. Washington DC: ACOG; 2006.

Hendrix N, et al. Cesarean delivery for nonreassuring fetal heart rate tracing. *Obstet Gynecol Clin N Am.* 2005;32:273–286.

Lagrew D, et al. Emergent (crash) cesarean delivery: Indications and outcomes. *Am J Obstet Gynecol.* 2006;194:1638–1643.

Landon M, et al. Maternal and perinatal outcomes associated with a trial of labor after prior cesarean delivery. *N Engl J Med.* 2004;351:2581–2589.

Silver R, et al. Maternal morbidity associated with multiple repeat cesarean deliveries. *Obstet Gynecol.* 2006;107:1226–1232.

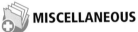 **MISCELLANEOUS**

CLINICAL PEARLS

- Review prenatal records on admission.
- Call for help early!
- Institute a protocol for team responsibilities in emergent deliveries.
- Communication between team members
- Call for blood products early; may need to activate massive transfusion protocol.

ABBREVIATIONS

- AF—Amniotic fluid
- CD—Cesarean delivery
- DIC—Disseminated intravascular coagulation
- DVT—Deep venous thrombosis
- FHT—Fetal heart tones
- IUPC—Intrauterine pressure catheter
- LMWH—Low-molecular-weight heparin
- PE—Pulmonary embolism
- PT—Prothrombin time
- PTT—Partial thromboplastin time

CODES

ICD9-CM

- 623.80 Vaginal bleeding
- 641.00 Placenta previa
- 641.20 Abruptio placenta
- 656.30 Abnormal fetal heart rate tracing (fetal distress)
- 663.00 Prolapsed umbilical cord
- 660.40 Shoulder dystocia
- 663.50 Vasa previa
- 666.00 Placenta accreta, increta, or percreta
- 669.71 Cesarean delivery with or without complication
- 763.89 Uterine rupture affecting the newborn

 PATIENT TEACHING

ACOG Patient Education Pamphlet: Cesarean Delivery. Available at http://www.acog.org

DEEP VEIN THROMBOSIS/PULMONARY EMBOLUS

Lisa Abaid, MD, MPH
Daniel Clarke-Pearson, MD

 BASICS

DESCRIPTION
Development of a partial or total thrombotic occlusion in the large veins of the extremities or pelvis, which may embolize to the pulmonary vasculature. This can result in limb-threatening vascular compromise from DVT or life-threatening hypoxia and cardiopulmonary collapse from PE. DVT and PE are collectively referred to as VTEs.

- System(s) affected: Cardiovascular, Pulmonary

DIFFERENTIAL DIAGNOSIS
- DVT:
  - Cellulitis
  - Lymphedema
  - Extrinsic venous compression due to mass or lymphadenopathy
  - Muscular or ligamentous injury
  - Compartment syndrome
  - Synovial cyst (Baker cyst)
- PE:
  - Pneumonia
  - Pulmonary edema
  - Pneumothorax/Pneumomediastinum
  - Asthma
  - Emphysema/COPD
  - Pleuritis
  - Airway obstruction:
    - Epiglottitis
    - Foreign body
  - Myocardial infarction
  - Angina
  - Pericarditis
  - Aortic dissection
  - Esophageal spasm or rupture
  - Musculoskeletal/Costochondritis
  - Anxiety

EPIDEMIOLOGY
- 2 million Americans are diagnosed with DVT each year.
- 1/3 of those with DVT will develop a clinically significant PE.
- 50–80% of those with a PE had no preceding clinical evidence of DVT.
- Mortality associated with PE is 10–40%; risk increases with advancing age.
- Thromboprophylaxis with low-dose heparin or LMWH can reduce incidence of DVT and PE by 50–70%.
- ≥1 risk factors can be identified in >80% of patients with VTE.

RISK FACTORS
- Increasing age >40
- Prior DVT or PE
- Surgery
- Major trauma/orthopedic trauma
- Pregnancy/Postpartum period
- Malignancy
- Obesity
- Prolonged immobility/paralysis
- Smoking
- Hormone use: OCP, HRT
- Central venous catheterization
- Inherited or acquired thrombophilia:
  - Most common: Factor V Leiden mutation and prothrombin gene mutation 20210A

 TREATMENT

MEDICAL MANAGEMENT
Diagnosis
- Physical Exam: Signs and symptoms:
  - DVT: Swollen, painful lower extremity, rarely massive edema with cyanosis and ischemia (phlegmasia cerulea dolens, a medical emergency)
  - PE: Pleuritic chest pain, shortness of breath, cough +/− hemoptysis, syncope, hypotension, tachypnea, tachycardia, hypoxia
- TESTS
  - DVT/PE:
    - D-dimer: Poor specificity, often elevated postoperatively, good negative predictive value
  - PE:
    - Arterial blood gas: Widened A-a oxygen gradient implies V/Q mismatch
    - Expected A-a gradient can be approximated by: 4 + patient age/4
- IMAGING
  - DVT:
    - Compression US: >90% sensitive for proximal clot, less sensitive for calf thrombosis
    - Contrast venography: Gold standard, invasive, expensive
  - PE:
    - CXR: Usually normal, rarely may show pulmonary infarct with effusion
    - EKG: Most common findings are tachycardia with nonspecific ST-segment and T-wave changes; classic (but infrequent) findings include atrial fibrillation, S1Q3T3 pattern, right ventricular strain, new incomplete right bundle branch block
    - V-Q scan: If normal, virtually excludes PE; however, in clinical practice has accuracy of 15–86%

- Helical (spiral) chest CT: Accuracy can be operator-dependent; with venous-phase imaging has sensitivity of 90%, specificity of 95%; cannot be performed in renal failure
- Pulmonary angiography: Gold standard, invasive, rarely used

Resuscitation
- Follow ACLS guidelines.
- Patient may require ventilatory support if profound hypoxia is present.
- If PE is suspected as cause of acute hypoxia or hypotension, and no absolute contraindications to anticoagulation exist, may initiate anticoagulation empirically.
- If persistent hypotension, consider thrombolysis or embolectomy.

Drugs
Anticoagulation:
- Initiate immediate therapeutic anticoagulation with LMWH:
  - Safer and equally effective as UFH
  - Daily weight-based dosing equivalent to b.i.d. administration
  - Typically does not require monitoring of antifactor Xa levels

> **ALERT**
> Consider checking antifactor Xa levels 4 hours after injection in patients with impaired renal function or severe obesity.

- Oral anticoagulation with vitamin K antagonists:
  - Warfarin most commonly used
  - Treatment of choice for long-term anticoagulation
  - May start simultaneously with LMWH or UFH
  - Goal INR: 2.0–3.0
  - Discontinue LMWH or UFH when INR stabilizes

> **ALERT**
> Warfarin is teratogenic and contraindicated during pregnancy. Consider LMWH or UFH until delivery.

- Thrombolytics:
  - Streptokinase, urokinase, or tissue-plasminogen activator
  - Indicated in DVT only for limb salvage
  - Indicated in acute PE with hemodynamic instability
  - Can be administered systemically or by catheter-directed infusion

SURGICAL MANAGEMENT
- IVC filters can prevent large emboli from the veins of the lower extremities or pelvis from reaching the lung.
- IVC filters are only indicated in the presence of a proximal DVT AND:
  – An absolute contraindication to anticoagulation (e.g., active bleeding)
  – Imminent major surgery
  – Recurrent PE on anticoagulation
- Embolectomy is rarely performed, and is indicated for massive PE with persistent hypotension when thrombolysis either fails or is contraindicated. It can be performed using a catheter or an open surgical approach.

 ## FOLLOW-UP

Length of anticoagulation:
- Idiopathic VTE: 3–6 months
- Trauma/Postsurgical: 3 months
- Recurrent VTE or hypercoagulable state (acquired, inherited, presence of malignancy, etc.): Minimum 12 months to life-long

PROGNOSIS
Recurrence:
- After 1st spontaneous DVT, annual recurrence risk is 5–15%
- Recurrence is low after postoperative DVT

COMPLICATIONS
- Clot sequelae:
  – Post-thrombotic syndrome occurs in 1/3 of patients after 1st proximal DVT, causing pain, swelling, skin changes:
    ○ Usually occurs within 2 years of clot
    ○ Reduced risk with thrombolytic therapy
    ○ Reduced risk with 2 years of below-knee graded compression stocking use
  – Large PE can cause chronic pulmonary HTN
- Complications of anticoagulation:
  – Risk of severe bleeding during 3-month course of warfarin is rare; in most studies ranges between 1% and 2%

BIBLIOGRAPHY

Blann AD, et al. Venous thromboembolism. *Br Med J.* 2006;332:215–219.

Geerts WH, et al. Prevention of venous thromboembolism: The 7th ACCP Conference on Antithrombotic and Thrombolytic Therapy. *Chest.* 2004;126:338S–400S.

Kyrle PA, et al. Deep vein thrombosis. *Lancet.* 2005;365:1163–1174.

Smith MI, et al. Preoperative Evaluation, Medical Management, and Critical Care. In: Berek JS, et al., ed. *Practical Gynecologic Oncology,* 4th ed. Philadelphia: Lippincott Williams & Wilkins; 2005:669–714.

 ## MISCELLANEOUS

SYNONYM(S)
- Deep vein thrombophlebitis (DVT)
- Venous thromboembolic events (VTE)

CLINICAL PEARLS
- Tachycardia is the most common presenting symptom of PE.
- Patients too unstable for helical chest CT may undergo bedside ECG; a massive PE is generally associated with increased RV size, decreased RV function, and tricuspid regurgitation.
- Virchow triad of abnormalities that promote thrombogenesis: Venous stasis, endothelial damage, and hypercoagulable state

ABBREVIATIONS
A-a oxygen gradient—Alveolar-arterial oxygen gradient
ACLS—Advanced cardiac life support
HRT—Hormone replacement therapy
IVC—Inferior vena cava filter
LMWH—Low molecular weight heparin
OCP—Oral contraceptive pills
RV—Right ventricle
UFH—Unfractionated heparin
VTE—Venous thromboembolic events

 ## CODES

ICD9-CM
- 289.81 Primary hypercoagulable state
- 289.82 Secondary hypercoagulable state
- 415.1 Pulmonary embolism and infarction
- 451.1 Phlebitis and thrombophlebitis of the deep vessels of the lower extremities
- 453.4 Venous embolism and thrombosis of the deep vessels of the lower extremities

PATIENT TEACHING

Warfarin levels can be significantly affected by dietary intake of vitamin K; patients taking warfarin should consume limited quantities of green, leafy vegetables. Levels may also be affected by homeopathic supplements and a number of prescription medications.

DISSEMINATED INTRAVASCULAR COAGULATION

Gary D. V. Hankins, MD
Nicole K. Ruddock, MD

 BASICS

DESCRIPTION
- Secondary systemic process associated with many comorbid conditions
- Prevalence 1–5% in chronic diseases states to 60–80% in acute obstetric complications/sepsis
- Pathophysiology is similar regardless of the underlying etiology.
- Activation of coagulation and fibrinolytic pathways
- Normal coagulation: A series of local reactions among blood vessels, platelets, and clotting factors

PATHOPHYSIOLOGY
- Activation of the coagulation system results in the circulation of thrombin and plasmin.
- Role of thrombin in DIC:
  – Circulating thrombin causes fibrin to cleave into fibrinopeptides leaving a fibrin monomer.
  – Fibrin monomer forms a fibrin clot resulting in thrombosis, impedance to blood flow, and ischemia.
  – Fibrin deposition causes platelet adhesion and consumption leading to thrombocytopenia.
- Role of plasmin in DIC:
  – Plasmin activates cleavage of fibrinogen into FDPs
  – FDPs:
    ○ Combine with fibrin monomers
    ○ FDP–monomer complexes interfere with normal polymerization and impair hemostasis.
    ○ Cause platelet dysfunction, resulting in significant hemorrhage
    ○ Induce synthesis of IL-1 and IL-6, inducing further endothelial damage, thrombus formation, and vascular occlusion
- Bradykinin increases vascular permeability and lowers BP
- Inflammatory and coagulation pathways interact and cause a vicious cycle of dysfunctional coagulation
- Acute DIC—uncompensated form:
  – *Hemorrhage* predominant clinical feature, which overshadows ongoing thrombosis
- Chronic DIC—compensated form:
  – *Thrombosis* predominant clinical feature

ETIOLOGY
- Precipitated by many disease states
- Complications of pregnancy:
  – IUFD (dead fetus syndrome)
  – AF embolism
  – Placental abruption (most common cause)
  – Abortion
  – Retained products of conception
  – Preeclampsia
  – Eclampsia
  – HELLP syndrome
  – Postpartum hemorrhage

- Sepsis
- Trauma
- Burns
- Malignancy:
  – Ovarian, uterine, breast
  – Metastatic disease
  – Leukemia
- Intravascular hemolysis:
  – Hemolytic transfusion reactions
  – Massive transfusion
  – Minor hemolysis
- Dilutional coagulopathy
- Thrombocytopenia:
  – TTP
  – ITP
- Acute liver disease
- Vascular disorders

DIFFERENTIAL DIAGNOSIS
- Inherited coagulation disorders:
  – Factor deficiencies
- Other acquired coagulation disorders:
  – Anticoagulant therapy
  – Drugs
  – Hepatic disease
- Hemolytic uremic syndrome
- Platelet dysfunction
- ITP/TTP

EPIDEMIOLOGY
- Incidence among obstetric patients: 1/1,355 deliveries
- Most common obstetric-associated conditions:
  – Placental abruption: 24%
  – Pregnancy-induced HTN: 20%
  – AF embolism: 16%
  – Acute fatty liver of pregnancy: 16%
  – HELLP syndrome: 12%

 DIAGNOSIS

SIGNS AND SYMPTOMS
Diagnosis and management of underlying condition causing DIC are paramount in management.

History
Of precipitating illness

Physical Exam
- Excessive bleeding:
  – From wounds/operative/IV sites
  – Purpura/Petechiae/Bullae
  – Mucosal/GI bleeding
- Excessive thrombosis:
  – Microvascular thrombosis and end-organ dysfunction
  – Cardiac, pulmonary, renal, hepatic, CNS
  – Thrombophlebitis
  – Pulmonary embolus

TESTS
Lab
- CBC/Peripheral smear
- Electrolytes/BUN/Creatinine
- Arterial blood gas
- PT, aPTT, Thrombin time
- Fibrinogen, FDPs, D-dimer
- Antithrombin III, fibrinopeptide A
- Decreased:
  – Platelets
  – Fibrinogen
  – Antithrombin III
- Elevated:
  – D-dimer
  – FDPs
  – Fibrinopeptide A
- Prolonged:
  – PT
  – aPTT
  – Thrombin time
- Peripheral smear:
  – Microangiopathic changes

Imaging
- CXR for suspected pneumonia
- Head CT for altered mental status

Diagnostic Procedures/Surgery
- Evacuation of uterus for retained fetus
- Hysterectomy for uncontrolled postpartum bleeding refractory to medical therapy

DIFFERENTIAL DIAGNOSIS
- Inherited coagulation disorders:
  – Factor deficiencies
- Other acquired coagulation disorders:
  – Anticoagulant therapy
  – Drugs
  – Hepatic disease
- Hemolytic uremic syndrome
- Platelet dysfunction

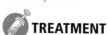 **TREATMENT**

MEDICAL MANAGEMENT
- Therapy of DIC should be individualized by:
  – Age
  – Hemodynamic status
  – Severity of hemorrhage
  – Severity of thrombosis
  – Precipitating disease

- Replacement therapy:
  - FFP:
    - For clotting factor deficiency
    - Use for PTT >54 seconds, PT >18 seconds, INR >1.6, fibrinogen <100 mg/dL
    - Provides clotting factors and volume replacement
    - Dose: 10–20 mL/kg (4–6 units)
    - 4–6 units increases clotting factors 20%
  - Platelets:
    - If platelet count <20,000 or platelet count <50,000 with ongoing bleeding
    - Dose: 1 U/10 kg
  - Cryoprecipitate:
    - Higher fibrinogen content than whole plasma
    - For severe hypofibrinogenemia (<50 mg/dL) or for active bleeding with fibrinogen <100 g/dL
    - Dose: 1 U/10 kg
    - I unit increases fibrinogen by 5–15 mg/dL
  - RBCs:
    - Nonclotting volume expanders

Resuscitation
- Airway management and resuscitation measures:
  - Control bleeding.
  - Establish IV access.
  - Restore and maintain circulating blood volume.
  - Maintain oxygenation.
- Initiate therapy of precipitating disease.

Drugs
- Heparin:
  - Use is controversial
  - Consider when thrombosis predominates (solid tumors, retained fetus)
  - Thromboembolic complications of large vessels
  - Low-dose regimen: 5–10 U/kg/h IV for chronic DIC
  - High-dose regimen: 10,000-U bolus followed by 1,000 U/h; 20–30,000 U q24h via constant infusion

- Antithrombin concentrates (controversial):
  - Used alone or in combination with heparin
- Fibrinolytic inhibitors:
  - Block secondary compensatory fibrinolysis that accompanies DIC
  - EACA, tranexamic acid
  - 10–15 mg/kg/h IV
  - Use complicated by severe thrombosis
  - Initiate in extreme cases only:
    - Profuse bleeding not responding to replacement therapy
    - Excessive fibrinolysis present (rapid whole blood lysis/short euglobulin lysis time)
- Newer agents:
  - Synthetic serine protease inhibitors:
    - Inhibits clotting cascade
    - Not approved for use in the USA
  - Activated protein C:
    - Inhibits factor V, VIII, activates fibrinolytic system

SURGICAL MANAGEMENT
Catastrophic obstetric hemorrhage with DIC requires aggressive fluid resuscitation and blood replacement and may require hysterectomy, as conservative procedures such as internal iliac-artery ligation are often ineffective.

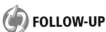 FOLLOW-UP

Severe precipitating illness in combination with DIC requires ICU admission or ICU-level care in obstetric unit.

BIBLIOGRAPHY

Bick RL. Disseminated intravascular coagulation: Current concepts of etiology, pathophysiology, diagnosis, and treatment. *Hematol Oncol Clin N Am*. 2003;17(1):149–176.

Dildy G, et al., eds. *Critical Care Obstetrics*, 4th ed. New York: Blackwell; 2004.

Franchini M. Pathophysiology, diagnosis and treatment of disseminated intravascular coagulopathy. *Clin Lab*. 2005;51:633–639.

Kobayashi T. Diagnosis and management of acute DIC. *Semin Thromb Hemostasis*. 2001;27(2):161–167.

Letsky E. Disseminated intravascular coagulation. *Best Practice Res Clin Obstet Gynecol*. 2001; 15(4):623–644.

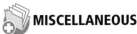 MISCELLANEOUS

ABBREVIATIONS
- aPTT—Activated partial thromboplastin time
- DIC—Disseminated intravascular coagulation
- EACAε—Aminocaproic acid
- FDP—Fibrin degradation products
- HELLP—Hemolytic anemia, elevated liver enzymes, low platelets
- IDP—Idiopathic thrombocytopenic purpura
- UIFD—Intrauterine fetal demise
- PT—Prothrombin time
- TTP—Thrombotic thrombocytopenic purpura

CODES

ICD9-CM
286.6 Disseminated intravascular coagulation

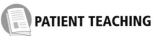 PATIENT TEACHING

Given the urgent and emergent care required and the critically ill patient:

- Brief, concise, and directive explanations are provided to patient and family at the time of decision making.
- Complete explanations of sequence, decision making, and course of care must be provided to the patient and family after stabilization.

ECLAMPSIA

Annette E. Bombrys, DO
Baha M. Sibai, MD

 BASICS

DESCRIPTION
- Eclampsia is defined as the development of convulsions and/or unexplained coma during pregnancy or postpartum in patients with signs and symptoms of preeclampsia.
- Other etiologies of seizures must be ruled out.

DIFFERENTIAL DIAGNOSIS
- Seizures:
  – Epilepsy presenting during pregnancy
  – Tumor
  – Other neurologic conditions
- Stroke, hemorrhagic or embolic
- Cerebral aneurysms
- Cerebral venous thrombosis

EPIDEMIOLOGY
- Incidence is 1 in 2,000 pregnancies.
- Incidence antepartum eclampsia is 38–53% and postpartum is 11–44%.

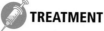 **TREATMENT**

MEDICAL MANAGEMENT
- Magnesium sulfate administration
- Maintain BP between 140–160 mm Hg systolic and 90–110 mm Hg diastolic
- Once stabilized, delivery should be expedited
- Diagnostic tests:
  – MRI is superior to CT in evaluation of eclampsia (imaging is not necessary in patients with uncomplicated eclampsia).

Resuscitation
- During seizure maintain respiratory and cardiovascular function (ABC).
- Prevent maternal injury during seizure by inserting tongue blade between teeth and padding bed rails.
- Administer oxygen at 8–10 L/min and apply pulse oximetry.
- To minimize risk of aspiration, place patient in the lateral decubitus position.

ALERT
- Fetal heart rate changes are common during an eclamptic seizure and include bradycardia, transient late decelerations, decreased beat-to-beat variability, and compensatory tachycardia.
- Fetal heart rate changes usually resolve spontaneously in 3–10 minutes.
- If bradycardia or recurrent late decelerations persist beyond 10–15 minutes, the patient should be delivered by cesarean section for possible abruption placentae or nonreassuring fetal status.

Drugs
- Medication for prevention of further seizures:
  – Magnesium sulfate (drug of choice) 6 g bolus IV/IM over 15–20 minutes with 2 g continuous infusion for the prevention of tonic-clonic seizures in severe preeclampsia. Magnesium is continued for 24 hours postpartum.

- 10% of eclamptic women will experience a 2nd convulsion with therapeutic magnesium levels. In these patients, another 2-g bolus may be given. Recurrent seizures may be treated with sodium amobarbital 250 mg IV over 3–5 minutes.
- Magnesium toxicity symptoms include loss of patellar reflex, feelings of warmth and flushing, somnolence, slurred speech, muscular paralysis, respiratory difficulty, and cardiac arrest:
  - Treat magnesium toxicity with calcium gluconate 10 mL of 10% solution
- Medication for BP control:
  - Hydralazine 5–10 mg IV q20min
  - Labetalol 20–40 mg IV q10min or 1 mg/kg as needed
  - Nifedipine 10–20 mg PO q20–30min

ALERT
Diuretic therapy is avoided in eclampsia because of the decreased intravascular volume. Diuretics are only used in cases where eclampsia is complicated by pulmonary edema.

 FOLLOW-UP

PROGNOSIS
Prognosis depends on GA at onset and at delivery, severity of disease, presence of multiple gestations, and presence of preexisting medical conditions.

COMPLICATIONS
- Aspiration pneumonia
- Pulmonary edema
- Cerebral hemorrhage
- Abruptio placentae
- Nonreassuring fetal status
- Maternal death
- Coma

BIBLIOGRAPHY

Dahmus MA, et al. Cerebral imaging in eclampsia: Magnetic resonance imaging versus computed tomography. *Am J Obstet Gynecol*. 1992;167: 935–941.

Sibai B. Diagnosis, prevention, and management of eclampsia. *Obstet Gynecol*. 2005;105:402–410.

Witlin et al. Magnesium sulfate in preeclampsia and eclampsia. *Obstet Gynecol*. 1998;92:883–889.

 MISCELLANEOUS

ABBREVIATIONS
GA—Gestational age

CODES

ICD9-CM
642.6X Eclampsia

 PATIENT TEACHING

- 25% risk of preeclampsia in subsequent pregnancy
- 2% risk eclampsia in subsequent pregnancy
- Subsequent pregnancies at increased risk for adverse perinatal outcome

ECTOPIC PREGNANCY

C. H. McCracken, III, MD

 BASICS

DESCRIPTION
Ectopic pregnancy is defined by the presence of the fertilized ovum outside of the endometrial cavity. The ectopic pregnancy may be ruptured or unruptured. Hemorrhage from ectopic pregnancy is the leading cause of pregnancy-related maternal death in the 1st trimester.

DIFFERENTIAL DIAGNOSIS
* Normal pregnancy
* Threatened abortion
* Missed abortion or blighted ovum
* Ruptured corpus luteum cyst
* Appendicitis
* Ovarian torsion
* Ovarian cyst

EPIDEMIOLOGY
* Occur in ~2% of all US pregnancies
* The highest rate of ectopic pregnancy occurs in women aged 35–44 years.
* The highest incidence of ectopic pregnancy is in women aged 20–29.

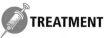 **TREATMENT**

MEDICAL MANAGEMENT
* Methotrexate, a folic acid antagonist, is the primary nonsurgical modality for treatment of ectopic pregnancy.
* Requirements for medical therapy:
  – Hemodynamically stable
  – No signs of hemoperitoneum or active bleeding
  – Patient is reliable and able to return for follow-up
  – No contraindications to methotrexate

* Relative indications:
  – Unruptured mass ≤3.5 cm
  – No fetal cardiac motion
  – hCG level <5,000
  – General anesthesia poses a significant risk
  – Nonlaparoscopic diagnosis
  – Desires future fertility
* Absolute contraindications:
  – Breastfeeding
  – Immunodeficiency
  – Alcoholism or alcoholic liver disease
  – Chronic liver disease
  – Preexisting blood dyscrasias
  – Known methotrexate sensitivity
  – Active pulmonary disease
  – Peptic ulcer disease
  – Hepatic, renal or hematologic dysfunction
* Relative contraindications:
  – Gestational sac ≥3.5 cm
  – Fetal cardiac motion

Regimens
* Single-dose:
  – Methotrexate 50 mg/m^2 IM injection on Day 0
  – No leucovorin rescue
  – 2nd dose if hCGs fail to decline 15% between days 4 and 7
* Multiple-dose:
  – Methotrexate 1.0 mg/kg on days 0, 2, 4, and 6
  – Leucovorin 0.1 mg/kg days 1, 3, 5, and 7
* Adverse drug effects:
  – Nausea
  – Vomiting
  – Stomatitis
  – Gastric distress
  – Dizziness
  – Severe neutropenia (rare)
  – Reversible alopecia (rare)
  – Pneumonitis

* Signs of treatment failure:
  – Significantly worsening abdominal pain
  – Hemodynamic instability
  – hCG levels that do not decline by at least 15% between day 4 and day 7
  – Increasing or plateauing hCG levels after the 1st week of treatment
* Patient instructions:
  – Some abdominal pain, vaginal bleeding, or spotting may occur.
  – Contact physician for sudden sever abdominal pain, heavy vaginal bleeding, dizziness, syncope, or tachycardia.
  – Avoid alcoholic beverages, folic acid–containing vitamins, NSAIDs, and sexual intercourse until the ectopic pregnancy has resolved.

Resuscitation
Initial stabilization and volume resuscitation is necessary for the hemodynamically unstable patient, followed expeditiously by surgical management.

> **ALERT**
> Hemodynamic instability is a contraindication to medical management, and surgical intervention is required.

Drugs
Pain medication may need to be provided. NSAIDs should be avoided.

> **ALERT**
> RhoGAM should be administered to all Rh negative patients once the ectopic pregnancy is diagnosed.

SURGICAL MANAGEMENT
Informed Consent
Patients should be informed of the alternatives of medical therapy (if appropriate) vs. surgical therapy, and the relative risks, benefits, and complications of the surgical procedure. These factors should be documented in the medical record.

Risks, Benefits

- In selected patients, laparoscopic and medical treatment are equally effective.
- Surgical treatment results in a faster resolution of hCGs, reducing the length of posttreatment follow-up.
- Medical treatment is less expensive.
- Surgical risks include:
  – Blood loss and transfusion risks
  – Infection
  – Surgical injury to pelvic organs
  – Anesthesia risks
  – Risk of salpingectomy or oophorectomy
  – Potential for conversion of laparoscopic procedure to laparotomy
  – Decreased fertility
  – Increased risk of subsequent ectopic pregnancy

Alternatives

Stable patients with low hCGs and without US confirmation of ectopic pregnancy may be followed expectantly with caution and close follow-up.

Surgical

- Laparoscopic or abdominal incision
- Salpingectomy
- Salpingostomy
- Cornual resection for cornual or interstitial pregnancies
- Cervical pregnancy:
  – D&C
  – Because of the risk of severe hemorrhage with cervical pregnancies, also consider the following adjuvants:
    ○ Shirodkar cerclage
    ○ Transvaginal ligation of the cervical branches of the uterine arteries
    ○ Uterine artery embolization
    ○ Intracervical vasopressin injection
    ○ Balloon tamponade
    ○ Hysterectomy (may be 1st line treatment if fertility not desired)

FOLLOW-UP

All patients, whether treated medically, surgically, or expectantly, require close follow-up.

- Weekly monitoring of hCG until the level is zero
- A decline of the hCG of <20% in 72 hours after surgical treatment is suggestive of incomplete treatment.
- Posttreatment tubal potency may be assessed with a hysterosalpingogram.

PROGNOSIS

- ~25% of conceptions after an ectopic pregnancy result in another ectopic pregnancy.
- 1/3 of nulliparous women with an ectopic pregnancy will have a subsequent ectopic pregnancy.

COMPLICATIONS

- Persistent ectopic pregnancy
- Tubal rupture
- Abdominal pregnancy
- Subfertility

BIBLIOGRAPHY

ACOG Practice Bulletin No. 3. Ory SJ. Medical Management of Tubal Pregnancy. Washington DC: ACOG; December 1998.

Mishell DR. Ectopic Pregnancy. In: Stenchever MA, et al., eds. *Comprehensive Gynecology*, 4th ed. St. Louis: Mosby; 2001:443–478.

Murray H, et al. Diagnosis and treatment of ectopic pregnancy. *Can Med Assoc J*. 2005;173(8): 905–912.

Seeber BE, et al. Suspected ectopic pregnancy. *Obstet Gynecol*. 2006;107:399–413.

Sowter MC, et al. Ectopic pregnancy: An update. *Curr Opin Obstet Gynecol*. 2004;16:289–293.

Stovall TG, et al. Single-dose methotrexate: An expanded trial. *Am J Obstet Gynecol*. 1993;168: 1759–1765.

MISCELLANEOUS

SYNONYM(S)

Tubal pregnancy

ABBREVIATIONS

hCG—Human chorionic gonadotropin

CODES

ICD9-CM

- 633.00 Abdominal pregnancy without intrauterine pregnancy
- 633.01 Abdominal pregnancy with intrauterine pregnancy
- 633.10 Tubal pregnancy without intrauterine pregnancy
- 633.11 Tubal pregnancy with intrauterine pregnancy
- 633.20 Ovarian pregnancy without intrauterine pregnancy
- 633.21 Ovarian pregnancy with intrauterine pregnancy
- 633.80 Other ectopic pregnancy without intrauterine pregnancy
- 633.81 Other ectopic pregnancy with intrauterine pregnancy
- 633.80 Unspecified ectopic pregnancy without intrauterine pregnancy
- 633.81 Unspecified ectopic pregnancy with intrauterine pregnancy

PATIENT TEACHING

- www.asrm.org/Patients/patientbooklets/ectopicpregnancy.pdf
- www.acog.org/publications/patient_education/bp155.cfm

GENITOURINARY INJURY, INTRAOPERATIVE

Eric R. Sokol, MD

BASICS

DESCRIPTION

ALERT

50–80% of all surgical complications to the lower urinary tract can be attributed to gynecologic surgery.

- Intraoperative injury to the female GU tract most commonly occurs during routine gynecologic surgery. Sites of injury can include:
  – Bladder
  – Ureter
  – Urethra
- The risk of GU injury is increased whenever normal anatomy is distorted or difficult to identify, such as with:
  – Congenital abnormalities
  – Endometriosis
  – Fibroids
  – Hemorrhage
  – Ovarian masses
  – Pelvic malignancy
  – Pregnancy
  – Previous pelvic radiation
  – Previous pelvic surgery
  – Prolapse

Pregnancy Considerations
The enlarged, gravid uterus can make identification of the ureters difficult and can distort normal bladder anatomy, increasing the likelihood of a GU injury.

EPIDEMIOLOGY
- 600,000 women undergo hysterectomies annually:
  – 75% of GU injuries that occur during gynecologic surgery occur during hysterectomy.
  – Overall rate of urinary tract injury is 1.6 per 1,000 major gynecologic cases.
  – 0.4–2.5% rate of ureteral injury during benign pelvic procedures
  – 0.4–1.8% bladder injury rate during benign pelvic procedures
  – Injury rates are under-reported.
- The type of hysterectomy influences the risk of GU injury:
  – Abdominal hysterectomy injury rates:
    ○ Bladder injury rate: 0.58%
    ○ Ureter injury rate: 0.35%
  – Vaginal hysterectomy injury rates:
    ○ Bladder injury rate: 1.86%
    ○ Ureter injury rate: <0.5%
  – Laparoscopic hysterectomy injury rates:
    ○ 13.9 per 1,000 cases

- Overall incidence of ureteral injury during laparoscopic surgery is 1–2%:
  – 20% of injuries occurred during laparoscopic-assisted vaginal hysterectomy
  – Only 8.6% of injuries recognized intraoperatively
  – Electrocoagulation accounts for ~25% of ureteral injuries during laparoscopic surgery:
    ○ Laparoscopic oophorectomy is the most common procedure in which thermal spread causes ureteral injury.
- Urogynecologic and pelvic reconstructive surgical procedures increase the risk of GU injury:
  – 5% of patients have unsuspected finding at cystoscopy.
  – 3% of patients have a finding at cystoscopy that prompts intervention:
    ○ Anterior colporrhaphy accounted for ~1/2 of the cases in which intervention was required.
  – 1.7% chance of ureteral compromise
  – Ureteral injury occurs in 1–11% of uterosacral plication and suspension procedures
- Obstetric procedures are associated with GU injuries:
  – Urologic consultation during cesarean section occurs in 0.3% of cases.
  – >90% of GU injuries occur during emergent cesarean delivery:
    ○ Dome of the bladder is the most common site of injury.
    ○ There is a 4-fold increase in bladder injury after repeat cesarean section compared to primary cesarean section.
  – Uterine rupture during attempted vaginal birth after cesarean delivery can lead to bladder and ureter injuries.

 TREATMENT

MEDICAL MANAGEMENT
- A careful preoperative history and physical exam can uncover factors that can predispose to GU injury, such as scarring from prior surgery or endometriosis, or a personal or family history of GU anomalies.
- Preoperative imaging studies can help identify altered anatomy, but have not been consistently shown to reduce rates of intraoperative GU injury.

SURGICAL MANAGEMENT
Informed Consent
- A discussion of the possibility of intraoperative GU injury should be part of the informed consent process for all gynecologic surgeries.
- Since GU injuries are unplanned and necessitate additional surgical time for repair, physician notification of family may be prudent.

Surgical
- The ureter should be routinely identified during hysterectomy and pelvic surgery.
- Preoperative placement of ureteral stents may help identify ureters in patients at high risk for injury, but stent placement has not been shown to decrease the overall rate of injury.
- The most common sites of ureter injury during gynecologic surgery are:
  – Where the ureter enters the pelvis near the pelvic brim, during ligation of the ovarian vessels
  – Where the ureter crosses medial to the bifurcation of the iliac vessels during pelvic lymph node dissection
  – Where the ureter crosses under the uterine vessels at the level of the cardinal ligament during ligation of the uterine vessels during hysterectomy
- The bladder is at risk for injury during dissection from the lower uterine segment and vagina during hysterectomy.
- Surgical strategies may be employed to avoid GU injury during pelvic surgery:
  – During abdominal hysterectomy, identify the ureter on the medial leaf of the broad ligament.
  – During vaginal hysterectomy, an adequate vesicouterine space should be developed to protect the bladder and ureters from injury.
  – During anterior colporrhaphy, sutures should not be placed too laterally or too deeply to avoid kinking the ureters or injuring the bladder.
  – During laparoscopic surgery, the ureter should be directly visualized through the peritoneum or via retroperitoneal exploration.
  – To avoid devascularization injuries during mobilization of the ureter, the mesentery of the ureter on the medial side of the peritoneum should be preserved to preserve vascular collaterals.
- Cystoscopy should be liberally used during pelvic surgery to confirm normal ureteral jets and bladder integrity.
- Surgical management of ureteral injury depends on the injury type:
  – For ligation, remove the offending suture.
  – For crush, immediately place ureteral stent to avoid stricture (if amenable) or resect crushed section and reanastomose ureter or reimplant ureter into the bladder.
  – For small injury, place ureteral stent and confirm integrity postoperatively by intravenous pyelogram prior to stent removal.
  – For transection, repair depends on the level of the injury:
    ○ For transaction of the abdominal ureter, ureteure terostomy may be performed.
    ○ For transaction below the mid-pelvis, ureteroneocystostomy may be performed.

- Ureteral stents should be placed and percutaneous nephrostomy tubes may be used to divert urine after ureteral repair, allowing the site of anastomosis to heal.
- Bladder injury can be recognized by cystoscopy or by retrograde filling of the bladder with methylene blue–stained fluid.
- Bladder injuries should be repaired with a 2-layered closure of fine, absorbable suture, and a Foley or suprapubic catheter should be left in place to allow for bladder healing.
- Urethral injuries that occur during vaginal surgery should be repaired with a 2-layered closure of fine, absorbable suture, and a Foley catheter should be left in place for 1–2 weeks to promote healing and prevent fistula formation.

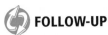 **FOLLOW-UP**

- Patients who have suffered an intraoperative GU injury should be discharged with urinary tract drainage, depending on the site of injury.
- Radiology imaging can be considered after GU injury to ensure complete healing before removing the ureteral stent or urinary catheter.
- Postoperative manifestations of unrecognized GU injury include hematuria, fever, flank pain, hyponatremia, and a rise of serum BUN or creatinine.

PROGNOSIS
The recognition, location and extent of injury, development of complications, and functional result determine prognosis.

COMPLICATIONS
GU fistulas can be late complications of unrecognized or improperly treated GU injuries.

BIBLIOGRAPHY

Carley ME, et al. Incidence, risk factors and morbidity of unintended bladder or ureter injury during hysterectomy. *Int Urogynecol J Pelvic Floor Dysfunct*. 2002;13(1):18–21.

Gilmour DT, et al. Lower urinary tract injury during gynecologic surgery and its detection by intraoperative cystoscopy. *Obstet Gynecol*. 1999;94(5):883–889.

Kwon CH, et al. The use of intraoperative cystoscopy in major vaginal and urogynecologic surgeries. *Am J Obstet Gynecol*. 2002;187(6):1466–1471.

Ostrzenski A, et al. A review of laparoscopic ureteral injury in pelvic surgery. *Obstet Gynecol Surv*. 2003;58(12):794–799.

Phipps MG, et al. Risk factors for bladder injury during cesarean delivery: Reply. *Obstet Gynecol*. 2005;105(4):901.

 MISCELLANEOUS

ABBREVIATIONS
GU—Genitourinary

CODES
ICD9-CM
- 56.82 Suture of laceration of ureter
- 56.86 Removal of ligature from ureter
- 57.32 Transurethral cystoscopy
- 57.81 Suture of laceration of bladder
- 57.82 Closure of cystostomy
- 58.41 Suture of laceration of urethra
- 75.61 Repair of current obstetric laceration (bladder or urethra)

PATIENT TEACHING

- Preoperative teaching and informed consent regarding potential risks of surgery, including GU injury
- Postoperative teaching regarding management of catheter helps alleviate anxiety
- Anticipatory guidance regarding catheter management and plans for removal

Section VIII

HELLP SYNDROME

Jason K. Baxter, MD, MSCP
Louis Weinstein, MD

 BASICS

DESCRIPTION

- HELLP syndrome is an acute, progressive, emergent obstetric condition whose sole therapy is delivery.
- An atypical severe variant of preeclampsia
- Mnemonic for hemolysis, elevated liver enzymes, and low platelets:
  - **Hemolysis**: Microangiopathic hemolytic anemia, with ≥ 2 of:
    - Schistocytes
    - Burr cells in peripheral smear
    - Serum bilirubin ≥ 1.2 mg/dL
    - Low serum haptoglobin
  - **Elevated liver enzymes**:
    - AST or ALT at least twice the level of normal, or ≥ 70 u/L
  - **Low platelets:**
    - Platelets $<100,000/mm^3$
  - 1st described >50 years ago
  - Coined by Weinstein 25 years ago

SIGNS AND SYMPTOMS

- HTN: 85%
- Proteinuria: 87%
- RUQ or epigastric pain: 40–90%
- Nausea or vomiting: 29–84%
- Headaches: 33–60%
- Visual changes: 10–20%
- Mucosal bleeding: 10%
- Jaundice: 5%

DIFFERENTIAL DIAGNOSIS

- HELLP syndrome is over- and underdiagnosed.
- Some acute, emergent conditions have been considered part of a spectrum of the same illness:
  - Severe preeclampsia
  - HELLP syndrome
  - Pregnancy-associated HUS
  - TTP
  - AFLP
  - Postpartum renal failure
- Preeclampsia or HELLP syndrome has been misdiagnosed as:
  - Viral hepatitis
  - Cholangitis
  - SLE
  - ITP
  - Detached retina
  - Gastric ulcer

- Significant medical and surgical conditions have initially mistakenly been diagnosed as HELLP syndrome, delaying appropriate therapy:
  - Cardiomyopathy
  - Dissecting aortic aneurysm
  - Cocaine abuse
  - Chronic renal disease
  - AFLP
  - Gangrenous gallbladder
  - Ruptured bile duct
  - Glomerulonephritis
  - Immune thrombocytopenia
  - SLE
  - Pheochromocytoma

EPIDEMIOLOGY

Incidence

- 10–20% of women with severe preeclampsia or eclampsia develop HELLP syndrome.
- With preeclampsia present, the incidence of HELLP syndrome varies between 2% and 12%.
- Timing:
  - Cases diagnosed antepartum: 72%
  - 28–36 weeks: 70%
  - >37 weeks: 20%
  - <28 weeks: 10%
  - Cases diagnosed postpartum: 28%
    - ≤ 48 hours postpartum: 80%
    - >48 hours postpartum: 20%

 TREATMENT

MEDICAL MANAGEMENT

- Delivery is the only cure for HELLP syndrome.
- Prompt delivery is indicated with HELLP syndrome:
  - Diagnosed at ≥ 34 weeks' gestation
  - Diagnosed <23 weeks' gestation
  - Fetal nonreassuring status
  - Maternal nonreassuring status:
    - Eclampsia
    - DIC
    - Renal failure
    - Abruptio placentae
    - Respiratory distress
    - Suspected liver hematoma
- Delivery can be delayed a maximum of 48 hours in stable preterm patients (24–34 weeks) to give course of steroids for fetal lung maturity.
- Preterm patients should be transferred to a tertiary care center once hemodynamically stable.

Drugs

- Magnesium sulfate:
  - Prophylactic drug of choice for prevention of eclampsia:
    - 59% reduction in the risk of eclampsia
    - 36% reduction in abruption
    - 46% reduction in maternal death
  - Given intravenously, 4–6-g load over 20 minutes, followed by 1–2 g/h
  - Usually started with HELLP diagnosis, but at least with onset of active labor
  - Continued at least 12–24 hours postpartum
- Antihypertensive medications for the treatment of severe "stroke range" HTN (>180/110 mm Hg):
  - Labetalol: 20 mg IV bolus, then 40 mg, 80 mg, 80 mg as needed, q10min, (maximum 220-mg total dose)
  - Nifedipine: 10–20 mg PO, may repeat in 30 minutes (caution with magnesium sulfate); (maximum 50-mg total dose)
  - Hydralazine: 5–10 mg IV (or IM) q20min (maximum 30-mg total dose)
  - Sodium nitroprusside (rarely needed): Start at 0.25 μg/kg/min to maximum of 5 μg/kg/min
- Steroids:
  - Indicated to improve perinatal complications associated with preterm birth <34 weeks
  - There is insufficient evidence to recommend the use of dexamethasone, betamethasone, or other steroids for therapy specific for HELLP syndrome:
    - No significant differences in maternal morbidity or mortality
    - No significant differences in perinatal morbidity or mortality
- Associated with a tendency to a greater platelet count increase over 48 hours, fewer days of maternal hospitalization, and longer interval to delivery

Other

- Route of delivery should be based on obstetric indications.
- HELLP syndrome is not an indication for cesarean delivery per se.
- Vaginal delivery is preferable if it can be obtained in a reasonable length of time.

- In a nulliparous patient with an unripe cervix <30 weeks' gestation, the incidence of cesarean delivery is high:
  - Regional anesthesia is usually preferred with platelet counts ≥75,000/mm³.
  - General anesthesia may be safer (if needed for cesarean delivery) with platelet counts <75,000/mm³:
    ○ Platelet transfusions are rarely needed, even with a platelet count of 25,000/mm³.

SURGICAL MANAGEMENT
- In cases of cesarean delivery, a peritoneal or suprafascial drain may be indicated.
- Liver hematomas are best managed conservatively, without surgery.
- If liver rupture occurs, get appropriate help for packing the liver.

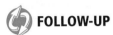 FOLLOW-UP

No follow-up is indicated after inpatient recovery (see "Prognosis").

PROGNOSIS
- Women with HELLP syndrome typically recover after delivery.
- Clinical and laboratory values typically start improving 48–72 hours after delivery.
- Risks in future pregnancies after HELLP syndrome:
  - HELLP syndrome recurrence: 5%
  - Preeclampsia: 25–30%
  - Preterm birth: 30–40%
  - SGA: 25%
  - Perinatal death: 5–10%
- An increased risk for cardiovascular disease exists in the future for women who have had preeclampsia or its complications.

COMPLICATIONS
- Preterm birth: 70%
- Perinatal death: 7–20%
- Pleural effusions: 10–15%
- Abruptio placentae: 10–15%
- DIC: 10–15%
- Marked ascites: 10–15%
- Pulmonary edema: 6–8%
- Acute renal failure: 3%
- Liver failure or hemorrhage: 1–2%
- Laryngeal edema: 1–2%
- ARDS: 1%
- Maternal death: 1%

BIBLIOGRAPHY

ACOG Practice Bulletin No. 33. Diagnosis and Management of Preeclampsia and Eclampsia. *Obstet Gynecol*. 2002;99:159–167.

Baxter JK, et al. HELLP syndrome: The state of the art. *Obstet Gynecol Survey*. 2005;59:838–845.

Report of the National High Blood Pressure Education Program Working Group on High Blood Pressure in Pregnancy. *Am J Obstet Gynecol*. 2000;183:S1–S22.

Sibai BM. A practical plan to detect and manage HELLP syndrome. *OBG Management*. 2005;17:52–69.

Weinstein L. Syndrome of hemolysis, elevated liver enzymes, and low platelet count: A severe consequence of hypertension in pregnancy. *Am J Obstet Gynecol*.1982;142:159–167.

MISCELLANEOUS

If only 1 or 2 criteria are present, some use the term "partial" or "evolving" HELLP syndrome to denote a better prognosis.

CLINICAL PEARLS
- ~15% of women with HELLP syndrome have no HTN or no proteinuria.
- Many HELLP syndrome maternal deaths have been prescribed antacids in the days preceding diagnosis.

ABBREVIATIONS
- AFLP—Acute fatty liver of pregnancy
- ARDS—Acute respiratory distress syndrome
- DIC—Disseminated intravascular coagulopathy
- GA—Gestational age
- HELLP—Hemolysis, elevated liver enzymes, low platelets
- HUS—Hemolytic uremic syndrome
- ITP—Idiopathic thrombocytopenic purpura
- RUQ—Right upper quadrant
- SGA—Small for gestational age
- SLE—Systemic lupus erythematsus
- TTP—Thrombotic thrombocytopenic purpura

CODES
ICD9-CM
642.5 Severe preeclampsia

PATIENT TEACHING

- HELLP syndrome is an atypical form of severe preeclampsia.
- Delivery is the only cure for HELLP syndrome:
  - Delivery should take place at a tertiary care center.
  - The baby's outcome depends on the GA at the time of delivery.
- Most mothers recover and have limited long-term effects:
  - The recurrence risk of HELLP syndrome in a subsequent pregnancy is ~5%.
- There is no proven therapy to prevent HELLP syndrome in pregnancy.

HEMORRHAGE: ACUTE UTERINE BLEEDING (NONGESTATIONAL)

Malcom G. Munro, MD
Eve S. Cunningham, MD

 BASICS

DESCRIPTION

Excessively heavy or prolonged bleeding of uterine origin in a nongravid patient sufficient in volume as to require urgent or emergent intervention. The bleeding may be associated with menarche, isolated in the context of historically normal menstrual function; may be superimposed on a background of chronic AUB, or, much less commonly, may occur in postmenopausal women.

ALERT

Always consider the possibility of pregnancy in a woman of reproductive age, even in young adolescents or mature women near the age of menopause.

Pregnancy Considerations

Acute uterine bleeding is managed differently from bleeding related to pregnancy.

DIFFERENTIAL DIAGNOSIS

Initial evaluation should confirm that the bleeding is of uterine origin and that there is no pregnancy. Possible causes or contributors to acute uterine bleeding include:

- Anovulation: Chronic or isolated with subsequent heavy bleeding secondary to the deficiency of endometrial hemostasis when the estrogen-primed endometrium is not exposed to progesterone
- Idiopathic HMB implies a history of heavy bleeding but regular, predictable onset of menses. These women usually do not present acutely, but may do so when they become anemic.
- Focal pathology in the endometrial cavity or cervical canal:
  - Polyps:
    ○ Probably uncommon causes of acute bleeding in themselves.
  - Leiomyomas:
    ○ May interfere with local endometrial hemostasis.
    ○ Usually an antecedent history of HMB.
  - Hyperplasia/Cancer:
    ○ More frequent in older women with a long history of anovulation or in postmenopausal women
  - Arteriovenous malformations of the myometrium:
    ○ Rare
    ○ May be explanation for uncontrollable bleeding without an obvious etiology
- Disorder of hemostasis (especially adolescents):
  - May 1st present at menarche
  - vWD, ITP, etc.
  - Cytotoxic chemotherapy, thrombocytopenia
  - Therapeutic anticoagulation
- Foreign body (IUD)
- Although endometritis has been related to acute bleeding, the evidence is rather weak.

EPIDEMIOLOGY

Most nongestational acute uterine bleeding occurs in the reproductive years, but severe cases may present at menarche, associated with anovulation and, in some instances, systemic disorders of hemostasis. Postmenopausal acute uterine bleeding is uncommon but when it occurs, often reflects the presence of underlying neoplasia.

Pediatric Considerations

Always consider systemic disorder of hemostasis as an underlying cause of acute uterine bleeding in adolescent patients.

Geriatric Considerations

Always consider endometrial hyperplasia, carcinoma, other malignant neoplasms as potential underlying causes of acute uterine bleeding in perimenopausal and postmenopausal women.

 TREATMENT

MEDICAL MANAGEMENT

- Assess appropriateness of inpatient or outpatient therapy based on clinical picture.
- Evaluate for the presence of focal lesions of the lower genital tract including neoplasms and lacerations, to confirm that bleeding is coming from the cervical canal or the endometrial cavity.

Resuscitation

- If evidence of hypovolemia, aggressive fluid hydration for hypotension:
  - Insert 2 large-bore IV catheters.
  - Run isotonic IV fluids (normal saline or Ringer's lactate) wide open; titrate to vital signs in context of overall medical condition.
  - Consider intrauterine tamponade (see below).
- If appropriate, transfuse packed RBCs for low hemoglobin, symptomatic anemia, or preparation for surgical intervention.

Drugs

- Specific pharmacologic approach depends on the acuity of the situation and the patient's overall clinical condition.
- For patients with a systemic disorder of hemostasis, specific therapy may be appropriate (e.g., DDAVP with vWD).
- IV pharmacologic agents are better suited for situations when in-hospital management is necessary.
- Oral regimens are suitable for office use (i.e., when the hemoglobin is above 7–8 g/dL and there is confidence that the clinical condition is stable).
- The role of pharmacologic agents in management of acute postmenopausal bleeding has not been established:
  - Therapeutic approaches involving tamponade and the opportunity to evaluate the endometrial cavity are preferred.

- Hemodynamically stable patients:
  - IV conjugated estrogen:
    ○ Conjugated equine estrogen (Premarin) 25 mg IV q4h for 24 hours or until bleeding stops:
      ■ 72% cessation of bleeding in 5 hours.
      ■ Convert to a progestin or combined OCP regimen once bleeding has stopped.
  - "High dose" oral progestins:
    ○ Medroxyprogesterone acetate: 20 mg PO t.i.d. or q.i.d. for 1 week, then daily for 3 weeks or satisfactory restoration of Hgb levels.
      ■ Bleeding stops in a mean of 3 days
  - COCs:
    ○ Norethindrone 1 mg/EE 0.35 mg t.i.d. for 1 week or until bleeding stops, then daily for 3 weeks or until satisfactory restoration of Hgb levels.
      ■ Bleeding stops in a mean of 3 days
  - Parenteral antifibrinolytic agents:
    ○ For patients with recalcitrant acute AUB or with known disorder of hemostasis
    ○ Aminocaproic acid:
      ■ 4–5 g IV over 60 minutes, then maintenance of 1 g IV/h. Up to 30 g/d. Stop infusion when bleeding stops.
  - DDAVP:
    ○ Patients with known vWD
    ○ 1 puff NAS (nasal) for 1 dose.

Other

- Intrauterine tamponade:
  - Large Foley catheter balloon (30 balloon on 16–20 G catheter) inflated to 50–80 mL within the endometrial cavity
  - Sengstaken-Blakemore tube
  - Packing uterus with long packing gauze
- Uterine artery compression/occlusion:
  - Placement of ring forceps on each uterine artery intravaginally by pinching the lateral fornices.
- Medical "tourniquet":
  - Intracervical injection of dilute vasopressin solution:
    ○ Avoid systemic injection.
    ○ 20 units vasopressin in 100 mL NS. Inject 4–5 mL deeply into the cervix at 4 and 8 o'clock.

SURGICAL MANAGEMENT

Informed Consent

- The need for informed consent can be suspended in an emergency situation, but certain criteria must be met 1st:
  - Patient must be unconscious or incapacitated, and suffering from a life-threatening condition requiring immediate treatment.
- Informed consent for surgical therapy depends on chosen procedure.

- D&C:
  - Should be reserved for patients who are inappropriate for or unresponsive to the use of medical therapy.
  - When performed, should preferably be accompanied by diagnostic hysteroscopy (see Endometrial Sampling, Dilation and Curettage).
- Hysteroscopically directed management:
  - Removal of focal lesion:
    - Myoma, polyp OR
  - Hysteroscopic endometrial ablation (See Hysteroscopy, Diagnostic and Operative.)
- Non-resectoscopic endometrial ablation:
  - Rarely appropriate for acute bleeding. Of some use in highly selected cases:
    - Poor medical condition, anticoagulated (See Endometrial Ablation.)
- Uterine artery embolization:
  - Use of tiny microspheres, coils, or gel foam to occlude uterine arteries bilaterally:
    - Impact on fertility not totally clear.
  - Performed by interventional radiologist under fluoroscopic guidance
- Hysterectomy:
  - Acute bleeding unresponsive to all other measures. This is a lifesaving procedure of last resort (see topics on Hysterectomy)

Patient Education
Refer to topics on specific procedures for patient counseling regarding postinterventional management.

Risks, Benefits
- All procedures carry risk of bleeding, infection, anesthesia risk, transfusion risk, and death. Other risks vary by procedure.
- Refer to chapters on specific procedures for patient counseling regarding risks and benefits.
- Decisions regarding surgical intervention should seriously consider patient's desire for future fertility.
  - Loss of reproductive function occurs with endometrial ablation and hysterectomy, whereas effect on reproduction is unknown in patients who undergo uterine artery embolization.

 FOLLOW-UP

Many patients with acute uterine bleeding have an underlying chronic disorder that requires systematic evaluation and, in many instances, chronic therapy, following the arrest of the acute phase of the process. See the appropriate topics on Heavy Menstrual Bleeding, Irregular Menstrual Bleeding, Oligomenorrhea, and Postmenopausal Bleeding.

COMPLICATIONS
- Anemia
- Complications related to the intervention or procedure

BIBLIOGRAPHY

DeVore GR, et al. Use of intravenous Premarin in the treatment of dysfunctional uterine bleeding—a double-blind randomized control study. *Obstet Gynecol*. 1982;59:285–291.

Goldrath MH. Uterine tamponade for the treatment of acute uterine bleeding. *Am J Obstet Gynecol*. 1983;147:869–872.

KP Southern California Acute Uterine Bleeding Guidelines. Available at: www.guideline.gov/browse/browsemode.aspx?node=27893&type=1

Munro MG, et al. Oral medroxyprogesterone acetate and combination oral contraceptives for acute uterine bleeding. *Obstet Gynecol*. 2006;108:924–929.

Oregon R, et al. Abnormal uterine bleeding. In: *Obstetric & Gynecologic Emergencies: Diagnosis and Management*. New York: McGraw Hill; 2004.

 MISCELLANEOUS

SYNONYM(S)
Acute Menorrhagia

ABBREVIATIONS
AUB—Abnormal uterine bleeding
COC—Combined oral contraceptive
EE—Ethinyl estradiol
Hgb—Hemoglobin
HMB—Heavy menstrual bleeding
ITP—Idiopathic thrombocytopenia
OCP—Oral contraceptive pill
vWD—von Willebrand disease

CODES
ICD9-CM
- 218.0A Benign neoplasm of uterus, submucous leiomyoma
- 218.1A Leiomyoma uterus, intramural
- 622.7B Polyp of cervix
- 626.2C Menorrhagia
- 626.6B Metrorrhagia

 PATIENT TEACHING

- If anemic, facilitate compliance with iron therapy, including discussion of side effects from iron ingestion such as constipation, GI upset, etc.
- Explain to the patient that acute uterine bleeding is often the result of a chronic condition that may require additional investigation and which may require long-term medical therapy or surgical intervention.

Section VIII

Phillip G. Stubblefield, MD

 BASICS

DESCRIPTION
- Heavy vaginal bleeding occurring to a woman in the 1st 12 weeks of pregnancy
- Diagnosis is based on the presence of profuse vaginal bleeding, a history of amenorrhea, a positive pregnancy test, and most importantly, on the physical findings of a somewhat enlarged uterus, dilated cervix, and the presence of pregnancy tissue extruding from the cervical os.

DIFFERENTIAL DIAGNOSIS
- Incomplete abortion is most likely.
- Missed abortion, threatened abortion, and inevitable abortion also present as bleeding, but the bleeding is usually less dramatic (see topics on other pregnancy complications).
- Ectopic pregnancy:
  – Cervical pregnancy can be confused with spontaneous abortion. It occurs rarely, but can be fatal if not recognized before instrumentation of the uterus.
- Molar pregnancy
- Twin gestation with 1 normal and 1 spontaneously aborting
- Vaginal or cervical lesion

EPIDEMIOLOGY
Incidence
In the interval from 1991–1999, an estimated 94 women died of SAB in the US. There were 7,882,974 miscarriages in this interval, representing 13.8% of pregnancy outcomes, and giving a death rate of 1.19 per 100,000 miscarriages. Hemorrhage is the most frequent cause of death from miscarriage.

RISK FACTORS
- Risk of SAB increases significantly with increasing maternal age. Bleeding is present with all abortions, but hemorrhage is not common. Risk of hemorrhages increases with GA.
- In early gestation, 8 weeks or less, the entire conceptus is usually expelled and intervention is not required. Beyond 8 weeks, gestational tissue is commonly retained and hemorrhages more likely.

ETIOLOGY
- Chromosomal abnormality is found in ~1/2 of abortuses when studied after expulsion from the uterus. CVS of missed abortions shows abnormal chromosomes in 75–90%.
- Other causes include uterine septum, maternal thrombophilia, maternal type I DM, and more.

 TREATMENT

MEDICAL MANAGEMENT
Medical management with misoprostol 800 μg given by the buccal or rectal route can be considered, but in acute hemorrhage, the best management is surgical vacuum curettage without delay.

Resuscitation
- Insert a large-bore intravenous line and start Ringer's lactate.
- Add oxytocin, 40 U/1,000 mL
- Monitor pulse and BP every 15 minutes

Labs
- Urine pregnancy test
- CBC
- Blood type and cross match 2 units of blood
- Administer nasal oxygen
- US can be considered, but treatment should not be delayed for this if patient continues to bleed heavily and uterine size by exam is ≤12 weeks.

Drugs
- Add oxytocin 40 U/1000 mL of IV fluid
- If Rh negative, give Rh-immune globulin before discharge from emergency department.

SURGICAL MANAGEMENT
- Prompt uterine evacuation by vacuum curettage is the preferred treatment. This can be accomplished under paracervical block and conscious sedation, in the emergency department or OR.
- Pregnancy tissue presenting at the cervical os is removed with a ring forceps, then the uterine content evacuated through a vacuum cannula:
  – Source of vacuum can be an electric uterine aspirator or manual vacuum aspiration (MVA) from a modified 60 mL syringe (IPAS, Chapel Hill, North Carolina or Mylex Corp, Chicago, IL)

Informed Consent
Describe procedure to patient:
- Type of anesthesia: Paracervical block and conscious sedation vs. general anesthesia
- Cervical dilatation (likely not needed)
- Use of vacuum cannula to evacuate uterus

Patient Education
- Causes of miscarriage:
  – Most commonly, aneuploid pregnancy
- Reassure that miscarriage is not the result of anything the patient did or did not do.
- Reassure of excellent probability of future normal pregnancy.

Risks, Benefits
- Benefits of vacuum curettage:
  – Prompt cessation of bleed and avoidance of blood transfusion
  – Prompt recovery
- Risks of vacuum curettage:
  – Possible cervical laceration
  – Possible uterine perforation with possible injury to internal organs, bowel, bladder
  – If perforation should occur, a 2nd procedure (laparoscopy) may be needed.

Alternative
- Observe patient in hospital (a poor choice in the face of continuing hemorrhage).
- Treat with misoprostol (expulsion of pregnancy tissue and cessation of bleeding may be delayed).
- Vacuum curettage (the best choice in this setting).

Medical
Misoprostol

Surgical
Vacuum curettage

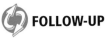

FOLLOW-UP

- Patient to take her temperature twice a day, call for temperatures >38°C.
- Patient to monitor bleeding; call if soaking a pad every hour.
- Mild, cramping lower abdominal pain is expected for a day or 2. Patient to call if severe or increasing pain is present.
- If Rh-negative and unsensitized be sure to give Rh-immune globulin before discharge.
- Arrange for follow up visit at 2 weeks.
- Offer contraceptive advice and prescribe if desired.
- Many patients want to try immediately to conceive. The conventional advice is to wait 3 months for physical recovery, and to rebuild essential nutrient stores.
- Prescribe multivitamin with folate to prepare for the next pregnancy.
- Refer for management of other illness, e.g.:
  – Type I diabetes
  – Thrombophilia
  – Other

PROGNOSIS

- Excellent chance of subsequent normal pregnancy for most patients.
- Patients for whom this is the 3rd spontaneous loss may be at higher risk for recurrence and should be evaluated for recurrent abortion.

COMPLICATIONS

- Hypovolemia
- Anemia
- Possible need for transfusion
- Postabortal endomyometritis
- Complications of vacuum curettage (see "Informed Consent")

BIBLIOGRAPHY

Grimes DA. Estimation of pregnancy-related mortality risk by pregnancy outcome, United States, 1991 to 1999. *Am J Obstet Gynecol.* 2006:194:92–94.

Nybo Andersen AM, et al. Maternal age and fetal loss: Population based register linkage study. *Br Med J.* 2000;320:1708–1712.

Strom C, et al. Analyses of 95 1st trimester spontaneous abortions by chorionic villus sampling and karyotype. *J Assist Reproduc Gene.* 1992;9: 458–461.

Stubblefield PG, et al. Complications of Induced Abortion. In: Pearlman MD, et al., eds. *Obstetric and Gynecologic Emergencies. Diagnosis and Management* 2nd ed. New York, McGraw-Hill; 2004:65–84.

Zhang J, et al. A comparison of medical management with misoprostol and surgical management for early pregnancy failure. *N Engl J Med.* 2005;353: 761–769.

MISCELLANEOUS

CLINICAL PEARLS

- In the 1st trimester of pregnancy, the most likely cause of vaginal hemorrhage is incomplete spontaneous abortion.
- The best treatment is vacuum curettage carried out with paracervical block and conscious sedation.
- This can be safely done in an emergency department with manual vacuum aspiration using a modified 60 mL syringe as vacuum source.

ABBREVIATIONS

- CVS—Chorionic villus sampling
- GA—Gestational age
- MVA—Manual vacuum aspiration
- SAB—Spontaneous abortion

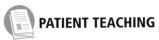

CODES

ICD9-CM
634.0 Spontaneous abortion

PATIENT TEACHING

See "Patient Education."

HEMORRHAGE, INTRAOPERATIVE

Matthew W. Guile, MD
Robert E. Bristow, MD

 BASICS

DESCRIPTION
- No strict definition of intraoperative hemorrhage
- Loss of >1 L blood, or blood loss requiring >1 L transfusion

Pelvic Blood Supply
- Hypogastric arteries:
  - Anterior division:
    - Uterine, superior vesical, middle hemorrhoidal, inferior hemorrhoidal, vaginal, obturator, inferior gluteal, internal pudendal
  - Posterior division:
    - Iliolumbar, lateral sacral, superior gluteal
- Ovarian arteries:
  - Direct branches of abdominal aorta
- Extensive collaterals allow for occlusion of hypogastric arteries

EPIDEMIOLOGY
Intraoperative hemorrhage during hysterectomy:
- Vaginal: 0.5–2.5%
- Abdominal: 0.2–3.7%

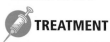 **TREATMENT**

MEDICAL MANAGEMENT
Concurrent with surgical management

Resuscitation
- Vascular access, IV fluids
- Blood products:
  - Packed RBCs increase Hct 3%/unit
  - FFP supplies clotting factors
  - Platelets increase platelet count by 5–10,000 plt/mm³/unit:
    - Intraoperative count should be kept above 50,000
  - Cryoprecipitate contains fibrinogen, Factors V, VIII, XIII, von Willebrand factor
  - Monitor acid/base status, electrolytes, PTTr, and INR

Drugs
- Many topical hemostatic products on the market:
  - Cellulose-, collagen-, gelatin-containing products
  - Fibrin glue
- Generally useful for venous oozing; work best in dry field

SURGICAL MANAGEMENT
Informed Consent
Separate consents are required for procedure and transfusion.
- Radical surgery involves greater risk of blood loss than surgery for benign conditions.

Risks, Benefits
Risk of blood transfusion, per unit transfused:
- Hepatitis C: 1:1.6 million
- Hepatitis B: 1:180,000
- HIV: 1:1.9 million
- Fatal red cell hemolytic reaction: 1:250,000–1.1 million
- Transfusion-related acute lung injury: 1:5,000
- Anaphylaxis: 1:150,000

Surgical
- Massive pelvic hemorrhage:
  - Bilateral hypogastric artery ligation:
    - Pelvic blood supply maintained through collaterals
    - Decreases pulse pressure 85%, MAP 24%
    - Allows visualization and thrombosis
    - Must identify ureter, iliac arteries, hypogastric vein
    - Ligated 2.5 cm distal to bifurcation of common iliac artery using nonabsorbable suture
    - Do not divide the vessels.
- Presacral hemorrhage:
  - Presacral venous plexus derived from middle sacral, lateral sacral, basivertebral veins:
    - At risk during sacral colpopexy, lymph node dissection:
    - Basivertebral veins originate in spongiosa of sacral body, very thin walled
    - Conventional measures often unsuccessful due to vessel retraction into sacrum
    - Initial management is packing for 5–7 minutes.
    - Persistent bleeding is treated using thumbtacks or bone wax pressed into sacral foramina.
- Obturator fossa hemorrhage:
  - Obturator neurovascular bundle follows pelvic sidewall and exits through obturator fossa
  - At risk during pelvic lymph node dissection
  - Direct visualization of obturator nerve essential
  - Obturator artery ligated or clipped
  - Venous bleeding of 2 types: Low flow—treated with compression, and high flow—requires suture ligation or clips

- Pelvic floor hemorrhage:
  - Major vessels include common, internal, and external iliac arteries and associated venous plexus
  - At risk during lymph node dissection, cytoreductive surgery, severe endometriosis resection, and lateral trocar placement
  - Coordinated, rapid response essential:
    - Immediate compression with laparotomy sponges
    - Visualization maximized through extension of incision, Trendelenburg position, adequate bowel packing, and extra suction
    - Repair requires meticulous dissection along injured vessel.
    - Vascular surgeon may be required.
- Internal iliac vein:
  - At risk during pelvic lymphadenectomy and hypogastric artery ligation
  - Relative immobility complicates management.
  - Initial management is packing for 5–7 minutes:
    - Small defects occluded with clips
    - Larger defects require running vascular stitch or ligation
- Pelvic venous plexus:
  - Initial management is packing for 5–7 minutes.
  - Continued bleeding requires packing for 48 hours:
    - Masterson method involves packing, closure with retention sutures.
    - Packing is pulled in 48 hours through wound
    - "Pack and go back" allows for surgical re-exploration in 48 hours after tightly packing with 5-cm gauze.
- External and common iliac veins:
  - At risk during lymph node dissection, especially on right side
  - Injuries are repaired using fine synthetic suture, delicate needles.
  - Do not ligate.
- External and common iliac arteries:
  - At risk during lymph node dissection, pelvic sidewall surgery, and lateral trocar placement
  - Essential for lower extremity perfusion:
    - Vascular clamps placed 2–3 cm distal/proximal to injury
    - Laceration repaired using monofilament polyethylene, 2-mm bites
    - Proximal clamp removed 1st, allowing egress of microemboli, air
    - Check distal pulses

- Infundibulopelvic ligament:
  – At risk during oophorectomy
  – Double-clamp technique diminishes risk of bleeding:
    ○ Minimize traction on vascular pedicle
    ○ Hematoma requires retroperitoneal dissection and identification of ipsilateral ureter.
    ○ Inspect pedicle immediately and before closure.
- Aorta and inferior vena cava:
  – At risk during lymph node dissection, and Veress needle and trocar placement
  – Vascular surgeon required
  – Immediate cross clamping of aorta below renal arteries can be life-saving.
  – Small tributary vein at risk during paraaortic lymph node dissection immediately above bifurcation of IVC:
    ○ Identify and clamp

Laparoscopic Surgery
- Vascular injuries comprise 30–50% of surgical trauma during laparoscopy.
- ~1/3 due to Veress needle, 1/3 from primary trocar, 1/3 auxiliary trocar
- Superficial epigastric artery:
  – At risk during lateral trocar placement
  – Occlusive pressure or ligation through small skin incision sufficient
- Inferior epigastric vessels:
  – At risk during lateral trocar placement
  – 20 Fr catheter placed through trocar sleeve, inflated with 10 mL water
  – Inflated balloon held taut against injury via Kelly clamp along anterior abdominal wall
  – Balloon removed, site inspected before closure
  – Keith needle passed medial to injury, inverted, passed out of peritoneum lateral to injury
  – Figure of 8 to occlude vessel
- Major retroperitoneal vessels:
  – At risk during Veress and trocar placement
  – Do not remove needle or trocar
  – Immediate exploratory laparotomy

FOLLOW-UP

Postoperative care:
- Routine care is appropriate for most patients.
  – Labs include hematocrit, coagulation indices, basic metabolic profile
  – Follow volume status, vital signs, urinary output
- Consider intensive care setting for the following:
  – Massive (>2,500 mL) blood loss/repletion
  – Coagulation abnormalities
  – Pelvic packing in place
  – Significant comorbidities

PROGNOSIS
Function of type of surgery, comorbidities

COMPLICATIONS
- Include both immediate and delayed sequelae
- Immediate:
  – End-organ damage including acute renal tubular necrosis, intestinal ischemia
  – Cardiovascular collapse, death
  – DIC
  – Metabolic alkalosis and free hypocalcemia secondary to massive blood transfusion
- Delayed:
  – Neurologic injury:
    ○ Obturator nerve injury leads to weakened abduction and sensory deficit inner thigh
    ○ Sciatic nerve injury leads to problems with ambulation and paresthesia
  – Vascular injury:
    ○ Common and external iliac vessel injury results in cool, congested lower extremity
  – Bleeding:
    ○ Retroperitoneal hematomas can occur secondary to inadequate infundibulopelvic ligament ligation.
    ○ Postoperative bleeding from inferior epigastric vessel can lead to rectus sheath hematomas.
  – Infectious:
    ○ Fevers in 1st 48 hours are likely cytokine-mediated.
  – Thromboembolic:
    ○ PE risk increased with major pelvic surgery, malignancy, immobility

BIBLIOGRAPHY

Finan MA, et al. Massive pelvic hemorrhage during gynecologic cancer surgery: "Pack and go back". *Gynecol Oncol*. 1996;62:390.

Thiel I, et al. Thumbtack application for control of presacral hemorrhage at pelvic lymphadenectomy: A case report. *J Pelvic Surg*. 2001;7(5):303–304.

Tomacruz RS, et al. Management of pelvic hemorrhage. *Surg Clin North Am*. 2001;81(4):925–948.

MISCELLANEOUS

CLINICAL PEARLS
- Use a right-angle clamp, passed lateral to medial, during hypogastric artery ligation to avoid the hypogastric vein.
- Avoid the presacral plexus by dissecting superficial to anterior sacral artery and vein.
- Limit dissection of obturator fossa to region superior to obturator nerve to avoid venous plexus.
- Always check infundibulopelvic ligament pedicle prior to abdominal closure.
- Inferior epigastric vessels can be avoided by placing the auxiliary trocar:
  – In midline
  – Lateral to external edge of rectus muscle
  – Under direct visualization, medial to obliterated umbilical artery or lateral to insertion of round ligament
- Insert primary trocar with patient in supine position, directing trocar toward hollow of sacrum.
- Auxiliary trocars should be directed toward uterine fundus to avoid common iliac vessels.
- Identification of bladder reflection adjacent to anterior vaginal wall is crucial to proper circumferential incision in vaginal hysterectomy:
  – Helps identify proper plane and decreases blood loss

ABBREVIATIONS
- DIC—Disseminated intravascular coagulation
- DVT—Deep venous thrombosis
- Hct—Hematocrit
- IVC—Inferior vena cava
- MAP—Mean arterial pressure
- PE—Pulmonary embolism
- PTTr—Partial thromboplastin time ratio

HEMORRHAGE, POSTPARTUM

Paula J. Adams Hillard, MD

 BASICS

DESCRIPTION

- PP hemorrhage is excessive bleeding after birth. The traditional definition of "excessive" includes EBL:
  - >500 mL for vaginal delivery
  - >100 mL for cesarean delivery
  - However, the average blood loss is close to these volumes, and EBL is frequently an underestimate.
- Alternative definition is decline of Hct of 10%, although this may not reflect hemodynamic status.
  - Typical symptoms and signs occurring with substantial blood loss (>10%) include:
    ○ Hypotension
    ○ Oliguria
    ○ Headache
    ○ Dizziness
    ○ Pallor
- Frequently occurs without warning, and thus all obstetric units should have the personnel and equipment, and maintain training to deal with this emergency.
- Risk factors for PP hemorrhage include:
  - Prolonged labor
  - Augmentation of labor
  - Rapid labor
  - Past history of PP hemorrhage
  - Episiotomy (Mediolateral > midline)
  - Preeclampsia
  - Uterine overdistension:
    ○ Multiple gestation
    ○ Macrosomia
    ○ Hydramnios
  - Forceps/Operative delivery
  - Asian or Hispanic ethnicity
  - Chorioamnionitis
  - Placenta accreta:
    ○ Increased risk from 0.2% for 1st CD through 7.7% for 6th CD
  - Placenta previa in current pregnancy, risk of placenta accreta from 3% with 1st CD to 67% with ≥5th CD
  - CD; risk of hysterectomy for hemorrhage in 0.7% 1st CD to 9% for ≥6th or greater
- If known or suspected placenta accreta:
  - Counsel about risk of hysterectomy.
  - Counsel about risk of transfusion.
  - Consider cell-saver technology.
  - Timing and availability of personnel for delivery
  - Anesthesia assessment

DIFFERENTIAL DIAGNOSIS

- Primary PP hemorrhage occurs in the 1st 24 hours, and is caused by uterine atony (80+%). Other causes include:
  - Retained placenta/ POCs
  - Coagulopathies
  - Uterine inversion

- Secondary PP hemorrhage occurs after 24 hours, but before 6 weeks postpartum in 1% of pregnancies, and is caused by:
  - Subinvolution of placental site
  - Retained POCs
  - Inherited coagulation defects:
    ○ Including vWD, present in ~1% of population
  - Bleeding often less heavy than primary PP hemorrhage

EPIDEMIOLOGY

- Worldwide, hemorrhage is the single largest cause of maternal death.
- >1/2 of all maternal deaths occur within 24 hours of delivery, and the most common cause is excessive bleeding. An estimated 140,000 women die of PP hemorrhage annually worldwide.

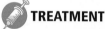 **TREATMENT**

MEDICAL MANAGEMENT

- Recognition of extent of hemorrhage is essential:
  - Bleeding may be concealed:
    ○ Hypotonic uterus filled with blood
    ○ Vaginal hematoma
    ○ Vulvar hematoma
- Immediately assess fundus to see if "boggy"—soft and not contracted
- Uterine massage and expression of clots with bimanual exam
- Labs:
  - CBC with platelets, repeat as indicated
  - Type and cross 4 units packed RBCs
  - Coagulation/Clotting labs, repeat as indicated:
    ○ PT, aPTT, fibrinogen
- Transfusion based on vital signs, labs, and assessment of EBL
- Suspect clotting abnormalities if:
  - Past history of PP hemorrhage
  - Family history of excessive bleeding
  - HELLP syndrome
  - Placental abruption
  - IUFD
  - Sepsis
  - Amniotic fluid embolism
  - Clotting abnormality can be caused by or exacerbated by the hemorrhage itself.
- Rule out lacerations by visualization and exam, in OR if needed to allow:
  - Positioning
  - Assistance
  - Lighting
  - Retractors (Sims, Simpson, Heaney, lateral vaginal)
  - Anesthesia
- US to assess for retained POCs

Resuscitation

- ABC:
  - Airway: Intubate or protect airway if necessary
  - Breathing: Supplemental O_2 5–7 L/min by tight face mask
  - Circulation:
    ○ Establish or maintain vascular access with 1–2 large-bore (14–16 G) IVs
- Crystalloid infusion:
  - RL solution or NS
- Foley catheter to measure output:
  - Careful record of I&O
- Notify:
  - Nursing
  - Anesthesia
  - Obstetric team

Drugs

- Conservative measures generally attempted 1st, especially if desire for future fertility
- At times, immediate surgery may be life-saving.
- Oxytocin 10–40 U/L NS or RL, continuous infusion
- Methylergonovine (Methergine) 0.2 mg IM, q2–4h:
  - Maximum 5 doses
  - Avoid if HTN
- 15 methyl prostaglandin F2-α (Hemabate) 250 μg IM, intramyometrial; repeat every 15–90 minutes:
  - Maximum 8 doses
  - Avoid if asthma or HTN
  - May cause diarrhea, fever, tachycardia
- Prostaglandin E2 suppositories (Dinoprostone, Prostin E2) 20 mg per rectum q2h:
  - Avoid with hypotension
  - Frozen for storage; thaw before use
- Misoprostol, PGE1 (Cytotec) 1,000 μg per rectum or sublingual (10 100-μg tablets or 5 200-μg tablets)

SURGICAL MANAGEMENT

Informed Consent

Inform patient of urgency and required surgical procedures that may include conservative measures or life-saving hysterectomy.

Alternatives

If fertility desired, attempt conservative measures, but may not be possible

Medical

- See Medical Management, Resuscitation, Drugs, which are typically used sequentially, effect assessed, and additional drugs given as required.
- Interventional radiology may be able to embolize bleeding pelvic vessel using Gelfoam, coils, glue; may also do balloon occlusion.

- Transfusion if significant or ongoing bleeding determined by clinical judgment:
  - EBL often inaccurate
  - Labs may not reflect equilibration or current status.
  - Signs and symptoms are late occurrence (blood loss >10–15%).
  - Replace RBC for oxygen-carrying capacity:
    ○ Volume 250 mL/unit increases Hct 3%; Hgb 1g/dL
  - Replace coagulation factors:
    ○ FFP 250 mL replaces fibrinogen, antithrombin III, factors V and VIII increase fibrinogen by 10 mg/dL
    ○ Cryoprecipitate 40 mL replaces fibrinogen, factors VIII and XIII, von Willebrand factor and increases fibrinogen by 10 mg/dL
  - Platelets:
    ○ 50 mL increases 5,000–10,000/mm^3/U

Surgical

- Hematoma may need incision and drainage:
  - Drain may be placed and left in situ.
  - Packing may be placed in hematoma or vagina.
- If retained POCs identified on US, curettage with blunt instrument: Banjo curette or ring forceps; US-guided, if needed, to reduce risk of perforation
- Uterine packing as temporizing measure; prepare for exploratory laparotomy:
  - 4-inch packing gauze; can be soaked with 5,000 units thrombin in 5 mL saline
  - Foley catheter (60–80 mL saline in bulb)
  - Sengstaken-Blakemore tube
  - SOS Bakri tamponade balloon with 300–400 mL saline
- If medical measures and/or packing do not control bleeding, exploratory laparotomy indicated. Surgical options:
  - Bilateral uterine artery ligation (O'Leary sutures)
  - Ligation of utero-ovarian ligaments
  - B-Lynch sutures to compress fundus
  - Hypogastric artery ligation:
    ○ Less successful than previously thought
    ○ Few clinicians technically experienced with this procedure
  - Hemostatic square suturing if atony, placenta previa, or accreta sutures anterior and posterior uterine wall together
- Uterine inversion as a cause of PP hemorrhage is diagnosed by firm mass below or near cervix with fundus not palpable abdominally:
  - If placenta not yet detached, leave in situ
  - Replace fundus by grasping fundus with palm and replacing through cervix
  - May require uterine relaxation with:
    ○ Terbutaline
    ○ Magnesium sulfate
    ○ Halothane or halogenated general anesthetics
    ○ Nitroglycerine
  - Laparotomy for uterine inversion rarely required

- Hemorrhage due to uterine rupture can occur after previous surgical procedures and requires surgical intervention to repair uterus and control hemorrhage.
- Hysterectomy may be indicated for intractable or life-threatening hemorrhage unresponsive to medical and conservative surgical measures.

 FOLLOW-UP

COMPLICATIONS

Sequelae of PP hemorrhage include:

- ARDS
- Coagulopathy
- Shock
- Sheehan syndrome, pituitary necrosis
- Loss of future fertility due to hysterectomy

BIBLIOGRAPHY

ACOG Practice Bulletin No. 76. Postpartum Hemorrhage. Washington, DC: ACOG; October 2006.

B-Lynch C, et al. The B-Lynch surgical technique for the control of massive postpartum haemorrhage: An alternative to hysterectomy? Five cases reported. *Br J Obstet Gynaecol*. 1997;104:372–375.

James AH. Von Willebrand disease. *Obstet Gynecol Surv*. 2006;61:136–145.

O'Leary JL, et al. Uterine artery ligation in the control of intractable postpartum hemorrhage. *Am J Obstet Gynecol*. 1966;94:920–924.

Joint Commission on Accreditation of Healthcare Organizations. Sentinel Event ALERT No. 30. Preventing infant death and injury during delivery. Available at: www.jointcommission.org/SentinelEvents/SentinelEventAlert/sea_30.htm. Accessed 06/12/06.

Stanco LM, et al. Emergency peripartum hysterectomy and associated risk factors. *Am J Obstet Gynecol*. 1993;168:879–883.

 MISCELLANEOUS

CLINICAL PEARLS

- Observe blood in red top tube:
  - Normally, clot forms in 8–10 minutes and remains.
  - If fibrinogen is low, clotting is delayed or dissolution of clot occurs in 30–60 minutes.
- Consider the possibility of vWD (present in ~1–2% of population) in patient with history of menorrhagia or with past history of PP hemorrhage.

ABBREVIATIONS

- aPPT—Activate partial thromboplastin time
- ARDS—Adult respiratory distress syndrome
- CD—Cesarean delivery
- EBL—Estimated blood loss
- FFP—Fresh frozen plasma
- HELLP—Hemolytic anemia, elevated liver enzymes, low platelets
- IUFD—Intrauterine fetal demise
- NS—Normal saline
- POCs—Products of conception
- PP—Postpartum
- PT—Prothrombin time
- RL—Ringer's lactate solution
- vWD—von Willebrand disease

CODES

ICD9-CM

- 666.1 Immediate postpartum hemorrhage
- 666.2 Delayed and secondary postpartum hemorrhage

 PATIENT TEACHING

- Postpartum iron replacement to maximize RBC production
- Erythropoietin not approved by FDA for postoperative anemia, and is expensive
- Counsel regarding 10% risk of PP hemorrhage in subsequent pregnancy

PREVENTION

Typical measures taken to minimize the risk of PP hemorrhage include:

- Oxytocin administered soon after delivery
- Careful monitoring of uterine tone with massage as needed postpartum

Section VIII

HEMORRHAGE, THIRD TRIMESTER

Reinaldo Figueroa, MD
Paul L. Ogburn, Jr., MD

BASICS

DESCRIPTION

- 3rd-trimester hemorrhage occurs in ~5% of all pregnancies. It is a major cause of maternal morbidity and mortality. The following clinical entities comprise the major cause of hemorrhage.
- Placenta previa:
  - Placenta covers or is close to the internal cervical os
  - Often presents as painless, bright-red bleeding
  - May be associated with contractions
  - Diagnosis is made with US:
    - Complete: Placenta completely covers the internal cervical os
    - Partial: Placenta partially covers the internal os
    - Marginal: Placenta reaches the internal os but does not cover it
- Placental abruption:
  - Premature separation of a normally implanted placenta
  - Clinical presentation ranges from minimally painful vaginal bleeding and uterine irritability to complete placental separation with fetal demise, maternal hypotension, and DIC.
  - Classic signs and symptoms include painful vaginal bleeding, abdominal pain, uterine hypertonicity and tenderness, as well as fetal heart rate abnormalities.
  - Concealed hemorrhage with no evident vaginal bleeding may occur in up to 20% of cases.
- Vasa previa:
  - Fetal vessels run through the chorioamnionic membranes over the cervical os and under the fetal presenting part.
  - High index of suspicion is necessary:
    - Acute bleeding with rupture of membranes
    - Fetal heart rate decelerations, fetal bradycardia, or sinusoidal pattern
  - Diagnosis:
    - Rarely during a digital cervical exam
    - Amnioscopy may allow direct visualization of vessels.
    - Apt test or Kleihauer-Betke test may detect fetal cells but not helpful when bleeding acutely (no time for the test).
    - Diagnosis is confirmed with inspection of placenta after delivery.

DIFFERENTIAL DIAGNOSIS

- Causes of 3rd-trimester hemorrhage:
  - Bloody show
  - Cervical neoplasm
  - Cervicitis
  - Circumvallate placenta
  - Genital tract trauma
  - Placenta previa
  - Placental abruption
  - Vaginal neoplasm
  - Vasa previa with differential diagnosis:
    - Amniotic band
    - Chorioamnionic membrane separation
    - Funic presentation
    - Marginal placental vascular sinus
    - Nuchal cord loop

EPIDEMIOLOGY

- Placenta previa:
  - Incidence: 0.3–0.5% of pregnancies
  - Risk factors:
    - Cocaine use
    - Increasing parity and maternal age
    - Multiple pregnancy
    - Previous CD
    - Previous curettage for spontaneous or induced abortion
    - Previous placenta previa
    - Previous uterine surgery
    - Smoking
  - Pathophysiology is unclear:
    - Endometrial damage (uterine scarring)
  - Increased risk of malpresentation, unstable lie
- Placental abruption:
  - Incidence: 0.8% of pregnancies
  - Risk factors:
    - Cigarette smoking
    - Cocaine abuse
    - HTN (chronic, pregnancy induced)
    - Increasing parity and maternal age
    - PROM
    - Rapid decompression of over distended uterus
    - Trauma
  - Pathophysiology:
    - Small arterial vessel bleeding into decidua basalis
  - Recurrence risk: 5–16%:
    - Increases to 25% after 2 previous abruptions
- Vasa previa:
  - Incidence: 0.04% deliveries
  - Risk factors:
    - IVF pregnancy
    - Multiple pregnancies
    - 2nd-trimester low-lying placenta
  - Pathophysiology:
    - Velamentous insertion of the cord
    - Alternatively, vessels running between a placental lobe and an accessory lobe
    - Fetal vessels rupture at time of spontaneous or artificial rupture of membranes

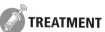

TREATMENT

MEDICAL MANAGEMENT

- Evaluate patient at the hospital.
- Assess hemodynamic (estimation of blood loss) and coagulation status.
- Assess GA, fetal viability and well-being.
- A large-bore intravenous catheter is placed:
  - Central venous access if hemodynamically unstable
- CBC, platelet count, and coagulation profile
- If considerable blood loss or coagulopathy:
  - Cross-match 2–4 units packed RBCs
  - Serum electrolytes and creatinine level
  - O-negative blood can be transfused if type-specific cross-matched blood is not available.
  - Oxygen supplementation by mask (or intubation, if needed)
  - Kleihauer-Betke test for quantification of fetal-maternal transfusion in Rh-negative mother

- Volume replacement with crystalloid (Ringer's lactate)
- Place a Foley catheter to assess urine output.
- Indication for immediate delivery:
  - Continued hemorrhage with maternal hemodynamic compromise or coagulopathy
  - Uncorrected fetal heart rate abnormalities
- If maternal hemodynamic status is stable and fetal status is reassuring:
  - Perform US to confirm GA and evaluate placental location:
    - Transabdominally 1st: Previa is excluded if placenta is fundal
    - Transvaginally: Superior in defining distance from the lower edge of placenta to internal cervical os
  - US evaluation usually is not useful for diagnosis of acute placental abruption:
    - Hematomas are isoechoic with respect to the placenta for up to 1 week
    - Hematomas become sonolucent in 2 weeks
- Continue fetal monitoring until delivery or maternal hemorrhage subsides.

ALERT

If placenta previa is diagnosed, avoid digital cervical exam to prevent bleeding.

- If placenta previa is ruled out, perform speculum exam to identify other causes of bleeding.
- Placenta previa: Decision to deliver:
  - Depends on persistent bleeding and GA at presentation
  - If remote from term, attempt conservative care to allow for fetal maturity
- Placental abruption: Decision to deliver:
  - Moderate to severe abruption:
    - Expeditious delivery
    - Careful maternal and fetal monitoring
  - Mild abruption:
    - Consider expectant management or tocolytic if premature fetus with stable fetal heart rate and no coagulopathy
  - Amniotomy may be useful:
    - In augmenting labor, anticipating vaginal delivery
    - To place fetal scalp electrode and IUPC
  - Continuous fetal monitoring
  - Careful hemostasis is mandatory.
  - Blood replacement:
    - To maintain BP, urinary output
    - To keep Hct >25%
    - If coagulopathy is present, give component therapy based on the etiology.
  - Heparin to prevent DIC is contraindicated.

Drugs

- Tocolytics for preterm uterine contractions if stable maternal and fetal status
- Corticosteroids for fetal lung maturation between 24 and 34 weeks

SURGICAL MANAGEMENT

Informed Consent
If CD is indicated, inform patient of the risks of ongoing bleeding to herself and the fetus, and of the need for expeditious delivery.

Patient Education
All patients must be educated about risks of vaginal bleeding in the 3rd trimester to assure prompt emergency medical attention.

Surgical
- Placenta previa:
  - Total or partial previa at term: CD
  - Marginal previa: Distance between the lower placental edge and internal cervical os:
    ○ If >2 cm: Attempt vaginal delivery
    ○ If <2 cm: CD
  - CD at 36–37 weeks after amniocentesis for fetal lung maturity
  - Regional anesthesia is preferable:
    ○ Less blood loss
    ○ Less uterine relaxation
  - CD: Low transverse incision:
    ○ Low vertical or classical incision if transverse lie or preterm infant
  - If placenta accreta, cesarean hysterectomy:
    ○ Fundal uterine incision
    ○ Leave placenta in place
- Placental abruption:
  - Vaginal delivery if fetal heart rate reassuring
  - CD if non-reassuring fetal heart rate pattern or arrest of labor
- Vasa previa:
  - Immediate cesarean delivery if bleeding
  - CD at 35–36 weeks without documentation of fetal lung maturity if diagnosed early and not bleeding

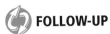 FOLLOW-UP

- Placenta previa:
  - Expectant management if stable at <36 weeks
  - Hospitalization usually after 1st bleed, but depends on clinical situation:
    ○ If continued bleeding, ongoing hospitalization for maternal and fetal monitoring until delivery
  - Bed rest with bathroom privileges
  - Typed and screened blood readily available:
    ○ If repeated transfusions are required, delivery should be considered
  - Corticosteroids for lung maturity if <34 weeks
  - Consider tocolytics if regular contractions and patient is hemodynamically stable.
  - Assess fetal growth and placental location every 2–3 weeks:
    ○ IUGR is more common.
    ○ Patients with placenta previa may have placenta accreta/increta/percreta.
    ○ MRI may be necessary for diagnosis.
  - Sonographic diagnostic criteria for placenta accreta/percreta/increta:
    ○ Irregularly shaped lacunae within placenta
    ○ Thinning of the myometrium overlying the placenta
    ○ Loss of the retroplacental clear space
    ○ Protrusion of placenta in the bladder
    ○ Increased vascularity of the uterine serosa-bladder interface
    ○ Turbulent blood flow through the lacunae on Doppler US

- If antepartum fetal testing is indicated:
  ○ NST or BPP
  ○ Contraction stress test is contraindicated
- If bleeding stops and patient is clinically stable, outpatient management can be considered:
  ○ Responsible adult and transportation available at all times
  ○ Lives within reasonable distance of hospital
  ○ Avoid intercourse and excessive activity.
- Delivery after 36 weeks of gestation because of increased risk of bleeding
- Placental abruption in the postpartum period:
  - Monitor resolution of coagulopathy
  - Correct anemia, fluid or electrolyte imbalance
  - Evaluate abdominal incision or episiotomy site for hematoma.
  - Strict intake and output
- Vasa previa:
  - Hospitalize at 30–32 weeks if detected early
  - Sonogram shows echolucent structure overlying the cervix:
    ○ Routinely evaluate the placental cord insertion when the placenta is low lying or has a succenturiate lobe.

PROGNOSIS
- Placenta previa:
  - Maternal mortality: 0.03% of cases
  - Perinatal mortality: Depends on GA
- Placental abruption:
  - Maternal mortality: 1–2/1,000 abruptions
  - Perinatal mortality: 0.9 per 1,000 births:
    ○ Due to appropriate intervention with CD
- Vasa previa:
  - Perinatal mortality: 60–80%
  - Prediction of neonatal survival is based on:
    ○ Prenatal diagnosis
    ○ GA at delivery

COMPLICATIONS
- Placenta previa:
  - Antepartum and postpartum hemorrhage
  - Blood transfusion
  - Increase in perinatal mortality and morbidity
  - Increase in preterm birth
  - Increase risk of congenital malformations
  - Maternal death
  - Need for hysterectomy
  - Placenta accreta:
    ○ Especially if anterior placenta covering the cesarean scar
    ○ Risk after 1 cesarean: 24%
    ○ Risk after ≥3 cesareans: 67%
  - Septicemia
  - Thrombophlebitis
- Placental abruption:
  - ARDS
  - DIC
  - Hypovolemic shock
  - Increase in perinatal mortality and morbidity
  - Increase in preterm birth
  - Increase risk of congenital malformations
  - Ischemic necrosis of kidney:
    ○ Acute tubular necrosis
    ○ Bilateral cortical necrosis
  - Maternal death
- Vasa previa:
  - Fetal asphyxia
  - Fetal death
  - Fetal exsanguination

BIBLIOGRAPHY

Clark SL. Placenta previa and abruptio placentae. In: Creasy RK, et al., eds. *Maternal-Fetal Medicine: Principles and Practice,* 5th ed. Philadelphia: Saunders; 2004:707–722.

Hladky K, et al. Placental abruption. *Obstet Gynecol Surv.* 2002;57:299–305.

Oyelese Y, et al. Vasa previa: The impact of prenatal diagnosis on outcomes. *Obstet Gynecol.* 2004;103:937–942.

Oyelese Y, et al. Placenta previa, placenta accreta, and vasa previa. *Obstet Gynecol.* 2006;107:927–941.

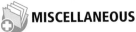 MISCELLANEOUS

SYNONYM(S)
- Marginal sinus hemorrhage
- Peripheral placental separation
- Placental abruption

CLINICAL PEARLS

> **ALERT**
> Digital exam of the cervix is absolutely contraindicated with 3rd-trimester bleeding until placenta previa is ruled out.

- Significant maternal hemodynamic changes are not seen until 25–30% of the intravascular volume has been lost.
- If placenta previa or placental abruption, increased risk for postpartum hemorrhage is possible.

ABBREVIATIONS
- ARDS—Acute respiratory distress syndrome
- BPP—Biophysical profile
- CD—Cesarean delivery
- DIC—Disseminated intravascular coagulation
- GA—Gestational age
- IUGR—Intrauterine growth restriction
- IUPC—Intrauterine pressure catheter
- IVF—In vitro fertilization
- NSS—Nonstress test
- PROM—Premature rupture of membranes

CODES
ICD9-CM
- 641.01 Placenta previa without hemorrhage, with delivery
- 641.03 Placenta previa without hemorrhage, antepartum
- 641.11 Hemorrhage from placenta previa, with delivery
- 641.13 Hemorrhage from placenta previa, antepartum
- 641.21 Premature separation of placenta, with delivery
- 641.23 Premature separation of placenta, antepartum
- 641.91 Unspecified antepartum hemorrhage, with delivery
- 663.53 Vasa previa, complicating labor and delivery, antepartum

Section VIII

OVARIAN CYST RUPTURE

Lisa Rahangdale, MD, MPH

 BASICS

DESCRIPTION

- Pelvic pain characterized by sudden, severe, unilateral onset secondary to rupture of ovarian cyst (CL cyst most common)
- Risk factors: Any ovulating woman is at risk.
- Diagnosis:
  - History:
    - Mid to late portion of the menstrual cycle, thus menstrual history/date of LMP is key
    - Recent intercourse or strenuous activity
    - Can be asymptomatic
    - Sudden onset of lower abdominal/pelvic pain. Pain is constant, dull, and aching. Can be worse with movement.
    - Light vaginal bleeding possible
    - Nausea, vomiting, or diarrhea possible
  - Physical exam:
    - Tachycardia, hypotension possible in cases of bleeding hemorrhagic cyst.
    - Low-grade fever may be present.
    - Abdominal exam: Tender lower abdomen, possible signs of peritoneal irritation—guarding, rebound
    - Pelvic exam: Tender adnexa, cervical motion tenderness. Possible palpable adnexal mass on pelvic or rectovaginal exam
  - Laboratory:
    - Hgb/Hct to evaluate for acute hemorrhage or serial studies to evaluate for a bleeding cyst
    - Type and cross-match blood if bleeding cyst suspected.
    - Consider coagulation studies if coagulopathy suspected or in women taking anticoagulant medications.
    - WBC may be elevated secondary to inflammation/peritoneal irritation or if infectious etiology is present.
    - Serum or urine pregnancy test to rule out ruptured ectopic pregnancy.
    - UA most likely normal, but WBCs or RBCs may be present secondary to peritoneal irritation.
    - If neoplasm is suspected, can check CA-125 but will likely be elevated secondary to peritoneal inflammation secondary to fluid and/or blood
  - Radiology:
    - US: To detect adnexal mass, characteristics of mass (solid/cystic/mixed echogenicity), volume of peritoneal fluid
    - CT scan: Findings similar to US, but can also rule out nongynecologic etiologies of pain

DIFFERENTIAL DIAGNOSIS

- Ectopic pregnancy
- PID
- Round ligament pain
- Endometriosis (endometrioma)
- Mittelschmerz
- Adnexal mass:
  - Paratubal cyst
  - Functional cyst (follicular, CL)
- Adnexal/Ovarian torsion
- Degenerating fibroid
- Neoplasm
- Appendicitis
- Diverticulitis
- IBD
- Renal colic

Geriatric Considerations
Must consider neoplasm in differential diagnosis of a postmenopausal woman with adnexal mass.

EPIDEMIOLOGY
Common in ovulating women. No exact prevalence or incidence established.

 TREATMENT

MEDICAL MANAGEMENT
Hemodynamically stable patient:

- Normotensive, normal pulse
- Stable Hgb/Hct on serial exams or no evidence of acute blood loss
- No radiologic evidence of expanding hemoperitoneum

Resuscitation
Fluid resuscitation may be required if evidence of large hemoperitoneum:

- 2 large-bore IVs
- Appropriate crystalloid
- Type and cross-match

Drugs
Pain management:

- Symptoms of CL cyst may take weeks to resolve.
- Appropriate and judicious use of narcotics, as pain is anticipated to be self-limited.

SURGICAL MANAGEMENT
Informed Consent
No benefit of laparotomy over laparoscopy in hemodynamically stable patient.

Risks, Benefits
- Standard surgical risk counseling for ovarian cystectomy.
- Review possibility of oophorectomy when obtaining consent for cystectomy procedure:
  - May be unable to remove cyst without removing ovary
  - May be neoplastic process or ovarian torsion

Alternatives
Medical
If patient is hemodynamically stable and menstrual history and US are characteristic of cyst, and exam suggests a CL or functional cyst, medical management is appropriate with:

- Appropriate analgesia, including narcotics
- Close follow-up for resolution/abatement of symptoms; symptoms that do not resolve with a few days to a week should suggest a reassessment of the diagnosis.
- Repeat US in next cycle to demonstrate resolution of this functional cyst.

Surgical
Surgical management recommended in cases of hemodynamically unstable patient or concern for neoplasm or torsion (see Adnexal Torsion).

Pediatric Considerations
- Similar medical and surgical management as in adult women, although pain tolerance may be lower than in adult woman.
- Attempt ovarian preservation if possible.
- Consider coagulopathy in differential diagnosis.

Pregnancy Considerations
If a CL cyst is removed, progesterone supplementation is needed until 10 weeks' gestation.

 FOLLOW-UP

- After establishing stable Hgb/Hct and excluding other surgical emergencies on differential diagnosis, patient may be managed as outpatient.
- Pain medications
- Follow-up US in 4–6 weeks to ensure resolution of cyst

PROGNOSIS
If pain is managed medically, anticipate resolution of cyst and pain over several weeks.

COMPLICATIONS
- Possible need for surgical exploration during outpatient management
- Unable to tolerate pain
- Continued bleeding of hemorrhagic cyst
- Chemical peritonitis secondary to sebaceous material from dermoid cyst

BIBLIOGRAPHY

Fritz MA, et al. *Clinical Gynecologic Endocrinology and Infertility,* 7th ed. Philadelphia: Lippincott Williams & Wilkins; 2005.

Hallatt JG, et al. Ruptured corpus luteum with hemoperitoneum. *Am J Obstet Gynecol.* 1984;149:5–9.

Hertzberg BS, et al. Ovarian cyst rupture causing hemoperitoneum: Imaging features and the potential for misdiagnosis. *Abdom Imaging.* 1999;24:304–308.

Mishell DR, et al, eds. *Comprehensive Gynecology,* 3rd ed. St. Louis: Mosby-Year Book; 1997.

Paajanen H, et al. Sensitivity of transabdominal ultrasonography in detection of intraperitoneal fluid in humans. *Eur Radiol.* 1999;9:1423–1425.

Takeda A, et al. Laparoscopic surgery in 12 cases of adnexal disease occurring in girls aged 15 years or younger. *J Minim Invasive Gynecol.* 2005;12:234–240.

Teng SW, et al. Comparison of laparoscopy and laparotomy in managing hemodynamically stable patients with ruptured corpus luteum with hemoperitoneum. *J Am Assoc. Gynecol LaparoSAC.* 2003;10:474–477.

MISCELLANEOUS

CLINICAL PEARLS
- Establish that patient is hemodynamically stable if diagnosis of ruptured hemorrhagic cyst suspected.
- Consider differential diagnosis for pelvic pain.
- The mere presence of an ovarian "cyst" on US, even if not pathologic (e.g., a 1-cm cystic follicle) often prompts the default diagnosis of "ruptured ovarian cyst":
  – Such findings are clearly not the cause of pain, and this diagnosis can cause considerable patient anxiety.
  – The diagnosis may become apparent in retrospect: Mittelschmerz as a diagnosis when the subsequent menstrual period occurs 14 days after the onset of pain.
- CL cysts can be painful without rupture, with the mechanism of pain being bleeding into the cyst rather than an intraperitoneal bleed.
  – Such cysts, even when symptomatic, should be managed medically.
  – Recurrent CL cysts may occur more frequently in young women with ovulatory dysfunction, as with PCOS:
    ○ Recurrence risk is not well established, although this is a common question from patients.
  – COCs, by preventing ovulation, markedly decrease the risk of painful CL cysts.

ABBREVIATIONS
- CL—Corpus luteum
- COC—Combined oral contraceptive
- IBD—Inflammatory bowel disease
- LMP—Last menstrual period
- PCOS—Polycystic ovary syndrome
- PID—Pelvic inflammatory disease

CODES

ICD9-CM
- 620.1 CL cyst or hematoma (CL hemorrhage or rupture lutein cyst)
- 620.1 Other and unspecified ovarian cyst
- 620.8 Other noninflammatory disorders of ovary, fallopian tube, and broad ligament (rupture of ovary or fallopian tube)

PATIENT TEACHING

ACTIVITY
No restrictions, but activity will be limited secondary to pain.

PREVENTION
Consider ovulation suppression through hormonal contraception to decrease likelihood of subsequent cyst formation by inhibiting ovulation and thus functional (follicular and CL) cysts.

Section VIII

SEPTIC ABORTION

Phillip G. Stubblefield, MD

 BASICS

ALERT
Septic abortion is highly lethal. Prompt evacuation of all infected gestational tissue is essential to patient survival.

DESCRIPTION
- Septic abortion is an infected abortion, complicated by fever, endometritis, and parametritis. It should be considered whenever a woman in the reproductive years presents with fever, lower abdominal pain, and vaginal bleeding.
- Where induced abortion is illegal, clandestine abortion using unsafe means is common, and maternal mortality from induced abortion is high. Septic abortion is the most common serious complication of unsafe abortion.
- Sepsis as a complication of SAB is rare.
- The earliest signs of infected abortion are pelvic pain, low-grade fever, and vaginal bleeding.
- If not adequately treated at this stage, the infection spreads and the patient may present with septic shock, septicemia, and rapidly develop ARDS.

DIFFERENTIAL DIAGNOSIS
- Other sources of pelvic infection:
  - PID
  - GI tract:
    - Ruptured appendix
    - Perforated diverticulum
  - Urinary tract:
    - Pyelonephritis
- Ectopic pregnancy

EPIDEMIOLOGY
- Risk of postabortion sepsis is greatest for younger and unmarried women, and more likely with induced abortion procedures that do not directly evacuate the uterine content.
- Most unsafe abortions occur in developing countries. An estimated 68,000 women die of this condition every year worldwide.
- Recently deaths from sepsis with toxic shock from *Clostridia sordellii* have occurred in the US after treatment with mifepristone/misoprostol for medical induction of early abortion.

Pediatric Considerations
Septic abortion must be considered as a possible source of sepsis in adolescent women.

TREATMENT

MEDICAL MANAGEMENT
- The principles of treatment are to eradicate the infection with antibiotics and prompt uterine evacuation, provide supportive care, and treat the complications of septic shock, ARDS, DIC, renal failure, and multiorgan system failure.
- Treatment of patients with early septic abortion:
  - Patients presenting with early infection have lower abdominal pain, low-grade fever ($<38°C$), and minimal vaginal bleeding. Pelvic exam reveals a tender, somewhat enlarged uterus.
  - At this stage of the illness, adequate treatment can be provided in the emergency department.
  - Eradicate the infection by:
    - Prompt evacuation of the uterus with vacuum curettage under paracervical block and conscious sedation
    - Treat with antibiotics as for outpatient management of PID
    - Levofloxacin 500 mg PO daily and metronidazole 500 mg b.i.d. for 14 days is 1 accepted regimen
    - See the patient in 48–72 hours to confirm significant improvement.
- Patients presenting with more severe infection will have higher fever, tachycardia, hypotension, severe prostration, and a tense tender abdomen.
- Treatment of severe septic abortion:
  - Stabilize the patient (see Resuscitation).
  - Monitor P, BP, temperature, oxygen saturation.
  - Evaluate for possible uterine perforation and bowel or bladder injury:
    - Obtain abdominal radiograph looking for free air in the abdomen.
    - Obtain pelvic US. Determine presence of tissue in uterus and possible pelvic abscess.
  - Eradicate the infection:
    - Obtain samples for blood, urine, and cervical cultures.
    - Perform endometrial biopsy with a flexible 3-mm catheter (Pipelle or similar) for immediate Gram stain and culture.
    - Begin high-dose IV antibiotic therapy as for severe PID.
    - 1 such regimen is clindamycin 900 mg IV q6h and gentamicin 2 mg/kg loading dose IV or IM, followed by 1.5 mg/kg q8h.

- Surgically evacuate the uterine content. Delay in evacuation can be fatal, even when appropriate antibiotics are used:
  - 1st trimester pregnancy, perform vacuum curettage
  - This can be accomplished under paracervical block and conscious sedation, in the emergency department or OR.
  - Source of vacuum can be an electric uterine aspirator or a manual vacuum from a modified 60 mL syringe (IPAS, Chapel Hill, North Carolina or Mylex Corp, Chicago, IL)
  - 2nd trimester: Perform dilatation and evacuation or induce labor with misoprostol 400 μg by buccal or rectal route q6h or high-dose oxytocin.
  - If the patient does not begin to improve within several hours of uterine evacuation, laparotomy and abdominal hysterectomy may be needed.
- Admit to hospital for supportive care:
  - These patients are best cared for in an ICU setting
  - Treat shock:
    - Provide fluid resuscitation (see below)
  - ARDS develops in 25–50% of patients with septic shock. Begin mechanical ventilation if oxygen saturation falls below 90%.

Resuscitation
- Fluid resuscitation is given to achieve a target MAP of 60 mm Hg without exceeding a PAWP of 12–15 mm Hg to maximize left ventricular performance. Initial resuscitation will require 200 mL/10 minutes and 15–20 L may be required in the 1st 24 hours.
- Vasopressors are added if the PAWP reaches 15 mm Hg before the target MAP of 60 is achieved. Dopamine and dobutamine are preferred. Initial therapy with dopamine is 1–3 μg/kg/min.
- Administer nasal oxygen.

Drugs
- High-dose IV antibiotic therapy as for severe PID:
  - 1 such regimen is ampicillin 2–3 gm IV q6h, clindamycin 900 mg IV q6h, and gentamicin 2 mg/kg loading dose IV or IM, followed by 1.5 mg/kg q8h.
  - Vasopressors are added if the PAWP reaches 15 mm Hg before the target MAP of 60 mm Hg is achieved.
  - Dopamine and dobutamine are preferred. Initial therapy with dopamine is 1–3 μg/kg/min.

- Adjunctive therapies:
  - Polyvalent IVIG has been of benefit in controlled trials of severe sepsis.
  - IV recombinant human activated protein C (drotrecogin-α) reduced the death rate in large randomized trial of patients with multiorgan system failure from sepsis.
- Unsensitized Rh-negative patients need Rh-immune globulin.

SURGICAL MANAGEMENT
Informed Consent
Explain risks and benefits.

Risks, Benefits
- The benefit is greater chance of survival.
- Risks of vacuum curettage or dilatation and evacuation include cervical laceration, uterine perforation with injury to bowel or bladder.
- Should perforation occur, laparoscopy and possibly laparotomy would be needed for treatment.

Alternatives
Unless infected tissue is promptly evacuated from the uterus, death is likely from disseminated sepsis.
Medical
For midtrimester pregnancies, labor induction with misoprostol or high-dose oxytocin can be used to produce evacuation of infected tissue.

Surgical
See above.
- 1st trimester: Vacuum curettage.
- 2nd trimester: Dilatation and evacuation

 FOLLOW-UP

- Patients with early infection recover quickly after treatment.
- All need contraceptive information and supplies.
- Patients who survive septic shock typically have been critically ill for weeks of intensive care and will need several months to recover to normal function.
- Survivors of ARDS may have chronic lung disease.

PROGNOSIS
Risk of death with septic shock exceeds 50% despite excellent treatment.

COMPLICATIONS
Complications of septic shock include ARDS, DIC, renal failure, multiorgan system failure, and death

BIBLIOGRAPHY

Alejandria MM, et al. Intravenous immunoglobulin for treating sepsis and septic shock. *Cochrane Database Syst Rev.* 2002;1111;CD001090.

Bernard GR, et al. Efficacy and safety of recombinant human activated protein C for severe sepsis. *N Engl J Med.* 2001;344:699–709.

Grimes DA, et al. Unsafe abortion: The preventable pandemic. *Lancet.* 2006;368:1908–1919.

Stubblefield PG, et al. Complications of Induced Abortion. In: Pearlman MD, et al., eds. *Obstetric and Gynecologic Emergencies. Diagnosis and Management* 2nd ed. New York: McGraw-Hill; 2004:65–84.

Stubblefield PG, et al. Septic abortion. *N Engl J Med.* 1994;331:310–314.

Workowski KA, et al. Sexually transmitted disease treatment guidelines, 2006. *MMWR.* 2006; 55(RR11):1–94.

 MISCELLANEOUS

CLINICAL PEARLS
Septic abortion is rare in the US. It must always be considered in women of reproductive age presenting with sepsis.

ABBREVIATIONS
- ARDS—Acute respiratory distress syndrome
- DIC—Disseminated intravascular coagulation
- IVIG—Intravenous immunoglobulin
- MAP—Mean arterial pressure
- PAWP—Pulmonary arterial wedge pressure
- PID—Pelvic inflammatory disease
- SAB—Spontaneous abortion

CODES
ICD9-CM
639.0 Genital and pelvic infection, infection following abortion

 PATIENT TEACHING

Provide contraceptive education and supplies.

Section VIII

SEPTIC SHOCK AND TOXIC SHOCK SYNDROME

Sebastian Faro, MD, PhD

 BASICS

DESCRIPTION

- Septic shock is an infection affecting multiple organs, causing organ dysfunction and eventual failure. If not treated aggressively, it can result in death:
  - Sepsis with hypotension in the face of adequate fluid resuscitation, inadequate tissue perfusion, lactic acidosis, oliguria, and alteration in mental status.
- A multisystem or multiorgan disease, it is most commonly caused by bacterial infection, but can result from a viral or fungal infection.
- TSS is a form of septic shock associated with menstruation and tampon use; it can also occur in anyone infected with *Staphylococcus aureus*:
  - Also be caused by *Streptococcus pyogenes*
  - Caused by exotoxin producing strains
- Infection: Microbe (bacteria, virus, fungus, parasite) gains entrance to the host, reproduces within the host, and causes local or systemic reaction.
- Bacteremia: Bacteria gain entrance into, and circulate in, the bloodstream.
- Sepsis: The inflammatory response to infection; same as SIRS.
  - Severe sepsis: Sepsis with hypotension or manifestations of hypoperfusion.
- SIRS: The host response to either infectious or noninfectious disease. A continuous process, depicted by abnormal inflammatory host response in organs distant from the initial site of infection.
- MODS: Physiologic derangements resulting from excessive activation of systemic inflammatory responses to infection, ischemia, injury, or immunologic activation.

EPIDEMIOLOGY

- Septic shock:
  - Most common cause of mortality in the intensive care unit
  - 10th leading cause of death in US, with mortality ranging from 15–60%
  - Most common form of shock; any organ can be affected
- 759,999 cases of sepsis occur annually in US:
  - 40% of sepsis cases progress to septic shock.
  - $5–10 billion annually in US

PATHOPHYSIOLOGY

- Microbiology of sepsis and septic shock:
  - Pelvis:
    - *Escherichia coli*
    - *Streptococcus agalactiae*
    - *S. pyogenes*
    - *S. aureus*
    - *Bacteroides fragilis*
    - *Fusobacterium*
    - *Prevotella bivia*

- Skin and soft tissue:
  - *S. aureus*
  - *Staphylococcus epidermidis*
  - *S. pyogenes*
  - *Clostridium*
- Gram-negative bacteria cause 50% of sepsis and are responsible for 115,000 deaths/year.
  - Gram-negative bacteria produce endotoxins, exotoxins, formyl peptides, and proteases that can initiate the cytokine cascade or proinflammatory response.
- Gram-positive bacteria cause 50% of the sepsis, but most are secondary to pneumonia and the presence of intravascular devices.
  - Gram-positive bacteria produce exotoxins, superantigens, enterotoxins, hemolysins, peptidoglycans, and lipoteichoic acids. *S. pyogenes* produces pyrogenic exotoxin A.
- Nosocomial pathogens:
  - Lung: Aerobic gram-negative bacilli.
  - Pelvis: Gram-negative and gram-positive facultative and obligate anaerobic bacteria derived mainly from endogenous vaginal microflora
  - Skin and soft tissue:
    - MRSA gram-negative facultative bacilli
  - Urinary tract: Gram-negative facultative bacteria, *Enterococcus*
  - CNS: *Pseudomonas aeruginosa, E. coli, Klebsiella, S. aureus*
- Source of anaerobes:
  - Lower genital tract
  - Instrumentation sites
  - IV fluids
  - Oropharynx
  - Inhalation equipment
  - Intestinal tract

RISK FACTORS

- Septic shock:
  - Altered vaginal endogenous microflora
  - Pelvic surgery
  - Chorioamnionitis
  - Pyelonephritis
  - Chemotherapy and radiation therapy
  - Increased use of systemic corticosteroids
  - Immune suppression
  - Increased use of devices (e.g., grafts, stents, long-term IV lines, indwelling catheters)
  - Chronic illness:
    - Neutropenia
    - Solid tumors
    - Leukemia
    - Dysproteinemia
    - Cirrhosis of the liver
    - Diabetes
    - AIDS
  - Prior drug therapy: Immunosuppressive agents, long-term corticosteroid use
  - Childbirth
  - Septic abortion
  - Intestinal ulceration
  - Inappropriate use of antibiotics

- Toxic shock syndrome:
  - Colonization and infection with *S. aureus* strain that produces TSST
  - Absence of antibody to TSST
  - Failure to change super-absorbent tampon frequently during the day when menstruating
  - Contraceptive diaphragm use, leaving diaphragm in vagina >24 hours
  - Nasal surgery with packing
  - Surgical site infections
  - Postpartum endometritis

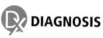 **DIAGNOSIS**

SIGNS AND SYMPTOMS

- Initial clinical presentation:
  - Temperature >38°C or <36°C
  - Tachycardia ≥90 bpm
  - Respiratory rate >20 breaths/minute
- Localized infection with systemic effect:
  - Skin/Soft tissue: Erythema, swelling, pain
  - Pelvic: Cervical and uterine tenderness
- WBC >12,000/uL, <4,000 uL, or ≥10% immature neutrophils (bands)
- Bacteremia
- Sepsis with ≥2 of the following:
  - Rectal temperature >38°C or <36°C
  - Tachycardia >90 bpm
  - Tachypnea >20 breaths/minute
- Evidence of dysfunction in at least 1 organ:
  - Change in mental state
  - Hypoxemia PaO_2 <72 mm Hg
  - Elevated plasma lactate level OR
  - Oliguria (<30 mL of urine/h)
- Severe sepsis; as above plus:
  - SIRS plus organ dysfunction:
    - Respiratory distress
    - Kidney failure
    - Cardiomyopathy
    - Hepatic dysfunction
    - Pancreatitis
  - Hypoperfusion
  - Hypotension (systolic BP <90 mm Hg or a decrease of >40 mm Hg from baseline)
  - Lactic acidosis
  - Oliguria
  - Altered mental state
  - Edema of extremities
- Toxic shock; as above plus:
  - Erythroderma
  - Diffuse macular rash
  - Skin desquamation appearing a few days after the rash develops
  - Nausea and vomiting
  - Headache
  - Purulent vaginal discharge
  - Pharyngeal erythema
  - Conjunctivitis
  - Strawberry tongue
  - Rarely present: Arthritis, hepatosplenomegaly, cardiomyopathy, pericarditis, seizures

TESTS

Lab

- CBC with differential
- Serum electrolytes
- BUN
- Creatinine
- Liver enzymes
- PT, PTT
- Fibrinogen
- Fibrin split products
- Protein/Albumin
- Lactic acid
- Calcium/Magnesium
- Total/Direct bilirubin
- UA
- Microbiology (obtain specimens):
  - Blood
  - Urine
  - If IV line, consider line infection:
    - Culture catheter tip.
  - Surgical site (if present and accessible)
  - Patient with suspected toxic shock:
    - Nares for *S. aureus*
    - Vagina for *S. aureus*

Imaging

- TSS: No benefit from imaging studies
- Postoperative patients:
  - US of abdomen and pelvis:
    - Free fluid in the abdomen or pelvis
    - Abscess: Pelvis or tubo-ovarian
    - Enlarged uterus: Endometrial fluid collection
    - Cesarean section: Fluid collection overlying anterior lower segment; dehiscence of uterine incision
  - CT:
    - Abscess
    - Inflammation of surgical site

 ## TREATMENT

MEDICAL MANAGEMENT

Resuscitation

- Admit to ICU
- IV fluids:
  - Crystalloids to maintain intravascular oncotic pressure
- Foley catheter
- Hourly I/Os
- Continuous cardiac monitoring
- Frequent BP determinations

- Continuous monitoring of oxygen saturation
- Vasoactive agents:
  - Dopamine – at <19 μg/kg/min increases myocardial contractility, lack of vasoconstriction maintains cardiac output; at doses <2 μg/kg/min, it increases blood flow to kidneys, spleen
  - Norepinephrine: 1–2 μg/kg/min
  - Dobutamine: 2–20 μg/kg/min

Drugs

- Broad-spectrum antibiotics
- Septic shock:
  - Clindamycin 900 mg or metronidazole 500 mg q8h
  - Ampicillin 2 mg q6h
  - Gentamicin 5 mg/kg of body weight q24h:
    - Determine trough levels
    - Calculate creatinine clearance to determine frequency of dosing
- Toxic shock:
  - Vancomycin 1 mg q12h:
    - Determine trough and peak levels
    - Calculate creatinine clearance to determine frequency of dosing
  - Alternative antibiotics:
    - Daptomycin
    - Linezolid
    - Tigecycline

Surgical

- Surgical site:
  - Drainage of abscess
  - Debridement of necrotic tissue (necrotizing fasciitis)
- Exploratory laparotomy:
  - Removal of necrotic tissue
  - Hysterectomy (post-cesarean section)
    - Diffuse microabscesses of the myometrium
    - Necrosis of the myometrium
  - Abscess drainage (percutaneous drainage can be considered)
  - Removal of TOA
- Drains:
  - Closed drains attached to suction device
  - Drain fluid:
    - Cloudy serous fluid: Gram stain and culture for aerobic, facultative, and anaerobic bacteria
    - Blood: Obtain serial hematocrit of fluid; rising indicates intraperitoneal bleeding
    - Green or brown particulate fluid indicates bowel injury

BIBLIOGRAPHY

Fein AM, et al. *Sepsis and Multiorgan Failure.* Baltimore: Williams & Wilkins; 1997.

Fitch SJ, et al. Optimal management of septic shock. Available at: www.postgradmed.com/issues/2002/03 02fitch 2.com.

Hotchkiss RS, et al. The pathophysiology and treatment of sepsis. *N Engl J Med.* 2003;348:138–150.

Rivers E, et al. Early goal directed therapy in the treatment of severe sepsis and septic shock. *N Engl J Med.* 2001;345:1368–1377.

Russell JA. Management of sepsis. *N Engl J Med.* 2006;355:1699–1713.

Schrier RW, et al. Acute renal failure and sepsis. *N Engl J Med.* 2004;351:159–169.

Sharma S, et al. Septic shock. Available at: www.emedicine.com/MED/topic2101.htm.

 ## MISCELLANEOUS

ABBREVIATIONS

- MODS—Multiple organ dysfunction syndrome
- MRSA—Methicillin-resistant *S. aureus*
- PT—Prothrombin time
- PTT—Partial thromboplastin time
- SIRS—Systemic inflammatory response system
- TOA—Tubo-ovarian abscess
- TSS—Toxic shock syndrome
- TSST—Toxic shock syndrome toxin

CODES

ICD9-CM

- 040.82 Toxic shock syndrome
- 785.52 Septic shock
- 995.92 Systemic inflammatory response syndrome due to infectious process with organ dysfunction

 ## PATIENT TEACHING

Toxic shock:

- Avoid prolonged use of tampons.
- Use sanitary napkins at night.
- Change tampons frequently.

GENERAL PREVENTION

- Early recognition of infection
- Administration of antibiotic for surgical prophylaxis
- Empiric administration of broad-spectrum antibiotics to treat infection
- Toxic shock:
  - Recognize and treat wounds and infected surgical incisions early.

Section VIII

SEXUAL ASSAULT

David Muram, MD

 BASICS

DESCRIPTION
- Legal definition varies from state to state.
- Usually defined as forced sexual contact without consent or if person is unable to give consent
- Continuum from unwanted touching, fondling, to forced penetration of vagina, anus, or oral cavity
- In many instances, the threat of force is sufficient to subdue the victim.

DIFFERENTIAL DIAGNOSIS
The diagnosis is based on the patient's statement that no consent was given. Delayed presentation is common, and some patients might not tell their physician of the assault.

Pediatric Considerations
Most children do not disclose abusive relationships, and the diagnosis may be suspected by the presence of findings indicative of abuse (e.g., STD).

EPIDEMIOLOGY
- 2005:191,670 victims of rape, attempted rape or sexual assault (National Crime Victimization Survey):
  - 44% of rape victims <18
  - 80% <30
  - Justice Department estimates 1/6 are <12
- 2/3 of all rapes were committed by someone who is known to the victim:
  - Even higher in assaults on children

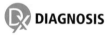 **DIAGNOSIS**

- Should be done in a suitable environment
- Adhere to local rape protocols
- Goals of the exam include:
  - Determine the extent of injuries.
  - Collect and properly handle forensic evidence.
  - Create a record of the medical findings.
  - Include full-body diagrams to denote areas of injury.
  - Consider medical photography.
  - Colposcopic pictures are expected as part of the record in child abuse cases.
  - Incomplete documentation may jeopardize legal proceedings.

SIGNS AND SYMPTOMS
History
- Obtain routine gynecologic history
- Ask the patient to describe the incident
- May reveal:
  - An unusual area of injury
  - Uncommon sites for evidence collection
  - Who is the perpetrator
- Record the incident using the patient's words.
- The patient should not be asked to repeat her account of the incident over and over.

Pediatric Considerations
Very young children may not be able to provide adequate history. This can then be obtained from adults. Clearly identify in the medical record the person who provided the history.

Physical Exam
- The primary objective of the exam is to attend to the medical needs of the victim.
- Examine the entire patient.
- Observe and document:
  - Extragenital injuries
  - Affect and behavior
  - Body language
- Perform a gynecologic exam.
- Most adults sustain only minor bruises and superficial lacerations with sexual assault.
- Adolescents subjected to blunt, forceful, penetrating vaginal trauma may sustain lacerations of the posterior portion of the hymen, between the 3 and 9 o'clock positions:
  - Deep lacerations of the vaginal mucosa may be seen in young adolescents.
- In addition to specimens collected for the medical management (e.g., cultures, pregnancy test), one must also collect samples to be used by the forensic laboratory.

Pediatric Considerations
- Most children can be fully evaluated in an office properly equipped to examine young patients. The evaluation is well-tolerated by most children.
- Consider EUA in all children with significant injuries to permit proper evaluation and repair of injuries. An EUA is also appropriate for the few children too anxious to permit adequate exam.
- Use of magnifying devices to enhance anogenital findings is well accepted:
  - Colposcopy most frequently used for exam of child victims of sexual abuse, and it is used in some facilities in all assault victims.
  - Colposcope camera attachment allows photos for the medical record. Such photos have become the standard of care in specialized clinics that see these young victims.
- The exam in most children is normal. Many abusive acts cause no injuries or only minor injuries that heal within days.
- However, vaginal penetration of a very young girl usually causes hymenal and vaginal lacerations. The thin, nonestrogenized vaginal mucosa, with its limited distensibility, is often lacerated along with the hymen. Penile pressure on the introitus is directed toward the posterior vaginal wall, and the hymen often tears between 4 and 8 o'clock. Secondarily, the laceration enlarges to involve the posterior vaginal wall and the perineum. With deeper penetration, the tear may extend into the rectum or into the peritoneal cavity.

Geriatric Considerations
A study of elderly victims of sexual assault showed these to be more likely to sustain a genital injury. Such injuries affected ~1/2 the patients and were severe enough to warrant surgical repair in ~1/2 of the injured women.

TESTS
- The decision to obtain genital or other specimens for STD diagnosis should be made on an individual basis. An initial exam should include the following:
  - Testing for *Neisseria gonorrhoeae* and *Chlamydia trachomatis*
  - Culture or FDA-cleared nucleic acid amplification tests for *N. gonorrhoeae* or *C. trachomatis*
  - Wet mount and culture of a vaginal swab specimen for *Trichomonas vaginalis* infection. The wet mount also should be examined for BV and candidiasis.
  - Collection of serum for HIV, hepatitis B, and syphilis
- Patients should be counseled regarding symptoms of STDs and the need for abstinence from sexual intercourse until STD prophylactic treatment is completed.

Lab
Collection of Evidence
Forensic evidence should be collected even if the patient states that she is not planning to pursue legal action. The rape kit is available and can be processed if and when the patient changes her mind. The following items should be collected:
- Patient's clothes. Place in a paper bag
- All foreign material on the patient's body
- Loose hairs on the skin
- Dried semen; use Wood's lamp to locate
- Fingernail scrapings, broken fingernail pieces
- Assailant's saliva if cunnilingus is reported.
- Semen from vagina
- Wet mount and Pap smear
- Vaginal fluid for acid phosphatase
- Screen for gonorrhea and *Chlamydia*
- Rectal washings for acid phosphatase (if sodomy occurred)
- Blood work:
  - For forensic lab and for serology
  - Drug and alcohol screen
  - Blood type
  - Syphilis and HIV screen

Pediatric Considerations
The examiner should decide if evidence collection is warranted based on the history, physical findings, and local protocols.

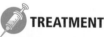 **TREATMENT**

MEDICAL MANAGEMENT
The following objectives must be addressed when treating a victim of sexual abuse:
- Repair of injuries
- Counsel and offer pregnancy interception if indicated
- Provide prophylaxis against STDs
- Emotional support services

SURGICAL MANAGEMENT
Repair of injuries
- Many victims do not sustain serious physical injury as a result of the assault, particularly if they have been sexually active prior to the assault.
- Superficial injuries (bruises, edema, local irritation) resolve within few days and require no special treatment.

- Meticulous perineal hygiene helps prevent secondary infections. Sitz-baths should be used to remove secretions and contaminants.
- With extensive skin abrasions, prophylactic broad-spectrum antibiotics can be used.
- Small vulvar hematomas do not require special treatment or can be controlled by pressure or with an ice pack.
- Large swelling of the vulva usually subsides with cold packs and external pressure.
- Large hematomas may continue to grow and should be incised, clots removed, and bleeding points identified and ligated.
- Irrigate bite wounds copiously, and debride necrotic tissue cautiously. Leave most open to heal by secondary intention. After 3–5 days, secondary debridement may be required.
  - Tetanus immunization should be given if immunization not up to date.
  - Use broad-spectrum antibiotics as therapy, not in a prophylactic manner.
- Vulvar lacerations often require surgical repair to control bleeding and to approximate tissues. These can be done using either local or regional anesthetics.
- Vaginal lacerations are often superficial, limited to the mucosal and submucosal tissues. If not bleeding, allow to heal spontaneously. When bleeding, use fine suture to gain hemostasis.
  - Vaginal wall hematomas may form; pressure created by the clot often controls bleeding.
  - If bleeding continues, incise overlying mucosa, evacuate clot, identify and ligate bleeding points.

Drugs
- STD prophylaxis:
  - Many specialists recommend routine preventive therapy after assault, as follow-up is often difficult. The following prophylactic regimen is suggested:
    - Hepatitis B vaccination if not previously vaccinated. Follow-up doses at 1–2 and 4–6 months after the 1st dose
    - An empiric antimicrobial regimen for chlamydia, gonorrhea, trichomonas, and BV.
- Pregnancy interception:
  - Many victims are concerned about an unwanted pregnancy.
  - Evaluate the probability of pregnancy:
    - Those using a reliable method of contraception (e.g., OCPs) are at very low risk.
  - Those seen within 72–120 hours from the assault should be appropriately counseled and provided medication to intercept pregnancy.
    - If such services are not provided at the facility, patient should be sent to a facility that provides this service.
    - A pregnancy test should be obtained prior to treatment, to exclude preexisting pregnancy.
    - Plan B should be provided if hCG negative.

Pediatric Considerations
- Strongly consider sexual abuse in children with STDs if nonsexual transmission cannot be identified.
- However, when STD is the only evidence of abuse, the findings should be confirmed with cultures, and the implications considered carefully.
- If a child has symptoms, signs, or evidence of infection, test for other common STDs before initiating therapy.
- Because of the legal and psychosocial consequences of a false-positive diagnosis, only tests with high specificities should be used.
- Defer presumptive treatment until a diagnosis has been confirmed by highly specific tests.

Emotional Support Services
- Supportive, careful history-taking may identify issues that are troubling the victim (e.g., her husband will not believe the story of the assault).
- Statements of disbelief are common (e.g., "I can't believe that this happened to me," as are statements of self-blame: e.g., "If I hadn't gone to the store to buy milk, this wouldn't have happened to me.")
- Fears of being alone or in the place of the assault (e.g., her own home or car) are common.
- The assailant may have threatened retaliation if the victim reports the assault.
- With time, victims often attempt to enhance their own security. It is common for victims to move from their homes, buy alarm systems, take self-defense classes, and often participate in counseling or attend meetings of support groups.
- Long-term reorganization is facilitated by early intensive intervention, with supportive counseling, crisis intervention, and follow-up instruction.

FOLLOW-UP
- Schedule a follow-up visit within 1–2 weeks to observe healing of injuries, evaluate for STDs, and to ensure the patient remains in the system and is receiving proper support services.
- The follow-up exam for STDs provides an opportunity to:
  - Detect new infections
  - Complete hepatitis B immunization
  - Provide counseling and treatment for STDs
  - Monitor side effects and adherence with treatment.
  - Serologic tests for syphilis and HIV infection should be repeated in 6 weeks, and 3 and 6 months after the assault if initial test results were negative and assailant's infection could not be ruled out.
  - Evaluate and provide counseling to determine if more intensive mental health services are required.

BIBLIOGRAPHY

Criminal Victimization, 2005. Bureau of Justice Statistics Bulletin, NCJ 214644. Washington, DC: Bureau of Justice; September 2006.

Hegar A, et al., eds. *Evaluation of the Sexually Abused Child*, 2nd ed. New York: Oxford University Press; 2000.

Muram D, et al. Adolescent victims of assault. *J Adolesc Health Care*. 1995;17:372–375.

Muram D, et al. Sexual assault of the elderly victim. *J Interpersonal Violence*. 1992;7:70–76.

Muram D. Child Sexual Abuse. Precis. [An update in Obstet Gynecol.] Washington DC: ACOG; 1998.

Sexually Transmitted Diseases Treatment Guidelines, 2006. *MMWR*. 2006;55 RR 11.

Sommers MS, et al. Using colposcopy in the rape exam: Health care, forensic, and criminal justice Issues. *J Forensic Nurs*. 2005;1;28–34.

US Department of Justice. A National Protocol for Sexual Assault Medical Forensic Examination. Office on Violence against Women. Washington DC: DOJ; September 2004.

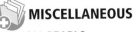 MISCELLANEOUS

CLINICAL PEARLS
- Expert medical testimony plays an important role in sexual assault litigation.
- Medical evidence of abuse is present in a relatively small number of cases:
  - When such evidence exists, it is generally admissible in court.
  - In cases where there is no physical evidence, the physician may explain to the jury that lack of physical findings is common and the patient could have been a victim of assault.
- Any examiner who sees victims of assault should be prepared to be part of the legal proceedings that follow (e.g., deposition, testimony):
  - When you provide testimony:
    - Be prepared. Review the record and the relevant literature you plan to cite.
    - Remain objective.
    - Use language the jury can understand.
    - Do not use legal terms. State your opinion in terms of the medical diagnosis.
    - Listen to the question asked. Make sure you understand the question.
    - Answer only the question asked. Do not use the witness stand to give a lecture.
    - If you do not know the answer to a question, just say "I do not know."

ABBREVIATIONS
- EUA—Exam under anesthesia
- hCG—Human chorionic gonadotropin
- OCP—Oral contraceptive pills
- STD—Sexually transmitted disease

CODES
ICD9-CM
- 995.53 Child rape
- 995.83 Adult rape
- V71.5 Alleged rape, observation or exam

PATIENT TEACHING
- ACOG Patient Flyer: Stay Alert, Stay Safe. Available at www.acog.org/departments/dept˙notice.cfm?recno=17&bulletin=295
- National Sexual Assault Hotline at 800–656–HOPE (4673)
- Womenshealth.gov. Sexual Assault. Available at http://4women.gov/faq/sexualassault.htm

SHOULDER DYSTOCIA

T. Murphy Goodwin, MD
J. Ingrid Lin, MD

 BASICS

DESCRIPTION

- Shoulder dystocia is generally defined as a delivery that requires additional obstetric maneuvers following failure of delivery of the fetal shoulder(s) with gentle traction on the fetal head.
- It is caused by the impaction of the anterior shoulder behind the maternal pubic symphysis, or, it is believed, from impaction of the posterior shoulder on the sacral promontory.
- Numerous risk factors have been used to predict shoulder dystocia, such as fetal macrosomia, maternal diabetes, operative vaginal delivery, abnormal labor, maternal weight, and previous shoulder dystocia.
- Shoulder dystocia often happens even in the absence of risk factors.
- Occasionally, a classic "turtle sign" may assist in the diagnosis.
- It is essentially unpredictable and unpreventable.
- The risk and expense of labor induction or CD for all women suspected of carrying a macrosomic fetus has not been shown to offer proportionate benefits in published studies.

DIFFERENTIAL DIAGNOSIS
Abdominal dystocia (rare)

EPIDEMIOLOGY

- The reported incidence ranges from 0.2–3.0% of all vaginal deliveries. This wide range can be attributed largely to the inherent subjectivity of the practitioner's definition of shoulder dystocia.
- Many studies have demonstrated an increased incidence of shoulder dystocia with increasing birth weight, but 40–60% of shoulder dystocias occur in infants who weigh <4,000 g.
- Maternal diabetes consistently is cited as a leading risk factor for shoulder dystocia as well because diabetic mothers tend to have a high incidence of macrosomia.
- Maternal obesity and maternal weight gain during pregnancy are associated with shoulder dystocia, largely because of their association with fetal macrosomia.

 TREATMENT

MEDICAL MANAGEMENT
Informed Consent

- Informed consent for attempting vaginal delivery should be obtained when the EFW is >5,000 g in a nondiabetic or 4,500 g in a diabetic mother. Some physicians may discuss the option of CD, in essence an informed consent for vaginal delivery, at a lower a lower EFW.
- When the condition of the patient and the clinical circumstances permit, informed consent for instrumental delivery should include mention of shoulder dystocia as a complication, if the fetus is thought to be large.

Patient Education

- Many risk factors are associated with shoulder dystocia, but their predictive value is low.
- The presence of both diabetes and macrosomia accurately predicted only 55% of cases of shoulder dystocia.
- A history of shoulder dystocia is associated with a recurrence rate ranging from 1–16.7%.
- Even though the use of EFW by US or the Leopold maneuver to plan delivery strategies, such as labor induction and prophylactic CD, has become common in practice, evidence is lacking that it can reduce permanent brachial plexus injury without incurring unacceptably large numbers of unnecessary CDs.

Risks, Benefits

- The principal risk of shoulder dystocia is brachial plexus injury; since most of these resolve completely, however, strategies for reducing shoulder dystocia must really focus on reducing the rare outcome of permanent brachial plexus injury.
- The benefit of CD in this setting is avoidance of brachial plexus injury in most cases.
- The risks of a strategy that increases cesarean births are associated, infection, transfusion, prolonged hospital stay, expense and even maternal death.

Alternatives

- McRoberts maneuver:
  - Sharp ventral flexion of maternal hips results in flattening of the sacrum and changing the angle of the symphysis pubis in relation to the fetus' anterior shoulder.
  - This maneuver alone may relieve >40% of all shoulder dystocias.
- Suprapubic pressure:
  - Apply downward pressure just above the maternal symphysis pubis.
  - Other techniques include applying pressure from either side of the maternal abdomen or alternating between sides using a rocking motion.
  - Resolves ~50% of shoulder dystocia when combined with McRoberts maneuver
- Episiotomy:
  - Episiotomy alone will not release the impacted shoulder since shoulder dystocia is considered to be a "bony dystocia."
  - Based on clinical circumstances, episiotomy may be needed to create more room for direct fetal rotational maneuvers.
- Rotational maneuvers:
  - Apply pressure to rotate the anterior or posterior shoulder to relieve the trapped shoulder from behind the symphysis pubis (e.g., Wood maneuver, Rubin maneuver, or combination of both)
- Delivery of posterior arm:
  - Flex the posterior fetal elbow, sweep the forearm across the chest, and deliver over the perineum.
  - Avoid grasping and pulling directly on the fetal arm to reduce risk of humerus fracture.
- Gaskin ("all fours") maneuver:
  - Patient rolls onto hands and knees to free the impacted anterior shoulder
- Maneuvers of last resort:
  - Deliberate clavicle fracture
  - Zavanelli maneuver
  - Symphysiotomy
  - Hysterotomy

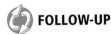

FOLLOW-UP

PROGNOSIS

- Most shoulder dystocia resolves without any complications.
- Among the most common fetal complications are brachial plexus injuries (palsies).
- Nearly all palsies resolve within 6–12 months, with <10% resulting in permanent injury.
- Although shoulder dystocia is the major risk factor for brachial plexus injury, many such injuries occur in the absence of apparent shoulder dystocia.

COMPLICATIONS

- Maternal complications:
  - Postpartum hemorrhage
  - 4th-degree lacerations
  - Rectovaginal fistula
  - Symphyseal separation or diathesis
  - Uterine rupture
- Neonatal complications:
  - Brachial plexus injuries
  - Fractures of clavicle and/or humerus
  - Hypoxic-ischemic encephalopathy
  - Neonatal death

BIBLIOGRAPHY

ACOG Practice Bulletin No. 40. Shoulder Dystocia. Washington, DC: ACOG; November 2002.

Gherman RB, et al. Shoulder dystocia: The unpreventable obstetric emergency with empiric management guidelines. *Am J Obstet Gynecol.* 2006;195(3):657–672.

Gobbo R, et al. Shoulder Dystocia. In: *ALSO: Advanced Life Support in Obstetrics Provider Course Syllabus.* Leawood KS: American Academy of Family Physicians; 2000.

Lerner HM. Shoulder dystocia: What is the legal standard of care? *OBG Management.* 2006;18(8):56–68.

MISCELLANEOUS

CLINICAL PEARLS

- Always be mentally prepared for possibility of shoulder dystocia.
- Empty the bladder when it is appropriate.
- Limit use of operative delivery when fetal macrosomia is suspected.
- Alert key personnel (e.g., nursing staff, pediatrician, anesthesiologist) when attempting to alleviate shoulder dystocia.
- The HELPERR mnemonic:
  - H Call for help
  - E Evaluate for episiotomy
  - L Legs (the McRoberts maneuver)
  - P Suprapubic pressure
  - E Enter maneuvers (internal rotation)
  - R Removal of the posterior arm
  - R Roll the patient
- Avoid harmful maneuvers:
  - Fundal pressure
  - More than the usual range of traction on fetal head or neck
  - Twisting or bending neck

- Detailed documentation of the shoulder dystocia is not essential for delivering excellent care, but it may be helpful for understanding and assessing the origin of fetal and maternal complications that may have occurred during the delivery. They may include:
  - How shoulder dystocia is diagnosed
  - Position of the shoulders
  - Assessment of the force applied
  - Duration of attempts to resolve the dystocia
  - Maneuvers performed
  - Length of each maneuver tried
  - Condition of the infant at delivery including Apgar, description of all injuries and bruises, cord pH if appropriate.
  - Documentation of the discussion with the patient following delivery

ABBREVIATIONS

- CD—Cesarean delivery
- EFW—Estimated fetal weight

CODES

ICD9-CM
660.4 Shoulder dystocia

UMBILICAL CORD PROLAPSE

Vern Katz, MD
Jacob Meyer, MD

 BASICS

DESCRIPTION
- UCP is an obstetric emergency that requires immediate fetal and maternal assessment and delivery.
- Overt: Umbilical cord presents visually between the presenting fetal part and the cervix following ROM or is in the vagina.
- Occult: Umbilical cord can only be palpated but not visualized between the fetal presenting part and the cervix.
- Funic cord presentation: Umbilical cord is between the fetal presenting part and the cervix before ROM.

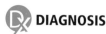 **DIAGNOSIS**

- Suspect UCP with the following:
  - Persistent fetal bradycardia
  - Moderate to severe variable decelerations on fetal heart monitor
- Definitive diagnosis is by palpating cord below fetal presenting part or visualizing the cord in the vagina during speculum exam.

ALERT
Obstetric emergency

PATHOPHYSIOLOGY
- Cord prolapse leads to either mechanical compression of the cord by the fetal presenting part or vasospasm from the lower extrauterine temperature. Either mechanism leads to decreased blood flow to the fetus, subsequent hypoxemia, eventual hypoxemic encephalopathy, and fetal demise.
- Funic presentation can be seen on US with color flow Doppler and thus diagnosed antepartum. This is mostly seen with malpresentation.

DIFFERENTIAL DIAGNOSIS
- Vasa previa:
  - Palpation of a cord-like structure upon cervical exam could also be vasa previa.
  - Vaginal bleeding is more common with vasa previa.
- Other causes of moderate to severe variable decelerations:
  - Hypoxemia
  - Cord compression
  - Nuchal cord
  - Knot in cord
- Other causes of prolonged fetal bradycardia:
  - Fetal acidosis
  - Prolonged cord compression
  - Paracervical block
  - Epidural or spinal anesthesia
  - Tetanic uterine contractions
  - Fetal arrhythmias

EPIDEMIOLOGY
Reported incidence ranges from 0.1–0.6% of births.

RISK FACTORS
- Malpresentation
- Prematurity, especially birth weight <1,500 g
- 2nd-born twin
- Multiparity
- Obstetric interventions:
  - Induction of labor
  - Amniotomy
  - External cephalic version
- Polyhydramnios

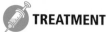 **TREATMENT**

MEDICAL MANAGEMENT
- Standard of care for management of UCP is delivery without delay. This means a CD unless VD is imminent. Several temporizing interventions can be done until delivery to relieve pressure on the cord:
- Call for assistance.
- Elevate the fetal presenting part:
  - Examiner pushes the presenting part up and out of the pelvis. Maintained until delivery can be accomplished.
  - Put bed in Trendelenburg and the mother in a knee-to-chest position.
  - Bladder filling: Filling the bladder will occupy space in the pelvis and take pressure off the cord. The bladder is filled with 500–700 mL of normal saline with a Foley catheter while the patient is prepared for CD. This technique can also be used with a tocolytic to decrease uterine contractions and assist in reducing pressure on the cord.
- Maintain cord at body temperature:
  - Decreased temperature inside the vagina leads to vasospasm and decreased delivery of oxygen to the fetus. Therefore, many providers have advocated keeping the cord warm with either warm gauze or towels.
- Reposition the cord:
  - In 1 series of 5 patients, the cord was positioned away from the fetal presenting part with successful VD. This is not recommended, as there is a worry for increased risk of vasospasm of the cord or continued compression with subsequent decreased oxygenation to the fetus leading to poor outcomes.

Drugs
Tocolysis in conjunction with bladder filling:
- Nifedipine
- Magnesium sulfate

Other
Mother may be started on oxygen by nasal canula and placed on her left side

SURGICAL MANAGEMENT
- Emergent delivery via CD or VD is indicated. Surgical approach will depend on fetal lie and GA.
- Prophylactic antibiotics should be given.

Informed Consent
Consent for a CD should be obtained as for any other surgical procedure.

Patient Education
Explain to mother the grave risk to fetus that UCP presents in terms of oxygenation, and the need for an emergency CD.

Risks, Benefits
- The risks to the fetus if CD is not done far outweigh the risks of CD.
- Infection:
  - Endometritis risk is higher with emergency CD
- All other surgical risks that come with a CD

Alternatives
See "Medical Management."
Medical
- Elevation of fetal presenting part
- Bladder-filling, with tocolysis
- Maintain cord at body temperature
- Repositioning of cord

Surgical
No surgical alternatives to CD exist.

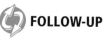 **FOLLOW-UP**

- Provided there is a good neonatal outcome, no extra follow-up is needed in addition to normal postpartum care.
- With poor neonatal outcomes, it is important to closely follow-up with the patient and assure she has adequate psychosocial support during her time of grieving.

PROGNOSIS
- Low birth weight and prematurity are associated with worse neonatal outcomes.
- Neonatal mortality in the most recent large series was 10%. This number is affected by type of prolapse, if it occurs in the hospital, GA, fetal weight, diagnosis to delivery time, and method of delivery.
- A recent community series of 52 patients had a mortality of 2/52; both deaths were related to extreme prematurity.
- FHR: Variable decelerations and persistent bradycardia are associated with UCP. Those fetuses with reassuring FHR at delivery have a low incidence of poor outcomes.
- CD has been associated with improved outcomes when compared to unassisted VD.

- Perinatal mortality is undoubtedly worse if UCP is diagnosed outside of the hospital.
- The interval from diagnosis to delivery is ideally as short as possible.
- 1 series showed that those cases of neonatal asphyxia associated with UCP had shorter diagnosis to delivery times than those infants with UCP and no asphyxia. This demonstrates that the diagnosis to delivery time, although important, is not the only determinant of outcome.
- Poorer Apgar scores have been associated with long diagnosis to delivery times.
- 1 long-term follow-up study was done of 13 infants whose delivery was complicated by UCP. 1 infant died from prematurity, and the 12 living infants had normal neurodevelopment at 2-year follow-up.

COMPLICATIONS
- Hypoxemic-ischemic encephalopathy
- Neonatal asphyxia and death

Pediatric Considerations
Another qualified physician must be present in the OR for neonatal resuscitation. Contact the appropriate personnel as soon as UCP is diagnosed.

BIBLIOGRAPHY

Boyle JJ, et al. Umbilical cord prolapse in current obstetric practice. *J Reprod Med*. 2005;50:303–306.

Lin MG. Umbilical cord prolapse. *Obstet Gynecol Survey*. 2006;61:269–277.

Nizard J, et al. Neonatal outcome following prolonged umbilical cord prolapse in preterm premature rupture of membranes. *Br J Obstet Gynaecol*. 2005;112:833–836.

Qureshi NS, et al. Umbilical cord prolapse. *Intern J Gynecol Obstet*. 2004;86:29–30.

Usta IM, et al. Current obstetrical practice and umbilical cord prolapse. *Am J Perinatol*. 1999; 16:479–484.

Uygur D, et al. Risk factors and infant outcomes associated with umbilical cord prolapse. *Intern J Obstet Gynecol*. 2002;78:127–130.

MISCELLANEOUS

SYNONYM(S)
- Cord presentation
- Prolapsed cord

ABBREVIATIONS
- CD—Cesarean delivery
- FHR—Fetal heart rate
- GA—Gestational age
- ROM—Rupture of membranes
- UCP—Umbilical cord prolapse
- VD—Vaginal delivery

CODES
ICD9-CM
663.0 Prolapse of cord

PATIENT TEACHING

Activity restrictions as normally advised following CD.

Section VIII

UTERINE PERFORATION

Lisa Keder, MD, MPH
Michelle M. Isley, MD

 BASICS

DESCRIPTION

- Uterine perforation is a transmural injury to the uterus, occurring when a instrument or object passes through the myometrium.
- The uterine sound and sharp curettes are the most common instruments to cause uterine perforation.
- Perforation can also be caused by suction curettes, forceps, cervical dilators, hysteroscopes, IUDs and their insertion tubes, or any instrument placed in the uterus.
- Uterine perforation can go unnoticed and be asymptomatic, or can involve damage to the bowel or bladder, or cause significant bleeding and hematoma formation.
- The most common sign of uterine perforation is insertion of an instrument beyond the expected depth of the uterine cavity. Uterine perforation may also present as excessive pain, intra- or postoperative hemorrhage, or loss of distension medium during hysteroscopy.
- The most common site of uterine perforation is the fundus (30–50%), but perforation can happen through any part of the uterus or cervix. If the lateral aspect of the uterus is perforated (<5%), the uterine vessels can be lacerated. An anterior uterine perforation can injure the bladder.
- Gynecologic procedures during which risk for uterine perforation occurs:
  - Hysteroscopy, diagnostic or operative
  - D&C:
    - Diagnostic
    - Control of postpartum hemorrhage
    - Evacuation of retained POC
  - Insertion of IUD:
    - Associated with the insertion procedure, either by the IUD itself, the sound, or the inserter
    - IUD perforations can be partial, resulting in uterine contractions that cause complete perforation
  - 1st- and 2nd-trimester abortion, both suction and extraction procedures
- Pelvic exam: Prior to any procedure in which the uterus will be instrumented, it is important to determine uterine position and size.

DIFFERENTIAL DIAGNOSIS

The differential diagnosis will vary depending of the type of procedure performed and may include the following conditions:
- Underestimation of uterine size
- Uterine atony
- Infection
- Retained products of conception
- Hematometra

EPIDEMIOLOGY

- Uterine perforation occurs during procedures in which the uterus is being instrumented.
- Predominant age:
  - Risk increases in postmenopausal women and in pregnancy with increasing GA.

Incidence

- True incidence may be underestimated since perforations may go unrecognized:
  - Hysteroscopy: 14.2 per 1,000 cases:
    - Highest perforation rates are during hysteroscopic myomectomy and resection of adhesions or uterine septa
    - Lowest perforation rates occur during hysteroscopic polypectomies and endometrial ablation
  - D&C: Rate of perforation varies with indication for the procedure:
    - 5.1% for control of postpartum hemorrhage
    - 0.3% in premenopausal and 2.6% in postmenopausal women undergoing diagnostic curettage
  - Placement of IUD, 0 to 1.3 per 1,000 insertions
  - Legal 1st- and 2nd-trimester abortion procedures: Incidence of uterine perforation is between 0.5 and 15 per 1,000 women
- Risk factors:
  - Nulliparity
  - Menopause
  - Advanced age
  - Previous cervical procedure, such as LEEP or cone biopsy
  - GnRH agonist use
  - Cervical stenosis
  - Markedly retroverted uterus
  - Undue force used
  - Clinician/Operator inexperience
  - Pregnancy:
    - Due to softening of the uterine wall and the increased size of endometrial cavity

TREATMENT

MEDICAL MANAGEMENT

- Management depends on the clinical setting. Recognition of uterine perforation and the mode of perforation are keys to management.
- Suspect uterine perforation during D&C, surgical abortion, or hysteroscopic procedures if:
  - Loss of resistance occurs during instrumentation of the uterus
  - An instrument extends into the uterine cavity further than expected
  - Unexpected pain occurs in an awake patient

- Quick fluid deficit develops during hysteroscopy, or there is inability to maintain uterine distension
- Severe uterine bleeding ensues, resulting in hemodynamic instability
- Abdominal viscera are brought through a perforation and visualized in the cervix/vagina
- Unrecognized perforation may cause symptoms several hours later:
  - Abdominal pain/distension
  - Hypotension
  - Tachycardia
  - Fever
  - Pelvic mass from broad ligament hematoma
  - If bowel injury, free air on an upright abdominal radiograph
- Suspect uterine perforation with IUD insertion if:
  - Persistent lower abdominal pain (most frequent symptom)
  - Heavy bleeding
  - Severe pain at insertion and during 1st 24 hours
  - Subsequent signs during contraceptive use:
    - Inability to identify IUD strings
    - Contraceptive failure

Resuscitation

Hemodynamic support with IV fluids and/or blood products as necessary

Other

- Fundal perforations that are recognized during sounding of uterus or during cervical dilation rarely produce significant hemorrhage or visceral trauma and can be managed with observation with serial hemoglobin measurements.
- Uterine perforation recognized at the time of IUD insertion:
  - Can attempt to gently pull on the IUD strings to remove the IUD

SURGICAL MANAGEMENT

Informed Consent

Patients undergoing uterine instrumentation should be informed of the risk of uterine perforation prior to the procedure. Consent for any patient undergoing a surgical procedure should include the possibility of additional surgery needed to repair injury to surrounding organs (bowel, bladder) caused by perforation.

Alternatives

Observation can be considered if the perforation occurs fundally with a blunt instrument, there is no evidence of hemorrhage, and the patient is clinically stable.

Surgical

- If visceral involvement is suspected or unknown, surgery is recommended to evaluate the perforation under direct visualization and to assess for any intraabdominal organ damage.
- Perforation with instruments other that the uterine sound or cervical dilators, or perforations located somewhere other than the fundus are more likely to be associated with hemorrhage or bowel/bladder injury.
- Surgical management allows for control of bleeding with cautery, sutures, or additional surgery.
- If perforation is suspected during suction evacuation of the uterus, the entire length of the bowel should be inspected, especially if abdominal contents were seen aspirated into the suction curette.
- The choice of diagnostic laparoscopy vs. laparotomy depends on:
  - Events leading up to the perforation
  - Extent and severity of the woman's symptoms
  - Experience of the surgeon:
    - An experienced laparoscopist may be able to accomplish both evaluation and repair using laparoscopic instruments.
- If uterine perforation occurs with IUD placement, and the IUD cannot be removed at the time of placement, laparoscopic removal is preferred.
  - If partial perforation with IUD occurs, hysteroscopy may be needed for removal.

 FOLLOW-UP

Outpatient or inpatient, depending on severity of symptoms

PROGNOSIS

- Good prognosis overall.
- If no surgery required, uterine myometrium heals well without intervention
- If surgery required, good prognosis if bowel thoroughly evaluated and bleeding evaluated and controlled

Pregnancy Considerations

- If the perforation was large, there may be an area of thin myometrium even after healing, and patients could be at increased risk of uterine rupture in future pregnancies.
- If uterine perforation occurs prior to complete evacuation of the uterus during a suction curettage, the uterus can be emptied of any remaining POCs under direct laparoscopic visualization.

COMPLICATIONS

A low cervical perforation can lacerate the descending branch of the uterine artery, which can lead to hysterectomy or need for uterine artery embolization.

BIBLIOGRAPHY

Amarin ZO, et al. A survey of uterine perforation following dilatation and curettage or evacuation of retained products of conception. *Arch Gynecol Obstet.* 2005;271:203–206.

Andersson K, et al. Perforations with intrauterine devices: Report from a Swedish study. *Contraception.* 1998;57:251–255.

Bradley LD. Complications in hysteroscopy: Prevention, treatment, and legal risk. *Curr Opin Obstet Gynecol.* 2002;14:409–415.

Van Houdenhoven K, et al. Uterine perforation in women using a levonorgestrel-releasing intrauterine system. *Contraception.* 2006;73:257–260.

 MISCELLANEOUS

To prevent or reduce the risk of uterine perforation:

- Predetermine the size and position of the uterus.
- Sound uterus cautiously.
- Introduce dilator only a short distance beyond the internal cervical os.
- Use preoperative cervical softening for hysteroscopy if cervical stenosis present:
  - 200 μg of misoprostol intravaginally inserted 9–10 hours prior to procedure
- Use preoperative osmotic cervical dilators or softening agents for 2nd-trimester abortion procedures.

CLINICAL PEARLS

A sharply anteflexed or retroflexed uterus is more vulnerable to anterior or posterior perforation:

- Cervical traction using a tenaculum will straighten the axis of the uterine cavity, decreasing the angle between the cervix and fundus, thus lowering the risk of perforation.

ABBREVIATIONS

- GA—Gestational age
- GnRH—Gonadotropin-releasing hormone
- LEEP—Loop electrosurgical excision procedure
- POC—Products of conception

 CODES

ICD9-CM

- 639 Complications following abortion and ectopic and molar pregnancies
- 869 Injury to unspecified organs (pelvic)

PATIENT TEACHING

Patients undergoing IUD insertion, D&C, surgical abortion, or hysteroscopy should report to a medical facility if they have persistent lower abdominal pain, unexpected heavy bleeding, or fever.

UTERINE RUPTURE

Jason N. Hashima, MD, MPH
Jeanne-Marie Guise, MD, MPH

 BASICS

DESCRIPTION

- Uterine rupture refers to a tear or separation of the uterine wall. Uterine rupture may occur with or without a prior uterine wall defect and may result in significant maternal and neonatal morbidity and mortality. Terminology and definitions have varied widely throughout medical practices and the literature.
- Anatomic definitions:
  - Incomplete: Uterine wall separation that does not completely extend through all layers of the uterine wall (e.g., serosa intact); this replaces the terminology "partial" or "dehiscence."
  - Complete: Separation of the entire thickness of the uterine wall with or without expulsion of the fetal-placental unit
- Clinical features:
  - Symptomatic: Rupture associated with related maternal or infant morbidity or mortality often signaled by fetal heart rate disturbances or maternal bleeding.
  - Asymptomatic: Rupture without clinical findings

DIFFERENTIAL DIAGNOSIS

- Abnormalities in fetal heart rate tracings (particularly fetal bradycardia) are the most common sign of uterine rupture in pregnancy. Other findings include vaginal bleeding, abdominal or pelvic pain, and abnormalities in contractions.
- The differential diagnosis includes:
  - Abdominal pain in pregnancy (see topic Acute Pelvic Pain):
    - Adnexal torsion
    - Appendicitis
    - Ectopic pregnancy
    - Infection/Abscess
    - Ovarian cyst
    - Trauma
  - Vaginal bleeding (see topic Hemorrhage, Third Trimester):
    - Cervicitis
    - Placental abruption
    - Placental previa
  - Abnormal fetal testing (see topic Abnormal Fetal Heart Tracing in Labor)

EPIDEMIOLOGY

Uterine rupture is an uncommon event, with a rate of 0–19 per 1,000 TOLACs. Despite advancements in medical practice, uterine rupture still remains associated with significant consequences.

Incidence

- 5.3 per 1,000 in unselected patients worldwide (e.g., not limited to TOLACs)
- Symptomatic uterine rupture: 0–7.8 per 1,000 TOLACs
- Asymptomatic uterine rupture: 0–19 per 1,000 TOLACs
- Overall risk for uterine rupture is <1%.

RISK FACTORS

- Prior uterine surgery
- Type of uterine incision: Classical, high vertical, T-shaped have greater risk
- Risk for rupture is as high as 4–9%
- Grand multiparity
- Uterine abnormalities
- Abnormal placentation
- Labor induction and/or augmentation—especially with prostaglandin agents
- TOLAC
- Assisted VD:
  - Forceps or vacuum
- Obstructed labor
- Maneuvers such as internal version
- Trauma

 TREATMENT

MEDICAL MANAGEMENT

- If there is concern for uterine rupture, the patient must be admitted for evaluation.
- Maternal assessment:
  - Physical exam: Rule out other causes of abdominal pain, including trauma:
    - Speculum exam to evaluate for vaginal bleeding
    - Cervical exam to determine stage of labor or possibly loss of station (possible sign of uterine rupture)
  - Labs: Hemoglobin/Hematocrit, coagulation studies, type and cross
  - Tocometry: Evaluate for labor or abruption

- Fetal assessment:
  - Fetal heart tracing: Fetal bradycardia is the most reliable finding with uterine rupture.
  - US: Evaluate fetal presentation and location (i.e., intrauterine vs. intraabdominal)

Resuscitation

If there is a concern for uterine rupture, immediate preparation for surgery must be made:

- Alert anesthesia
- NPO
- 2 large-bore IVs
- IV fluid/bolus
- Labs (as listed above)
- Availability of blood products

SURGICAL MANAGEMENT

If there is the concern for uterine rupture, or if there is a compromise of either maternal or fetal status, immediate surgical management is required.

Patient Education

Inform the patient that her symptoms may be due to a rupture of the uterine wall and that if a cesarean is not performed immediately, this can put both her and her fetus in danger of significant morbidity and mortality. Informed consent must be obtained for general anesthesia and CD.

Risks, Benefits

- Maternal risks:
  - Hemorrhage
  - Infection
  - Organ injury
  - Hysterectomy
  - Infertility
  - Increased future risk of uterine rupture
  - Death
- Fetal risks:
  - Asphyxia
  - Hypoxia
  - Encephalopathy
  - Other neurologic sequelae
  - Death

Alternatives

None

Medical

None

Surgical

- Immediate CD
- Exploratory surgery for abdominal organ injury

FOLLOW-UP

PROGNOSIS

Delays in diagnosis and delivery by CD can result in significant morbidity and mortality.

COMPLICATIONS

- Abdominal organ injury
- Intraabdominal adhesions
- Infection
- Future pregnancy risks:
  – Uterine rupture
  – Placentation abnormalities
  – Loss of fertility

BIBLIOGRAPHY

ACOG Practice Bulletin No. 54. Vaginal Birth after Previous Cesarean Delivery. Washington DC: ACOG; July 2004.

AHRQ Publication No. 033-E018. Vaginal Birth After Cesarean. Rockville, MD: AHRQ; March 2003.

Guise J-M, et al. Safety of vaginal birth after cesarean: A systematic review. *Obstet Gynecol*. 2004;103(3): 420–429.

Guise J-M, et al. Systematic review of the incidence and consequences of uterine rupture in women with prior cesarean delivery. *Br Med J*. 2004;329(7456): 19–23.

Hofmeyr GJ, et al. WHO systematic review of maternal mortality and morbidity: The prevalence of uterine rupture. *Br J Obstet Gynaecol*. 2005;112: 1221–1228.

 MISCELLANEOUS

SYNONYM(S)

- Uterine or scar disruption
- Uterine or scar dehiscence
- Uterine window

CLINICAL PEARLS

- Patients with risk factors for uterine rupture, especially prior uterine surgery, should be informed of the warning signs for uterine rupture. These include, but are not limited to:
  – Abdominal or incisional pain
  – Vaginal bleeding
  – Decreased fetal movement
- The overall risk of uterine rupture is <1%.
- Fetal bradycardia is often associated with symptomatic complete uterine rupture.
- Immediate CD is required to reduce maternal and fetal morbidity and mortality.

ABBREVIATIONS

- CD—Cesarean delivery
- TOLAC—Trial of labor after cesarean
- VBAC—Vaginal birth after cesarean
- VD—Vaginal delivery

CODES

ICD9-CM

- 665.0 Uterus rupture before onset of labor
- 665.1 Uterus rupture unspecified
- 674.1 Disruption of uterine wound
- 763.89 Uterus rupture affecting fetus or newborn

 PATIENT TEACHING

Patients, particularly those with prior cesarean, should be instructed to call with any questions or concerns regarding abdominal or incisional pain, vaginal bleeding, or decreased fetal movement. These are potential signs of uterine rupture or other significant obstetric condition, which may require immediate treatment and management.

Section VIII

VULVAR AND VAGINAL TRAUMA

Diane F. Merritt, MD
Michelle Moniz, BA

BASICS

DESCRIPTION

Female genital trauma includes: Injury to the labia, vulva or vagina. Worldwide, the most common cause of genital trauma in postmenarcheal women is injury sustained during childbirth.

- Ranges from minor bruising/cuts that heal rapidly to serious coitus-related injuries.
- Profuse bleeding can occur due to rich vascular supply.
- Genital injuries alone rarely result in death.
- In certain populations, FGM, also called "female circumcision," comprises procedures with partial or total removal of the external female genitalia or other injury for cultural, religious, or other nontherapeutic reasons.
  – This intentionally mutilative practice is strongly discouraged by the WHO and women's rights groups.

Types of genital injuries:

- Straddle injury (with or without penetration):
  – Fall onto an object such as bicycle frame, fence, playground equipment, swimming pool edge, or furniture resulting in a laceration, or hematoma or other trauma.
  – Typical features of accidental straddle injuries include anterior and unilateral location.
  – Lacerations are classically linear, vertically oriented, and superficial.
- Accidental penetrating injury falling onto fixed object, impaling vagina or rectum.
  – Commonly results in lacerations to the posterior aspect of the hymen.
  – Lateral vaginal wall or posterior fornix lacerations can perforate abdomen, with cervical avulsion, evisceration of bowel, omentum or fallopian tube into vagina.
- Insufflation injury:
  – Fall while water skiing, riding Jet Ski, water sliding, or direct contact with pool/spa jet.
  – Significant blood loss without external trauma can occur if branches of anterior division of the internal iliac artery, which supply the vagina, are avulsed.
  – Insufflation injuries can occur with oral genital sex in pregnant and nonpregnant patients.
- Crush or shearing injury: MVAs (often associated with pelvic fracture), fall while inline skating, building collapse
- Animal bite
- Thermal burn: Scalding and immersion in children; flames more likely mechanism in adults
- Chemical burn: Work-related, caustic agent used for douching, abortifacients, foreign object (i.e., batteries)
- FGM/Female circumcision
- Sexual abuse: Coerced or forced vaginal or anal fondling or penetration (see topic)

Pediatric Considerations

Minors have a greater frequency of anogenital injuries than adult victims.

- Common sites of injury in adolescents included the labia minora, hymen, fossa navicularis, and fourchette.

DIFFERENTIAL DIAGNOSIS

- Dermatologic complaints: Lichen Sclerosis, Lichen Simplex Chronicus, Lichen Planus
- Urethral prolapse
- Medical conditions: Autoimmune thrombocytopenia
- Infections: Genital impetigo, group A streptococcal vaginitis, pinworms, perianal dermatitis
- STIs: Gonorrhea, chlamydia, syphilis, herpes, chancroid, lymphogranuloma venereum, granuloma inguinale, genital warts
- Vaginal foreign objects: Various objects have been inserted into the vagina, and many patients are too embarrassed to seek medical assistance in retrieving them and so will wait and try to remove them on their own. Vaginal foreign bodies of long duration might be complicated by vesicovaginal fistulae.
- Initial, consensual intercourse
- Tumor: Benign or malignant

EPIDEMIOLOGY

- Increased incidence during the summer months particularly in temperate climates, due to increased outdoor activities like bicycle riding, swimming, and climbing activities, while wearing light weight clothing.
- Risk factors for sexual abuse or assault:
  – Developmental delay
  – Alcohol and drug use, history of previous sexual victimization
  – Risk factors for injury include 1st experience of coitus, coitus after long abstinence, congenital vaginal anomalies, deep penetration, substance abuse, brutality, violence, or insertion of foreign objects.

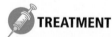 DIAGNOSIS

SIGNS AND SYMPTOMS
History

A detailed history is key to determining the cause of injury. In any case of genital trauma, the mechanism of injury should be consistent with the documented physical findings.

> **ALERT**
> Inconsistencies between the history and physical examination, or the presence of a vaginal laceration without external injury, should arouse suspicion of sexual assault or abuse.

Physical Exam

- Stabilize patient and determine the status of coexistent injuries.
- Examine genital and anal regions for erythema, bruising, abrasions, lacerations, and vulvar hematomas. Topical 2% lidocaine and irrigation with warm water can help in visualization of active bleeding sites.

- To assess vaginal injury in adults, a digital exam is insufficient. A speculum-guided inspection is indicated.
- If unable to assess the extent of injury, examine under general anesthesia.

Pediatric Considerations

All children with genital trauma must be evaluated for possible abuse. If unattended, exsanguinating blood loss may occur in children with significant genital trauma.

- Follow your institution's protocol for obtaining a history from a child with genital injury. It is paramount to determine whether the history provided is compatible with the proposed mechanism of injury.
- Sedation may be indicated to fully assess the extent of injury. Anesthesia is always indicated for internal vaginal exam of a prepubertal child. Never restrain or force a frightened or resistant child to complete a genital exam.

Geriatric Considerations

A high incidence of genital trauma in elderly sexual assault victims has been reported and is attributed to thinning and atrophy of the vulvovaginal tissues and decreased lubrication increasing susceptibility to injury. The skin is easily traumatized and slow to heal.

TESTS
Lab

Urinalysis for blood:

- Gross hematuria is the hallmark of urethral or bladder injury.
- Patients with gross hematuria, multiple associated injuries, or significant abnormalities are most likely to benefit from urological consult and lower urinary tract imaging.

> **ALERT**
> In cases of alleged sexual assault, follow institutional protocol for collection of forensic evidence and provide photo documentation.

Imaging

Pelvic fracture warrants imaging.

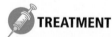 TREATMENT

MEDICAL MANAGEMENT

- Treat with a multidisciplinary team.
- There are multiple psychological consequences to genital trauma, particularly after sexual abuse. A psychiatrist or social worker should be involved in evaluation and treatment.
- Superficial lacerations that are not actively bleeding can be observed.
- Small nonexpanding vulvar hematomas can be managed with ice, pain medication, and rest.
- Use urethral or suprapubic catheter if dysuria, local swelling, or urethral spasm prevent voiding, depending on location and severity of injury.
  – Catheterization is generally sufficient for urethral contusion; more severe injuries necessitate surgical management.
  – Controversy over whether repair of urethral injuries should be immediate or delayed until swelling and hemorrhage resolve.

- Sitz baths are helpful for discomfort, and to remove bloody drainage for hygiene; significant injuries may respond to whirlpool therapy for debridement.
- Topical triple antibiotic ointment or petroleum jelly and good hygiene is sufficient for superficial injuries. Actively bleeding vaginal lacerations require either packing or suturing.
- Genital and perianal burns managed by topical application of antimicrobials (silver sulfadiazine) and estrogen cream to minimize scarring. Contractures can be prevented with thigh abduction, hip exercises, early ambulation, and pressure garments.

Resuscitation

Initial first aid at the scene for external genital and vaginal injuries is compression of bleeding to suppress blood loss and hematoma expansion. Ice packs and vaginal packing with tampons or sterile gauze can be used as temporizing measures preceding a professional gynecologic exam.

- Lavage with warm water; direct inspection to identify active bleeding. Irrigation to neutralize and dilute agents implicated in chemical burns.

Drugs

- Phenazopyridine as local bladder analgesic, to alleviate pain, irritation, discomfort, or urgency caused by urinary tract injury.
- Application of vaginal estrogen cream daily for 3–7 days to promote healing and decrease scarring.
- Oral NSAIDs and narcotics may be indicated.

SURGICAL MANAGEMENT

- Repair deepest vaginal injuries first and conclude with introital lacerations.
- Treat superficial vaginal injuries with packing rather than suturing. Premoistened packing with estrogen cream or petroleum jelly to ease removal. Moisten dry packing with saline to remove.
- Large vulvar hematomas can dissect into the loose areolar tissue along vaginal wall and fascial planes over the symphysis and abdominal wall, and may result in necrosis of overlying skin.
  - Incise large vulvar hematomas at the medial mucosal surface, near the vaginal orifice.
  - Debride devitalized tissue, ligate bleeding vessels, and place absorbable sutures.
  - Place closed suction drain to prevent fluid accumulation, ease pain, and hasten recovery.
- Remove foreign objects from vagina.
  - Lavage small, soft items (e.g., toilet paper) or removed by twirling moistened cotton-tipped applicator in the vagina.
  - Small objects can sometimes be milked out with a finger in the rectum.
  - Remove larger or metallic items with forceps.
  - For difficult to remove items, insert Foley catheter past the object, inflate to remove.
  - If sharp edges, remove carefully.
  - Use vaginal lubricants and manipulation to break suction if tightly wedged.
  - General anesthesia may be indicated.
- Urethral transection or bladder disruption should be repaired by an expert professional.
- With penetrating injuries of vagina or anus, monitor for signs of peritoneal irritation or ongoing hemodynamic instability. Penetrating injuries may be associated with intra-abdominal extension requiring laparoscopy or laparotomy.

Pediatric Considerations

Vaginoscopy is an important tool used by the pediatric gynecologist. Use of a cystoscope or hysteroscope provides fluid distension allowing full visualization of the vaginal vault. The labia should be gently opposed to enable the fluid to distend the vagina and enhance visualization.

 FOLLOW-UP

- Disposition: Generally outpatient care
- Patient monitoring: A child victim of sexual abuse must be protected from further abuse.
- STDs should be treated.
- Assess minor genital injuries at 3–4 days to ensure healing. Daily reassessment if more extensive.
- Sitz baths or whirlpool therapy, with rinsing after bowels movements for perianal hygiene
- Discuss future sexual function and reproduction with the patient (and her family, if age appropriate). This is almost always a major source of anxiety for the patient and family. Reassurance from the medical professional can substantially alleviate these fears and concerns.
- Genital trauma can create significant short-term anxiety for the patient and her family, particularly after sexual assault, as well as long-term medical sequelae. Intensive support and counseling must be provided. Psychiatric care should be offered to both victim and family.

PROGNOSIS

Children and teens recovering from an isolated genital trauma rarely have long-standing psychological trauma from the event.

- Victims of sexual assault may experience a multitude of psychological complications.

COMPLICATIONS

- Scarring or vaginal stenosis (i.e., with extensive burns)
- Vesicovaginal fistula (obstructed labor, vaginal foreign body, failure to successfully repair injuries to bladder or urethra)
- Long-standing psychological trauma
- The victim of female genital mutilation may suffer severe pain, shock, hemorrhage, urine retention, ulceration of the genital region and injury to adjacent tissue. Hemorrhage and infection can cause death. Long-term sequelae include cysts, abscesses, keloids, damage to the urethra with incontinence, dyspareunia, sexual dysfunction and difficulties with childbirth.

BIBLIOGRAPHY

Corriere JN, et al. Diagnosis and Management of Bladder Injuries. *Urol Clin N Am.* 2006;33:67–71.

Danielson CK, et al. Adolescent sexual assault: An update of the literature. *Curr Opin Obstet Gynecol.* 2004;16:383–388.

Heger A, et al. Children referred for possible sexual abuse: Medical findings in 2384 children. *Child Abuse Negl.* 2002;26(6-7):645–659.

Jones JS, et al. Comparative analysis of adult versus adolescent sexual assault: Epidemiology and patterns of anogenital injury. *Acad Emerg Med.* 2003;10:872–877.

Lacy J et al. Vaginal Laceration from a high-pressure water jet in a prepubescent girl. *Pediatr Emerg Care.* 2007;23(2):113–114.

Merritt DF, et al. Genital Injuries in Pediatric and Adolescent Patients. In: *Pediatric and Adolescent Gynecology.* 2nd edition. Philadelphia: W.B. Saunders Company; 2002:539–549.

Merritt, DF. Vulvar and genital trauma in pediatric and adolescent gynecology. *Curr Opin Obstet Gynecol.* 2004;16:371–381.

Muram D, et al. Genital Injuries. *J Pediatr Adolesc Gynecol.* 2003;16(3):149–155.

Templeton DJ. Sexual assault of a postmenopausal woman. *J Clin Forensic Med.* 2005;12:98–100.

Yacobi Y, et al. Emergent and surgical interventions for injuries associated with eroticism: A review. *J Trauma.* 2007;62:1522–1530.

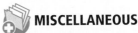 **MISCELLANEOUS**

ABBREVIATIONS

- FMG—Female genital mutilation
- STD—Sexually transmitted disease
- STI—Sexually transmitted infection

CODES

ICD9-CM

- 623.6 Vaginal hematoma
- 624.5 Vulvar hematoma
- 629.2 Female genital mutilation status
- 867 Injury to pelvic organs
- 878 Open wound of genital organs
- 926.0 Crushing injury of external genitals
- 939 Foreign body in genitourinary tract
- 942.05 Burn, genitourinary organ(s), external
- 959.14 Other injury of external genitals

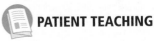 **PATIENT TEACHING**

Age-appropriate patient education may be useful:

- Young children: Parents can teach appropriate names for genital structures and help a child understand that private parts (areas covered by underwear) should not be touched by strangers. Childproofing includes hot temperatures <100° F.
- Adolescents: Protective clothing, such as jeans or a neoprene, for water sport activities. Caution about alcohol and drug-associated rape.
- The practice of FGM is to be discouraged by raising awareness and enhancing patient education.

Section VIII

WOUND DEHISCENCE AND DISRUPTION

Snehal M. Bhoola, MD
Donald G. Gallup, MD

 BASICS

DESCRIPTION
- Wound disruption/dehiscence is the postoperative separation of one or more abdominal musculoaponeurotic layers.
- WI is the separation of suprafascial layers, including skin and subcutaneous tissue.
  - WI may result from infection or aseptic failure of suture or staples.
- WD involves separation of fascia and muscle and may be with or without evisceration.
  - WD usually occurs between postoperative days 5 and 10.
  - WD with or without evisceration is a surgical emergency.
  - Recent reviews quote a 25% average mortality rate.
  - Most common cause of death is cardiorespiratory compromise (50%); peritonitis is the second most common cause (15%).

DIFFERENTIAL DIAGNOSIS
Wound failure can be associated with multiple factors. Clinical evaluation should confirm or exclude one of the following:
- Superficial wound separation without fascial disruption
- Wound infection without fascial separation
- Aseptic fascial separation without evisceration
- Aseptic fascial separation with evisceration
- Fascial infection with or without evisceration

EPIDEMIOLOGY
Incidence
- Up to 2.5% of patients undergoing clean contaminated surgeries, and up to 20% undergoing intra-abdominal operations will develop surgical site infections.
- In studies conducted since 1985, incidence of WD ranged from 0.4–2.3%, average 1.2%.
- Overall incidence in gynecologic surgery is 0.4%.

RISK FACTORS
- Recent studies show NO increased risk in the following:
  - Midline over transverse incision
  - Male sex
  - Controlled diabetes

- Patient factors with known increased risk of fascial disruption include:
  - Advanced age >65
  - Anemia related to malnutrition
  - Broncopulmonary disease
  - Poorly controlled diabetes mellitus
  - Intra-abdominal or wound infection
  - Jaundice
  - Chronic corticosteroid use
  - Severe malnutrition
- Patient factors with presumed increased risk, but conflicting studies:
  - Obesity
  - Radiation therapy
  - Abdominal distention
  - Renal failure
  - Cancer
- Closure technique to reduce risk includes:
  - Short stitch interval
  - Nonstrangulating tension
  - Wide tissue bites
- Strongest closure is at suture length to wound length ratio of 4:1. This translates to stitch interval and tissue bite of 1 cm each.
- Continuous mass closure provides strongest wound.
- For greatest risk reduction, perform closure with no. 1 or no. 2 delayed absorbable monofilament suture. Alternatively, a polyglactin (Vicryl) or polyglycolic acid (Dexon) suture may be used.

 TREATMENT

MEDICAL MANAGEMENT
- Examine patient's wound to narrow differential diagnosis:
  - Remove appropriate staples around disrupted site to allow adequate assessment of wound.
  - Visually examine fascia for visible defects or bowel evisceration.
  - Gently probe small or deep separation with Q-tip to test fascial integrity.
  - Culture wound if infection suspected.
- Examine overall patient status:
  - Assess vital signs and urine output.
  - Evaluate for signs of distress.
- Obtain initial laboratory studies:
  - CBC with differential, serum electrolytes, type and screen

- Pack wound at bedside:
  - Superficial wound disruption without infection may be closed at bedside if within 1st 6 hours
  - If closure is delayed for >6 hours, pack wound with saline-moistened gauze and perform secondary closure in 4–5 days.
  - If infection is noted, open and pack wound.
  - If evisceration is noted, pack wound gently with saline-moistened gauze and prepare for surgical closure.

Resuscitation
Initiate the following if wound evisceration or fascial separation is noted.
- Initiate NPO status
- Start IV fluids
- Place foley catheter

Drugs
Initiate broad-spectrum antibiotics only for clinical signs of infection, including fever, hypotension, purulent discharge from wound, or necrotic or malodorous wound.

Other
May need NG tube placement if distended bowel or ileus noted.

SURGICAL MANAGEMENT
Informed Consent
Obtain consent for the following:
- Wound closure with repair of fascia
- Possible wound debridement

Patient Education
- Inform patient of clinical findings.
- Discuss potential risk of repeat wound disruption and possible hernia formation.
- If wound is packed, educate patient and family on appropriate wound care and dressing changes.

Risks, Benefits
- Inform patient of possible open, packed wound after fascial closure.
- With complete evisceration, inform patient of possible ICU stay.
- Inform patient on possible need for mesh placement to close fascia.

Surgical

- With WD, surgery is only option.
  - If a delay in taking the patient to the OR is anticipated, dress wound and cover with a sterile plastic drape and an abdominal binder.
- Administer prophylactic antibiotics.
- Explore wound after prep and drape.
- Replace bowel within abdomen.
- Remove any foreign material, clot or suture and debride wound (if needed).
- Close fascia with no. 1 or no. 2 nylon monofilament suture in a running mass closure.
- Close skin of a clean wound primarily.
- If wound infection is noted, pack SC space after debridement and irrigation with saline-moistened gauze.
- If fascial edges will not come together, insert Dexon mesh to reinforce the fascia and allow closure.

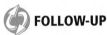 **FOLLOW-UP**

- Check wound daily while in hospital.
- Examine and pack open wound twice daily while in hospital.
- If patient has an open packed wound, follow-up 1 week postdischarge to assure wound is healing.
- Routine follow-up for any WD closed primarily

PROGNOSIS

- Mortality in recent studies of wound dehiscence is 25%.
- Excellent prognosis if closure performed in appropriate and timely manner

COMPLICATIONS

- Sepsis
- Cardiopulmonary failure in unrecognized wound evisceration
- Persistent wound infection

BIBLIOGRAPHY

Carlson MA. Acute wound failure. *Surgical Clin North Am*. 1997;77(3):607.

Blatzler DW, et al. Antimicrobial prophylaxis for surgery: An advisory statement from the national surgical infection prevention project. *Clin Infect Dis*. 2004;38:1706.

Jenkins TN. The burst abdominal wound: A mechanical approach. *Br J Surg*. 1976;63:873.

Jenkins TN. Incisional hernia repair. A mechanical approach. *Br J Surg*. 1980;67:335.

Gallup DG, et al. Primary mass closure of midline incisions with a continuous polyglyconate monofilament absorbable suture. *Obstet Gynecol*. 1990;76:872.

 MISCELLANEOUS

SYNONYM(S)

Burst abdomen

ABBREVIATIONS

- ICU—Intensive care unit
- NG tube—Nasogastric tube
- WI—Wound disruption without fascial separation
- WD—Wound dehiscence with fascial separation

CODES

ICD9-CM

- 674.14 Postpartum disruption of cesarean wound
- 998.31 Disruption of internal operation wound (dehiscence)
- 998.5 Postoperative wound infection

 PATIENT TEACHING

- Postoperative wound care by family member with supervision/surveillance by home visiting nurse if possible
- Instructions for all post-op patients to call if significant wound redness or drainage

WOUND INFECTION/NECROTIZING FASCIITIS

Donald G. Gallup, MD

 BASICS

DESCRIPTION

- NF is a severe soft tissue infection that is often mistaken for a wound infection in early stages.
- NF is a polymicrobial infectious process that spreads along fascial planes.
- The bacteria causing these infections was originally identified as hemolytic streptococci, but subsequent studies have implicated aerobic and anaerobic bacteria, often acting synergistically.

ALERT

- Mortality rates for this rapidly spreading infection range from 6–76%, and NF involving the vulva and perineum has generally been associated with a graver prognosis.
- Prompt medical and especially surgical intervention decrease mortality.

DIFFERENTIAL DIAGNOSIS

- Several clinical findings differentiate NF from a wound infection:
  - Local soft tissue edema and discoloration
  - Severe agonizing pain, particularly in postpartum patients
  - Sensory deficits in only 10–15%
- Serial examinations are mandatory.
  - Draw a "circle" around affected area with indelible marker and re-examine in 2–4 hours.
  - Progression of edema or discoloration should lead to immediate surgery.
- Gram stains of aspirations may reveal a paucity of WBCs
- CT or MRI may help in distinguishing NF from cellulitis and lead to earlier intervention.
- If the diagnosis is unclear, emergency wound exploration to find necrosis is indicated.

EPIDEMIOLOGY

- Predisposing factors:
  - Although ~10% of cases of NF have no predisposing factors, the following are often cited:
    ○ Diabetes, obesity, heart disease, hypertension, chronic renal disease, alcoholism, malnutrition, older age, history of recent radiation or chemotherapy
- Other less often associated conditions:
  - Steroid use, HIV, IV drug use, history of organ transplants
  - Suspect NF in women with vulvar infections or postoperative patients with predisposing conditions.

 TREATMENT

MEDICAL MANAGEMENT

- Obtain initial laboratory studies:
  - CBC, serum electrolytes and calcium
  - Aerobic and anaerobic blood cultures
  - Gram stain of wound
- Initiate broad-spectrum antibiotics early:
  - Include a penicillin
  - Add an aminoglycoside with or without clindamycin
  - Efficacious single agent antibiotics include:
    ○ Imipenem
    ○ Meropenem
    ○ Piperacillin and tazobactam (Zosyn)
  - May add ciprofloxacin or clindamycin to Zosyn

Resuscitation

Monitoring:

- Foley catheter
- Central line insertion

Drugs

- Clindamycin (Cleocin) 600–900 mg IV q6–8h
- Ciprofloxacin (Cipro) 400 mg IV q8–12h
- Gentamicin (Garamycin) 5 mg/kg/d:
  - IV in 3 divided doses
- Meropenem (Merrem) 1 g IV q8h
- Imipenem and Cilastatin (Primaxim) 500 mg IV q6h to 1g IV q8h:
  - Piperacillin and Tazobactam (Zosyn) 3.375 g IV q6h

Other

- Consider TPN or enteral alimentation given need for multiple surgeries
- Hyperbaric oxygen may benefit select patients:
  - Controversial as it may increase cost
- May need ICU

SURGICAL MANAGEMENT

Informed Consent

Should include possibilities of:

- Extensive debridement
- Need for second or third operation
- Need for flaps (rotational or myocutaneous)
- Need for colostomy with posterior perineal disease

Patient Education

Better self-management of underlying morbidities such as diabetes and obesity.

Risks, Benefits

- Patient should be informed of possibilities outlined in an informed consent.
- Without aggressive surgical management, she is likely to die from the disease process.

Alternatives

There are no alternatives to aggressive medical and surgical management.

Medical as outlined in initial paragraph

May require ICU admission or change in antibiotics, depending on course and cultures

Surgical

- Prompt radical debridement:
  - Resection of all necrotic tissue until bleeding ensues
- Consult with gynecologic oncologist and/or a plastic surgeon during original procedure.
- Colostomy for posterior perineal disease may be necessary:
  - Can do laparoscopic loop colostomy or loop ileostomy
- Reoperate and débride as necessary.

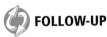 **FOLLOW-UP**

Depends on what was done surgically:

- Plastic surgery if flaps done
- Gynecologic oncology or surgery for colostomy take down
- Internist for management comorbidities

PROGNOSIS

- Mortality in recently managed patients ranges between 13% and 50% (9 series)
- Mortality is less if operated with 24 hours of suspected diagnosis.

COMPLICATIONS

- Sepsis
- Candidemia in immunocompromised patients
- Malnutrition

BIBLIOGRAPHY*

Stephenson H, et al. Droegemuller W. Necrotizing fasciitis of the vulva. *Am J Obstet Gynecol.* 1992;166:324–327.

Schorge JD, et al. Postpartum and vulvar necrotizing fasciitis. Early clinical diagnosis and histopathologic correlation. *J Repro Med.* 1998;43:586–590.

Goepfert AR, et al. Necrotizing fasciitis after cesarean delivery. *Obstet Gynecol.* 1997;89:409–412.

Gallup DG, et al. Necrotizing fasciitis in gynecologic and obstetric patients: A surgical emergency. *Am J Obstet Gynecol.* 2002;187:305–311.

Wysoki MG, et al. Necrotizing fasciitis: CT characteristics. *Radiology.* 1997;203:859–863.

Bochud PV, et al. Antimicrobial therapy for patients with severe sepsis and septic shock: An evidence based review. *Crit Care Med.* 2004;32(suppl): S495–S512.

Mindrup SR, et al. Hyperbaric oxygen for the treatment of Fournier's gangrene. *J Urol.* 2005;173: 1975–1977.

*Due to the rarity of the condition, very few reports meet the criteria for a high level of evidence rating.

 MISCELLANEOUS

SYNONYM(S)

- Hemolytic streptococcal gangrene
- Synergistic bacterial gangrene
- Fournier's gangrene

CLINICAL PEARLS

- Be aware of vulvar or abdominal soft tissue infections in patients with comorbidities such as diabetes or obesity.
- Early aggressive surgical debridement is the key to successful management.

ABBREVIATIONS

- CT—Computed tomography
- ICU—Intensive care unit
- MRI—Magnetic resonance imaging
- NF—Necrotizing fasciitis
- TPN—Total parental nutrition

CODES

ICD9-CM
728.86 Necrotizing fasciitis

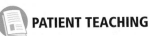 **PATIENT TEACHING**

- The disease is unlikely to reoccur.
- Management of comorbidities such as diabetes and obesity should be emphasized.
- Ambulation instructions and diet instructions will be based on defect incurred by the surgery.

Section IX
Appendices

APPENDIX I: SCREENING FOR CERVICAL CANCER

	ACS[1]	ACOG[2]	USPSTF[3]
When to initiate screening	~3 years after the onset of vaginal intercourse. Screening should begin no later than 21 years of age.	~3 years after initiation of sexual intercourse, but no later than age 21 years	Within 3 years of onset of sexual activity, or age 21, whichever comes 1st
When to stop screening	Age ≥70 with an intact cervix and who have had ≥3 documented, consecutive, technically satisfactory normal/negative cervical cytology tests, and no abnormal/positive cytology tests within the 10-year period prior to age 70		Age 65 if they have had adequate recent screening with normal Pap smears and are not otherwise at high risk for cervical cancer
Screening after hysterectomy	Screening following total hysterectomy (with removal of the cervix) for benign gynecologic disease is not indicated	Women who have had a total hysterectomy and have no prior history of high-grade CIN may discontinue screening	Recommends against screening for women who have had a hysterectomy for benign disease
Frequency of screening	Annually with conventional cervical cytology smears OR every 2 years using liquid-based cytology; after age 30, women who have had 3 consecutive, technically satisfactory normal/negative cytology results may be screened every 2–3 years (unless high risk)	Based on cytology testing method and/or use of ancillary HPV in women ≥30. Annual for women <30. Women ≥30 with 3 consecutive negative tests may be screened every 2–3 years. More frequent screening: HIV, immunosuppression, DES exposure in utero	At least every 3 years

1. Saslow D, et al. American Cancer Society guideline for the early detection of cervical neoplasia and cancer. *CA Cancer J Clin*. 2002;52(6):342–362.
2. ACOG Practice Bulletin No. 45. Cervical Cytology Screening. *Obstet Gynecol*. 2003;102:417–427.
3. Screening for Cervical Cancer. Systematic Evidence Review, January 2002. Available at: www.ncbi.nlm.nih.gov/books/bv.fcgi?rid=hstat3.chapter.4180. Accessed 09/22/07.

APPENDIX II: CANCER STAGING

FIGO STAGING BY DISEASE

Vulvar Cancer

FIGO stages

0	Carcinoma in situ (preinvasive carcinoma)
I	Tumor confined to vulva or vulva and perineum, ≤2 cm in greatest dimension
IA	Tumor confined to vulva or vulva and perineum, ≤2 cm in greatest dimension and with stromal invasion no greater than 1.0 mm*
IB	Tumor confined to vulva or vulva and perineum, ≤2 cm in greatest dimension and with stromal invasion greater than 1.0 mm*
II	Tumor confined to the vulva or vulva and perineum, >2 cm in greatest dimension
III	Tumor invades any of the following: Lower urethra, vagina, anus, and/or unilateral regional node metastasis
IV	
IVA	Tumor invades any of the following: Bladder mucosa, retal mucosa, upper urethral mucosa, or is fixed to bone and/or bilateral regional node metastases
IVB	Any distant metastasis, including pelvic lymph nodes

*The depth of invasion is defined as the measurement of the tumor from the epithelial-stromal junction of the adjacent most superficial dermal papilla to the deepest point of invasion.

Vaginal Cancer

Stage 0	Carcinoma in situ: Intraepithelial neoplasia grade 3
Stage I	The carcinoma is limited to the vaginal wall
Stage II	The carcinoma has involved the subvaginal tissue but has not extended to the pelvic wall
Stage III	The carcinoma has extended to the pelvic wall
Stage IV	The carcinoma has extended beyond the true pelvis or has involved the mucosa of the bladder or rectum; bullous edema as such does not permit a case to be allotted to stage IV
IVA	Tumor invades bladder and/or rectal mucosa and/or direct extension beyond the true pelvis
IVB	Spread to distant organs

Cervical Cancer

Stage	Characteristics
0	Carcinoma in situ, cervical intraepithelial neoplasia Grade III.
I	The carcinoma is strictly confined to the cervix (extension to the corpus should be disregarded).
IA	Invasive cancer identified only microscopically. All gross lesions, even with superficial invasion, are stage IB cancers. Invasion is limited to measured stromal invasion with maximum depth of 5.0 mm, taken from the base of the epithelium, and a horizontal extension of not >7.0 mm. Depth of invasion should not be >5.0 mm taken from the base of the epithelium of the either surface or glandular, from which it originates. Vascular space involvement, either venous or lymphatic, should not alter the staging.
IA1	Measured stromal invasion no greater than 3.0 mm in depth and extension of not >7.0 mm
IA2	Measured stromal invasion more than 3.0 mm and not more than 5.0 mm with an extension of not >7.0 mm
IB	Clinically visible lesions confined to the cervix or preclinical lesions >IA
IB1	Clinically visible lesions not >4.0 cm.
IB2	Clinically visible lesions >4.0 cm.
II	The carcinoma extends beyond the cervix, but has not extended onto the pelvic wall or to the lower third of vagina.
IIA	No obvious parametrial involvement
IIB	With parametrial involvement
III	The carcinoma has extended to the pelvic wall. On rectal exam, there is no cancer-free space between the tumor and the pelvic wall. The tumor involves the lower third of the vagina. All cases with a hydronephrosis or nonfunctioning kidney should be included, unless they are known to be due to other causes.
IIIA	Tumor involves lower third of the vagina, with no extension to the pelvic wall.
IIIB	Extension to the pelvic wall and/or hydronephrosis or nonfunctioning kidney
IV	The carcinoma has extended beyond the true pelvis or has involved (biopsy proven) the mucosa of the bladder or rectum. A bullous edema as such, does not permit a case to be allotted to Stage IV.
IVA	Spread of the growth to adjacent organs
IVB	Spread to distant organs

Cancer of the Uterine Corpus

FIGO stages

0	Carcinoma in situ (preinvasive carcinoma)
I	Tumor confined to the corpus uteri
IA	Tumor limited to endometrium
IB	Tumor invades up to <1/2 of myometrium
IC	Tumor invades to ≥1/2 of myometrium
II	Tumor invades cervix but does not extend beyond uterus
IIA	Endocervical glandular involvement only
IIB	Cervical stromal invasion
III	Local and/or regional spread as specified in IIIA, B, C
IIIA	Tumor involves serosa of the corpus uteri and/or adnexa (direct extension or metastasis) and/or cancer cells in ascites or peritoneal washings
IIIB	Vaginal metastases
IIIC	Metastasis to pelvic and/or para-aortic lymph nodes
IVA	Tumor invades bladder mucosa and/or bowel mucosa
IVB	Distant metastasis, including intra-abdominal metastasis and/or inguinal lymph nodes

Cancer of the Fallopian Tube

FIGO

0	No evidence of primary tumor
	Carcinoma in situ (proinvasive carcinoma)
I	Tumor confined to fallopian tubes
IA	Tumor limited to 1 tube, without penetrating the serosal surface; no ascites
IB	Tumor limited to both tubes, without penetrating the serosal surface no ascites
IC	Tumor limited to 1 or both tubes, with extension onto/through the tubal serosa; or with positive malignant cells in the ascites or positive peritoneal washings
II	Tumor involves 1 or both fallopian tubes with pelvic extension
IIA	Extension and/or metastasis to uterus and/or ovaries
IIB	Extension to other pelvic organs
IIC	IIB/C with positive malignant cells in the ascites or positive peritoneal washings
III	Tumor involves 1 or both fallopian tubes with peritoneal implants outside the pelvis and/or positive regional lymph nodes
IIIA	Microscopic peritoneal metastasis outside the pelvis
IIIB	Macroscopic peritoneal metastasis outside the pelvis ≤2 cm in greatest dimension
IIIC	Peritoneal metastasis >2 cm in greatest dimension and/or positive regional lymph nodes
IV	Distant metastasis beyond the peritoneal cavity

Cancer of the Ovary

FIGO

0	No evidence of primary tumor
I	Tumor confined to ovaries
IA	Tumor limited to 1 ovary capsule intact
	No tumor on ovarian surface
	No malignant cells in the ascites or peritoneal washings
IB	Tumor limited to both ovaries, capsules intact
	No tumor on ovarian surface
	No malignant cells in the ascites or peritoneal washings
IC	Tumor limited to 1 or both ovaries, with any of the following: Capsule ruptured, tumor on ovarian surface, positive malignant cells in the ascites, or positive peritoneal washings
II	Tumor involves 1 or both ovaries with pelvic extension
IIA	Extension and/or implants in uterus and/or tubes
	No malignant cells in the ascites or peritoneal washings
IIB	Extension to other pelvic organ
	No malignant cells in the ascites or peritoneal washings
IIC	IIA/B with positive malignant cells in the ascites or positive peritoneal washings
III	Tumor involves 1 or both ovaries with microscopically confirmed peritoneal metastasis outside the pelvis and/or regional lymph nodes metastasis
IIIA	Microscopic peritoneal metastasis beyond the pelvis
IIIB	Macroscopic peritoneal metastasis beyond the pelvis ≤2 cm in greatest dimension
IIIC	Peritoneal metastasis beyond pelvis >2 cm in greatest dimension and/or regional lymph nodes metastasis
IV	Distant metastasis beyond the peritoneal cavity

APPENDIX III: WHEN TO INDUCE AMENORRHEA

Paula J. Adams Hillard, MD

- Hematologic conditions:
  - Inherited anemias:
    - Sickle cell disease
    - Thalassemia
    - Fanconi's anemia
  - Inherited bleeding disorders:
    - von Willebrand disease
    - Hemophilia, other clotting factor deficiencies
  - Anticoagulation
  - Hematologic or other malignancy requiring chemotherapy:
    - Bone marrow transplant for recurrent malignancy
  - Other hematologic conditions:
    - Thrombocytopenia/Idiopathic thrombocytopenia purpura
  - Afibrinogenemia
- Neurologic disease:
  - Seizure disorders
  - Menstrual or other migraine headaches
- Blood-borne infectious diseases:
  - HIV/AIDS
  - Hepatitis B, C
- Gynecologic conditions:
  - Endometriosis
  - Premenstrual syndrome
  - Menorrhagia:
    - Uterine leiomyomata
    - Anemia due to anovulatory bleeding
  - Dysmenorrhea
  - Preprocedure:
    - Hysteroscopy
    - Endometrial ablation
- Developmental disabilities:
  - Moderate-to-severe mental retardation
- Other:
  - Mobilized military personnel

APPENDIX IV: COMPLEMENTARY AND ALTERNATIVE MEDICINE USED FOR GYNECOLOGIC AND WOMEN'S HEALTH INDICATIONS

Paula J. Adams Hillard, MD

Category	Indication	Drug or Treatment	Evidence of benefit	Evidence of harm
Gynecology	Dysmenorrhea	Chiropracty	No significant difference between manipulative therapy and mimic [1]	Reports of stroke [2]
		Vitamin E	Decreased primary dysmenorrhea in adolescents [3]	
	PMS	Vitamin E	Reduced symptoms of anxiety, craving, and depression [3]	
		Chasteberry/Chaste tree	Comparable to Fluoxetine in one study; more effective for physical symptoms (breast tenderness, swelling, cramps, food cravings) [4]	Avoid in pregnancy, theoretical adverse impact on pregnancy and lactation [4]
		Gingko biloba	Significant relief of breast tenderness and neuropsychological symptoms [5]	
	Cystitis	Cranberry products	Promising studies suggest *prevention* of UTIs [4]; components of cranberries may prevent *E. coli* from adhering to uroepithelium [3]	
	Yeast vulvovaginitis	Boron (boric acid)	Intravaginal boric acid may treat candidiasis and other vaginal fungal infections, but low-quality studies; possibly effective for azole-resistant infections [4]	
	Mastalgia	Evening primrose oil	Relief of cyclic and noncyclic mastalgia and in 27% less effective than Danazol, similar effectiveness to bromocriptine [4]	
		Gingko biloba	Relief in premenstrual breast symptoms [5]	
		Chasteberry/Chaste tree	Insufficient reliable data [4]	
	Nausea in pregnancy	Ginger	More effective than placebo and comparable to vitamin B_6 [6]	Caution re lack of safety data [7]
	Postsurgery nausea	Ginger	Reduced incidence post-op nauseas and vomiting (PONV) at 24 hours, but not at 3 hours; possibly not in those with low rate PONV [6]	
	Labor pain	Acupuncture	RCT significantly reduced need for epidural [8]	
Women's health	Depression	St. John's wort	No more effective than placebo for treating moderate severity major depression [9]	Interaction with medication, including oral contraceptives [10]
	Anxiety, age-related memory impairment, cognitive function	Gingko biloba	Some benefit in cognitive function, mild-moderate age-related memory impairment	
	Osteoarthritis pain	Glucosamine/Chondroitin	Did not provide significant relief from pain; subgroup with moderate-severe pain showed relief [11]	
	Ovarian cancer, cervical dysplasia, colorectal cancer	Green tea	Women who regularly consume tea appear to have lower risk of ovarian cancer compared to those who don't drink tea [12]; no effect on colon cancer risk [12]; possible reduced risk of cervical dysplasia [12]	
		Flaxseed	May improve mild menopausal symptoms 35% for hot flashes, and 44% for night sweats; unknown if effective for moderate-severe symptoms [13]	
	Colorectal cancer	Vitamin E	RCT show vitamin E alone or in combination with beta-carotene does not prevent development of colorectal adenomas [3]	

(continued)

Category	Indication	Drug or Treatment	Evidence of benefit	Evidence of harm
Women's health	Menopause	Black cohosh	Mixed results for relief of menopause symptoms; specific commercial extract reduces hot flash frequency compared to placebo; other formulations and extracts mixed or negative [14]	Possible liver toxicity
		Phytoestrogens/Soy/Red clover	No consistent or conclusive evidence that red clover reduces hot flashes [3]	
		Kava	May decrease anxiety; no evidence of benefit for hot flashes [3]	Serious liver toxicity and potential drug interactions [15] FDA warning
		Ginseng	Not helpful for hot flashes, but may help mood symptoms, sleep disturbances and sense of well-being [3]	
		Vitamin E	No reduction in hot flashes in women who have had breast cancer [3]	
		DHEA	One RCT showed no benefit for hot flashes; small nonrandomized trials suggest some benefit, not confirmed [3]	Long-term safety not established; unclear if impact on risk of breast cancer [3]
		Dong Quai root	One RCT—not useful in reducing hot flashes [3]	
		Evening Primrose oil	RCT no benefit over placebo [4]	
		Wild yam	No better than placebo in relieving vasomotor symptoms of hot flashes and night sweats [16]	
		St. John's wort	Insufficient reliable evidence regarding menopausal symptoms [17]	
		Liu Wei Di Huang Tang	Not effective in relieving menopausal symptoms [18]	

1. Hondras MA, et al. Spinal manipulative therapy versus a low force mimic maneuver for women with primary dysmenorrhea: A randomized, observer-blinded, clinical trial. *Pain.* 1999;81(1–2):105–114.
2. Di Fabio RP. Manipulation of the cervical spine: Risks and benefits. *Phys Ther.* 1999;79(1):50–65.
3. National Center for Complementary and Alternative Medicine. Do CAM therapies help menopausal symptoms? Available at: http://nccam.nih.gov/health/menopauseandcam. Accessed 11/26/2007.
4. Natural medicines comprehensive database. *Cranberry, effectiveness.* 2007.
5. Natural medicines comprehensive database. *Ginko biloba, effectiveness.* 2007.
6. Natural medicines comprehensive database. *Ginger, effectiveness.* 2007.
7. Marcus DM, et al. Do no harm: Avoidance of herbal medicines during pregnancy. *Obstet Gynecol.* 2005;105(5 Pt 1):1119–1122.
8. Ramnero A, et al. Acupuncture treatment during labour—a randomised controlled trial. *BJOG.* 2002;109(6):637–644.
9. Effect of Hypericum perforatum (St John's wort) in major depressive disorder: A randomized controlled trial. *JAMA.* 2002;287(14):1807–1814.
10. Murphy PA, et al. Interaction of St. John's Wort with oral contraceptives: Effects on the pharmacokinetics of norethindrone and ethinyl estradiol, ovarian activity and breakthrough bleeding. *Contraception.* 2005;71(6):402–408.
11. Clegg DO, et al. Glucosamine, chondroitin sulfate, and the two in combination for painful knee osteoarthritis. *N Engl J Med.* 2006;354(8):795–808.
12. Natural medicines comprehensive database. *Green tea, effectiveness.* 2007.
13. Natural medicines comprehensive database. *Flaxseed, effectiveness.* 2007.
14. Natural medicines comprehensive database. *Black cohosh, effectiveness.* 2007.
15. Clouatre DL. Kava kava: Examining new reports of toxicity. *Toxicol Lett.* 2004;150(1):85–96.
16. Natural medicines comprehensive database. *Wild yam, effectiveness.* 2007.
17. Natural medicines comprehensive database. *St. John's wort, effectiveness.* 2007.
18. Sidani M, et al. *Gynecology: Select topics. Primary Care.* 2002;29(2):297–321, vi.

Section IX

Office Environment

- Have a nondiscrimination policy visible to patients.
- Provide reading materials (magazines, health education pamphlets) that address the specific needs of lesbian patients.
- Ensure that the staff are comfortable with lesbian patients and their families.
- Ensure confidentiality.
- Make sure intake forms include options for nonmarried partners.

Interviewing

- Use gender-neutral language:
  - "Do you have a significant other?"
- Use language free of heterosexist assumptions. Avoid questions like:
  - "Are you married?"
  - "What form of birth control do you use?"
- Ask about prior heterosexual intercourse and assess safe sex behavior:
  - "Have you ever been sexually active with men, women, or both?"
  - "Are you presently in a sexual relationship with a woman or a man or both?"
- Ask with whom the patient lives, who is important to her, who would care for her if she were sick.
- Ask the patient how she would like to be referred to and/or how to refer to her partner.
- Encourage lesbians to have legal documents regarding who can make medical and/or legal decisions for them (Durable Power of Attorney for Healthcare and Finances).

From McGarry KA, et al. Lesbian Health. In: McGarry KA, et al., eds. *The 5-Minute Consult Clinical Companion to Women's Health*. *Philadelphia: Lippincott Williams & Wilkins; 2007:166–167*.

APPENDIX VI: ACOG SCREENING BY AGE

PERIODIC ASSESSMENT
AGES 13–18 YEARS

SCREENING
History

- Reason for visit
- Health status: Medical, menstrual, surgical, family
- Dietary/Nutrition assessment
- Physical activity
- Use of complementary and alternative medicine
- Tobacco, alcohol, other drug use
- Abuse/Neglect
- Sexual practices

Physical Examination

- Height
- Weight
- Body mass index (BMI)
- Blood pressure
- Secondary sexual characteristics (Tanner staging)
- Pelvic examination (when indicated by the medical history)
- Skin*

Laboratory Testing

Periodic

- Cervical cytology (annually beginning at approximately 3 years after initiation of sexual intercourse)
- Chlamydia and gonorrhea testing (if sexually active)

High-Risk Groups*

- Hemoglobin level assessment
- Bacteriuria testing
- Sexually transmitted disease testing
- Human immunodeficiency virus (HIV) testing
- Genetic testing/counseling
- Rubella titer assessment
- Tuberculosis skin testing
- Lipid profile assessment
- Fasting glucose testing
- Hepatitis C virus testing
- Colorectal cancer screening[†]

EVALUATION AND COUNSELING
Sexuality

- Development
- High-risk behaviors
- Preventing unwanted/unintended pregnancy:
  – Postponing sexual involvement
  – Contraceptive options, including emergency contraception

- Sexually transmitted diseases:
  – Partner selection
  – Barrier protection

Fitness and Nutrition

- Dietary/Nutrition assessment (including eating disorders)
- Exercise: Discussion of program
- Folic acid supplementation (0.4 mg/d)
- Calcium intake

Psychosocial Evaluation

- Suicide: Depressive symptoms
- Interpersonal/Family relationships
- Sexual identity
- Personal goal development
- Behavioral/Learning disorders
- Abuse/Neglect
- Satisfactory school experience
- Peer relationships
- Date rape prevention

Cardiovascular Risk Factors

- Family history
- Hypertension
- Dyslipidemia
- Obesity
- Diabetes mellitus

Health/Risk Behaviors

- Hygiene (including dental), fluoride supplementation*
- Injury prevention:
  – Safety belts and helmets
  – Recreational hazards
  – Firearms
  – Hearing
  – Occupational hazards
  – School hazards
  – Exercise and sports involvement
- Skin exposure to ultraviolet rays
- Tobacco, alcohol, other drug use

IMMUNIZATIONS
Periodic

- Tetanus–diphtheria–pertussis booster (once between ages 11 years and 16 years)
- Hepatitis B vaccine (one series for those not previously immunized)
- Human papillomavirus vaccine (one series for those not previously immunized)
- Meningococcal conjugate vaccine (before entry into high school for those not previously immunized)

High-Risk Groups*

- Influenza vaccine
- Hepatitis A vaccine
- Pneumococcal vaccine
- Measles–mumps–rubella vaccine
- Varicella vaccine

Leading Causes of Death[‡]

1. Accidents
2. Malignant neoplasms
3. Homicide
4. Suicide
5. Congenital anomalies
6. Diseases of the heart
7. Chronic lower respiratory diseases
8. Influenza and pneumonia
9. Septicemia
10. Pregnancy, childbirth, and puerperium

Leading Causes of Morbidity[‡]

- Acne
- Asthma
- Chlamydia
- Headache
- Mental disorders, including affective and neurotic disorders
- Nose, throat, ear, and upper respiratory infections
- Obesity
- Sexual assault
- Sexually transmitted diseases
- Urinary tract infections
- Vaginitis

*See Table 1.

[†]Only for those with a family history of familial adenomatous polyposis or 8 years after the start of pancolitis. For a more detailed discussion of colorectal cancer screening, see Smith RA, von Eschenbach AC, Wender R, Levin B, Byers T, Rothenberger D, et al. ACS American Cancer Society guidelines for the early detection of cancer: Update of early detection guidelines for prostate, colorectal, and endometrial cancers. Also: Update 2001—testing for early lung cancer detection. Prostate Cancer Advisory Committee, ACS Colorectal Cancer Advisory Committee, ACS Endometrial Cancer Advisory Committee [published erratum appears in *CA Cancer J Clin.* 2001;51:150]. *CA Cancer J Clin.* 2001;51:38–75; quiz 77–80.

[‡]See box.

PERIODIC ASSESSMENT AGES 19–39 YEARS

SCREENING

History

- Reason for visit
- Health status: Medical, surgical, family
- Dietary/Nutrition assessment
- Physical activity
- Use of complementary and alternative medicine
- Tobacco, alcohol, other drug use
- Abuse/Neglect
- Sexual practices
- Urinary and fecal incontinence

Physical Examination

- Height
- Weight
- Body mass index (BMI)
- Blood pressure
- Neck: Adenopathy, thyroid
- Breasts
- Abdomen
- Pelvic examination
- Skin*

Laboratory Testing

Periodic

- Cervical cytology (annually beginning no later than age 21 years; every 2–3 years after 3 consecutive negative test results if age 30 years or older with no history of cervical intraepithelial neoplasia 2 or 3, immunosuppression, human immunodeficiency virus [HIV] infection, or diethylstilbestrol exposure in utero)†
- Chlamydia testing (if aged 25 years or younger and sexually active)
- Human immunodeficiency virus (HIV) testing‡

High-Risk Groups*

- Hemoglobin level assessment
- Bacteriuria testing
- Mammography
- Fasting glucose testing
- Sexually transmitted disease testing
- Genetic testing/counseling
- Rubella titer assessment
- Tuberculosis skin testing
- Lipid profile assessment
- Thyroid-stimulating hormone testing
- Hepatitis C virus testing
- Colorectal cancer screening
- Bone density screening

EVALUATION AND COUNSELING

Sexuality and Reproductive Planning

- High-risk behaviors
- Discussion of a reproductive health plan§

- Contraceptive options for prevention of unwanted pregnancy, including emergency contraception
- Preconception and genetic counseling
- Sexually transmitted diseases:
  - Partner selection
  - Barrier protection
- Sexual function

Fitness and Nutrition

- Dietary/Nutrition assessment
- Exercise: Discussion of program
- Folic acid supplementation (0.4 mg/d)
- Calcium intake

Psychosocial Evaluation

- Interpersonal/Family relationships
- Intimate partner violence
- Work satisfaction
- Lifestyle/Stress
- Sleep disorders

Cardiovascular Risk Factors

- Family history
- Hypertension
- Dyslipidemia
- Obesity
- Diabetes mellitus
- Lifestyle

Health/Risk Behaviors

- Hygiene (including dental)
- Injury prevention:
  - Safety belts and helmets
  - Occupational hazards
  - Recreational hazards
  - Firearms
  - Hearing
  - Exercise and sports involvement
- Breast self-examination‖
- Chemoprophylaxis for breast cancer (for high-risk women aged 35 years or older)¶
- Skin exposure to ultraviolet rays
- Suicide: Depressive symptoms
- Tobacco, alcohol, other drug use

IMMUNIZATIONS

Periodic

- Human papillomavirus vaccine (1 series for those aged 26 years or less and not previously immunized)
- Tetanus–diphtheria–pertussis booster (every 10 years)

High-Risk Groups*

- Measles–mumps–rubella vaccine
- Hepatitis A vaccine
- Hepatitis B vaccine
- Influenza vaccine
- Meningococcal vaccine
- Pneumococcal vaccine
- Varicella vaccine

Leading Causes of Death**

1. Malignant neoplasms
2. Accidents
3. Diseases of the heart
4. Suicide
5. Human immunodeficiency virus (HIV) disease
6. Homicide
7. Cerebrovascular diseases
8. Diabetes mellitus
9. Chronic liver diseases and cirrhosis
10. Chronic lower respiratory diseases

Leading Causes of Morbidity**

- Acne
- Arthritis
- Asthma
- Back symptoms
- Cancer
- Chlamydia
- Depression
- Diabetes mellitus
- Gynecologic disorders
- Headache/Migraine
- Hypertension
- Joint disorders
- Menstrual disorders
- Mental disorders, including affective and neurotic disorders
- Nose, throat, ear, and upper respiratory infections
- Obesity
- Sexual assault/domestic violence
- Sexually transmitted diseases
- Substance abuse
- Urinary tract infections

*See Table 1.

†For a more detailed discussion of cervical cytology screening, including the use of human papillomavirus DNA testing and screening after hysterectomy, see Cervical cytology screening. ACOG Practice Bulletin No. 45. American College of Obstetricians and Gynecologists. *Obstet Gynecol*. 2003;102:417–427.

‡Physicians should be aware of and follow their states' HIV screening requirements. For a more detailed discussion of HIV screening, see Branson BM, Handsfield HH, Lampe MA, Janssen RS, Taylor AW, Lyss SB, et al. Revised recommendations for HIV testing of adults, adolescents, and pregnant women in health care settings. Centers for Disease Control and Prevention. *MMWR Recomm Rep*. 2006;55(RR-14):1–17; quiz CE1–4.

§For a more detailed discussion of the reproductive health plan, see The importance of preconception care in the continuum of women's health care. ACOG Committee Opinion No. 313. American College of Obstetricians and Gynecologists. *Obstet Gynecol*. 2005;106:665–666.

‖Despite a lack of definite data for or against breast self-examination, breast self-examination has the potential to detect palpable breast cancer and can be recommended.

¶For a more detailed discussion of risk assessment and chemoprevention therapy, see Selective estrogen receptor modulators. ACOG Practice Bulletin No. 39. American College of Obstetricians and Gynecologists. *Obstet Gynecol*. 2002;100:835–843.

**See box.

PERIODIC ASSESSMENT AGES 40–64 YEARS

SCREENING
History

- Reason for visit
- Health status: Medical, surgical, family
- Dietary/Nutrition assessment
- Physical activity
- Use of complementary and alternative medicine
- Tobacco, alcohol, other drug use
- Abuse/Neglect
- Sexual practices
- Urinary and fecal incontinence

Physical Examination

- Height
- Weight
- Body mass index (BMI)
- Blood pressure
- Oral cavity
- Neck: Adenopathy, thyroid
- Breasts, axillae
- Abdomen
- Pelvic examination
- Skin*

Laboratory Testing

Periodic

- Cervical cytology (every 2–3 years after three consecutive negative test results if no history of cervical intraepithelial neoplasia 2 or 3, immunosuppression, human immunodeficiency virus [HIV] infection, or diethylstilbestrol exposure in utero)†
- Mammography (every 1–2 years beginning at age 40 years, yearly beginning at age 50 years)
- Lipid profile assessment (every 5 years beginning at age 45 years)
- Colorectal cancer screening (beginning at age 50 years), using one of the following options:
  1. Yearly patient-collected fecal occult blood testing†
  2. Flexible sigmoidoscopy every 5 years
  3. Yearly patient-collected fecal occult blood testing‡ plus flexible sigmoidoscopy every 5 years
  4. Double contrast barium enema every 5 years
  5. Colonoscopy every 10 years
- Fasting glucose testing (every 3 years after age 45 years)
- Thyroid-stimulating hormone screening (every 5 years beginning at age 50 years)
- Human immunodeficiency virus (HIV) testing§

High-Risk Groups*

- Hemoglobin level assessment
- Bacteriuria testing
- Fasting glucose testing
- Sexually transmitted disease testing
- Tuberculosis skin testing
- Lipid profile assessment
- Thyroid-stimulating hormone testing
- Hepatitis C virus testing
- Colorectal cancer screening

EVALUATION AND COUNSELING
Sexuality‖

- High-risk behaviors
- Contraceptive options for prevention of unwanted pregnancy, including emergency contraception
- Sexually transmitted diseases:
  – Partner selection
  – Barrier protection
- Sexual function

Fitness and Nutrition

- Dietary/Nutrition assessment
- Exercise: Discussion of program
- Folic acid supplementation (0.4 mg/d before age 50 years)
- Calcium intake

Psychosocial Evaluation

- Family relationships
- Intimate partner violence
- Work satisfaction
- Retirement planning
- Lifestyle/Stress
- Sleep disorders

Cardiovascular Risk Factors

- Family history
- Hypertension
- Dyslipidemia
- Obesity
- Diabetes mellitus
- Lifestyle

Health/Risk Behaviors

- Hygiene (including dental)
- Hormone therapy
- Injury prevention:
  – Safety belts and helmets
  – Occupational hazards
  – Recreational hazards
  – Exercise and sports involvement
  – Firearms
  – Hearing
- Breast self-examination¶
- Chemoprophylaxis for breast cancer (for high-risk women)**
- Skin exposure to ultraviolet rays
- Suicide: Depressive symptoms
- Tobacco, alcohol, other drug use

IMMUNIZATIONS
Periodic

- Influenza vaccine (annually beginning at age 50 years)
- Tetanus-diphtheria-pertussis booster (every 10 years)

High-Risk Groups*

- Measles–mumps–rubella vaccine
- Hepatitis A vaccine
- Hepatitis B vaccine
- Influenza vaccine

- Meningococcal vaccine
- Pneumococcal vaccine
- Varicella vaccine

Leading Causes of Death‡

1. Malignant neoplasms
2. Diseases of the heart
3. Cerebrovascular diseases
4. Chronic lower respiratory diseases
5. Accidents
6. Diabetes mellitus
7. Chronic liver disease and cirrhosis
8. Septicemia
9. Suicide
10. Human immunodeficiency virus (HIV) disease

Leading Causes of Morbidity‡

- Arthritis/Osteoarthritis
- Asthma
- Cancer
- Cardiovascular disease
- Depression
- Diabetes mellitus
- Disorders of the urinary tract
- Headache/Migraine
- Hypertension
- Menopause
- Mental disorders, including affective and neurotic disorders
- Musculoskeletal symptoms
- Nose, throat, ear, and upper respiratory infections
- Obesity
- Sexually transmitted diseases
- Ulcers
- Vision impairment

*See Table 1.

†For a more detailed discussion of cervical cytology screening, including the use of human papillomavirus DNA testing and screening after hysterectomy, see Cervical Cytology screening. ACOG Practice Bulletin No. 45. American College of Obstetricians and Gynecologists. *Obstet Gynecol.* 2003;102:417–427.

‡Fecal occult blood testing (FOBT) requires 2 or 3 samples of stool collected by the patient at home and returned for analysis. A single stool sample for FOBT obtained by digital rectal examination is not adequate for the detection of colorectal cancer.

§Physicians should be aware of and follow their states' HIV screening requirements. For a more detailed discussion of HIV screening, see Branson BM, Handsfield HH, Lampe MA, Janssen RS, Taylor AW, Lyss SB, et al. Revised recommendations for HIV testing of adults, adolescents, and pregnant women in health care settings. Centers for Disease Control and Prevention. *MMWR Recomm Rep.* 2006;55(RR-14):1–17; quiz CE1–4.

‖Preconception and genetic counseling is appropriate for certain women in this age group.

¶Despite a lack of definitive data for or against breast self-examination, breast self-examination has the potential to detect palpable breast cancer and can be recommended.

**For a more detailed discussion of risk assessment and chemoprevention therapy, see Selective estrogen receptor modulators. ACOG Practice Bulletin No. 39. American College of Obstetricians and Gynecologists. *Obstet Gynecol.* 2002;100:835–843.

‡See box.

PERIODIC ASSESSMENT AGES 65 YEARS AND OLDER

SCREENING
History

- Reason for visit
- Health status: Medical, surgical, family
- Dietary/Nutrition assessment
- Physical activity
- Use of complementary and alternative medicine
- Tobacco, alcohol, other drug use, and concurrent medication use
- Abuse/Neglect
- Sexual practices
- Urinary and fecal incontinence

Physical Examination

- Height
- Weight
- Body mass index (BMI)
- Blood pressure
- Oral cavity
- Neck: Adenopathy, thyroid
- Breasts, axillae
- Abdomen
- Pelvic examination
- Skin*

Laboratory Testing
Periodic

- Cervical cytology (every 2–3 years after three consecutive negative test results if no history of cervical intraepithelial neoplasia 2 or 3, immunodeficiency virus [HIV] infection, or diethylstilbestrol exposure in utero)[†]
- Urinalysis
- Mammography
- Lipid profile assessment (every 5 years)
- Colorectal cancer screening using one of the following methods:
  1. Yearly patient-collected fecal occult blood testing[†]
  2. Flexible sigmoidoscopy every 5 years
  3. Yearly patient-collected fecal occult blood testing[‡] plus flexible sigmoidoscopy every 5 years
  4. Double contrast barium enema every 5 years
  5. Colonoscopy every 10 years
- Fasting glucose testing (every 3 years)
- Bone density screening[§]
- Thyroid-stimulating hormone screening (every 5 years)

High-Risk Groups*

- Hemoglobin level assessment
- Sexually transmitted disease testing
- Human immunodeficiency virus (HIV) testing

- Tuberculosis skin testing
- Thyroid-stimulating hormone screening
- Hepatitis C virus testing
- Colorectal cancer screening

EVALUATION AND COUNSELING
Sexuality

- Sexual function
- Sexual behaviors
- Sexually transmitted diseases:
  – Partner selection
  – Barrier protection

Fitness and Nutrition

- Dietary/Nutrition assessment
- Exercise: Discussion of program
- Calcium intake

Psychosocial Evaluation

- Neglect/Abuse
- Lifestyle/Stress
- Depression/Sleep disorders
- Family relationships
- Work/Retirement satisfaction

Cardiovascular Risk Factors

- Hypertension
- Dyslipidemia
- Obesity
- Diabetes mellitus
- Sedentary lifestyle

Health/Risk Behaviors

- Hygiene (including dental)
- Hormone therapy
- Injury prevention:
  – Safety belts and helmets
  – Prevention of falls
  – Occupational hazards
  – Recreational hazards
  – Exercise and sports involvement
  – Firearms
- Visual acuity/glaucoma
- Hearing
- Breast self-examination[||]
- Chemoprophylaxis for breast cancer (for high-risk women)[¶]
- Skin exposure to ultraviolet rays
- Suicide: Depressive symptoms
- Tobacco, alcohol, other drug use

IMMUNIZATIONS
Periodic

- Tetanus–diphtheria booster (every 10 years)
- Influenza vaccine (annually)
- Pneumococcal vaccine (once)

High-Risk Groups*

- Hepatitis A vaccine
- Hepatitis B vaccine
- Meningococcal vaccine
- Varicella vaccine

Leading Causes of Death**

1. Diseases of the heart
2. Malignant neoplasms
3. Cerebrovascular diseases
4. Chronic lower respiratory diseases
5. Alzheimer's disease
6. Influenza and pneumonia
7. Diabetes mellitus
8. Nephritis, nephrotic syndrome, and nephrosis
9. Accidents
10. Septicemia

Leading Causes of Morbidity**

- Arthritis/Osteoarthritis
- Asthma
- Cancer
- Cardiovascular disease
- Chronic obstructive pulmonary diseases
- Diabetes mellitus
- Diseases of the nervous system and sense organs
- Hearing and vision impairment
- Hypertension
- Mental disorders
- Musculoskeletal symptoms
- Nose, throat, ear, and upper respiratory infections
- Obesity
- Osteoporosis
- Pneumonia
- Ulcers
- Urinary incontinence
- Urinary tract infections
- Vertigo

*See Table 1.

[†]For a more detailed discussion of cervical cytology screening, including the use of human papillomavirus DNA testing and screening after hysterectomy, see Cervical Cytology screening. ACOG Practice Bulletin No. 45. American College of Obstetricians and Gynecologists. *Obstet Gynecol*. 2003;102:417–427.

[‡]Fecal occult blood testing (FOBT) requires 2 or 3 samples of stool collected by the patient at home and returned for analysis. A single stool sample for FOBT obtained by digital rectal examination is not adequate for detection of colorectal cancer.

[§]In the absence of new risk factors, subsequent bone density screening should not be performed more frequently than every 2 years.

[||]Despite a lack of definitive data for or against breast self-examination, breast self-examination has the potential to detect palpable breast cancer and can be recommended.

[¶]For a more detailed discussion of risk assessment and chemoprevention therapy, see Selective estrogen receptor modulators. ACOG Practice Bulletin No. 39. American College of Obstetricians and Gynecologists. *Obstet Gynecol*. 2002;100:835–843.

**See box.

Table 1. High-Risk Factors

Intervention	High-risk factor
Bacteriuria testing	Diabetes mellitus
Bone density screening*	Postmenopausal women <65 years: history of prior fracture as an adult; family history of osteoporosis; Caucasian; dementia; poor nutrition; smoking; low weight and BMI; estrogen deficiency caused by early (<45 years) menopause, bilateral oophorectomy or prolonged (>1 year) premenopausal amenorrhea; low lifelong calcium intake; alcoholism; impaired eyesight despite adequate correction; history of falls; inadequate physical activity
	All women: Certain diseases or medical conditions and those who take certain drugs associated with an increased risk of osteoporosis
Colorectal cancer screening†	Colorectal cancer or adenomatous polyps in 1st-degree relative <60 years or in 2 or more 1st-degree relatives of any ages; family history of familial adenomatous polyposis or hereditary nonpolyposis colon cancer; history of colorectal cancer, adenomatous polyps, inflammatory bowel disease, chronic ulcerative colitis, or Crohn's disease
Fasting glucose testing	Overweight (BMI ≥25); family history of diabetes mellitus; habitual physical inactivity; high-risk race/ethnicity (e.g., African American, Hispanic, Native American, Asian, Pacific Islander); have given birth to a newborn weighing >9 lb or have a history of gestational diabetes mellitus; hypertension; high-density lipoprotein cholesterol level ≤35 mg/dL; triglyceride level ≥250 mg/dL; history of impaired glucose tolerance or impaired fasting glucose; polycystic ovary syndrome; history of vascular disease
Fluoride supplementation	Live in area with inadequate water fluoridation (<0.7 ppm)
Genetic testing/counseling	Considering pregnancy and: Patient, partner, or family member with history of genetic disorder or birth defect; exposure to teratogens; or African, Cajun, Caucasian, European, Eastern European (Ashkenazi) Jewish, French Canadian, Mediterranean, or Southeast Asian ancestry
Hemoglobin level assessment	Caribbean, Latin American, Asian, Mediterranean, or African ancestry; history of excessive menstrual flow
HAV vaccination	Chronic liver disease, clotting factor disorders, illegal drug users, individuals who work with HAV-infected nonhuman primates or with HAV in a research laboratory setting, individuals traveling to or working in countries that have high or intermediate endemicity of hepatitis A
HBV vaccination	Hemodialysis patients; patients who receive clotting factor concentrates; health care workers and public safety workers who have exposure to blood in the workplace; individuals in training in schools of medicine, dentistry, nursing, laboratory technology, and other allied health professions; injecting drug users; individuals with more than one sexual partner in the previous 6 months; individuals with a recently acquired STD; all clients in STD clinics; household contacts and sexual partners of individuals with chronic HBV infection; clients and staff of institutions for the developmentally disabled; international travelers who will be in countries with high or intermediate prevalence of chronic HBV infection for >6 months; inmates of correctional facilities
HCV testing	History of injecting illegal drugs; recipients of clotting factor concentrates before 1987; chronic (long-term) hemodialysis; persistently abnormal alanine aminotransferase levels; recipients of blood from donors who later tested positive for HCV infection; recipients of blood or blood-component transfusion or organ transplant before July 1992; occupational percutaneous or mucosal exposure to HCV-positive blood
HIV testing	More than 1 sexual partner since most recent HIV test or a sex partner with more than 1 sexual partner since most recent HIV test, seeking treatment for STDs, drug use by injection, history of prostitution, past or present sexual partner who is HIV positive or bisexual or injects drugs, long-term residence or birth in an area with high prevalence of HIV infection, history of transfusion from 1978 to 1985, invasive cervical cancer, adolescents who are or ever have been sexually active, adolescents entering detention facilities. Offer to women seeking preconception evaluation.
Influenza vaccination	Anyone who wishes to reduce the chance of becoming ill with influenza; chronic cardiovascular or pulmonary disorders, including asthma; chronic metabolic diseases, including diabetes mellitus, renal dysfunction, hemoglobinopathies, and immunosuppression (including immunosuppression caused by medications or by HIV); residents and employees of nursing homes and other long-term care facilities; individuals likely to transmit influenza to high-risk individuals (e.g., household members and caregivers of the elderly, children aged from birth to 59 months, and adults with high-risk conditions); those with any condition (e.g., cognitive dysfunction, spinal cord injury, seizure or other neuromuscular disorder) that compromises respiratory function or the handling of respiratory secretions, or that increases the risk of aspiration; health care workers
Lipid profile assessment	Family history suggestive of familial hyperlipidemia; family history of premature (age <50 years for men, age <60 years for women) cardiovascular disease; diabetes mellitus; multiple coronary heart disease risk factors (e.g., tobacco use, hypertension)
Mammography	Women who have had breast cancer or who have a 1st-degree relative (i.e., mother, sister, or daughter) or multiple other relatives who have a history of premenopausal breast or breast and ovarian cancer
Meningococcal vaccination	Adults with anatomic or functional asplenia or terminal complement component deficiencies, 1st-year college students living in dormitories, microbiologists routinely exposed to Neisseria meningitidis isolates, military recruits, travel to hyperendemic or epidemic areas
MMR vaccination	Adults born in 1957 or later should be offered vaccination (one dose of MMR) if there is no proof of immunity or documentation of a dose given after 1st birthday; individuals vaccinated in 1963–1967 should be offered revaccination (2 doses); health care workers, students entering college, international travelers, and rubella-negative postpartum patients should be offered a 2nd dose.
Pneumococcal vaccination	Chronic illness, such as cardiovascular disease, pulmonary disease, diabetes mellitus, alcoholism, chronic liver disease, cerebrospinal fluid leaks, functional asplenia (e.g., sickle cell disease) or splenectomy; exposure to an environment where pneumococcal outbreaks have occurred; immunocompromised patients (e.g., HIV infection, hematologic or solid malignancies, chemotherapy, steroid therapy). Revaccination after 5 years may be appropriate for certain high-risk groups.
Rubella titer assessment	Childbearing age and no evidence of immunity
STD testing	History of multiple sexual partners or a sexual partner with multiple contacts, sexual contact with individuals with culture-proven STD, history of repeated episodes of STDs, attendance at clinics for STDs, women with developmental disabilities; routine screening for chlamydial infection for all sexually active women aged ≤25 years and other asymptomatic women at high risk for infection; routine screening for gonorrheal infection for all sexually active adolescents and other asymptomatic women at high risk for infection; sexually active adolescents who exchange sex for drugs or money, use intravenous drugs, are entering a detention facility, or live in a high prevalence area should also be tested for syphilis.

(continued)

Table 1. High-Risk Factors (*continued*)

Intervention	High-risk factor
Skin examination	Increased recreational or occupational exposure to sunlight; family or personal history of skin cancer; clinical evidence of precursor lesions
Thyroid-stimulating hormone testing	Strong family history of thyroid disease; autoimmune disease (evidence of subclinical hypothyroidism may be related to unfavorable lipid profiles)
Tuberculosis skin testing	HIV infection; close contact with individuals known or suspected to have tuberculosis; medical risk factors known to increase risk of disease if infected; born in country with high tuberculosis prevalence; medically underserved; low income; alcoholism; intravenous drug use; resident of long-term care facility (e.g., correctional institutions, mental institutions, nursing homes and facilities); health professional working in high-risk health care facilities
Varicella vaccination	All susceptible adults and adolescents, including health care workers; household contacts of immunocompromised individuals; teachers; daycare workers; residents and staff of institutional settings, colleges, prisons, or military installations; adolescents and adults living in households with children; international travelers; nonpregnant women of childbearing age

Abbreviations: BMI, body mass index; HAV, hepatitis A virus; HBV, hepatitis B virus; HCV, hepatitis C virus; HIV, human immunodeficiency virus; MMR, measles–mumps–rubella; STD, sexually transmitted disease.

*For a more detailed discussion of bone density screening, see Osteoporosis. ACOG Practice Bulletin 50. American College of Obstetricians and Gynecologists. *Obstet Gynecol*. 2004;103:203–216.

†For a more detailed discussion of colorectal cancer screening, see Smith RA, von Eschenbach AC, Wender R, Levin B, Byers T, Rothenberger D, et al. American Cancer Society guidelines for the early detection of cancer: Update of early detection guidelines for prostate, colorectal, and endometrial cancers. Also: update 2001—testing for early lung cancer detection. Prostate Cancer Advisory Committee, ACS Colorectal Cancer Advisory Committee, ACS Endometrial Cancer Advisory Committee [published erratum appears in *CA Cancer J Clin*. 2001;51:150]. *CA CancerJ Clin*. 2001;51:38–75; quiz 77–80.

SOURCES OF LEADING CAUSES OF MORTALITY AND MORBIDITY

Leading causes of mortality are provided by the Mortality Statistics Branch at the National Center for Health Statistics. Data are from 2002, the most recent year for which final data are available. The causes are ranked.

Leading causes of morbidity are unranked estimates based on information from the following sources:

- National Health Interview Survey, 2004
- National Ambulatory Medical Care Survey, 2004
- National Health and Nutrition Examination Survey, 2003–2004
- National Hospital Discharge Survey, 2004
- National Nursing Home Survey, 1999
- U.S. Department of Justice National Violence Against Women Survey, 2006
- U.S. Centers for Disease Control and Prevention Sexually Transmitted Disease Surveillance, 2004
- U.S. Centers for Disease Control and Prevention HIV/AIDS Surveillance Report, 2004

Source: Primary and preventive care: Periodic assessments. ACOG Committee Opinion No. 357. American College of Obstetricians and Gynecologists. *Obstet Gynecol*. 2006;108:1615–1622.

APPENDIX VII: SCREENING: US PREVENTIVE SERVICES TASK FORCE

Michelle Berlin, MD, MPH

 BASICS

DESCRIPTION

USPSTF:

- Conducts scientific evidence reviews of a broad array of clinical preventive services, including screening, counseling, and preventive medications
- Recommendations are considered the gold standard for clinical preventive services.
- Leading independent panel of private-sector experts in prevention and primary care, supported by the AHRQ

ALERT

- Look to USPSTF 1st for screening recommendations.
- Recommendations of other groups and societies are not always evidence-based.

Services

- EPSS:
  - Useful to help identify appropriate screening, counseling, and preventive medication services for patients
  - Search for the most current recommendations by age, sex, and behavioral risk factors
  - http://epss.ahrq.gov/PDA/learnmore.jsp for web-based and PDA-compatible software
- Pocket Guide to Clinical Preventive Services, 2006:
  - Most recent version, containing short explanation of guidelines
  - www.ahrq.gov/clinic/pocketgd.htm
- USPSTF recommendations:
  - Full reports supporting recommendations
  - www.ahrq.gov/clinic/uspstfix. htm#Recommendations
    ○ Listed in "Topic Index" and by "Clinical Categories"

BIBLIOGRAPHY

AHRQ. U.S. Preventive Services Task Force. Available at: www.ahrq.gov/clinic/uspstfix.htm. Accessed 09/07/07.

ABBREVIATIONS

- USPSTF—US Preventive Services Task Force
- AHRQ—Agency for Healthcare Research and Quality
- EPSS—Electronic Preventive Services Selector

Recommended Adult Immunization Schedule

Note: These recommendations must be read with the footnotes that follow.

**Figure 1. Recommended adult immunization schedule, by vaccine and age group
United States, October 2007 – September 2008**

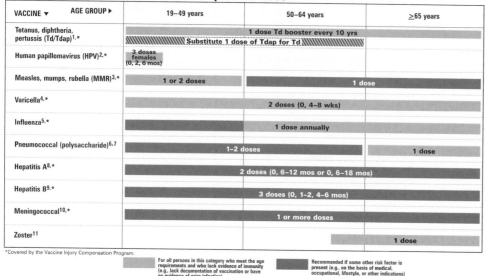

*Covered by the Vaccine Injury Compensation Program.

For all persons in this category who meet the age requirements and who lack evidence of immunity (e.g., lack documentation of vaccination or have no evidence of prior infection)

Recommended if some other risk factor is present (e.g., on the basis of medical, occupational, lifestyle, or other indications)

Report all clinically significant postvaccination reactions to the Vaccine Adverse Event Reporting System (VAERS). Reporting forms and instructions on filing a VAERS report are available at www.vaers.hhs.gov or by telephone, 800-822-7967.

Information on how to file a Vaccine Injury Compensation Program claim is available at www.hrsa.gov/vaccinecompensation or by telephone, 800-338-2382. To file a claim for vaccine injury, contact the U.S. Court of Federal Claims, 717 Madison Place, N.W., Washington, D.C. 20005; telephone, 202-357-6400.

Additional information about the vaccines in this schedule, extent of available data, and contraindications for vaccination is also available at www.cdc.gov/vaccines or from the CDC-INFO Contact Center at 800-CDC-INFO (800-232-4636) in English and Spanish, 24 hours a day, 7 days a week.

Use of trade names and commercial sources is for identification only and does not imply endorsement by the U.S. Department of Health and Human Services.

**Figure 2. Vaccines that might be indicated for adults based on medical and other indications
United States, October 2007 – September 2008**

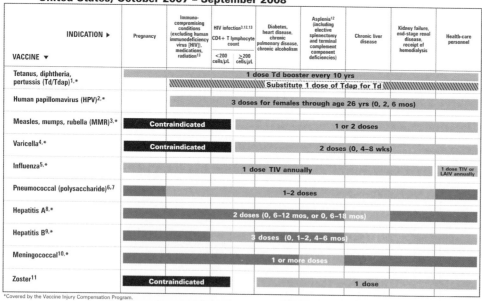

*Covered by the Vaccine Injury Compensation Program.

For all persons in this category who meet the age requirements and who lack evidence of immunity (e.g., lack documentation of vaccination or have no evidence of prior infection)

Recommended if some other risk factor is present (e.g., on the basis of medical, occupational, lifestyle, or other indications)

These schedules indicate the recommended age groups and medical indications for which administration of currently licensed vaccines is commonly indicated for adults ages 19 years and older, as of October 1, 2007. Licensed combination vaccines may be used whenever any components of the combination are indicated and when the vaccine's other components are not contraindicated. For detailed recommendations on all vaccines, including those used primarily for travelers or that are issued during the year, consult the manufacturers' package inserts and the complete statements from the Advisory Committee on Immunization Practices (www.cdc.gov/vaccines/pubs/acip-list.htm).

The recommendations in this schedule were approved by the Centers for Disease Control and Prevention's (CDC) Advisory Committee on Immunization Practices (ACIP), the American Academy of Family Physicians (AAFP), the American College of Obstetricians and Gynecologists (ACOG), and the American College of Physicians (ACP).

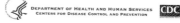

DEPARTMENT OF HEALTH AND HUMAN SERVICES
CENTERS FOR DISEASE CONTROL AND PREVENTION

CS115143

Footnotes

Recommended Adult Immunization Schedule · United States, October 2007 – September 2008

For complete statements by the Advisory Committee on Immunization Practices (ACIP), visit www.cdc.gov/vaccines/pubs/ACIP-list.htm.

1. Tetanus, diphtheria, and acellular pertussis (Td/Tdap) vaccination

Tdap should replace a single dose of Td for adults aged <65 years who have not previously received a dose of Tdap. Only one of two Tdap products (Adacel® [sanofi pasteur]) is licensed for use in adults.

Adults with uncertain histories of a complete primary vaccination series with tetanus and diphtheria toxoid–containing vaccines should begin or complete a primary vaccination series. A primary series for adults is 3 doses of tetanus and diphtheria toxoid–containing vaccines; administer the first 2 doses at least 4 weeks apart and the third dose 6–12 months after the second. However, Tdap can substitute for any one of the doses of Td in the 3-dose primary series. The booster dose of tetanus and diphtheria toxoid–containing vaccine should be administered to adults who have completed a primary series and if the last vaccination was received ≥10 years previously. Tdap or Td vaccine may be used, as indicated.

If the person is pregnant and received the last Td vaccination ≥10 years previously, administer Td during the second or third trimester; if the person received the last Td vaccination in <10 years, administer Tdap during the immediate postpartum period. A one-time administration of 1 dose of Tdap with an interval as short as 2 years from a previous Td vaccination is recommended for postpartum women, close contacts of infants aged <12 months, and all health-care workers with direct patient contact. In certain situations, Td can be deferred during pregnancy and Tdap substituted in the immediate postpartum period, or Tdap can be administered instead of Td to a pregnant woman after an informed discussion with the woman.

Consult the ACIP statement for recommendations for administering Td as prophylaxis in wound management.

2. Human papillomavirus (HPV) vaccination

HPV vaccination is recommended for all females aged ≤26 years who have not completed the vaccine series. History of genital warts, abnormal Papanicolaou test, or positive HPV DNA test is not evidence of prior infection with all vaccine HPV types; HPV vaccination is still recommended for these persons.

Ideally, vaccine should be administered before potential exposure to HPV through sexual activity; however, females who are sexually active should still be vaccinated. Sexually active females who have not been infected with any of the HPV vaccine types receive the full benefit of the vaccination. Vaccination is less beneficial for females who have already been infected with one or more of the HPV vaccine types.

A complete series consists of 3 doses. The second dose should be administered 2 months after the first dose; the third dose should be administered 6 months after the first dose.

Although HPV vaccination is not specifically recommended for females with the medical indications described in Figure 2, "Vaccines that might be indicated for adults based on medical and other indications," it is not a live-virus vaccine and can be administered. However, immune response and vaccine efficacy might be less than in persons who do not have the medical indications described or who are immunocompetent.

3. Measles, mumps, rubella (MMR) vaccination

Measles component: Adults born before 1957 can be considered immune to measles. Adults born during or after 1957 should receive ≥1 dose of MMR unless they have a medical contraindication, documentation of ≥1 dose, history of measles based on health-care provider diagnosis, or laboratory evidence of immunity.

A second dose of MMR is recommended for adults who 1) have been recently exposed to measles or are in an outbreak setting; 2) have been previously vaccinated with killed measles vaccine; 3) have been vaccinated with an unknown type of measles vaccine during 1963–1967; 4) are students in postsecondary educational institutions; 5) work in a health-care facility; or 6) plan to travel internationally.

Mumps component: Adults born before 1957 can generally be considered immune to mumps. Adults born during or after 1957 should receive 1 dose of MMR unless they have a medical contraindication, history of mumps based on health-care provider diagnosis, or laboratory evidence of immunity.

A second dose of MMR is recommended for adults who 1) are in an age group that is affected during a mumps outbreak; 2) are students in postsecondary educational institutions; 3) work in a health-care facility; or 4) plan to travel internationally. For unvaccinated health-care workers born before 1957 who do not have other evidence of mumps immunity, consider administering 1 dose on a routine basis and strongly consider administering a second dose during an outbreak.

Rubella component: Administer 1 dose of MMR vaccine to women whose rubella vaccination history is unreliable or who lack laboratory evidence of immunity. For women of childbearing age, regardless of birth year, routinely determine rubella immunity and counsel women regarding congenital rubella syndrome. Women who do not have evidence of immunity should receive MMR vaccine upon completion or termination of pregnancy and before discharge from the health-care facility.

4. Varicella vaccination

All adults without evidence of immunity to varicella should receive 2 doses of single-antigen varicella vaccine unless they have a medical contraindication. Special consideration should be given to those who 1) have close contact with persons at high risk for severe disease (e.g., health-care personnel and family contacts of immunocompromised persons) or 2) are at high risk for exposure or transmission (e.g., teachers; child care employees; residents and staff members of institutional settings, including correctional institutions; college students; military personnel; adolescents and adults living in households with children; nonpregnant women of childbearing age; and international travelers).

Evidence of immunity to varicella in adults includes any of the following: 1) documentation of 2 doses of varicella vaccine at least 4 weeks apart; 2) U.S.-born before 1980 (although for health-care personnel and pregnant women birth before 1980 should not be considered evidence of immunity); 3) history of varicella based on diagnosis or verification of varicella by a health-care provider (for a patient reporting a history of or presenting with an atypical case, a mild case, or both, health-care providers should seek either an epidemiologic link with a typical varicella case or to a laboratory-confirmed case or evidence of laboratory confirmation, if it was performed at the time of acute disease); 4) history of herpes zoster based on health-care provider diagnosis; or 5) laboratory evidence of immunity or laboratory confirmation of disease.

Assess pregnant women for evidence of varicella immunity. Women who do not have evidence of immunity should receive the first dose of varicella vaccine upon completion or termination of pregnancy and before discharge from the health-care facility. The second dose should be administered 4–8 weeks after the first dose.

5. Influenza vaccination

Medical indications: Chronic disorders of the cardiovascular or pulmonary systems, including asthma; chronic metabolic diseases, including diabetes mellitus, renal or hepatic dysfunction, hemoglobinopathies, or immunosuppression (including immunosuppression caused by medications or human immunodeficiency virus [HIV]); any condition that compromises respiratory function or the handling of respiratory secretions or that can increase the risk of aspiration (e.g., cognitive dysfunction, spinal cord injury, or seizure disorder or other neuromuscular disorder); and pregnancy during the influenza season. No data exist on the risk for severe or complicated influenza disease among persons with asplenia; however, influenza is a risk factor for secondary bacterial infections that can cause severe disease among persons with asplenia.

Occupational indications: Health-care personnel and employees of long-term care and assisted-living facilities.

Other indications: Residents of nursing homes and other long-term care and assisted-living facilities; persons likely to transmit influenza to persons at high risk (e.g., in-home household contacts and caregivers of children aged 0–59 months, or persons of all ages with high-risk conditions); and anyone who would like to be vaccinated. Healthy, nonpregnant adults aged ≤49 years without high-risk medical conditions who are not contacts of severely immunocompromised persons in special care units can receive either intranasally administered live, attenuated influenza vaccine (FluMist®) or inactivated vaccine. Other persons should receive the inactivated vaccine.

6. Pneumococcal polysaccharide vaccination

Medical indications: Chronic pulmonary disease (excluding asthma); chronic cardiovascular diseases; diabetes mellitus; chronic liver diseases, including liver disease as a result of alcohol abuse (e.g., cirrhosis); chronic alcoholism, chronic renal failure or nephrotic syndrome; functional or anatomic asplenia (e.g., sickle cell disease or splenectomy [if elective splenectomy is planned, vaccinate at least 2 weeks before surgery]); immunosuppressive conditions; and cochlear implants and cerebrospinal fluid leaks. Vaccinate as close to HIV diagnosis as possible.

Other indications: Alaska Natives and certain American Indian populations and residents of nursing homes or other long-term care facilities.

7. Revaccination with pneumococcal polysaccharide vaccine

One-time revaccination after 5 years for persons with chronic renal failure or nephrotic syndrome; functional or anatomic asplenia (e.g., sickle cell disease or splenectomy); or immunosuppressive conditions. For persons aged ≥65 years, one-time revaccination if they were vaccinated ≥5 years previously and were aged <65 years at the time of primary vaccination.

8. Hepatitis A vaccination

Medical indications: Persons with chronic liver disease and persons who receive clotting factor concentrates.

Behavioral indications: Men who have sex with men and persons who use illegal drugs.

Occupational indications: Persons working with hepatitis A virus (HAV)–infected primates or with HAV in a research laboratory setting.

Other indications: Persons traveling to or working in countries that have high or intermediate endemicity of hepatitis A (a list of countries is available at wwwn.cdc.gov/travel/contentdiseases.aspx) and any person seeking protection from HAV infection.

Single-antigen vaccine formulations should be administered in a 2-dose schedule at either 0 and 6–12 months (Havrix®), or 0 and 6–18 months (Vaqta®). If the combined hepatitis A and hepatitis B vaccine (Twinrix®) is used, administer 3 doses at 0, 1, and 6 months.

9. Hepatitis B vaccination

Medical indications: Persons with end-stage renal disease, including patients receiving hemodialysis; persons seeking evaluation or treatment for a sexually transmitted disease (STD); persons with HIV infection; and persons with chronic liver disease.

Occupational indications: Health-care personnel and public-safety workers who are exposed to blood or other potentially infectious body fluids.

Behavioral indications: Sexually active persons who are not in a long-term, mutually monogamous relationship (e.g., persons with more than 1 sex partner during the previous 6 months); current or recent injection-drug users; and men who have sex with men.

Other indications: Household contacts and sex partners of persons with chronic hepatitis B virus (HBV) infection; clients and staff members of institutions for persons with developmental disabilities; international travelers to countries with high or intermediate prevalence of chronic HBV infection (a list of countries is available at wwwn.cdc.gov/travel/contentdiseases.aspx); and any adult seeking protection from HBV infection.

Settings where hepatitis B vaccination is recommended for all adults: STD treatment facilities; HIV testing and treatment facilities; facilities providing drug-abuse treatment and prevention services; health-care settings targeting services to injection-drug users or men who have sex with men; correctional facilities; end-stage renal disease programs and facilities for chronic hemodialysis patients; and institutions and nonresidential daycare facilities for persons with developmental disabilities.

Special formulation indications: For adult patients receiving hemodialysis and other immunocompromised adults, 1 dose of 40 μg/mL (Recombivax HB®), or 2 doses of 20 μg/mL (Engerix-B®) administered simultaneously.

10. Meningococcal vaccination

Medical indications: Adults with anatomic or functional asplenia, or terminal complement component deficiencies.

Other indications: First-year college students living in dormitories; microbiologists who are routinely exposed to isolates of *Neisseria meningitidis*; military recruits; and persons who travel to or live in countries in which meningococcal disease is hyperendemic or epidemic (e.g., the "meningitis belt" of sub-Saharan Africa during the dry season [December–June]), particularly if their contact with local populations will be prolonged. Vaccination is required by the government of Saudi Arabia for all travelers to Mecca during the annual Hajj.

Meningococcal conjugate vaccine is preferred for adults with any of the preceding indications who are aged ≤55 years, although meningococcal polysaccharide vaccine (MPSV4) is an acceptable alternative. Revaccination after 3–5 years might be indicated for adults previously vaccinated with MPSV4 who remain at increased risk for infection (e.g., persons residing in areas in which disease is epidemic).

11. Herpes zoster vaccination

A single dose of zoster vaccine is recommended for adults aged ≥60 years regardless of whether they report a prior episode of herpes zoster. Persons with chronic medical conditions may be vaccinated unless a contraindication or precaution exists for their condition.

12. Selected conditions for which *Haemophilus influenzae* type b (Hib) vaccine may be used

Hib conjugate vaccines are licensed for children aged 6 weeks–71 months. No efficacy data are available on which to base a recommendation concerning use of Hib vaccine for older children and adults with the chronic conditions associated with an increased risk for Hib disease. However, studies suggest good immunogenicity in patients who have sickle cell disease, leukemia, or HIV infection or who have had splenectomies; administering vaccine to these patients is not contraindicated.

13. Immunocompromising conditions

Inactivated vaccines are generally acceptable (e.g., pneumococcal, meningococcal, and influenza [trivalent inactivated influenza vaccine]), and live vaccines generally are avoided in persons with immune deficiencies or immune suppressive conditions. Information on specific conditions is available at www.cdc.gov/vaccines/pubs/acip-list.htm.

APPENDIX IX: FOOD SOURCES OF SELECTED NUTRIENTS

Seppidek Sami, MS, RD, LDN

CALCIUM: A SAMPLE LIST OF FOODS CONTAINING CALCIUM

Food Sources

Item	Amount	Calcium content (mg)
Apple	1 medium, raw	10
Broccoli	1 C cooked	72
Cabbage	1 C raw shredded	32
Cheddar cheese	1 oz	204
Kidney beans	1 C canned	62
Milk or yogurt	8 oz nonfat	302
Muenster cheese	1 oz	203
Oysters	1 C raw	111
Romano cheese	1 oz	301
Salmon	3 oz canned + bones	204
Salmon	3 oz meat only	6
Sardines	3 oz canned + bones	324
Sirloin steak	3 oz cooked, lean	7
Turnip greens	1 C cooked	198

FIBER: A SAMPLE LIST OF FOODS CONTAINING FIBER

Food Sources

Item	Amount	Fiber content (g)
Fruits, with skins provide about 2–3 g fiber per serving:		
Apple	1 small	
Banana	1 small, ~4 oz	
Berries	3/4 C	
Cantaloupe	1/2 small melon, no skin	
Pear	1/2 small	
Prune	2	
Grains and cereals provide about 2–4 g fiber per serving (depending on brand):		
Barley	1/2 C	
Oatmeal	1 C cooked	
Grape-Nuts	1/3 C	
Popcorn	2 C popped	
Whole-wheat bread	1 slice	
Legumes	**1/2 C cooked**	**6–8**
(Baked beans, chick peas, kidney beans, lentils, lima beans)		
Vegetables	**1/2 C cooked**	**2**
Vegetables	**1 C raw**	**2**
Peanuts	7	1
Peanut butter	2½ teaspoon	1
Walnuts	1/2 C	1

FOLATE: A SAMPLE LIST OF FOODS CONTAINING FOLATE

Natural Sources

Item	Amount	Folate content (μg)
Asparagus	1/2 C	125
Apple	1 medium, raw	4
Avocado	1/4 C	35
Banana	1 medium (~6–8 oz)	24
Beets	1/2 C cooked	46
Cheddar cheese	1 oz (114 cal)	5
Chickpeas	1/2 C cooked	145
Lentils	1/2 C cooked	180
Lima beans	1 C cooked	156
Liver, beef	3 oz cooked	185
Milk or yogurt	8 oz nonfat	14
Peas	1/2 C cooked	51
Pinto beans	1/2 C cooked	145
Potato	1 medium baked	22
Spinach	1 C raw	115
Turnip greens	1 C cooked (27 cal)	171
Whole-wheat bread	1 slice (1 oz)	20

Fortified Sources

Item	Amount	Folate content (μg)
Bagel	2 oz	50
Bread, white	1 slice	8–20, depending on brand
Kellogg's corn flakes	1 C	100
Kellogg's bran flakes	1 C	100
English muffin	1 whole	22
Multi Grain Cheerios	1/2 C	69
Plus	1 C	400
Pasta	1 C cooked	110
Product 19 cereal	1 C	400

IRON: A SAMPLE LIST OF FOODS CONTAINING IRON

Food Sources, Heme

Item	Amount	Iron content (mg)
Liver, beef	3 oz fried	5.3
Milk or yogurt	8 oz nonfat	0.1
Oysters	1 C raw	16.6
Sirloin steak, lean	2 oz cooked	2.1

Food Sources, Nonheme

(Note: The nonheme sources of iron must be consumed along with foods rich in vitamin C for optimal absorption of iron.)

Item	Amount	Iron content (mg)
Bran flakes	1 C	11.0
Legumes	**1/2 C cooked:**	
Black-eyed beans		2.6
Chick peas		6.2
Kidney beans		2.2
Lentils		3.2
Lima beans		2.2
Navy beans		2.5
Nuts/Seeds	**2 Tablespoons:**	
Almond		1.3
Pumpkin seeds		2.5
Sesame seeds		1.2
Sunflower seeds		1.2
Oatmeal	1 packet	6.3
Peach halves	10 dried	5.3
Potato	1 large	1.4
Prune juice	4 oz	1.5
Semolina/Cream of Wheat	1/2 C cooked	5.5
Soy foods	**1/2 C cooked:**	
Soybeans		4.4
Soybeans		0.9
Tempeh		1.8
Tofu		6.6
Vegetables	**1/2 C cooked:**	
Sea vegetables		18.1–42.0
Spinach		3.2
Swiss chard		2.0
Turnip greens		1.6
Wheat germ	2 Tablespoons	1.2
Whole-wheat bread	1 slice	0.9

VITAMIN C: A SAMPLE LIST OF FOODS CONTAINING VITAMIN C

Food Sources

Item	Amount	Vitamin C content (mg)
Apple	1 medium, raw	8
Broccoli	1 C cooked	116
Brussels sprouts	1 C cooked	97
Cantaloupe	1/2 small	113
Cheddar cheese	1 oz	0
Green pepper	1 whole (18 cal)	66
Milk or yogurt	1 C nonfat	2
Orange juice	1 C fresh	124
Tomato juice	8 oz canned	45
Whole-wheat bread	1 slice	0

REFERENCES

Pennington JAT, et al. *Bowes & Church's Food Values of Portions Commonly Used*. Philadelphia: Lippincott Williams & Wilkins;

USDA National Nutrient Database for Standard Reference. Nutrient Data Laboratory. Agricultural Research Service. Available at: www.nal.usda.gov/fnic/foodcomp/search/. Accessed 08/30/07.

Section IX

APPENDIX X: SAMPLE OF MENU-PLANNING GUIDELINES

Seppidek Sami, MS, RD, LDN

A wide spectrum of menu-planning guidelines and recommendations have been made available through government agencies as well as private groups and organizations. This is a mere sample.

THE PLATE METHOD

The Plate Method is most appropriate for individuals who need simple guidelines to begin their menu planning while they are waiting to meet with a registered dietitian for an in-depth, individualized menu plan. The Plate Method has been used as part of treatment for obesity and diabetes. It typically asks that the plate be divided into 4 quarters. For breakfast: 1 quarter of the plate will be filled with high-fiber starchy foods (if weight loss is not of concern, 2 quarters) and 1 quarter with low-fat protein foods. For lunch and dinner: 2 quarters (1/2) of the plate will be filled with nonstarchy vegetables, 1 quarter with high-fiber (low glycemic index) starchy foods, and 1 quarter with lean, protein-rich foods and healthy fats (~5%). The fat will most likely be used as salad dressing on your vegetables or as nuts/seeds mixed in with the salad. For each meal, a serving of fruit and 4–8 oz of low-fat milk or yogurt are also permitted. It is worth mentioning that a smaller plate (33 square inches) vs. a larger plate (36 square inches) will need to be used. Also, it is a good idea to serve the food on the plate from the stove so that you are not tempted with seconds. For an in-depth presentation of the Plate Method please visit: www.bettycjung.net/Pdfs/Denverplatemethod.pdf.

MY PYRAMID

In 2005, the Food Guide Pyramid (originally introduced in 1992) was replaced by MyPyramid. This was a new menu-planning and guidance system that focused on the need for a more individualized approach to improving a person's eating plan as well as over-all lifestyle. MyPyramid incorporated recommendations from the USDA's *2005 Dietary Guidelines for Americans*. MyPyramid, with its motto "One size doesn't fit all," allows a personal meal plan to be developed with food choices and portions that are based on an in-depth assessment of the individual's activity and general calorie needs, using an interactive technology tool. The MyPyramid symbol refers to the various food groups and the recommended portions from each group. The significance of making healthy choices from each food group is strongly emphasized. Also, physical activity is a new element in the symbol. The interactive activities make it easy for individuals to use the system with or without the help of their healthcare professional. MyPyramid's food and activity patterns are meant for the general population, >2 years of age, and are not meant to be used for the treatment of specific health conditions, or during pregnancy and lactation. It has been recommended that those with specific health conditions work with their provider to develop a specific menu plan that fits their specific health needs. Please visit www.MyPyramid.gov for more information on: MyPyramid Plan, MyPyramid Tracker, and Inside MyPyramid, plus tips, resources, and worksheets.

THE NEW 4 FOOD GROUPS

The old 4 food groups were meat, dairy, grains, and fruits/vegetables. In 1992, Physician's Committee for Responsible Medicine unveiled The New Four Food Groups, which presented a nutrition plan founded upon high-fiber plant foods. The development of The New 4 Food Groups was founded upon evidence that high-cholesterol, high-fat, and protein-rich animal products (as found in the old Four Food Groups and the Food Guide Pyramid) contributed significantly to degenerative diseases such as cardiovascular diseases, some cancers, and osteoporosis. The New Four Food Groups are:

1. **Fruit** ($\geq$3 servings/day). Fruits are rich in fiber, vitamin C, and beta-carotene. Be sure to include at least 1 serving each day of fruits that are high in vitamin C—citrus fruits, melons, and strawberries are all good choices. Choose whole fruit over fruit juices, which do not contain very much fiber.
   Serving size: 1 medium piece of fruit • 1/2 cup cooked fruit • 4 ounces juice

2. **Legumes** ($\geq$2 servings/day). Legumes, which is another name for beans, peas, and lentils, are all good sources of fiber, protein, iron, calcium, zinc, and B vitamins. This group also includes chickpeas, baked and refried beans, soy milk, tempeh, and texturized vegetable protein.
   Serving size: 1 cup cooked beans • 4 ounces tofu or tempeh • 8 ounces soy milk

3. **Whole grains** ($\geq$5 servings/day). This group includes bread, rice, tortillas, pasta, hot or cold cereal, corn, millet, barley, and bulgur wheat. Build each of your meals around a hearty grain dish—grains are rich in fiber and other complex carbohydrates, as well as protein, B vitamins, and zinc.
   Serving size: 1/2 cup rice or other grain • 1 ounce dry cereal • 1 slice bread

4. **Vegetables** ($\geq$4 servings/day). Vegetables are packed with nutrients; they provide vitamin C, beta-carotene, riboflavin, iron, calcium, fiber, and other nutrients. Dark-green leafy vegetables, such as broccoli, collards, kale, mustard and turnip greens, chicory, or cabbage, are especially good sources of these important nutrients. Dark-yellow and orange vegetables such as carrots, winter squash, sweet potatoes, and pumpkin provide extra beta-carotene. Include generous portions of a variety of vegetables in your diet.
   Serving size: 1 cup raw vegetables • 1/2 cup cooked vegetables

Please Note: It is important to include a good source of vitamin B$_{12}$ in your diet, such as fortified cereals or vitamin supplements.

To download a copy of the New Four Food Groups please visit www.pcrm.org/health/veginfo/vsk/food_groups.html; to obtain accurate information on vegetarian eating plans please visit www.pcrm.org or www.vrg.org.

Contraceptive Efficacy: WHO

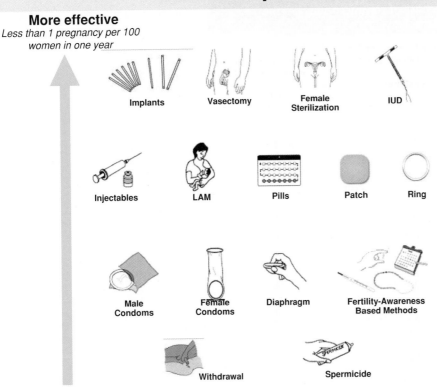

More effective

Less than 1 pregnancy per 100 women in one year

Implants   Vasectomy   Female Sterilization   IUD

Injectables   LAM   Pills   Patch   Ring

Male Condoms   Female Condoms   Diaphragm   Fertility-Awareness Based Methods

Withdrawal   Spermicide

Less effective

About 30 pregnancies per 100 women in 1 year

How to make your method most effective

After procedure, little or nothing to do or remember
<u>Vasectomy</u>: Use another method for 1st 3 months

<u>Injections</u>: Get repeat injections on time
<u>LAM</u> (for 6 months): Breast-feed often, day and night
<u>Pills</u>: Take a pill each day

<u>Patch, ring</u>: Keep in place, change on time

<u>Condoms, diaphragm</u>: Use correctly every time you have sex
<u>Fertility-awareness based methods</u>: Abstain or use condoms on fertile days.
Newest methods (Standard Days Method and TwoDay Method) may be easier to use.

<u>Withdrawal, spermicide</u>: Use correctly every time you have sex

Source: WHO, 2007.

**SUMMARY TABLE OF
CONTRACEPTIVE EFFICACY**

Percentage of US women experiencing an unintended pregnancy during the 1st year of typical use, the 1st year of perfect use of contraception, and the percentage continuing use at the end of the 1st year.

Method (1)	% of women experiencing an unintended pregnancy within the 1st year of use		% of women continuing use at 1 year[3] (4)
	Typical use[1] (2)	Perfect use[2] (3)	
No method[4]	85	85	–
Spermicides[5]	29	18	42
Withdrawal	27	4	43
Fertility awareness-based methods	25	–	51
Standard Days method[6]	–	5	–
2-Day method[6]	–	4	–
Ovulation method[6]	–	3	–
Sponge	–	–	–
Parous women	32	20	46
Nulliparous women	16	9	57
Diaphragm[7]	16	6	57
Condom[8]	–	–	–
Female (Reality)	21	5	49
Male	15	2	53
Combined pill and progestin-only pill	8	0.3	68
Evra Patch	8	0.3	68
NuvaRing	8	0.3	68
Depo-Provera	3	0.3	56
IUD	–	–	–
ParaGard (copper T)	0.8	0.6	78
Mirena (LNG-IUS)	0.2	0.2	80
Implanon	0.05	0.05	84
Female Sterilization	0.5	0.5	100
Male Sterilization	0.15	0.10	100

Emergency Contraceptive Pills: Treatment initiated within 72 hours after unprotected intercourse reduces the risk of pregnancy by at least 75%.[9]

Lactational Amenorrhea Method: LAM is a highly effective, *temporary* method of contraception.[10]

Source: Trussell J. Contraceptive Efficacy. In Hatcher RA, et al., eds. *Contraceptive Technology, 19th revised ed. New York NY: Ardent Media; 2007.*

1. Among *typical* couples who initiate use of a method (not necessarily for the 1st time), the percentage who experience an accidental pregnancy during the 1st year if they do not stop use for any other reason. Estimates of the probability of pregnancy during the 1st year of typical use for spermicides, withdrawal, periodic abstinence, the diaphragm, the male condom, the pill, and Depo-Provera are taken from the 1995 National Survey of Family Growth, corrected for underreporting of abortion; see the text for the derivation of estimates for the other methods.

2. Among couples who initiate use of a method (not necessarily for the 1st time) and who use it *perfectly* (both consistently and correctly), the percentage who experience an accidental pregnancy during the 1st year if they do not stop use for any other reason. See the text for the derivation of the estimate for each method.

3. Among couples attempting to avoid pregnancy, the percentage who continue to use a method for 1 year.

4. The percentages becoming pregnant in columns (2) and (3) are based on data from populations in which contraception is not used and from women who cease using contraception in order to become pregnant. Among such populations, ~89% become pregnant within 1 year. This estimate was lowered slightly (to 85%) to represent the percentage who would become pregnant within 1 year among women now relying on reversible methods of contraception if they abandoned contraception altogether.

5. Foams, creams, gels, vaginal suppositories, and vaginal film

6. The Ovulation and TwoDay methods are based on evaluation of cervical mucus. The Standard Days method avoids intercourse on cycle days 8–19.

7. With spermicidal cream or jelly

8. Without spermicides

9. The treatment schedule is 1 dose within 120 hours after unprotected intercourse, and a 2nd dose 12 hours after the 1st dose. Both doses of Plan B can be taken at the same time. Plan B (1 dose is 1 white pill) is the only dedicated product specifically marketed for emergency contraception. The FDA has, in addition, declared the following 22 brands of oral contraceptives to be safe and effective for emergency contraception: Ogestrel or Ovral (1 dose is 2 white pills), Levlen or Nordette (1 dose is 4 light-orange pills), Cryselle, Levora, Low-Ogestrel, Lo/Ovral or Quasence (1 dose is 4 white pills), Tri-Levlen or Triphasil (1 dose is 4 yellow pills), Jolessa, Portia, Seasonale, or Trivora (1 dose is 4 pink pills), Seasonique (1 dose is 4 light-blue-green pills), Empresse (1 dose is 4 orange pills), Alesse, Lessina, or Levlite (1 dose is 5 pink pills), Aviane (1 dose is 5 orange pills), and Lutera (1 dose is 5 white pills).

10. However, to maintain effective protection against pregnancy, another method of contraception must be used as soon as menstruation resumes, the frequency or duration of breast-feeds is reduced, bottle feeds are introduced, or the baby reaches 6 months of age.

APPENDIX XIII: INHERITED THROMBOPHILIAS AND THEIR ASSOCIATION WITH VTE IN PREGNANCY

Charles J. Lockwood, MD

Thrombophilia	Prevalence	% of VTE in pregnancy	Probability of VTE without personal or family history	Probability of VTE with a personal or family history
FVL (homozygous)	<0.1%	<1%	1.5%	17%
FVL (heterozygous)	5%	44%	0.26%	10%
PGM (homozygous)	<0.1%	<1%	2.8%	>17%
PGM (heterozygous)	3%	17%	0.37%	>10%
FVL/PGM (compound heterozygous)	0.2%	<1%[+]	4.7%	>20%
Antithrombin (<60% functional activity)	0.2%	1–8%	7.2%	>40%
Protein S (<55% free antigen-nonpregnant)	0.5%	12.4%	0.1%	0–22%
Protein C (<50% functional activity)	0.3%	<14%	0.8%	4–17%

FVL, factor V Leiden; PGM, prothrombin G202–1A promoted mutation

Patricia A. Lohr, MD, MPH
Beatrice A. Chen, MD

Brand	Company	First dose[b]	Second dose[b] (12 hours later)	Ethinyl estradiol per dose (μg)	Levonorgestrel per dose (mg)[c]
Progestin-only pills					
Plan-B	Barr/Duramed	2 white pills	None[b]	0	1.5
Combined progestin and estrogen pills					
Alesse	Wyeth-Ayerst	5 pink pills	5 pink pills	100	0.50
Aviane	Barr/Duramed	5 orange pills	5 orange pills	100	0.50
Cryselle	Barr/Duramed	4 white pills	4 white pills	120	0.60
Enpresse	Barr/Duramed	4 orange pills	4 orange pills	120	0.50
Jolessa	Barr/Duramed	4 pink pills	4 pink pills	120	0.60
Lessina	Barr/Duramed	5 pink pills	5 pink pills	100	0.50
Levlen	Berlex	4 light-orange pills	4 light-orange pills	120	0.60
Levlite	Berlex	5 pink pills	5 pink pills	100	0.50
Levora	Watson	4 white pills	4 white pills	120	0.60
Lo/Ovral	Wyeth-Ayerst	4 white pills	4 white pills	120	0.60
Low-Ogestrel	Watson	4 white pills	4 white pills	120	0.60
Lutera	Watson	5 white pills	5 white pills	100	0.50
Nordette	Wyeth-Ayerst	4 light-orange pills	4 light-orange pills	120	0.60
Ogestrel	Watson	2 white pills	2 white pills	100	0.50
Ovral	Wyeth-Ayerst	2 white pills	2 white pills	100	0.50
Portia	Barr/Duramed	4 pink pills	4 pink pills	120	0.60
Quasense	Watson	4 white pills	4 white pills	120	0.60
Seasonale	Barr/Duramed	4 pink pills	4 pink pills	120	0.60
Seasonique	Barr/Duramed	4 light-blue-green pills	4 light-blue-green pills	120	0.60
Tri-Levlen	Berlex	4 yellow pills	4 yellow pills	120	0.50
Triphasil	Wyeth-Ayerst	4 yellow pills	4 yellow pills	120	0.50
Trivora	Watson	4 pink pills	4 pink pills	120	0.50

Used with permission from http://ec.princeton.edu/. Accessed 12/28/06.

Notes:

[a] Plan-B is the only dedicated product specifically marketed for emergency contraception. Alesse, Aviane, Cryselle, Enpresse, Jolessa, Lessina, Levlen, Levlite, Levora, Lo/Ovral, Low-Ogestrel, Lutera, Nordette, Ogestrel, Ovral, Portia, Quasense, Seasonale, Seasonique, Tri-Levlen, Triphasil, and Trivora have been declared safe and effective for use as ECPs by the United States Food and Drug Administration. Outside the United States, more than 50 emergency contraceptive products are specifically packaged, labeled, and marketed. For example, Gedeon Richter and HRA Pharma are marketing in many countries the levonorgestrel-only products Postinor-2 and NorLevo, respectively, each consisting of a two-pill strip with each pill containing 0.75 mg levonorgestrel. Levonorgestrel-only ECPs are available either over-the-counter or from a pharmacist without having to see a clinician in 43 countries. On August 24, 2006, the FDA approved Plan B for nonprescription sale to women and men 18 and older.

[b] The label for Plan B says to take one pill within 72 hours after unprotected intercourse, and another pill 12 hours later. However, recent research has found that both Plan B pills can be taken at the same time. Research has also shown that that all of the brands listed here are effective when used within 120 hours after unprotected sex.

[c] The progestin in Cryselle, Lo/Ovral, Low-Ogestrel, Ogestrel, and Ovral is norgestrel, which contains two isomers, only one of which (levonorgestrel) is bioactive; the amount of norgestrel in each tablet is twice the amount of levonorgestrel.

PREGNANCY CATEGORY A:
Adequate and well-controlled studies have failed to demonstrate a risk to the fetus in the 1st trimester of pregnancy (and there is no evidence of risk in later trimesters).

PREGNANCY CATEGORY B:
Animal reproduction studies have failed to demonstrate a risk to the fetus, and there are no adequate and well-controlled studies in pregnant women OR animal studies that have shown an adverse effect, but adequate and well-controlled studies in pregnant women have failed to demonstrate a risk to the fetus in any trimester.

PREGNANCY CATEGORY C:
Animal reproduction studies have shown an adverse effect on the fetus, and there are no adequate and well-controlled studies in humans, but potential benefits may warrant use of the drug in pregnant women despite potential risks.

PREGNANCY CATEGORY D:
There is positive evidence of human fetal risk based on adverse reaction data from investigational or marketing experience or studies in humans, but potential benefits may warrant use of the drug in pregnant women despite potential risks.

PREGNANCY CATEGORY X:
Studies in animals or humans have demonstrated fetal abnormalities and/or there is positive evidence of human fetal risk based on adverse reaction data from investigational or marketing experience, and the risks involved in use of the drug in pregnant women clearly outweigh potential benefits.

Source: US Food and Drug Association (FDA)

APPENDIX XVI: HYPERTENSION IN PREGNANCY

Bryan E. Freeman, MD
Kathryn L. Reed, MD

 BASICS

DESCRIPTION

Hypertension existing prior to the onset of pregnancy, hypertension diagnosed prior to 20 weeks estimated gestational age, or persistent postpartum hypertension (>12 weeks postpartum). Hypertension diagnosed during pregnancy may be categorized as:

- Mild: BP >140/90
- Severe: BP >160/110

EPIDEMIOLOGY

5% of all pregnancies, but may be population dependent.

- Incidence is higher in African Americans, Hispanics, and Native Americans

RISK FACTORS

- Obesity
- Smoking
- Family history of HTN (especially parents)
- Sedentary lifestyle
- Ethnicity
- Stress
- Drugs (e.g., cocaine, methamphetamine)

Genetics

Family history of chronic hypertension is a risk factor.

PATHOPHYSIOLOGY

This varies greatly between patients; assess each patient according to identifiable risk factors. Many cases of essential hypertension are idiopathic; those that are not may be attributed to an extensive range of etiologies including renal disease, endocrine abnormalities, vascular disease, and dietary factors, among others.

ASSOCIATED CONDITIONS

Depends upon duration and severity of disease.May include end-organ damage, such as:

- Renal (glomerulonephritis, interstitial nephritis)
- Retinal (retinopathy)
- Cardiac (cardiomegaly, LVH)

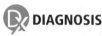 **DIAGNOSIS**

SIGNS AND SYMPTOMS

History

Documented history of chronic hypertension; with or without medical management.

Physical Exam

Diagnosis and monitoring are based upon vital signs.Physical examination findings, such as clonus, may signal a transition to chronic hypertension with superimposed preeclampsia

TESTS

- ECG
- ECHO (if indicated)

Lab

Because the diagnosis is made based on the patient's BP, laboratory tests are of more use to either confirm or rule out other related conditions such as superimposed preeclampsia.

- Baseline labs (at presentation) to assess renal function:
  – 24-hour urine for protein and creatinine clearance
  – Electrolytes
  – BUN
  – Creatinine
  – Uric acid
- UA
- If suspicion of preeclampsia or HELLP is developing:
  – CBC, differential, platelets
  – AST, ALT
  – LDH
- Acute episodes of hypertension, labs for other potential etiologies may be considered:
  – Check urine drug screen (especially cocaine and methamphetamine)
  – Pheochromocytoma: Check for urinary metanephrines and VMA

Imaging

Fetal: Regular assessment of fetal growth by ultrasound.
Maternal: Imaging assessment is only necessary in cases of suspected complications such as CVA, chest pain, dyspnea, cardiac failure or hypertrophy.

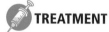 **TREATMENT**

GENERAL MEASURES

- Treatment options are outlined in the medications section below.
- Recommendations for fetal monitoring are variable. For patients with stable chronic hypertension, without evidence of IUGR or superimposed preeclampsia, a targeted ultrasound (at ~18 weeks EGA) followed by a subsequent growth ultrasound at 28–32 weeks (or earlier if clinically indicated) is recommended.Ultrasounds for interval growth (and Doppler studies, if indicated) should be performed monthly thereafter, or more frequently if growth curves indicate.
- Complications such as IUGR or superimposed preeclampsia warrant weekly or twice weekly antenatal testing (BPP or NST).

PREGNANCY-SPECIFIC ISSUES

Women with chronic hypertension are at increased risk for preeclampsia–eclampsia.

By Trimester

- 1st: Baseline labs; referrals to ophthalmology, nephrology, cardiology if indicated (these may be done preconceptionally as well)
- 2nd: Targeted ultrasound at approximately 18 weeks
- 3rd: Follow-up ultrasound for interval fetal growth (and Doppler studies if indicated):
  – Monthly ultrasounds for growth (and Doppler studies) until delivery
  – Antenatal testing if complications arise

Risks for Mother

- CVA or other sequelae of hypertension
- Preeclampsia-eclampsia
- HELLP Syndrome
- Cesarean delivery

Risks for Fetus

- IUGR
- IUFD
- Abruptio placentae
- Spontaneous abortion
- Preterm delivery due to:
  – Preterm labor
  – Deterioration of maternal or fetal status

MEDICATION (DRUGS)

- Discontinue ACE inhibitors. These have been associated with such fetal complications as fetal renal dysplasia, IUGR, IUFD, neonatal renal failure, and oligohydramnios when used in the second and third trimesters, and more recent evidence demonstrates an increase in other congenital malformations when used in the 1st trimester.
- There is no consensus outlining a single, ideal regimen. The following medications have been used with success in pregnant patients:
  – Methyldopa (most common in pregnant women, but not in nonpregnant population); starting dose = 250 mg PO b.i.d.; maximum dose = 4 g/d
  – Labetalol: Good initial agent; starting dose = 100 mg PO b.i.d.; maximum dose = 2,400 mg/d
  – Nifedipine: Starting dose = 10 mg PO b.i.d.; maximum dose = 120 mg/d
  – Thiazide diuretics: Starting dose = 12.5 mg PO BID; maximum dose = 50 mg/day (However, these should be used with caution, especially in patients who develop preeclampsia, as intravascular volume depletion is already an issue and should not be exacerbated.)

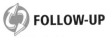

FOLLOW-UP

DISPOSITION

Issues for Referral

- Ophthalmology examination (examine for evidence of retinopathy)
- Cardiology (abnormal ECG or ECHO)
- Renal (if evidence of preexisting nephropathy)

PROGNOSIS

If blood pressure is well controlled, and patient's condition does not progress to preeclampsia or other disease, the outcome of the pregnancy should be normal for both mother and fetus. Delivery can be anticipated at term, unless complications develop.

COMPLICATIONS

- Potential for development of preeclampsia
- Sequelae are the same for any nonpregnant chronic hypertensive (risks of CVA, cardiac disease, end-organ damage)

PATIENT MONITORING

- Prenatal visits with regular blood pressure checks and screening for preeclampsia
- Home BP monitoring
- Antenatal testing (BPP or NST) if IUGR or suspicion of preeclampsia

Mother

Postpartum: If the patient's BPs are still well-controlled, she may continue her pregnancy regimen or may resume her prepregnancy regimen. If prior control was adequate with ACE inhibitor, this may be resumed.

Fetus

Potential issues associated with prematurity (if preterm delivery occurred) or growth restriction.

BIBLIOGRAPHY

Chronic Hypertension in Pregnancy. ACOG Practice Bulletin Number 29, July 2001.

Cooper WO, et al. Major congenital malformations after first-trimester exposure to ACE inhibitors. *N Engl J Med*. 2006;2443–2451.

Ferrer RL, et al. Management of mild chronic hypertension during pregnancy: A review. *Obstet Gynecol*. 2000;96:849–860.

Sibai BM. Chronic hypertension in pregnancy. *Obstet Gynecol*. 2002;100(2):369–377.

Sibai BM. Hypertension. In: Gabbe SG, et al., eds. *Obstetrics: Normal and Problem Pregnancies*. 4th ed. Philadelphia: Churchill Livingstone; 2002:945–1004.

 MISCELLANEOUS

CLINICAL PEARLS

The management goal for the pregnant patient with chronic hypertension is not necessarily to reach a "normal pregnancy blood pressure." The fetoplacental unit will adapt to the increased maternal blood pressure, and reduction of this blood pressure may compromise placental perfusion.

Since there is a natural physiologic decrease in blood pressure in pregnancy, some patients with mild chronic hypertension may not require medication during pregnancy, and some women who are actually hypertensive may not be diagnosed.

ABBREVIATIONS

- ACE—Angiotensin-converting enzyme
- b.i.d.—Twice a day
- BP—Blood pressure
- BUN—Blood urea nitrogen
- ECG—Electrocardiogram
- ECHO—Echocardiogram
- EGA—Estimated gestational age
- HELLP syndrome—Hemolysis, elevated liver enzymes, low platelets syndrome
- IUFD—Intrauterine fetal demise
- IUGR—Intrauterine growth restriction
- LDH—Lactate dehydrogenase
- LVH—Left ventricular hypertrophy
- PO—Oral administration
- VMA—Vanillylmandelic acid
- UA—Urinalysis

CODES

ICD9-CM

- 642 Hypertension complicating pregnancy, childbirth, and the puerperium

PATIENT TEACHING

- Emphasize importance of adherence to medical regimen
- Regular prenatal visits
- Home blood pressure monitoring
- Education regarding signs and symptoms of preeclampsia

PREVENTION

- Exercise
- Weight reduction (if indicated)
- Abstinence from drugs
- Avoidance of stress

Section IX

INDEX